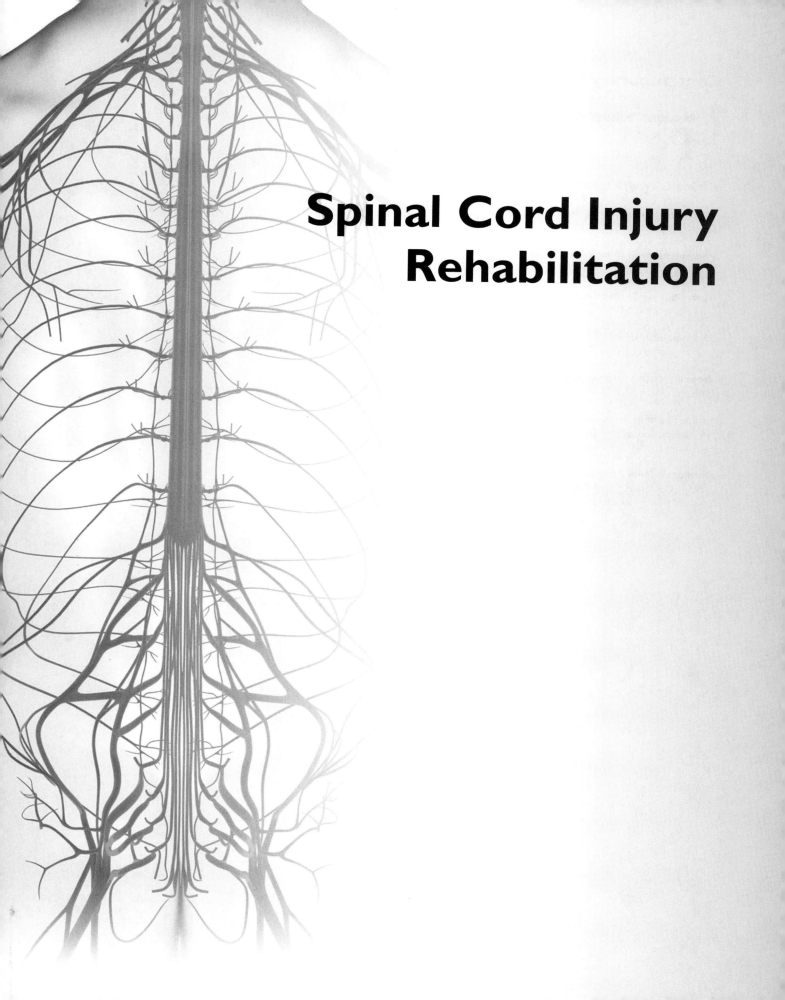

Spinal Cord Injury Rehabilitation

Contemporary Perspectives in Rehabilitation

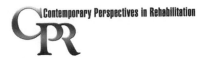

Steven L. Wolf, PT, PhD, FAPTA, Editor-in-Chief

Vestibular Rehabilitation, 3rd Edition
Susan J. Herdman, PT, PhD, FAPTA

Pharmacology in Rehabilitation, 4th Edition
Charles D. Ciccone, PT, PhD

Modalities for Therapeutic Intervention, 4th Edition
Susan L. Michlovitz, PT, PhD, CHT and Thomas P. Nolan, Jr., PT, MS, OCS

Fundamentals of Musculoskeletal Imaging, 2nd Edition
Lynn N. McKinnis, PT, OCS

Wound Healing: Alternatives in Management, 3rd Edition
Luther C. Kloth, PT, MS, CWS, FAPTA and Joseph M. McCulloch, PT, PhD, CWS, FAPTA

Evaluation and Treatment of the Shoulder:
An Integration of the Guide to Physical Therapist Practice
Brian J. Tovin, PT, MMSc, SCS, ATC, FAAOMPT and Bruce H. Greenfield, PT, MMSc, OCS

Cardiopulmonary Rehabilitation: Basic Theory and Application, 3rd Edition
Frances J. Brannon, PhD, Margaret W. Foley, RN, MN, Julie Ann Starr, PT, MS, CCS, and
Lauren M. Saul, MSN, CCRN

For more information on each title in the *Contemporary Perspectives in Rehabilitation* series, go to www.fadavis.com.

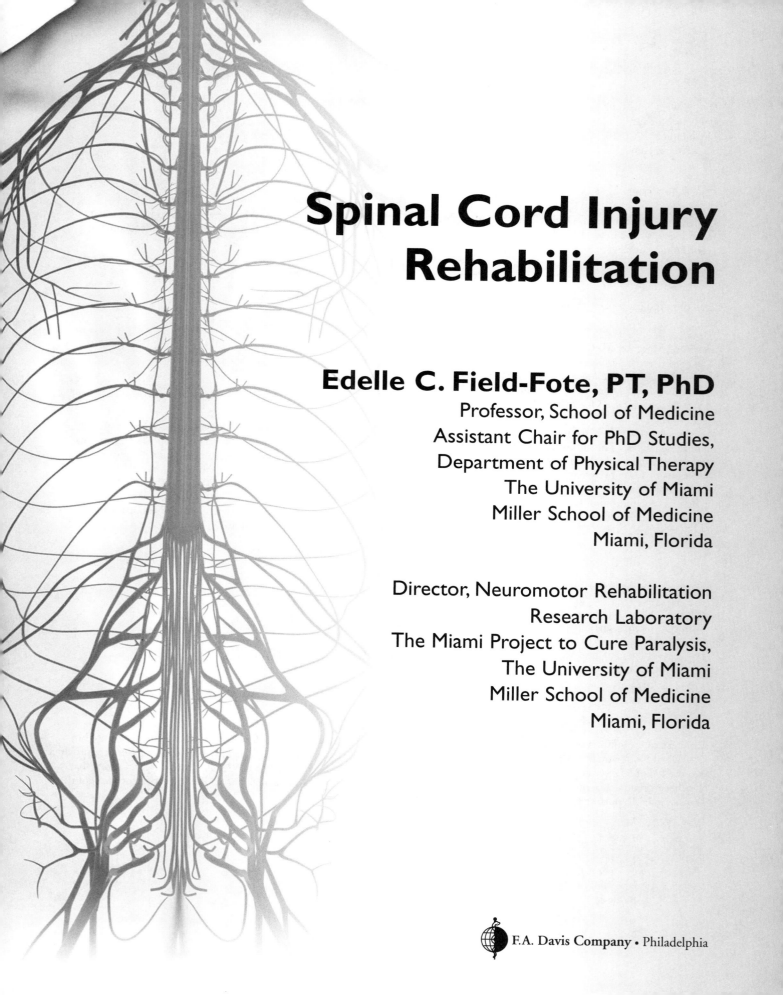

Spinal Cord Injury Rehabilitation

Edelle C. Field-Fote, PT, PhD

Professor, School of Medicine
Assistant Chair for PhD Studies,
Department of Physical Therapy
The University of Miami
Miller School of Medicine
Miami, Florida

Director, Neuromotor Rehabilitation
Research Laboratory
The Miami Project to Cure Paralysis,
The University of Miami
Miller School of Medicine
Miami, Florida

F.A. Davis Company • Philadelphia

F. A. Davis Company
1915 Arch Street
Philadelphia, PA 19103
www.fadavis.com

Printed in the United States of America

Last digit indicates print number: 10 9 8 7 6 5 4 3 2 1

Publisher: Margaret M. Biblis
Manager, Creative Development: George W. Lang
Senior Developmental Editor: Jennifer A. Pine
Production Manager: Samuel A. Rondinelli
Art & Design Manager: Carolyn O'Brien

As new scientific information becomes available through basic and clinical research, recommended treatments and drug therapies undergo changes. The author(s) and publisher have done everything possible to make this book accurate, up to date, and in accord with accepted standards at the time of publication. The author(s), editors, and publisher are not responsible for errors or omissions or for consequences from application of the book, and make no warranty, expressed or implied, in regard to the contents of the book. Any practice described in this book should be applied by the reader in accordance with professional standards of care used in regard to the unique circumstances that may apply in each situation. The reader is advised always to check product information (package inserts) for changes and new information regarding dose and contraindications before administering any drug. Caution is especially urged when using new or infrequently ordered drugs.

Library of Congress Cataloging-in-Publication Data

Spinal cord injury rehabilitation / [edited by] Edelle C. Field-Fote.
    p. ; cm.
  Includes bibliographical references and index.
  ISBN-13: 978-0-8036-1717-9
  ISBN-10: 0-8036-1717-8
  1. Spinal cord—Wounds and injuries—Patients—Rehabilitation. I. Field-Fote, Edelle C.
  [DNLM: 1. Spinal Cord Injuries—rehabilitation. WL 400 S757765 2009]
  RD594.3.S66945 2009
  617.4'820441—dc22

2009001369

This book is dedicated to all the individuals with spinal cord injury who have donated their time to participate in the research studies in my laboratory—I owe you a sincere debt of gratitude. And to my husband Alek and my son Tray, who allowed me to use "their time" to complete this text.

Foreword

Perhaps there is no greater need for the concept of a team meeting or team rounds in rehabilitation than when we are confronted with the multitude of problems faced by the person who has sustained a catastrophic injury. This reality is particularly compelling in the case of spinal cord injury (SCI), especially in light of the comparative youth of such survivors and the need to maximize a quality of life for many years. At times, the physical, functional, behavioral, environmental, and social problems facing these patients appear insurmountable. Coupled with this reality is another inescapable fact. The time allocated for team meetings has often become constricted by a need to provide multiple services over less time, often with fewer resources. Accordingly, all team members being better positioned to understand their respective roles as well as the roles of others becomes an imperative.

In this context, students in health-related professions, as well as physicians from multiple specialties, are not optimally prepared to engage in dialogue with other team members. Indeed, some of us may never have learned how to do so. If there is a modicum of truth to these suppositions or if the image portrayed is remotely familiar to some, then a compendium that provides comprehensive information written for all rehabilitationists charged with the remarkable responsibility of optimizing the potential for the SCI survivor has long been needed. Edelle Field-Fote, PT, PhD., is passionate in her commitment to understand the mechanisms underlying SCI, exploiting the potential for inducing plasticity in the nervous system following such injuries, and tracking the evidence underlying the best practice amongst all members of the rehabilitation team. Her commitment to the SCI survivor to assure the best that rehabilitationists can offer is now approaching two decades. She believes fervently in the need to provide treatment to these patients through assembling the very best information at our disposal based upon critical reviews of the literature. Indeed, *Spinal Cord Rehabilitation* offers the most comprehensive treatment on this subject ever written for the rehabilitation community. She has painstakingly remained true to the philosophy underlying the *Comprehensive Perspectives in Rehabilitation* by assuring that all contributors have searched the literature to support the information provided, whether it be fundamental science or treatment approaches. The work is presented as an evidence-based approach to best practice more than a cookbook on how

to treat. Thus the philosophy of the CPR series is preserved. Moreover, empiricism, while often important, plays a secondary role in the detailed accounts offered throughout this text.

Each chapter outlines what is to be accomplished within its pages, summarizes key points, and often is supplemented with relevant case histories, thus affording the reader some insights into how the presenter thinks. In fact, students and clinicians alike should realize that Dr. Field-Fote, by dint of shear effort complemented by a well-earned international respect, has assembled an uncontested "who's who" in SCI management. So, whether it is the student who needs to better understand multiple perspectives in the treatment of the SCI patient or the clinical specialist needing to catch up on the latest information within any aspect of patient management, the cast assembled herein would comprise a "dream team" that could easily surpass even the most accomplished in-hospital treatment team. The book is divided into three logical sections that first offer a contemporary overview of fundamental science and, as such, represents an excellent compilation of science related to SCI, expressed in a manner that is easily comprehensible to student and clinician alike. The second section addresses perspectives on treatment that are written with the intent to yield the maximal function achievable. Simply reading the specificity of the title for each chapter provides an expectation of the uniqueness of content. The last section approaches components that are so very important to the patient, but for which we sometimes claim ignorance or discomfort. Thus, participation in sports, relearning to drive, sexuality, and fertility are essential topics recognized by all of us, but which we are often unprepared to address or even understand.

There can be no greater contribution made by students of the rehabilitation process to the care of SCI patients than a proactive effort to absorb information from a myriad of issues that consume the thoughts of many of these patients. An appreciation for how other professionals manage essential aspects of care can have a profound impact on how your treatment plan is implemented and, more importantly, on the empathy you express toward your patients. 1To the experienced clinician whose time seems progressively more consumed by the rigors of administrative tasks at the expense of exercising the compassion and problem solving that directed their interests toward the SCI survivor, this book will foster the opportunity to absorb important and documented information. This opportunity can certainly occur within the treatment environment, but, more importantly, outside of it, when time permits reflection on the glorious commitment you have made to these courageous individuals.

STEVEN L. WOLF, Ph.D., PT, FAPTA, FAHA
Editor-in Chief, *Contemporary Perspectives in Rehabilitation Series*
Atlanta, Georgia
January 2009

Preface

We live in a time that is ripe with possibilities. Advances in technology, pharmacology, and biomedical sciences have positioned us on the brink of unparalleled discoveries that are sure to transform the lives of individuals with disability. Then again, we are not quite there. In the past 15 years, in the field of spinal cord injury research alone, there have been countless millions of dollars spent on basic and clinical trials of pharmacological and cellular transplantation approaches aimed at restoration of neural function. Studies of stem cells, fetal tissue transplants, activated macrophages, and olfactory ensheathing glial cells, just to name a few. Despite amazing progress, there are still critical pieces to the puzzles of neurologic restoration that remain mysterious.

And yet, there is one form of intervention for which research across disciplines and across animal species has concluded, time and time again, promotes recovery of function—that intervention is rehabilitation: practice, training, and motor experience. To date, there have been no reproducible pharmacological or cellular transplantation studies showing restoration of function in individuals with SCI that equal the functional improvements that have been shown by studies of rehabilitation interventions.

When spinal cord injury affects a high profile actor or athlete, it captures the attention of the public. The inability to move without a wheelchair informs the world that the individual can no longer move his arms and legs. However, save for the individual, family, and caregivers, few people understand the full impact of damage to the spinal cord—how it affects functions that so many of us take for granted: breathing, sexuality, bowel and bladder function, and many others. Even small improvements in functional status can make tremendous differences in quality of life, such as the ability to use a fork without an assistive device, to stand and walk into bathroom that is not accessible to a wheelchair, to step up a short flight of stairs—these things make a tremendous difference to quality of life. In many cases, such functions can be regained to some extent even many years after SCI. Individuals with SCI merit access to rehabilitation professionals who can assist them in reaching their fullest potential.

One day scientists will find the right combination of strategies to improve function—be it stem cells, transplantations of activated macrophages, or a drug that promotes remyelination—but these strategies will never realize their maximum potential unless they are combined with rehabilitation. The individual with a cellular transplant is not going to jump up from the operating table and run down the hallway. These strategies will only be effective when combined with rehabilitation. Just as the developing nervous system requires activity and experience for cells to differentiate into the right cell type, to find their target end organ, and to form the necessary connections with their targets, newly transplanted cells will only be maximally functional if they are in an optimal environment—a body that is healthy and provided with opportunities for practice, training, and motor experience.

This book is intended for my colleagues and future colleagues in rehabilitation who work in partnership with individuals with spinal cord injury either in the clinical setting to maximize function in an individual or in the research setting to gather evidence that will influence clinical practice to improve function in all individuals with SCI. My goal is that the chapters will be sufficiently comprehensive to meet the needs of the rehabilitation professional, the nonclinician researcher desiring to learn about how spinal cord injury affects human beings, and the individual with SCI who wants a broader understanding of their injury. Across chapters, the material is presented at different levels—basic, intermediate, and advanced—depending on the content area. While some chapters answer basic questions related to rehabilitation management, other chapters are unapologetically scientific, delving into complex topics for which many answers are not yet known. In all chapters, the emphasis has been on summarizing the evidence that is available in the literature, identifying areas of controversy where they exist, and providing information to the reader who wishes to explore the topic further.

EDELLE C. FIELD-FOTE

Contributors

Maria J. Amador, BSN, RN, CRRN
Director of Education
The Miami Project to Cure Paralysis
University of Miami Miller School of Medicine
Miami, Florida

Andrea L. Behrman, PT, PhD
Associate Professor
Department of Physical Therapy
University of Florida
Research Scientist
VA Brain Rehabilitation Research Center, Malcom
Randall VAMC
Gainesville, Florida

Kendra L. Betz, MS, PT, ATP
Prosthetics Clinical Coordinator
Prosthetics and Sensory Aids Service
Veterans Health Administration
Washington, DC

Amy Bohn, OTR/L
Therapist/Coordinator
Hand and Upper Extremity Rehabilitation Clinic
Shepherd Center
Atlanta, Georgia

Laurent J. Bouyer, PhD
Associate Professor
Department of Rehabilitation
Center for Interdisciplinary Research in Rehabilitation
and Social Integration
University of Laval
Quebec City, Quebec
Canada

Nancy L. Brackett, PhD, HCLD
Associate Professor
The Miami Project to Cure Paralysis
Departments of Neurological Surgery and Urology
University of Miami Miller School of Medicine
Miami, Florida

Diana D. Cardenas, MD, MS, MHA, FACRM
Professor and Chair
Department of Rehabilitation Medicine
University of Miami Miller School of Medicine
Miami, Florida

Thomas Cesarz, MD
Department of Physical Medicine and Rehabilitation
University of Rochester Medical Center
University of Rochester School of Medicine and
Dentistry
Rochester, New York

Kathleen A. Curtis, PT, PhD
Dean
College of Health Sciences, Charles H. and Shirley T.
Leavell Chair in Health Sciences
The University of Texas at El Paso
El Paso, Texas

Denise Dixon, PhD
Assistant Professor
Stony Brook University Hospital
Department of Pediatrics
Stony Brook, New York

Shauna Dudley-Javoroski, PT
Research Physical Therapist
Graduate Program in Physical Therapy &
Rehabilitation Science
University of Iowa
Iowa City, Iowa

Valerie Eberly, PT, NCS
Pathokinesiology Laboratory
Rancho Los Amigos National Rehabilitation Center
Downey, California

Stacy L. Elliot, MD
Director, BC Center for Sexual Medicine
Clinical Professor, Departments of Psychiatry and
Urological Sciences
University of British Columbia Faculty, ICORD
Vancouver, British Columbia
Canada

Edelle C. Field-Fote, PT, PhD
Professor
Department of Physical Therapy
Director, Neuromotor Rehabilitation Research
Laboratory
The Miami Project to Cure Paralysis
University of Miami Miller School of Medicine
Miami, Florida

Manuel Gonzalez-Brito, DO
Assistant Professor
Department of Pediatrics
University of Miami Miller School of Medicine
Miami, Florida

Judi Hamelburg, PT, CDRS
Director
Advanced Driver Rehabilitation, Inc.
Biscayne Park, Florida

Jennifer Hastings, PT, PhD, NCS
Clinical Associate Professor and Director of Clinical
Education
School of Physical Therapy
University of Puget Sound
Tacoma, Washington

Allen W. Heinemann, PhD, ABPP(Rp), FACRM
Professor, Physical Medicine and Rehabilitation
Feinberg School of Medicine, Northwestern University
Director, Center for Rehabilitation Outcomes Research
Rehabilitation Institute of Chicago
Chicago, Illinois

Larisa Hoffman, PT, PhD
Assistant Professor
Department of Physical Therapy
Regis University
Denver, Colorado

Emad Ibrahim, MD
Assistant Scientist
The Miami Project to Cure Paralysis
Department of Neurological Surgery
University of Miami Miller School of Medicine
Miami, Florida

Heakyung Kim, MD
Assistant Professor
Physical Medicine and Rehabilitation and Pediatrics
Children's Hospital of Philadelphia
University of Pennsylvania School of Medicine
Philadelphia, Pennsylvania

Kelley L. Kubota, PT, MS, NCS, ATP
PT Supervisor, Adult Brain Injury and Neurology Services
Rancho Los Amigos National Rehabilitation Center
Downey, California
Adjunct Faculty, University of Southern California
Division of Biokinesiology and Physical Therapy
Los Angeles, California

John Kuluz, MD
Associate Professor
Department of Pediatrics
University of Miami Miller School of Medicine
Miami, Florida

Susan Magasi, PhD, OTR
Research Assistant Professor
Department of Physical Medicine and Rehabilitation
Feinberg School of Medicine, Northwestern University
Research Scientist, Center for Outcomes,
Research and Education
NorthShore University Health Systems—
Research Institute
Chicago, Illinois

Sarah Morrison, PT
Director
Spinal Cord Injury Services
Shepherd Center, Inc.
Atlanta, Georgia

Mary Jane Mulcahey, PhD, OTR\L
Director of Rehabilitation Services and Clinical
Research
Shriners Hospitals for Children
Philadelphia, Pennsylvania

Sara Mulroy, PT, PhD
Director
Pathokinesiology Laboratory
Rancho Los Amigos National Rehabilitation Center
Adjunct Faculty, University of Southern California
Division of Biokinesiology and Physical Therapy
Los Angeles, California

Mark S. Nash, PhD, FACSM
Professor
Departments of Neurological Surgery, Rehabilitation
Medicine, and Physical Therapy
Principal Investigator, The Miami Project to Cure Paralysis
Director of Research, Department of Rehabilitation
Medicine
University of Miami Miller School of Medicine
Miami, Florida

Allan E. Peljovich, MD, MPH
Attending Surgeon
Hand and Upper Extremity Rehabilitation Clinic,
Shepherd Center
The Hand & Upper Extremity Center of Georgia
Atlanta, Georgia

Kanakadurga R. Poduri, MD
Department of Physical Medicine and Rehabilitation
University of Rochester Medical Center
University of Rochester School of Medicine and Dentistry
Rochester, New York

Arthur Prochazka, PhD
Professor
Centre for Neuroscience
University of Alberta
Edmonton, Alberta, Canada

Amer Samdani, MD
Director Pediatric Spine Service
Shriners Hospital for Children
Philadelphia, Pennsylvania

Richard K. Shields, PT, PhD, FAPTA
Director and Professor
Graduate Program in Physical Therapy &
Rehabilitation Science
University of Iowa
Iowa City, Iowa

Christine K. Thomas, PhD
Professor
The Miami Project to Cure Paralysis
Department of Neurological Surgery
University of Miami Miller School of Medicine
Miami, Florida

Catherine Warms, PhD, ARNP, CRRN
Assistant Professor
School of Nursing
University of Washington
Seattle, Washington

Jane L. Wetzel, PT, PhD
Assistant Professor
Rangos School of Health Science
Duquesne University
Pittsburgh, Pennsylvania

Eva Widerstrom-Noga, PhD, DDS
Associate Professor
The Miami Project to Cure Paralysis
Department of Neurological Surgery
University of Miami Miller School of Medicine
Miami, Florida

Catherine S. Wilson Psy D., ABPP (Rp)
Instructor
Department of Physical Medicine and Rehabilitation
Rehabilitation Institute of Chicago
Chicago, Illinois

Acknowledgments

It is good to have an end to journey toward, but it is the journey that matters in the end

~ URSULA K. LEGUIN

There are so many people to whom I am grateful for their guidance, support and encouragement. To my mentors Paul SG Stein, whose enthusiasm for science was contagious, and Blair Calancie, whose brilliant work gave me hope that there really was a human application for my turtle research. To my colleagues Sherri Hayes who is always there to give me a push when I need it, Susan Herdman who unbeknownst to me set the stage for me to succeed, Carol Davis and Meryl Cohen who are always ready with words of encouragement, and Steve Wolf who, for as long as I can remember, has been someone to whom I can ask the hard questions and discuss the possibilities even when there are no answers. I have been fortunate to grow up in physical therapy with peers in the APTA Section on Research and the Neurology Section whose achievements are a constant source of inspiration and whose friendship is a light in my life. I am grateful for the many opportunities I have had to exchange ideas with my outstanding basic science and clinical colleagues at The Miami Project to Cure Paralysis. To the members of my laboratory team who make every day an exciting adventure. To my dear friend Juliana Mares-Guia who, now with 20-plus years in a wheelchair, gives real meaning to the adage "attitude is everything," and reminds me about what is really important in life. And to my mother, Mirta Field, whose love and life-long pursuit of knowledge have left their marks on me.

Contents

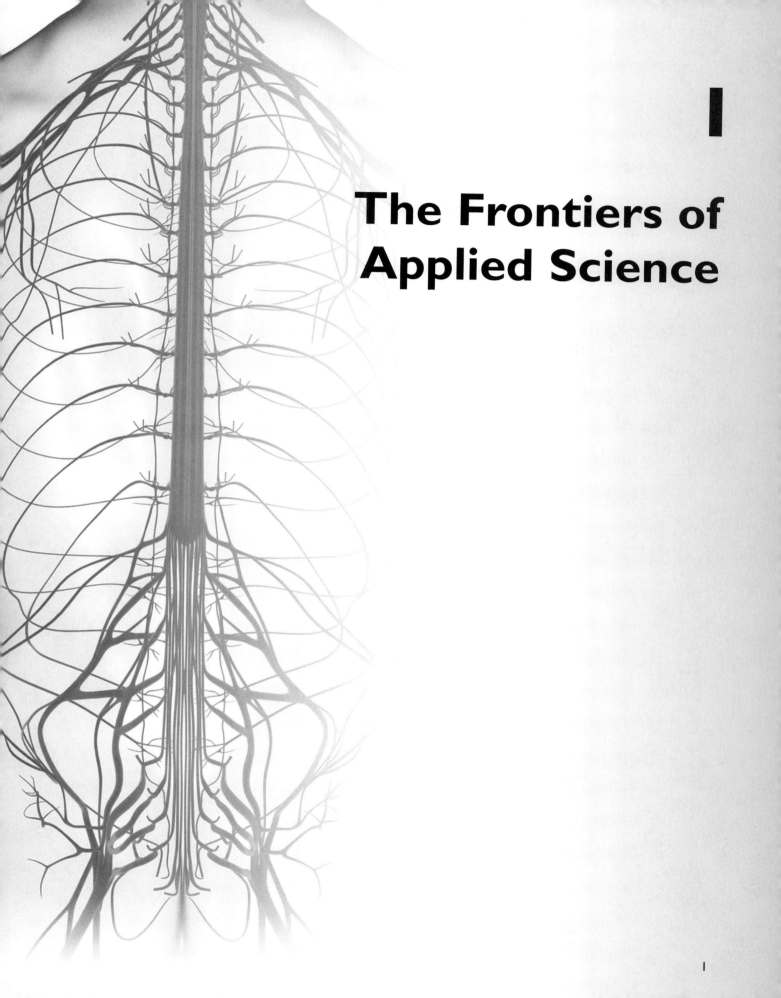

The Frontiers of Applied Science

Spinal Cord Injury: An Overview

Edelle Field-Fote, PT, PhD

After reading this chapter, you will be able to:

OBJECTIVES

- Differentiate between traumatic and nontraumatic causes of spinal cord injury (SCI) and describe the most common of these
- Discuss how level of injury and severity of injury contribute differently to the disability associated with SCI
- Compare and contrast the different syndromes that may be associated with incomplete SCI
- Describe the indicators that may assist in predicting functional outcomes in individuals with SCI
- Describe the secondary conditions that may occur after SCI and identify those that are preventable

Introduction

We live in a time when there are tremendous resources available to assist individuals with spinal cord injury (SCI) in living long and productive lives. While injury to the spinal cord frequently results in impairments of function that have a significant impact on the life of the individual, progress in the care of individuals with SCI has resulted in near-normal life expectancy. This outlook represents a radical reversal from the view expressed in the earliest known records describing SCI, dating back almost 4 millennia, which indicate that the ancient Egyptians characterized vertebral fracture as "an ailment not to be treated." From that time and even through World War II, individuals typically died from the initial trauma that injured the spinal cord or suffered severe morbidity from secondary conditions such as respiratory problems[1] or circulatory problems.[2] Since then, there have been dramatic steps forward, particularly in the 1970s. At that time, the routine use of intermittent bladder catheterization[3-5] resulted in a dramatic decrease in the mortality due to renal failure. Improvements in emergency medical care[6] meant that precautions were taken to prevent further damage to the spinal cord during transport to emergency medical facilities, resulting in a decrease in the proportion of complete injuries.

Most of the time we give little thought to the spinal cord, but it is truly an amazing structure. Descending and ascending communications between our brain and spinal cord allow our wish to move to become a reality, and allow us to experience the world through touch and other tactile sensations. Far from being a simple conduit for information going to and coming from the brain, the spinal cord is critical for modulating descending motor commands and ascending sensory signals. Interestingly, the spinal cord can generate complex, elegant motor output via spinal central pattern generators (this concept is discussed further in chapter 13, "Locomotor Training"). When the spinal cord is damaged due to trauma or disease, the loss of these important mechanisms results in disruption of motor, sensory, and autonomic functions. Because sensory organs, muscles, and visceral organs are innervated by distinct segments of the spinal cord, there is an associated relationship between the level and severity of injury and the residual sensory, motor, and autonomic function.

Today excellent emergency care and progressive rehabilitation strategies mean that individuals with SCI can benefit from interventions that will optimize their functional capacity and their ability to participate in society. Unfortunately, the constraints on rehabilitation practice, in terms of short lengths of stay in rehabilitation facilities, means that, following SCI, individuals are likely to be discharged from the hospital long before their neural recovery is complete. For this reason, early in the acute phase of injury, therapists focus on teaching compensatory movement strategies to allow the individual to be as functional as possible in the shortest possible time. The latest research suggests that the nervous system has an amazing capacity to recover from damage as long as the appropriate experiences are provided. The potential to improve function persists long after the acute phase, and there is much evidence to indicate that individuals with chronic SCI can make significant functional gains if given the opportunity to participate in these interventions. Many of the following chapters in this text will focus on the use of training to improve function in individuals with chronic SCI.

Demographics of SCI

According to the best available estimates from the Spinal Cord Injury Information Network,[7] approximately 11,000 individuals experience a SCI each year in the United States, and there are between 225,000 to 296,000 individuals living with SCI. When the last formal studies of the incidence of SCI were conducted in the 1970s, the mean age of individuals experiencing SCI was 28.7 years. More recent data (since 2000) indicate the mean age of individuals experiencing SCI has risen to 38 years. These data reflect both the increasing median age of the population, as well as an increase in the number of elderly individuals diagnosed with SCI. The incidence of SCI is greater in men (77.8%) than in women (22.2%). Functional outcomes are thought to be better in women, although the differences do not appear to be statistically significant.[8] Still, there is some evidence to suggest that female hormones such as estrogen[9-11] and progesterone[12-14] may have a neuroprotective effect that accounts for the lessened severity in women, but these views are not without controversy.[15,16]

Along with the increasing proportion of individuals in the United States belonging to minority groups, minority representation among those with SCI has increased as well. Caucasians, African Americans, Hispanics, and other ethnic/racial groups accounted for 63%, 22.7%, 11.8%, and 2.4%, respectively, of individuals experiencing SCI since 2000. Comparatively, these groups accounted for 76.8%, 14.2%, 6%, and 3%, respectively, of those with SCI who were injured between 1973 and 1979.[7]

Etiology of SCI

The majority of spinal cord injuries occur secondary to trauma. Rarely, except in the case of a penetrating injury (e.g., knife or gunshot wound), is there complete disruption of the spinal cord. Additionally, while the primary trauma damages neural tissue and disrupts the blood supply to the spinal cord, death of neural tissue is largely due to secondary damage. Inflammatory processes are accompanied by edema, leading to compression of spinal cord tissue within the confined dimensions of the vertebral canal. In addition to the forces placed in the vulnerable tissue, the edema increases the distance between cells and blood vessels supplying vital oxygen and nutrients. In addition to edema, injury-induced alterations in cellular metabolism result in excitotoxicity that further damages vulnerable neural structures.

The etiology of SCI from traumatic causes comes in many forms. According to a National Spinal Cord Injury Database query in 1995, the primary cause of traumatic SCI was motor vehicle accidents (44.5%), followed by falls (18.1%), assault (16.6%), sports (12.7%), and other (8.1%).[17] These figures are consistent with a more recent regional study.[18] There is limited information available regarding the etiology of nontraumatic sources of SCI. Likewise, there are few available studies comparing demographics, deficits, and outcomes in individuals with traumatic versus nontraumatic SCI. Some of the more common forms of nontraumatic SCI are noted in Box 1-1.

One study of individuals admitted to a SCI rehabilitation unit indicates that there may be differences between those with nontraumatic (42%) versus traumatic SCI (58%). On average, individuals admitted with nontraumatic SCI were significantly older than those with traumatic SCI (55 years and 39 years, respectively), had a lower incidence of neurologically complete injury (5.3% and 45.6%, respectively), and had a shorter length of rehabilitation stay (26.4 days vs. 43.0 days, respectively). In regard to secondary conditions, the incidence of deep vein thrombosis, pressure ulcers, autonomic dysreflexia, pneumonia, orthostatic hypotension, and spasticity was significantly lower in those with nontraumatic SCI. There were no differences between those with nontraumatic versus traumatic SCI in rates of depression, urinary tract infections, heterotopic ossification, or pain.[19] A retrospective study conducted in Turkey suggests that admissions to a rehabilitation hospital for nontraumatic SCI comprise approximately 32% of all SCI admissions. As might be expected, the proportion of women and men is more evenly distributed among those with

nontraumatic SCI compared to traumatic injuries wherein the rate of SCI is greater in men. While on admission the functional test scores were significantly better in the group with nontraumatic SCI, there were no differences between the groups in functional test scores at discharge.[20]

Characterization of SCI

The spinal cord is a column of neural tissue that begins at the base of the brain stem where it exits the skull through the foramen magnum. The spinal cord is contained within and protected by the vertebral canal. Along the length of the spinal cord, paired spinal nerves, containing both sensory and motor fibers, emerge from the vertebral column through the intervertebral foramen formed by adjacent vertebrae. The spinal cord is described as having 31 segmental levels, however, this notion is somewhat inaccurate as the spinal cord is not a segmented structure. The segments and paired spinal nerves are named for the level of the vertebral column at which the spinal nerves exit (see Fig. 1-1). Note that above C7 the nerves exit above their respective vertebra, while the C8 nerve exits below the C7 vertebra and all nerves below C8 exit below their respective vertebra. By this convention, the 31 spinal segments are made up of 8 cervical, 12 thoracic, 5 lumbar, 5 sacral, and 1 coccygeal segment.

Level of Injury

The impact of SCI depends on a number of factors, with the two most influential factors being the spinal level at which the injury occurs and the amount of damage or severity of injury sustained by the spinal cord. To an inexperienced observer, the most obvious consequence of injury is impairment of upper and/or lower extremity function. In terms of level of injury, damage to the cervical spinal cord results in impairment of both upper and lower extremity function, termed tetraplegia (formerly, the term quadriplegia was often used). Likewise, injury to the thoracic, lumbar, or sacral spinal cord results in impairment of lower extremity function, termed paraplegia. SCI can affect any level of the cervical (C1–C8), thoracic (T1–T12), lumbar (L1–L5), or sacral (S1–S5) spinal cord segments.

Often there is a difference between the vertebral level of injury and the spinal cord (segmental) level of injury. This is particularly true for injuries below the cervical level. In the cervical region the spinal cord segmental levels and the spinal vertebra are at the same or similar levels, but in more distal regions of the spinal cord, there is a large discrepancy between the vertebral level and the spinal cord segmental level. For example, in the adult the cervical enlargement (i.e., the region of the spinal cord containing the motor neurons that innervate the upper extremities) is comprised of spinal segments C3–T1 and is located anatomically at approximately vertebral levels

---

BOX 1-1
Nontraumatic causes of spinal cord injury

Multiple sclerosis
Spinal cord tumor (metastatic or intrinsic)
Degenerative disease (e.g., disk herniation, cervical spondylosis)
Ischemia
Hemorrhage, including spinal subdural/epidural and hematomyelia
Infectious/inflammatory pathologies
  Meningitis
  Myelitis
  Herpes zoster/Herpes simplex
  Tuberculosis
  Syphilis

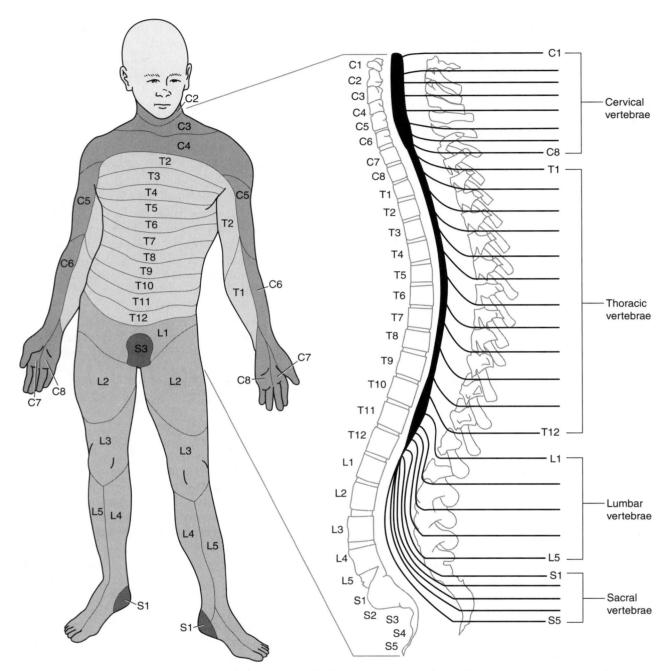

Figure 1-1. The spinal cord and key anatomical/dermatomal landmarks. The cervical spinal nerves C1–C7 exit above the vertebrae for which they are named, cervical spinal nerve C8 exits below the C7 vertebra, and below this level the spinal nerves exit below the vertebrae for which they are named. The boney protuberance at the base of the neck is the spinal process of C7. Note that the adult spinal cord ends in the conus medullaris at approximately the level of the L1 or L2 vertebra. Below this level the spinal nerves comprise the cauda equina, traversing caudally in the vertebral canal to exit below the vertebra for which each is named.

C3–T1. However, the lumbar enlargement (i.e., the region of the spinal cord containing the motor neurons that innervate the lower extremities) is comprised of spinal segments L1–S3 and is located anatomically at approximately vertebral levels T9–T12. The reason for this discrepancy is that while the spinal cord extends the entire length of the vertebral canal in the first few months of development (*see* Fig. 1-2a), thereafter the

vertebral column grows at a much faster rate than the spinal cord itself. As a result, by adulthood the spinal cord extends only to the level of the first or second lumbar vertebrae (*see* Fig. 1-2b).

Therefore, damage to the C4 vertebrate likely results in damage at or near the C4 segment of the spinal cord, because the C4 root originates in the C4 spinal cord and exits near the C4 vertebra. However, if damage to the

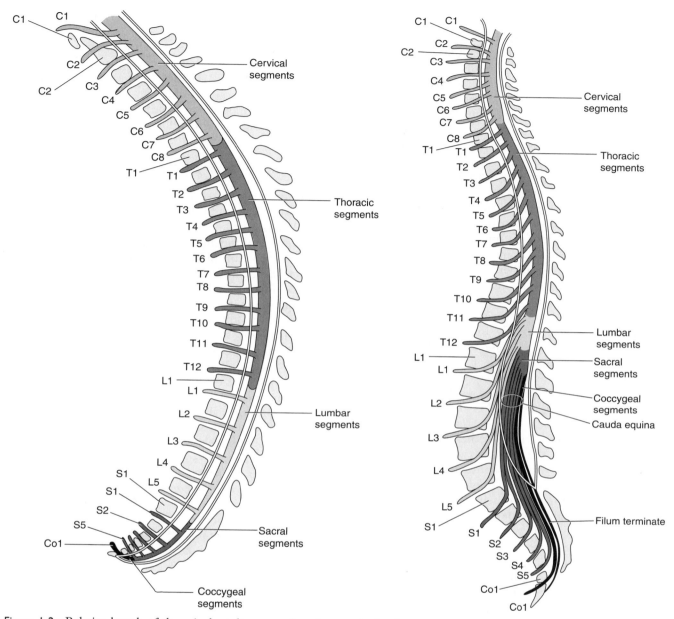

Figure 1-2. Relative length of the spinal cord compared to the vertebral column. A. The spinal cord occupies the entire length of the vertebral column in a 3-month-old fetus. B. In an adult, the cervical spinal segmental nerves exit at approximately the same vertebral level, but in more caudal regions the spinal segmental nerves occupy a more rostral location relative to their respective vertebrate.

L1 vertebra results in injury to the neural structures, it will likely affect the sacral spinal segments as well as the roots of the spinal nerves related to L1 through S5. This concept will be revisited later in the section on Spinal Cord Injury Syndromes.

Severity of Injury

Spinal cord injuries are often referred to as being "complete" or "incomplete," and while the term "complete" seems to suggest that there is no transmission of descending motor information or ascending sensory information below the level of injury, spinal injuries are usually not so straightforward. The American Spinal Injury Association (ASIA) has developed a system for classification of SCI [21] that defines injury level and severity of impairment (i.e., the ASIA Impairment Scale [AIS]) in unambiguous terms that provides a common language for use among clinicians and individuals with SCI, allowing identification of the motor and sensory level of injury, and a motor and a sensory score that indicates severity of injury to the motor and sensory pathways, respectively. The frequency of the different categories of SCI is incomplete tetraplegia (34.1%), complete paraplegia (23.0%), complete tetraplegia (18.3%), and incomplete paraplegia (18.5%).[7] This classification system is introduced below to provide necessary terminology, but will be discussed in greater detail in chapter 6, "Assessment of Function."

Using the ASIA classification system,[21] the motor level is determined by assessing the strength of the key muscles for each spinal level using a standard manual muscle test with muscle force rated on a scale of 0–5. The motor level is defined by the most caudal muscle that has a manual muscle test score of at least 3/5, as long as the immediately rostral muscle segment has a muscle test score of 5/5. Because muscles typically receive innervation from more than one spinal segment, damage to a specific spinal level will result in impairment of muscles innervated by that segment. However, if the muscle also receives innervation from more rostral spinal levels in the uninjured region of the spinal cord there may be preservation of some function. The bilateral muscles scores from the key five upper extremity and five lower extremity muscles are summed for a total motor score (maximum = 100), or may be considered separately for an upper extremity motor score (maximum = 50) and lower extremity motor score (maximum = 50). Assessment of voluntary function in the anal sphincter is important, as the ability (yes or no) to voluntarily contract this muscle results in classification of motor incomplete injury (AIS C at minimum) regardless of other findings.

The sensory score as rated by the ASIA classification system[21] is based on the extent to which an individual is able to perceive a wisp of cotton and/or a pinprick, representing the functional roles of the ascending dorsal columns (discriminative touch, vibration) and the anterolateral funiculus (crude touch, pain, temperature), respectively. The bilateral sensory scores for each dermatome are summed (maximum = 112 for each of light touch and pinprick). The most caudal dermatome to have intact sensation for both light touch and pinprick on both sides of the body defines the sensory level. Assessment of anal sensation (S4-5 dermatome) is important, as presence of sensory function (yes or no) in this dermatome results in classification of *incomplete injury* (AIS B at minimum) regardless of other findings.

Despite the standardized definition of the term "incomplete spinal cord injury," as having preserved anal sensation in the S4-5 dermatomal distribution, and the term "motor incomplete injury" as having preserved voluntary anal sphincter contraction, many people continue to use both the terms "incomplete injury" and "motor incomplete injury" to characterize an injury in which there is some remaining voluntary motor function of the extremities. In addition to the use of the terms "complete" and "incomplete" to describe remaining motor function, the terms *paralysis* and *paresis*, are also used, meaning loss of voluntary activation and impaired voluntary activation (weakness), respectively, of the muscles at or below the level of injury. For this reason, determining neurological classification by actually performing the assessment oneself rather than

relying on a prior assessment is advisable. However, if relying on an available prior assessment is necessary, one should bear in mind that assessments performed early post-injury may not reflect the most current status of an individual with SCI who is seen at a later date, as significant spontaneous motor recovery occurs within the first post-injury year. More detailed information regarding assessment of neurological level will be addressed in chapter 6, "Assessment of Function."

Chronicity of Injury

While the majority of motor return occurs within the first post-injury year, it is not uncommon for individuals with long-standing injury to report modest improvements in motor function years after injury. The literature indicates that an individual with incomplete SCI is likely to experience substantial improvements in motor function following acute SCI, as well as modest degrees of improvements in sensory function. A study of 21 individuals followed over the first three years after injury found that motor scores were significantly different between the acute phase (0–50 days post-injury) and the chronic phase (301–400 days post-injury) increasing about 36 points (from a score of approximately 42/100 to approximately 78/100).[22] Sensory function, however, did not change appreciably between the acute phase and the chronic phase, increasing only about 15 points (from score of approximately 72/112 to approximately 85/112). The large amount of spontaneous motor recovery that occurs within the first post-injury year makes determining the effectiveness of interventions that are applied during this period difficult. Without large numbers of study participants, differentiating between the improvements related to the intervention and those which occur as part of the natural course of recovery from the neural injury is not an easy task.

Upper Versus Lower Motor Neuron Injuries

Damage to descending pathways results in impairment or loss of the ability to voluntarily activate muscles that are innervated by spinal segments below the level of injury, due to disruption of the neural pathways that carry signals from motor neurons in the brain and brainstem (i.e., the upper motor neurons) to the spinal cord motor neurons (i.e., the lower motor neurons).

Below the level of injury, the lower motor neurons, motor nerves, and sensory nerves remain functional. Because the reflex loop (sensory nerve → spinal motor neuron → motor nerve → muscle activation) is therefore intact, muscles innervated by segments of the spinal cord below the level of injury may be activated by involuntary reflex mechanisms when sensory input (such as muscles stretch, noxious input, pressure, etc.) evokes in a reflex response. In fact, the reflex responses evoked by sensory input may be exaggerated. These exaggerated responses arise because damage to the descending tracts impairs not only transmission of the commands for voluntary movement, but also transmission of descending commands that normally modulate spinal reflex activity. This loss of descending modulation results in *hyperreflexia* and *spasticity* (these concepts will be explored further in chapter 18, "Spasticity After Spinal Cord Injury: Etiology and Management") in which responses to sensory input are exaggerated. The combination of hyperreflexia and weak voluntary muscle control is referred to as *spastic paresis* (or *spastic paralysis* in cases in which there is no remaining voluntary muscle control). Spastic paresis and paralysis are indications of *upper motor neuron damage* as they reflect a loss of input to the motor neurons from areas of the central nervous system above the level of injury. The muscles below the level of injury will undergo *disuse atrophy* as their innervation remains intact but voluntary control is diminished or lost; however, muscle bulk may be maintained to some extent because of the reflex-driven muscle activation (i.e., spasticity) described previously.[24]

In addition to the damage inflicted upon the descending upper motor neuron pathways (and ascending sensory pathways), injury to the spinal cord typically results in *lower motor neuron damage* at the spinal level of injury. The peripheral nerves in the region of injury may also be damaged. In a study investigating the integrity of the peripheral motor nerves in individuals with cervical SCI, more than 50% had reduced or absent muscle responses to maximal stimulation of the motor nerve,[23] indicating that the peripheral nerve function was impaired.

The consequence of damage to lower motor neurons in the spinal cord is diminished or absent reflex activation of the affected muscles. Lower motor neuron damage in combination with weak voluntary muscle control is referred to as *flaccid paresis* (or *flaccid paralysis* in cases in which there is no remaining voluntary muscle control). Muscles formerly innervated by the damaged lower motor neurons or nerves undergo *denervation atrophy* as their motor innervation is impaired or lost.[24]

Because trauma to the spinal cord may involve damage to both the descending upper motor neuron pathways and the lower motor neurons in the spinal cord, individuals with SCI often have signs associated with both upper and lower motor neuron pathology.[24] For example, an individual with injury classified according the ASIA system as being at the C6 motor level will have intact motor neurons at the C5 level, but likely has damage to at least some of the motor neurons at the C6 level. In such a case, the individual will have both impaired voluntary control and impaired reflex-driven activation of muscles formerly innervated by the lost lower motor neurons. If damage to the spinal cord extends more than a single segment (as is often the case), then the same may be true to varying degrees for muscles that are innervated by C7, C8, T1, and so on.

Incomplete SCI Syndromes

Information descending to the spinal cord from supraspinal centers, and ascending from the spinal cord to supraspinal centers travels in discrete tracts within the spinal cord. Incomplete SCI results in some areas of the spinal cord experiencing relatively more or less damage than other areas. For this reason, incomplete spinal cord injuries can be further characterized according to the distribution of functions that are relatively more or less spared and those that are more or less impaired. The incomplete SCI syndromes include central cord syndrome, Brown-Sequard syndrome, and anterior cord syndrome.[25,26] Conus medullaris syndrome and cauda equina syndrome may be either complete or incomplete, with the latter being most likely to be incomplete due to the nature of the injury (see the following sections). Earlier versions of the International Standards for Neurological Classification of Spinal Cord Injury also included posterior cord syndrome and mixed syndrome, but these were eliminated due to the low incidence of posterior cord syndrome and indefinable nature of mixed syndrome.[25] Among individuals with incomplete SCI, those individuals classified as having either central cord syndrome or Brown-Sequard syndrome have the best prognosis for recovery.[27]

Anterior Cord Syndrome

Anterior cord syndrome is characterized by loss of function of ventral pathways (including motor function and sensation of pain and temperature), but relative preservation of the dorsal columns (including proprioception, light touch, and deep pressure)[25] (see Fig. 1-3). Among individuals whose injuries are classified as incomplete cervical SCI syndrome, those with anterior cord syndrome demonstrate less functional recovery than other incomplete syndrome classifications.[27]

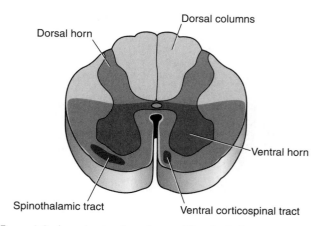

Figure 1-3. Anterior cord syndrome. The shaded area represents the general region damaged in individuals with anterior cord syndrome. The severity and extent of damage vary greatly.

Central Cord Syndrome

Central cord syndrome is characterized by greater upper extremity than lower extremity dysfunction.[25] The injury is typically characterized by a central area of injury, which selectively affects the medially located motor fibers that control distal upper extremity function (*see* Fig. 1-4). Many individuals with injuries that fall into this classification make dramatic improvements in their sensorimotor scores.[28] One investigation of 112 individuals with central cord syndrome found that two years post-injury, the average motor score was 92 out of a total 100.[28] While the prognosis for functional recovery is good for individuals with central cord syndrome, the pattern is such that in individuals who make good recovery intrinsic hand function is the last to recover[29,30] and in many cases fine motor control does not recover completely. Consequently, many individuals with only minor impairment in sensorimotor scores demonstrate moderate to severe limitations in the performance of functional activities.[28] In individuals with central cord syndrome, many factors influence the amount of motor recovery, return of functional skills, and perceived health quality life. Factors that predict recovery in individuals with central cord syndrome include level of education, presence of spasticity, and age; wherein a higher level of education, absence of spasticity, and younger age is positively correlated with improved functional outcome.[28] This form of injury often occurs in elderly individuals with spinal stenosis who experience a hyperextension injury.

Brown-Sequard Syndrome

An individual with a pure Brown Sequard Injury has damage that affects one-half of the spinal cord to a significantly greater extent than it does the other half (*see* Fig. 1-5). The clinical presentation of this syndrome is spastic paresis and loss of light touch and vibration sensation on the side of damage and loss of pain and temperature sensation on the contralateral side. These

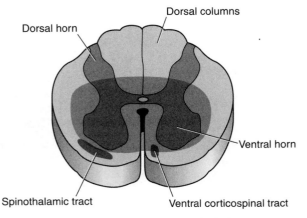

Figure 1-4. Central cord syndrome. The shaded area represents the general region damaged in individuals with central cord syndrome. The severity and extent of damage vary greatly.

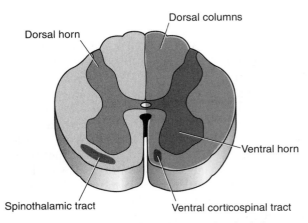

Figure 1-5. Brown-Sequard syndrome. The shaded area represents the general region damaged in individuals with Brown-Sequard syndrome. The severity and extent of damage vary greatly.

clinical findings can be explained by the organization of the spinal pathways. While the corticospinal tract and the dorsal column-medial lemniscus pathways decussate at the level of the brainstem, the spinothalamic pathway decussates at or near the root level where the sensory nerves enter. Thus, for an individual whose injury is characterized as Brown-Sequard syndrome, the pathways that carry light touch, deep pressure, and proprioceptive information, as well as those that carry motor information will be disrupted on the same side as the injury; whereas the pathways that carry pain and temperature will be disrupted on the side opposite the injury. Brown-Sequard syndrome is frequently caused by a penetrating injury.[25] Most individuals with this syndrome have a relative asymmetry of symptoms and not a pure form of Brown-Sequard syndrome.[25] One of the most important factors impacting functional recovery in individuals with Brown-Sequard syndrome is the preservation of motor function in the dominant hand.[31]

Conus Medullaris Syndrome

The conus medullaris is the terminal end of the spinal cord located anatomically at approximately vertebral levels T12–L2 in adults (*see* Fig. 1-6). The conus medullaris contains the motor neurons of the S4 and S5 spinal segments. Because the motor neurons of this segment innervate the bowel and bladder, damage to this region has important implications for control of these functions, as well as for some sexual functions (these concepts will be explored in detail in later chapters). Other characteristic signs and symptoms of conus medullaris syndrome include decreased sensation (particularly in the perianal area) and diminished Achilles reflexes. Involvement is usually bilateral and symmetric. There is also likely to be mixed upper and lower motor neuron damage, with the lower motor neuron damage being due both to injury of the motor neurons and trauma to the spinal roots that are descending in the

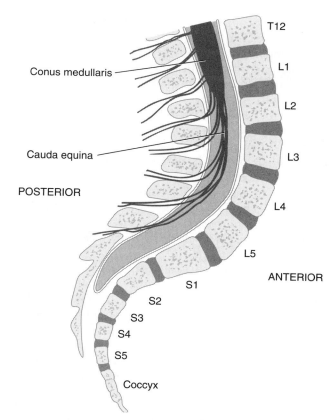

Figure 1-6. Injury to the distal spinal cord may result in conus medullaris syndrome, cauda equina syndrome, or a combination of these two syndromes.

vertebral canal to exit more caudally (i.e., cauda equina involvement—see the following section).

Cauda Equina Syndrome

The cauda equina (i.e., horse's tail) is the bundle of nerve roots (consisting of the nerves from spinal segmental levels L2–S5) that extend through the vertebral canal below the level of the conus medullaris. Trauma or compressive forces that result in narrowing of the vertebral canal can compress the nerves resulting in cauda equina syndrome. In the presence of progressive compression (e.g., from disc herniation or lumbar spondylosis), the onset of cauda equina syndrome may be gradual. This syndrome is characterized by low back pain, radicular pain (typically in the sciatic nerve distribution), lower extremity paresis or paralysis, sensory deficit or loss in the perineal area and in affected dermatomal distributions in the lower extremities, bowel and/or bladder dysfunction, and diminished or absent patellar and Achilles reflexes. As such, with traumatic injury to lumbar levels L2–L5, the spinal cord may be spared, but the nerves in the cauda equina are damaged, resulting in lower motor neuron injuries. With damage to the nerves there is impairment or loss of the reflex pathway, such that individuals with cauda equina injuries do not exhibit spastic hyperreflexia and therefore have denervation atrophy of

the deafferented muscles. Cauda equina syndrome may accompany conus medullaris injury.

The distribution of traumatic forces is variable in all forms of SCI, but because of the mobile nature of the nerve roots the variability may be even greater in cauda equina injuries compared to those that affect the spinal cord itself. Cauda equina injuries are typically asymmetrical and incomplete as not all nerve roots are likely to be damaged to an equal extent. As with injury to the spinal cord, the neurological outcomes associated with damage to the cauda equina depend to a large extent on the severity of the injury.[32] However, because peripheral nerves have greater potential for spontaneous regrowth than do tracts in the central nervous system, there is a possibility of regeneration of the peripheral nerves damaged in this type of injury.

Prognosis for Functional Recovery in Individuals with SCI

Early Clinical Measures Correlated with Neurological Outcomes

For individuals with cervical SCI, factors used to identify prognosis of recovery of arm and hand function include severity of injury and the neurological level of injury.[33] As would be expected, individuals with an initial diagnosis of incomplete cervical SCI demonstrate greater motor recovery than individuals with an initial diagnosis of complete SCI.[34,35] Recovery of upper limb function is almost two times greater in individuals with incomplete SCI than in individuals with complete SCI.[35] There are a number of early clinical assessment measures that have been shown to correlate with longer-term functional outcomes. Most notably, the presence of sensation at a motor level improves the probability of motor return at that level, especially if perception of pain is intact.[36] The close proximity of the spinothalamic tract to the corticospinal tract may indicate that if one of these tracts is preserved the other tract is also likely to be preserved. Thus, preservation of the perception of pain (ability to sense pinprick; a modality relayed through the spinothalamic pathway) may indicate that other pathways that travel in the anterolateral columns may also be preserved.[31] Motor function at 3 months post-injury is better predicted by muscle test scores obtained at 72 hours post-injury compared to scores obtained earlier (i.e., at 24 hours post-injury).[37] In addition, radiographical evidence (e.g., MRI) of edema and hemorrhage in the spinal cord, and significant spinal cord compression have some predictive value, as these factors are associated with poorer prognosis for neurological recovery.[38]

Recovery of Hand and Arm Function

Individuals with complete cervical SCI frequently recover at least one level of sensory or motor function, with the greatest rate of recovery occurring within the first 3 months.[35] In individuals with cervical SCI, functional recovery of upper limb function begins to plateau around 12–18 months.[39,40] For this reason, the chronic phase of SCI is considered to begin at 12 months post-injury. The level of injury may determine the relative amount of sensory or motor recovery in individuals with complete tetraplegia.

Individuals with complete C4 injury have a lower likelihood of regaining sensorimotor function at the C5 level compared to the likelihood of individuals with a complete C5 injury regaining sensorimotor function at the C6 level.[40] Further, the early presence of even small amounts of voluntary muscle activation indicates greater probability of achieving antigravity muscle strength for that muscle.[35] Ninety-seven percent of individuals initially classified with complete cervical SCI who had a motor score of 1/5 or 2/5 at one month post-injury regained antigravity muscle strength (3/5) by the end of the first post-injury year. Conversely, of individuals with complete cervical SCI who at one month post-injury had a motor score of 0/5 at the level caudal to the last level of normal motor function, only 27% regained antigravity muscle strength at that level by 1 year post-injury.[39]

Individuals with motor incomplete cervical SCI have the greatest potential for recovery of upper extremity function,[33,35,41] and recovery of function at the next caudal level occurs much faster in individuals with motor incomplete SCI.[42] Waters et al.[33] found that in individuals with motor incomplete cervical SCI, muscles having an initial score of 2/5 had a 100% likelihood of being able to move against gravity at 1 year post-injury. Further, 73% of muscles having an initial score of 1/5 were able to move against gravity at one year post-injury, and 20% of muscles having an initial score of 0/5 were able to move against gravity at 1 year post-injury.[33] In these individuals, functional recovery of the upper extremities begins to plateau around 9–12 months.[28,41]

Recovery of Walking Function

In individuals with incomplete paraplegia, lower extremity motor scores (derived from the five key lower extremity muscles tested as part of the AIS[21] increased significantly between 1 month and 1 year post-injury, with the average increase being 12/50 points. The rate of recover is greatest in the first 6 months post-injury and then begins to plateau.[43] As expected, there is a significant correlation between walking function and the lower extremity motor score. Those individuals who at 1 month post-injury had lower extremity motor scores of at least 10/50 and scores of at least 2/5 in either the hip flexors or knee extensors, were able to achieve community ambulation with walking aides and lower extremity orthoses.[44] These data were compiled prior to 1994, at which time aggressive locomotor training for individuals with motor incomplete SCI was a far less common practice than it is today.

Therefore, locomotor outcomes in individuals with incomplete SCI may be better than what has been reported in the literature.

In both individuals with complete SCI and those with incomplete SCI, the spontaneous recovery of function that occurs as the nervous system recovers from the edema and trauma of the acute injury may be augmented by sprouting of new axon collaterals from the remaining lower motor neurons.[45] However, this sprouting results in the creation of large motor units as the motor neurons must innervate a greater number of muscle fibers than normal, thereby decreasing the ratio of motoneurons per muscle fiber.[46,47] Maintaining a high ratio of motoneurons to muscle fibers is vital for grading muscle force,[48] therefore, altering the proportion of muscle fibers to motor neurons results in the inability to grade movement.[49]

While aggressive physical and occupational therapy clearly impact long-term functional outcomes, there is often little agreement regarding the optimal approach. This is especially true in individuals with motor incomplete injury. While the lack of definitive data is largely due to a paucity of comparative studies, the situation is further complicated by the lack of standardization in outcome measures that would allow comparisons to be made among the results of different studies.[50,51]

Secondary Conditions Associated with SCI

Autonomic Dysreflexia

Autonomic dysreflexia (AD) is a potentially life-threatening hypertensive condition that occurs in individuals with SCI above the level of T6 as a result of the loss of supraspinal regulation of autonomic function in the control of blood pressure. The incidence of AD is higher in individuals with motor complete SCI (i.e., AIS A or B) but may also occur in those with motor incomplete SCI (i.e., AIS C) with the first incident typically occurring within 1–6 months of the injury.[52]

In nondisabled individuals, noxious sensory inputs excite the sympathetic portion of the autonomic nervous system (T6–T12; also called the splanchnic outflow). This excitation is associated with vasoconstriction and increased cardiac output resulting in elevation of blood pressure. Activation of the sympathetic nervous system evokes a balancing response from the parasympathetic nervous system. Receptors in the aortic arch and carotid sinus sense the increased blood pressure, triggering a reflex response (the baroreceptor reflex) mediated by the brainstem. This reflex normally decreases the sympathetic drive to the blood vessels, thereby decreasing vasoconstriction and subsequently reducing blood pressure. In individuals with SCI above the level of T6, the normal balance of excitation and inhibition between the sympathetic and parasympathetic portions of the autonomic nervous systems is disrupted. Noxious input below the level of injury is transmitted rostrally to the sympathetic neurons in the intermediolateral cell column of the spinal cord. As with nondisabled individuals, this results in reflex sympathetic discharge that induces elevation of blood pressure. However, among individuals with SCI, the descending signals that would typically counteract the increased blood pressure cannot be transmitted to the levels below the injury. In contrast, above the level of the injury reflex-driven vasodilation does occur, resulting in headache and skin flushing. Unless the precipitating noxious input is removed, the excitatory drive to the sympathetic nervous system persists, and the blood pressure continues to rise. Episodes of hypertension are often accompanied by bradycardia due to vagal parasympathetic stimulation, especially for individuals in whom the injury is caudal to the spinal segments providing control of cardiac output (T1-6).

The ability to recognize the signs and symptoms of AD is critical as AD has the potential to develop into an acute medical emergency with cerebral hemorrhage and (rarely) death resulting from extremely high levels of blood pressure. Other serious medical complications may include seizures, myocardial infarction, and renal hemorrhage. Signs and symptoms associated with AD include headache, sweating, increased blood pressure (systolic pressure 20 mm–40 mm Hg above baseline), and decreased heart rate. The individual may exhibit flushing of the face and neck, sweating, and piloerection above the level of the lesion. Below the level of the lesion, there may be pallor of the skin. Other signs and symptoms are given in Table 1-1. Identification and removal of the offending stimulus should be the immediate response to suspected AD. The individual should be assisted to an upright position to facilitate lowering of the blood pressure.

Table 1-1
Recognizing the Causes and Signs/Symptoms of Autonomic Dysreflexia

Common Causes	Common Signs/Symptoms[53]
Gastrointestinal Irregularities Bladder distension (most common) Urinary tract infection Urinary retention Blocked catheter Overfilled urine bag or kink in catheter tube Bowel distension Constipation/impaction Hemorrhoids Acute abdominal conditions (gastric ulcer, colitis, peritonitis)	High blood pressure Severe headache Bradycardia (may be a relative slowing so that the heart rate is still within the normal range) Profuse sweating above the level of the lesion, especially in the face, neck, and shoulders, or possibly below the level of the lesion
Skin-related Disorders Pressure ulcers Ingrown toenails Burns Restrictive clothing	Piloerection or goose bumps above or possibly below the level of the lesion Cardiac arrhythmias, atrial fibrillation, premature ventricular contractions, and atrioventricular conduction abnormalities
Sexual Activity Over stimulation during sexual activity (stimuli to the pelvic region which would ordinarily be painful if sensation were present) Menstrual cramps Labor and delivery	Flushing of the skin above the level of the lesion, especially in the face, neck, and shoulders, or possibly below the level of lesion Blurred vision Appearance of spots in the patient's visual fields
Other Bone fractures (including occult fractures) Heterotopic ossification Electrical stimulation	Nasal congestion Feelings of apprehension or anxiety over an impending physical problem Minimal or no symptoms, despite a significantly elevated blood pressure (silent autonomic dysreflexia)

From the perspective of rehabilitation, it is important to note the high intensities of electrical stimulation that are frequently used with functional electrical stimulation can, and do, evoke AD in some individuals. The most common sources of noxious and nonnoxious stimuli are also given in Table 1-1.

If the offending stimulus cannot be promptly identified and removed, and if blood pressure continues to be elevated, then emergency medical attention with administration of fast-acting vasodilators (such as nifedipine[53]) may be critical in preventing serious medical complications. All individuals involved in the care of the person with SCI should be knowledgeable about the signs and symptoms of AD, and should be prepared to respond appropriately. Individuals who experience frequent episodes of AD should be counseled to wear a medical alert bracelet or carry a medical alert card, and may be prescribed fast-acting vasodilators for episodic use. Published guidelines for acute management of autonomic dysreflexia in individuals with SCI are available from, the Consortium for Spinal Cord Medicine.[53]

Deep Vein Thrombosis

Deep vein thrombosis (DVT) is the result of coagulation of blood resulting in a thrombus in the venous system in areas below the level of injury. The incidence of DVT in individuals with acute SCI is highest in the initial two weeks after injury, and it has been recommended that weekly screening for DVT be performed during the first 13 weeks post-SCI.[8] There is disagreement in the literature regarding the incidence of DVT. While pooled estimates suggest an incidence rate of approximately 17%,[8] some investigators have reported rates over 60%.[54] In those admitted for acute hospitalization following SCI, there appears to be an increased incidence of DVT depending on level and severity of injury with greater risk among those having motor complete paraplegia compared to those with motor incomplete tetraplegia.[55] However, following the initial hospitalization, among individuals admitted for rehabilitation there is no evident relationship between development of DVT and level of injury (i.e., tetraplegia, paraplegia), severity of injury (i.e., motor complete, motor incomplete), or cause of injury (i.e., traumatic, nontraumatic).[56] There is some evidence to suggest that SCI in combination with long bone fracture increases the risk for DVT.[57]

Venous thromboembolism results when a portion of a thrombus breaks free and travels to another location in the venous system. Pulmonary emboli occur when the thrombus becomes lodged in the pulmonary venous system, and is the most serious complication of SCI as it represents a critical medical situation that may result in death. While some reports estimate the incidence of pulmonary embolism in individuals with acute SCI to be just less than 5%,[8] others have suggested that the rate may be over 18%.[54]

Clinical signs and symptoms for the diagnosis of DVT may be different than in noninjured patients and DVTs may also be much more difficult to identify in those with SCI. Rapid onset of swelling in one lower extremity is the characteristic symptom of DVT, but swelling may also occur bilaterally. In individuals with preserved sensation, there may be lower extremity pain. There may also be increased temperature of one or both lower extremities and/or tenderness upon compression of the muscles over the course of the veins in the calf or thigh.

Medical management with pharmacological thromboprophylaxis as anticoagulation therapy is the primary preventive measure and treatment; however, there is evidence to suggest that pharmacological prophylaxis may actually increase the risk of DVT.[56] Other noninvasive forms of prophylaxis include intermittent pneumatic compression devices and graduated compression stockings. Vena cava filters may be implanted early after SCI to prevent pulmonary emboli.[57,58] However, these filters may not be warranted as a form of routine prophylaxis for those who respond well to anticoagulation therapy[57] In addition, filters may be indicated for individuals who develop pulmonary embolus while on anticoagulation therapy, those with contraindications for anticoagulation therapy who have a history of pulmonary embolus, and those with documented free-floating ileofemoral thrombus[58] or with long bone fractures.[57]

Pressure Ulcers

Pressure ulcers are lesions of the skin and underlying tissue. They represent a preventable complication that results from prolonged immobilization or poor handling during transfers or bed mobility activities. Pressure ulcers are usually the result of prolonged compression of a bony prominence against a support surface resulting in decreased tissue perfusion, ischemia, and in the worst cases, tissue necrosis. While pressure ulcers occur most commonly over bony prominences, they also frequently occur at sites where skin is folded, such as at joint creases (e.g., as in cases of joint contractures where the two surfaces approximate each other) and under breast tissue in women. Friction forces between skin and the support surface can also result in damage to the epidermal and dermal layers of the skin, resulting in a pressure ulcer. Additionally, shear forces between the skin and underlying fascial and bony tissue can result in pressure ulcers if the vascular supply is compromised. Finally, excessive moisture can exacerbate the effects of interface forces making skin more prone to breakdown.

Pressure ulcers are a significant source of morbidity after SCI; therefore, skin care is a critical component of lifetime health maintenance. It is essential that the individual with SCI be educated in self-management of a complete skin care regimen. There are some excellent published guidelines available from the Paralyzed Veterans of America[59] and from the Consortium for

Spinal Cord Medicine Clinical Practice Guidelines.[60] The skin care regimen may be accomplished independently by individuals with adequate motor function to move sufficiently and frequently enough to allow tissue perfusion in areas of pressure, and to perform skin inspections. As might be expected, individuals with greater disability who require more assistance with activities of daily living are more likely to develop pressure ulcers.[61] Individuals with SCI who lack the necessary motor function to relieve areas of pressure and adequately perform skin inspections, must take responsibility for managing their own skin care by directing others to perform the necessary pressure relief activities and inspection.

Prevention of pressure ulcers should be a primary goal. The individual with SCI must be taught to perform or guide a caregiver through thorough visual and tactile skin inspections on a daily basis. Close attention should be given to inspection of the weight-bearing prominences that are most prone to the development of pressure ulcers, including the ischial tuberocities, sacrum/coccyx, greater trochanters, calcaneae, inion, and ears. The individual must also be taught to avoid prolonged positional immobilization, and to seek assistance and instruct others in pressure-relief techniques if necessary, including turning in bed every 2 hours. When moving or being moved, care should be taken to minimize friction and shearing of the skin, and when positioned, care must be taken to avoid stretching or folding of the skin. Pillows and cushions should be positioned to bridge bony prominences and relieve areas of tissue contact with the support surface. However, doughnut cushions should not be used as these create a ring of pressure surrounding the central area that restricts blood flow. The appropriate pressure-reducing support surfaces (e.g., wheelchair cushions, mattresses, pillows) should be acquired and maintained in optimally effective condition. Care should be taken to minimize moisture and elevated temperatures at the interface between the skin and the support surface.[59,60] Finally, proper nutrition is essential for skin health, the individual's diet should be evaluated by qualified professionals to insure adequate dietary intake of calories, fluids, protein, vitamins, and minerals.

Heterotopic Ossification

Heterotopic ossification (HO) is ectopic bone formation in the soft tissues surrounding a joint. In individuals with SCI it occurs only caudal to the level of injury. While incompletely understood, the pathophysiology of HO is thought to involve an inflammatory process following trauma to soft tissue wherein bone morphogenic proteins act on mesenchymal stem cells in the soft tissue activating them to differentiate into osteoblasts.[62] Whether the mesenchymal cells originate in the soft tissue or migrate there from distance sites is unknown.

Heterotopic ossification represents the most frequent orthopedic complication associated with SCI, with

incidence rates reported to be as high as 53%, but the incidence of clinically significant HO is lower at approximately 27%. While HO most typically occurs within the first 4 months after injury, later onsets are not uncommon. HO may limit joint mobility and may make mobility painful in those with sensation. In these cases, surgical resection of the ectopic bone may be considered. In extreme cases, ankylosis may occur, but this is rare (5% or less of cases). In situations where surgical resection of HO is deemed warranted, this occurs after the bone has reached maturity (usually 12 to 18 months after onset). In these individuals, radiation therapy may prevent recurrence of HO postoperatively.[62]

The sooner the onset of HO is detected the more can be done to prevent its progression. While the hip is the most common site for the formation of HO, it may also occur in knee, shoulder, and elbow. The first sign is often an observation of limited range of motion at the involved joint, despite consistent range of motion exercise, with joint limitation frequently accompanied by hyperemia, warmth, and/or swelling. Early range of motion exercise (either active or passive as indicated) is important for maintaining joint function. In early HO, medical management may include administration of etidronate to prevent calcium from being deposited in the bone matrix, but there is controversy regarding whether etidronate prevents or simply delays mineralization of the bony matrix.[63] Because HO is accompanied by various degrees of inflammation, prophylactic use of nonsteroidal anti-inflammatory agents may reduce the incidence of HO. In the initial inflammatory phase of HO formation, if etidronate is prescribed, it may be useful to supplement etidronate with nonsteroidal anti-inflammatory agents.[62]

A study of individuals with HO who were within 6 months of injury indicated that range of motion exercises were sufficient to maintain joint range of motion in the presence of immature ectopic bone.[64] A small study suggests that in individuals in whom range of motion exercises are delayed after SCI (such that muscle contracture begins to develop before exercises are initiated) the subsequent application of range of motion exercises may traumatize the soft tissue and increase the risk for HO.[65] Consistent with this concept is that there appears to be an association between the degree of spasticity and the development of HO.[66] It is important to minimize pressure over prominences created by the presence of heterotopic bone in seating and bed positioning to reduce the risk of pressure ulcer development at these sites.

Urinary Tract Infections and Renal Complications

Urinary tract infections (UTIs) are a common occurrence in individuals with SCI, particularly in those individuals who use intermittent catheterization for bladder management. Education and good personal hygiene are essential to reduce the occurrence of UTIs in individuals with SCI. Factors that increase the risk of UTI includes large residual urine volumes after voiding, bladder overdistention, voiding via high-pressure bladder evacuation techniques, outlet obstruction, and stones in the urinary system. Prevention of UTIs is a key to preventing kidney damage. Renal complications at one time represented the most common and serious of secondary conditions after SCI, and were a significant source of mortality. The widespread use of intermittent catheterization by individuals with SCI has greatly reduced the number of deaths due to renal failure in the USA, but this remains a significant problem for individuals with SCI who live in the developing world. There is some evidence that the risk for development of UTIs is lower in those who engage in weekly exercise.[61] Current concepts regarding bladder management in individuals with SCI is discussed in detail in chapter 15, "Bowel and Bladder Function and Management."

Bone Fracture

Individuals with SCI usually experience some degree of bone demineralization (i.e., osteopenia or osteoporosis) following the injury. Reduced bone density in individuals with SCI is associated with the occurrence of fractures when mechanical stress and strain is applied, such as occurs during transfers. Multiple factors contribute to bone demineralization in individuals with SCI, including changes in hormonal regulation, as well as neural and vascular factors.[67]

In those with motor complete SCI, the annual incidence of fracture is approximately 2%, and the likelihood of fracture increases over time, with the time between injury and first fracture averaging approximately 9 years.[68] Fracture thresholds for the femur and distal tibia have been established through comparison of bone mineral density values in a group of individuals with motor complete SCI who experienced bone fracture to a group who did not. These fracture threshold values may allow the identification of those who are at risk for fracture with minor trauma.[69]

The reduced or absent muscle activity in paretic or paralyzed muscles results in significantly decreased muscular load on the underlying bone. The reduction of mechanical stimuli to the bone from muscle contraction is thought to be an important contributor to bone demineralization.[70] There is some evidence to suggest that while physical activity level and spasticity do not greatly influence bone mineral density, there may be some benefit to regular intensive loading activities in the early stages of rehabilitation.[71] While individuals with tetraplegia experience decreased density of bones in both the upper and lower extremities, only the bones of the lower extremities exhibit decreased density in individuals with paraplegia, and demineralization of lower extremity bones does not differ between these groups.[71] Current

concepts related to the preservation of bone density in individuals with SCI are discussed in detail in chapter 3 "Musculoskeletal Plasticity after SCI."

Syringomyelia

Following traumatic injury, hemorrhage and infarction within the spinal cord may lead to formation of a cavity within the spinal cord. A spinal cord cyst is a small, oval-shaped cavity that is restricted to the level at which the vertebrate protrude most prominently into the spinal cord.[72] MRI evidence suggests that approximately 10% of individuals injured longer than 20 years have a spinal cord cyst.[73] A syrinx is a tapered, fluid-filled cavity within the spinal cord (i.e., syringomyelia) that may extend for multiple spinal levels.

Syringomyelia is thought to occur in just over 3% of individuals with traumatic SCI,[74] but it can cause considerable reduction in functional capacity as well as be a source of pain. Symptoms of syrinx development include increased severity of neurological deficits (e.g., weakness, sensory loss), ascending neurological level, pain, and increasing reflex activity such as spasticity and spasms. The syrnix may be stable, in which case functional loss plateaus. Alternatively, if the cavity is unstable, there is progressive loss of neural tissue as the cavity enlarges over multiple spinal segments. The etiology of syrinx formation is not completely understood, and these may develop years after the acute injury.

The placement of a shunt to move the fluid from the cavity to the subarachnoid space has been reported to reduce symptoms or at least limit their progression.[75] In some cases, the development of a syrinx is thought to be associated with the tethering of the spinal cord (in which the spinal cord tissue becomes adhered or "tethered" to the dural tube)[73] resulting in disruption of the normal flow of cerebrospinal fluid. The alteration in the fluid pressures is thought to contribute to the formation of the syrinx. In some situations, surgical untethering of the dural tissue, with or without a syringosubarachnoid shunt, may halt or slow the enlargement of the syrinx and reverse or halt the progression of functional loss.[76] However, this option must be weighed against the additional trauma and scarring associated with the surgery, which may in itself contribute to subsequent tethering. The apparent increase in the incidence of syringomyelia may simply reflect improved ability to identify this condition because of increased awareness of the problem, longer post-injury survival times, and improved imaging techniques.

Spasticity

Early after injury the spinal cord may be relatively unresponsive to stimuli that would typically evoke a reflex motor response. This period has been referred to as "spinal shock" suggesting that the spinal cord is unresponsive, but evidence suggests reflexes can be elicited even in individuals with acute SCI.[77] This period of relative areflexia is usually followed by the development of spastic paresis or spastic paralysis in those who do not have purely lower motor neuron damage. Spasticity is a complex phenomenon that is thought to be due, in large part, to the aberrant processing of incoming sensory information by the spinal cord. However, there are also known to be changes to the mechanical properties of the muscle associated with spasticity.[78–81] It has been suggested that spasticity arises as a default level of neural control to maximize functional movement following damage to the central nervous system.[82,83] Current concepts regarding the etiology and management of spasticity in individuals with SCI is discussed in detail in chapter 18, "Management of Spasticity after SCI."

Pain

Pain is a common and often persistent secondary complication associated with SCI. Pain is a problem for many individuals with SCI, as it impacts their quality of life and ability to function in activities of daily living.[84,85] There are two different types of pain that primarily affect those with SCI: nociceptive pain and neuropathic pain.

Nociceptive pain is the type of pain experienced by everyone at one time or another. This type of pain is part of the body's normal protective mechanisms, it has an identifiable cause. Sensory input arising from sensory receptors in the soft tissue indicates actual or impending tissue damage. These signals are transmitted to the spinal cord and higher centers of the central nervous system. At the level of the spinal cord, these signals may elicit a reflex response (such as reflex withdrawal from the painful stimulus), and signals reaching the higher centers impart conscious awareness of the painful stimulus. In individuals with spastic paresis or paralysis, the reflex response to painful input is often exaggerated, resulting in a reflex spasm that may involve the whole limb or the entire body. Nociceptive pain can also be persistent, as in the case of bone fractures, back pain from prolonged sitting, or repeated musculoskeletal microtrauma (e.g., overuse syndromes of the shoulder).

Neuropathic pain is pain or sensory disturbance that occurs due to abnormal processing of afferent input following damage to the peripheral or central nervous system. Neuropathic pain is characterized by the location or region of sensory disturbance and by its quality (e.g., sharp, shooting, electric, burning, and stabbing). Neuropathic pain can be further described by where the pain or sensory disturbance occurs relative to the level of SCI. "Below level" neuropathic pain is present at least three segments below the level of injury; it is usually diffuse pain that may be described as burning, tingling, aching, shooting, or stabbing. "At level" neuropathic pain occurs in a segmental distribution at or within two segments of the level of the spinal injury; this type of neuropathic pain can be further classified as radicular (due to changes in the peripheral nervous system; i.e., nerve or nerve root) or central (due to changes within the central nervous system; i.e., spinal or supraspinal structures).[86,87] "Above level" neuropathic pain is located above the level of injury. This type of pain includes complex regional pain syndrome (formerly referred to as causalgia or reflex sympathetic dystrophy) and is experienced by both individuals with and without SCI. Current concepts regarding the etiology, assessment, and management of pain in individuals with SCI is discussed in detail in chapter 17, "Pain after SCI: Etiology and Management."

Summary

The care of individuals with SCI at the emergency, acute, and rehabilitation stages has improved dramatically in recent decades. However, SCI continues to affect people of all ages, backgrounds, and lifestyles. The average age of SCI has been increasing in recent years, but men continue to experience traumatic SCI in higher proportions than do women. While most epidemiological and outcomes research has focused on individuals with traumatic injury, a fair proportion of spinal cord injuries are nontraumatic in nature and there are some differences in secondary conditions in traumatic versus nontraumatic SCI.

There are a number of factors that contribute to the neurological and functional status after SCI. Chief among these are the level and severity of injury. Level of injury determines what muscles will and will not be affected by the injury as well as the location and extent of sensory and autonomic deficits. Severity of injury indicates whether some motor, sensory, and /or autonomic functions are spared (i.e., less severe injuries) or lost (i.e., more severe injuries). Injuries to the spinal cord usually result in both upper and lower motor neuron signs and symptoms, as the injury affects the descending pathways from upper motor neurons as well as the lower motor neurons located in the spinal cord itself. Because different regions of the spinal cord contain different types of ascending and descending pathways, incomplete injury may be associated with one of several incomplete SCI syndromes.

While it is frequently not possible in the early stages after SCI to offer a definitive prognosis regarding eventual functional outcomes, there are a number of prognostic signs that can give some indication of what may be expected in terms of recovery of upper extremity function and for return of walking capacity. There are a number of secondary conditions associated with SCI, several of which can be life-threatening. Fortunately, many of these are preventable with education, awareness, and a healthy lifestyle.

REVIEW QUESTIONS

1. List the top four most common causes of traumatic SCI in the United States.
2. You are working in the rehab gym with two individuals, one with a motor complete injury (AIS A) at the level of T10 compared and the other with a motor complete (AIS A) injury at L2. They want to know why one of them has involuntary muscle spasms in the legs and the other does not. What would you tell them?
3. Describe the motor deficits that will be observed in an individual with C6 anterior cord syndrome. Compare and contrast these with the deficits observed in an individual with central cord syndrome at the same neural level.
4. Describe three clinical assessments performed early after SCI that may assist in predicting functional outcomes.
5. You are working on transfers with an individual who was transferred to the rehab unit 2 days ago. You notice that his face appears flushed and sweaty. What should you be concerned about? What questions would you ask him, and what assessments would you perform to determine whether your inference is correct? What action would you take?

REFERENCES

1. Botterell EH, Jousse AT, Kraus AS, Thompson MG, WynneJones M, Geisler WO. A model for the future care of acute spinal cord injuries. *Can J Neurol Sci.* 1975;2:361–380.
2. National Institute of Neurological Disorders and Stroke. Spinal Cord Injury: Hope Through Research. http://www.ninds.nih.gov/disorders/sci/detail_sci.htm NIH Publication No. 03-160. 2006. National Institutes of Health. 11-12-2007.
3. Bors E. Intermittent catheterization in paraplegic patients. *Urol Int.* 1967;22:236–249.
4. Firlit CF, Canning JR, Lloyd FA, Cross RR, Brewer R, Jr. Experience with intermittent catheterization in chronic spinal cord injury patients. *J Urol.* 1975;114:234–236.
5. Sperling KB. Intermittent catheterization to obtain catheter-free bladder function in spinal cord injury. *Arch Phys Med Rehabil.* 1978;59:4–8.
6. Lorenzi ME, Berzins E, Webb SB, Jr. Emergency medical care and transportation of spinal cord injured patients in Connecticut, 1973–1977. *Emerg Med Serv.* 1982;11:26, 28, 30-26, 28, 33.
7. Spinal Cord Injury Information Network. Spinal Cord Injury Facts and Figures at a Glance—June 2006. http://www.spinalcord.uab.edu/show.asp?durki=19679. 2007. 5-17-2007.
8. Furlan JC, Fehlings MG. Role of screening tests for deep venous thrombosis in asymptomatic adults with acute spinal cord injury: An evidence-based analysis. *Spine.* 2007;32:1908–1916.
9. Regan RF, Guo Y. Estrogens attenuate neuronal injury due to hemoglobin, chemical hypoxia, and excitatory amino acids in murine cortical cultures. *Brain Res.* 1997;764:133–140.
10. Sribnick EA, Matzelle DD, Ray SK, Banik NL. Estrogen treatment of spinal cord injury attenuates calpain activation and apoptosis. *J Neurosci Res.* 2006;84:1064–1075.
11. Sribnick EA, Wingrave JM, Matzelle DD, Wilford GG, Ray SK, Banik NL. Estrogen attenuated markers of inflammation and decreased lesion volume in acute spinal cord injury in rats. *J Neurosci Res.* 2005;82:283–293.
12. Labombarda F, Gonzalez SL, Deniselle MC et al. Effects of injury and progesterone treatment on progesterone receptor and progesterone binding protein 25-Dx expression in the rat spinal cord. *J Neurochem.* 2003;87:902–913.
13. Gonzalez SL, Labombarda F, Deniselle MC et al. Progesterone neuroprotection in spinal cord trauma involves up-regulation of brain-derived neurotrophic factor in motoneurons. *J Steroid Biochem Mol Biol.* 2005;94:143–149.
14. Thomas AJ, Nockels RP, Pan HQ, Shaffrey CI, Chopp M. Progesterone is neuroprotective after acute experimental spinal cord trauma in rats. *Spine.* 1999;24:2134–2138.
15. Fee DB, Swartz KR, Joy KM, Roberts KN, Scheff NN, Scheff SW. Effects of progesterone on experimental spinal cord injury. *Brain Res.* 2007;1137:146–152.
16. Swartz KR, Fee DB, Joy KM et al. Gender differences in spinal cord injury are not estrogen-dependent. *J Neurotrauma.* 2007;24:473–480.
17. Stover S, DeLisa J, Whiteneck G. *Spinal Cord Injury: Clinical Outcomes from the Model Systems.* Gaitherville, MD: Aspen; 1995.
18. Burke DA, Linden RD, Zhang YP, Maiste AC, Shields CB. Incidence rates and populations at risk for spinal cord injury: A regional study. *Spinal Cord.* 2001;39:274–278.
19. McKinley WO, Tewksbury MA, Godbout CJ. Comparison of medical complications following nontraumatic and traumatic spinal cord injury. *J Spinal Cord Med.* 2002;25:88–93.
20. Ones K, Yilmaz E, Beydogan A, Gultekin O, Caglar N. Comparison of functional results in non-traumatic and traumatic spinal cord injury. *Disabil Rehabil.* 2007;29:1185–1191.
21. American Spinal Injury Association. International Standards for Neurological Classification of Spinal Cord Injury. 2002. Chicago, ASIA.
22. Smith HC, Savic G, Frankel HL et al. Corticospinal function studied over time following incomplete spinal cord injury. *Spinal Cord.* 2000;38:292–300.
23. Curt A, Keck ME, Dietz V. Clinical value of F-wave recordings in traumatic cervical spinal cord injury. *Electroencephalogr Clin Neurophysiol.* 1997;105:189–193.
24. Gordon T, Mao J. Muscle atrophy and procedures for training after spinal cord injury. *Phys Ther.* 1994;74:50–60.
25. Hayes KC, Hsieh JT, Wolfe DL, Potter PJ, Delaney GA. Classifying incomplete spinal cord injury syndromes: Algorithms based on the International Standards for Neurological and Functional Classification of Spinal Cord Injury Patients. *Arch Phys Med Rehabil.* 2000;81:644–652.
26. Maynard FM, Jr., Bracken MB, Creasey G et al. International Standards for Neurological and Functional Classification of Spinal Cord Injury. American Spinal Injury Association. *Spinal Cord.* 1997;35:266–274.
27. Pollard ME, Apple DF. Factors associated with improved neurologic outcomes in patients with incomplete tetraplegia. *Spine.* 2003;28:33–39.
28. Dvorak MF, Fisher CG, Hoekema J et al. Factors predicting motor recovery and functional outcome after traumatic central cord syndrome: a long-term follow-up. *Spine.* 2005;30:2303–2311.

29. Merriam WF, Taylor TK, Ruff SJ, McPhail MJ. A reappraisal of acute traumatic central cord syndrome. *J Bone Joint Surg Br.* 1986;68:708–713.

30. Roth EJ, Lawler MH, Yarkony GM. Traumatic central cord syndrome: Clinical features and functional outcomes. *Arch Phys Med Rehabil.* 1990;71:18–23.

31. Kirshblum SC, O'Connor KC. Predicting neurologic recovery in traumatic cervical spinal cord injury. *Arch Phys Med Rehabil.* 1998;79:1456–1466.

32. Thongtrangan I, Le H, Park J, Kim DH. Cauda equina syndrome in patients with low lumbar fractures. *Neurosurg Focus.* 2004;16:e6.

33. Waters RL, Sie I, Adkins RH, Yakura JS. Injury pattern effect on motor recovery after traumatic spinal cord injury. *Arch Phys Med Rehabil.* 1995;76:440–443.

34. Curt A, Keck ME, Dietz V. Functional outcome following spinal cord injury: Significance of motor-evoked potentials and ASIA scores. *Arch Phys Med Rehabil.* 1998;79:81–86.

35. Kirshblum S, Millis S, McKinley W, Tulsky D. Late neurologic recovery after traumatic spinal cord injury. *Arch Phys Med Rehabil.* 2004;85:1811–1817.

36. Crozier KS, Graziani V, Ditunno JF, Jr., Herbison GJ. Spinal cord injury: Prognosis for ambulation based on sensory examination in patients who are initially motor complete. *Arch Phys Med Rehabil.* 1991;72:119–121.

37. Brown PJ, Marino RJ, Herbison GJ, Ditunno JF, Jr. The 72-hour examination as a predictor of recovery in motor complete quadriplegia. *Arch Phys Med Rehabil.* 1991;72:546–548.

38. Miyanji F, Furlan JC, Aarabi B, Arnold PM, Fehlings MG. Acute cervical traumatic spinal cord injury: MR imaging findings correlated with neurologic outcome—prospective study with 100 consecutive patients. *Radiology.* 2007;243:820–827.

39. Waters RL, Adkins RH, Yakura JS, Sie I. Motor and sensory recovery following complete tetraplegia. *Arch Phys Med Rehabil.* 1993;74:242–247.

40. Ditunno JF, Jr., Stover SL, Freed MM, Ahn JH. Motor recovery of the upper extremities in traumatic quadriplegia: A multicenter study. *Arch Phys Med Rehabil.* 1992;73:431–436.

41. Ditunno JF, Jr., Cohen ME, Hauck WW, Jackson AB, Sipski ML. Recovery of upper-extremity strength in complete and incomplete tetraplegia: A multicenter study. *Arch Phys Med Rehabil.* 2000;81:389–393.

42. Mange KC, Ditunno JF, Jr., Herbison GJ, Jaweed MM. Recovery of strength at the zone of injury in motor complete and motor incomplete cervical spinal cord injured patients. *Arch Phys Med Rehabil.* 1990;71:562–565.

43. Waters RL, Adkins RH, Yakura JS, Sie I. Motor and sensory recovery following incomplete paraplegia. *Arch Phys Med Rehabil.* 1994;75:67–72.

44. Waters RL, Adkins R, Yakura J, Vigil D. Prediction of ambulatory performance based on motor scores derived from standards of the American Spinal Injury Association. *Arch Phys Med Rehabil.* 1994;75:756–760.

45. Thomas CK, Zijdewind I. Fatigue of muscles weakened by death of motoneurons. *Muscle Nerve.* 2006;33:21–41.

46. Thomas CK, Broton JG, Calancie B. Motor unit forces and recruitment patterns after cervical spinal cord injury. *Muscle Nerve.* 1997;20:212–220.

47. Thomas CK, Nelson G, Than L, Zijdewind I. Motor unit activation order during electrically evoked contractions of paralyzed or partially paralyzed muscles. *Muscle Nerve.* 2002;25:797–804.

48. Totosy de Zepetnek JE, Zung HV, Erdebil S, Gordon T. Innervation ratio is an important determinant of force in normal and reinnervated rat tibialis anterior muscles. *J Neurophysiol.* 1992;67:1385–1403.

49. Bodine SC, Roy RR, Eldred E, Edgerton VR. Maximal force as a function of anatomical features of motor units in the cat tibialis anterior. *J Neurophysiol.* 1987;57:1730–1745.

50. Ditunno JF, Jr., Burns AS, Marino RJ. Neurological and functional capacity outcome measures: Essential to spinal cord injury clinical trials. *J Rehabil Res Dev.* 2005;42:35–41.

51. Kleim JA. III STEP: A basic scientist's perspective. *Phys Ther.* 2006;86:614–617.

52. Helkowski WM, Ditunno JF, Jr., Boninger M. Autonomic dysreflexia: incidence in persons with neurologically complete and incomplete tetraplegia. *J Spinal Cord Med.* 2003;26:244–247.

53. Consortium for Spinal Cord Medicine. Acute management of autonomic dysreflexia: individuals with spinal cord injury presenting to health care facilities [clinical practice guideline]. 2nd edition. 2001. Washington, DC, The Consortium, Paralyzed Veterans of America.

54. Spinal Cord Injury Thromboprophylaxis Investigators. Prevention of venous thromboembolism in the acute treatment phase after spinal cord injury: A randomized, multicenter trial comparing low-dose heparin plus intermittent pneumatic compression with enoxaparin. *J Trauma.* 2003;54:1116–1124.

55. Waring WP, Karunas RS. Acute spinal cord injuries and the incidence of clinically occurring thromboembolic disease. *Paraplegia.* 1991;29:8–16.

56. Powell M, Kirshblum S, O'Connor KC. Duplex ultrasound screening for deep vein thrombosis in spinal cord injured patients at rehabilitation admission. *Arch Phys Med Rehabil.* 1999;80:1044–1046.

57. Maxwell RA, Chavarria-Aguilar M, Cockerham WT et al. Routine prophylactic vena cava filtration is not indicated after acute spinal cord injury. *J Trauma.* 2002;52:902–906.

58. Johns JS, Nguyen C, Sing RF. Vena cava filters in spinal cord injuries: Evolving technology. *J Spinal Cord Med.* 2006;29:183–190.

59. Paralyzed Veterans of America. Pressure ulcer prevention and treatment following spinal cord injury: A clinical practice guideline for health care professionals. 2000. Washington, DC, Paralyzed Veterans of America.

60. Consortium for Spinal Cord Medicine Clinical Practice Guidelines. Pressure ulcer prevention and treatment following spinal cord injury: A clinical practice guideline for health-care professionals. *J Spinal Cord Med.* 2001;24 Suppl 1:S40–S101.

61. Kroll T, Neri MT, Ho PS. Secondary conditions in spinal cord injury: results from a prospective survey. *Disabil Rehabil.* 2007;29:1229–1237.

62. Banovac K, Sherman AL, Estores IM, Banovac F. Prevention and treatment of heterotopic ossification after spinal cord injury. *J Spinal Cord Med.* 2004;27:376–382.

63. Haran M, Bhuta T, Lee B. Pharmacological interventions for treating acute heterotopic ossification. *Cochrane Database Syst Rev.* 2004;CD003321.

64. Hsu JD, Sakimura I, Stauffer ES. Heterotopic ossification around the hip joint in spinal cord injured patients. *Clin Orthop Relat Res.* 1975;165–169.

65. Daud O, Sett P, Burr RG, Silver JR. The relationship of heterotopic ossification to passive movements in paraplegic patients. *Disabil Rehabil.* 1993;15:114–118.

66. Dai L. Heterotopic ossification of the hip after spinal cord injury. *Chin Med J (Engl).* 1998;111:1099–1101.

67. Maimoun L, Lumbroso S, Paris F et al. The role of androgens or growth factors in the bone resorption process in recent spinal cord injured patients: A cross-sectional study. *Spinal Cord.* 2006.

68. Zehnder Y, Luthi M, Michel D et al. Long-term changes in bone metabolism, bone mineral density, quantitative ultrasound parameters, and fracture incidence after spinal cord injury: A cross-sectional observational study in 100 paraplegic men. *Osteoporos Int.* 2004;15:180–189.

69. Eser P, Frotzler A, Zehnder Y, Denoth J. Fracture threshold in the femur and tibia of people with spinal cord injury as determined by peripheral quantitative computed tomography. *Arch Phys Med Rehabil.* 2005;86:498–504.

70. Lanyon LE. Using functional loading to influence bone mass and architecture: Objectives, mechanisms, and relationship with estrogen of the mechanically adaptive process in bone. *Bone.* 1996;18 (Suppl):37S–43S.

71. Frey-Rindova P, de Bruin ED, Stussi E, Dambacher MA, Dietz V. Bone mineral density in upper and lower extremities during 12 months after spinal cord injury measured by peripheral quantitative computed tomography. *Spinal Cord.* 2000;38:26–32.

72. Potter K, Saifuddin A. Pictorial review: MRI of chronic spinal cord injury. *Br J Radiol.* 2003;76:347–352.

73. Wang D, Bodley R, Sett P, Gardner B, Frankel H. A clinical magnetic resonance imaging study of the traumatised spinal cord more than 20 years following injury. *Paraplegia.* 1996;34:65–81.

74. el Masry WS, Biyani A. Incidence, management, and outcome of post-traumatic syringomyelia. In memory of Mr. Bernard Williams. *J Neurol Neurosurg Psychiatry.* 1996;60:141–146.

75. Asano M, Fujiwara K, Yonenobu K, Hiroshima K. Post-traumatic syringomyelia. *Spine.* 1996;21:1446–1453.

76. Lee TT, Alameda GJ, Camilo E, Green BA. Surgical treatment of post-traumatic myelopathy associated with syringomyelia. *Spine.* 2001;26:S119–S127.

77. Calancie B, Broton JG, Klose KJ, Traad M, Difini J, Ayyar DR. Evidence that alterations in presynaptic inhibition contribute to segmental hypo- and hyperexcitability after spinal cord injury in man. *Electroencephalogr Clin Neurophysiol.* 1993;89:177–186.

78. Mirbagheri MM, Barbeau H, Ladouceur M, Kearney RE. Intrinsic and reflex stiffness in normal and spastic, spinal cord injured subjects. *Exp Brain Res.* 2001;141:446–459.

79. Mirbagheri MM, Settle K, Harvey R, Rymer WZ. Neuromuscular abnormalities associated with spasticity of upper extremity muscles in hemiparetic stroke. *J Neurophysiol.* 2007;98:629–637.

80. Friden J, Lieber RL. Spastic muscle cells are shorter and stiffer than normal cells. *Muscle Nerve.* 2003;27:157–164.

81. Lieber RL, Runesson E, Einarsson F, Friden J. Inferior mechanical properties of spastic muscle bundles due to hypertrophic but compromised extracellular matrix material. *Muscle Nerve.* 2003;28:464–471.

82. Dietz V. Proprioception and locomotor disorders. *Nat Rev Neurosci.* 2002;3:781–790.

83. Dietz V, Sinkjaer T. Spastic movement disorder: Impaired reflex function and altered muscle mechanics. *Lancet Neurol.* 2007;6:725–733.

84. Widerstrom-Noga EG, Felipe-Cuervo E, Broton JG, Duncan RC, Yezierski RP. Perceived difficulty in dealing with consequences of spinal cord injury. *Arch Phys Med Rehabil.* 1999;80:580–586.

85. Turner JA, Cardenas DD, Warms CA, McClellan CB. Chronic pain associated with spinal cord injuries: A community survey. *Arch Phys Med Rehabil.* 2001;82:501–509.

86. Siddall PJ, Taylor DA, Cousins MJ. Classification of pain following spinal cord injury. *Spinal Cord.* 1997;35:69–75.

87. Bryce TN, Ragnarsson KT. Pain after spinal cord injury. *Phys Med Rehabil Clin N Am.* 2000;11:157–168.

Translating Animal Research to Humans with Spinal Cord Injury

2

Laurent J. Bouyer, PhD

OBJECTIVES

After reading this chapter, you will be able to:

- Understand the roadblocks inherent in translating animal research in spinal cord injuries (SCI) to humans
- Review the neural structures involved in the control of locomotion
- Evaluate the relevance of a study based on an animal model to individuals with SCI
- Critique the extent and the limits of questions that can be answered using models of SCI
- Discuss the different types of models currently used (complete transection, contusion, partial transections) and the answers that each model can provide

OUTLINE

INTRODUCTION

THE BASICS OF THE NEURAL CONTROL OF LOCOMOTION

   Pattern and Rhythm Generation

   Responding to the Environment

INFLUENCE OF SEVERITY OF INJURY

RETRAINING AVAILABLE NEURAL STRUCTURES

   Complete Spinal Cord Transections

     Training-induced improvement versus spontaneous recovery

     Locomotor training: Beyond the treadmill

     Specificity of training

     Retention of training effects

   Partial Transection or Incomplete Injury

     Effect of Lesion Location and Severity

   Influence of Lesion Type on Response to Interventions

SUMMARY

REVIEW QUESTIONS

Introduction

When attempting to understand the mechanisms underlying central nervous system (CNS) compensation after spinal cord injury, animal models have many advantages. Among other issues, humans with spinal cord injury (SCI) frequently have damage to structures other than the spinal cord that may confound the results of an experimental intervention. Humans may have associated conditions (e.g., traumatic brain injury), additional physical damage (damage to peripheral nerve, muscle, joints, etc.), trauma that makes it difficult to assess the

21

extent and stability of the lesion (partial sparing of descending tracts, temporary demyelinization that partly recovers, etc.), as well as issues related to psychological responses to injury and the influence of social and environmental factors. It is for these reasons and others that using animal models is valuable. Using animal models allows researchers to separate the complex problem of SCI into simpler parts that they can study one aspect at a time. While some may consider this approach to be too reductionist, the great conservation of basic anatomy and physiology across species (including humans) has, since the late 1980s, allowed scientists to improve the locomotor recovery of individuals with SCI based on evidence obtained from animal models, for example, using weight-supported treadmill training. While in many areas of spinal cord injury research it remains to be seen whether the new discoveries are directly applicable to humans, locomotor function is one area in which evidence from animal models has already lead to the development of valuable new technologies such as robotics and spinal cord stimulation. For this reason, this chapter will use evidence from studies of locomotion in animal models of SCI as the basis for the discussion of translational studies.

The Basics of the Neural Control of Locomotion

When observing an able-bodied individual walking across a room, the movement appears to be fluid and effortless. To achieve this graceful displacement of the whole body, many different components of the central nervous system must be activated and coordinated to precisely time dozens of interacting muscles across a multiarticular system that is inherently unstable.

Animal models of locomotor control have allowed scientists to identify two important principles describing the neural control of walking: (1) control is distributed across the CNS, and (2) control is hierarchical. The walking movement can be decomposed into several elements, summarized here under two categories:

1. *Pattern and rhythm generation:* Rhythmic alternating activation of leg muscles, interlimb coordination adjusted to speed of progression, support of body weight, and stumbling recovery.
2. *Responding to the environment:* Navigation (path planning to get where you want), walking initiation, postural control, obstacle avoidance, anticipation of difficult terrains.

One of the elegant features of the control of locomotion is that a separate neural structure (or group of structures) can be associated with each of the elements described above. Box 2-1 summarizes the different types of animal preparations that are used to study the neural elements involved in locomotor function. The basic rhythmicity is generated by spinal interneurons (also called the locomotor network or central pattern generator) located in the gray matter lumbar enlargement of the spinal cord.[1,2] Using spinal cats (i.e., animals with transection of the spinal cord) walking on a treadmill, it was possible to demonstrate that the spinal control of locomotion is quite sophisticated.[3-5] Indeed, after a complete spinal cord transection at low thoracic level (i.e., above the lumbar enlargement), spinal cats can generate an alternating movement of the hind limbs with proper paw placement, bear the weight of their hindquarters, recover from a stumble,[6] adjust to different belt speeds,[7] and compensate for added load.[8,9] These movements are very similar to those made by intact animals.[10] However, spinal animals also have major deficits: they cannot initiate walking voluntarily, have no postural control, and are unable to anticipate obstacles placed on their walking path.

Progressing rostrally in the CNS, the next level of interest above the spinal cord is in the brainstem. Electrical stimulation of a brainstem area called the mesencephalic locomotor region (MLR) initiates locomotion.[11,12] Furthermore, as the intensity of stimulation is increased, the type of movement changes from walk, to trot, to gallop.[13] Therefore, this center is also involved in the interlimb coordination necessary to adapt to higher speeds of walking. In humans, this area is likely to be involved in the initiation of walking as well as in transitioning from walking to running. The MLR neurons activate interneurons in the medial reticular formation, which in turn activate the spinal central pattern generator. Axons from these reticular neurons travel from the brainstem to the lumbar spinal cord in the ventrolateral quadrant of the spinal cord bilaterally.[14] Therefore, a ventrolateral lesion will have a major impact on the ability to initiate walking. The brainstem is also where the vestibular nuclei are located. The vestibular system is involved in balance control during walking. Therefore, a lesion below the brainstem will also affect the ability to control balance during walking. The vestibulospinal pathway also runs through the ventral aspect of the spinal cord.

The brain is the rostral-most aspect of the CNS. Little is known about the role of the deep brain nuclei in the control of locomotion. The fact that the basal ganglia projects to the MLR is clinically evident in individuals with Parkinson's disease, one of the associated symptoms of which is difficulty with voluntary gait initiation.[15] The role of the cerebral cortex in locomotor function is better understood. Lesion studies,[16] as well as recordings[17]/stimulations[18] in awake behaving animals have shown that the main role of the motor cortex/red nucleus complex during locomotion is to coordinate visuomotor tasks such as obstacle avoidance. The corticospinal tract travels in the dorsolateral quadrant of the spinal cord. Lesions to this area of the cord result in inability to accurately adjust movement to the environment due to inadequate limb flexion when the animal tries to step over an obstacle during walking.

BOX 2-1
The Types of Locomotor Preparations

The CNS comprises the brain *and* the spinal cord. Lesion experiments performed over the last 100 years have been used to demonstrate the essential contribution of several centers within the CNS, including in the isolated spinal cord, to the control of walking. They can be grouped into five categories, depending on the site and extent of the lesion (see Table 2-1).

Decorticate: Only the cerebral cortex is removed. The animal can continue to use deep brain nuclei, brainstem, spinal centers, and sensory feedback to control the movement.

Decerebrate: A lesion is made at the level of the mammillary bodies, leaving the brainstem intact.

High spinal: A lesion is made in the cervical spinal cord below the centers controlling autonomic functions (heart rate, blood pressure, respiration). The animal becomes functionally quadriplegic and therefore requires a significant amount of care. This preparation is therefore rarely used. Experimentally, the interactions between the spinal cord gray matter and sensory feedback from all four limbs can be tested. Propriospinal interneurons, a class of interneurons located in the gray matter of the spinal cord that have long processes extending from the cervical to the lumbar enlargement, convey information back and forth between these two integration centers and are important for interlimb coordination.

Low spinal: A lesion is made at the low thoracic level, above the lumbar enlargement. The animal becomes functionally paraplegic and therefore requires much less care than does the high spinal preparation. This preparation is therefore more commonly used. Experimentally, only interactions between the lower part of the spinal cord gray matter and sensory feedback from the hind limbs remain.

Fictive: The preparations described so far all retain both a central (e.g., cortex, spinal cord gray matter) and a peripheral (sensory feedback from the limbs) component. To understand the neural control of locomotion, it is sometimes necessary to determine which component of a movement results from a reflex (i.e., a response to external sensory stimuli) versus what component is generated by the CNS (i.e., centrally generated). The term *reflex* is often misused to include any movement that is not voluntary. However, the strict definition of the word *reflex* is a movement in reaction to an external stimulus. Therefore, in the hierarchy of movement types, at least three categories must be defined: voluntary, automatic, and reflex. This distinction between automatic and reflex movements is key to our understanding of the control of locomotion. Indeed, the finding that a low spinal cat could start walking with its hind limbs when put on a treadmill lead to a divergence of opinion between early investigators regarding the origin of the locomotor movements as being a reflex or an automatic act. As can be seen in Table 2-1, low spinal cats could produce locomotion either through stimuli coming from sensory feedback or through automatic movement generation by the spinal cord gray matter. To address this question, a new animal preparation was required wherein the spinal cord would be separated from sensory feedback from the limbs. Initially, this posed a problem because the spinal cord is a myelinated structure, and therefore it could not simply be extracted surgically and studied in a dish (as it would rapidly die due to the inability of oxygen to diffuse through myelin). To solve this problem, in 1911 the Scottish physiologist Thomas Graham Brown cut dorsal roots in a low spinal cat, thereby eliminating what was believed at the time to be all sensory afferents. The fact that he still observed rhythmic, locomotor-like activity in the hind limbs after such a procedure led him to believe that locomotion was therefore an automatic movement generated by the CNS (in this case the spinal cord gray matter) and not a reflex.

While this experiment was a breakthrough in the early 20th century, refined anatomical techniques later showed that cutting the dorsal roots did not completely abolish sensory feedback, as a small fraction of afferents enter the spinal cord through the ventral roots. It was therefore necessary to improve the preparation. In the late 1970s, the group of Sten Grillner at the Karolinska Institute in Sweden developed the "fictive" locomotion preparation.[2] Its principle is very simple: instead of cutting the sensory afferents, the animal is paralyzed with curare to block the neuromuscular junction, eliminating all movements and therefore any *movement-related* sensory feedback. With this preparation, these authors were able to show rhythmic, locomotor-like activity in hind limb nerves (remember that the neuromuscular junction is blocked by curare) of low spinal cats. This experiment unequivocally demonstrates that locomotion is not a reflex, but rather is an automatic movement generated by interneurons located in the spinal cord. These authors coined the term *central pattern generator* to describe such interneurons.

The fictive locomotion preparation is complex, as the motor output of the spinal cord must be recorded directly from the motor nerve instead of from the muscle, but it offers several advantages: for example, as afferents are still intact, the preparation offers the opportunity to experimentally manipulate sensory feedback during a fictive locomotion episode and better understand how sensorimotor processing occurs during walking. In addition, several central lesions may be tested in the fictive state (decerebrate, high spinal, and low spinal) to study the role of several descending systems and their interaction with the central pattern generator.

Table 2-1
Animal Preparations in Studies of Locomotion

Preparation name	Cerebral cortex	Deep brain nuclei	Brainstem	Propriospinal	Sensory feedback	Spinal cord gray matter
Intact	√	√	√	√	√	√
Decorticate		√	√	√	√	√
Decerebrate			√	√	√	√
High spinal				√	√	√
Low spinal					√	√
Fictive			*	*	Experimentally controlled	√

*These levels can be spared in the fictive preparation for specific experiments above.

While there are no direct pathways from the cerebellum to the spinal interneurons, the cerebellum nevertheless contributes to the control of locomotion. As with other movements, the cerebellum can monitor and finely tune locomotor output through its projections to the MLR, the motor cortex, the red nucleus, the vestibular nuclei, and the reticular formation (reviewed in Armstrong[16,19]). Recordings in awake walking cats show that the cerebellum is most active when locomotion has to be adapted to environmental demands (such as during visuomotor tasks) similarly to the motor cortex.[20,21] In addition, the cerebellum receives sensory inputs from the limbs through axons ascending in the dorsal spinocerebellar tract and also receives spinal locomotor network output through axons ascending in the ventral spinocerebellar tract. By comparing these two inputs, the cerebellum can also fulfill its role as a comparator of expected and actual movement trajectory. The cerebellum is therefore involved in all aspects of locomotor control, from gait initiation to the adjustment of fine distal movements. Finally, the association areas of the parietal cortex seem to be involved in more complex tasks, such as navigation. This area does not project directly down to the spinal cord, but among other functions, it helps coordinate the visual information coming from the visual cortex with activity in the motor cortex for the negotiation of obstacles.

The foregoing makes it clear that the neural control of locomotion involves many structures, located at all levels of the CNS, from the spinal cord to the cortex. The figure in Box 2-2 illustrates the spinal cord targets of the various supraspinal structures involved in the neural control of locomotion. Residual function is therefore largely determined by which areas of the spinal cord are damaged and which are spared. For this reason, deficits to motor control will vary widely among individuals with SCI, depending on the particular injury.

Efforts to restore locomotor function in individuals with incomplete SCI are complicated both by the individual variability in spared neural structures, was well as by the fact that locomotion is partly automatic (basic movement generation at the spinal level) and partly voluntary (requiring descending motor commands to traverse the area of injury in order to reach the spinal cord). These factors contribute to the challenge of determining the optimal type and dosage of intervention required for retraining. To address this issue it is necessary to know the adaptive capacity of each of the remaining structures and pathways. These issues will be addressed in the next section of this chapter.

Influence of Severity of Injury

In the context of locomotion, the spinal cord serves three main functions: (1) *automatic movement generation*: interneurons in the lumbar enlargement generate the basic locomotor rhythm; (2) *integration*: the spinal cord processes information from sensory receptors and adjusts motor output based on the phase of the step cycle; (3) *high-speed information transfer*: the white matter of the spinal cord conveys sensory and central pattern generator

Box 2-2
The Spinal White Matter "Map"

Considering the number of brain structures involved in the control of locomotion and the anatomy of the spinal cord, it is clear that partial lesions to the spinal cord will cause different deficits, depending on their location. The figure below shows the localization of the different ascending and descending tracts. Along with the information presented in the section entitled "The Basics of the Neural Control of Locomotion" in this chapter, it allows us to draw a functional map of the spinal cord for locomotion.

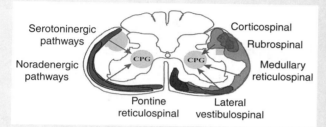

Schematic view of the spinal cord. Right. Location of the descending pathways from the brain to the lumbar spinal cord in the cat. Left. Neurotransmitters used by the different pathways shown on the right. (From Dr. E. Brustein, PhD Thesis. University of Montreal, Montreal, Canada.)

The Spinal Cord is Smart

While the white matter of the spinal cord is composed of axons conveying information up from the sensory receptors to the brain and down from the brain to the motoneurons, its gray matter is a minibrain. On the motor side, less than 10% of the descending neurons make direct contact with motoneurons. The vast majority of the descending neurons synapse with local interneurons and therefore undergo integration before reaching the motoneurons. On the sensory side, somatosensory afferents divide into several branches (collaterals) as they enter the cord. One branch goes directly up toward the nuclei gracilis and cuneatus by way of the dorsal columns, but the others enter the gray matter and are responsible for segmental and suprasegmental reflexes. Interneurons of several types are also found in the spinal cord, including long propriospinal interneurons conveying information between the cervical and lumbar enlargements. Other types of processing done by the spinal cord include reciprocal inhibition, presynaptic inhibition, pattern generation (see text), and reflex modulation.

Stepping Versus Walking

While spinal cats can generate alternating weight-bearing hind limb movements when they are held by the tail over a motorized treadmill, they will immediately loose balance if the experimenter releases the tail. This shows that after spinalization, rhythmic control is preserved, but balance control is not. This is not surprising considering that balance control is performed by the vestibular system, located supraspinally in the inner ear. Axons from vestibulospinal neurons travel from the brainstem vestibular nuclei to the lower spinal cord by way of the ventral spinal white matter to provide the necessary information for dynamic balance control during walking. When the spinal cord is severed at the thoracic level, these neurons can no longer reach their target, and balance control is permanently lost. It is clear, however, that walking requires both rhythmic stepping and balance control to be functional for ambulation. Due to this separate control of balance and rhythmic information, complete spinal animals can be retrained to "step," but not to walk independently, and a postural aid (such as crutches or a walker) will always be required to compensate for the loss of balance information.

(CPG) information up to higher integration centers and motor commands down to interneurons.

From the point of view of rehabilitation interventions, the functional anatomy of the spinal cord dictates that the *size* and the *location* of a spinal injury will have a major impact on the *type* and *extent* of the initial deficit, as well as on the potential for functional recovery. The number and nature of possible deficits is so large that one can appreciate how diverse will be the cases to be treated in the clinic. This illustrates one of the advantages of using animal models of spinal cord injury; they allow the study of damage to specified areas of the spinal cord while at the same time controlling the severity of this damage. Injuries that are restricted to known areas of the spinal cord can be produced in laboratory animals to represent

the main questions one faces when rehabilitating a person with SCI. Obviously, humans usually have more complex injuries. The goal in the following section of the chapter is to show the best case rehabilitation scenario in order to extract general concepts. Once these concepts are well understood, the reader will be able to combine the information from the different examples presented and have a better understanding of real-life human situations. As will be seen, animal models do not provide all the answers, but they can provide guidelines to better understand the deficits and residual capacity in SCI, and they may suggest avenues from which to develop intervention strategies.

It bears repeating that the control of locomotion is only partly voluntary.[22] While this concept will be clearly demonstrated using animal models throughout this chapter, experimental data indicate that the same is true for humans. For example, Crenna and Inverno[23] have shown that in some children with cerebral palsy, while *voluntarily* contracting the tibialis anterior muscle is not possible, the same muscle can be recruited normally during walking. The reverse was also observed in other children; while they were capable of voluntary contraction, the muscle was not activated during walking. Additional evidence comes from the work of Peiper,[24] who reported "stepping" in babies born without a brain (anencephaly). In this situation, only the spinal cord is available to provide movement control. Taken together, these examples of human pathology strongly support the notion of a non-voluntary contribution to the control of human walking. However, they do not address the relative contribution of spinal and supraspinal structures, which differs across species. Nevertheless, two levels of control coexist, and understanding the adaptive capacity of nervous structures located above and below the lesion will be of paramount importance for improving the efficiency of our treatment strategies.

Retraining Available Neural Structures

After immediate care to limit secondary damage has been given (e.g., reducing swelling), there are only two ways to promote recovery of function after spinal cord injury: neural regeneration, to reconnect structures on either side of the lesion, and retraining, to improve functional recovery using the adaptive capacity and plasticity of remaining nervous structures. As neural regeneration techniques are still in their infancy (see Basso[25]), the best available approach for rehabilitation is to push the remaining nervous structures to their full potential.

To describe the adaptive potential of neural structures, two experimental preparations will be presented: complete and incomplete spinal cord transections. The complete transection model addresses the adaptive capacity of the spinal nervous system in isolation from higher centers. As will be seen, the spinal cord is capable of important training-induced functional improvement (also called *adaptive plasticity*). Comparing the results obtained in complete spinal animals to those with incomplete lesions, the contribution of supraspinal structures can be inferred.

Complete Spinal Cord Transections

Training-Induced Improvement versus Spontaneous Recovery

In the late 1980s, Barbeau and Rossignol trained adult cats with complete spinal transection to walk on a motorized treadmill.[7] In the first few days after the lesion, no stepping could be induced when the hind limbs were placed on a treadmill. However, over the following 2–3 weeks, if treadmill training was provided, stepping with proper foot placement and weight bearing gradually returned. Figure 2-1 shows the large improvement in locomotor function that was obtained over time. This experiment revealed two important concepts: (1) training can help to improve stepping and (2) the adult spinal cord is capable

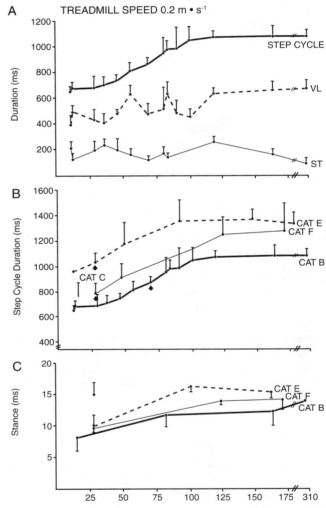

Figure 2-1. (A) Step cycle, vastus lateralis (VL), and semitendinosus (ST) duration as a function of time following spinalization for a constant treadmill speed of 0.2 m/s. Each point represents the mean of 10 to 15 cycles, and the vertical bar represents one standard deviation. (B) The step cycle duration in three spinal cats versus time following spinalization. In another cat (cat C), only the initial point is illustrated. Arrows indicate the day of documented digitigrade placing and weight bearing for each cat. (C) Stance length measured from video recordings in relation to the time following spinalization. For cat E, one point at day 29 indicates step cycles, with weight bearing obtained only 2 days after the points that lie on the main curve for that cat. Horizontal axes represent days after spinalization. (From Barbeau H, Rossignol S. Recovery of locomotion after chronic spinalization in the adult cat. *Brain Research*. 1987; 412:84–95.)

of relearning to walk. This study had a major impact on the field of human locomotor rehabilitation, serving as the basis for the development of body weight-supported treadmill training[26,27] (discussed in detail in the chapter on locomotor training), now used in clinics all over the world.

The complete spinal cord transection represents one type of experimentally induced spinal cord injury, and it is a powerful model as it demonstrates the capacity of the mammalian spinal cord that has been completely disconnected from supraspinal influences. In addition to the complete spinal cord transection injury, there are various types of partial spinal cord transection injuries that leave specific pathways intact. These injuries allow an assessment of the influence of the transected pathways based on the deficits observed after they have been removed. However, it has been argued that the transection injury does not correspond to the types of injuries that are most common inindividuals with SCI, as human SCI most often involves contusion and compression injuries rather than transection (the exception being cases of penetrating injuries such as gunshot wounds). Box 2-3 summarizes the most common types of experimentally induced

spinal cord injury; each type of injury has its unique attributes.

In addition to the various types of experimentally induced spinal cord injury, there are various animal models in which the influence of spinal cord injury has been studied. As with injury type, each animal model has its own unique characteristics; these are summarized in Box 2-4. Cats and mice are animal models that can develop what is called *spinal locomotion*, that is, alternated, rhythmic stepping on a motorized treadmill after complete cord transection, without receiving drug therapy. These animals can also spontaneously recover some rhythmic hindlimb movements over time.[28,29] However, this rhythmic movement is of poor quality when compared to stepping in spinal animals that are exposed to training. For example, cats trained to walk on a treadmill for several weeks can bear more weight, walk at faster speeds, and produce on average three times more successful steps per unit of time[29,30] than can untrained controls. Comparisons between training and spontaneous recovery suggest that exposure to movement-related (or "phasic") sensory feedback that is present during treadmill walking may retrain the

---

Box 2-3
Types of Experimentally Induced Spinal Cord Injuries

Complete Transections
Procedure: A complete transection is performed by cutting the spinal cord with a sharp object (scalpel or small scissors) under general anesthesia and aseptic conditions.

Consequences: This method permanently disconnects spinal neural circuits and motoneuron pools located below the lesion from supraspinal influences. It causes minimal secondary damage. Usually, a complete transection is performed at the cervical (high-spinal) or thoracic (low-spinal) level.

Animal models: A complete transection can be performed on essentially all animal models; it has been done in monkeys, cats, rats, mice, dogfish, lamprey, etc.

Partial Spinal Lesions
Over 90% of the partial spinal lesions performed to study SCI in rodents have been obtained either by contusion (30%), compression (20%), or transection (40%), according to a survey of the literature published between October 2002 and November 2003.[63] The other 10% include chemical lesions and injury to in vitro preparations.

Transections
Procedure: As with complete cord transections, this method involves cutting the cord with a sharp instrument. To spare some of the vasculature in smaller

animals such as rodents, suction is sometimes used in addition to, or instead of, a sharp object.[63]

Consequences: This method interrupts only some of the connections between supraspinal structures and spinal interneurons. The location of the lesion (ventral/dorsal/lateral) can be targeted to either spare or remove only specific pathways (see Box 2-2). It causes minimal secondary damage.

Animal models: This method can be performed on essentially all animal models.

Contusions and Compressions
Procedure: A blunt object is used to damage the spinal cord. The concept underlying this procedure is that it will produce an injury similar to what is experienced by humans after a traumatic injury. Several methods have been validated and are reproducible. They include dropping weights,[69] moving a solenoid-driven device onto the cord,[70] inflating a balloon subdurally,[71] squeezing the cord with a modified aneurysm clip,[72] etc. (see Rosenzweig and McDonald[63] for a more complete list).

Consequences: The initial injury is more diffuse than those induced by transection. Secondary damage is important. After contusion or compression injury, there is often partial sparing of axons in the injured area. Because of the partial sparing of axons, this model is often less appropriate than others in the study of the adaptive capacity of neural centers in the recovery of locomotion. Its main role is to study neural regrowth after SCI.[63]

Animal models: This method is used mainly in rodents.

Box 2-4

Adult Mammalian Animal Models to Study Locomotor Recovery After SCI

There are three main animal models used today to study locomotor recovery after SCI: cats, rats, and mice. Experiments in primates with complete SCI have also been attempted, but have been rare and have had mixed success in producing spinal locomotion.[73–76] This model will therefore not be considered in this chapter. More studies involving different species of monkeys will be required before this model can be used reliably.[77]

Cat:

To study the neural control of locomotion, the cat is probably the animal model with the longest history. It was already in use at the beginning of the 20th century by Sherrington and his colleagues (see Bouyer and Rossignol for a review[78]). It is by far the best-documented animal model of locomotion.

Time to locomotor recovery after a complete SCI:
Locomotor recovery occurs after less than 21 days of training.[7,10,79]

Mouse:

Over the last several years, mice models have gained popularity. This is mainly due to the fact that knockout animals, in which specific genes have been altered or deleted, express specific motor deficits. Studying these mutants will help our understanding of the role of specific interneurons in the control of locomotion (see for example Kullander et al.[80]).

Time to locomotor recovery after a complete SCI:
Locomotor recovery occurs after 14 days of training.[81]

Rat:

While cats and mice can be readily trained to walk after a complete spinal transection, rats do not exhibit such good locomotor recovery. Work by Antri et al.[82] shows that out of 10 rats used in their study, only 4 exhibited rhythmicity after 28 days of training. And even in these animals, rhythmicity was poor, alternation between the two limbs disorganized, paw placement rare, and body weight support never obtained. However, if drug therapy was given in combination with training, rhythmic stepping with paw placement and weight bearing was obtained within 15 days. If drug therapy was then stopped, walking ability started to degrade within 10 to 15 days, reinforcing the concept that spinal transected rats are poor walkers.

Time to locomotor recovery after a complete SCI:
Locomotor recovery does not always occur after training; spinal transected rats are poor walkers after SCI.

---

spinal cord to produce the pre-lesion locomotor pattern.[31] This is supported by measurements of the locomotor pattern in trained spinal animals by using electromyography and showing that the pattern that was present before spinalization is re-expressed after training in the spinal state.[10]

Locomotor Training: Beyond the Treadmill

With recent advances in technology, several methods are now available (or will soon be) to supplement treadmill training for locomotor rehabilitation. Some of these methods have been tested in animal models.

Robotic Orthoses

If treadmill training improves locomotion by increasing the amount of appropriate phasic sensory feedback, then moving the limbs in a way that mimics normal locomotor kinematics may promote faster and/or more extensive recovery of function. This is the hypothesis at the base of using assistive robotic orthoses as a complement to treadmill training.[31–35] In spinal rats, a robotic assistive device was tested using three different force profiles: downward force during stance, upward force during swing, and imposed "normal" ankle trajectory.[33] Training under conditions that imposed these forces

modified locomotor output in the rats. By assisting movement, such a device may be useful early in the rehabilitation process in subjects with severe impairments.[36,37] However, it must be clearly understood that using a robot to provide movement assistance will likely have limitations during actual training. In an extreme case, the individual could decide to stay completely passive and let the robot execute the "ideal" limb trajectory on its own. Used this way, the robotic orthosis simply becomes a sophisticated walking aid. Conversely, during manually assisted treadmill training, the trainer assisting the movement is there only to augment the active contribution made by the individual, thereby allowing the person to always train to full potential. This empowerment of the subject is especially necessary at later stages of rehabilitation as has been shown in individuals with stroke.[38]

Robotic orthoses could also be used to promote active participation in movement generation. If instead of assisting leg movements, the machine was to generate a force impeding movement, individuals with some motor capacity could be trained to modify their locomotor pattern by trying to overcome the imposed force. Preliminary results show that this type of training results in modifications of the locomotor pattern that are specific to the forces used. Furthermore, these modifications persist for several step cycles after removing the force; that is, the modified patterns are carried over to unassisted walking.[39,40] This locomotor training approach is in its infancy, beginning to be tested in animals[33] and humans,[40,41] but appears promising. In studies done for the upper limb, robotic devices have already been used for several years, and training is retained for at least 3 years.[42]

Drug Therapy

Information is transmitted in the CNS by action potentials. For example, consider a neuron located in the brain. Action potentials travel along the axon of this neuron to the presynaptic terminals located at the end of the axon. When the action potentials reach the presynaptic terminals, neurotransmitter is released and diffuses across the synaptic cleft. The neurotransmitter contacts receptors in the dendrites of a second neuron (in the spinal cord, for example), opening its ion channels and causing depolarization in, and activation of, the second neuron. After spinal cord injury, neurons in the brain may no longer be connected to neurons in the spinal cord. However, if a neurotransmitter that is typically used by the brain to communicate with neurons in the spinal cord was to be artificially injected near the cell bodies of neurons in the spinal cord (as illustrated in Fig. 2-2), then the latter would become activated *and carry out their normal function*. This is the manner by which drug therapies improve CNS function.

In the specific case of cat locomotion, noradrenaline (NA) is the neurotransmitter used by supraspinal neurons to "turn on" spinal locomotor centers.

Therefore, when NA is injected into the spinal cord shortly after a complete spinalization (i.e., during the period where no movement can be induced just by placing the animal on the treadmill; between 3 days and 2 weeks postlesion), then locomotion on a treadmill can be triggered.[28] This effect occurs through receptors on the spinal neurons known as alpha-2 adrenergic receptors. The alpha-2 adrenergic agonist clonidine, is usually used for triggering locomotion instead of NA, as it only binds to the alpha-2 receptors.

Based on evidence that clonidine could readily initiate locomotion so early after a complete spinal lesion, Chau et al.[43] used this drug in combination with treadmill training to determine whether recovery of walking function could be accelerated. Locomotor performance was measured each day over the course of the 2-week study using kinematic and electromyographic (EMG) recordings before and after drug application. Clonidine not only initiated locomotion, but also allowed the daily training sessions to be much longer. The results were quite compelling; not only did the cats walk better after drug injection each day, but this improvement carried over from day to day. Cats could bear weight and place the paw on the plantar surface after only 9 days of combined drug administration and training, compared to 14–21 days with treadmill training alone.[10] The conclusion reached based on this study is that by initiating locomotion earlier after SCI and increasing daily training duration, adrenergic drugs seem to have the potential to enhance the effects of treadmill training and allow for a faster expression of spinal stepping in cats with *complete* spinal cord transection.

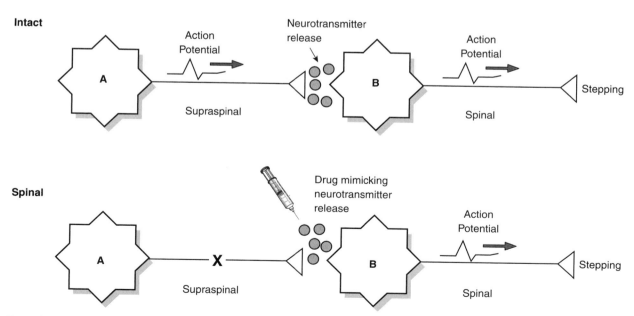

Figure 2-2. Principle of action of drug therapy. After spinal cord lesion, supraspinal neurons (A) normally activating spinal neurons (B) are no longer available. Injecting drugs that are similar to the endogenous neurotransmitter can activate the spinal neurons.

Neural Prostheses

Enhancement of locomotor activity through activation of spinal structures is not restricted to the use of drugs. Another approach is to use stimulators to depolarize the neuron pools below the lesion (see Fig. 2-3), either directly with microelectrodes implanted in the spinal cord or indirectly with larger electrodes placed on the dura.

Intraspinal Microstimulation. Studies carried out in anesthetized frogs by Bizzi et al.[44–46] have shown that microstimulation of specific areas in the spinal cord can generate what these authors named *movement primitives.* Combining limited numbers of these primitives gave rise to complex limb movements. The possibility of using spinal cord microstimulation to produce and/or enhance walking movements by eliciting such movement primitives has been tested in cats (reviewed in Prochazka et al.[47]). Microelectrode arrays are first implanted in the spinal cord, through the dura matter. Single electrodes on the array are then stimulated alternatively during locomotion. This procedure allows locomotor-like movements to occur.[48]

This approach is still under development, but pros and cons are already emerging:[49]

Pros:

- Only a limited number of stimulation sites are necessary to produce complex movements.
- Low-intensity stimulation can be used to lower the threshold of residual voluntary movements.

Cons:

- Low precision during electrode placement (~1 mm) prevents its use in humans for now.

- Movements obtained under anesthesia don't necessarily match those obtained in the awake state.
- Due to their low reliability and fragility, the number of electrodes implanted at this time remains large (~20), and their long-term stability is unknown.
- For the near future, this approach may turn out to be more practical for bladder control than as a tool to assist training of endogenous neural circuits for the control of locomotion. [47,50]

Epidural Stimulation. Rather than trying to artificially control individual movement primitives, another approach attempts to electrically trigger the network of spinal cord interneurons that is normally responsible for the generation of the walking pattern. Studies using pharmacological agents[49] or lesions[51] have determined that these interneurons are located in the midlumbar segments. Therefore, stimulating nonspecifically over this region of the spinal cord should increase the excitability of locomotor interneurons and produce stepping. This can be achieved simply by placing a large stimulation electrode in the epidural space on the dorsal side of the spinal cord, on top of the midlumbar segments.[52] This approach, called *epidural stimulation,* is less invasive and avoids the problems associated with implanted electrodes. Early evidence is very supportive of epidural stimulation both in animals[52] and humans.[53].

Optimizing Sensory Feedback

While the discussion of approaches to activating the spinal locomotor networks has thus far been limited to the use of artificial means, there is evidence that such mechanisms can also be activated via more natural

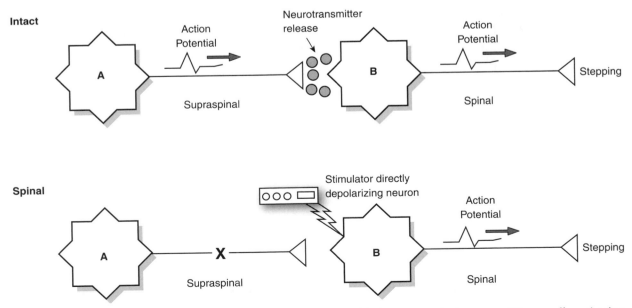

Figure 2-3. Principle of action of neural prostheses. After spinal cord lesion, supraspinal neurons (A) normally activating spinal neurons (B) are no longer available. The spinal neurons can be depolarized by local electrical stimulation.

approaches. Sensory feedback from skin,[54] muscle, [8,9,55] and tendons[56] are normally involved in the generation of the locomotor movement. Enhanced activation of these pathways may be useful for rehabilitation. After spinal cord injury, with the loss of descending influences, it seems that the role of sensory receptors (skin receptors in particular) becomes of paramount importance for the quality of the walking movement. This has been shown in two animal models. Muir and Steeves[57,58] have compared the swimming movements of young chicks with spinal hemisections that were trained under two conditions: swimming in an ordinary pool or swimming in a pool containing neutrally buoyant tubes that provide increased sensory input to the limbs during swimming (as illustrated in Fig. 2-4). Spinal chicks trained with the tubes recovered better than chicks trained in water only, suggesting that phasic cutaneous inputs, independent of loading, helps to improve swimming recovery after SCI.

In cats, Bouyer and Rossignol[41] have cut all five cutaneous nerves relaying sensory input from the skin of the hind paws. They have shown that while intact cats can walk almost normally in the absence of these inputs, after complete spinalization, the same animals entirely lost the ability to place the paw normally or to bear weight on their hind limbs (see Fig. 2-5).[59] Treadmill training for more than 2 months could not reverse this effect. If spinalization is performed prior to cutting the cutaneous nerves, and the cat is trained to walk on the treadmill, subsequent denervation of the skin still leads to abnormal paw placement and loss of weight-bearing ability. These experiments suggest that inputs from hind paw skin receptors, while of use for the normal control of locomotion, become essential after SCI for the complete expression of the stepping pattern. Taken together, these studies suggest that cutaneous inputs from the paw should not be neglected during locomotor training. They seem to be part of the "natural" feedback used by the spinal locomotor circuits to relearn to walk and to maintain the expression of the spinal locomotor pattern. The corollary in human locomotion, however, is not known.

Specificity of Training

When designing a new training paradigm, it is important to know how task-specific the training approach needs to be. For example, for proper spinal stepping on a treadmill, two elements of locomotion must be trained: weight bearing and rhythmic alternation. Is weight-bearing training sufficient to improve locomotion? To address this question, spinal cats have been trained to stand for several weeks. They developed full weight-bearing standing ability within 12 weeks of training.[60] When tested on a treadmill after training, these animals did not walk as well as step-trained cats.[32] If the same animals were then exposed to a locomotor-training regimen, they gradually learned to re-express locomotion, but lost their ability to stand. These results emphasize the need for training specificity in locomotor rehabilitation, a need that is already well-known for other motor tasks.

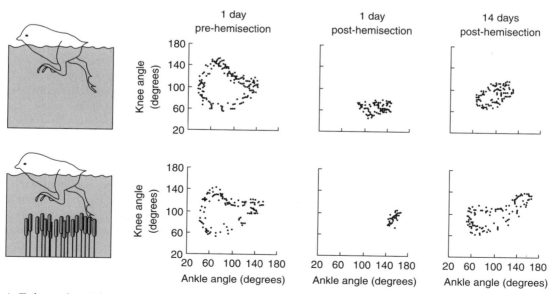

Figure 2-4. Enhanced peripheral stimulation improves limb action during training. Provision of phasic cutaneous stimulation improves motor recovery after lateral thoracic hemisection in chicks. After hemisection (upper panels), measurement of knee- and ankle-joint angles during swimming demonstrates that the ipsilateral leg moves through a limited range of motion, which does not recover. Physical stimulation of the footpads (lower panels), in the form of non-weight-supporting plastic tubes, provokes greater leg extension during swim-training sessions and results in an increased range of leg motion after 2 weeks of training. This enhanced leg action is retained after stimulation is removed. (From: Muir GD, Steeves JD. Phasic cutaneous input facilitates locomotor recovery after incomplete spinal injury in the chick. *J Neurophysiol.* 1995; 74:358–368.)

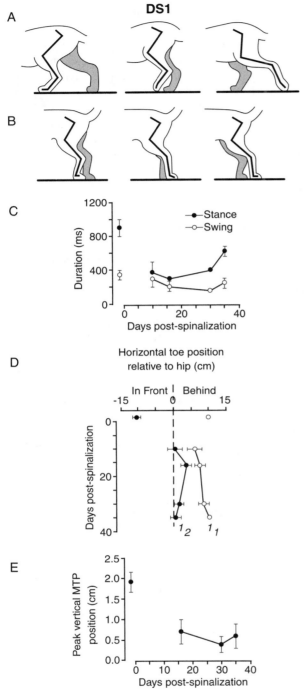

Figure 2-5. Locomotion in completely denervated cat DS1 before and 35 days after spinalization. (A, B) Line drawings from video images at onset, midway, and end of swing phase. (C) Time course of swing (open circles) and stance (filled circles) duration. (D) Horizontal toe position at onset of swing (l_1) and foot contact (l_2). (E) Toe clearance, expressed as peak vertical metatarsal phalangeal joint distance relative to treadmill belt surface during swing. All data points represent mean ± 1 SD. Data points not linked by a line and displayed before day 0 represent pre-spinalization values in denervated cat. (From: Bouyer LJ, Rossignol S. Contribution of cutaneous inputs from the hindpaw to the control of locomotion. II. Spinal cats. *J Neurophysiol.* 2003; 90:3640–3653.)

Retention of Training

While it is interesting that spinal animals can be trained to step, for this training to have functional relevance for humans, its effects must be retained. How long are training effects retained after training stops? Does it remain indefinitely? After how long do effects start to fade? To address these questions, spinal cats were trained to walk for 6 to 12 weeks and were then left in their cages for 6 to 12 weeks before being retested on the treadmill.[61] After 6 weeks, no significant losses in maximum speed or in stepping success were measured. However, both of these parameters were significantly degraded after 12 weeks of inactivity. While this work clearly suggests that retention of locomotor training after spinal cord transection can last for several weeks after training stops, it also has important limitations. For example, muscle atrophy due to inactivity during the 6 to 12 weeks between locomotor tests undoubtedly contributed to the degradation in performance. It is therefore difficult to accurately determine the retention time. In any event, it seems that the effects are retained for a period on the order of weeks rather than days or hours, a finding that has positive implications for the clinical relevance of this type of training.

Partial Transection or Incomplete Injury

When observing the trends in severity of SCI in humans over recent decades, there is a growing proportion of incomplete SCIs, while the proportion of complete injuries has declined. In fact, more than 50% of the new cases are incomplete. The evidence related to the locomotor activity in animals with complete spinal lesions makes it clear that there is an extensive capacity for plasticity in the neural circuits located below the lesion.

When considering incomplete lesions of the cord, questions immediately come to mind: how are the neural circuits located above and below the lesion reorganized after the injury? Is the neural plasticity similar or totally different from complete transections? To address these questions, animal models with incomplete spinal lesions are used. Unfortunately, much less is known at the moment about the neural plasticity after incomplete lesions. Part of this is due to the methodology used to quantify locomotion. In many studies using rats and mice with incomplete spinal lesions, walking ability has been measured using only the open field locomotor test[62] (see Rosenzweig and McDonald[63]). The advantage of this test is that it is very effective for comparing groups of animals evaluated by different observers. However, having only a single score that characterizes all walking parameters is not sufficient to understand the neural changes underlying the recovery of locomotor function. A more complete analysis of the walking movement, using kinematic and EMG recordings, is necessary (e.g., Kaegi et al.[64]; see Box 2-5).

The following section summarizes the key points related to the neural control of locomotion after partial SCI based on the limited number of available studies with electromyography and kinematics of the movement.

Effect of Lesion Location and Severity

Depending on the location and extent of the spinal damage, very different deficits, and potential extent of recovery, can be expected, a fact that can be appreciated by examining the figure in Box 2-2. Two models summarize the main principles: ventral lesions and dorsal lesions.

BOX 2–5
Method of Kinematics and EMG Recordings

To best describe the motor deficits and time course of recovery after a spinal lesion, methods had to be developed to record kinematics and EMG from the same animals over time periods of months. This represented a technical challenge because the electrodes used for the recording of muscle EMG activity had to remain at the exact same place in the muscle and their electrical properties had to stay stable over a long period of time. Implanted chronic electrodes made from Teflon-coated stainless steel wires turned out to be the answer. Such wires were led subcutaneously from a head-mounted connector to the muscles of interest. Teflon was then removed from the extremity, and the wires were sown into the muscle belly. Pairs of wires were used for differential recording. These wires are sufficiently small and flexible to interfere minimally with walking. Connective tissue rapidly grows over the muscle–wire interface, securing and isolating the recording site from its environment. The result is a high-quality EMG signal that is stable for periods extending to more than 1 year. (Photo courtesy of Dr. Serge Rossignol's laboratory.)

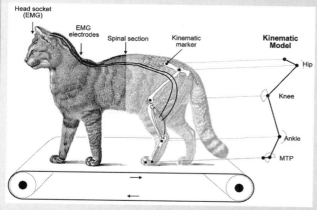

Schematic view of the method used for the chronic recording of muscle EMG activity and hind limb kinematics in cats. (Courtesy of Dr. Serge Rossignol's laboratory.)

Lesions of the Ventral Spinal Cord

Of interest in ventral and ventrolateral lesions is that they interrupt several descending (motor) tracts while causing little damage to ascending (sensory) pathways. For example, cutaneous and proprioceptive information from the hind limbs that travels in the dorsal columns remains able to reach the cortex to provide data about limb position, ground contact, etc. However, vestibulospinal and reticulospinal tracts are interrupted. Referring to the figure in Box 2-2 and to the section on the basics of the neural control of locomotion (above), it is clear that ventral and ventrolateral lesions will simultaneously affect posture, walking initiation, and interlimb coordination. Using kinematics and electromyography, Brustein and Rossignol[65] documented the recovery of eight cats after ventral and ventrolateral spinal transection lesions of graded severity. Figure 2-6a illustrates the location and extent of the lesion in each of the cats.

While amount of training that was required increased with lesion severity, as Figure 2-6b illustrates, all animals eventually recovered voluntary quadrupedal locomotion, both on the treadmill and over ground after treadmill training. This is quite remarkable, considering that one cat had only a small section of the dorsolateral cord intact. These results suggest that after interruption of both the pathway normally responsible for initiation of walking and of vestibulospinal pathway, the remaining structures involved in the control of locomotion (such as the motor cortex and red nucleus) can be trained to compensate. The result is a re-expression of the ability to voluntarily trigger walking, an element of prime importance for independent ambulation. Some deficits remained, however, such as poor lateral stability and variable coupling between the forelimbs and hind limbs, but this is considered to be of lesser importance compared to the ability to voluntarily initiate walking.

Lesions of the Dorsal Spinal Cord

In contrast to ventral lesions, dorsal lesions interrupt sensory information ascending via the dorsal columns to the thalamus and cortex and motor commands descending through the dorsal funiculus, conveying information originating from the motor cortex and the red nucleus. Jiang and Drew[66] made transection lesions of graded severity to the dorsal side of the spinal cord in five cats. Lesions varied from complete interruption to partial sparing of the dorsal columns and dorsolateral funiculus bilaterally. Recovery was documented using kinematics and EMG. In contrast to ventral lesions, quadrupedal locomotion returned very rapidly; within 10 days, cats could walk for extended periods of time on the treadmill, *regardless of the extent of the lesion.* The remaining deficits were also much smaller; only animals with dorsolateral funiculus lesions presented a

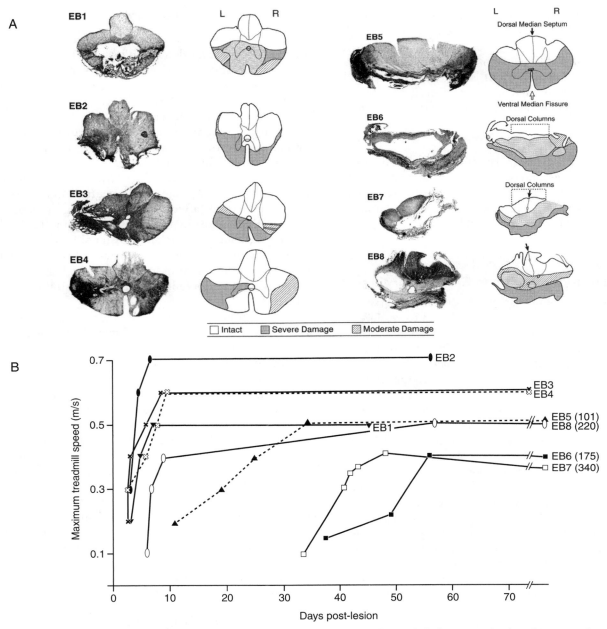

Figure 2-6. (A) Extent of the spinal lesions for all eight cats: the histology of all the cats is displayed in two columns. On the left, photomicrographs of the cross-sections taken from the spinal site of lesion, stained with cresyl violet or with Kluver-Barrera, to demonstrate the maximal extent of the lesion. To the right of the photomicrographs, a schematic reconstruction of the site of lesion, evaluated using light microscope. For cats EB1 to EB5, the total extent of the lesion is projected on a spinal cord section taken more rostrally after inspecting several consecutive sections, whereas for cats EB6 to EB8 the schemes illustrate the maximal site of lesion to emphasize the deformation of the spinal cord. The various shades identify the extent of damage. Intact: myelinated axons (or axonal profiles) appeared normal under the microscope; severe damage: absent or highly fibrotic tissue; moderate damage: some myelinated axons (or axonal profiles) of normal appearance within fibrotic and gliotic tissue; syrinx: cyst. L = left; R = right. (B) Recovery of treadmill locomotion following spinal lesion for each one of the eight cats; graph illustrates the maximal treadmill speed each cat could attain and maintain at least for a few step cycles, as a function of days after spinal lesion.

persistent paw drag on the same side as the lesion during swing. When compared to ventral lesions, these experiments suggest that dorsal spinal lesions produce much milder initial locomotor deficits and the recovery of function is faster and more complete.

Influence of Lesion Type on Response to Intervention

When considering the neural circuitry available to control locomotion after a spinal injury, it is important to bear in mind that intact neurons in all remaining structures will likely influence the neural reorganization underlying the recovery of function. This means that the spinal cord circuitry that is entirely isolated from descending influence (such as after a complete SCI) may reorganize differently compared to what occurs in an incomplete injury in which some descending influence remains (such as after an incomplete SCI). While this statement may seem obvious, its implications become of primary importance when attempting to transfer drug therapy protocols based on studies of complete SCI to those with incomplete SCI. As discussed earlier, after a complete SCI, drugs can be used to "replace" the neurotransmitter normally activating the postsynaptic neurons. After an incomplete SCI, the situation is different. As Figure 2-7 illustrates, there are two conditions under which function may be restored after incomplete SCI: (1) some neurotransmitter may still be liberated by the remaining descending neurons, or

(2) other descending neurons, normally not involved, may take on a new role and become part of the activating system. Both of these cases will profoundly affect the efficiency of the drug therapy.

Considering the heterogeneity in the presentation of incomplete SCI, the number of possible interactions between descending and spinal connections is extremely large and as yet is not well-described and understood. The following is an example that illustrates the complexity of finding a "miracle drug" to enhance locomotor performance after partial spinal injury. Using the two most severely lesioned cats with ventrolateral lesions from their initial study (cf Fig. 2-6a), Brustein and Rossignol[67] tested the effects of noradrenaline and clonidine after the lesion. Noradrenaline did improve the regularity of stepping and stabilized interlimb coupling. However, clonidine, the alpha-2 adrenergic agonist that promoted good-quality walking in completely spinalized

1) Partly spared pathway

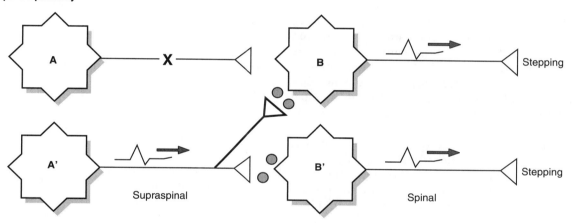

2) Reorganized pathway

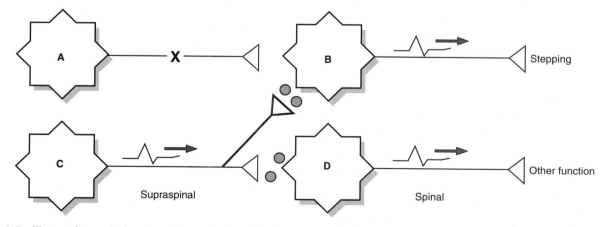

Figure 2-7. Types of neural plasticity. After spinal cord lesion, supraspinal neurons (A) normally activating spinal neurons involved in stepping (B) are no longer available. Spinal neurons B therefore become deafferented. Two types of reorganization in the CNS can result in a reactivation of these spinal neurons: (1) If the axonal projections originating from the supraspinal center controlling locomotion was not completely severed, supraspinal neurons (A') projecting to adjacent spinal neurons also involved in stepping (B') could sprout to also activate the deafferented spinal neurons (B). (2) If instead the entire axon bundle was severed, supraspinal neurons normally having a different function (C) and normally projecting onto other types of spinal neurons (D) could sprout distally to activate the deafferented spinal neurons (B).

cats, *deteriorated* the walking performance of the partially lesioned cats. Clonidine is a drug that shares many similarities with noradrenaline; yet, their effect is very different, depending on the type of spinal lesion. These findings suggest that while drugs can be used to improve locomotion after both partial or complete SCI, different classes or combinations of drugs may be required depending on the SCI type.[68]

Summary

The control of walking results from an interaction of voluntary and automatic neural centers distributed across the whole CNS, from the spinal cord (central pattern generator) to the motor cortex (voluntary gait modifications based on visual information), by way of the brainstem (gait initiation). Such a distributed system of control is extremely efficient in healthy individuals, allowing for a complex movement to be properly executed and adapted to the context of walking while requiring minimal conscious attention. However, distributed control also means that damage to any of the structures involved or to the integrity of the pathways from the supraspinal to the spinal structures will result in some form of locomotor deficit. SCI is one example in which the control of locomotion can be dramatically affected.

Using models of complete spinal cord transections, we have seen that substantial adaptive capacity is present in the spinal neural circuits controlling locomotion and that recovery can be faster and more extensive if task-specific locomotor training is provided. This is true even in the adult animal and even if other tasks have been learned previously. However, the spinal cord circuitry seems to be capable of remembering only one task at a time: standing or walking. This training effect lasts for several weeks after training cessation. Treadmill training can be further accelerated if clonidine, a drug that mimics the action of the neurotransmitter involved in initiating voluntary locomotion, is given along with training in the early days after the lesion. Other methods that are still in their infancy may eventually also be used to enhance recovery, such as intraspinal/peridural stimulation and robotic orthoses. While these methods are already being tested in humans, their mechanisms of action remain to be elucidated through animal model experiments if they are to be used to their full potential during rehabilitation.

Using models of incomplete spinal transections, we have explored the complexities of incomplete injury by discussing how numerous possible forms of neural reorganization can arise from the plasticity occurring simultaneously above and below the site of injury. Cats seem to recover much faster and more extensively from dorsal lesions compared to ventral lesions. Yet, even after a complete section of the ventrolateral pathway normally responsible for voluntary gait initiation, several weeks of training are sufficient to regain this ability through the remaining dorsolateral pathways. This provides great possibilities for the rehabilitation of individuals with incomplete lesions. Finally, we have emphasized the fact that our understanding of the effects of drug therapy is much more advanced in models of complete SCI than in incomplete injury. It is necessary to consider the type and extent of a spinal lesion before being convinced that a new "miracle drug" tested in complete spinal models will have the same effect after partial lesions.

Taken into perspective, this chapter demonstrates the tremendous capacity of the neural control of locomotion for training-induced modification and recovery of function. It also shows that only a small amount of descending control is necessary for gait initiation. Taken together, these findings are very exciting, providing evidence upon which to base the training of individuals with partial spinal lesions and suggesting that the nervous system likely has great potential for functional recovery after injury, provided the appropriate feedback signals for training are identified and methods to capitalize on the innate locomotor networks are established.

REVIEW QUESTIONS

1. It is Christmas and you have to buy last minute presents for your family. From the moment you leave your car in the parking lot to the moment you reach the gift shop inside the shopping center, what parts of your CNS will you need to use for locomotion and why? (Cue: Decompose the movement sequence.)
2. What are the challenges associated with locomotor training after SCI?
3. What is spinal locomotion?
4. What is the functional consequence of a bilateral ventral/ventrolateral lesion of the spinal cord?

REFERENCES

1. Grillner S. Control of locomotion in bipeds, tetrapods, and fish. *Handbook of Physiology USA.* 1981:1179–1236.
2. Grillner S, Zangger P. On the central generation of locomotion in the low spinal cat. *Exp Brain Res.* 1979;34:241–261.
3. Rossignol S, Bouyer L, Langlet C et al. Determinants of locomotor recovery after spinal injury in the cat. *Prog Brain Res.* 2004;143:163–172.
4. Rossignol S, Bouyer L, Barthelemy D et al. Recovery of locomotion in the cat following spinal cord lesions. *Brain Res Brain Res Rev.* 2002;40:257–266.
5. Rossignol S, Chau C, Giroux N et al. The cat model of spinal injury. *Prog Brain Res.* 2002;137:151–168.

6. Forssberg H, Grillner S, Rossignol S. Phasic gain control of reflexes from the dorsum of the paw during spinal locomotion. *Brain Res.* 1977;132:121–139.

7. Barbeau H, Rossignol S. Recovery of locomotion after chronic spinalization in the adult cat. *Brain Res.* 1987;412:84–95.

8. Dietz V, Duysens J. Significance of load receptor input during locomotion: A review. *Gait Posture.* 2000;11:102–110.

9. Duysens J, Pearson KG. Inhibition of flexor burst generation by loading ankle extensor muscles in walking cats. *Brain Res.* 1980;187:321–332.

10. Belanger M, Drew T, Provencher J et al. A comparison of treadmill locomotion in adult cats before and after spinal transection. *J Neurophysiol.* 1996;76:471–491.

11. Shik ML, Severin FV, Orlovskii GN. [Control of walking and running by means of electric stimulation of the midbrain]. *Biofizika.* 1966;11:659–666.

12. Shik ML, Severin FV, Orlovsky GN. Control of walking and running by means of electrical stimulation of the mesencephalon. *Electroencephalogr Clin Neurophysiol.* 1969;26:549.

13. Shik ML, Orlovskii GN, Severin FV. [Organization of locomotor synergism]. *Biofizika.* 1966;11:879–886.

14. Mori S, Matsuyama K, Kohyama J et al. Neuronal constituents of postural and locomotor control systems and their interactions in cats. *Brain Dev.* 1992;14 Suppl: S109–S120.

15. Jordan LM. Initiation of locomotion in mammals. *Ann N Y Acad Sci.* 1998;860:83–93.

16. Armstrong DM. Supraspinal contributions to the initiation and control of locomotion in the cat. *Prog Neurobiol.* 1986;26:273–361.

17. Widajewicz W, Kably B, Drew T. Motor cortical activity during voluntary gait modifications in the cat. II. Cells related to the hindlimbs. *J Neurophysiol.* 1994;72:2070–2089.

18. Rho MJ, Lavoie S, Drew T. Effects of red nucleus microstimulation on the locomotor pattern and timing in the intact cat: A comparison with the motor cortex. *J Neurophysiol.* 1999;81:2297–2315.

19. Armstrong DM. The supraspinal control of mammalian locomotion. *J Physiol.* 1988;405:1–37.

20. Armstrong DM, Marple-Horvat DE. Role of the cerebellum and motor cortex in the regulation of visually controlled locomotion. *Can J Physiol Pharmacol.* 1996;74:443–445.

21. Drew T, Jiang W, Widajewicz W. Contributions of the motor cortex to the control of the hindlimbs during locomotion in the cat. *Brain Res Brain Res Rev.* 2002;40:178–191.

22. Duysens J, Van de Crommert HW. Neural control of locomotion: The central pattern generator from cats to humans. *Gait Posture.* 1998;7:131–141.

23. Crenna P, Inverno M, Fedrizzi E et al. Objective detection of pathophysiological factors contributing to gait disturbance in supraspinal lesions. *Motor Development in Children.* London: John Libbey & Company Ltd; 1994:103–118.

24. Peiper A. *Cerebral functions in infancy and childhood.* New York: Consultants Bureau; 1961.

25. Basso DM. Neuroanatomical substrates of functional recovery after experimental spinal cord injury: Implications of basic science research for human spinal cord injury. *Phys Ther.* 2000;80:808–817.

26. Wernig A, Nanassy A, Muller S. Laufband (LB) therapy in spinal cord lesioned persons. *Prog Brain Res.* 2000;128:89–97.

27. Wernig A, Muller S. Laufband locomotion with body weight support improved walking in persons with severe spinal cord injuries. *Paraplegia.* 1992;30:229–238.

28. Barbeau H, Julien C, Rossignol S. The effects of clonidine and yohimbine on locomotion and cutaneous reflexes in the adult chronic spinal cat. *Brain Res.* 1987;437:83–96.

29. Smith JL, Smith LA, Zernicke RF et al. Locomotion in exercised and nonexercised cats cordotomized at two or twelve weeks of age. *Exp Neurol.* 1982;76:393–413.

30. De Leon RD, Hodgson JA, Roy RR et al. Locomotor capacity attributable to step training versus spontaneous recovery after spinalization in adult cats. *J Neurophysiol.* 1998;79:1329–1340.

31. Edgerton VR, Leon RD, Harkema SJ et al. Retraining the injured spinal cord. *J Physiol.* 2001;533:15–22.

32. Hodgson JA, Roy RR, de Leon R et al. Can the mammalian lumbar spinal cord learn a motor task? *Med Sci Sports Exerc.* 1994;26:1491–1497.

33. De Leon RD, Kubasak MD, Phelps PE et al. Using robotics to teach the spinal cord to walk. *Brain Res Brain Res Rev.* 2002;40:267–273.

34. Edgerton VR, Tillakaratne NJ, Bigbee AJ et al. Plasticity of the spinal neural circuitry after injury. *Annu Rev Neurosci.* 2004;27:145–167.

35. Timoszyk WK, De Leon RD, London N et al. The rat lumbosacral spinal cord adapts to robotic loading applied during stance. *J Neurophysiol.* 2002;88:3108–3117.

36. Colombo G, Joerg M, Schreier R et al. Treadmill training of paraplegic patients using a robotic orthosis. *J Rehabil Res Dev.* 2000;37:693–700.

37. Colombo G, Wirz M, Dietz V. Driven gait orthosis for improvement of locomotor training in paraplegic patients. *Spinal Cord.* 2001;39:252–255.

38. Carr J, Shepherd R. *Stroke Rehabilitation: Guidelines for Exercise and Training to Optimize Motor Skill.*: Edinburgh: Butterworth-Heinemann, 2003.

39. Bouyer LJ, DiZio P, Lackner JR. Adaptive modification of human locomotion by Coriolis force. *Soc Neurosci Abstracts.* 2003;29:494.

40. Tremblay E, Bouyer LJG. Modifications of locomotor output during and after exposure to an elastic force applied to the leg. *Soc Neurosci Abstracts.* 2003;29:494.

41. Bouyer LJ, Rossignol S. Contribution of cutaneous inputs from the hindpaw to the control of locomotion. I. Intact cats. *J Neurophysiol.* 2003;90:3625–3639.

42. Volpe BT, Krebs HI, Hogan N et al. Robot training enhanced motor outcome in patients with stroke maintained over 3 years. *Neurology.* 1999;53:1874–1876.

43. Chau C, Barbeau H, Rossignol S. Early locomotor training with clonidine in spinal cats. *J Neurophysiol.* 1998;79:392–409.

44. Giszter SF, Mussa-Ivaldi FA, Bizzi E. Convergent force fields organized in the frog's spinal cord. *J Neurosci.* 1993;13:467–491.

45. Loeb EP, Giszter SF, Saltiel P et al. Output units of motor behavior: An experimental and modeling study. *J Cogn Neurosci.* 2000;12:78–97.

46. Tresch MC, Bizzi E. Responses to spinal microstimulation in the chronically spinalized rat and their relationship to

spinal systems activated by low threshold cutaneous stimulation. *Exp Brain Res.* 1999;129:401–416.

47. Prochazka A, Mushahwar VK, McCreery DB. Neural prostheses. *J Physiol.* 2001;533:99–109.

48. Mushahwar VK, Gillard DM, Gauthier MJ et al. Intraspinal micro stimulation generates locomotor-like and feedback-controlled movements. *IEEE Trans Neural Syst Rehabil Eng.* 2002;10:68–81.

49. Marcoux J, Rossignol S. Initiating or blocking locomotion in spinal cats by applying noradrenergic drugs to restricted lumbar spinal segments. *J Neurosci.* 2000;20:8577–8585.

50. Shefchyk SJ. Sacral spinal interneurones and the control of urinary bladder and urethral striated sphincter muscle function. *J Physiol.* 2001;533:57–63.

51. Langlet C, Leblond H, Rossignol S. Mid-lumbar segments are needed for the expression of locomotion in chronic spinal cats. *J Neurophysiol.* 2005;93:2474–2488.

52. Gerasimenko Y., Musienko P, Ishiyama RM, Zhong H, Roy RR, Edgerton VR. Peripheral feedback plays a key role in stepping during epidural spinal cord stimulation in decerebrated or spinalized animals. Abstract. Conference Proceedings 2005. San Diego.

53. Dimitrijevic MR, Gerasimenko Y, Pinter MM. Evidence for a spinal central pattern generator in humans. *Ann N Y Acad Sci.* 1998;860:360–376.

54. Duysens J, Pearson KG. The role of cutaneous afferents from the distal hindlimb in the regulation of the step cycle of thalamic cats. *Exp Brain Res.* 1976;24:245–255.

55. Pearson KG. Proprioceptive regulation of locomotion. *Curr Opin Neurobiol.* 1995;5:786–791.

56. Whelan PJ, Hiebert GW, Pearson KG. Stimulation of the group I extensor afferents prolongs the stance phase in walking cats. *Exp Brain Res.* 1995;103:20–30.

57. Muir GD, Steeves JD. Phasic cutaneous input facilitates locomotor recovery after incomplete spinal injury in the chick. *J Neurophysiol.* 1995;74:358–368.

58. Muir GD, Steeves JD. Sensorimotor stimulation to improve locomotor recovery after spinal cord injury. *Trends Neurosci.* 1997;20:72–77.

59. Bouyer LJ, Rossignol S. Contribution of cutaneous inputs from the hindpaw to the control of locomotion. II. Spinal cats. *J Neurophysiol.* 2003;90:3640–3653.

60. De Leon RD, Hodgson JA, Roy RR et al. Full weight-bearing hindlimb standing following stand training in the adult spinal cat. *J Neurophysiol.* 1998;80:83–91.

61. De Leon RD, Hodgson JA, Roy RR et al. Retention of hindlimb stepping ability in adult spinal cats after the cessation of step training. *J Neurophysiol.* 1999;81:85–94.

62. Basso DM, Beattie MS, Bresnahan JC. A sensitive and reliable locomotor rating scale for open field testing in rats. *J Neurotrauma.* 1995;12:1–21.

63. Rosenzweig ES, McDonald JW. Rodent models for treatment of spinal cord injury: Research trends and progress toward useful repair. *Curr Opin Neurol.* 2004;17:121–131.

64. Kaegi S, Schwab ME, Dietz V et al. Electromyographic activity associated with spontaneous functional recovery after spinal cord injury in rats. *Eur J Neurosci.* 2002;16:249–258.

65. Brustein E, Rossignol S. Recovery of locomotion after ventral and ventrolateral spinal lesions in the cat. I. Deficits and adaptive mechanisms. *J Neurophysiol.* 1998;80:1245–1267.

66. Jiang W, Drew T. Effects of bilateral lesions of the dorsolateral funiculi and dorsal columns at the level of the low thoracic spinal cord on the control of locomotion in the adult cat. I. Treadmill walking. *J Neurophysiol.* 1996;76:849–866.

67. Brustein E, Rossignol S. Recovery of locomotion after ventral and ventrolateral spinal lesions in the cat. II. Effects of noradrenergic and serotoninergic drugs. *J Neurophysiol.* 1999;81:1513–1530.

68. Rossignol S, Giroux N, Chau C et al. Pharmacological aids to locomotor training after spinal injury in the cat. *J Physiol.* 2001;533:65–74.

69. Gruner JA. A monitored contusion model of spinal cord injury in the rat. *J Neurotrauma.* 1992;9:123–126.

70. Beattie MS. Anatomic and behavioral outcome after spinal cord injury produced by a displacement controlled impact device. *J Neurotrauma.* 1992;9:157–159.

71. Martin D, Schoenen J, Delree P et al. Experimental acute traumatic injury of the adult rat spinal cord by a subdural inflatable balloon: Methodology, behavioral analysis, and histopathology. *J Neurosci Res.* 1992;32:539–550.

72. Rivlin AS, Tator CH. Effect of duration of acute spinal cord compression in a new acute cord injury model in the rat. *Surg Neurol.* 1978;10:38–43.

73. Eidelberg E, Walden JG, Nguyen LH. Locomotor control in macaque monkeys. *Brain.* 1981;104:647–663.

74. Fulton JF, Sherrington CS. State of the flexor reflex in paraplegic dog and monkey respectively. *J Physiol.* 1932;75:17–22.

75. Vilensky JA, O'Connor BL. Stepping in humans with complete spinal cord transection: A phylogenetic evaluation. *Motor Control.* 1997;1:284–292.

76. Hultborn H, Petersen RN, Brownstone RM et al. Evidence of fictive spinal locomotion in the marmoset (*Callithrix jacchus*). *Soc Neurosci Abstracts.* 1993;19:539.

77. Vilensky JA, O'Connor BL. Stepping in nonhuman primates with a complete spinal cord transection: Old and new data, and implications for humans. *Ann N Y Acad Sci.* 1998;860:528–530.

78. Bouyer L, Rossignol S. Spinal cord plasticity associated with locomotor compensation to peripheral nerve lesions in the cat. In: Patterson MM, Grau JW, eds. *Spinal Cord Plasticity: Alterations in Reflex Function.* Boston, Massachusetts: Kluwer Academic Publishers; 2001:207–224.

79. Lovely RG, Gregor RJ, Roy RR et al. Weight-bearing hindlimb stepping in treadmill-exercised adult spinal cats. *Brain Res.* 1990;514:206–218.

80. Kullander K, Butt SJ, Lebret JM et al. Role of EphA4 and EphrinB3 in local neuronal circuits that control walking. *Science.* 2003;299:1889–1892.

81. Leblond H, L'Esperance M, Orsal D et al. Treadmill locomotion in the intact and spinal mouse. *J Neurosci.* 2003;23:11411–11419.

82. Antri M, Orsal D, Barthe JY. Locomotor recovery in the chronic spinal rat: Effects of long-term treatment with a 5-HT2 agonist. *Eur J Neurosci.* 2002;16:467–476.

Musculoskeletal Plasticity after SCI: A Conceptual Framework Based on Plasticity, Adaptation, and Outcome

Richard K. Shields, PT, PhD, FAPTA and
Shauna Dudley-Javoroski, PT, MPT

OBJECTIVES

After reading this chapter, the reader will be able to:

- Enumerate the protein categories that underlie the plastic potential of skeletal muscle
- Summarize the major muscular adaptations to reduced use after SCI
- Discuss the adaptations of paralyzed muscle to the reintroduction of loads via electrical stimulation
- Describe how mechanotransduction and osteoclast/osteoblast activity underlie skeletal plasticity
- Summarize the adaptations of trabecular versus cortical bone to reduced use after SCI, along with consequences for bone strength and fracture risk
- Discuss the concept of dose of loading in research protocols designed to preserve bone density after SCI
- Discuss the subject-safety considerations of using electrical muscle stimulation to preserve musculoskeletal integrity after SCI (especially autonomic dysreflexia and fractures)

OUTLINE

Introduction

Musculoskeletal Deterioration After SCI

Given the catastrophic nature of traumatic spinal cord injury (SCI), the degree of adaptation made by many people with paralysis is remarkable. Despite sensory and motor loss, secondary medical complications, social adjustments, and financial and emotional challenges, many people with SCI regain partial or complete functional independence. Some individuals with SCI return to their former vocations or begin new occupations, and many return to busy, productive lives. Even individuals with high quadriplegia may, with the necessary adaptive assistance, fully participate in a broad range of vocational, academic, and social activities. People with SCI today can expect to live full lives, a credit to the resilience of people with SCI and to the success of modern rehabilitation interventions. In the broadest view, it would appear that the contemporary standard of SCI rehabilitation care has greatly advanced over time.

However, even very high-functioning people with SCI will be the first to remark on the difficulty of living with the secondary complications of paralysis. Joint contractures, spasms, pain, and urinary and bowel complications can be inconvenient, health limiting, or even life threatening. Muscle atrophy below the level of the lesion impairs weight distribution over bony prominences, leading to pressure ulcers even in people who try to conscientiously perform pressure-relief measures. As paralyzed muscles atrophy, the loss of muscular loading through the skeleton precipitates severe osteoporosis in paralyzed limbs. Fractures reportedly occur in the paralyzed extremities of 1% to 6% of people with SCI,[1-3] but this figure may be grossly underestimated because many fractures may go undetected.[4] Undetected fractures likely lead to increased spasms, functional limitations, and decreased independence. These interrelated secondary complications represent various levels of *musculoskeletal deterioration.*[5] Modern rehabilitation has yet to devise therapeutic interventions to fully prevent the wide range of secondary complications that emerge after complete SCI.

Both individuals with SCI and the rehabilitation community eagerly await the development of a cure for SCI, which may reasonably emerge within the life spans of people living with SCI today. However, people with severe musculoskeletal deterioration may miss opportunities for reintroduction to standing mobility if bone and muscle deterioration are allowed to progress. (Post-SCI osteoporosis, in particular, may be irreversible once established.[6,7]) Moreover, any future cure is likely to require a protracted rehabilitation phase during the neural regenerative process. Numerous animal studies indicate that spinal regeneration is hastened (and may even be predicated upon) muscular activity (for reviews see Vaynman and Gomez-Pinilla and Edgerton et al.[8,9]). Atrophied muscles and brittle bones will be poorly suited for the therapeutic exercise regimens that will be required during the neural recovery process.

Thus, two compelling lines of reasoning support the development of rehabilitation interventions to limit musculoskeletal deterioration after SCI. First, such interventions could limit the noisome secondary complications that develop after SCI. Secondly, these interventions may also increase the probability that people who currently have SCI could fully capitalize upon a forthcoming cure. Contemporary research efforts strive to develop highly efficacious rehabilitation strategies to prevent musculoskeletal deterioration after SCI. Any efforts to develop rehabilitation strategies, however, are necessarily limited by what adaptations may or may not be possible in the paralyzed musculoskeletal system. Thus, a thorough understanding of the **plasticity** of the paralyzed musculoskeletal system must provide the theoretical framework for rehabilitation research in this area.

Plasticity, Adaptation, and Outcome

In our own clinical and research efforts, we have adopted a conceptual framework called the *plasticity-adaptation-outcome (PAO)* model (Fig. 3-1).[10] The

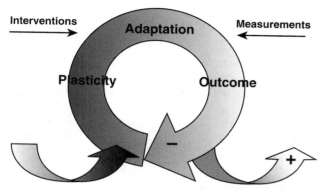

Figure 3-1. Plasticity-adaptation-outcome model. Rehabilitation interventions capitalize upon the intrinsic plasticity of the paralyzed musculoskeletal system to yield desirable adaptations. If the measured outcomes of these adaptations are favorable, intervention is withdrawn. Unfavorable outcomes trigger continued attempts to instigate adaptations.

plasticity of the neuromusculoskeletal system is defined as its underlying capacity to change, largely determined by its physiological processes and cellular and histochemical characteristics. A great body of basic research has revealed the potential mutability of the paralyzed musculoskeletal system. Upon this foundation of plastic potential, **adaptations** occur in response to various imposed stimuli. In the case of SCI, a disuse stimulus sometimes followed by an increased use stimulus (depending on the rehabilitation approach) powerfully affects the underlying plastic musculoskeletal substrate. Adaptations in response to stimuli are the specialty of applied research, which must parse the interrelationships among type, frequency (dose), and duration of the applied stimuli. The **outcome** of the applied stimulus incorporates a broader view, using a range of metrics to determine the importance or impact of the adaptations that emerge. Although applied research routinely uses these metrics, clinical research also plays an important role in determining the significance of outcomes across broad groups of individuals with SCI. Thus, SCI rehabilitation research, when conceptualized according to the PAO model, spans the continuum from basic, applied, clinical, and broad-spectrum outcomes research, each component working synergistically to provide a more complete picture.

Our primary goal in this chapter is to describe in detail the underlying capacity of the paralyzed musculoskeletal system to change (plasticity), summarizing findings from a wide variety of basic research studies. We will frame this summary in light of the adaptations and outcomes that are possible, given the inherent musculoskeletal plasticity that exists after SCI. In our experience, the PAO model has revealed two important guidelines that bear upon the success of various strategies that tap into the adaptive capacity of the paralyzed musculoskeletal system. First, the paralyzed musculoskeletal system retains plastic capabilities that are not so very different from the neurologically intact model.

Much of rehabilitation research in the non-SCI model, therefore, is germane to the study of the paralyzed musculoskeletal system. SCI-specific interventions can therefore be designed to be congruent with well-established physiologic and rehabilitation principles; we conceptualize this as the **feasibility** of an intervention that strives to adapt the tissue. Secondly, the **dose** of an intervention is usually a critical factor in not only the outcome of the tested intervention, but also in the heuristic value of the eventual clinical research conclusion. For example, if dose is not carefully quantified, a researcher or clinician cannot know if a failed intervention is fundamentally flawed or was merely administered at an inadequate dose. If dose is precisely quantified, however, a researcher, and ultimately the clinician, can more confidently rule out an unsuccessful intervention. Although this may be is a disappointing result, this knowledge can be tremendously important in the long, costly, iterative process of developing effective rehabilitation strategies.

Thus, we will review the wide body of basic research that deals first with muscular, then skeletal plasticity after SCI, following each with a summary of adaptations that occur in response to various research interventions. Although we will not offer a comprehensive discussion of clinical outcomes, we will evaluate many studies in terms of their feasibility and their adherence to careful quantification of dose. By using these two criteria, we hope that practitioners and scientists will be able to integrate the outcomes of the studies we summarize into their own knowledge of practical rehabilitation approaches after SCI.

Muscular Plasticity and Adaptation
Muscular Plasticity: Potential Loci of Change

Skeletal muscle is an amazingly versatile tissue that has the ability to adapt in response to the demands it encounters. Routine activity, such as exercise or disuse, is a powerful determinant of the structural and functional characteristics of muscle. The muscle adaptations that emerge are specific to the characteristics of the imposed stimulus. For example, the muscles of powerlifters undergo extreme hypertrophy, but the muscles of marathoners transform in ways that maximize endurance. In cases of extreme disuse, such as SCI, muscles adapt in other ways.

The localized hypoxia and mechanical stress associated with exercise are likely candidates for the physiologic signal that triggers muscle adaptation.[11] Although it remains uncertain exactly how these signals are transduced, the net result is that the nuclei of muscle cells upregulate or downregulate the expression of genes involved in muscle adaptation. These gene expression products (mRNA) facilitate the production of a wide range of proteins. These proteins are then incorporated into the existing muscle structure. Sometimes, these proteins magnify a certain characteristic of the muscle, as when individual fibers hypertrophy (they "pack on" protein). Other times, the proteins instigate a transformation of a particular aspect of the muscle, as the new proteins are incorporated and old versions are degraded and removed. Thus, the key element to skeletal muscle plasticity is genetic control of protein transcription and degradation, which is finely tuned to the demands routinely (or in some cases, even sporadically) placed upon the muscle. A discussion of skeletal muscle plasticity, therefore, largely centers on proteins. Because proteins can be added, subtracted, or substituted, skeletal muscle is a supremely plastic tissue. Where exactly does this plastic potential reside?

Fiber Cross-Sectional Area

The most obvious way that muscle adapts to increased or decreased use is to become larger or smaller. Although in some species, increases in muscle size can occur by the splitting of existing fibers (hyperplasia), in humans, size increases occur by the thickening of existing muscle fibers (hypertrophy). Muscle cells ("fibers") contain bundles of *myofibrils*, all of which comprise contractile proteins (to be described in detail below) arranged in units called *sarcomeres*. Sarcomeres are positioned end to end in series along the length of the myofibril. In hypertrophy, contractile proteins are added circumferentially within myofibrils, increasing the myofibril's cross-sectional area (Fig. 3-2).

The summed cross-sectional area of all contractile proteins in the muscle is a key determinant of the muscle's force-generating capacity. This is clearly illustrated in situations of decreased use when protein degradation occurs; the muscle shrinks (atrophies) and force production declines. Although hypertrophy generally requires several weeks of prolonged increased activity, atrophy may occur in a matter of days in cases of SCI or other neurologic insult (denervation, etc).

Contractile Filaments

The two main contractile proteins in skeletal muscle, actin and myosin, are the key players in generation of muscle force. Actin filaments are arranged in a hexagonal array about the myosin filament (Fig. 3-2, inset). In the presence of calcium, each myosin head bonds with actin, creating a *cross-bridge*. A complex series of chemical reactions causes a configuration change of the cross-bridge, causing the myosin fiber to slide past the actin fiber (for a detailed description, see Lieber, chapter 2[12]). This small movement, summed along many thousands of actin-myosin cross-bridges in series down the length of the muscle, causes the muscle to shorten by as much as several centimeters. On the other hand, this same cross-bridge movement, summed *across* many thousands of cross-bridges in parallel,

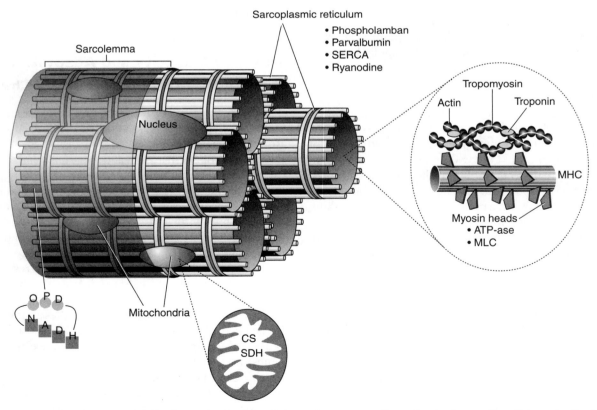

Figure 3-2. Sources of skeletal muscle plasticity. Schematic representation of a single muscle cell (muscle fiber) surrounded by the sarcolemmal membrane. Abbreviations are as described in the chapter text.

largely determines the overall force of the muscular contraction.

A major source of skeletal muscle plasticity is that multiple types (isoforms) of myosin protein molecules can be produced in response to the demands the muscle encounters. Over time, the new myosin type is gradually incorporated into the contractile filaments, causing the filaments to be hybrids of new and old proteins. Eventually, new myosin proteins may completely replace the old isoforms, causing the myosin filament to once again express a single type of myosin protein. In other cases, hybrid fibers may be a persistent feature.[13] Myosin type varies considerably among muscles with different functions. For example, the majority of myosin in the soleus, a postural muscle, is a different isoform from myosin in the adjacent gastrocnemius muscle, which mainly performs high-velocity phasic contractions.

Several other proteins associated with actin and myosin have regulatory roles in the process of contraction and may be additional potential sources of plasticity in skeletal muscle. Proteins called *myosin light chains* exist within the myosin head. (The remainder of the myosin head and tail is called the *heavy chain*.) They are believed to play a role in the speed of contraction[14] and in restoration of muscular force during fatigue.[15–17] Different myosin light chain isoforms exist in muscles with different physiologic functions, suggesting a possible role for light chains in muscular plasticity. Tropomyosin and troponin, two proteins that wind along the actin filament, regulate the interaction of calcium, actin, and myosin. In animal experiments, the neural input to a muscle is one factor that determines the troponin isoforms contained within the muscle.[18] It therefore seems possible that exercise or disuse, other modes of altered neuromuscular input, could yield similar troponin adaptations.

Enzymes

Another class of proteins, called *enzymes*, serves to catalyze chemical substrates into metabolic end products. An important way that muscles adapt to task demands, particularly those involving muscle endurance, is to alter the genetic transcription of enzymes, thus increasing or decreasing their concentration, which in turn alters the rate at which the relevant physiologic process occurs. In addition, muscle cell nuclei may trigger the production of alternate enzyme isoforms in order to change catalyzing rates within the muscle cell. Both of these strategies serve to regulate skeletal muscle cell function according to external demands (plasticity).

The myosin molecule has an enzymatic subunit that acts upon adenosine triphosphate (ATP), the primary energy molecule in skeletal muscle (Fig. 3-2, inset).[19] Different myosin ATPase isoforms possess different ATP catalyzing rates, and as such, some allow faster cross-bridge cycling than others. As will be described in a later section, altered ATPase activity of myosin is a cardinal

way in which skeletal muscle adapts to increased or decreased task demands.

Two other enzymes, succinate dehydrogenase (SDH) and citrate synthase (CS), reside within the mitochondria of muscle cells and catalyze the production of ATP in the presence of oxygen (Fig. 3-2, lower inset). In response to increased or decreased activity, genetic transcription for these proteins changes, leading to a measurable elevation or decline in enzyme levels in muscle tissue. Muscle fibers with superior fatigue resistance have high levels of these two oxidative enzymes, an important adaptation when routine activities demand good muscle endurance.

Another enzyme, α-glycerophosphate dehydrogenase (GPD), resides in the cytoplasm of muscle cells, where it transports nicotinamide adenine dinucleotide (NADH), an energy-storing molecule, into the mitochondria. (NADH, like SDH and CS, is another commonly measured marker of oxidative function.) Higher levels of GPD in a cell indicate faster transport of NADH, which reflects upon the glycolytic (anaerobic metabolism) capacity of the cell, another potential source of skeletal muscle plasticity.

A final cellular structure, the sarcoplasmic reticulum (SR), is a muscle membrane that transports calcium to and from the contractile proteins of the muscle (Fig. 3-2). In response to nerve impulses traveling over the muscle sarcolemma, several SR membrane enzymes (dihydropyridine, ryanodine, phospholamban, parvalbumin[20]) instigate and regulate calcium release. Calcium ions flood into the muscle cytoplasm, causing troponin to slide away from "active sites" on the actin molecule, making them available for cross-bridge formation with myosin. The rate of calcium release influences the rate at which the muscle generates force and is therefore generally proportional to the time to peak force during an isometric single twitch. Calcium ions must be resequestered (taken up), both for the cessation of the present contraction and in preparation for subsequent contractions. The rate at which calcium is resequestered determines how fast the muscle relaxes and is generally proportional to the time it takes the isometric twitch force to decline to half of its peak value. Resequestration of calcium is accomplished by sarco(endo)-plasmic reticulum calcium ATPase (SERCA), an enzyme that resides in the SR membrane. Various isoforms of SERCA exist in muscles based on whether they have fast or slow contractile properties. The presence of multiple isoforms supports that SERCA, like the many other proteins described in this section, adapts according to the stresses placed upon skeletal muscle.

Muscular Adaptations: Response to Reduced Use

According to the PAO model, adaptations arise in response to a stimulus that taps into the underlying plasticity of a cell, tissue, organ, or organism. Decreased muscular activity represents an important stimulus that causes rapid and extensive structural and physiologic changes in the muscle(s) under consideration. In the context of human studies, a neurological insult such as SCI typically results in reduced use. The health of any muscle depends on its connection to an intact peripheral nerve, which is the case after an upper motor neuron injury. Most people with SCI have skeletal muscles with normal peripheral nerve innervation below the level of the injury. However, the trauma associated with SCI often severely damages alpha motor neurons at the level of the injury, causing denervation of certain muscles. For the purpose of this review, we will concentrate only on the more common upper motor neuron conditions. Differences between upper motor neuron injuries and lower motor neuron injuries are discussed in detail in Chapter 1.

Animal models have taught us much about the effects of reduced use on skeletal muscle. However, the results of animal studies must be interpreted carefully, because most animal models do not reproduce the type of reduced activity observed in humans with SCI. Importantly, the degree of neural and musculoskeletal plasticity as well as the necessary post-SCI management is quite different in quadruped animals compared to biped humans. All of these factors are important to consider when striving to understand the plasticity of skeletal muscle following SCI in humans.

Under normal conditions, the majority of whole human muscles comprise a mixture of fast fatigable (FF), fast fatigue-resistant (FFR), and slow (S) motor units. Fast muscle fibers, which are associated with FF and FFR motor units, demonstrate a greater capacity for glycolytic metabolism, as befits their prevalent use in short-duration, high-intensity contractions. Slow muscle fibers, which are associated with S motor units, demonstrate a greater capacity for aerobic metabolism, which is necessary for long-duration, sustained types of contractions. In humans, the soleus muscle, which is active at a low level even during quiet standing, uniquely contains more than 70% slow muscle fibers. In general, S motor units are recruited first by the nervous system because they can continue contracting for a prolonged period of time, allowing muscular tasks to be completed without fatigue. If the muscular tasks require greater force output, the nervous system may increase the firing frequency of slow motor units and may then recruit FFR and, eventually, FF motor units. However, because they fatigue quickly, FF motor units are normally recruited briefly for high-force tasks. In the event that FF motor units and the associated fast muscle fibers are activated repetitively, the associated fatigue and contractile property changes are dramatic. These changing properties of fast skeletal muscle with fatigue create significant problems for the activation of muscles with an external control system (electrical stimulation).

Chronic disuse from a variety of sources, notably SCI, triggers a transformation from slow, fatigue-resistant muscle to fast, fatigable muscle in humans,[21–24] in cats,[25] and in rats.[26] During this transformation, proteins that typify slow muscle are gradually replaced by proteins that typify fast muscle. The rate and extent of this transformation differs according to the protein in question, according to the muscle being studied, according to the duration of reduced activity, and according to species. Associated with the transformation from slow to fast muscle fibers is a loss of mitochondria and associated muscle blood flow (capillary reduction).

Myosin Adaptations

During normal levels of use, human muscle fibers contain one of three myosin heavy chain (MHC) isoforms, denoted IIx, IIa, and I. Fibers containing type IIx fibers generally have the highest contractile speed, followed by type IIa and type I fibers.[27,28] The proportion of each isoform present depends on the type of muscular activity typically required (phasic versus postural). During decreased use after SCI (and in many other disuse scenarios), slow myosin production is downregulated in favor of faster myosin isoforms. The time course of these adaptations is currently under investigation. Few MHC adaptations have been observed in the human vastus lateralis (a mixed fiber-type muscle) in the early phase of SCI (<1 month).[23] After 6 months post-SCI, hybrid fibers appeared that coexpressed MHC type IIa and IIx myosin.[29] At the same time, the relative proportion of pure type IIa fibers decreased,[29] and the proportion of pure IIx fibers increased.[30] This suggests that new type IIx MHC proteins were gradually incorporated into the contractile filaments, replacing the original type IIa myosin proteins. In other studies, minimal MHC transformation was observed at 4 weeks post-SCI, but hybrid fibers appeared at about 4.7 months.[23] Conversely, Talmadge et al.[31] reported increased MHC-IIx expression by 6 weeks, whereas measurable hybrid MHCs were not observed until 24 weeks. The period of hybrid fiber expression may last as long as 20 months.[23]

Adaptations in the proportion of type I fibers occur along an even more uncertain time course. By 6 months post-SCI, no reduction in type I fibers has been observed,[29,30] but hybrid fibers coexpressing types I and IIa myosin begin to appear.[30] Because type I myosin is almost absent in the vastus lateralis[32] several years post-SCI, the presence of hybrid I/IIa fibers at 6 months may hint that the shift away from type I myosin occurs around that time. Another study has reported quite extensive loss of type I fibers in paralyzed vastus lateralis by only 4 months post-SCI.[33] Additional studies are necessary to more clearly delineate the time course of MHC changes in the human vastus lateralis after SCI. However, it is clear that paralyzed muscles with intact peripheral nerves move toward a faster MHC phenotype as a result of prolonged paralysis.

Little is known about the time course of MHC adaptations in the paralyzed human soleus, a functionally slow muscle. Before molecular methods of analysis were available, earlier studies stained the whole muscle fiber cells for the density of myosin ATPase enzyme. This method classifies muscle fibers as type I, type IIa, or type IIb and closely approximates the molecular classification MHC-I, MHC-IIa, and MHC-IIx. After chronic paralysis, the human soleus expresses nearly 100% type IIb fibers.[21,34] A small study by Lotta and coauthors[35] suggested that soleus myosin ATPase adaptations may not appear until 9 to 10 months post-SCI. (Recall that in the vastus lateralis studies mentioned above, MHC adaptations appeared as early as 4 to 6 months.) In cats, 6 months of SCI causes MHC-IIa and -IIx levels to rise from ~ 0% to 17% and 14%, respectively,[25] at the expense of MHC-I (usually 99% of fibers). The decline of soleus MHC-I is even more dramatic in rats, falling from 90% to 18% after 3 months[36] and to 12% after 1 year.[13] Hybrid fibers coexpressing two MHC types are common in animal models of SCI.[13,36,37] Overall, animal studies confirm that SCI leads to the transformation of muscle fibers from slow to fast, albeit to different extents across species.

Although future molecular studies are needed to quantify post-SCI soleus MHC changes in humans, the physiological changes that occur after SCI suggest that myosin adaptations are extensive. Myosin heavy chain type is generally believed to regulate the speed of muscular contraction. Muscles consisting of predominantly MHC-I, such as the soleus, contract and relax more slowly than muscles that contain a greater proportion of MHC-IIa and -IIx (such as the gastrocnemius and the quadriceps). In the human soleus, MHC-I is gradually (and almost completely) replaced by MHC-IIa and -IIx (Fig. 3-3). As would be expected, the paralyzed soleus contracts very slowly in the acute post-SCI stage, but demonstrates faster contractile speeds as time passes post-SCI.[21,38] This adaptation has also been observed in the paralyzed cat soleus.[39,40] In chronic SCI, therefore, the soleus functions as a composite of fast fibers, retaining few of its original contractile speed characteristics.

Fiber Size Adaptations

During reduced use, muscle size visibly declines due to the atrophy of individual muscle fibers. The time course and extent of muscle fiber atrophy has been well-characterized after human SCI, particularly in the vastus lateralis muscle. Castro and coauthors reported significant atrophy of all fiber types (MHC-I, -IIa, -IIx) between 6 and 11 weeks post-SCI.[29] Type IIa fibers showed continued cross-sectional area (CSA) decline at 24 weeks. Between 4 and 20 weeks post-SCI, Crameri and coauthors reported CSA declines of 62%, 68%, and 49% for type I, IIa, and IIx fibers, respectively.[33] Many other studies of individuals with chronic SCI (>1 year) report fiber type-specific CSA values that are commensurate with the CSA values listed above for

subacute SCI subjects.[41–44] Post-SCI muscle fiber atrophy, therefore, occurs rapidly after SCI and may be complete after just 4 to 6 months, well ahead of MHC isoform transformations.[45] Human post-SCI studies cannot commence until subjects are medically stable; therefore, little is known about the very earliest stages of post-SCI muscle fiber atrophy. Evidence of type I and IIa fiber atrophy appears in rat soleus after just 5 days of paralysis.[46] Although human muscle systems generally adapt more slowly than animal models, it seems likely that humans with SCI experience extensive muscle fiber atrophy during their acute hospitalization and rehabilitation phase.

As mentioned previously, muscle cross-sectional area is an important determinant of force output. Atrophied muscles post-SCI would not be expected to generate high forces during electrical stimulation. However, in some cases, single-twitch forces remain quite high in nonfatigued paralyzed muscle.[21,38] Some evidence suggests that fibers containing MHC-IIa and IIx have a higher specific tension (innate force-generating capacity) than fibers expressing MHC-I.[28,47] As MHC expression shifts away from MHC-I after SCI, an increased average specific tension per muscle fiber may partially offset the force reductions imposed by muscle fiber atrophy.[38] Additionally, muscle atrophy

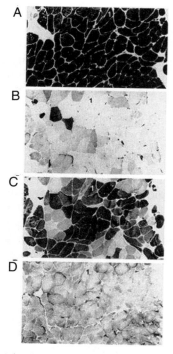

Figure 3-3. Serial soleus muscle biopsy sample stained for the myosin ATPase enzyme with a preincubation at pH 9.4 (A), pH 4.2 (B), and pH 4.6 (C), as well as the stain for the NADH reductase (D). The 1 represents the same cell across stains. (Reprinted from Shields RK. Fatigability, relaxation properties and electromyographic responses of the human paralyzed soleus muscle *J. Neurophys.* 1995, 73(6); 2195–2206.

after SCI may be accompanied by a proliferation of inelastic tissues within the muscle.[38,48,49] We have previously suggested that connective tissue extensibility may decrease after SCI, which acts to "take up the slack" in the musculotendinous unit,[38] allowing the atrophied muscle to function on a different portion of the length-tension curve.[50] Such adaptations may facilitate the transmission of muscular forces, which could further offset force losses due to atrophy. Thus, although paralyzed, atrophied muscle generally demonstrates impaired force-generating capacity, particularly after repetitive stimulation, single twitch forces may occasionally be unexpectedly high.

Regulatory Protein Adaptations

The extent to which actin-myosin regulatory proteins (troponin, tropomyosin, myosin light chains) adapt in humans with SCI is not known. Animal data are scarce but do suggest that troponin isoforms may be moderated by neural input.[18] Chronic low-frequency stimulation (CLFS) is a method used to induce fast-to-slow fiber phenotypic changes in animal studies. The adaptations that occur with CLFS are generally in the opposite "direction" from the adaptations that occur after SCI (slow to fast). However, the extent to which CLFS studies can be instructive for the study of post-SCI adaptations remains unclear. CLFS causes myosin isoforms to gradually skew toward the slow end of the MHC continuum (MHC-I).[51] Concurrent with this change, but not necessarily in lockstep fashion, myosin regulatory light chains and various forms of troponin shift from fast to slow isoforms.[52,53] The physiological significance of these adaptations remains unclear. Further work is necessary to determine the effects of reduced use on all regulatory proteins of the contractile filaments.

Enzyme Adaptations

Following SCI, skeletal muscle demonstrates a reduced ability to resist fatigue during repetitive electrical stimulation. Even very fatigue-resistant postural muscles such as the soleus demonstrate poor endurance when tested after long-term SCI (>2 years), generating only 20% to 30% of the initial peak torque after a bout of repetitive activation.[6] Adaptations of the enzymes of energy metabolism likely play a key role in this process. Myosin ATPase enzymatic activity does not appear to decline in the acute and subacute post-SCI phase (up to 6 months) for any fiber type in cats[54] and humans.[55] However, in chronic SCI, absolute enzymatic activity for myosin ATPase in both type I and II fibers is reduced by as much as 40%.[56] The time course of myosin ATPase adaptations after SCI therefore warrants further investigation.

Enzymatic activity levels of citrate synthase (CS), a marker of oxidative metabolic capacity, also decline in humans after SCI. Vastus lateralis CS activity has been reported to be ~ 6 to 6.9 units/g in individuals with chronic SCI[42,44] compared to 11.6 units/g in sedentary individuals without SCI.[57] Moderate correlations (r = 0.44) exist between CS activity and fatigue resistance.[57] Fatigability has also been shown to correlate with decreased SDH activity.[58] However, this relationship generally appears only in the late stages of SCI. In rats at 1, 3, and 6 months post-SCI, both SDH and GPD were elevated, suggesting enhancements to oxidative and glycolytic capacities.[59] MHC types demonstrated the expected slow-to-fast transition during this same time period, underscoring the different timelines by which post-SCI adaptations of various protein populations are orchestrated. A similar preservation of post-SCI SDH activity has been reported in the spinal cat.[54] In humans, SDH activity of type I, IIa, and IIx fibers increased from 6 to 11 weeks post-SCI. SDH activity in type I fibers continued to increase at 24 weeks. Similarly, GPD enzymatic activity increased in all fiber types from 6 to 11 weeks, with further increases in type IIx fibers at 24 weeks. Despite early increases in SDH, however, it appears that the activity of this enzyme may decline with long-standing SCI. Grimby and coauthors reported low SDH levels in the soleus, gastrocnemius, and vastus lateralis of individuals with chronic SCI.[34] Martin and coauthors reported that tibialis anterior type I fiber SDH activity was 48% lower in SCI than in non-SCI individuals.[56] In type II fibers, SDH activity was 67% lower in people with SCI.

Sarcoplasmic reticulum enzymes, which regulate the release and reuptake of calcium ions in the process of muscular contraction, show varying degrees of adaptation during post-SCI disuse. The adaptations of phospholamban and parvalbumin have not been studied in post-SCI humans. Because phospholamban is present only in slow-twitch fibers, the post-SCI transformation from slow to fast fibers may suggest that phospholamban expression declines after SCI. In contrast, because parvalbumin is present only in fast fibers, one might expect its expression to be upregulated after SCI. Neither of these hypotheses has been tested to date. SERCA, on the other hand, is known to exist in two distinct isoforms in skeletal muscle: SERCA1a in fast fibers and SERCA2a in slow fibers. Talmadge and coauthors showed that SERCA isoform adaptations begin quickly after SCI in humans (within 24 weeks).[30] SCI caused MHC-I and MHC-IIa vastus lateralis fibers to coexpress both SERCA1a and 2a, at the expense of fibers expressing only SERCA2a (slow SERCA). Hybrid MHC fibers did not similarly emerge. Such mismatches between MHC and SERCA type were rare in non-SCI muscles. As with MHC, SCI causes SERCA to skew from the slow to the fast isoforms; however, these changes did not occur in synchrony with MHC changes. As illustrated by Talmadge and coauthors, SERCA adaptations appeared to precede MHC adaptations.[30] The physiologic consequences of SERCA adaptations are unclear but may impact skeletal muscle fatigability after SCI. Because SERCA has primary responsibility for calcium resequestration during muscle contraction, changes in SERCA isoform expression could alter ATP utilization rates, a primary determinant of muscle fatigue resistance.

Ultrastructure Adaptations

The extensive decline in fatigue resistance observed after SCI may be partially attributable to decreased capillary density in paralyzed muscle. The cause of capillary decline is uncertain; it may reflect the loss of normal autonomic input from supraspinal centers, or it may simply be an atrophic process related to muscular disuse. As stated by Chilibeck and coauthors,[60] muscle capillarization is related to both maximal oxygen uptake[61] and recovery from exercise.[62]

Several studies have measured capillary density in paralyzed human vastus lateralis muscle. Early after SCI (6 to 24 weeks), capillary density did not differ from non-SCI subjects.[29] However, in individuals with chronic SCI (>2 years), the number of capillaries per muscle fiber ranged from 0.75 to 2.6,[41,42,60] well below non-SCI values (>3.5).[57] Interestingly, however, chronically paralyzed vastus lateralis demonstrated the same pattern of capillarization by fiber type as neurologically intact muscle. Crameri and coauthors identified 2.6, 2.0, and 1.9 capillaries per fiber for type I, IIa, and IIx fibers, respectively.[41] Though sedentary non-SCI adults had more capillaries per fiber, the distribution by fiber type was the same; 4.35, 4.13, and 3.56 capillaries per fiber for types I, IIa, and IIx.[57]

Summary of Adaptations to Reduced Use

Human skeletal muscle exhibits a general conversion from a slower phenotype (MHC, regulatory proteins, enzymes of metabolism, and ultrastructure) to a faster phenotype after spinal cord injury. These adaptations capitalize on the plasticity inherent in the collection of proteins that compose skeletal muscle. Physiological consequences of these molecular adaptations are profound; torque production diminishes, fatigue resistance declines, and contractile speed characteristics change, rending paralyzed skeletal muscle a very ineffective generator of muscle forces. Functional electric stimulation protocols that aim to employ paralyzed muscle for tasks such as standing, ambulation, or upper extremity reaching and grasping are invariably limited by the poor physiologic performance of paralyzed muscle. Additionally, as mentioned in the introduction, paralyzed muscle atrophy has its own noxious sequelae; decreased protection over bony prominences, poor cosmesis, and strain on the renal system due to protein degradation by-products. A rehabilitation method to arrest the progress of skeletal muscle deterioration after SCI could have broad-ranging benefits. Fortunately, paralyzed skeletal muscle retains a great degree of plasticity in the anabolic, not just the catabolic, mode. The next section will explore the adaptations of

paralyzed skeletal muscle to increased use in the context of therapeutic electrical muscle stimulation.

Muscular Adaptations: Response to Increased Use

Exercise taps into the extensive plasticity of the musculoskeletal system, eliciting adaptations that enhance the muscle's ability to cope with routine demands. This process has quite rightly been compared to rebuilding the engine of a car while speeding down the interstate.[12] Fortunately for spinal cord injury rehabilitation specialists, this remarkable plastic potential persists to a large degree after SCI. In complete SCI, electrical muscle stimulation, rather than volitional exercise, can serve as a stimulus to elicit desirable adaptations. Although the specific adaptations differ according to the stimulation parameters and the muscle being trained, we can broadly state that electrical stimulation training attenuates the normal post-SCI deterioration of muscle. Electrical muscle stimulation can even reverse certain deleterious adaptations after they have become well-established in chronic SCI. Thus, in the most general sense, electrical muscle stimulation can help ameliorate or reverse the slow-to-fast functional transformation of paralyzed skeletal muscle. The content of the previous section on disuse adaptations, therefore, should help the reader predict how paralyzed muscle may react to increased use during electrical stimulation training. In many instances, the adaptations to increased use are simply the opposite of what occurs in disuse, a rather logical outcome, given our understanding of the protein changes that underlie skeletal muscle plasticity.

As mentioned in the chapter introduction, our focus will be on muscular adaptations to increased use, not on the broad outcomes of these adaptations (such as improved function, quality of life, or health). However, we will remark upon how certain studies rate in *feasibility*, which is in congruence with well-established exercise and rehabilitation principles, and in *dose*, which must be closely quantified if the adaptations to an intervention are to be truly understood. For the clinician, many of the electrical stimulation protocols we review would be difficult to translate to clinical reality. However, by considering feasibility and dose, we may be able to gauge the "real world" prospects of the protocol. If feasibility and dose are within reasonable parameters, then the adaptations observed in the study protocols might be replicable in clinical research studies. Clinical research, in turn, will illuminate the therapeutic potential of electrical stimulation interventions after SCI.

Myosin Adaptations

With muscle disuse, MHC expression gradually shifts from the slow to the fast end of the MHC spectrum. We might posit, therefore, that exercise training could elicit the opposite adaptations, that MHC-I might become more prevalent in highly trained muscles. Although endurance athletes may indeed have a greater proportion of MHC-I in their muscles than untrained individuals,[63] we must be careful about inferring causality. Perhaps a selection bias is in operation; individuals with genetically determined high MHC-I levels may excel at endurance sports, reinforcing future participation and training, while individuals with more average MHC profiles may have greater difficulty in reaching elite training levels. Although enhancements to MHC-I do indeed occur in response to intensive endurance training,[64] far greater plasticity seems to exist among the faster myosin isoforms. A great number of studies suggest that the most common adaptation of muscle myosin to endurance training,[64] strength training,[65,66] and sprint training[67] is a reduction of MHC-IIx fibers and an increase in fibers expressing MHC-IIa.

This pattern of adaptation has been observed frequently in electrical stimulation training studies in individuals with SCI. Both short-term (10 weeks)[41,42] and long term (6 to 12 months)[32,48] electrically assisted cycling protocols elicited reductions in IIx fibers and proliferation of IIa fibers in paralyzed vastus lateralis muscle. This shift is nearly 100% complete by 1 year of training.[32] On the other hand, we are aware of no cycling intervention published to date, whether using electrical muscle stimulation or passive motion, that has yielded a statistically significant increase in MHC-I fibers.[32,41,42,48,60,68,69] However, increases in MHC-I fibers or mRNA expression have been reported in studies that use isometric muscle training.[42,70] Additionally, the pre-SCI percentages of MHC isoforms (including MHC-I) can largely be maintained with timely introduction of isometric electrical stimulation (within 4 weeks post-SCI).[33] The mechanical stresses developed within isometrically contracting muscles are likely to be higher than in muscles engaged in cycling. Recalling that local mechanical stress is believed to be an important instigating stimulus for muscular adaptation,[11] we may be tempted to conclude that isometric forces are the key element required to elicit increases in MHC-I expression. Indeed, a protocol that allowed quasi-isometric contractions (designed with an elastic resistance device that limited the magnitude of the evoked muscle forces) showed no changes in MHC-I, even though subjects trained 7 days a week.[58] However, a study of tibialis anterior stimulation demonstrates that even with very low muscular load (free joint rotation), electrical stimulation training can elicit MHC-I increases if the duration of stimulation is very high (8 hours per day).[56] The concept of *dose* of muscular load, therefore, is multidimensional, encompassing the total duration of stimulation as well as mechanical stress. However, the *feasibility* of 8 hours of daily stimulation in a clinical population is questionable. Though a viable research methodology, long-duration muscle stimulation is unlikely to be an acceptable therapeutic intervention for the majority of people with SCI, particularly if multiple muscles are to receive stimulation. For this reason, and because it induces fast-to-slow transformations for *all* MHC isoforms, short-duration isometric muscle training emerges as a particularly appealing strategy for eliciting MHC adaptations after SCI. (Conversely, this approach may be less feasible in those with deconditioned musculoskeletal systems, due to the danger of placing large loads through osteoporotic limbs. The reader is encouraged to note this issue in the skeletal adaptations section to follow.

Fiber Size Adaptations

Hypertrophy of muscle fibers (and of total muscle size) is one of the most conspicuous adaptations to exercise made by neurologically intact skeletal muscle. Paralyzed skeletal muscle maintains a considerable degree of this plastic potential. As with MHC adaptations, muscular load appears to be a crucial determinant of whether muscle fiber CSA adaptations will emerge. Tibialis anterior stimulation with free joint rotation yielded no improvements in fiber CSA, even though training duration was high (8 hours per day).[56] Quadriceps stimulation against elastic resistance was similarly ineffective.[58] Electrically stimulated cycling led to a 23% mean increase in fiber CSA in one study[60] and a 129% increase in another.[41] Muscle torque outputs were not quantified in either study, making the estimation of dose of muscle loading difficult. However, we speculate that the individuals who demonstrated greater adaptations also generated higher loads. Isometric muscle contractions, with concomitant high muscle loads, may more readily trigger hypertrophy of paralyzed muscle (Fig. 3-4). This conjecture is supported by two isometric muscle-stimulation studies that reported striking CSA adaptations to training (likely at higher loads than the cycling studies). Isometric quadriceps stimulation in subjects with recent SCI (<4 weeks) prevented muscle fiber atrophy of all fiber types.[33] In another study by the same investigators, subjects cycled with one leg and performed isometric training with the other. No CSA adaptations occurred in the cycling leg, whereas fiber CSA more than doubled for all fiber types in the isometrically trained leg.[42] Only isometric training demonstrated the potential to enhance the CSA of type I fibers.[33,41,42] Once again, isometric electrical stimulation training may uniquely tap into the plastic potential of all muscle fiber types.

Regulatory Protein Adaptations

No previous human studies have examined whether contractile filament regulatory proteins adapt during electrical stimulation training after SCI. In animal studies, chronic low-frequency stimulation leads to a fast-to-slow shift in myosin light chain and troponin isoforms.[51,52,71,72] The timing of shifts in MHC and myosin light chains is complex.[53,71] As proteins are degraded and replaced in the myosin heavy filament, hybrid filaments with slow heavy chains and fast light chains appear (or vice versa). Similar

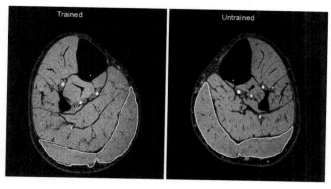

Figure 3-4. MRI of a subject who performed >3 years of soleus electrical stimulation training. The trained soleus was substantially larger (~28%) than the untrained soleus (shaded regions denoted "S"). Gastrocnemius area did not appreciably differ between limbs ("G"). Because the gastrocnemius is placed on slack during training in a knee-bent position, it received electrical current but little isometric loading. Conversely, all deep single-joint muscles (which *did* experience isometric loading) hypertrophied ("D"). Thus, electrical activation of muscle yielded hypertrophy when muscle loads were high, but not in muscles that contracted against low resistance (gastrocnemius).

hybrid subunit combinations likely occur within troponin molecules.[51] The contractile filament regulatory proteins are generally believed to modulate the speed of contraction; as such, changes in contractile speed might be expected to emerge in muscle trained with electrical stimulation. However, because contractile speed is also determined by MHC expression and the fatigue state of the muscle,[38] the role of regulatory protein adaptations remains unclear.

Enzyme Adaptations

In the neurologically intact muscular system, adaptations to metabolic enzyme levels occur rapidly in response to exercise. In sedentary individuals, as little as 6 weeks of electrical stimulation training can double CS levels.[57] In paralyzed muscle, electrically stimulated cycling for 10 weeks led to no significant increase in CS activity[42] or to a doubling of CS activity[41] in various studies. Stimulation frequency and exercise duration were similar in these studies; however, the cycling resistance appeared to be lower in the study that noted no CS adaptations.[42] In two other studies, CS activity increased rapidly during 3 months of electrically stimulated cycle training, with no further increases for 9 additional months.[48,73] Adaptations in SDH, another enzyme of oxidative metabolism, have been observed even when evoked muscle forces are low. Long-duration (8 hour) tibialis anterior stimulation with free joint rotation increased SDH activity by 49% to 340%.[56] Post-training SDH levels matched non-SCI normative values for four of the five subjects tested. Likewise, 12 weeks of quadriceps stimulation against elastic resistance led to a 72% increase in SDH without concomitant increases in GPD (a marker of glycolytic capacity).[58]

No previous studies have examined the effects of electrical stimulation training on SR enzymes (SERCA, phospholamban, parvalbumin, ryanodine) in individuals with SCI. Recall that after SCI, fast-slow mismatches appear between SERCA and MHC isoforms, eventually leading to a predominant expression of fast SERCA (SERCA1a).[30] We might hypothesize that, similar to adaptations in MHC and metabolic enzymes, electrical stimulation after SCI would instigate a return to the slow SERCA isoform (SERCA2a). Animal models of chronic low-frequency muscle stimulation support this hypothesis. Chronically stimulated rabbit muscle demonstrated a coordinated transition toward MHC-I and slow SERCA.[74] Phospholamban expression, a characteristic of slow muscle, appears after chronic stimulation,[75,76] and parvalbumin, found only in fast muscle, ceases to be expressed.[77–79] The expression of ryanodine decreases, but changes in isoform expression have not been observed.[80,81] Although chronic muscle stimulation has feasibility limitations for humans with SCI, the results of animal studies support that SR enzyme adaptations may be possible during electrical muscle stimulation after SCI.

The physiologic outcomes of SR enzyme adaptations remain uncertain. Endurance-trained athletes showed a reduction of SERCA1 (fast SERCA).[82] Rat plantaris muscles subjected to chronic overload conditions demonstrate robust hypertrophy and coordinated shifts toward MHC-I and slow SERCA2a[83,84] and increased expression of phospholamban.[84] A theoretical link exists, therefore, between SR protein fast-to-slow adaptations and improved muscular performance. However, because muscle physiologic status also closely correlates with myosin expression,[63] it is difficult to delineate the role of SR proteins alone. Future studies are needed to determine whether SR proteins adapt due to electrical stimulation after SCI, and if so, what the physiological outcomes of these adaptations may be.

Precautions: Monitoring for Episodes of Dysreflexia

Many studies demonstrate the ability of electrical muscle stimulation to prevent or reverse deleterious cellular and physiologic changes after SCI. In the future, large-scale randomized controlled clinical trials will determine the outcome of these adaptations on post-SCI function, health quality, and secondary medical complications. In the meantime, clinicians should be aware of the risk for autonomic dysreflexia during electrical stimulation protocols. The level of stimulation in most protocols is sufficiently noxious to elicit excessive sympathetic activity in many subjects, particularly in those with lesions above T4. For this reason, it is important to monitor responses to stimulation to identify the onset of autonomic dysreflexia should it occur. Signs and Symptoms of autonomic dysreflexia are discussed in detail in Chapter 1.

Summary: Physiologic Outcomes of Protein Adaptations

As outlined above, certain post-SCI adaptations to electrical muscle stimulation are well-understood (MHC, fiber CSA, metabolic enzymes). In contrast, hardly anything is known about adaptations of other protein groups (regulatory proteins, SERCA). Muscle biopsies carry risks for people with SCI (due to insensate skin around surgical wounds), increasing the difficulty of directly measuring protein adaptations post-SCI. Muscle physiology experiments, however, are far less invasive and more feasible to perform. As such, the physiologic responses of muscle to electrical stimulation training have been well-characterized. Long-term (>2 years) electrical stimulation training begun shortly after SCI (within 6 weeks) largely preserves the torque, fatigue resistance, and contractile speed properties of the paralyzed soleus.[38] Adaptations in postfatigue torque potentiation hint that electrical stimulation training may affect the muscle's excitation-contraction coupling system (possibly at the level of SERCA or other regulatory proteins) or the expression of myosin regulatory light chains.[85] Fatigue resistance readily improves during long-duration training of the wrist extensors,[86] tibialis anterior,[87] quadriceps,[88,89] and soleus.[38] These improvements in fatigue resistance occurred in protocols that generated both high[38] and low[87] muscular loads. Recall that increases in SDH activity (an oxidative enzyme that helps determine fatigue resistance) have also been observed in protocols that generate low loads.[56,58] Conversely, improvements in muscle force output generally only appear in protocols that involve high muscle forces[38,42,86] and not in those that involve low forces.[42,86,87] Once again, this observation is congruent with the adaptations seen in muscle fiber CSA, a primary determinant of muscle force, which increases most readily during high-force protocols.[33,42] Although one-to-one correlations between physiologic adaptations and protein adaptations are tenuous at best, in general, gross physiologic adaptations to electrical stimulation training mirror the fast-to-slow transitions observed in muscle cell-level studies.

The broad outcomes of these interventions to preserve muscle integrity after SCI are only beginning to be studied. As basic and applied researchers report what physiologic adaptations are possible, clinical rehabilitation researchers are exploring how these adaptations affect the health-related quality of life of individuals with SCI. For example, preserving muscle CSA could reduce renal complications by limiting protein degradation by-products that must be filtered by the kidneys. Preserving muscle bulk could also reduce the incidence of pressure ulcers by normalizing weight distribution over bony prominences. Such medical benefits, if they did indeed occur, would address two of the most bothersome secondary complications reported by people with

SCI.[90] Maintenance of muscle properties after SCI could also affect post-SCI joint contractures, spasms/spasticity, pain, and perhaps most importantly, post-SCI fractures (discussed in the next section). Interventions that yield measurable muscle adaptations but that do not more broadly improve post-SCI outcomes are unlikely to be valued by individuals with SCI. Rehabilitation researchers must work steadily in the upcoming decades to develop therapeutic interventions that offer global benefits to the health-related quality of life of people with SCI.

Skeletal Plasticity and Adaptation

In the neurologically intact musculoskeletal system, muscles operate at a considerable mechanical disadvantage against externally applied resistance. Imagine holding a bowling ball out at arm's length, then bending forward at the lumbar spine. The weight of the bowling ball multiplied by its distance from the spine creates a torque that tends to tip the body forward. The erector spinae muscles, in contrast, lie at a very short distance from the spine (the moment arm), no more than a centimeter. To create an equal and opposite torque (to avoid tipping forward), the erector spinae muscles must exert a tremendously high force through a very small moment arm. These forces are transmitted as compressive loads through the vertebrae over which the erector spinae cross. This very important principle operates in nearly every muscle and bone system in the body; while compensating for their extreme mechanical disadvantage, muscles deliver sizable loads to the skeletal system. Muscular contraction, in fact, loads the skeletal system to a far greater degree than weight-bearing forces.[91] The concept of moment arms is discussed in detail in Chapter 7.

As described previously, skeletal muscle becomes highly fatigable and atrophied after SCI, with limited functional usefulness for standing,[92-95] grasping,[94,96] or ambulating,[94,97,98] with electrical stimulation. Additionally, the loss of volitional muscular loads deprives the skeletal system of an important stimulus for maintenance of bone mineral density (BMD). Complete unloading of the limbs, such as in SCI, yields bone loss that is 5 to 20 times greater than losses from purely metabolic etiologies.[99] Post-SCI osteoporosis has a multifactorial pathophysiology, including hormonal, neural, and vascular components[100,101]; however, the diminution of mechanical stimuli to the bone is considered to be a powerful contributor to bone demineralization.[102,103]

For this reason, the reintroduction of mechanical loads after SCI, particularly via electrical muscle stimulation, may be a promising strategy to prevent post-SCI osteoporosis. We will first summarize the plastic capabilities of bone, followed by the adaptations that occur in response to post-SCI unloading. Next, we will describe the adaptations that occur when load is reintroduced to the skeletal system of paralyzed extremities, either by reintroduction of weight bearing, by loads generated with electrically elicited muscle contraction, or by vibration training. Finally, we will discuss the feasibility of reintroducing loads to osteoporotic extremities, as well as the dose-response nature of loading interventions.

Skeletal Plasticity: Mechanotransduction

An engineering analogy is often a useful aid for illustrating how mechanical forces are transmitted through the skeletal system. In some ways, long bones such as the femur and tibia resemble hollow cylinders, with a thin cortical shell surrounding a marrow cavity. Squeezing the top and bottom of the cylinder between two hands would deliver a compressive load through the material composing the cylinder wall (Fig. 3-5). A three-point bending force (like snapping a pencil) applied to the cylinder may cause compression on one side of the cylinder and tension on the opposite side. One could also wring the cylinder with both hands to deliver a torsional force or could apply a strong vibration to the cylinder. In any of these loading scenarios, if the cylinder walls are thin or made of weak material, the cylinder could break. This analogy is a gross oversimplification, but itillustrates the variety of load modalities that bones must be able to withstand.

In addition to a hollow, roughly cylindrical shaft (the diaphysis), long bones flare outward at each end to form articulating surfaces, the epiphyses. Unlike the tightly packed cortical bone present in diaphyseal walls, epiphyseal

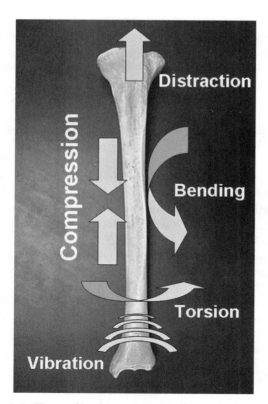

Figure 3-5. Types of loads routinely experienced by bone.

bone is organized into trabeculae, which fill the epiphysis like a web of struts and columns. A very thin shell of cortical bone surrounds the trabecular envelope at the epiphysis. Animal experiments have recently shown that during development, trabeculae form along the principal lines of strain within bone epiphyses.[104] That is, bone is laid down where it is needed most in response to the routine stresses the bone encounters. The amount of bone mineral present (bone density), as well as the orientation of trabeculae and the thickness of the cortical walls (bone architecture), both contribute to the overall strength of bone. As will be described in this section, bone is a remarkably plastic tissue, able to remake itself in response to a wide variety of loading stimuli. The first step in the adaptation of bone is *mechanotransduction*, the conversion of mechanical stimuli into a cellular response.

Mechanical loading yields physical deformation of the bone surface and fluid flow within the bone lacuno-canalicular system (a series of pores and conduits for nerves and blood vessels).[105] Although osteoblasts (bone-building cells) at the bone surface may respond directly to mechanical deformation,[106] the primary mechanotransducing cells may be the osteocytes (quiescent bone cells) embedded deep within the cortical shell.[105,107] Osteocyte cytoplasmic projections form a network with many other neighboring osteocytes via the canaliculi.[108] Fluid shear stress at the surface of these projections may be a primary way that bone remodeling cells detect mechanical stimuli.[109,110] This fluid shear stress appears to trigger a cascade of metabolic activity that promotes osteoblast proliferation.[111] Because embedded osteocytes are ideally positioned to sense deformation of the mineralized bone surrounding them,[112] and because they communicate with a great many other osteocytes (via gap junctions and cell-to-cell electrical communication[113]), transduced mechanical signals can be rapidly transmitted to bone remodeling cells at the bone's surface. (Note that this may be on the periosteal or endosteal surface of the bone or, just as commonly, on the surface of trabeculae within epiphyses.) In this way, the transduction of mechanical loads and subsequent cellular signaling yield specific anabolic or catabolic responses at the sites of bone adaptation.

In response to transduced mechanical stimuli, bone remodeling cells begin the work of depositing or removing bone material. (Hormonal changes, particularly estrogen decline after menopause, also offer a strong stimulus for bone adaptation, but these changes will not be covered in this review.) Bone resorption is the first step in bone remodeling.[114] In response to transduced mechanical signals and hormonal factors, osteoclasts attach to the bone surface and dissolve the exposed bone minerals. Lysosomal enzymes degrade the collagenous latticework, and the mineral and collagen degradation products are transported out of the osteoclast. The osteoclast moves on, leaving a small pit called a *resorptive lacuna* to mark the site of bone degradation. Next, bone deposition occurs when osteoblasts secrete collagen fibers, glycoproteins, and proteoglycans to create an organic lattice-work at the site of bone remodeling. Osteoblasts then deposit calcium phosphate granules into the collagenous framework, orienting the mineral crystals in a parallel fashion. As more mineral granules are added, the bone structure becomes more and more dense, translating into greater strength (for a more complete review of bone remodeling, refer to Downey and Siegel[115]). Under normal loading and hormonal conditions, the activities of osteoblasts and osteoclasts are in balance, leading to no net change in the density of bone. Architectural features may shift as bone modeling proceeds,[116] but this occurs primarily during childhood and adolescent growth. However, in the adult skeletal system, either disuse or excessive loading can lead to profound anabolic or catabolic changes in bone mineral density and bone architecture.

Skeletal Adaptations to Reduced Load

When weight bearing and muscular contraction diminish or cease after SCI, the loss of mechanical loading yields an imbalance between osteoclastic and osteoblastic activity. Bone resorption outpaces bone formation, eventually yielding neurogenic osteoporosis.[117] This term has been coined to acknowledge the likelihood that lost neural connectivity, and not just lost mechanical loading, may contribute to post-SCI osteoporosis. Bone has an extensive sympathetic and sensory nerve supply,[118–120] which may sense local demands or may stimulate bone remodeling by several locally acting neuropeptides.[121,122] However, almost nothing is known about bone–neural interactions after SCI; this intriguing area has only just begun to be investigated. Much more work is needed to determine what role the nervous system itself plays in the establishment of osteoporosis after SCI.

Bone Mineral Density Decline

Within the first few months after SCI, bone mass begins to decline at a rate of 2% to 4% per month,[123] particularly at sites rich in trabecular bone.[124] The rate of bone loss varies across anatomical sites, but it generally stabilizes at 3 to 8 years post-SCI.[125] BMD declines by as much as 58% in the epiphyses of long bones after 3 to 5 years.[125] At its nadir, post-SCI trabecular BMD may be 50% to 70% lower than non-SCI BMD, depending on the anatomic location, severity and chronicity of SCI.[38,125,126] The most common locations for post-SCI fracture are the distal and proximal femur and tibia epiphyses.[1,127–130] Even small impacts to the limbs have the potential to cause a fracture.[4] Consequently, fractures frequently occur during routine, necessary activities of daily living, such as dressing, bathing, and transferring to and from a wheelchair. Treatment options for fractures in individuals with SCI are limited. Casting is often contraindicated because of the high risk of skin breakdown in insensate

extremities. (Paralyzed extremities also tend to have impaired vascular supply, another contraindication for casting.) Internal or external fixation of fractures is often required, adding surgical risk and multiplying the individual's health-care costs manyfold. Surgical fixation may be undermined by the difficulty of adequately securing metal components to very porous bone with bone screws. Complications of fracture healing such as malunion or bone infection may fail to be detected in insensate limbs unless they trigger autonomic symptoms (noxious input leading to autonomic hyperreflexia). Between 1% and 6% of people with SCI will sustain fractures in their paralyzed extremities,[1–3] approximately double the risk for the non-SCI population.[131] Rehabilitation interventions to prevent post-SCI osteoporosis are therefore in great demand.

In the epiphyses, post-SCI BMD decline is accompanied by (or just as accurately, is driven by) gradual destruction of the epiphyseal trabecular lattice. The trabecular lattice is replaced by fatty marrow until, with long-term SCI, almost no intact trabeculae survive in the epiphyseal trabecular envelope (Fig. 3-6). With time, the architectural strength afforded by the trabecular "struts" is almost wholly lost.

Interestingly, BMD of diaphyseal regions stays relatively high after SCI.[38,125] Instead, osteoclastic activity at the surface of the marrow cavity gradually thins the cortical shell from the inside out (endosteal absorption) (Fig. 3-6).[125,132–134] Although the surviving bone is almost completely mineralized (that is, BMD values are near non-SCI norms), the cortical shell of long-bone diaphyses may be as much as 47% thinner than non-SCI values.[125,133] Due to these adaptations to disuse, the bending stiffness of long bones after SCI has been estimated to be as much as 33% lower than that in non-SCI individuals.[132] Although historically the precipitous post-SCI drop in BMD has received the most attention, the destruction of bone architecture is now believed to play an equal role in undermining bone strength after SCI.[132,135] The thinness of the diaphyseal cortical wall severely reduces overall *bone strength*, typically estimated by the second moment of inertia of the cortical shell (an estimate of the eccentricity of the bone mineral: how far it is positioned from the center of the "cylinder"). Bone strength, perhaps the ultimate factor that determines whether or not a bone will fracture, can also be estimated by a BMD-normalized bone stress-strain index (SSI).[136–139] SSI combines density and architecture-related parameters and may therefore offer better predictions of bone-breaking strength than BMD alone.[139,140] Tibia SSIs may be 25% to 31% lower in individuals with SCI than in age-matched controls.[125]

Specificity of Osteogenic Stimuli

It is worth mentioning that not all skeletal sites below the level of a spinal cord lesion develop neurogenic osteoporosis. Even after many years of SCI, lumbar spine BMD often remains within age-normal parameters.[127,141–145]

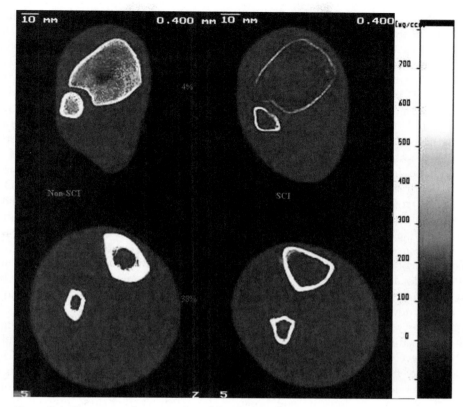

Figure 3-6. Representative examples of distal tibia BMD in a non-SCI (left) and a SCI individual (right; 22 years post-SCI) at two percentages of tibia length. (pQCT scan normalized to fat density = 0 mg/cm³).

Although the cause of this preservation of BMD is not known with certainty, it may be the case that unlike the paralyzed extremities, the lumbar spine receives a relatively normal dose of compressive load during wheelchair use. The spine also experiences a significant level of vibration during wheelchair use,[146] another likely osteogenic stimulus. While it is true that the hips and possibly even the entire lower extremity also receive vibratory input, it is important to note that bone is an *anisotropic* material. Bone most readily responds to mechanical forces imposed from a narrow range of directions. Forces imposed from other directions elicit a far smaller adaptive response than forces arriving from the "typical" direction. Thus, during wheelchair use, the lumbar spine receives compressive and vibratory loads in the typical pre-SCI loading direction, which may help preserve BMD at normal levels. In the seated position, however, the compressive and vibratory forces are 90 degrees askew from the typical loading direction of the hips and lower extremities, likely negating the effectiveness of these loads for maintaining BMD after SCI. Thus, the example of wheelchair use offers three important insights into skeletal adaptations to decreased loading after SCI. First, maintenance of relatively physiologic levels of load may help minimize bone demineralization after SCI (as is postulated to occur in the lumbar spine). Second, the precise stimulus for osteogenesis is not known with certainty. As will be described in a later section, low-magnitude, seemingly trivial vibratory loads may play a key role in the maintenance of bone density and architecture. Third, the dose of load delivered to the skeletal system includes not just considerations of magnitude, frequency, and duration, but also load orientation. These three insights are germane not only to a discussion of bone's adaptive response to disuse, but also to the consideration of rehabilitation efforts to reintroduce osteogenic loads to paralyzed extremities.

Skeletal Adaptations to Increased Load

Animal Studies: Well-Controlled Load Dose

Bone adaptations to increased mechanical loading can be quite remarkable. Proximal tibia BMD in triple jumpers, for example, is 41% higher than in untrained individuals.[147] These athletes likely experience the highest impact loads of any voluntary activity,[148] and their bones illustrate perhaps the maximum adaptive capacity of the human skeletal system.[147] Animal studies also underscore the adaptive capacity of bone in response to mechanical loading. Compressive loads introduced via vertebral pins,[149] external fixators,[150] and external loading devices[139,151,152] have yielded notable bone adaptations. Likewise, torsional loads,[150] bending,[153] and impact loading[154] have all elicited bone anabolism in animal models.

In animal studies, the use of bone-mounted strain gauges facilitates a detailed understanding of the relationships between load dose and bone adaptation. Protocols employing external compressive loading of the rat or mouse ulna have helped to illustrate the roles of strain magnitude,[155,156] strain rate,[151] and loading bout frequency and duration.[157] In general, bone adaptations exhibit a positive dose-response relationship with peak strain magnitude.[155,156,158,159] *Peak strain magnitude*, however, refers only to the highest forces delivered in any given protocol and does not imply that strains must be excessive to trigger bone formation. In general, peak strains need only approximate the high end of normal physiologic values to trigger bone formation.[155,156] Protocols with short, frequent loading bouts[157] conducted at a high strain rate[151] and interspersed with rest periods[160] may yield the greatest bone adaptations. In addition, bone may be particularly attuned to the "error-rich" components of the loading environment.[102,105] Even small strains may engender an osteogenic response if they are presented at a novel strain rate, distribution, frequency, or duration.

To simulate SCI unloading, animal models of limb unloading have been developed, including hind limb unloading[161-163] and the functionally isolated avian ulna.[150] In these animal models, the pattern of bone loss resembles the trends observed in human long bones after SCI (trabecular BMD decline, reduction of cortical thickness). Small doses of load interspersed within prolonged unloading protocols appear sufficient to preserve BMD in animal models.[150,164] These results suggest that reintroduction of physiologic loads may be a useful strategy for preserving bone density and architecture after SCI.

Human Studies: Problematic Load Dose

The direct measurement of bone adaptation in humans is fraught with difficulty. Direct measurement of strain with bone-mounted strain gauges is ethically problematic, hindering the direct estimation of loading dose. Biomechanical models offer a method to indirectly estimate load,[165-167] but historically have not been included in most studies. Several common rehabilitation strategies to address neurogenic osteoporosis after SCI in humans have appeared to be ineffective. Previous dual x-ray absorptiometry (DEXA)-based studies of passive standing,[168] standing with low-level electrical stimulation,[169,170] body weight-supported treadmill training,[171] and electrically stimulated cycling[172,173] revealed no BMD effects due to resumption of loading. Cortical bone, because it generally does not demineralize after SCI, might not be expected to show BMD adaptations to loading, but trabecular bone, which is much more metabolically active than cortical bone,[174] would be expected to respond readily to a loading stimulus of sufficient magnitude. However, mechanical loads delivered to the skeletal system during these studies were not estimated and may have been insufficient to exceed bone's remodeling threshold.[175,176] The importance of dose of load was illustrated in a study of electrically stimulated cycling, in which a subset of subjects who worked at a higher intensity (and ostensibly, a higher mechanical load) showed small BMD increases at the distal femur.[177] Mohr and colleagues showed that SCI subjects who substantially increased their cycling work capacity (and again, perhaps their dose of loading) experienced a small (10%) increase in BMD at the proximal tibia.[178] The site of BMD increases in these studies (the distal femur and proximal tibia) are both rich in trabecular bone; exactly the regions that would be expected to have the greatest plastic potential during loading interventions.

If mechanical loads in the aforementioned unsuccessful loading strategies[169-173] were indeed below the threshold necessary to elicit a response, then no adaptations to trabecular bone likely occurred. However, because DEXA (a two-dimensional imaging method) cannot differentiate between cortical and trabecular bone, trabecular adaptations may have been overlooked.[135] Again, without quantification of mechanical loads and without three-dimensional analysis of trabecular bone, it is unclear whether these interventions induced trabecular anabolism that remained hidden or whether the loads delivered to the skeletal system simply were sub-threshold. Three-dimensional imaging methods such as peripheral quantitative computed tomography (pQCT) can differentiate the responses of trabecular and cortical bone to loading interventions. In a report by de Bruin and colleagues, 25 weeks of weight bearing yielded attenuation of trabecular BMD decline in the distal tibiae of people with SCI.[179] Our recent work shows that trabecular bone vigorously responds to the reintroduction of physiologic mechanical loads early after SCI.[38,144] Unilateral soleus electrical stimulation training delivered repetitive compressive loads approximating 1.5 times body weight to the tibia. After 3 years of training, pQCT revealed that trabecular BMD at the distal tibia was 31% higher in trained limbs than in untrained limbs.[38] No BMD difference was apparent in cortical bone, nor did cortical bone substantially demineralize, in accordance with previous studies. Sites that experienced no mechanical loading (hips and the untrained tibia) showed the expected degree of post-SCI demineralization.[144] Interestingly, the bone-sparing effect of soleus contraction was limited to the posterior half of the tibia (see Case Study 3-1), underscoring that load orientation is part of the "equation" of loading dose.

In individuals with chronic SCI (>2 years) this same muscle/bone loading protocol had no effect on tibia BMD.[6] As mentioned in the previous section, long-term SCI leads to endosteal absorption and destruction of the trabecular lattice. Bone deposition due to osteoblast activity must occur on a preexisting bone surface, such as on trabeculae. We posit that in chronic SCI, so little surface for osteoblastic activity survives that the adaptive response of bone is severely blunted. Our findings concur with other authors[7] who suggest that trabecular BMD loss after chronic SCI may be irreversible. A window of opportunity may therefore exist for preserving bone density and architecture in paralyzed extremities.

Skeletal Adaptations to Vibration

Low-intensity, usually imperceptible vibratory loads dominate bone's daily strain history.[180] Although large-amplitude loads undoubtedly lead to bone adaptation, it is possible that pervasive vibratory loads play an equally important osteoregulatory role. The loss of routine small-amplitude postural contractions after SCI may therefore play a critical role in the development of neurogenic osteoporosis. The reintroduction of low-magnitude mechanical signals (vibration) is being investigated as a way to preserve BMD after SCI and other disuse conditions (spaceflight, etc).

Flieger and coauthors found that a strong vibratory stimulus (50 Hz, two times gravitational acceleration [2 g]) prevented early bone loss in ovariectomized rats.[181] In hind limb-suspended rats, 10 minutes per day of a much less intense vibratory input (90 Hz, 0.25 g) completely offset a 92% reduction in bone formation rate (BFR).[182] Rats that were allowed to bear weight on their extremities for 10 minutes per day still demonstrated a 61% reduction in BFR. In sheep femora, 12 months of vibration training (30 Hz, 0.3 g) yielded a 34% difference in trabecular BMD between trained and untrained animals, as measured by pQCT.[183] Cortical BMD demonstrated no such training effect. Two-dimensional imaging (DEXA) of the same animals revealed only a 5.4% total BMD difference due to training, masking the significant divergent effects that occurred in the trabecular and cortical envelopes. This underscores the necessity of employing three-dimensional densitometric techniques such as pQCT when exploring the training effects of mechanical loading interventions.

Results from human studies have been difficult to interpret. Training effects, when they have appeared, have generally been small, leading to questions about the eventual clinical usefulness of vibration training. In postmenopausal women, 4 minutes of vibration per day in conjunction with alendronate treatment offered no BMD benefit over alendronate treatment alone.[184] A similar protocol in young adults likewise failed to yield differences in BMD or serum markers of bone turnover.[185] Several other studies demonstrated more promising results. Postmenopausal women who performed knee exercises while standing on a high-amplitude (2.28 to 5.09 g) vibration platform experienced a small but significant increase

in hip BMD after 6 months.[186] Another cohort of post-menopausal women who demonstrated high compliance with a standing vibration protocol experienced a 2.17% relative BMD benefit over a placebo group (that is, placebo subjects lost bone whereas vibration subjects did not).[187] Heavier subjects and those with low protocol compliance experienced less relative benefit. Young women with very low BMD demonstrated a 3.9% increase in lumbar spine trabecular BMD with short bouts (2 minutes per day) of vibration for 12 months.[188] The most successful demonstration to date of vibration training in human subjects (children with cerebral palsy or muscular dystrophy) demonstrated a 17.7% relative difference in tibia trabecular BMD over placebo treatment after 6 months of vibration during standing (90 Hz, 0.3 g).[189] Just as was observed in sheep,[183] cortical bone parameters were unresponsive to vibration. No previous studies have investigated vibration training in individuals with SCI. However, the notable success of vibration training in children with neuromuscular impairment suggests that investigation of vibration training after SCI is warranted.

Feasibility of Loading Interventions

Vibration training, if efficacious, could be a particularly feasible rehabilitation intervention after SCI. Electrical muscle stimulation protocols, while effective, do carry a risk of autonomic hyperreflexia that would likely be minimized in vibration training. Similarly, the risks of limb fracture associated with vibration are likely to be quite low. Fracture risk can certainly be minimized in muscular loading protocols by applying biomechanical principles to reduce shear forces through loaded bones.[165,166] Some commonly studied muscle stimulation training paradigms, however, appear to inadequately implement this safeguard. Modeled shear forces in electrically stimulated cycling suggest that knee joint kinetics may be sufficient to cause fracture in subjects with SCI.[167] In the case of quadriceps stimulation in 90 degrees of knee flexion, another commonly studied intervention, shear forces across the femoral condyle are considerable. At least one fracture has been reported during such a quadriceps stimulation research protocol.[190] Muscle force output adapts reasonably quickly after SCI (usually a few weeks),[42] while bone adaptations appear on a considerably slower time scale (usually several months).[144] Thus, in the early phases of electrical stimulation training, muscular strength gains may outpace adaptations in bone density or architecture, exacerbating the risk for fracture. For this reason, and because trabecular lattice destruction may be irreversible after chronic SCI, we advocate further study of **early** interventions to prevent neurogenic osteoporosis. Muscle stimulation training in individuals with acute SCI (and hence, nearly normal BMD), conducted with a physiologic dose of load in a methodology that limits biomechanical shear forces, can offer both efficacy and subject safety. In our experience, subjects rapidly acclimate to the applied electrical stimulation, and signs and symptoms of autonomic hyperreflexia diminish within 4 to 6 weeks. During standing interventions with applied electrical stimulation, we have observed orthostasis more commonly than hyperreflexia. This symptom also resolves quickly as subjects develop standing tolerance. Thus, although electrical muscle stimulation after SCI appears to be an efficacious way to attenuate BMD decline over time, supervision of research protocols by rehabilitation specialists is absolutely critical. The vagaries and complexities of the paralyzed neuromusculoskeletal system require a clinician's judgment, especially during the subject acclimatization phase, to ensure that subject safety risks are minimized. With

this safeguard in place, however, we believe that electrical stimulation of muscle will find widespread applicability for the treatment of both muscular and skeletal deterioration after SCI.

Precautions: Awareness of Fracture Risk

Muscle adaptations to electrical stimulation readily outstrip bone anabolic adaptations to loading. Muscle forces during electrical stimulation therefore pose a fracture risk for osteoporotic extremities. Clinicians should consider the force-generating capacity of the muscle, the bone density status of the skeletal system, and the biomechanical orientation of muscular loads before undertaking electrical muscle stimulation after SCI. Load orientations that reduce shear forces should be rigorously implemented.

CASE STUDY 3-1:   Electrical stimulation training for preservation of bone mineral density

A 21-year-old male sustained T4 complete paraplegia as a result of a gunshot wound.[192] At 7 weeks post-SCI he enrolled in a longitudinal study of soleus electrical stimulation training. The subject stimulated the right soleus muscle while the left soleus muscle served as a within-subject control. The subject completed an average of 8000 isometric soleus contractions per month at home using a custom-designed stimulator equipped with data-logging and compliance-monitoring software. At 1.4 years post-SCI (1.25 years of training), the subject underwent pQCT assessment of the

distal tibia. At this point, BMD differed by only 4.7% between limbs (Fig 3-7, left). A more robust soleus training effect emerged over time, with trained limb BMD at 4.6 years exceeding untrained limb BMD by 44.9%. The bone-sparing effect of soleus loading was largely restricted to the posterior half of the tibia. At 4.6 years post-SCI, BMD of the posterior half of the trained tibia (258.3 mg/cm³) remained within the range of non-SCI normative values (~250 mg/cm³),[191] a 79.1% difference from the untrained limb posterior region (144.2 mg/cm³; Fig. 3-7, right).

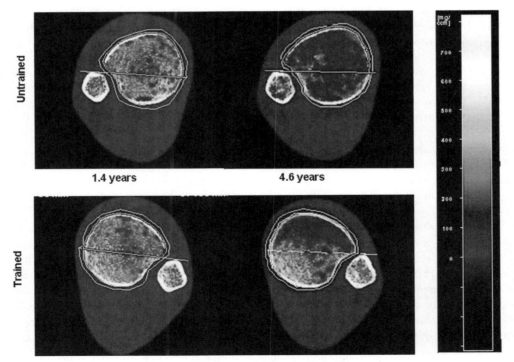

Figure 3-7. Progression of muscle adaptation with controlled dose of muscular loading after SCI for the subject described in Case Study 3-1.

Summary

Muscular and skeletal adaptations to disuse after SCI can, at least in part, be prevented or reversed by electrical muscle stimulation training. Vibration training may be an additional strategy to address skeletal adaptations to disuse. The feasibility and dose of post-SCI rehabilitation protocols are important considerations for their eventual viability as therapeutic interventions. Preserving muscle and bone integrity after SCI may yield immediate benefits in reduction of secondary complications due to SCI. In the future, individuals who have taken steps to preserve muscle and skeletal integrity may be optimally poised to capitalize upon a cure for SCI. Clinical studies are urgently needed to determine the outcomes of therapeutic interventions to address musculoskeletal deterioration after SCI.

REVIEW QUESTIONS

1. Enumerate the protein categories that underlie the plastic potential of skeletal muscle.
2. Summarize the major muscular adaptations to reduced use after SCI.
3. Discuss the adaptations of paralyzed muscle to the reintroduction of loads via electrical stimulation.
4. Describe how mechanotransduction and osteoclast/osteoblast activity underlie skeletal plasticity.
5. Summarize the adaptations of trabecular versus cortical bone to reduced use after SCI, along with consequences for bone strength and fracture risk.
6. Discuss the concept of dose of loading in research protocols designed to preserve bone density after SCI.
7. Discuss the subject-safety considerations of using electrical muscle stimulation to preserve musculoskeletal integrity after SCI (especially autonomic dysreflexia and fractures).

REFERENCES

1. Comarr AE, Hutchinson RH, Bors E. Extremity fractures of patients with spinal cord injuries. *Am J Surg* 1962;103:732–739.
2. Eichenholtz SN. Management of long-bone fractures in paraplegic patients. *Journal of Bone & Joint Surgery—American Volume* 1963;45-A:299–310.
3. Ragnarsson KT, Sell GH. Lower extremity fractures after spinal cord injury: A retrospective study. *Arch Phys Med Rehabil* 1981;62(9):418–423.
4. Keating JF, Kerr M, Delargy M. Minimal trauma causing fractures in patients with spinal cord injury. *Disabil Rehabil* 1992;14(2):108–109.
5. Shields RK, Dudley-Javoroski S. Musculoskeletal deterioration and hemicorporectomy after spinal cord injury. *Phys Ther* 2003;83(3):263–275.
6. Shields RK, Dudley-Javoroski S. Musculoskeletal adaptation in chronic spinal cord injury: Effects of long-term soleus electrical stimulation training. *Journal of Neurorehabilitation and Neural Repair* 2007;21:169–179.
7. Parfitt AM. Trabecular bone architecture in the pathogenesis and prevention of fracture. *Am J Med* 1987;82(1B):68–72.
8. Vaynman S, Gomez-Pinilla F. License to run: Exercise impacts functional plasticity in the intact and injured central nervous system by using neurotrophins. *Neurorehabil Neural Repair* 2005;19(4):283–295.
9. Edgerton VR, Leon RD, Harkema SJ, Hodgson JA, London N, Reinkensmeyer DJ, Roy RR, Talmadge RJ, Tillakaratne NJ, Timoszyk W, Tobin A. Retraining the injured spinal cord. *J Physiol* 2001;533(Pt 1):15–22.
10. Shields RK. Rehabilitation medicine summit: Building research capacity—Invited commentary. *Phys Ther* 2006;86(2): 299–300.
11. Fluck M. Functional, structural and molecular plasticity of mammalian skeletal muscle in response to exercise stimuli. *J Exp Biol* 2006;209(Pt 12):2239–2248.
12. Lieber RL. *Skeletal Muscle Structure, Function, & Plasticity.* Baltimore, MD: Lippincott Williams & Wilkins; 2002.
13. Talmadge RJ, Roy RR, Edgerton VR. Persistence of hybrid fibers in rat soleus after spinal cord transection. *Anat Rec* 1999;255(2):188–201.
14. Bottinelli R, Reggiani C. Force-velocity properties and myosin light chain isoform composition of an identified type of skinned fibres from rat skeletal muscle. *Pflugers Arch* 1995;429(4):592–594.
15. Tubman LA, MacIntosh BR, Maki WA. Myosin light chain phosphorylation and posttetanic potentiation in fatigued skeletal muscle. *Pflugers Archiv-European Journal of Physiology* 1996;431(6):882–887.
16. Tubman LA, Rassier DE, MacIntosh BR. Attenuation of myosin light chain phosphorylation and posttetanic potentiation in atrophied skeletal muscle. *Pflugers Archiv-European Journal of Physiology* 1997;434(6):848–851.
17. Vandenboom R, Houston ME. Phosphorylation of myosin and twitch potentiation in fatigued skeletal muscle. *Can J Physiol Pharmacol* 1996;74(12):1315–1321.
18. Obinata T, Saitoh O, Takano-Ohmuro H. Effect of denervation on the isoform transitions of tropomyosin, troponin T, and myosin isozyme in chicken breast muscle. *J Biochem (Tokyo)* 1984;95(2):585–588.
19. Weiss A, Schiaffino S, Leinwand LA. Comparative sequence analysis of the complete human sarcomeric myosin heavy chain family: Implications for functional diversity. *J Mol Biol* 1999;290(1):61–75.
20. Heizmann CW, Berchtold MW, Rowlerson AM. Correlation of parvalbumin concentration with relaxation speed in mammalian muscles. *Proc Natl Acad Sci USA* 1982;79(23):7243–7247.
21. Shields RK. Fatigability, relaxation properties, and electromyographic responses of the human paralyzed soleus muscle. *J Neurophysiol* 1995;73(6):2195–2206.
22. Shields RK, Law LF, Reiling B, Sass K, Wilwert J. Effects of electrically induced fatigue on the twitch and tetanus of paralyzed soleus muscle in humans. *J Appl Physiol* 1997;82(5):1499–1507.
23. Burnham R, Martin T, Stein R, Bell G, MacLean I, Steadward R. Skeletal muscle fibre type transformation following spinal cord injury. *Spinal Cord* 1997;35(2):86–91.
24. Gerrits HL, De Haan A, Hopman MT, van Der Woude LH, Jones DA, Sargeant AJ. Contractile properties of the quadriceps muscle in individuals with spinal cord injury. *Muscle Nerve* 1999;22(9):1249–1256.
25. Talmadge RJ, Roy RR, Edgerton VR. Myosin heavy chain profile of cat soleus following chronic reduced activity or inactivity. *Muscle Nerve* 1996;19(8):980–988.

26. Talmadge RJ, Roy RR, Caiozzo VJ, Edgerton VR. Mechanical properties of rat soleus after long-term spinal cord transection. *J Appl Physiol* 2002;93(4):1487–1497.

27. Harridge SD, Bottinelli R, Canepari M, Pellegrino MA, Reggiani C, Esbjornsson M, Saltin B. Whole-muscle and single-fibre contractile properties and myosin heavy chain isoforms in humans. *Pflugers Arch* 1996;432(5):913–920.

28. Larsson L, Moss RL. Maximum velocity of shortening in relation to myosin isoform composition in single fibres from human skeletal muscles. *J Physiol* 1993;472:595–614.

29. Castro MJ, Apple DF, Jr., Staron RS, Campos GE, Dudley GA. Influence of complete spinal cord injury on skeletal muscle within 6 mo of injury. *J Appl Physiol* 1999;86(1): 350–358.

30. Talmadge RJ, Castro MJ, Apple DF, Jr., Dudley GA. Phenotypic adaptations in human muscle fibers 6 and 24 wk after spinal cord injury. *J Appl Physiol* 2002;92(1):147–154.

31. Talmadge RJ. Myosin heavy chain isoform expression following reduced neuromuscular activity: Potential regulatory mechanisms. *Muscle Nerve* 2000;23(5):661–679.

32. Andersen JL, Mohr T, Biering-Sorensen F, Galbo H, Kjaer M. Myosin heavy chain isoform transformation in single fibres from m. vastus lateralis in spinal cord injured individuals: Effects of long-term functional electrical stimulation (FES). *Pflugers Archiv-European Journal of Physiology* 1996;431(4):513–518.

33. Crameri RM, Weston AR, Rutkowski S, Middleton JW, Davis GM, Sutton JR. Effects of electrical stimulation leg training during the acute phase of spinal cord injury: A pilot study. *European Journal of Applied Physiology* 2000;83(4–5):409–415.

34. Grimby G, Broberg C, Krotkiewska I, Krotkiewski M. Muscle fiber composition in patients with traumatic cord lesion. *Scand J Rehabil Med* 1976;8(1):37–42.

35. Lotta S, Scelsi R, Alfonsi E, Saitta A, Nicolotti D, Epifani P, Carraro U. Morphometric and neurophysiological analysis of skeletal muscle in paraplegic patients with traumatic cord lesion. *Paraplegia* 1991;29(4):247–252.

36. Houle JD, Morris K, Skinner RD, Garcia-Rill E, Peterson CA. Effects of fetal spinal cord tissue transplants and cycling exercise on the soleus muscle in spinalized rats. *Muscle Nerve* 1999;22(7):846–856.

37. Talmadge RJ, Roy RR, Edgerton VR. Prominence of myosin heavy chain hybrid fibers in soleus muscle of spinal cord-transected rats. *J Appl Physiol* 1995;78(4):1256–1265.

38. Shields RK, Dudley-Javoroski S. Musculoskeletal plasticity after acute spinal cord injury: Effects of long-term neuromuscular electrical stimulation training. *J Neurophysiol* 2006;95:2380–2390.

39. Zhong H, Roy RR, Hodgson JA, Talmadge RJ, Grossman EJ, Edgerton VR. Activity-independent neural influences on cat soleus motor unit phenotypes. *Muscle Nerve* 2002;26(2):252–264.

40. Roy RR, Zhong H, Hodgson JA, Grossman EJ, Siengthai B, Talmadge RJ, Edgerton VR. Influences of electromechanical events in defining skeletal muscle properties. *Muscle Nerve* 2002;26(2):238–251.

41. Crameri RM, Weston A, Climstein M, Davis GM, Sutton JR. Effects of electrical stimulation-induced leg training on skeletal muscle adaptability in spinal cord injury. *Scand J Med Sci Sports* 2002;12(5):316–322.

42. Crameri RM, Cooper P, Sinclair PJ, Bryant G, Weston A. Effect of load during electrical stimulation training in spinal cord injury. *Muscle Nerve* 2004;29(1):104–111.

43. Chilibeck PD, Bell G, Jeon J, Weiss CB, Murdoch G, MacLean I, Ryan E, Burnham R. Functional electrical stimulation exercise increases GLUT-1 and GLUT-4 in paralyzed skeletal muscle. *Metabolism* 1999;48(11): 1409–1413.

44. Stewart BG, Tarnopolsky MA, Hicks AL, McCartney N, Mahoney DJ, Staron RS, Phillips SM. Treadmill training-induced adaptations in muscle phenotype in persons with incomplete spinal cord injury. *Muscle Nerve* 2004;30(1):61–68.

45. Round JM, Barr FM, Moffat B, Jones DA. Fibre areas and histochemical fibre types in the quadriceps muscle of paraplegic subjects. *J Neurol Sci* 1993;116(2):207–211.

46. Dupont-Versteegden EE, Houle JD, Gurley CM, Peterson CA. Early changes in muscle fiber size and gene expression in response to spinal cord transection and exercise. *Am J Physiol* 1998;275(4 Pt 1):C1124–C1133.

47. Maganaris CN, Baltzopoulos V, Ball D, Sargeant AJ. In vivo specific tension of human skeletal muscle. *J Appl Physiol* 2001;90(3):865–872.

48. Mohr T, Andersen JL, Biering-Sorensen F, Galbo H, Bangsbo J, Wagner A, Kjaer M. Long-term adaptation to electrically induced cycle training in severe spinal cord injured individuals.[erratum appears in Spinal Cord 1997 Apr;35(4):262]. *Spinal Cord* 1997;35(1):1–16.

49. Scelsi R, Marchetti C, Poggi P, Lotta S, Lommi G. Muscle fiber type morphology and distribution in paraplegic patients with traumatic cord lesion. Histochemical and ultrastructural aspects of rectus femoris muscle. *Acta Neuropathol (Berl)* 1982;57(4):243–248.

50. McDonald MF, Garrison MK, Schmit BD. Length-tension properties of ankle muscles in chronic human spinal cord injury. *J Biomech* 2005;38:2344–2353.

51. Pette D. Training effects on the contractile apparatus. *Acta Physiol Scand* 1998;162(3):367–376.

52. Leeuw T, Pette D. Coordinate changes in the expression of troponin subunit and myosin heavy-chain isoforms during fast-to-slow transition of low-frequency-stimulated rabbit muscle. *Eur J Biochem* 1993;213(3):1039–1046.

53. Brown WE, Salmons S, Whalen RG. The sequential replacement of myosin subunit isoforms during muscle type transformation induced by long term electrical stimulation. *J Biol Chem* 1983;258(23):14686–14692.

54. Jiang B, Roy RR, Edgerton VR. Expression of a fast fiber enzyme profile in the cat soleus after spinalization. *Muscle Nerve* 1990;13(11):1037–1049.

55. Castro MJ, Apple DF, Jr., Melton-Rogers S, Dudley GA. Muscle fiber type-specific myofibrillar Ca(2+) ATPase activity after spinal cord injury. *Muscle Nerve* 2000;23(1):119–121.

56. Martin TP, Stein RB, Hoeppner PH, Reid DC. Influence of electrical stimulation on the morphological and metabolic properties of paralyzed muscle. *J Appl Physiol* 1992;72(4):1401–1406.

57. Theriault R, Boulay MR, Theriault G, Simoneau JA. Electrical stimulation-induced changes in performance and fiber type proportion of human knee extensor muscles. *Eur J Appl Physiol Occup Physiol* 1996;74(4):311–317.

58. Gerrits HL, Hopman MT, Offringa C, Engelen BG, Sargeant AJ, Jones DA, Haan A. Variability in fibre properties in paralysed human quadriceps muscles and effects of training. *Pflugers Arch* 2003;445(6):734–740.

59. Otis JS, Roy RR, Edgerton VR, Talmadge RJ. Adaptations in metabolic capacity of rat soleus after paralysis. *J Appl Physiol* 2004;96(2):584–596.

60. Chilibeck PD, Jeon J, Weiss C, Bell G, Burnham R. Histochemical changes in muscle of individuals with spinal cord injury following functional electrical stimulated exercise training. *Spinal Cord* 1999;37(4):264–268.

61. Ingjer F. Maximal aerobic power related to the capillary supply of the quadriceps femoris muscle in man. *Acta Physiol Scand* 1978;104(2):238–240.

62. Tesch PA, Wright JE. Recovery from short term intense exercise: Its relation to capillary supply and blood lactate concentration. *Eur J Appl Physiol Occup Physiol* 1983;52(1):98–103.

63. Li JL, Wang XN, Fraser SF, Carey MF, Wrigley TV, McKenna MJ. Effects of fatigue and training on sarcoplasmic reticulum Ca(2+) regulation in human skeletal muscle. *J Appl Physiol* 2002;92(3):912–922.

64. Baumann H, Jaggi M, Soland F, Howald H, Schaub MC. Exercise training induces transitions of myosin isoform subunits within histochemically typed human muscle fibres. *Pflugers Arch* 1987;409(4-5):349–360.

65. Staron RS, Karapondo DL, Kraemer WJ, Fry AC, Gordon SE, Falkel JE, Hagerman FC, Hikida RS. Skeletal muscle adaptations during early phase of heavy-resistance training in men and women. *J Appl Physiol* 1994;76(3):1247–1255.

66. Staron RS, Leonardi MJ, Karapondo DL, Malicky ES, Falkel JE, Hagerman FC, Hikida RS. Strength and skeletal muscle adaptations in heavy-resistance-trained women after detraining and retraining. *J Appl Physiol* 1991;70(2):631–640.

67. Allemeier CA, Fry AC, Johnson P, Hikida RS, Hagerman FC, Staron RS. Effects of sprint cycle training on human skeletal muscle. *J Appl Physiol* 1994;77(5):2385–2390.

68. Willoughby DS, Priest JW, Jennings RA. Myosin heavy chain isoform and ubiquitin protease mRNA expression after passive leg cycling in persons with spinal cord injury. *Arch Phys Med Rehabil* 2000;81(2):157–163.

69. Hjeltnes N, Galuska D, Bjornholm M, Aksnes AK, Lannem A, Zierath JR, Wallberg-Henriksson H. Exercise-induced overexpression of key regulatory proteins involved in glucose uptake and metabolism in tetraplegic persons: Molecular mechanism for improved glucose homeostasis. *FASEB J* 1998;12(15):1701–1712.

70. Harridge SD, Andersen JL, Hartkopp A, Zhou S, Biering-Sorensen F, Sandri C, Kjaer M. Training by low-frequency stimulation of tibialis anterior in spinal cord-injured men. *Muscle Nerve* 2002;25(5):685–694.

71. Leeuw T, Pette D. Coordinate changes of myosin light and heavy chain isoforms during forced fiber type transitions in rabbit muscle. *Dev Genet* 1996;19(2):163–168.

72. Bozzo C, Spolaore B, Toniolo L, Stevens L, Bastide B, Cieniewski-Bernard C, Fontana A, Mounier Y, Reggiani C. Nerve influence on myosin light chain phosphorylation in slow and fast skeletal muscles. *Febs J* 2005;272(22):5771–5785.

73. Kjaer M, Mohr T, Biering-Sorensen F, Bangsbo J. Muscle enzyme adaptation to training and tapering-off in spinal-cord-injured humans. *European Journal of Applied Physiology* 2001;84(5):482–486.

74. Hamalainen N, Pette D. Coordinated fast-to-slow transitions of myosin and SERCA isoforms in chronically stimulated muscles of euthyroid and hyperthyroid rabbits. *J Muscle Res Cell Motil* 1997;18(5):545–554.

75. Leberer E, Hartner KT, Brandl CJ, Fujii J, Tada M, MacLennan DH, Pette D. Slow/cardiac sarcoplasmic reticulum Ca2+-ATPase and phospholamban mRNAs are expressed in chronically stimulated rabbit fast-twitch muscle. *Eur J Biochem* 1989;185(1):51–54.

76. Briggs FN, Lee KF, Wechsler AW, Jones LR. Phospholamban expressed in slow-twitch and chronically stimulated fast-twitch muscles minimally affects calcium affinity of sarcoplasmic reticulum Ca(2+)-ATPase. *J Biol Chem* 1992;267(36):26056–26061.

77. Leberer E, Pette D. Neural regulation of parvalbumin expression in mammalian skeletal muscle. *Biochem J* 1986;235(1):67–73.

78. Leberer E, Seedorf U, Pette D. Neural control of gene expression in skeletal muscle. Calcium-sequestering proteins in developing and chronically stimulated rabbit skeletal muscles. *Biochem J* 1986;239(2):295–300.

79. Huber B, Pette D. Dynamics of parvalbumin expression in low-frequency-stimulated fast-twitch rat muscle. *Eur J Biochem* 1996;236(3):814–819.

80. Hicks A, Ohlendieck K, Gopel SO, Pette D. Early functional and biochemical adaptations to low-frequency stimulation of rabbit fast-twitch muscle. *Am J Physiol* 1997;273(1 Pt 1):C297–C305.

81. Ohlendieck K, Briggs FN, Lee KF, Wechsler AW, Campbell KP. Analysis of excitation-contraction-coupling components in chronically stimulated canine skeletal muscle. *Eur J Biochem* 1991;202(3):739–747.

82. Green HJ, Ballantyne CS, MacDougall JD, Tarnopolsky MA, Schertzer JD. Adaptations in human muscle sarcoplasmic reticulum to prolonged submaximal training. *J Appl Physiol* 2003;94(5):2034–2042.

83. Kandarian SC, Peters DG, Taylor JA, Williams JH. Skeletal muscle overload upregulates the sarcoplasmic reticulum slow calcium pump gene. *Am J Physiol* 1994;266(5 Pt 1):C1190–1197.

84. Talmadge RJ, Roy RR, Chalmers GR, Edgerton VR. MHC and sarcoplasmic reticulum protein isoforms in functionally overloaded cat plantaris muscle fibers. *J Appl Physiol* 1996;80(4):1296–1303.

85. Shields RK, Dudley-Javoroski S, Littmann AE. Post-fatigue potentiation of paralyzed soleus muscle: Evidence for adaptation with long-term electrical stimulation training. *J Appl Physiol* 2006;101:556–565.

86. Hartkopp A, Harridge SD, Mizuno M, Ratkevicius A, Quistorff B, Kjaer M, Biering-Sorensen F. Effect of training on contractile and metabolic properties of wrist extensors in spinal cord-injured individuals. *Muscle Nerve* 2003;27(1):72–80.

87. Stein RB, Gordon T, Jefferson J, Sharfenberger A, Yang JF, de Zepetnek JT, Belanger M. Optimal stimulation of paralyzed muscle after human spinal cord injury. *J Appl Physiol* 1992;72(4):1393–1400.

88. Gerrits HL, de Haan A, Sargeant AJ, Dallmeijer A, Hopman MT. Altered contractile properties of the quadriceps muscle in people with spinal cord injury following functional electrical stimulated cycle training. *Spinal Cord* 2000;38(4):214–223.

89. Gerrits HL, Hopman MT, Sargeant AJ, Jones DA, De Haan A. Effects of training on contractile properties of paralyzed quadriceps muscle. *Muscle Nerve* 2002;25(4):559–567.

90. Dudley-Javoroski S, Shields RK. Assessing health-related quality of life and secondary complications after complete spinal cord injury. *Disabil Rehabil* 2006;28(2):103–110.

91. Lu TW, Taylor SJ, O'Connor JJ, Walker PS. Influence of muscle activity on the forces in the femur: An in vivo study. *J Biomech* 1997;30(11–12):1101–1106.

92. Cybulski GR, Penn RD, Jaeger RJ. Lower extremity functional neuromuscular stimulation in cases of spinal cord injury. *Neurosurgery* 1984;15(1):132–146.

93. Jaeger RJ. Lower extremity applications of functional neuromuscular stimulation. *Assist Technol* 1992;4(1):19–30.

94. Yarkony GM, Roth EJ, Cybulski G, Jaeger RJ. Neuromuscular stimulation in spinal cord injury: I: Restoration of functional movement of the extremities. *Arch Phys Med Rehabil* 1992;73(1):78–86.

95. Yarkony GM, Jaeger RJ, Roth E, Kralj AR, Quintern J. Functional neuromuscular stimulation for standing after spinal cord injury. *Arch Phys Med Rehabil* 1990;71(3):201–206.

96. Billian C, Gorman PH. Upper extremity applications of functional neuromuscular stimulation. *Assist Technol* 1992;4(1):31–39.

97. Goodship AE, Lanyon LE, McFie H. Functional adaptation of bone to increased stress. An experimental study. *Journal of Bone & Joint Surgery—American Volume* 1979;61(4):539–546.

98. Kralj AR, Bajd T. *Functional Electrical Stimulation: Standing and Walking after Spinal Cord Injury.* Boca Raton, FL: CRC; 1989.

99. Mazess RB, Whedon GD. Immobilization and bone. *Calcif Tissue Int* 1983;35(3):265–267.

100. Maimoun L, Lumbroso S, Paris F, Couret I, Peruchon E, Rouays-Mabit E, Rossi M, Leroux JL, Sultan C. The role of androgens or growth factors in the bone resorption process in recent spinal cord injured patients: A cross-sectional study. *Spinal Cord* 2006; 44(12):791–797.

101. Chantraine A, van Ouwenaller C, Hachen HJ, Schinas P. Intra-medullary pressure and intra-osseous phlebography in paraplegia. *Paraplegia* 1979;17(4):391–399.

102. Lanyon LE. Using functional loading to influence bone mass and architecture: Objectives, mechanisms, and relationship with estrogen of the mechanically adaptive process in bone. *Bone* 1996;18(1 Suppl):37S–43S.

103. Schultheis L. The mechanical control system of bone in weightless spaceflight and in aging. *Exp Gerontol* 1991; 26(2–3):203–214.

104. Biewener AA, Fazzalari NL, Konieczynski DD, Baudinette RV. Adaptive changes in trabecular architecture in relation to functional strain patterns and disuse. *Bone* 1996;19(1):1–8.

105. Ehrlich PJ, Lanyon LE. Mechanical strain and bone cell function: A review. *Osteoporos Int* 2002;13(9):688–700.

106. Jones DB, Nolte H, Scholubbers JG, Turner E, Veltel D. Biochemical signal transduction of mechanical strain in osteoblast-like cells. *Biomaterials* 1991;12(2):101–110.

107. Cowin SC. Mechanosensation and fluid transport in living bone. *J Musculoskelet Neuronal Interact* 2002;2(3):256–260.

108. Palumbo C, Palazzini S, Marotti G. Morphological study of intercellular junctions during osteocyte differentiation. *Bone* 1990;11(6):401–406.

109. Bakker AD, Soejima K, Klein-Nulend J, Burger EH. The production of nitric oxide and prostaglandin E(2) by primary bone cells is shear stress dependent. *J Biomech* 2001;34(5):671–677.

110. Weinbaum S, Cowin SC, Zeng Y. A model for the excitation of osteocytes by mechanical loading-induced bone fluid shear stresses. *J Biomech* 1994;27(3):339–360.

111. Gronowicz GA, Fall PM, Raisz LG. Prostaglandin E2 stimulates preosteoblast replication: An autoradiographic study in cultured fetal rat calvariae. *Exp Cell Res* 1994;212(2):314–320.

112. Lanyon LE. Osteocytes, strain detection, bone modeling and remodeling. *Calcif Tissue Int* 1993;53 Suppl 1: S102–S106; discussion S106–S107.

113. Zhang D, Cowin SC, Weinbaum S. Electrical signal transmission and gap junction regulation in a bone cell network: A cable model for an osteon. *Ann Biomed Eng* 1997;25(2):357–374.

114. Teitelbaum SL. Bone resorption by osteoclasts. *Science* 2000;289(5484):1504–1508.

115. Downey PA, Siegel MI. Bone biology and the clinical implications for osteoporosis. *Phys Ther* 2006;86(1):77–91.

116. Adami S, Gatti D, Braga V, Bianchini D, Rossini M. Site-specific effects of strength training on bone structure and geometry of ultradistal radius in postmenopausal women.[comment]. *J Bone Miner Res* 1999;14(1):120–124.

117. Garland DE, Adkins RH, Kushwaha V, Stewart C. Risk factors for osteoporosis at the knee in the spinal cord injury population. *J Spinal Cord Med* 2004;27(3):202–206.

118. Serre CM, Farlay D, Delmas PD, Chenu C. Evidence for a dense and intimate innervation of the bone tissue, including glutamate-containing fibers. *Bone* 1999;25(6):623–629.

119. Mach DB, Rogers SD, Sabino MC, Luger NM, Schwei MJ, Pomonis JD, Keyser CP, Clohisy DR, Adams DJ, O'Leary P, Mantyh PW. Origins of skeletal pain: Sensory and sympathetic innervation of the mouse femur. *Neuroscience* 2002;113(1):155–166.

120. Hohmann EL, Elde RP, Rysavy JA, Einzig S, Gebhard RL. Innervation of periosteum and bone by sympathetic vasoactive intestinal peptide-containing nerve fibers. *Science* 1986;232(4752):868–871.

121. Konttinen Y, Imai S, Suda A. Neuropeptides and the puzzle of bone remodeling. State of the art. *Acta Orthop Scand* 1996;67(6):632–639.

122. Bjurholm A, Kreicbergs A, Brodin E, Schultzberg M. Substance P- and CGRP-immunoreactive nerves in bone. *Peptides* 1988;9(1):165–171.

123. Wilmet E, Ismail AA, Heilporn A, Welraeds D, Bergmann P. Longitudinal study of the bone mineral content and of soft tissue composition after spinal cord section. *Paraplegia* 1995;33(11):674–677.

124. Frey-Rindova P, de Bruin ED, Stussi E, Dambacher MA, Dietz V. Bone mineral density in upper and lower extremities during 12 months after spinal cord injury measured by peripheral quantitative computed tomography. *Spinal Cord* 2000;38(1):26–32.

125. Eser P, Frotzler A, Zehnder Y, Wick L, Knecht H, Denoth J, Schiessl H. Relationship between the duration of paralysis and bone structure: A pQCT study of spinal cord injured individuals. *Bone* 2004;34:869–880.

126. Shields RK, Dudley-Javoroski S, Boaldin KM, Corey TA, Fog DB, Ruen JM. Peripheral quantitative computed tomography (pQCT): Measurement sensitivity in individuals with and without spinal cord injury. *Archives of Physical Medicine and Rehabilitation* 2006 (in press).

127. Biering-Sorensen F, Bohr HH, Schaadt OP. Longitudinal study of bone mineral content in the lumbar spine, the forearm and the lower extremities after spinal cord injury. *Eur J Clin Invest* 1990;20(3):330–335.

128. Garland DE, Stewart CA, Adkins RH, Hu SS, Rosen C, Liotta FJ, Weinstein DA. Osteoporosis after spinal cord injury. *J Orthop Res* 1992;10(3):371–378.

129. Uebelhart D, Demiaux-Domenech B, Roth M, Chantraine A. Bone metabolism in spinal cord injured individuals and in others who have prolonged immobilisation. A review. *Paraplegia* 1995;33(11):669–673.

130. Eser P, Frotzler A, Zehnder Y, Denoth J. Fracture threshold in the femur and tibia of people with spinal cord injury as determined by peripheral quantitative computed tomography. *Arch Phys Med Rehabil* 2005;86(3):498–504.

131. Vestergaard P, Krogh K, Rejnmark L, Mosekilde L. Fracture rates and risk factors for fractures in patients with spinal cord injury. *Spinal Cord* 1998;36(11):790-796.

132. de Bruin ED, Herzog R, Rozendal RH, Michel D, Stussi E. Estimation of geometric properties of cortical bone in spinal cord injury. *Arch Phys Med Rehabil* 2000;81(2):150–156.

133. Modlesky CM, Slade JM, Bickel CS, Meyer RA, Dudley GA. Deteriorated geometric structure and strength of the midfemur in men with complete spinal cord injury. *Bone* 2005;36(2):331–339.

134. Lee TQ, Shapiro TA, Bell DM. Biomechanical properties of human tibias in long-term spinal cord injury. *J Rehabil Res Dev* 1997;34(3):295-302.

135. Jarvinen TL, Kannus P, Sievanen H. Have the DXA-based exercise studies seriously underestimated the effects of mechanical loading on bone?[comment]. *J Bone Miner Res* 1999;14(9):1634–1635.

136. Ferretti JL, Capozza RF, Zanchetta JR. Mechanical validation of a tomographic (pQCT) index for noninvasive estimation of rat femur bending strength. *Bone* 1996;18(2):97–102.

137. Haapasalo H, Kontulainen S, Sievanen H, Kannus P, Jarvinen M, Vuori I. Exercise-induced bone gain is due to enlargement in bone size without a change in volumetric bone density: A peripheral quantitative computed tomography study of the upper arms of male tennis players. *Bone* 2000;27(3):351–357.

138. Kontulainen S, Sievanen H, Kannus P, Pasanen M, Vuori I. Effect of long-term impact-loading on mass, size, and estimated strength of humerus and radius of female racquet-sports players: A peripheral quantitative computed tomography study between young and old starters and controls. *J Bone Miner Res* 2003;18(2):352–359.

139. Jamsa T, Jalovaara P, Peng Z, Vaananen HK, Tuukkanen J. Comparison of three-point bending test and peripheral quantitative computed tomography analysis in the evaluation of the strength of mouse femur and tibia. *Bone* 1998;23(2):155–161.

140. Augat P, Reeb H, Claes LE. Prediction of fracture load at different skeletal sites by geometric properties of the cortical shell. *J Bone Miner Res* 1996;11(9):1356–1363.

141. Szollar SM, Martin EM, Parthemore JG, Sartoris DJ, Deftos LJ. Densitometric patterns of spinal cord injury associated bone loss. *Spinal Cord* 1997;35(6):374–382.

142. Leslie WD, Nance PW. Dissociated hip and spine demineralization: A specific finding in spinal cord injury. *Arch Phys Med Rehabil* 1993;74(9):960–964.

143. Garland DE, Foulkes GD, Adkins RH, Stewart CA, Yakura JS. Regional osteoporosis following incomplete spinal cord injury. *Contemp Orthop* 1994;28(2):134–139.

144. Shields RK, Dudley-Javoroski S, Frey Law L. Electrically-induced muscle contractions influence bone density decline after spinal cord injury. *Spine* 2006;31(5):548–553.

145. Garland DE, Adkins RH, Stewart CA, Ashford R, Vigil D. Regional osteoporosis in women who have a complete spinal cord injury. *Journal of Bone & Joint Surgery—American Volume* 2001;83-A(8):1195–1200.

146. DiGiovine CP, Cooper RA, Fitzgerald SG, Boninger ML, Wolf EJ, Guo S. Whole-body vibration during manual wheelchair propulsion with selected seat cushions and back supports. *IEEE Trans Neural Syst Rehabil Eng* 2003;11(3):311–322.

147. Heinonen A, Sievanen H, Kyrolainen H, Perttunen J, Kannus P. Mineral mass, size, and estimated mechanical strength of triple jumpers' lower limb. *Bone* 2001;29(3):279–285.

148. Hay JG. Citius, altius, longius (faster, higher, longer): The biomechanics of jumping for distance. *J Biomech* 1993;26 Suppl 1:7–21.

149. Chow JW, Jagger CJ, Chambers TJ. Characterization of osteogenic response to mechanical stimulation in cancellous bone of rat caudal vertebrae. *Am J Physiol* 1993;265(2 Pt 1):E340–347.

150. Rubin C, Gross T, Qin YX, Fritton S, Guilak F, McLeod K. Differentiation of the bone-tissue remodeling response to axial and torsional loading in the turkey ulna. *Journal of Bone & Joint Surgery—American Volume* 1996;78(10):1523–1533.

151. Mosley JR, Lanyon LE. Strain rate as a controlling influence on adaptive modeling in response to dynamic loading of the ulna in growing male rats. *Bone* 1998;23(4):313–318.

152. Lanyon LE. Experimental support for the trajectorial theory of bone structure. *J Bone Joint Surg Br* 1974;56(1):160–166.

153. O'Connor JA, Lanyon LE, MacFie H. The influence of strain rate on adaptive bone remodelling. *J Biomech* 1982;15(10):767–781.

154. Jarvinen TL, Kannus P, Sievanen H, Jolma P, Heinonen A, Jarvinen M. Randomized controlled study of effects of sudden impact loading on rat femur. *J Bone Miner Res* 1998;13(9):1475–1482.

155. Mosley JR, March BM, Lynch J, Lanyon LE. Strain magnitude related changes in whole bone architecture in growing rats. *Bone* 1997;20(3):191–198.

156. Lee KC, Maxwell A, Lanyon LE. Validation of a technique for studying functional adaptation of the mouse ulna in response to mechanical loading. *Bone* 2002;31(3):407–412.

157. Robling AG, Hinant FM, Burr DB, Turner CH. Shorter, more frequent mechanical loading sessions enhance bone mass. *Med Sci Sports Exerc* 2002;34(2):196–202.

158. Hsieh YF, Robling AG, Ambrosius WT, Burr DB, Turner CH. Mechanical loading of diaphyseal bone in vivo: The strain threshold for an osteogenic response varies with location. *J Bone Miner Res* 2001;16(12):2291–2297.

159. De Souza RL, Matsuura M, Eckstein F, Rawlinson SC, Lanyon LE, Pitsillides AA. Non-invasive axial loading of mouse tibiae increases cortical bone formation and modifies trabecular organization: A new model to study cortical and cancellous compartments in a single loaded element. *Bone* 2005;37(6):810–818.

160. Robling AG, Burr DB, Turner CH. Partitioning a daily mechanical stimulus into discrete loading bouts improves the osteogenic response to loading. *J Bone Miner Res* 2000;15(8):1596–1602.

161. Bloomfield SA, Allen MR, Hogan HA, Delp MD. Site- and compartment-specific changes in bone with hindlimb unloading in mature adult rats. *Bone* 2002;31(1):149–157.

162. Allen MR, Bloomfield SA. Hindlimb unloading has a greater effect on cortical compared with cancellous

bone in mature female rats. *J Appl Physiol* 2003;94(2): 642–650.

163. David V, Lafage-Proust MH, Laroche N, Christian A, Ruegsegger P, Vico L. Two-week longitudinal survey of bone architecture alteration in the hindlimb-unloaded rat model of bone loss: Sex differences. *Am J Physiol Endocrinol Metab* 2006;290(3):E440–447.

164. Fluckey JD, Dupont-Versteegden EE, Montague DC, Knox M, Tesch P, Peterson CA, Gaddy-Kurten D. A rat resistance exercise regimen attenuates losses of musculoskeletal mass during hindlimb suspension. *Acta Physiol Scand* 2002;176(4):293–300.

165. Frey Law L, Shields RK. Femoral loads during passive, active, and active-resistive stance after spinal cord injury: A mathematical model. *Clinical Biomechanics* 2004;19:313–321.

166. Rittweger J, Gerrits K, Altenburg T, Reeves N, Maganaris CN, de Haan A. Bone adaptation to altered loading after spinal cord injury: A study of bone and muscle strength. *J Musculoskelet Neuronal Interact* 2006;6(3):269–276.

167. Franco JC, Perell KL, Gregor RJ, Scremin AM. Knee kinetics during functional electrical stimulation induced cycling in subjects with spinal cord injury: A preliminary study. *J Rehabil Res Dev* 1999;36(3):207–216.

168. Kunkel CF, Scremin AM, Eisenberg B, Garcia JF, Roberts S, Martinez S. Effect of "standing" on spasticity, contracture, and osteoporosis in paralyzed males. *Arch Phys Med Rehabil* 1993;74(1):73–78.

169. Needham-Shropshire BM, Broton JG, Klose KJ, Lebwohl N, Guest RS, Jacobs PL. Evaluation of a training program for persons with SCI paraplegia using the Parastep 1 ambulation system: Part 3. Lack of effect on bone mineral density. *Arch Phys Med Rehabil* 1997;78(8): 799–803.

170. Thoumie P, Le Claire G, Beillot J, Dassonville J, Chevalier T, Perrouin-Verbe B, Bedoiseau M, Busnel M, Cormerais A, Courtillon A. Restoration of functional gait in paraplegic patients with the RGO-II hybrid orthosis. A multicenter controlled study. II: Physiological evaluation. *Paraplegia* 1995;33(11):654–659.

171. Giangregorio LM, Hicks AL, Webber CE, Phillips SM, Craven BC, Bugaresti JM, McCartney N. Body weight supported treadmill training in acute spinal cord injury: Impact on muscle and bone. *Spinal Cord* 2005;43(11): 649–657.

172. Leeds EM, Klose KJ, Ganz W, Serafini A, Green BA. Bone mineral density after bicycle ergometry training. *Arch Phys Med Rehabil* 1990;71(3):207–209.

173. BeDell KK, Scremin AM, Perell KL, Kunkel CF. Effects of functional electrical stimulation-induced lower extremity cycling on bone density of spinal cord-injured patients. *Am J Phys Med Rehabil* 1996;75(1):29–34.

174. Snyder WS, editor. *Report of the Task Group on Reference Man.* Oxford, New York: Pergamon; 1975. 75 p.

175. Frost HM. Bone's mechanostat: A 2003 update. *Anat Rec* 2003;275A(2):1081–1101.

176. Frost HM. A 2003 update of bone physiology and Wolff's Law for clinicians. *Angle Orthod* 2004;74(1):3–15.

177. Bloomfield SA, Mysiw WJ, Jackson RD. Bone mass and endocrine adaptations to training in spinal cord injured individuals. *Bone* 1996;19(1):61–68.

178. Mohr T, Podenphant J, Biering-Sorensen F, Galbo H, Thamsborg G, Kjaer M. Increased bone mineral density after prolonged electrically induced cycle training of paralyzed limbs in spinal cord injured man. *Calcif Tissue Int* 1997;61(1):22–25.

179. de Bruin ED, Frey-Rindova P, Herzog RE, Dietz V, Dambacher MA, Stussi E. Changes of tibia bone properties after spinal cord injury: Effects of early intervention. *Arch Phys Med Rehabil* 1999;80(2):214–220.

180. Fritton SP, McLeod KJ, Rubin CT. Quantifying the strain history of bone: Spatial uniformity and self-similarity of low-magnitude strains. *J Biomech* 2000;33(3):317–325.

181. Flieger J, Karachalios T, Khaldi L, Raptou P, Lyritis G. Mechanical stimulation in the form of vibration prevents postmenopausal bone loss in ovariectomized rats. *Calcif Tissue Int* 1998;63(6):510–514.

182. Rubin C, Xu G, Judex S. The anabolic activity of bone tissue, suppressed by disuse, is normalized by brief exposure to extremely low-magnitude mechanical stimuli. *FASEB J* 2001;15(12):2225–2229.

183. Rubin C, Turner AS, Mallinckrodt C, Jerome C, McLeod K, Bain S. Mechanical strain, induced noninvasively in the high-frequency domain, is anabolic to cancellous bone, but not cortical bone. *Bone* 2002;30(3):445–452.

184. Iwamoto J, Takeda T, Sato Y, Uzawa M. Effect of whole-body vibration exercise on lumbar bone mineral density, bone turnover, and chronic back pain in post-menopausal osteoporotic women treated with alendronate. *Aging Clin Exp Res* 2005;17(2):157–163.

185. Torvinen S, Kannus P, Sievanen H, Jarvinen TA, Pasanen M, Kontulainen S, Nenonen A, Jarvinen TL, Paakkala T, Jarvinen M, Vuori I. Effect of 8-month vertical whole body vibration on bone, muscle performance, and body balance: A randomized controlled study. *J Bone Miner Res* 2003;18(5):876–884.

186. Verschueren SM, Roelants M, Delecluse C, Swinnen S, Vanderschueren D, Boonen S. Effect of 6-month whole body vibration training on hip density, muscle strength, and postural control in postmenopausal women: A randomized controlled pilot study. *J Bone Miner Res* 2004;19(3):352–359.

187. Rubin C, Recker R, Cullen D, Ryaby J, McCabe J, McLeod K. Prevention of postmenopausal bone loss by a low-magnitude, high-frequency mechanical stimuli: A clinical trial assessing compliance, efficacy, and safety. *J Bone Miner Res* 2004;19(3):343–351.

188. Gilsanz V, Wren TA, Sanchez M, Dorey F, Judex S, Rubin C. Low-level, high-frequency mechanical signals enhance musculoskeletal development of young women with low BMD. *J Bone Miner Res* 2006;21(9):1464–1474.

189. Ward K, Alsop C, Caulton J, Rubin C, Adams J, Mughal Z. Low magnitude mechanical loading is osteogenic in children with disabling conditions. *J Bone Miner Res* 2004;19(3):360–369.

190. Hartkopp A, Murphy RJ, Mohr T, Kjaer M, Biering-Sorensen F. Bone fracture during electrical stimulation of the quadriceps in a spinal cord injured subject. *Arch Phys Med Rehabil* 1998;79(9):1133–1136.

191. Shields RK, Dudley-Javoroski S, Boaldin KM, Corey TA, Fog DB, Ruen JM. Peripheral quantitative computed tomography: Measurement sensitivity in persons with and without spinal cord injury. *Arch Phys Med Rehabil* 2006;87(10):1376–1381.

192. Dudley-Javoroski S, Shields RK. Dose estimation and surveillance of mechanical loading interventions for bone loss after spinal cord injury. *Phys Ther* 2008;88:387–396.

Contemporary Experimental Procedures for Individuals with Spinal Cord Injury

4

Maria J. Amador, BSN, CRRN

After reading this chapter, the reader will be able to:

- Outline the pathophysiology of spinal cord injury (SCI), identifying potential targets for neuroprotective and regenerative treatments
- Describe priorities in SCI research
- Describe past, present, and impending clinical trials and experimental procedures directed at neuroprotection, neural cell replacement, and axon repair
- Discuss the rationale and preclinical experience for each intervention
- Discuss the importance of scientific rigor for advancing the field of SCI research
- Outline current issues important for the translation of preclinical procedures to clinical trials
- Apply knowledge gained from this chapter to current clinical practice

OBJECTIVES

OUTLINE

Introduction

In recent decades, progress in the field of neurobiology has led to new knowledge suggesting that regeneration of the central nervous system (CNS) might be an attainable goal. Today, one of the greatest challenges faced by researchers is that of achieving functional repair of the injured spinal cord. Scientists have developed several transplantation strategies that promote axonal regrowth and partial recovery in experimental models of spinal cord injury (SCI). Because these preclinical experimental strategies demonstrate some extent of axonal regeneration, translating them into human clinical trials is expected in the not too distant future.

Though several trials directed at promoting recovery after SCI have been carried out in humans over the years, an effective treatment has been elusive. Some studies have used pharmacological interventions, while others have included cellular transplantation approaches based on a variety of promising strategies that induced regeneration and functional improvements in experimental models of SCI. As new treatment strategies are designed and advanced to clinical trial, the prospect of recovering lost spinal cord functions seems tantalizingly close. Media reports and the Internet are revealing enticing news of possible functional improvements to the community of people with SCI. Some people are acting on the opportunity to undergo various experimental procedures that, in the opinion of some in the SCI scientific community, have not been subjected to valid clinical trials. An expectation that an effective treatment is imminent is presenting new challenges to health care professionals providing education and care to their clients.

This chapter will examine several interventions recently subjected to clinical trial so readers can become more savvy consumers of the research literature related to SCI. Readers can also use the knowledge to help clients gauge their expectations of current clinical trials and decide if they will participate. Clinical trials of interventions for SCI have been abundant, with more than 300 peer-reviewed articles published between 1999 and 2003.[1] Most of those trials were directed at chronic complications associated with SCI, such as bowel, bladder, and sexual problems; exercise; locomotion; and muscle spasticity and control. The focus of this chapter is on clinical trials that involve pharmacological or invasive experimental procedures and that have the goal of improving neurological recovery in people with SCI. Past, current, and impending clinical trial experiences documented in the scientific literature will be described. A brief review of the pathophysiology of SCI and a description of available preclinical evidence will provide background for the rationale of each experimental intervention. Since a constantly growing number of unsubstantiated experimental treatments are becoming available to people with SCI, a goal of this review is to provide information to help readers recognize reputable and well-designed clinical trials. It will conclude with a discussion of current issues confronting clinical trials and the needs that must be addressed to move forward with valid clinical trials.

Pathophysiology of SCI

In humans, the most common mechanism of SCI is contusion and compression caused by fracture and dislocation of vertebrae. The mechanical insult triggers a cascade of biological events that leads to a complex state of tissue disrepair. While the primary injury directly disrupts a small area of spinal cord tissue and its surrounding vasculature, more damaging secondary events that occur over the course of several weeks often further the destruction. These secondary injury events include swelling, ischemia, excitotoxicity, and inflammation (Fig. 4-1A).

Within minutes of trauma, broken blood vessels cause swelling in the spinal cord that prevents the normal delivery of nutrients and oxygen to the cells. Cells become damaged or die due to ischemia (restriction in blood supply). In addition, damaged cells and vessels release higher than normal amounts of the neurotransmitter glutamate that results in a disruptive process known as *excitotoxicity*. Overexcited cells release highly reactive molecules that attack the cell membranes of healthy neurons, causing their deaths. Later, with the influx and activation of immune system cells, inflammation produces the further release of toxic substances. The initial trauma and these secondary injury mechanisms lead to anatomical changes that include loss of neurons located in the central gray matter. Tissue damage also extends out from the epicenter of the lesion to the surrounding white matter that houses the vital circuitry

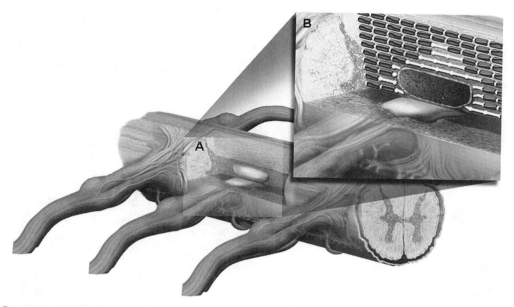

Figure 4-1. Pathophysiology of Spinal Cord Injury: Injury Events A. Primary injury (compression or contusion) leads to secondary injury mechanisms (swelling, ischemia, excitotoxicity, inflammation) that leaves a state of complex neural disrepair. (B) Tissue damage extends outward from the epicenter of the injury, forming a cystic cavity. Neurons and neural glia are lost. Myelin is stripped from the axons. Severed axons retract. Physical and inhibitory neurochemical barriers form on borders of cavities.

for motor and sensory function. Ascending and descending axons become dysfunctional, losing their physical connection due to axotomy, or their conduction capacity due to demyelination. (Fig. 4-1B). Extensive axonal degeneration also occurs as the axon dies back at the lesion site and Wallerian degeneration extends over long distances of the cord (Fig. 4-1B). This degeneration can be seen along the entire length of the affected tract (Fig. 4-2).[2] Postmortem studies also reveal that demyelination in white matter tracts occurs following compressive injury.[3,4]

In addition to damage of the fundamental components that make up the vital circuitry of the spinal cord, the injury also leads to physical and chemical barriers that prevent regeneration. As seen in postmortem pathological studies of human spinal cords, contusive injury often leads to the formation of a cystic cavity, called a *syrinx*, at and around the epicenter of the lesion (Fig. 4-3).[3,4] A physical gap results as a football-shaped cavity gradually extends over several segments above and below the lesion site. In addition to the formation of a physical gap, an inhibitory chemical barrier is produced by the astrocytes, microglia, and oligodendrocytes found within the borders of the cavity.[5] Astrocytes express proteoglycans, and oligodendrocytes release proteins, such as Nogo-A, myelin-associated glycoprotein, and oligodendrocyte-myelin glycoprotein, which inhibits axon regrowth.

When the major ascending and descending pathways that connect the spinal and supraspinal centers are interrupted or become dysfunctional, paralysis and loss of sensation occur. To restore voluntary motor control and sensation, the white matter pathways involved in long-distance communication will likely need to be reestablished. In addition, because SCI also damages

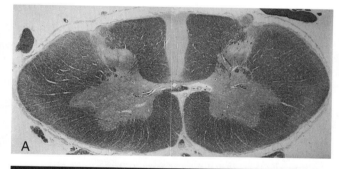

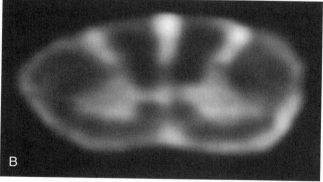

Figure 4-2. Correlation of histology and magnetic resonance images showing Wallerian degeneration in a human 11 years after injury. (A) This low-power image of a section from C8 clearly demonstrates the loss of myelin staining from the Wallerian degenerated pathway in the dorsal columns of this 38-year-old male 11 years after a complete lesion at T12 cord level. (B) The magnetic resonance (MR) image from the same cord shows increased signal intensity in the posterior columns corresponding to the Wallerian degeneration demonstrated by the histology. (Images and postmortem case description courtesy The Miami Project to Cure Paralysis/University of Miami Miller School of Medicine.)

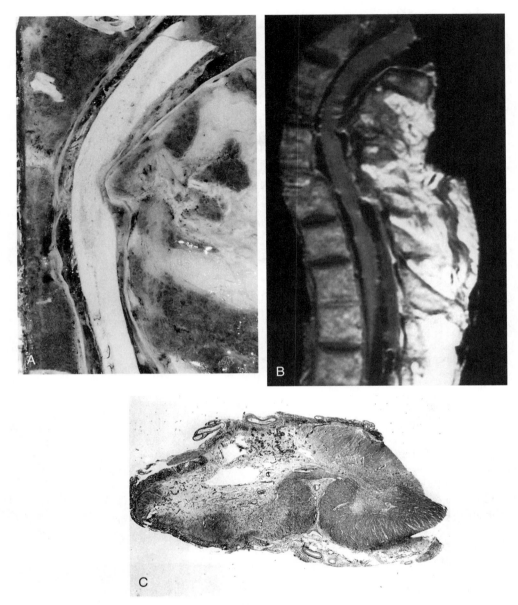

Figure 4-3. These images demonstrate the displacement of a large fragment of bone into the vertebral canal, which has caused damage to one side of the spinal cord. The cryomacrocut preparation (A) can be directly compared to the MR image (B) and correlated with a histological cross section at the level of the fracture (C). This 67-year-old male was injured in a fall, sustaining damage at neurological level C4; his cord was compressed by fractured vertebrae. The MR image and histological sections reveal the loss of neuronal tissue and formation of a cavity in the spinal cord. (Reprinted with permission, The Miami Project to Cure Paralysis/University of Miami Miller School of Medicine. Spring 1994, The Project.)

motoneurons residing in the gray matter of the spinal cord, the injured segment of the spinal cord may need to be restored. Thus, the major hurdles researchers face in their quest for a "cure" are to design treatment strategies that replace damaged or lost neural cells, promote the regrowth and remyelination of axons, and restore vital circuitry.

Potential Strategies for Spinal Cord Repair

Since the early 1980s, as the breadth and depth of new scientific discoveries relevant to SCI have expanded, so

have the possibilities for developing new treatments. An improved understanding of the cellular and molecular biology of SCI as well as the discovery that peripheral nervous system (PNS) tissue could promote axonal regeneration of CNS neurons,[6,7] have dismissed the dogma that the CNS cannot regenerate. In addition to treatment strategies that target regeneration, the possibility of designing cell replacement strategies has come about from studies since the late 1990s showing the potential usefulness of human stem cells.[8-11] These advances have helped to identify therapeutic targets and provide a more positive view regarding the possibility of repairing the damaged spinal cord.

With an improved understanding of the complex state of disrepair after SCI (see Fig. 4-1), researchers are devising a set of strategies directed at protecting and repairing the spinal cord to improve or restore function. In 2005, a review of SCI research was provided when the Institute of Medicine (IOM)[1] convened a 13-member committee made up of experts in neuroscience, clinical research, trauma surgery, health care, physiology, and biomedical engineering. The goal of this review was to assess the full scope of research related to SCI, as well as propose future research directions and provide recommendations for advancing and accelerating progress in the treatment of spinal cord injuries. As a result, the IOM proposed priorities in SCI research aimed at developing neuroprotection therapies, promoting axonal sprouting and growth, steering axonal growth, reestablishing essential neuronal and glial circuitry, preventing acute and chronic complications, and maintaining maximal potential for recovery.[1] Various basic science review papers have proposed strategies that could lead to the goal of protecting and repairing the spinal cord.[5,12-14] The potential targets proposed for future repair generally include (1) preventing further tissue loss, (2) replacing cells that have died, and (3) growing and myelinating axons.

With the completion of several clinical trials, experience has already been gained in some of these areas. An objective of this chapter is to review neuroprotective and repair strategies that have come under evaluation in the clinical arena and for which documentation in scientific proceedings or peer-reviewed journals is available. While a number of neurosurgical and rehabilitative interventions have been or are under investigation, this review will focus on pharmacological approaches and cellular transplantation strategies. Some past, ongoing, and impending experiences with experimental approaches to SCI repair that target preventing neural loss, replacing cells and promoting axon repair will be described.

Clinical Trials Experience Directed at Preventing Further Neural Loss

Over the last quarter century, several experimental neuroprotective therapies have undergone clinical trial in people with acute SCI. These treatments target the neural loss associated with secondary injury mechanisms, which include ischemia, calcium influx, the formation of free radicals, inflammation, and tissue loss. So far, the therapies evaluated for their neuroprotective impact in subjects with acute SCI include the pharmacologic compounds methylprednisolone, GM-1 ganglioside, and gacyclidine, and the cellular implantation of activated macrophages.

Completed Studies in Acute SCI

Methylprednisolone

Methylprednisolone (MP) is a glucocorticoid steroid that exerts an anti-inflammatory effect and may promote neuroprotection by reducing posttraumatic CNS tissue inflammation. Positive preclinical findings showing improved recovery after administration of MP in animals with SCI led to extensive studies of MP in four separate clinical trials. The first trial, the National Acute Spinal Cord Injury Studies (NASCIS),[15] was initiated in 1979. The study enrolled 330 subjects who received either a low dose or a high dose of MP. The results showed no differences in functional outcomes between the two groups. At the same time, however, continued animal research shed some light on the mechanism for action of MP and showed the desired neuroprotective effect may require higher doses of MP than were used in the first clinical study.[16] Thus, NASCIS 2 began in 1985 and was a randomized double-blind, placebo-controlled study that used the dose and timing of treatment based on the new preclinical data. In this trial, Bracken and colleagues[17] assessed American Spinal Injury Association (ASIA) impairment scale (AIS) motor and sensory scores[18] and observed an improvement in those subjects treated within 8 hours of injury. NASCIS 3 commenced to determine if there was a therapeutic window for treatment. Outcomes were compared in subjects who received MP over a 24-hour period (as in NASCIS 2) versus one of two regimens of MP administered over a 48-hour period.[19,20] The results led the study authors to conclude that the treatment regimen should be maintained for 24 hours if administration of MP occurs within 3 hours of injury and for 48 hours if MP is initiated between 3 and 8 hours. Beside the NASCIS studies, several review papers[16,21] report that a Japanese study evaluating MP essentially corroborate the findings of NASCIS 2 but in a smaller number of subjects.

While these trials suggested neurological improvements, the NASCIS studies generated marked controversy. In NASCIS 2, the investigators saw a treatment effect in a subgroup of subjects who received the drug within 8 hours, but not in the overall treatment group. When the investigators compared this subgroup to those treated with placebo, changes in scores reached significance for motor function (16.0 versus 11.2), pinprick sensation (11.4 versus 6.6), and light touch (8.9 versus 4.3).[17] Because this subgroup analysis was not part of the original study design, critics considered these observations to be a post-hoc analysis, thus weakening the significance of the findings.[22,23] Further work by others suggests that possible serious complications occur when MP is administered over prolonged periods[24-26] and that MP is not effective in penetrating spinal injuries.[27,28] More recent evidence suggests that MP causes myopathy, and the improvements in motor and sensory function reported in the NASCIS studies may actually be a recovery from this adverse effect once the MP regimen was completed.[29] Because of these concerns, the American Association of Neurological Surgeons and the Congress of Neurological Surgeons[30] have taken the position that insufficient evidence exists to support the use of MP in acute SCI as a treatment standard. The use of MP remains a treatment option prescribed at the discretion of the treating physician.

GM-1 ganglioside

GM-1 ganglioside is a naturally occurring glycolipid that integrates into the outer membranes of cells, including nerve cells. While the specific mechanism of action of GM-1 is unclear, laboratory studies have suggested that gangliosides prevent apoptosis (programmed cell death) and induce neuronal sprouting. When applied in animal models of CNS injury, this drug had been shown to enhance neuronal plasticity[31] and regeneration,[32] and it also has neuroprotective effects.[33] Following clinical trials of GM-1 in subjects with stroke,[34] a single-center study involving individuals with SCI was initiated.[35] Geisler and colleagues[36] reported a significant treatment effect in a trial with 37 subjects with acute SCI randomized to receive either GM-1 or placebo. They observed two grades of improvement on the Frankel scale[37] in 50% of subjects in the GM-1 group versus 7.1% of subjects in the placebo group. Based on these findings and others,[38] a multicenter study of GM-1 in acute SCI commenced and accrued a total of 760 subjects.[39-41] To date, this has been the largest clinical trial ever conducted for an SCI intervention. The randomized, double-blind trial compared low-dose and high-dose GM-1 to placebo. Outcomes included the ASIA motor, sensory, and impairment scales and the Modified Benzel Classification.[42] In an a priori design, the investigators defined "marked recovery" as a two-grade improvement, as had been seen in the first study. Overall results showed no differences in the ASIA assessments between treatment and placebo groups at the 6-month end point. GM-1-treated subjects, however, showed earlier recovery at the 8-week follow-up than placebo-treated subjects, and those with incomplete injuries appeared to benefit when subgroup analyses were performed. Even though significance and efficacy were not established and U.S. Food and Drug Administration (FDA) approval was not attained, these studies generated considerable and valuable data that Fawcett and colleagues[43] recently analyzed to examine the natural history of spontaneous recovery.

Gacyclidine

Gacyclidine is a receptor blocker that may reduce excitotoxic cell death by antagonizing N-methyl D-aspartate (NMDA) receptors. After CNS trauma, the concentration of the excitatory neurotransmitter glutamate increases dramatically. Glutamate activates NMDA receptors leading to an excitotoxic influx of calcium into neurons. The hypothesis that gacyclidine might prevent nerve cell death by blocking NMDA receptors was examined in preclinical studies.[44,45] After a neuroprotective effect in spinally injured rodents had been demonstrated, Tadie and colleagues[46] in France tested gacyclidine in a large SCI clinical trial. While no peer-reviewed reports have been published, the study has been discussed at scientific conferences and described in various review articles.[16,21,47] The trial enrolled 280 subjects with acute SCI who received intravenous administration of gacyclidine or placebo within 2 hours of injury. All subjects were randomized and underwent surgical decompression or fixation if indicated. The investigators assessed neurological outcomes over a 1-year period using the ASIA scores. The overall results indicated no statistically significant neurologic benefit in the treatment group, although the findings in a subgroup of subjects with incomplete cervical injury suggest improvements in motor scores both at 1-month and at 1-year follow-up. Despite these benefits, further development of gacyclidine was suspended.[21]

In general, the aforementioned studies did not definitively demonstrate the efficacy of MP, GM-1 ganglioside, and gacyclidine. They have shown, however, that large multicenter randomized SCI trials involving individuals with acute SCI can be performed. The experience gained from these trials calls attention to the complexities of clinical trials and shows that successful implementation of future clinical trials will require considerable planning and attention to study design.

Ongoing Studies in Acute SCI

Procord

Procord (activated macrophages) is a treatment approach for acute SCI that uses macrophages, the immune system cells that show wound-healing properties in most tissues. Macrophages may help in repair of injured tissue by removing damaging tissue debris and secreting growth factors that promote the early phases of the wound healing.[48] While macrophages serve this function in the PNS and tissues outside the CNS, they do not play a robust role in wound-healing within the CNS.[49] Researchers hypothesize that a compromised recruitment of macrophages into the CNS may contribute to the lack of neurological recovery after CNS injury.[50,51]

To potentiate a beneficial immune response within the spinal cord, Michal Schwartz and colleagues at the Weizman Institute in Israel designed a treatment to enhance macrophage activity.[48] The goal of this treatment is to produce a neuroprotective effect and facilitate axonal regeneration. To activate the macrophages, the investigators co-cultured them with peripheral nerve. In preclinical experiments in adult rats with complete spinal cord transection, injection of activated macrophages resulted in partial motor recovery.[52]

The clinical evaluation of the Procord (activated macrophage) treatment represents one of the first major studies of cellular transplantation in acute human SCI. Sponsored by Proneuron Biotechnologies, Ltd., the first Phase 1 trial started in 2000 and had study sites in Israel and Belgium. For the human studies, the authors developed a clinically feasible procedure to activate the cells. Instead of using injured peripheral nerve, the source of activating tissue was an autologous skin biopsy.[53] Activating the macrophages by exposure to the skin appears to enhance the synthesis of trophic factors that may promote neuroprotection and axon regeneration.[53,54] The first trial enrolled 16 subjects with complete AIS A neurologic injuries at spinal levels C5 to T11.[55] To meet the inclusion criteria, subjects had to be screened, enrolled, and treated within 14 days of their injury. The day before treatment, the subject's macrophages obtained from blood samples were co-cultured with a full-thickness skin sample derived from the subject. On the day of implantation, the investigators surgically exposed the spinal cord and injected four divided doses of activated macrophages just caudal to the spinal cord lesion. Assessments of the research subjects took place over a 1-year period using outcome measures that included the ASIA sensory and motor assessment, Functional Independence Measure (FIM), a modified Ashworth spasticity index, Quality of Life scales, somatosensory evoked potentials (SSEP), motor evoked potentials (MEP), and magnetic resonance imaging (MRI). All the study subjects were classified as AIS A at enrollment, and the results showed modest improvements in five individuals: three improved from AIS A to C, and two improved from AIS A to B.[55]

This small Phase 1 study led to Phase 2 trials at five centers in the United States.[56] The specific inclusion criteria for this study were traumatic SCI within 14 days and an injury level between C5 and T11. Subjects were between the ages of 16 and 65, had neurologically complete AIS A injuries, and were randomized into treatment and control groups. The subjects in the control group received standard rehabilitative care but were not subjected to a surgical transplantation procedure. The study included follow-up assessments carried out over 12 months. Proneuron had been enrolling subjects for this Phase 2 trial until early 2006, when they announced suspension of the study, making it clear the suspension was not for clinical or safety reasons.[56] Clinical follow-up of individuals enrolled at that time was to continue for the full 12-month follow-up.

Clinical Trials Experience Directed at Replacing Cells

One component of SCI pathology is neuronal cell death that occurs primarily by mechanical impact or secondarily by apoptosis, inflammation, or necrotic mechanisms. In addition, the nonneuronal cells that have a supportive role in the nervous system—astrocytes, microglia and oligodendrocytes—may die. Several clinical trials have or are using tissue or cellular transplantations to target this cell loss.

Completed Studies in Chronic SCI

Human Fetal Tissue Transplantation

Human fetal tissue transplantation was the first SCI cellular transplant study documented in the United States. In the early 1990s, Reier and colleagues at the University of Florida in Gainesville[57,58] and Falci and colleagues at the Karolinska Institute in Sweden[59] evaluated the use of human fetal tissue grafts in nine subjects with chronic SCI and clinical symptoms of syringomyelia. This treatment approach was based on extensive experience with grafting embryonic and fetal tissue in animal models of SCI.[60-62] Fetal neural tissue gathered from multiple fetuses was transplanted into the fluid-filled cysts. The subjects were followed for at least 2 years to determine if the size of the cavity was reduced and whether the disease process stabilized. The results showed the cysts were smaller and the subjects experienced no serious adverse effects.[57,58] While questions remain regarding the survival of the graft tissue, and the therapeutic and long-term benefits, the study authors report the procedure appears safe.[51] The study was suspended before reaching its full enrollment of 10 subjects when in November 2000, the FDA served notice that cell and tissue transplantation required, from that point on, an Investigational New Drug (IND) application. For this and other reasons, the investigators suspended the study.[51]

Porcine Fetal Oligodendrocyte Precursor Implants

The use of porcine fetal oligodendrocyte precursor implants, initiated in 2001 by McDonald and Becker[63] and supported by Diacrin, Inc., was another transplant trial carried out in the United States in subjects with SCI. Oligodendrocyte precursors may give rise to oligodendrocytes, the myelin-forming cells of the CNS. The rationale for their use is based on the assumption that surviving axons at the injury site are chronically demyelinated[64,65] and might be repaired by transplanting myelinating cells.[66,67] The study, carried out at Washington University in St. Louis, Missouri and Albany Medical Center in Albany, New York, included six subjects with traumatic SCI who were one year or more post-injury. The subjects received transplants of fetal porcine oligodendrocyte precursor cells into the spinal cord and were followed for several years. According to reports at scientific conferences,[47] collection of the final outcome data was scheduled for completion in 2004 and publication of the results was to follow. So far, however, peer-reviewed reports of the study results have yet to be published.

Ongoing Studies in Acute and Chronic SCI

Bone Marrow Stromal Cells

Bone marrow stromal cells (BMS) are hemopoietic cells that have characteristics similar to stem cells. Various research studies suggest they have the ability to give rise to neurons and glia.[68,69] Thus, BMS cells may serve as a source of cells to replace lost or damaged neural cells. In addition to their potential differentiation into neural components, BMS cells are appealing because they can be harvested easily and cultivated for autologous transplantation.

Several preclinical studies of bone marrow stromal cells transplants in spinal cord contusion models have shown some degree of locomotor recovery. Chopp and colleagues[70] injected BMS cells into the epicenter of spinal lesions of rats 1 week after contusive injury. Significant motor function improvements were noted in the treatment group compared with the control group. Similarly, Hofstetter and colleagues[71] injected BMS cells into three sites: the epicenter, and rostral and caudal to the lesion site. The injections were done either immediately after contusion or 1 week after injury. Only animals that received the injections at 1 week showed significant improvements in the motor function. While these studies demonstrate functional improvements, the mechanism for the outcomes is still unclear. Investigators hypothesize the transplanted cells integrate into the spinal cord and replace damaged cells or they express factors that promote repair.[70] Other studies using MRI imaging to visualize the transplanted cells[72,73] have confirmed the BMS cells have an ability to migrate to the lesion site.[74] These experiences appear to confirm the feasibility of this treatment approach and have led to a clinical application.

Initiation of autologous BMS cell treatments in subjects with SCI was announced by Sykova and colleagues from the Czech Republic at a scientific conference in 2004.[51,75] At that time, two subjects with paraplegia and seven subjects with tetraplegia had been treated with the cells delivered via angiography to the vertebral artery. The subjects were in two groups: an early group (between 11 and 30 days post-injury) and a late group (2 and 17.5 months post-injury). Six of the nine subjects showed varying degrees of improvement. The initial description of the procedure at scientific conferences was then followed by a published report in 2006 in which the investigators summarize the results in 20 subjects with complete traumatic SCI.[75] This report included 20 subjects divided into subacute (n = 8) and chronic (n = 12) groups. Some received injection of the cells via the vertebral artery and others intravenously. While the report indicates that ASIA and Frankel scores and MEP and SEPs were assessed, the individual outcome measures were not documented in this publication. The investigators report partial improvement in ASIA scores stating, "the improved ASIA outcome was mostly from a score of A to B, in one case from B to D."[75] They also report recovery of MEP and SEP in four of four subacute subjects receiving the cells via the vertebral artery and in one subacute subject receiving the cells intravenously. The authors recognize that conclusions about efficacy will require a larger study population. Based on their current experience, however, they have concluded implantation of autologous BMS cells is safe and that implantation within 3 to 4 weeks of injury and via the vertebral artery may be important for better outcome.[75]

At a scientific meeting, Barros and colleagues in Brazil described their experience with the infusion of autologous bone marrow cells into the anterior spinal artery in 32 people with chronic complete SCI.[47] Based on outcome measures that included SSEPs, this group reported that 15 of 32 people showed improvement in lower extremity SSEPs and some modest functional improvements. The account of the scientific meeting did not provide details about the tools used to measure outcomes nor how the investigators concluded there were modest improvements. To date, no peer-reviewed published results are available from Barros and colleagues. Meanwhile, other investigators in Brazil have announced their experience in using an alternative and less invasive route for delivery of the cells. Callera and colleagues[76] conclude from observations in 10 subjects that delivery of BMS cells via lumbar puncture is feasible though the therapeutic effects of the implant remain to be elucidated.

Park and colleagues[77] in South Korea have also injected BMS cells in humans with complete cervical SCI and deem the procedure safe. In addition to the BMS cells, granulocyte macrophage colony-stimulating factor (GM-CSF) was administered. GM-CSF is a factor that stimulates hematopoietic stem cell proliferation and differentiation. In the nervous system, it activates macrophages that may remove myelin debris that is inhibitory to axon regeneration. Five of six subjects in the study received injection of the cells in six locations surrounding the spinal contusion site. All subjects received subcutaneous injections of GM-CSF given in five doses over the course of a month. Four subjects improved from AIS A to C, one subject from AIS A to B, and one subject remained AIS A. Some sensory improvements were also noted. While no serious adverse effects were noted, the preliminary data are insufficient to determine the efficacy of BMS cell and

GM-CSF treatment, but do support further study in a more comprehensive multicenter study.[77]

Impending Study in Acute SCI

Human Embryonic Stem Cells

Human embryonic stem cells (hESCs) may serve as a source of cells to replace the neuronal and glial cells lost in SCI. Since demyelination is a component of the pathology in human SCI, a potential treatment strategy involves transplantation of hESCs from which myelin-producing oligodendrocytes may be derived. Treatment strategies such as this are based on the increasing body of knowledge concerning hESCs.[11] Keirstead and colleagues[10] have shown enhanced remyelination and significant functional improvement after transplantation of the hESCs into spinal cord-injured rats 7 days after injury. However, animals transplanted at 10 months post injury showed no improvements. Based on these studies, plans to initiate a clinical trial to evaluate the safety of human embryonic oligodendrocyte progenitor cell transplants in subjects with acute SCI have been made by Geron, Inc.[78] After four years of discussion with the FDA and completion of recommended preclinical animal toxicology and efficacy studies, Geron filed an IND application. As of May 2008, the FDA had put the clinical trial on hold.[79]

Clinical Trials Experience Directed at Growing and Myelinating Axons

Reestablishment of critical spinal circuitry is a major goal in SCI "cure" research. Enhancing regeneration and remyelination of severed or damaged CNS axons is a first step in restoring connectivity. Many approaches to improve the function of damaged axons are under evaluation in basic science studies and include administration of agents and cellular components to improve nerve conduction, promote regeneration, and counteract the inhibitory CNS environment. Some of these approaches are now being applied in experimental procedures in humans.

Completed Studies in Chronic SCI

4-Aminopyridine

In preclinical studies, the potassium channel blocker 4-aminopyridine (4-AP) was associated with enhanced action potential conduction across chronically damaged axons at the site of spinal cord injury. [80,81] Demyelination, a component of human injury, causes potassium to leak from axons thereby preventing transmission of the action potentials. Investigators hypothesized that blocking the loss of potassium with administration of 4-AP (fampridine) would enhance conduction and improve function.

Several SCI clinical trials sponsored by Acorda Therapeutics evaluated the effect of 4-AP in subjects with chronic incomplete injuries. In some studies, the results were positive and included gains in motor function, sensation, and independence, as well as decreased spasticity. [82-84] Other studies,[85,86] however, report no benefit in functional status and no changes in muscle force or improvements in gait analysis. Because the clinical trials have not provided sufficient or definitive evidence of efficacy, the FDA has not given approval and Acorda has suspended the trials in SCI.[87] One possible explanation for the diversity in results is the difficulty in determining which subjects have intact but chronically dysfunctioning axons across their injury site that could potentially respond to 4-AP.

Ongoing Studies in Acute SCI

Oscillating Field Stimulation

Oscillating field stimulation (OFS) is an experimental intervention for acute SCI that involves implantation of a device that emits a weak electrical field across a spinal lesion. Studies in developmental biology suggest electrical field gradients guide cranial-to-caudal neural tube development. In vivo studies in sea lamprey have shown the negative pole of an electric field cathode can attract regenerating axons.[88] In guinea pigs, application of an electric field for a period of 3 weeks promoted axonal regeneration and led to functional improvements.[89] The findings also suggest an electric field reduces the number of astrocytes in the injury, which may reduce formation of glial scars. Thus, OFS is a potential treatment to stimulate axon growth.

To promote regeneration in both ascending and descending neurons, the investigators hypothesized that oscillation of the polarity of the electrical field may be needed. The OFS device was designed to change the polarity every 15 minutes. In a preclinical randomized controlled trial, Borgens and colleagues[90] at Purdue University in Indiana implanted the OFS device within 18 days of onset of paraplegia into 20 dogs with complete paralysis by natural causes. The OFS-treated dogs were compared to 14 sham-operated dogs. Over a 6-month period, the outcomes were measured by various neurological assessments including standard reflex testing, urologic tests, urodynamic testing, tests for deep and superficial pain appreciation, proprioceptive placing of the hind limbs, ambulation, and evoked potential testing. The data showed that OFS-treated dogs had greater improvement in functional outcomes than the sham-treated animals. These studies laid the foundation for a recent human trial.

A Phase 1 trial of OFS was carried out by Shapiro and colleagues[91] at Indiana University Medical Center in Indianapolis, Indiana. The study was designed to assess safety in 10 subjects with complete injuries. The newly injured participants were between the ages of 18 and 65 years old, had injuries ranging from the C5 to T10, and had no cord transection as confirmed by MRI. Before OFS implantation, subjects received customary acute care with methylprednisolone and surgical intervention for cord compression or vertebral instability. Then, in a separate operation within 18 days of injury, the subjects had implantation of the cylindrical OFS device into their paraspinal musculature. Two sets of three electrodes extending from the device were sutured to the spinous process and facets at one segment above and below the injury site.

The subjects underwent assessments of the incision site, pain levels, the function of the OFS device, and neurological function every 2 weeks. At 15 weeks after implantation, the device was removed. Formal neurological testing using ASIA scores, visual analog scale (VAS) pain scores, and SSEPs were done at 6 weeks, 6 months, and 1 year. Statistically significant improvements in ASIA scores were noted in the areas of light touch, pinprick sensation, and motor function. Because no control subjects were included in this Phase 1 study, the overall efficacy could not be directly evaluated. Since some recovery is routine during the post-injury period, the improvements in OFS-treated subjects were compared to improvements noted in subjects included in the third NASCIS trial. At the 12-month assessment, OFS-treated subjects compared to subjects in the NASCIS 3 study showed a mean increase of 25.5 versus 0.5 points in light touch sensation, an increase of 20.4 versus 0.6 points for pinprick sensation, and an increase of 6.3 points versus 3.0 in motor function. According to the study authors, this comparison strongly suggested that OFS therapy exerts beneficial effects after acute injury in humans and warranted further study.[91] As no complications were noted in any of the subjects and the outcomes measured suggest a beneficial effect, the OFS device is expected to be taken to market if an application to classify it as a Humanitarian Use Device is accepted by the FDA.[92]

Cethrin

The drug Cethrin has the potential to offset the inhibitory environment that is characteristic of the CNS and that contributes to the failure of axons to regenerate. When neurons send out new axons in an attempt to regenerate, their growing tips (growth cones) are influenced by various molecular and receptor-mediated signals. An important signal pathway for turning axon growth on or off is one associated with the intracellular enzyme, Rho. In a developing neuron, when Rho is inactive, growth cones extend to find their paths. When Rho is active, growth cones collapse.

Recent investigations provide evidence that CNS injury dramatically increases activation of Rho[93] and thus, any attempts for regeneration by injured neurons are thwarted. Rho activation also occurs when inhibitory proteins outside the cell act on receptors on the neuron. CNS myelin contains inhibitory proteins such as Nogo, myelin-associated glycoprotein, and oligodendrocyte-myelin glycoprotein. When these proteins bind to the receptors, Rho is activated. In addition to serving as a switch for collapse of growth cones, Rho activation has been associated with apoptosis. Therefore, the Rho signaling pathway is thought to be a good target for the prevention of cell death and promotion of regeneration.

Various basic science studies have been conducted to identify factors and treatments to block the inhibition of axon growth.[94,95] One approach targets Rho and was developed by McKerracher and colleagues[94] at the University of Montreal. In their preclinical study involving mice, a Rho antagonist, C3 transferase, was used to treat acute spinal cord lesions. C3 transferase is a naturally occurring protein that specifically inhibits Rho. The investigators administered C3 transferase immediately following a dorsal hemisection of the spinal cord at T7. Results showed inhibition and even reversal of abnormal Rho activation, significant reduction of apoptosis at the site of injury, promotion of axonal regeneration, and functional recovery in animals after SCI as measured by hind limb movements using a common locomotor rating scale.[94]

A clinical trial currently sponsored by Alseres Pharmaceuticals, Inc. was initiated in 2005 and is ongoing with the drug Cethrin.[96] Cethrin is a combination of fibrin sealant with BA-210, a form of C3 transferase engineered to enhance its ability to enter mammalian cells. The initial study enrolled men and women between the ages of 16 and 70 years who have acute AIS A spinal cord injury. Cethrin is administered at the site of the spinal cord lesion in subjects undergoing spinal stabilization or decompression surgery within 7 days of injury. The purpose of this study was to determine the safety and tolerability of Cethrin when administered as a single extradural application. Enrollment included 48 subjects at nine clinical sites in Canada and the United States. After analyzing the 12-month data, Alseres Pharmaceuticals announced that the treatment is well-tolerated and appears safe, and the data suggests a trend toward efficacy. Based on these findings, they are planning for a double-blind, randomized, placebo-controlled, multi-center, Phase 2 study to further test efficacy.[97]

Ongoing studies in Chronic SCI

Peripheral Nerve Grafts

Peripheral nerve grafts may provide a supportive scaffold for regenerating axons and help reestablish important circuitry. It has long been known the peripheral nerve environment is permissive for axonal regeneration. Research in rats in the early 1980s by Richardson, Aguayo, and colleagues[6] showed when peripheral nerve segments were inserted into the gap of severed spinal cord, the cut axons from both sides of the transaction regrew into the implanted nerve. For recovery of function following chronic SCI, it is likely that regeneration of long fiber tracts that extend through and beyond the lesion site is required. Beside peripheral nerve grafts, several experimental studies have shown that regenerating axons can grow beyond a lesion site when an appropriate PNS environment is provided. For example, studies from the laboratory of Bunge and colleagues[98,99] at The Miami Project to Cure Paralysis have long focused on transplantation of Schwann cells and/or olfactory ensheathing glia.[100,101]

Autologous peripheral nerve grafts may serve as bridges to foster axonal regeneration across transected regions of SCI. A highly publicized preclinical study in 1996 by Cheng and Olson[102] at the Karolinska Institute in Sweden, provided the basis for this approach. In this study, the investigators placed peripheral nerve grafts in rats with complete spinal cord transection. The grafts were aligned to route regenerating white matter tract axons into gray matter, believed to be more permissive for axonal regeneration. The grafts were also combined with acidic fibroblast growth factor (aFGF)-impregnated fibrin glue and rigid spinal column fixation. A normal component of the spinal cord, aFGF is thought to enhance nerve fiber development. During the first 6 months after the procedure, the rat's hind limb function improved progressively, and corticospinal tract fibers regenerated through the grafted area to the lumbar enlargement. The results of this study generated much enthusiasm, and several research groups attempted to replicate it.[103,104] While no group has fully replicated the dramatic results reported, the study by Lin and colleagues[103] corroborates the use of peripheral grafts with the aFGF fibrin glue.

The clinical application of peripheral nerve grafts has been initiated by several clinicians. Cheng and colleagues[105] in Taiwan published a case report in which significant motor recovery was achieved in a subject with T11 partial SCI from a stab wound 4 years prior to transplantation. The report describes the use of four autologous sural nerve grafts transplanted to span across the gap in the spinal cord. The grafted area was sealed with fibrin glue mixed with aFGF. Interestingly, this subject was classified as an AIS C injury prior to the surgery. Motor scores on the right and left legs were 12 and 0, respectively. Two and a half years after the surgery, motor scores improved to 15 and 12. Sensory scores also improved. The subject recovered to AIS D, becoming ambulatory with a walker. In addition to this formal case report, unconfirmed Internet reports suggest Cheng and colleagues have performed the procedure in more than 50 individuals. Further peer-reviewed accounts, however, have not yet surfaced.

Other investigators have reported the use of different surgical approaches to bypass the lesion site with peripheral nerve grafts.[106,107] The approach involves implantation of nerve grafts to connect sites above the lesion to ventral nerve roots below thoracic lesions. In a 52-year old subject with T9 complete paralysis for 3 years, Tadie and colleagues[106] in France report implantation of autologous sural nerves into the right and left ventral horn of the cord at T7–8 levels. The other end of the sural nerve was then connected to L2–4 lumbar ventral roots. Eight months after the surgery, the subject had voluntary contractions of the bilateral adductors and the left quadriceps. Motor-evoked potentials from these muscles were recorded by transcranial magnetic stimulation and confirmed when the subject attempted to contract the muscles. In another case, Brunelli and colleagues[107] in Italy describe a similar procedure performed in a young woman 4 months after her T9 complete injury. Voluntary movements of the targeted muscles were first seen 17 months after the procedure, and 27 months after the procedure she was able to walk with the help of a walker.

The peripheral nerve graft procedures described above involve obtaining explanted autologous peripheral nerve tissue for implantation. Zhang and colleagues[108] describes using a different approach in which they reroute peripheral nerves from above the spinal lesion and connect them to nerves or nerve roots below the injury. For example, after releasing an intercostal nerve from its normal location near the rib cage, the distal end is transferred to the vertebral canal through a submuscle tunnel and sutured into the target nerve roots below the injury. If the intercostal nerve was not long enough to reach the intended nerve root below the injury, a sural nerve was isolated and grafted to the intercostal nerve. Zhang reports that 23 subjects with injuries between T9 and T12 received this surgical approach, and 18 regained an ability to walk with crutches or other assistive devices. Some of these data obtained from the experimental application of peripheral nerve grafts suggest that delayed surgical reconstruction of motor pathways may contribute to partial functional recovery.[108]

Olfactory Ensheathing Cells

Specialized glial cells, olfactory ensheathing cells (OEC), are housed in the olfactory bulb. They are attractive cellular transplant candidates for SCI because under normal circumstances they help to support regeneration of axons from the olfactory bulb *into* the CNS throughout life.[109] One of the challenges in regeneration research is not only sufficient elongation of regenerating axons, but also their reentry into host tissue caudal to the lesion. While long-tract regeneration has been achieved in preclinical studies, the reentry of fibers into the inhibitory environment of the host spinal cord presents a problem. In addition to supporting regeneration, OECs might enhance reentry of fibers because of their unique ability to migrate and integrate within the CNS.[13,100,110]

Several groups have transplanted OECs into experimental spinal cord injury models and reported recovery of function after lesions of the corticospinal tract,[111] and recovery of coordinated walking after complete cord transection.[101,112] In rodent studies, the primary OECs are fairly easy to harvest from the olfactory bulb. In humans, however, harvesting OECs would require intracranial surgery and thus is not very feasible. An alternative approach, lending to a more realistic application in humans, is to harvest and culture OECs from the olfactory mucosa. Lu and colleagues[113,114] demonstrated that OECs derived from the mucosa and transplanted into the completely transected spinal cord of the adult rat promoted improved locomotor function. This group also reported regeneration and recovery in rodents after a delayed transplantation of the mucosal cells.

Based on these favorable preclinical experiments, Feron and colleagues[115] in Australia initiated a Phase 1 clinical trial of adult-derived mucosal OEC transplants. The study enrolled six male subjects between the ages of 18 and 55 who had complete injuries between T4 and T10 and were between 18 and 32 months post-injury. Three subjects were treated with a surgical implantation of autologous mucosal OECs. Another three subjects served as the control group. Nasal biopsies were obtained from the subjects and OECs were isolated, purified, and expanded in a 6-week process for autotransplantation. When there were enough cells, a laminectomy was performed and the dura opened. The investigators inserted the cells into the spinal cord by multiple injections around and within the injury area. They scheduled collection of outcome data at 3-month intervals over 2 years and again at 3 years. The study and control subjects underwent physical, medical, and psychosocial assessments in a blinded fashion. X-rays, MRIs, neurological and electrophysiological testing were also performed. After collecting the 1-year follow-up data, a preliminary peer-reviewed published report indicated no medical, surgical, or other complications and the authors concluded that this method for transplantation of OECs is feasible and safe.[115] Final results are pending completion of the final third-year assessment to confirm the long-term safety and whether neurological function was affected.

According to Internet reports,[116] Lima and colleagues in Portugal have also performed transplants since July 2001 in 70 or more people with chronic SCI. In a slightly different surgical approach, autologous olfactory mucosal tissue is harvested from the nasal cavity and minced. During the same operation and after debridement of scar tissue in the injury area, the minced mucosal tissue is implanted into the spinal cord. In 2004 at a scientific conference, Lima gave an account of his experience with the procedure and outcomes that included ASIA scores, MEP, SSEP, and MRI scans.[47] The surgeon reported that subjects experienced decreased spasticity, and had some improvements in autonomic and bladder function. No improvements in touch, pinprick, or motor function were noted.[47] Later, Lima and colleagues[117] offered their first

peer-reviewed account describing the procedure in seven subjects with injury levels between C6 and T6, who were classified as AIS A or B. Subjects were between the ages of 18 and 32 and between 6 months and 6.5 years post-injury. The results showed the transplanted tissue, via visualization on MRI, survived and filled cavities within the spinal cord. Improvements in AIS motor scores were noted in all subjects, and ASIA sensory scores increased in all but one subject. Two of seven subjects improved from AIS A to AIS C. Two subjects reported a return of sensations in the bladder. Based on these findings and because they saw no serious adverse effects, the authors suggest further investigation.

In evaluating this pilot study,[118] Kirshblum offered commentary on its design and pointed out its limitations. The study was not blinded, and did not include placebo-controlled comparisons. Limited conclusions can be made because it included subjects with both tetraplegia and paraplegia, with both AIS A and B classifications, and varying times post-injury. While Lima reports subjects had improvements in quality of life, Kirshblum notes that no quality of life assessment tools were used to measure a change. Similarly, the reported changes in bladder function were not substantiated with urodynamic testing. While there were limitations in this study, Kirshblum asserted publication of Lima's data was important stating, "It is hoped that much can be learned from this trial and a randomized controlled trial can be discussed after analysis of the patients who have already undergone the treatment."

Another experimental procedure using fetal olfactory tissue has been performed in more than 400 people with varying levels and degrees of chronic injury by Huang of Beijing, China. In a scientific presentation,[47] the procedure was described as an injection of transplant material cultured from the olfactory bulb of a human fetus at 12 to 16 weeks gestation. The olfactory bulb-derived material is processed over a 10- to 14-day period and 1 million cells are injected rostral and caudal to the injury site. Although the identity of the transplanted cells has not been established nor published, the surgeon claims the transplanted cells are OECs.

This experimental treatment has been of particular interest for several reasons. First, papers published by Huang and colleagues in 2003[119] and 2006[120] note rapid improvements in the motor and sensory function within 2 to 3 days of transplantation. They observed this in 300 people with chronic SCI with duration ranging from 6 months to 31 years. After publication of the findings in 2003, other scientists visited this clinic and were allowed to observe a limited number of cases. Guest and colleagues[121] documented a single case report of an 18-year-old C3 AIS A motor and sensory complete who was neurologically stable at 18 months post-injury. These authors found the subject had improved to C5 motor and C4 sensory AIS A within

48 hours following transplantation of cultured fetal olfactory bulb-derived cells.

Another reason for heightened interest in this particular treatment series is the report of postoperative complications and unconfirmed neurological benefits. A case series published in 2006 reports postoperative meningitis in five of seven people assessed by independent investigators.[122] In this small case series, Dobkin and colleagues found no motor, sensory, or functional changes in six of seven subjects after at least a 3-month follow-up. The paper was critical of the lack of control groups and systematic long-term follow-up and was referenced in a recent warning about the procedure published in the journal *Nature*.[123] In April 2006, in a Chinese journal, Huang documented a 38-month follow-up of 16 subjects with chronic SCI who received the OEC procedure. He reported no cell-related adverse effects from the procedure and concludes long-term safety.[124]

Whereas large numbers of people have undergone procedures involving the use of OECs, currently, the experience of the clinicians with the largest number of subjects is difficult to evaluate because of a lack of control groups and systematic follow-up, which limits the ability to derive objective data.[47,122,123]

Newly Initiated Trials in Acute SCI

IN-1

The antibody IN-1 neutralizes the myelin-associated protein Nogo-A. Nogo-A is a strong inhibitor of nerve growth that is expressed mainly by oligodendrocytes in the CNS. After first identifying Noga-A in the late 1980s, Schwab and colleagues[125,126] at the University of Zurich, Switzerland, developed a monoclonal antibody IN-1 to neutralize the inhibitory effect of Noga-A. Experiments performed on rats with SCI showed sprouting of corticospinal fibers and recovery of locomotor function.[127,128] A humanized form of IN-1 administered to rats also showed long-distance axonal regeneration through and beyond the lesion.[129] As the presence of Noga-A has been confirmed in humans,[130,131] neutralization of this nerve growth inhibitor is a potential treatment option for subjects with SCI. To assess the feasibility of IN-1 treatment in humans, Schwab and colleagues[132] administered IN-1 to adult Marmoset monkeys with partial hemisection. As in previous results with rats, they found the treatment enhanced regeneration of the lesioned corticospinal tract. Based on this preclinical work, the pharmaceutical company Novartis is supporting a clinical trial in Europe directed at evaluating the safety and efficacy of IN-1 (the clinical trial drug is referred to as *ATI355*) in acute SCI. The trial commenced in 2006 and expects to complete enrollment in late 2009.[133]

Future Directions: Accelerating Progress with Scientific Rigor

Exciting new findings from basic science laboratories are revealing and will continue to reveal new treatment possibilities. An increasing number of experimental procedures, as may be seen by a current search of the Internet, are now available to people with SCI. Unfortunately, some of these procedures are based on little or no scientific evidence or, in the opinion of some scientists, bear little resemblance to valid or well-designed studies. Questions are arising about which promising preclinical strategies should advance to clinical trial, when this should occur, and what study design should be used. To advance and accelerate the science of SCI research, committed and coordinated interactions between basic, translational and clinical scientists will be required. Experience gained from previous and current clinical trials confirm the importance of scientific rigor and the need to safely convert promising preclinical findings into new treatments.

Within the international SCI research community, serious discussions are underway regarding the essential principles for planning and developing a clinical trial for SCI.[47,134] The impetus for this effort came from meetings organized in 2003 and 2004 by the National Institute of Neurological Disorders and Stroke (NINDS)[12] and the ICCP (International Campaign for Cures for Spinal Cord Paralysis).[47] These collective international discussions have identified several important issues for the future of clinical trials in SCI, some of which are reviewed below.

Need for Sufficient Evidence

One concern regarding the translation of a preclinical treatment to the clinical setting is whether sufficient evidence has been obtained and documented to justify advancing with a clinical trial.[1] Groups of international colleagues in SCI research have proposed guidelines for the conduct of studies of human subjects with SCI.[43,134-137] Published in 2005 and 2007, the guidelines offer recommendations for planning and carrying out clinical research studies. In general, the documents suggest that clinical studies should be designed only after preclinical animal studies establish efficacy, findings are presented in peer-reviewed meetings and publications, and results are replicated. An example of an experimental therapy for SCI that lacked substantiated preclinical evidence, replication and documentation is the transplantation of embryonic shark cells in humans with SCI. This procedure, in which cells from the blue shark are inserted into the spinal cord lesion, was initiated in the early 1990s and is still being offered in Tijuana, Mexico.[138] No rationale for this treatment approach has been documented in the scientific literature. While the procedure has been carried out for more than a decade, no peer-reviewed documentation of the clinical procedures, methods used to evaluate outcomes, or the results have been generated. Anecdotally, reports of improvements of function in over 30 people with SCI have been made via Internet accounts.[138]

Recommended guidelines also suggest clinical trials performed in people with chronic injury should be validated in preclinical studies in animals with chronic injury. Preclinical studies should also mimic both the type of injury—whether contusive, ischemic or penetrating—and the exact treatment proposed for human trial. In addition to clearly demonstrating benefit, the proposed treatment should be replicated independently by other investigators in the field.[134] While clinical procedures with fetal olfactory bulb-derived cells continue to be carried out in humans, little preclinical data on the specific use of these cells exists. Neither is there published experimental studies showing efficacy of such fetal cells in a contusion SCI model. Investigators have documented, however, the specific use of mucosal-derived OECs[113] including a study of transplantation of the cells in rodents with chronic injury.[114]

Need for Safety

In addition to sufficient preclinical evidence, the safety of any proposed treatment before its use in a clinical trial is a chief concern. Preclinical studies should evaluate the potential toxicity of the intervention and should be of sufficient duration to assess for adverse effects, such as pain, tumors, or loss of function. A common view in the scientific community is preclinical testing should move to large animals before trials in humans, especially if interventions such as cellular transplantations are highly invasive or pose high or unknown risk.[47,134] Of the studies reviewed here, only two interventions have been evaluated in larger animals prior to their application in humans: the oscillating field stimulation study tested in dogs,[90] and the study of IN-1 antibody tested in nonhuman primates.[132] Once in clinical trial, a continued assessment of the safety of an intervention is the primary goal of any Phase 1 study. Even with prerequisite safety testing in large animals, the safety of an intervention in humans is not assured until testing in humans is carried out. Thus, particular attention to the potential for adverse effects must be considered in the design of any clinical trial.

Need for Well-Designed Studies

To properly assess potential treatments, rigorous, well-designed clinical trials will be important. All clinical trials should have clearly defined protocols that outline the specific goals and details of the studies before their initiation. They should also include appropriate control groups for comparison with a treatment group. Studies that lack controls are of limited value because many factors can influence outcomes and definitive conclusions are difficult to make. Another important factor that must be considered is the rate of spontaneous recovery that could be expected. Fawcett and colleagues[43] recently analyzed data from several published studies that revealed approximately 20% of patients diagnosed as AIS A at time of injury had converted to AIS B, C, or D within 1 year after injury. In patients with AIS B, the rate of conversion to AIS C or D was as much as 40%. Because recovery in subjects undergoing experimental treatments could be attributed to spontaneous recovery, investigators need to include appropriate numbers of subjects for the study to show statistical significance.

Besides controlling for spontaneous recovery, clinicians responsible for evaluation of the measured end-points of the study should be blinded to which treatment group the subject is assigned. It is also advantageous if the subject does not know if he or she received the treatment. This double-blinded design is ideal as it allows for detection of placebo effects and other sources of bias. Randomized and controlled study design is also important to help limit the effect of psychological factors that could powerfully influence a person's and family's perception of benefit. As shown in the examples in Box 4-1, subjects who expect benefits from an intervention may be inclined to perceive benefits following the intervention.[122]

Of the ongoing experimental procedures discussed in this chapter and summarized in Table 4-1, only a few would meet the suggested guidelines[43,134-137] or the standards set by the U.S. Food and Drug Administration or European regulatory agencies. Some should be viewed as clinical treatment series rather than clinical trials, as might be the case with some treatments that involve transplantation of OECs and BMS cells. Some studies do little to generate information that advances the field, and definitive conclusions are difficult to make when the study design fails to compare study subjects to control groups or document long-term assessment of neurological function, complications, or risk.

Need for Sensitive and Standardized Outcome Measures

The SCI research community is currently discussing the need for accurate and sensitive outcome measures to detect small functional changes that may result from future treatment strategies.[140] The widely used American Spinal Injury Association (ASIA) International Standards for Neurological Classifications scale is internationally accepted and standardized,[18] however, ASIA scores alone do not sufficiently detect subtle changes in neurological function.[1,47] A key issue for future clinical trials, especially multicenter trials, is development of more sensitive and standardized outcome measures.

While ASIA scores provide an assessment of neurological function, other objective clinical assessments are under development to more meaningfully measure changes in function. Some of the available outcome

Table 4-1

Intervention	Status	Randomized	Controlled	Blinded	Long-Term Assessment
Pharmacological					
NASCIS 2	Completed	Yes	Yes	Double-blind	Yes
GM-1 ganglioside	Completed	Yes	Yes	Double-blind	Yes
Gacyclidine	Competed	Yes	Yes	Double-blind	Yes
4-aminopyridine	Competed Phase 3	Yes	Yes	Double-blind	Yes
Cell/Tissue Transplantation					
Human fetal tissue	Completed	No	No	No	Yes
Porcine fetal oligodendrocyte precursor implants	Completed	No	No	No	
ProCord (activated macrophages)	Phase 2 www. Proneuron.com	Yes, in second Phase 2 trial	Yes	Single-blind	Yes, 1 year
Bone marrow stromal cells	Phase 1 Sykova, Barros, Park	No	No	No	Yes, 1 year (Sykova) 7 months (Park)
Peripheral nerve grafts	Treatment Series, Zhang case reports, Cheng, Barros, Tadie, von Wild	No	No	No	
Olfactory ensheathing cells	Phase 1, Feron, et al.	Yes	Yes	Single-blind	Yes, 3 years
	Experimental series Lima, Huang	No	No	No	
Other interventions					
Oscillating field stimulation	Phase 1 www.Andaratrials.com	No, but planned if second Phase 1 indicates	No, but planned if second Phase 1 indicates	No	Yes, 1 year
Cethrin	Phase 1 www.Alseres.com	No	No	No	

BOX 4-1
Examples: Biased Perception of Benefit

Subjects who had undergone a cellular transplantation perceive benefit. Is this a treatment effect or a placebo effect?

Case 1 was a subject with high tetraplegia whose right elbow flexor strength score139 was 2 of 5 on examination before receiving the cellular transplantation. Three months after surgery, the motor score was unchanged. It was the subject's perception, however, that elbow flexion had improved. While the motor score had not improved, the subject had been practicing elbow flexion with gravity eliminated and could perform 12 instead of 10 flexions in 30 seconds. Functional MRI showed a wider recruitment of activity in the bilateral primary sensorimotor cortex. The family also interpreted an improvement in wrist extension; however, on both preoperative and postoperative examinations, rather than wrist extension, the investigators noted a slight involuntary motion of several fingers caused by fasciculation of the intrinsic hand muscles.122

Case 2 was a subject with no motor function below C3 who required ventilation assistance of at least 12 mm Hg inspiratory pressure before surgery. On returning home from the cell transplantation procedure, the family decreased the ventilator inspiratory pressure to 8 mm Hg because they believed the subject's respiratory function was improving. The subject was hospitalized for pneumonia and atelectasis 2 days later and upon recovery was maintained at the presurgery inspiratory pressures. In the months after surgery, the subject perceived improvements in the strength of the neck and trapezius muscles above the level of injury. He attributed these improvements to the surgery; however, they were likely due to his new daily program of physical therapy.122

assessment tools developed and validated for use in individuals with SCI are given in Table 4-2. To evaluate the effect of a study's intervention, new trials for SCI repair are also likely to include functional MRI (fMRI), neuroelectrophysiologic tests such as SSEPs, MEPs, and tests of bladder, rectal sphincter, and respiratory function. In addition, the SCI research community considers it necessary to include objective pain assessment measures.[12,47] A challenge is arriving at a consensus on which assessment tools would be suitable and for what kinds of studies. Another challenge is to acquire sufficiently trained clinical researchers to achieve standardization of the selected assessments.

Need for SCI Research Networks

To hasten progress in SCI research and reach the goal of moving promising preclinical findings to clinical trial, the SCI research community has urged development of coordinated, focused, and collaborative research networks.[1,140] As noted above, there is a need to establish consistency in collection of outcome data, especially across multiple clinical trial sites. In addition, developing collaborative research networks and centers of excellence focused on SCI will provide an infrastructure to facilitate trials involving multidisciplinary approaches.[1] Such networks will improve the speed and efficiency of trials, access to participants, and acceptance of effective therapies into standard practice.

One international collaborative effort is underway to develop an international data set for classification and assessment of SCI.[149] This internationally accepted set of data is expected to facilitate comparisons regarding injuries, treatments, and outcomes in future clinical trials. An international committee has proposed a core data set consisting of 24 variables, which include basic demographic characteristics, cause of injury, dates and place of admission and discharge from care, presence of vertebral fractures and associated injuries, occurrence of spinal surgery, and measures of neurological and ventilator status.[150] Assessing and comparing worldwide outcomes of people with SCI will be enhanced by using a common international data set.

Other collaborative efforts include a European Clinical Trial Network supported by the International Spinal Research Trust[140] and the North American Clinical Trials Network supported by the Christopher and Dana Reeve Foundation.[151] These two groups are cooperating to define the natural history of SCI and to develop standard measures for treatment success. In addition, the China Spinal Cord Injury Network is a large network bringing eight Chinese medical centers together to bring SCI therapies to clinical trial.[152] Researchers expect that establishing these types of networks will lead to a common framework for the design and analysis of clinical trials that can be used by researchers throughout the world.

Impact on Rehabilitation Professional Practice

Of the invasive experimental interventions described in this chapter, only a few have undergone rigorous evaluation via randomized, blinded, and placebo-controlled study design (*see* Table 4-1). This review was limited to studies that have had some form of peer review and have the potential to offer some evidence to enhance scientific knowledge. Currently, however, people with SCI have the opportunity to consider other experimental procedures, some that have yet to be refereed by the SCI scientific community. Media reports, Internet searches, and visits to SCI community bulletin boards reveal various cell transplantation opportunities offered by organizations such as XCell Center at the Institute of Regenerative Medicine[153] (Germany), Medra, Inc.[154] (Santo Domingo), and Beike Biotechnologies, Inc.[156] (China). An individual's choice to participate in any experimental treatment is ultimately up to them. Their point of view is naturally focused on the personal gains from participation in an experimental procedure and their primary questions will be: Does this treatment have the potential to help? What are the potential risks? What are the costs? The perspective of scientists and clinical professionals, however, focuses on the process by which a treatment has been readied for and how it will be evaluated in clinical trial. As the field advances in scientific knowledge, other promising treatment strategies will be brought to clinical trial and offered to people with SCI. Therefore, clinical professionals have a responsibility to

| Table 4-2 | |
Measurement	Assessment
Impairment	ASIA
Functional limitation	Grasp and release test[141]
	Capabilities of Upper Extremities Instrument (CUE)[142]
Ambulation	Walking Index for Spinal Cord Injury (WISCI)[143]
	Timed up-and-go (TUG)[144]
	The Spinal Cord Injury Functional Ambulation Inventory (SCI-FAI)[145]
Activity	Functional Independence Measure (FIM)[146]
	Quadriplegia Index of Function (QIF)[147]
	Spinal Cord Independence Measure (SCIM)[148]

educate their clients on the clinical trial process so they become educated consumers who can make truly informed choices regarding undergoing an experimental intervention.[122,156] By incorporating discussions into inpatient and outpatient rehabilitation programs, clients will be better equipped to discern the reputation of an organization, its clinical personnel, and their study design, as well as weigh the potential risks of undergoing procedures that might not be under the scrutiny of a well-designed clinical trial.

To aid in educating clients, the International Campaign for the Cures for spinal cord injury Paralysis (ICCP) sponsored the creation of a guide entitled, "Experimental Treatments for Spinal Cord Injury: What You Should Know."[157] The guide is based on published scientific papers and the professional opinion of two dozen scientists and doctors from around the globe who served on a panel to develop and publish a set of guidelines for the conduct of clinical trials for SCI.[43,135-137] The guide is written for people living with SCI and their families and friends, and summarizes some of the current concerns about experimental treatments. It outlines appropriate SCI clinical trials procedures and, perhaps most importantly, offers a set of questions that people should ask before agreeing to undergo an experimental procedure. As shown in Box 4-2, the questions fall under seven categories: safety, possible benefits, preclinical evidence, clinical trial protocol, participation in other trials, payment and costs, and independent assessment of the treatment and investigators.

BOX 4-2
What Should You Ask Before Agreeing to Take Part in a Clinical Trial

Category 1. Safety
a. Are there safety risks associated with this experimental treatment?
b. Could my condition or my health get worse after this experimental treatment?
c. If so, can you describe the possible risks associated with this experimental treatment?

Category 2. Possible benefits
a. Can you describe the possible specific benefits of this experimental treatment?
b. Can you describe the maximum level of recovery I might see after this treatment?
c. Can you describe how any potential benefit will be measured?
d. Is this outcome measure accurate and sensitive as an assessment tool?

Category 3. Preclinical evidence
a. Can you describe the preclinical evidence that demonstrates this experimental treatment is beneficial (i.e., in animals with SCI)?
b. Have these findings been independently replicated?
c. If they have been replicated, is there a consensus among the scientists that this treatment addresses a valid therapeutic target for improving my functional outcomes?
d. Are there any dissenting opinions, and do these arguments have some validity for not going forward with this treatment?

Category 4. Clinical trial protocol
a. Is this human study registered as a clinical trial with an appropriate qualified regulatory body?
b. Can you describe what clinical trial phase this particular human study falls within?
c. Is there a control group in this study?
d. Could I be randomly assigned to the control group?
e. Can you tell me how long I will be assessed for any change in outcome?
f. Will I be blinded to whether I have received the experimental or control treatment?
g. Will the investigators and examiners be blind to what treatment I have received?

Category 5. Participation in other trials
a. Will my participation in this clinical trial limit my participation in other SCI clinical trials?
b. If I am assigned to the control group and the experimental treatment is subsequently validated as an effective therapy for my type of SCI by this clinical trial program, will I be eligible to receive this treatment later?

Category 6. Payment and costs
a. Do I have to pay for this treatment?
b. Are there any other costs associated with my participation in this study?
c. Will my expenses associated with participating in this study be paid (e.g., travel to center for follow-up assessment)?

Category 7. Independent assessment of the treatment and investigator
a. Can you provide me several names of scientists and clinicians (not involved with this study) who can provide me independent advice about this treatment and your reputation?

From "Experimental Treatments for Spinal Cord Injury: What You Should Know," a guide from: International Campaign for Cures of Spinal Cord Injury Paralysis (ICCP).[157]

As more individuals opt to undergo experimental procedures, they return to their communities with an expectation for improvement in their condition. How will the field of SCI rehabilitation adjust its practices as it strives for evidence-based practice and the goal of advancing the science of SCI and improving client care? Clinical professionals treating clients who have undergone experimental procedures could consider documenting case studies, especially in cases where the client is not part of a well-designed study with adequate follow-up. Some scientific knowledge may be gained for the research community from accurately reported experiences of individual cases, though the level of evidence is limited in individual case studies.

With more and more clinical trials in SCI under design and poised for implementation, more rehabilitation professionals with knowledge of and experience in implementation of clinical trials will need to integrate research into their practices. As discussed previously, sensitive and standardized outcome measures that more clearly measure benefits are needed to strengthen clinical trials in SCI and advance the field. Rehabilitation professionals will likely have the opportunity, with the organization of clinical trial networks, to contribute to the development and standardization of these new measures. In addition, they will need to acquire this new knowledge and incorporate the new measures into their practices.

In the last few years, basic science and clinical researchers in the field of SCI have initiated serious international discussions. Coordinated efforts to carefully and efficiently translate promising findings into well-designed clinical trials are expected to come about because of these discussions. While these international efforts require a tremendous amount of work and commitment, they are important if we are to see experimental treatments become evidence-based standard treatments for SCI. It is an exciting time for rehabilitation professionals, in which they will not only follow the progress of these efforts but also contribute to them, whether as an educator of clients or as an active contributor to the research effort.

Summary

This chapter has offered a description of recent clinical research experience of various pharmacological and invasive interventions directed at spinal cord repair and recovery. Strategies directed at preventing further neural loss, replacing neural components, regrowing and remyelinating damaged axons have been undertaken in clinical trials and experimental series. Though none have been successful in substantially improving the recovery of people with SCI, the experiences identify some important issues for the sound conduct of clinical trials. The experiences also provide a framework for the future translation of promising preclinical findings into successful clinical trials.

Most in the SCI research community agree on the need to perform rigorous preclinical studies that provide evidence of benefit and safety prior to introducing a treatment in clinical trials. These preclinical studies should be done in animal models that are relevant and appropriate for the level of risk that might be associated with the experimental intervention. When a procedure or drug is ready for clinical trial, those trials should use a rigorous study design that, when possible, randomizes subjects, includes blinded assessments, and employs controls. The controls should consider the power of placebo effects as well as the influences that hope—on the part of the subject, family, and even clinician—can have on the study.

Some experimental procedures have been carried out that do not meet the current standards for clinical trials. These experiences have stimulated discussion in the scientific community that has prompted coordinated and collaborative international efforts to develop clinical trial guidelines. These international discussions have also inspired efforts to establish international data sets, develop and standardize more sensitive outcome measures, and organize clinical trial networks to prepare the field of SCI research for implementation of successful clinical trials.

No longer is there the dogma that the damaged CNS is unamenable to repair. The prospect of recovering lost spinal cord functions has brought us to an exciting but challenging time in the history of SCI medicine. Evidence-based practice is increasingly emphasized within the SCI rehabilitation community and should remain a standard for all SCI clinical trials. The rehabilitation professional can have a role in furthering this standard by educating clients and their significant others on the characteristics of and need for sound scientific practices and by incorporating research into their practices.

It is an encouraging fact that this chapter will become outdated rather quickly as new information about current, impending, and upcoming clinical trials is made known at scientific meetings and with the publication of study outcomes. The clinical trials summarized in this chapter serve as examples for readers to become savvy consumers of the research literature related to SCI and to assist clients in gauging their expectations of current clinical trials. Promising new preclinical findings will continue to be revealed and will lead to new clinical trials. While much more needs to be accomplished, the current collaborative efforts can do nothing but move the field forward.

REVIEW QUESTIONS

1. Describe at least two pathological events occurring in SCI that researchers have targeted in recent clinical trials.
2. Compare and contrast two interventions described in this chapter.
3. When considering an experimental treatment for clinical trial, what guidelines should be met prior to initiation of a trial? Explain why.
4. What role can rehabilitation professionals take in advancing the field of SCI research?
5. Describe how you will incorporate the information in this chapter into your clinical practice.

ACKNOWLEDGMENT

Support for the preparation of this chapter was provided by The Miami Project to Cure Paralysis/University of Miami Miller School of Medicine.

REFERENCES

1. *Spinal Cord Injury: Progress, Promise, and Priorities.* Washington, D.C.: The National Academies Press; 2005.
2. Becerra JL, Puckett WR, Hiester ED et al. MR-pathologic comparisons of wallerian degeneration in spinal cord injury. *AJNR Am J Neuroradiol* 1995;16(1):125–133.
3. Kakulas BA. Neuropathology: The foundation for new treatments in spinal cord injury. *Spinal Cord* 2004;42(10): 549–563.
4. Bunge RP, Puckett WR, Becerra JL, et al. Observations on the pathology of human spinal cord injury. A review and classification of 22 new cases with details from a case of chronic cord compression with extensive focal demyelination. *Adv Neurol* 1993;59:75–89.
5. Cheng H, Lee YS. Spinal Cord Repair Strategies. In: Lin VW, Cardenas DD, Cutter NC, et al., editors. *Spinal Cord Medicine: Principles and Practice.* New York: Demos Medical Publishing, Inc.; 2003. pp. 801–816.
6. Richardson PM, McGuinness UM, Aguayo AJ. Axons from CNS neurons regenerate into PNS grafts. *Nature* 1980;284(5753):264–265.
7. Hopkins JM, Bunge RP. Regeneration of axons from adult human retina in vitro. *Exp Neurol* 1991;112(3):243–251.
8. McDonald JW, Becker D, Holekamp TF et al. Repair of the injured spinal cord and the potential of embryonic stem cell transplantation. *J Neurotrauma* 2004;21(4):383–393.
9. Lakatos A, Franklin RJ. Transplant mediated repair of the central nervous system: An imminent solution? *Curr Opin Neurol* 2002;15(6):701–705.
10. Keirstead HS, Nistor G, Bernal G et al. Human embryonic stem cell–derived oligodendrocyte progenitor cell transplants remyelinate and restore locomotion after spinal cord injury. *J Neurosci* 2005;25(19):4694–4705.
11. Faulkner J, Keirstead HS. Human embryonic stem cell–derived oligodendrocyte progenitors for the treatment of spinal cord injury. *Transpl Immunol* 2005;15(2):131–142.
12. Kleitman N. Keeping promises: Translating basic research into new spinal cord injury therapies. *J Spinal Cord Med* 2004;27(4):311–318.
13. Keirstead H, Stewart L. Recent Advances in Neural Regeneration. In: Lin VW, Cardenas DD, Cutter NC, et al., editors. *Spinal Cord Medicine: Principles and Practice.* New York: Demos Medical Publishing, Inc.; 2003. pp. 785–800.
14. Ramer LM, Ramer MS, Steeves JD. Setting the stage for functional repair of spinal cord injuries: a cast of thousands. *Spinal Cord* 2005;43(3):134–161.
15. Bracken MB, Collins WF, Freeman DF et al. Efficacy of methylprednisolone in acute spinal cord injury. *JAMA* 1984;251(1):45–52.
16. Lammertse DP. Update on pharmaceutical trials in acute spinal cord injury. *J Spinal Cord Med* 2004;27(4):319–325.
17. Bracken MB, Shepard MJ, Collins WF et al. A randomized, controlled trial of methylprednisolone or naloxone in the treatment of acute spinal-cord injury. Results of the Second National Acute Spinal Cord Injury Study. *N Engl J Med* 1990;322(20):1405–1411.
18. American Spinal Injury Association. International Standards for Neurological Classification of Spinal Cord Injury. 2000. Chicago, ASIA. 2000.
19. Bracken MB, Shepard MJ, Holford TR et al. Administration of methylprednisolone for 24 or 48 hours or tirilazad mesylate for 48 hours in the treatment of acute spinal cord injury. Results of the Third National Acute Spinal Cord Injury Randomized Controlled Trial. National Acute Spinal Cord Injury Study. *JAMA* 1997;277(20):1597–1604.
20. Bracken MB, Shepard MJ, Holford TR et al. Methylprednisolone or tirilazad mesylate administration after acute spinal cord injury: 1-year follow up. Results of the Third National Acute Spinal Cord Injury Randomized Controlled Trial. *J Neurosurg* 1998;89(5):699–706.
21. Fehlings MG, Baptiste DC. Current status of clinical trials for acute spinal cord injury. *Injury* 2005 July; 36 Suppl 2:B113–B122.
22. Nesathurai S. Steroids and spinal cord injury: Revisiting the NASCIS 2 and NASCIS 3 trials. *J Trauma* 1998;45(6): 1088–1093.
23. Coleman WP, Benzel D, Cahill DW et al. A critical appraisal of the reporting of the National Acute Spinal Cord Injury Studies (II and III) of methylprednisolone in acute spinal cord injury. *J Spinal Disord* 2000;13(3):185–199.
24. Galandiuk S, Raque G, Appel S, Polk HC, Jr. The two-edged sword of large-dose steroids for spinal cord trauma. *Ann Surg* 1993;218(4):419–425.
25. Gerndt SJ, Rodriguez JL, Pawlik JW et al. Consequences of high-dose steroid therapy for acute spinal cord injury. *J Trauma* 1997;42(2):279–284.
26. Qian T, Campagnolo D, Kirshblum S. High-dose methylprednisolone may do more harm for spinal cord injury. *Med Hypotheses* 2000;55(5):452–453.
27. Prendergast MR, Saxe JM, Ledgerwood AM, et al. Massive steroids do not reduce the zone of injury after penetrating spinal cord injury. *J Trauma* 1994;37(4):576–579.
28. Heary RF, Vaccaro AR, Mesa JJ et al. Steroids and gunshot wounds to the spine. Neurosurgery 1997;41(3):576–583.
29. Qian T, Guo X, Levi AD, Vanni S, Shebert RT, Sipski ML. High-dose methylprednisolone may cause myopathy in acute spinal cord injury patients. *Spinal Cord* 2005 April;43(4):199–203.

30. Pharmacological therapy after acute cervical spinal cord injury. *Neurosurgery* 2002;50 Suppl 3:S63–S72.

31. Gorio A. Ganglioside enhancement of neuronal differentiation, plasticity, and repair. *CRC Crit Rev Clin Neurobiol* 1986;2(3):241–296.

32. Bose B, Osterholm JL, Kalia M. Ganglioside-induced regeneration and reestablishment of axonal continuity in spinal cord-transected rats. *Neurosci Lett* 1986 16;63(2):165–169.

33. Skaper SD, Leon A. Monosialogangliosides, neuroprotection, and neuronal repair processes. *J Neurotrauma* 1992 May;9 Suppl 2:S507–S516.

34. Braune S. Is ganglioside GM1 effective in the treatment of stroke? *Drugs Aging* 1991;1(1):57–66.

35. Geisler FH, Dorsey FC, Coleman WP. GM1 gangliosides in the treatment of spinal cord injury: Report of preliminary data analysis. *Acta Neurobiol Exp (Wars)* 1990;50(4–5):515–521.

36. Geisler FH, Dorsey FC, Coleman WP. Recovery of motor function after spinal-cord injury-a randomized, placebo-controlled trial with GM-1 ganglioside. *N Engl J Med* 1991 27;324(26):1829–1838.

37. Frankel HL, Hancock DO, Hyslop G et al. The value of postural reduction in the initial management of closed injuries of the spine with paraplegia and tetraplegia. I. *Paraplegia* 1969;7(3):179–192.

38. Geisler FH. GM-1 ganglioside and motor recovery following human spinal cord injury. *J Emerg Med* 1993;11 Suppl 1:49–55.

39. Geisler FH, Coleman WP, Grieco G, Poonian D. The Sygen multicenter acute spinal cord injury study. *Spine* 2001 15;26(24 Suppl):S87–S98.

40. Geisler FH, Coleman WP, Grieco G, Poonian D. Measurements and recovery patterns in a multicenter study of acute spinal cord injury. *Spine* 2001;26 Suppl 24:S68–S86.

41. Geisler FH, Coleman WP, Grieco G, Poonian D. Recruitment and early treatment in a multicenter study of acute spinal cord injury. *Spine* 2001;26 Suppl 24:S58–S67.

42. Benzel EC, Larson SJ. Functional recovery after decompressive spine operation for cervical spine fractures. *Neurosurgery* 1987;20(5):742–746.

43. Fawcett JW, Curt A, Steeves JD et al. Guidelines for the conduct of clinical trials for spinal cord injury as developed by the ICCP panel: Spontaneous recovery after spinal cord injury and statistical power needed for therapeutic clinical trials. *Spinal Cord* 2007;45(3):190–205.

44. Gaviria M, Privat A, D'Arbigny P, Kamenka JM, Haton H, Ohanna F. Neuroprotective effects of gacyclidine after experimental photochemical spinal cord lesion in adult rats: dose-window and time-window effects. *J Neurotrauma* 2000;17(1):19–30.

45. Gaviria M, Privat A, D'Arbigny P, Kamenka J, Haton H, Ohanna F. Neuroprotective effects of a novel NMDA antagonist, Gacyclidine, after experimental contusive spinal cord injury in adult rats. *Brain Res* 2000;874(2):200–209.

46. Tadie M, D'Arbigny P, Mathe JF. Acute spinal cord injury: Early care and treatment in a multicenter study with gacyclidine. *Soc Neurosci Abstr , 1090.* 1999.

47. Steeves J, Fawcett J, Tuszynski M. Report of international clinical trials workshop on spinal cord injury February 20–21, 2004, Vancouver, Canada. *Spinal Cord* 2004;42(10):591–597.

48. Lazarov-Spiegler O, Solomon AS, Zeev-Brann AB, et al.. Transplantation of activated macrophages overcomes central nervous system regrowth failure. *FASEB J* 1996;10(11):1296–1302.

49. Zeev-Brann AB, Lazarov-Spiegler O, Brenner T, et al. Differential effects of central and peripheral nerves on macrophages and microglia. *Glia* 1998;23(3):181–190.

50. Lazarov-Spiegler O, Solomon AS, Schwartz M. Link between optic nerve regrowth failure and macrophage stimulation in mammals. *Vision Res* 1999;39(1):169–175.

51. Reier PJ. Cellular transplantation strategies for spinal cord injury and translational neurobiology. *NeuroRx* 2004;1(4):424–451.

52. Rapalino O, Lazarov-Spiegler O, Agranov E et al. Implantation of stimulated homologous macrophages results in partial recovery of paraplegic rats. *Nat Med* 1998;4(7):814–821.

53. Bomstein Y, Marder JB, Vitner K et al. Features of skin-coincubated macrophages that promote recovery from spinal cord injury. *J Neuroimmunol* 2003;142(1–2):10–16.

54. Bubis M, Ziona N, Sarel I et al. Characterization of Procord macrophage cell therapy for spinal cord injury. *J Spinal Cord Med* 2004;27(4).

55. Knoller N, Auerbach G, Fulga V et al. Clinical experience using incubated autologous macrophages as a treatment for complete spinal cord injury: Phase I study results. *J Neurosurg Spine* 2005;3(3):173–181.

56. Proneuron BioTechnologies. ProCord-An Experimental Procedure for Spinal Cord Injuries. Available at: http://www.proneuron.com/ClinicalStudies/index.html. Accessed July 31, 2008.

57. Thompson FJ, Reier PJ, Uthman B et al. Neurophysiological assessment of the feasibility and safety of neural tissue transplantation in patients with syringomyelia. *J Neurotrauma* 2001;18(9):931–945.

58. Wirth ED, III, Reier PJ, Fessler RG et al. Feasibility and safety of neural tissue transplantation in patients with syringomyelia. *J Neurotrauma* 2001;18(9):911–929.

59. Falci S, Holtz A, Akesson E et al. Obliteration of a post-traumatic spinal cord cyst with solid human embryonic spinal cord grafts: First clinical attempt. *J Neurotrauma* 1997;14(11):875–884.

60. Reier PJ, Bregman BS, Wujek JR. Intraspinal transplantation of embryonic spinal cord tissue in neonatal and adult rats. *J Comp Neurol* 1986 15;247(3):275–296.

61. Reier PJ, Stokes BT, Thompson FJ, Anderson DK. Fetal cell grafts into resection and contusion/compression injuries of the rat and cat spinal cord. *Exp Neurol* 1992;115(1):177–188.

62. Stokes BT, Reier PJ. Fetal grafts alter chronic behavioral outcome after contusion damage to the adult rat spinal cord. *Exp Neurol* 1992;116(1):1–12.

63. McDonald JW, Becker D. Spinal cord injury: Promising interventions and realistic goals. *Am J Phys Med Rehabil* 2003;82(10 Suppl):S38–S49.

64. Blakemore WF, Smith PM, Franklin RJ. Remyelinating the demyelinated CNS. *Novartis Found Symp* 2000;231:289–298.

65. McDonald JW, Howard MJ. Repairing the damaged spinal cord: A summary of our early success with embryonic stem cell transplantation and remyelination. *Prog Brain Res* 2002;137:299–309.

66. Bambakidis NC, Miller RH. Transplantation of oligodendrocyte precursors and sonic hedgehog results in improved function and white matter sparing in the spinal cords of adult rats after contusion. *Spine J* 2004;4(1):16–26.

67. Hill CE, Proschel C, Noble M et al. Acute transplantation of glial-restricted precursor cells into spinal cord contusion injuries:Survival, differentiation, and effects on lesion environment and axonal regeneration. *Exp Neurol* 2004;190(2): 289–310.

68. Deng W, Obrocka M, Fischer I, Prockop DJ. In vitro differentiation of human marrow stromal cells into early progenitors of neural cells by conditions that increase intracellular cyclic AMP. *Biochem Biophys Res Commun* 2001 23;282(1):148–152.

69. Sanchez-Ramos J, Song S, Cardozo-Pelaez F et al. Adult bone marrow stromal cells differentiate into neural cells in vitro. *Exp Neurol* 2000;164(2):247–256.

70. Chopp M, Zhang XH, Li Y et al. Spinal cord injury in rat: Treatment with bone marrow stromal cell transplantation. *Neuroreport* 2000 11;11(13):3001–3005.

71. Hofstetter CP, Schwarz EJ, Hess D et al. Marrow stromal cells form guiding strands in the injured spinal cord and promote recovery. *Proc Natl Acad Sci USA* 2002;99(4): 2199–2204.

72. Jendelova P, Herynek V, DeCroos J et al. Imaging the fate of implanted bone marrow stromal cells labeled with superparamagnetic nanoparticles. *Magn Reson Med* 2003;50(4):767–776.

73. Jendelova P, Herynek V, Urdzikova L et al. Magnetic resonance tracking of transplanted bone marrow and embryonic stem cells labeled by iron oxide nanoparticles in rat brain and spinal cord. *J Neurosci Res* 2004;76(2):232–243.

74. Sykova E, Jendelova P. Magnetic resonance tracking of implanted adult and embryonic stem cells in injured brain and spinal cord. *Ann N Y Acad Sci* 2005;1049:146–160.

75. Sykova E, Jendelova P, Urdzikova L, Lesny P, Hejcl A. Bone marrow stem cells and polymer hydrogels-two strategies for spinal cord injury repair. *Cell Mol Neurobiol* 2006;26(7–8):1111–1127.

76. Callera F, do Nascimento RX. Delivery of autologous bone marrow precursor cells into the spinal cord via lumbar puncture technique in patients with spinal cord injury: A preliminary safety study. *Exp Hematol* 2006;34(2):130–131.

77. Park HC, Shim YS, Ha Y et al. Treatment of complete spinal cord injury patients by autologous bone marrow cell transplantation and administration of granulocyte-macrophage colony stimulating factor. *Tissue Eng* 2005;11(5–6):913–922.

78. Geron Corporation. hESC-Derived Oligodendrocytes - GRNOPC1. Available at: http://www.geron.com/products/ productinformation/spinalcordinjury.aspx. Accessed July 31, 2008.

79. Geron Corporation. News Release: FDA Places Geron's GRNOPC1 IND on Clinical Hold. Available at: http://www.geron.com/media/pressview.aspx?id=840, Accessed July 31, 2008.

80. Blight AR. Effect of 4-aminopyridine on axonal conduction-block in chronic spinal cord injury. *Brain Res Bull* 1989;22(1):47–52.

81. Shi R, Kelly TM, Blight AR. Conduction block in acute and chronic spinal cord injury: Different dose-response characteristics for reversal by 4-aminopyridine. *Exp Neurol* 1997;148(2):495–501.

82. Hansebout RR, Blight AR, Fawcett S et al. 4-Aminopyridine in chronic spinal cord injury: A controlled, double-blind, crossover study in eight patients. *J Neurotrauma* 1993;10(1):1–18.

83. Segal JL, Brunnemann SR. 4-Aminopyridine alters gait characteristics and enhances locomotion in spinal cord injured humans. *J Spinal Cord Med* 1998;21(3): 200–204.

84. Grijalva I, Guizar-Sahagun G, Castaneda-Hernandez G et al. Efficacy and safety of 4-aminopyridine in patients with long-term spinal cord injury: A randomized, double-blind, placebo-controlled trial. *Pharmacotherapy* 2003;23(7): 823–834.

85. van der Bruggen MA, Huisman HB, Beckerman H et al. Randomized trial of 4-aminopyridine in patients with chronic incomplete spinal cord injury. *J Neurol* 2001;248(8): 665–671.

86. Deforge D, Nymark J, Lemaire E et al. Effect of 4-aminopyridine on gait in ambulatory spinal cord injuries: a double-blind, placebo-controlled, crossover trial. *Spinal Cord* 2004;42(12):674–685.

87. Hayes KC. The use of 4-aminopyridine (fampridine) in demyelinating disorders. *CNS Drug Rev* 2004;10(4):295–316.

88. Borgens RB, Roederer E, Cohen MJ. Enhanced spinal cord regeneration in lamprey by applied electric fields. *Science* 1981;213(4508):611–617.

89. Borgens RB, Blight AR, Murphy DJ et al. Transected dorsal column axons within the guinea pig spinal cord regenerate in the presence of an applied electric field. *J Comp Neurol* 1986;250(2):168–180.

90. Borgens RB, Toombs JP, Breur G et al. An imposed oscillating electrical field improves the recovery of function in neurologically complete paraplegic dogs. *J Neurotrauma* 1999;16(7):639–657.

91. Shapiro S, Borgens R, Pascuzzi R et al. Oscillating field stimulation for complete spinal cord injury in humans: a phase 1 trial. *J Neurosurg Spine* 2005;2(1):3–10.

92. Cyberkinetics Neurotechnology Systems, Inc. Medical Products: Andara™ OFS™ Therapy. Available at: http:// www.cyberkinetics.com/content/medicalproducts/andara ofs.jsp. Accessed July 31, 2008.

93. Dubreuil CI, Winton MJ, McKerracher L. Rho activation patterns after spinal cord injury and the role of activated Rho in apoptosis in the central nervous system. *J Cell Biol* 2003;162(2):233–243.

94. Dergham P, Ellezam B, Essagian C et al. Rho signaling pathway targeted to promote spinal cord repair. *J Neurosci* 2002;22(15):6570–6577.

95. Lehmann M, Fournier A, Selles-Navarro I et al. Inactivation of Rho signaling pathway promotes CNS axon regeneration. *J Neurosci* 1999;19(17):7537–7547.

96. Alseres Pharmaceuticals, Inc. Regenerative Therapeutics Program: Cethrin(r), a Rho Inhibitor. Available at: http://www.alseres.com/product-pipeline/product-candidates/ cethrin.asp. Accessed July 31, 2008

97. Alseres Pharmaceuticals, Inc. Alseres Pharmaceuticals Announces 12Month Interim Results from the Phase I/IIa Cethrin® Clinical Trial in Acute Spinal Cord Injury. Available at: http://ir.alseres.com/releasedetail.cfm? ReleaseID+309749. Accessed July 31, 2008.

98. Xu XM, Zhang SX, Li H et al. Regrowth of axons into the distal spinal cord through a Schwann-cell-seeded

mini-channel implanted into hemisected adult rat spinal cord. *Eur J Neurosci* 1999;11(5):1723–1740.

99. Guest JD, Rao A, Olson L et al. The ability of human Schwann cell grafts to promote regeneration in the transected nude rat spinal cord. *Exp Neurol* 1997;148(2):502–522.

100. Ramon-Cueto A, Plant GW, Avila J, Bunge MB. Long-distance axonal regeneration in the transected adult rat spinal cord is promoted by olfactory ensheathing glia transplants. *J Neurosci* 1998;18(10):3803–3815.

101. Ramon-Cueto A, Cordero MI, Santos-Benito FF, Avila J. Functional recovery of paraplegic rats and motor axon regeneration in their spinal cords by olfactory ensheathing glia. *Neuron* 2000;25(2):425–435.

102. Cheng H, Cao Y, Olson L. Spinal cord repair in adult paraplegic rats: Partial restoration of hind limb function. *Science* 1996;273(5274):510–513.

103. Lee YS, Hsiao I, Lin VW. Peripheral nerve grafts and aFGF restore partial hindlimb function in adult paraplegic rats. *J Neurotrauma* 2002;19(10):1203–1216.

104. Onifer SM, Loor KE, Cannon AB et al. Combining methylprednisolone, peripheral nerves, FGF1, Fibrin and vertebral wiring for spinal cord repair. *Soc Neurosci Abstr* 1999;25:492. (Abstr.)

105. Cheng H, Liao KK, Liao SF, Chuang TY, Shih YH. Spinal cord repair with acidic fibroblast growth factor as a treatment for a patient with chronic paraplegia. *Spine* 2004;29(14):E284–E288.

106. Tadie M, Liu S, Robert R et al. Partial return of motor function in paralyzed legs after surgical bypass of the lesion site by nerve autografts three years after spinal cord injury. *J Neurotrauma* 2002;19(8):909–916.

107. von Wild KR, Brunelli GA. Restoration of locomotion in paraplegics with aid of autologous bypass grafts for direct neurotisation of muscles by upper motor neurons—the future: Surgery of the spinal cord? *Acta Neurochir Suppl* 2003;87:107–112.

108. Zhang S, Johnston L, Zhang Z et al. Restoration of stepping-forward and ambulatory function in patients with paraplegia: Rerouting of vascularized intercostal nerves to lumbar nerve roots using selected interfascicular anastomosis. *Surg Technol Int* 2003;11:244–248.

109. Mackay-Sim A. Olfactory ensheathing cells and spinal cord repair. Keio J Med 2005;54(1):8–14.

110. Li Y, Field PM, Raisman G. Repair of adult rat corticospinal tract by transplants of olfactory ensheathing cells. *Science* 1997;277(5334):2000–2002.

111. Keyvan-Fouladi N, Raisman G, Li Y. Functional repair of the corticospinal tract by delayed transplantation of olfactory ensheathing cells in adult rats. *J Neurosci* 2003;23(28):9428–9434.

112. Santos-Benito FF, Ramon-Cueto A. Olfactory ensheathing glia transplantation: a therapy to promote repair in the mammalian central nervous system. *Anatomical Record Part B, New Anatomist* 2003;271(1):77–85.

113. Lu J, Feron F, Ho SM et al. Transplantation of nasal olfactory tissue promotes partial recovery in paraplegic adult rats. *Brain Res* 2001;889(1–2):344–357.

114. Lu J, Feron F, Mackay-Sim A et al. Olfactory ensheathing cells promote locomotor recovery after delayed transplantation into transected spinal cord. *Brain* 2002;125(Pt 1):14–21.

115. Feron F, Perry C, Cochrane J et al. Autologous olfactory ensheathing cell transplantation in human spinal cord injury. *Brain* 2005 r;128(Pt 12):2951–2960.

116. SCI Recovery Center. Stem Cell Research in Pursuit of Spinal Cord Injury Treatments, Available at: http://www.sci-recovery.org/stem1.htm. Accessed July 31, 2008.

117. Lima C, Pratas-Vital J, Escada P et al. Olfactory mucosa autografts in human spinal cord injury: a pilot clinical study. *J Spinal Cord Med* 2006;29(3):191–203.

118. Kirshblum S. Commentary: "A Start" Olfactory Mucosa Autografts in Human Spinal Cord Injury. *J Spinal Cord Med* 2006;29(3):204–206.

119. Huang H, Chen L, Wang H et al. Influence of patients' age on functional recovery after transplantation of olfactory ensheathing cells into injured spinal cord injury. *Chin Med J (Engl)* 2003;116(10).

120. Huang H, Wang H, Chen L et al. Influence factors for functional improvement after olfactory ensheathing cell transplantation for chronic spinal cord injury. *Zhongguo Xiu Fu Chong Jian Wai Ke Za Zhi* 2006;20(4): 434–438.

121. Guest J, Herrera LP, Qian T. Rapid recovery of segmental neurological function in a tetraplegic patient following transplantation of fetal olfactory bulb-derived cells. *Spinal Cord* 2006;44(3):135–142.

122. Dobkin BH, Curt A, Guest J. Cellular transplants in China: Observational study from the largest human experiment in chronic spinal cord injury. *Neurorehabil Neural Repair* 2006;20(1):5–13.

123. Cyranoski D. Patients warned about unproven spinal surgery. *Nature* 2006 13;440(7086):850–851.

124. Huang H, Chen L, Wang H et al. Safety of fetal olfactory ensheathing cell transplantation in patients with chronic spinal cord injury. A 38-month follow-up with MRI. *Zhongguo Xiu Fu Chong Jian Wai Ke Za Zhi* 2006;20(4): 439–443.

125. Caroni P, Schwab ME. Antibody against myelin-associated inhibitor of neurite growth neutralizes nonpermissive substrate properties of CNS white matter. *Neuron* 1988;1(1):85–96.

126. Schnell L, Schwab ME. Sprouting and regeneration of lesioned corticospinal tract fibres in the adult rat spinal cord. *Eur J Neurosci* 1993;5(9):1156–1171.

127. Bregman BS, Kunkel-Bagden E, Schnell L et al. Recovery from spinal cord injury mediated by antibodies to neurite growth inhibitors. *Nature* 1995;378(6556):498–501.

128. Merkler D, Metz GA, Raineteau O, Dietz V, Schwab ME, Fouad K. Locomotor recovery in spinal cord-injured rats treated with an antibody neutralizing the myelin-associated neurite growth inhibitor Nogo-A. *J Neurosci* 2001;21(10): 3665–3673.

129. Brosamle C, Huber AB, Fiedler M, Skerra A, Schwab ME. Regeneration of lesioned corticospinal tract fibers in the adult rat induced by a recombinant, humanized IN-1 antibody fragment. *J Neurosci* 2000;20(21): 8061–8068.

130. Spillmann AA, Amberger VR, Schwab ME. High molecular weight protein of human central nervous system myelin inhibits neurite outgrowth: An effect which can be neutralized by the monoclonal antibody IN-1. *Eur J Neurosci* 1997;9(3):549–555.

131. Prinjha R, Moore SE, Vinson M et al. Inhibitor of neurite outgrowth in humans. *Nature* 2000;403(6768): 383–384.

132. Fouad K, Klusman I, Schwab ME. Regenerating corticospinal fibers in the Marmoset (Callitrix jacchus) after spinal cord lesion and treatment with the anti-Nogo-A antibody IN-1. *Eur J Neurosci* 2004;20(9):2479–2482.

133. ClinicalTrials.gov. Acute Safety, Tolerability, Feasibility and Pharmacokinetics of Intrath. Administered ATI355 in Patients With Acute SCI. Available at: http://www. clinicaltrials.gov/ct2/show/NCT00406016? term=ATI355&rank=1. Accessed July 30, 2008.

134. Anderson DK, Beattie M, Blesch A et al. Recommended guidelines for studies of human subjects with spinal cord injury. *Spinal Cord* 2005;43(8):453–458.

135. Steeves JD, Lammertse D, Curt A et al. Guidelines for the conduct of clinical trials for spinal cord injury (SCI) as developed by the ICCP panel: Clinical trial outcome measures. *Spinal Cord* 2007;45(3):206–221.

136. Tuszynski MH, Steeves JD, Fawcett JW et al. Guidelines for the conduct of clinical trials for spinal cord injury as developed by the ICCP Panel: Clinical trial inclusion/ exclusion criteria and ethics. *Spinal Cord* 2007;45(3): 222–231.

137. Lammertse D, Tuszynski MH, Steeves JD et al. Guidelines for the conduct of clinical trials for spinal cord injury as developed by the ICCP panel: clinical trial design. *Spinal Cord* 2007;45(3):232–242.

138. International Spinal Cord Regeneration Center. The Treatment: Reconstructive Surgery . Available at: http:// spinal.siteutopia.net/treat.htm. Accessed July 31, 2008.

139. Maynard FM, Jr., Bracken MB, Creasey G et al. International Standards for Neurological and Functional Classification of Spinal Cord Injury. American Spinal Injury Association. *Spinal Cord* 1997;35(5):266–274.

140. Ellaway PH, Anand P, Bergstrom EM et al. Towards improved clinical and physiological assessments of recovery in spinal cord injury: a clinical initiative. *Spinal Cord* 2004;42(6):325–337.

141. Wuolle KS, Van Doren CL, Thrope GB et al. Development of a quantitative hand grasp and release test for patients with tetraplegia using a hand neuroprosthesis. *J Hand Surg [Am]* 1994;19(2):209–218.

142. Marino RJ, Shea JA, Stineman MG. The Capabilities of Upper Extremity instrument: Reliability and validity of a measure of functional limitation in tetraplegia. *Arch Phys Med Rehabil* 1998;79(12):1512–1521.

143. Ditunno JF, Jr., Ditunno PL, Graziani V et al. Walking index for spinal cord injury (WISCI): An international multicenter validity and reliability study. *Spinal Cord* 2000;38(4):234–243.

144. van Hedel HJ, Wirz M, Dietz V. Assessing walking ability in subjects with spinal cord injury: Validity and reliability

of 3 walking tests. *Arch Phys Med Rehabil* 2005;86(2): 190–196.

145. Field-Fote EC, Fluet GG, Schafer SD et al. The Spinal Cord Injury Functional Ambulation Inventory (SCI-FAI). *J Rehabil Med* 2001;33(4):177–181.

146. Stineman MG, Shea JA, Jette A et al. The Functional Independence Measure: tests of scaling assumptions, structure, and reliability across 20 diverse impairment categories. *Arch Phys Med Rehabil* 1996;77(11):1101–1108.

147. Gresham GE, Labi ML, Dittmar SS et al. The Quadriplegia Index of Function (QIF): Sensitivity and reliability demonstrated in a study of thirty quadriplegic patients. *Paraplegia* 1986;24(1):38–44.

148. Catz A, Itzkovich M, Agranov E, Ring H, Tamir A. SCIM— Spinal Cord Independence Measure: A new disability scale for patients with spinal cord lesions. *Spinal Cord* 1997;35(12):850–856.

149. Biering-Sorensen F, Charlifue S, DeVivo M et al. International Spinal Cord Injury Data Sets. *Spinal Cord* 2006;44(9):530–534.

150. DeVivo M, Biering-Sorensen F, Charlifue S et al. International Spinal Cord Injury Core Data Set. *Spinal Cord* 2006;44(9):535–540.

151. Christopher Reeve Foundation. Christopher Reeve Foundation – North American Clinical Trials Network. Available at: http://www.christopherreeve.org/site/ c.geIMLPOpGjF/b.1048737/k.322D/North_American_ Clinical_Trials_Network_NACTN.htm. Accessed on July 31, 2008.

152. HKU Spinal Cord Injury Fund – China Network. Lighting the Way to a Cure. Available at: http://www.hku.hk/hkuscif/ wise.htm. Accessed July 31, 2008.

153. XCell-Center at the Institute for Regenerative Medicine-Stem cell treatment of Spinal Cord Injuries. Available at: http://www.xcell-center.com/treatments/diseases-treated/spinal-cord-injuries.aspx. Accessed July 31, 2008.

154. Medra, Inc. Medra, Inc. Human Fetal Stem Cells Treatment Available Today. Available at: www.medra.com. Accessed July 31, 2008.

155. China Stem Cell News. China Stem Cell News – Beike Biotechology Company. Available at: http://www.stem-cellschina.com/content/view/6/22/lang,en/. Accessed July 31, 2008.

156. Amador MJ, Guest JD. An appraisal of ongoing experimental procedures in human spinal cord injury. *J Neurol Phys Ther* 2005;29(2):70-86.

157. International Campaign for Cures of Spinal Cord Paralysis. Experimental Treatments for Spinal Cord Injury: What You Should Know if You are Considering Participation in a Clinical Trial. Available at: http:// www.icord.org/iccp.html. Accessed July 31, 2008.

Neuroprosthetics

5

Arthur Prochazka, PhD

Introduction

Definition

Neuroprostheses (NPs) are electronic devices that stimulate nerves in order to improve bodily functions lost as a result of damage to the peripheral or central nervous system. This approach is also called functional electrical stimulation (FES) or functional neuromuscular stimulation (FNS). NPs include both surface stimulators, which deliver current through the skin to target nerves, and implanted stimulators, which deliver current directly to the target nerves. NPs range from simple "muscle" stimulators used to increase muscle bulk to complex devices implanted in the spinal cord and brain. The aim of this chapter is to describe the numerous types of NPs that have been developed since the early days of therapeutic electrical stimulation (TES), with a particular emphasis on those NPs that are useful in functional restoration after spinal cord injury (SCI). The spectacular advances that have occurred in the neurosciences and in biomedical engineering in the last two decades have led to numerous technical advances and innovations. Surface and implanted NPs are now available to assist with a wide variety of functions, including hand function, postural control, standing, walking, respiration, micturition, and pain control. This chapter will address issues related to the benefits and limitations of these devices and factors affecting the choice of an NP for a particular individual.

History

Electrostatic machines capable of generating single high-voltage pulses were invented in the 1740s. Clinicians very soon began using them to apply single stimuli through pairs of surface electrodes, more to impress than to provide therapy.[1,2] Michael Faraday's invention of the induction coil in the mid-19th century allowed continuous trains of stimuli to be delivered to nerves and muscles. *Faradic stimulation* quickly became an important means of experimentally stimulating the brain, spinal cord, and peripheral nerves (see "Mechanisms" below).

The first detailed manual of motor points, that is, locations at which faradic stimulation through the skin activated muscles at the lowest thresholds, was published in 1867.[3] Electrical stimulation continued to be used at the fringes of medicine until the 1960s, when the advent of the transistor allowed stimulators to become portable enough to be used in activities of daily life (ADL).

Mechanisms

Electrical Stimulation of Nerves

Faradic stimulation consists of delivering trains of very brief pulses of electrical current through pairs of electrodes applied to bodily tissues. Electrodes applied to the skin surface are made of a conductive material, for example, metal or carbonized rubber, often with a soft conductive material such as a moistened cloth pad or a gel coating that forms an intimate and even contact with the skin surface to prevent hot spots of high-current density. Implanted electrodes are insulated leads with small conductive terminals made of a biologically compatible metal such as stainless steel or platinum-iridium. The terminals are usually built into a nonconductive substrate such as a silastic button (epimysial electrodes), a silastic nerve cuff, or an insulated cannula (brain or epidural spinal cord stimulation).

The voltage produced by a stimulator is the product of current and resistance ($V = IR$). To understand current and voltage, the analogy of water being pushed through a showerhead is useful. In this analogy, the flow of water per second is equivalent to current (I). The pressure drop from inside to outside the showerhead is equivalent to voltage (V). The smaller the holes in the showerhead, the greater the resistance to flow (R) and so the smaller the current. You can force the same amount of water through

smaller holes by increasing the pressure inside the showerhead. So flow (current) clearly depends on both the pressure drop (voltage) and resistance. Each pulse of current lasts from 50 to 300 microseconds. Surface stimulation requires currents ranging from 10 to 100 mA and voltages ranging from 10 to 100 V, depending on the electrode surface area. Implanted electrodes can activate the nerves they contact with currents in the range 0.1 to 2 mA and voltages in the range 0.1 to 2 V between the electrode terminals. This is because implanted electrodes allow the current to be delivered directly to the nerve rather than being dispersed through a large volume of tissue.

The amount of current required to activate muscle fibers is more than 10 times greater than that required to activate the *nerve* that innervates them, so *muscle* stimulators are really nerve stimulators. Denervated muscles cannot be activated with the pulse amplitudes normally used in FES, so individuals with lesions that have destroyed the relevant motoneuron pools in the gray matter of the spinal cord, or the motoneuronal axons in spinal nerves (as occurs in cauda equina lesions), unfortunately often do not benefit from FES. A single pulse delivered to a motor nerve causes the muscle to twitch once. Repeated pulses cause repeated twitches. Each twitch lasts about 1/20th of a second, so when pulses are repeated at a rate greater than 20 per second, the twitches fuse and the muscle contracts smoothly (this is called a *tetanic contraction* or *tetany*). More force can be produced at higher rates, but the increase levels off at around 35 to 45 pulses/second. Fatigue sets in more rapidly the faster the pulse rate. A good compromise between force and fatigue is usually reached between 30 and 40 pulses/second.

NP stimulators have electronic circuitry that controls either the voltage or current using feedback. If the current is feedback controlled, the voltage is automatically adjusted on a moment-to-moment basis so that the same current is delivered, regardless of the impedance presented by the electrodes and tissue. The result is that if the electrode contact is poor (as an analogy, smaller holes in the showerhead), impedance is high, and so the stimulator automatically increases the voltage to maintain current flow through the smaller contact area. This procedure ensures a constant level of activation of the target nerves but can cause skin burns. On the other hand, if voltage is feedback controlled and electrode contact is poor, the amount of current pushed through is less and the nerve may not be adequately stimulated, but there is little risk of skin burns.

The advantage of current-controlled stimulators is that the device always attempts to deliver the same current regardless of the impedance, thereby ensuring stimulation, but this carries the risk of local tissue damage. Voltage-controlled stimulators always try to deliver the desired voltage. Therefore, if the electrodes make poor contact, less current will flow. There is no risk of damage to the tissue, but the nerve may not be activated. Often in less-sophisticated stimulators, neither voltage nor current are feedback controlled. On the other hand, in advanced current-controlled stimulators, impedance is monitored and current is limited when the impedance is high.

Therapeutic Carryover Effects

Electrical stimulation of muscles has long been known to have carryover or therapeutic effects,[4-6] especially in conjunction with voluntary exercise training.[7-10] Surface stimulators triggered during attempted functional tasks (Fig. 5-1a) or by voluntary electromyographic (EMG) activity (Fig. 5-1b[11]) have been used in some clinics for FES-assisted motor retraining of the upper extremity.[9,12] The mechanism of carryover is poorly understood. Short-term carryover lasting less than a few hours may result from short-term changes in the energetics of neuromuscular activation, whereas long-term carryover lasting weeks or months is usually attributed to muscle strengthening, neural plasticity, or both.[13-15]

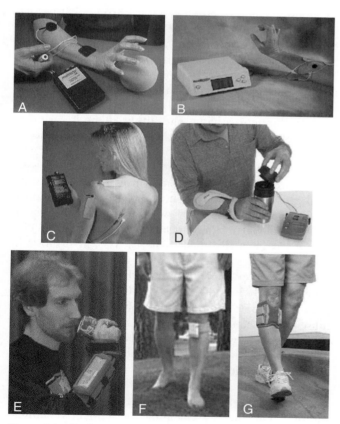

Figure 5-1. Surface NPs. (A) Medtronic, Inc. Respond physiotherapy stimulator; (B) Neuromove EMG-triggered stimulator; (C) Stimulation of trapezius muscle to prevent shoulder subluxation; (D) Ness Handmaster; (E) University of Alberta Bionic Glove; (F) Innovative Neurotronics WalkAide; (G) Bioness L300.

Types of Neuroprostheses

Surface FES Devices

Surface Stimulation Devices for Enhancing Walking Function

The first portable FES device was a surface stimulator that delivered trains of stimuli to the common peroneal nerve to correct foot drop in hemiparetic people.[16] This invention was further developed and commercialized in Europe in the 1960s by a group in Ljubljana, Slovenia (then Yugoslavia) led by Lojze Vodovnik (the FEPO, or functional electrical peroneal orthosis[17]). Since then, portable foot-drop stimulators of various designs have been used by well over 10,000 people worldwide. Most users have been individuals with stroke, though some people with SCI have successfully used them, too. Standard physical therapy stimulators equipped with under-heel sensors to trigger stimulation (and hence muscle activation) appropriately timed to the gait cycle have also been used as foot-drop stimulators in clinics for many years (e.g., the original Medtronic Respond unit and currently the Empi 300PV). By the year 2000, there had been three successful initiatives in countries with public health-care systems to provide foot-drop stimulators to hemiparetic people on a routine basis: Yugoslavia,[18] Denmark,[19] and the United Kingdom.[20] In the United States, a ruling by the Centers of Medicare and Medicaid Services (CMS)[20a] in the 1980s precluded reimbursement of neuromuscular stimulators prescribed for neurological disorders (although paradoxically, reimbursement is available when the same devices are used for treating back pain, which generally involves the neuromuscular system). Consequently, adoption of foot-drop stimulators in the United States has been slow and patchy. Currently the three main foot-drop stimulators available in North America on a self-pay basis are the Odstock[21], the WalkAide (Fig. 5-1f[22]), and the Bioness L300 (Fig. 5-1g). They are proving popular and effective, so pressure may increase on CMS to provide a reimbursement code for these aids. They can be effective in individuals with SCI whose main locomotor problem is foot drop.

The Parastep, a multielectrode bilateral FES stimulator used in conjunction with a walker and controlled by hand switches, was introduced commercially in the 1980s. Up to six muscles were stimulated, three in each leg (foot dorsiflexors, quadriceps, and gluteus medius). The device is primarily used by individuals who have complete paraplegia. These individuals have the arm and hand function required to control the device, and they lack sensation in the legs that would preclude the use of high levels of stimulation. Users must have intact lower motor neuron function in the legs (see Chapter 1). Studies have shown that although ambulation was enabled or improved by this system, the metabolic costs were generally high.[23-25] A study in France came to the following conclusion: "In spite of its ease of operation and good cosmetic acceptance, the Parastep approach has very limited applications for mobility in daily life because of its modest performance associated with high metabolic cost and cardiovascular strain. However, the Parastep can be proposed as a resource to keep physical and psychological fitness in patients with SCI".[26]

Starting in the late 1990s, surface FES has been combined with treadmill training and body weight support for locomotor training. In the first study of its kind on 19 individuals with chronic incomplete SCI (ASIA C), over-ground and treadmill gait speed more than doubled after 3 months of 1.5 hours, 3 days per week, FES plus partial weight-support training.[27] The overall conclusion reached in the SCIRE metastudy[28] on surface FES for gait post-SCI was that "FES-assisted walking can enable walking or enhance walking speed in incomplete SCI or complete (T4–T11) SCI. Regular use of FES in gait training or activities of daily living can lead to improvement in walking even when the stimulator is not in use."

Surface Stimulation Devices for Enhancing Hand Function

As with many early FES studies, the first experiments exploring FES for upper extremity function were performed by Vodovnik and colleagues in Ljubljana, Slovenia.[29,30] In the late 1970s, a group at Rancho Los Amigos in Los Angeles, California, developed a therapeutic program for hand function within their clinic, involving dozens of individuals performing daily FES-assisted biofeedback exercises.[31] In the 1990s, two designs of surface stimulator for hand function were developed for people with C6–C7 quadriplegia: the Handmaster (Fig. 5-1d[32,33]) and the Bionic Glove (Fig. 5-1e[34,35]). A clinic-based device, the ETHZ-Paracare, was developed in Switzerland and has undergone two pilot studies.[36,37]

The Handmaster, manufactured by Ness Ltd. in Israel, was medically reimbursed in Holland for several years for use as a functional splint. Recently, this device has been sold to clinics and private users in the United States under the proprietary name Bioness H200. Bioness H200 comprises a hinged wrist-forearm splint with a stimulator box electrically connected to the splint via a cable. Electrodes deployed on detachable panels inside the splint deliver trains of stimuli to combinations of three or four motor points. Stimulation is controlled by a push button on the stimulator or a switch on the part of the orthosis overlying the medial heel of the hand. A recent study in eight individuals with C5–C6 SCI reported significant improvements in hand function after using the Handmaster daily for 3 weeks.[38] Both size and rigid structure make the H200 suitable mainly for use in the clinic as a therapeutic, rather than as an orthotic, device.

The Bionic Glove comprises a fingerless flexible garment with an inbuilt stimulator and electrode contacts. The device is controlled by wrist position (flexion and extension) to augment tenodesis grasp and release. In a pilot study on nine individuals with C6–C7 SCI using the Bionic Glove as part of their usual ADL, grasp force increased fourfold and performance of manual tasks improved significantly during stimulation.[35] In an independent study in 12 individuals with C5–C7 SCI, after 6 months of using the Bionic Glove, voluntary hand function in the absence of the device had improved.[39] Individuals with C6–C7 SCI benefited the most; however, higher functioning individuals were less likely to use the device in ADL because the glove required about 5 minutes to don. Furthermore, even though the Bionic Glove was more formfitting and compliant than the Handmaster, it was still considered too bulky to wear during daily life by some individuals. Various other technical problems were encountered during this 6-month study that led to the overall conclusion that, much like the Handmaster, the Bionic Glove was more useful as a therapeutic/training device than as a permanent orthosis.

A new, more formfitting version of the Bionic Glove is currently being used in a trial involving in-home telesupervised hand exercise therapy in chronic SCI participants in Edmonton, Canada. The device has a smaller inbuilt stimulator approximately the size of an iPod Nano, which is triggered by a wireless transmitter worn behind the ear like a hearing aid. The device detects small voluntary tooth clicks, allowing the user to activate hand opening and grasp independently of wrist position and without involving the other hand.[40] Another improvement is that rather than requiring self-adhesive electrodes to be attached to the skin to make contact with metal mesh panels inside the glove, low-tack gel electrodes are now attached to the inside of the garment. With this new configuration, the system can be donned within approximately 30 seconds. A commercial version will be available to clinical researchers in early 2008. This device has been designed to be used as an orthosis in ADL as well as for therapeutic training.

Multichannel upper extremity FES has been tested experimentally in individuals with C3–C7 SCI.[10] A programmable multichannel stimulator was used to activate muscles in a sequence that allowed reach and grasp. One of the problems with surface stimulation of large muscles such as biceps and triceps brachii is that during activity, the motor points of these muscles can move several centimeters under the skin. This fact changes the relationship between the stimulating electrode and the motor nerve, thereby changing the amount of muscle activation as the elbow flexes and extends. This, in turn, results in problems of control. Nevertheless, encouraging therapeutic results were reported in this study.

Arguably, transcutaneous electrical nerve stimulators (TENS) are NPs too. The mechanism of TENS analgesia is thought to be inhibition of nociceptive transmission in the spinal dorsal horn by the activation of large sensory axons (the gate theory of pain:[41]). One popular version of electrical stimulation for pain relief is interferential stimulation.[42] The mechanism of interferential stimulation is to set up a rotating electric field that activates large afferents deep within bodily tissues by delivering alternating current through several pairs of electrodes and cyclically varying the currents through each pair independently. This approach is also known as "current steering" or "field steering," when used in implanted dorsal column and cochlear stimulators.[43,44] Interferential devices are usually large, expensive and therefore confined to clinics.

Implanted NPs

General: Cochlear, Phrenic Nerve, Deep Brain, and Sacral Stimulators

In the late 1950s and early 1960s, the first implantable cardiac pacemakers were developed.[45] According to the National Institutes of Health, over 3 million cardiac pacemakers have since been implanted, and the number may be in excess of 5 million. Cardiac pacemakers stimulate specialized cardiac muscle cells; thus, according to the above definition, they are not NPs. However, they are implanted stimulators that must remain functional in the hostile environment of the human body for many years. The development of the technology needed to achieve this quality led to a proliferation of a wide range of NPs in the late 1960s and early 1970s.

Individuals with diverse types of impairment and disability have benefited from the technology associated with the development of the cardiac pacemaker. Thousands of dorsal column stimulators have since been implanted for pain control and spasticity.[46] Dorsal column stimulators activate large sensory afferents in posterior spinal roots and in the dorsal columns. As mentioned above, according to the gate theory of pain, input from large afferents inhibits nociceptive transmission. Modified versions of dorsal column stimulators were later introduced for use as deep-brain stimulators (DBS).[47–49] Several thousand patients have been implanted with DBS devices. DBS is often effective in counteracting tremor and bradykinesia in Parkinson's disease and reducing essential tremor by affecting the firing of neurons in the basal ganglia. Several competing theories have been proposed to explain these effects.[50–52] Phrenic nerve NPs that activate the diaphragm have also been implanted in the thousands (Fig. 5-2b),[53,54] as have vagus nerve stimulators for epilepsy (Fig. 5-2d). Radio-frequency-controlled NPs that stimulated the bladder detrusor muscle were implanted in a small number of individuals in the 1960s.[55,56] In 1997, the Medtronic, Inc. (Minneapolis, Minnesota) InterStim sacral root stimulator (Fig. 5-2c) was approved by the FDA to treat urge incontinence, and since then, according to Medtronic, Inc.,[56a] 40,000 InterStim devices have been implanted. The InterStim has also been implanted off-label in a small number of SCI individuals in attempts to facilitate voiding (see below).

The most successful NP remains the cochlear stimulator.[57] In its 2007 Annual Report,[57a] Cochlear Corporation (Lane Cove, NSW, Australia) disclosed that by 2006, 100,000 of its stimulators had been implanted. Advanced Bionics had implanted 3,000 of its own cochlear stimulators by 1999. Cochlear stimulators and their associated external sound and speech processors and stimulus synthesizers are now at an advanced stage and provide a model for a new generation of NPs for motor control.

Implanted Devices for Enhancing Walking Function

Progress in restoring limb movement with implantable NPs has been slow. The technical challenge of delivering trains of pulses to nerves innervating one or more muscle groups for several hours a day for many years is formidable. A small number of individuals were implanted with foot-drop stimulators in pilot studies in the 1970s and 1980s.[58–60] The Waters and McNeal study[59] commenced in 1968 and led Medtronic, Inc. to develop a sophisticated device called the Neuromuscular Assist, which included an under-heel sensor that wirelessly triggered a portable external receiver/stimulator. This delivered power and stimulus commands through an external antenna taped to the skin to an implanted passive receiver. The receiver delivered pulse trains through a pair of electrodes in a silicone rubber flap wrapped around branches of the common peroneal nerve distal to the knee. Fifteen individuals were implanted. The system worked well in most of the recipients, in some cases for many years, but Medtronic, Inc. decided not to pursue commercialization. Recently, two models of implantable peroneal nerve stimulator have become available commercially in Europe, the Finetech Medical Ltd. (Welwyn Garden City, UK) STIMuSTEP[61] and the Neurodan ActiGait (Fig. 5-2a). In a Phase 2 safety study, 15 individuals with foot drop due to stroke were implanted with the ActiGait system and showed improvements in gait.[62] From a safety point of view, the nerve cuffs in the device was reported not capable of producing detectable reductions in nerve conduction velocity. Technical problems occurred, but were resolved at follow-up.[62] Like the Medtronic, Inc. device, the STIMuSTEP and ActiGait stimulators are triggered from an under-heel sensor. A new innovation still at the experimental stage is the use of signals recorded in sensory nerves to trigger stimulation[63,64] (Fig. 5-1).

Only a small minority of individuals with incomplete SCI benefit enough from the correction of foot drop alone to warrant the implantation of these devices. Multichannel NPs that stimulate up to 16 muscles of the legs through percutaneous or fully implanted leads have been experimented with over the years,[65–68] but they are not commercially available. However, research in this area continues, and recent results have been encouraging, particularly in relation to posture, standing, and the avoidance of pressure ulcers (bedsores).[69–73]

Intraspinal Microstimulation

A radically different approach to NPs, namely intraspinal microstimulation (ISMS) has been explored in animal experiments.[74] The method consists of implanting up to 16 microwires in the lumbosacral enlargement of the spinal cord (the region containing motoneurons innervating leg muscles). Stimulation through these microwires can activate single muscles or muscle synergies in normal animals.[75] After some initial promise,[76] several implants in spinalized animals revealed the technical limitations of the approach.[77] The implant surgeries took up to 12 hours. Manually positioning the electrodes in the right parts of the spinal cord to obtain the full set of desired synergies was difficult, and it was rarely completely successful. After days or weeks, the elicited movements changed, indicating migration of the microwires. In a trial in chronically implanted monkeys, co-contraction responses were often seen,[78] which would make it difficult or impossible to control movement in an NP application. The overall impression is that with current electrode technology,

ISMS is invasive, insufficiently reliable, and therefore not ready for clinical application (Fig. 5-2).

Implanted Devices for Enhancing Hand Function

Regarding the upper extremity, after proof-of-principle trials with percutaneous leads, a fully implanted stimulator was developed at Case Western Reserve University (CWRU) in Cleveland, Ohio.[79] The stimulator was approved by the FDA in 1997 and marketed by NeuroControl as the Freehand System (Fig. 5-2e). About 200 of these systems were implanted in individuals with C4–C5 quadriplegia. Shoulder or wrist movements were used to control the stimulation of muscles in the forearm. An external control unit and antenna wirelessly activated an implanted receiver to generate pulse trains and stimulate the muscles selected by the external controller to produce different types of hand movement. Though all aspects of the technology and surgery were highly advanced, and many recipients benefited significantly with improved hand function,[80] the Freehand System was ultimately withdrawn from the market in 2002. A fascinating analysis of the history of this and other NPs that showed clinical efficacy but did not survive commercially is to be found in a Princeton University thesis by Samuel

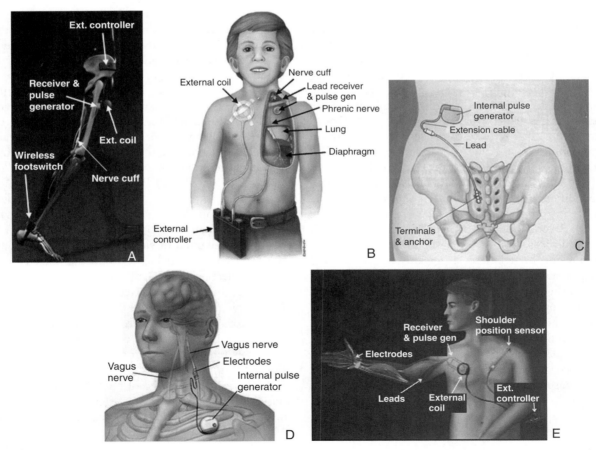

Figure 5-2. Implantable NPs. (A) Neurodan; (B) Avery phrenic nerve pacer; (C) Medtronic, Inc. InterStim sacral nerve stimulator; (D) Cyberonics vagal nerve stimulator; (E) NeuroControl Freehand System.

W. Hall.[81] Hall concludes, "While the over-exuberant health care spending of the 1970s and early 1980s has taught policymakers a valuable lesson, the vicious cost-containment initiatives characteristic of current Medicare policy are outdated and have far-reaching negative effects on public health. The Centers for Medicare and Medicaid Services should replace their anti-technology bias with a payment system capable of recognizing the profound health economic benefits of neuroprostheses."

An improved multichannel version of the CWRU device has recently been implanted in seven individuals with SCI.[82] The new device is controlled myoelectrically (i.e., via signals picked up from voluntarily activated muscles) and activates the biceps muscle as well as muscles controlling hand opening and grasp. Other recent research into novel implantable NPs for hand function include the Finetech Medical Ltd. STIMuGRIP[83] and an implantable system called the Stimulus Router, which requires only the leads to be implanted, using pulse trains coupled through the skin from a wireless-triggered wristlet stimulator[84] (Fig. 5-3). The Stimulus Router system was tested intraoperatively in January 2008 and the first permanent implant took place on June 10, 2008 in a quadriplegic man.[85]

Bladder Control

Bladder control is ranked the second most significant problem after loss of sex function among individuals with paraplegia and the fourth priority of individuals with quadriplegia.[86] SCI can cause incontinence due to a loss of external urethral sphincter (EUS) contraction and/or an inability to void due to bladder–sphincter hyperactivity (dyssynergia). Untreated, this condition can lead to very high bladder pressures, vesicoureteral reflux, and eventual renal failure. It once was the leading cause of death in people with SCI, but dropped to fourth place after the widespread adoption of clean intermittent catheterization.[87]

Electrical stimulation for bladder control has been explored for over 40 years. Stimulation has been delivered variously to the inside of the bladder, bladder wall, thigh, pelvic floor, dorsal penile nerve, pelvic nerve, tibial nerve, sacral roots, sacral nerves, and spinal cord. The successes and failures of these numerous approaches have recently been described in a detailed review.[88]

The first commercially available NP for bladder control derived from experiments in which voiding was elicited in spinalized animals by stimulation of sacral anterior roots.[89–91] Human trials of a sacral anterior root stimulator implant (SARSI) followed shortly thereafter.[92] Brindley's device was commercialized as the Finetech-Brindley Bladder System (Finetech Medical Ltd). The device has been implanted in over 2500 people, in some cases for over 20 years.[93] The main disadvantage of this device is that dorsal rhizotomies (cutting sensory nerves

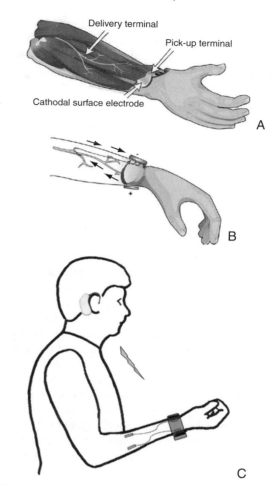

Figure 5-3. Stimulus router system. (A) Cutaway view showing a surface electrode, implanted pick-up electrode, passive conductor, and nerve cuff. (B) Cross-section showing current flowing between two surface electrodes, some being diverted through the implanted conductor to the nerve cuff and returning via forearm tissues. (C) Schematic showing stimulator cuff containing surface electrodes that deliver current to hand opening and closing nerves via the implanted leads. The cuff is triggered from a wireless earpiece that detects small voluntary tooth clicks.

to the spinal cord) are required, resulting in an irreversible loss of sensory input from the genital organs. Another drawback is that anterior root stimulation activates the EUS as well as the bladder. Voiding is achieved in bursts by taking advantage of the slower relaxation time of the detrusor (bladder) muscle after short trains of stimuli. A recent study has shown that trapezoidal pulse waveforms can activate the bladder more selectively, thus improving the performance of SARSI implants.[94] The permanent nature of procedures that require dorsal rhizotomies have lead many individuals to decline these types of interventions. However, techniques such as pudendal nerve blockade and neuromodulation may soon provide alternative NP types that do not require rhizotomies.

Regarding incontinence, implanted sacral root stimulators (e.g., the Medtronic, Inc. InterStim) are currently the most successful implantable NPs for bladder control in a variety of neural disorders, including SCI.[95]

ISMS has been explored as an alternative means of eliciting voiding, but as in the case of locomotion, ISMS so far has not lived up to initial expectations. Pilot experiments in animals and humans in the 1970s showed that stimulation through pairs of relatively large intraspinal electrodes could elicit bladder contractions, but not without coactivating the EUS.[96,97] More recent experiments have been performed with microwires implanted in the dorsal commissure of the spinal cord, which contains interneurons that inhibit EUS motoneurons.[98] Although reductions in intraurethral pressure could be elicited in some implants, the more common outcome was activation.[88,99] The dorsal commissure was subsequently shown to probably contain more interneurons that excite EUS motoneurons than those that inhibit them.[100,101] In a report published in October 2007, McCreery's group reported success in eliciting bladder contraction, concomitant EUS inhibition, and voiding in two of three spinally transected cats by stimulating mainly within the dorsal columns.[102] However, the voiding trials were performed during deep propofol anesthesia. Urinary tract responses are suppressed by propofol.[103] Bladder and EUS responses to ISMS and pudendal nerve stimulation under deep anesthesia in spinal cord-transected cats can change dramatically when the same animals are awake.[104] Stimuli that relax the EUS under anesthesia are no longer as effective under normal awake conditions. Further evidence in awake SCI animals would be needed before clinical trials could be justified.

Other experimental approaches to bladder control with NPs include neuromodulation of sacral roots;[105,106] activation of reflexes evoked by selective stimulation of specific branches of the pudendal nerve,[107–111] and high-frequency blockade of the pudendal nerve to inhibit the EUS.[112–118] Recently, activation and blockade of the pudendal nerve has been demonstrated with the stimulus router system in the awake SCI cat. This may provide a low-cost type of NP for either maintaining continence or eliciting voiding, as only two leads would be implanted.[117,118]

Factors Influencing Choice

Level of Injury

The level and completeness of SCI will determine the relevance of NPs to a particular individual. Phrenic nerve pacers are only relevant for high cervical injuries, typically at C3 and above. Upper extremity NPs are usually only effective for injuries in the range C4 to C7. Importantly, NPs activate muscles via their nerves. Often motoneurons are destroyed at the epicenter of an injury. This fact is particularly troublesome at segmental level C7,

because denervation can make eliciting hand opening and grasping virtually impossible. NPs for restoring locomotion can be useful in incomplete injuries at nearly all levels and also in complete injuries at low thoracic and lumbar levels where postural control is partially preserved. Likewise, bladder control NPs can be useful for nearly all levels of SCI, with the exception of cauda equina injuries, again because these are associated with denervation of the target muscles, in particular the EUS for bladder control.

Time After Injury

There is little evidence-based consensus on the appropriate time after injury at which to commence the use of the various types of commercially available NPs. The same could, of course, be said of conventional physiotherapy. For example, 20 years ago, the accepted wisdom was that gait training should only start at an absolute minimum of 6 weeks after stroke, whereas today it starts as soon as such training is judged clinically to be safe, which can be within a few days in mild cases. Some NPs (e.g., surface muscle stimulators applied to the forearm or shoulder) can be used within a week or two of SCI to maintain muscle bulk and to ward off spasticity, contractures, and shoulder subluxation (see Fig. 5-1c). Others (e.g., SARSI implants requiring rhizotomies) should be considered only after natural recovery has been allowed to run its full course (typically 1 year or more after injury).

Risks and Contraindications

Certain side effects or risks of electrical stimulation should always be taken into account when considering the use of NP devices. FES in people with SCI at T6 level and above can trigger autonomic dysreflexia.[119] Originally, this was attributed to nociceptive stimulation of the skin, but topical anesthesia did not change the response to FES, so muscle activation was thought to be the cause.[121] The larger the muscles stimulated, the greater the chance of triggering an episode of dysreflexia. Other side effects include pain or discomfort at high stimulus levels. There is a very wide range of tolerance between individuals in this regard. As to the cost–benefit ratio, although NP design is constantly improving, some devices still tend to be cumbersome and awkward to don and doff. The financial cost can be high, particularly in the case of implantable NPs. Having a clear idea of the functional gains that can reasonably be expected, and weighing these against cost and inconvenience are important.

Supramaximal stimulation of large leg muscles has caused patellar dislocation and even bone breakage in rare cases. Dried-out or faulty electrodes can cause skin burns, particularly in users with poor or lacking skin sensation. Implanted NPs carry a risk of postimplant infection. The risk is well established for cardiac pacemakers (~ 1%[122]) but not so for NPs, which vary considerably in size and design. Generally, the larger the stimulator and the greater the number of leads, the greater is the risk of infection. Lead breakage and migration tend to occur more in NPs than in cardiac pacemakers, necessitating relocation or explantation and replacement. Implanted microstimulators such as the Bion may also migrate, though how often this might happen cannot as yet be determined.

Despite the growing numbers of implantable NPs and, in some cases, excellent clinical outcomes, some technical and physiological concerns remain. For example, difficulties and risks are involved in implanting multiple electrodes to activate widely distributed peripheral nerves. The long-term effects of chronic stimulation of populations of neurons in the brain, spinal cord, or peripheral nerves remain to be fully explored.

Summary

In this chapter, the historical origins of electrotherapy were briefly reviewed. The basic mechanism of electrical stimulation of nerves was described. Some of the key advances in the development of NPs were identified. The main types of NP used in the management of SCI were considered, and the successes, limitations, and failures of the NP approach were discussed. Finally, some of the factors influencing an SCI individual's choice of NP treatment were reviewed.

It is now recognized that when the use of NPs is combined with other treatments, such as task-related exercise therapy,[27] significant improvements in function can result. In the near future, NPs are likely to be used increasingly in conjunction with surgical procedures such as tendon transfers, pharmacological interventions that reduce spasticity, such as Botox injections and devices that promote exercise training, such as partial weight-support robots and in-home telerehabilitation devices that allow remote supervision and game-playing to improve compliance.[123]

The treatment of incontinence has been one of the success stories of NPs. The control of bladder voiding in people with SCI remains a very important and elusive goal of NP research, but there have been some promising developments in this regard since 2003.

The last decade has seen a big increase in the number of researchers around the world developing new NP devices and approaches. There has also been a significant increase in interest and investment on the part of government agencies and the medical electronics industry in this area. The next decade should see a significant increase in the range and availability of NPs, a lowering of their cost, and an increase in the number and variety of clinical problems they can address.

REVIEW QUESTIONS

1. How effective are NPs in the control of bladder function?
2. Can present-day NPs for the upper extremity provide clinically significant benefits, and if so, does this depend on the cervical level of the SCI?
3. NPs seem very hi-tech. Are therapists and clinicians who have little or no training in electronics, math, or physics likely to understand and use them?
4. What percentage of people with SCI find electrical stimulation uncomfortable or painful?
5. NPs are often very expensive, particularly implantables. What are the payment and reimbursement options?

ACKNOWLEDGMENTS

This work was supported by the NIH, Canadian Institutes of Health Research, Alberta Heritage Foundation for Medical Research, and the International Spinal Research Trust.

REFERENCES

1. Licht SH. *Electrodiagnosis and Electromyography*. 3rd ed. New Haven,: Licht, E.; 1971.
2. McNeal D. 2000 years of electrical stimulation. In: Hambrecht FT, Reswick, J.B., eds. *Functional Electrical Stimulation*. Vol 3. New York: Dekker; 1977:3–35.
3. Duchenne G-B. *Physiology of Motion Demonstrated by Means of Electrical Stimulation and Clinical Observation and Applied to the Study of Paralysis and Deformities*. 1959 ed. Philadelphia: W. B. Saunders; 1867.
4. Vodovnik L. Therapeutic effects of functional electrical stimulation of extremities. *Med Biol Eng Computing*. 1981;19(4):470–478.
5. Andrews BJ, Wheeler GD. Functional and therapeutic benefits of electrical stimulation after spinal injury. *Curr Opinion Neurol*. 1995;8(6):461–466.
6. Shealy CN. The viability of external electrical stimulation as a therapeutic modality. *Med Instrum*. 1975;9(5):211–212.
7. Cauraugh JH, Kim SB. Chronic stroke motor recovery: duration of active neuromuscular stimulation. *J Neurol Sci*. Nov 15 2003;215(1–2):13–19.
8. Cauraugh JH, Kim SB, Duley A. Coupled bilateral movements and active neuromuscular stimulation: Intralimb transfer evidence during bimanual aiming. *Neurosci Lett*. Jul 1 2005;382(1–2):39–44.
9. de Kroon JR, Ijzerman MJ, Chae J, Lankhorst GJ, Zilvold G. Relation between stimulation characteristics and clinical outcome in studies using electrical stimulation to improve motor control of the upper extremity in stroke. *J Rehabil Med*. Mar 2005;37(2):65–74.
10. Popovic MR, Thrasher TA, Adams ME, Takes V, Zivanovic V, Tonack MI. Functional electrical therapy: retraining grasping in spinal cord injury. *Spinal Cord*. Mar 2006;44(3):143–151.

11. Hansen GvO. EMG-controlled functional electrical stimulation of the paretic hand. *Scand J Rehabil Med.* 1979; 11:189–193.

12. Heckmann J, Mokrusch T, Kroeckel A, Warnke S, von Stockert T, Neundoerfer B. Electromyogram-triggered neuromuscular stimulation for improving the arm function of acute stroke survivors: a randomized pilot study. *Eur J Phys Med Rehabil.* 1997;7:138–141.

13. Stein RB, Gordon T, Jefferson J, et al. Optimal stimulation of paralyzed muscle after human spinal cord injury. *J Appl Physiol.* 1992;72(4):1393–1400.

14. Field-Fote EC. Electrical stimulation modifies spinal and cortical neural circuitry. *Exerc Sport Sci Rev.* Oct 2004;32(4): 155–160.

15. Thomas SL, Gorassini MA. Increases in corticospinal tract function by treadmill training after incomplete spinal cord injury. *J Neurophysiol.* Oct2005;94(4):2844–2855.

16. Liberson WT, Holmquest HJ, Scott D, Dow M. Functional electrotherapy: stimulation of the peroneal nerve synchronized with the swing phase of the gait of hemiplegic patients. *Arch Phys Med Rehabil.* 1961;42: 101–105.

17. Vodovnik L, Kralj A, Stanic U, Acimovic R, Gros N. Recent applications of functional electrical stimulation to stroke patients in Ljubljana. *Clin Orthop Related Res.* 1978(131): 64–70.

18. Kralj AR, Bajd T. *Functional Electrical Stimulation: Standing and Walking after Spinal Cord Injury.* Boca Raton, FL: CRC Press; 1989.

19. Dr. Benny Klemar, personal communication.

20. Taylor P, Burridge J, Dunkerley A, et al. Clinical audit of 5 years provision of the Odstock dropped foot stimulator. *Artif Organs.* 1999;23(5):440–442.

20a. CMS; Ruling 160.12, www.cms.hhs.gov/manuals/downloads/ ncd103cl_Part2.pdf [accessed 12/20/2008].

21. Taylor PN, Burridge JH, Dunkerley AL, et al. Patients' perceptions of the Odstock Dropped Foot Stimulator (ODFS). *Clin Rehabil.* 1999;13(5):439–446.

22. Stein RB, Chong S, Everaert DG, et al. A multicenter trial of a footdrop stimulator controlled by a tilt sensor. *Neurorehabil Neural Repair.* Sep 2006;20(3):371–379.

23. Gallien P, Brissot R, Eyssette M, et al. Restoration of gait by functional electrical stimulation for spinal cord injured patients. *Paraplegia.* 1995;33:660–664.

24. Klose KJ, Jacobs PL, Broton JG, et al. Evaluation of a training program for persons with SCI paraplegia using the Parastep 1 ambulation system: part 1. Ambulation performance and anthropometric measures. *Arch Phys Med Rehabil.* Aug 1997;78(8):789–793.

25. Spadone R, Merati G, Bertocchi E, et al. Energy consumption of locomotion with orthosis versus Parastep-assisted gait: a single case study. *Spinal Cord.* Feb 2003;41(2): 97–104.

26. Brissot R, Gallien P, Le Bot MP, et al. Clinical experience with functional electrical stimulation-assisted gait with Parastep in spinal cord-injured patients. *Spine.* Feb 15 2000;25(4):501–508.

27. Field-Fote EC. Combined use of body weight support, functional electric stimulation, and treadmill training to improve walking ability in individuals with chronic incomplete spinal cord injury. *Arch Phys Med Rehabil.* Jun 2001;82(6):818–824.

28. Lam T, Wolfe DL, Hsieh JTC, Whittaker MW, Eng JJ. *Lower Limb Rehabilitation Following Spinal Cord Injury.*

29. Vodovnik L, Crochetiere WJ, Reswick JB. Control of a skeletal joint by electrical stimulation of antagonists. *Med Biol Eng.* 1967;5(2):97–109.

30. Rebersek S, Vodovnik L. Proportionally controlled functional electrical stimulation of hand. *Arch Phys Med Rehabil.* 1973;54(8):378–382.

31. Waters R, Bowman B, Baker L, Benton L, Meadows P. Treatment of hemiplegic upper extremity using electrical stimulation and biofeedback training. In: Popovic DJ, ed. *Advances in External Control of Human Extremities.* Vol 7. Belgrade: Yugoslav Committee for Electronics and Automation; 1981:251–266.

32. Nathan RH. US Patent #5,330,516. Device for generating hand function. *US Patent Office.* 1994:15 claims, 16 drawing sheets.

33. Snoek GJ, MJ IJ, in 't Groen FA, Stoffers TS, Zilvold G. Use of the NESS handmaster to restore handfunction in tetraplegia: clinical experiences in ten patients. *Spinal Cord.* 2000;38(4):244–249.

34. Prochazka A, Wieler M, Kenwell Z, Prochazka A, Wieler M, Kenwell ZProchazka A, Wieler M, Kenwell Zs. Garment for applying controlled electrical stimulation to restore motor function. US patent 5,562,707, 1996.

35. Prochazka A, Gauthier M, Wieler M, Kenwell Z. The bionic glove: an electrical stimulator garment that provides controlled grasp and hand opening in quadriplegia. *Arch Phys Med Rehabil.* 1997;78(6):608–614.

36. Mangold S, Keller T, Curt A, Dietz V. Transcutaneous functional electrical stimulation for grasping in subjects with cervical spinal cord injury. *Spinal Cord.* Jan 2005;43(1): 1–13.

37. Popovic MR, Keller T. Modular transcutaneous functional electrical stimulation system. *Med Eng Phys.* Jan 2005;27(1): 81–92.

38. Alon G. Use of neuromuscular electrical stimulation in neurorehabilitation: a challenge to all. *J Rehabil Res Dev.* Nov–Dec 2003;40(6):ix–xii.

39. Popovic D, Stojanovic A, Pjanovic A, et al. Clinical evaluation of the bionic glove. *Arch Phys Med Rehabil.* 1999;80(3): 299–304.

40. Prochazka A, Prochazka AProchazka As; Prochazka, A., assignee. Method and Apparatus for controlling a device or process with vibrations generated by tooth clicks. US patent 6,961,623. Priority: October 17 2002, filing: 16 October 2003, 2005.

41. Melzack R, Wall PD. Pain mechanisms: a new theory. *Science.* 1965;150(699):971–979.

42. Nemec H. [Endogenous electrostimulation with middle frequencies and interference zones]. *Rehabil (Bonn).* 1967;20(1):1–11.

43. Manola L, Holsheimer J, Veltink PH, Bradley K, Peterson D. Theoretical Investigation Into Longitudinal Cathodal Field Steering in Spinal Cord Stimulation. *Neuromodulation 10.* 2007;10:120–132.

44. Firszt JB, Koch DB, Downing M, Litvak L. Current steering creates additional pitch percepts in adult cochlear implant recipients. *Otol Neurotol.* Aug 2007;28(5): 629–636.

45. Chardack WM, Gage AA, Greatbatch W. Treatment of complete heart block with an implantable and selfcon-

Vancouver, BC: iCord (International Collaboration on Research Discoveries) www.icord.org/scire/home.php; 2006.

tained pacemaker. *Bull Soc Int Chir.* Jul–Aug 1962;21: 411–432.

46. Waltz JM. Spinal cord stimulation: a quarter century of development and investigation. A review of its development and effectiveness in 1,336 cases. *Stereotactic Funct Neurosurg.* 1997;69(1–4 Pt 2):288–299.

47. Benabid AL, Pollak P, Hommel M, Gaio JM, de Rougemont J, Perret J. [Treatment of Parkinson tremor by chronic stimulation of the ventral intermediate nucleus of the thalamus]. *Rev Neurol (Paris).* 1989;145(4):320–323.

48. Rezai AR, Kopell BH, Gross RE, et al. Deep brain stimulation for Parkinson's disease: surgical issues. *Mov Disord.* Jun 2006;21 Suppl 14:S197–218.

49. Benabid AL, Chabardes S, Seigneuret E. Deep-brain stimulation in Parkinson's disease: long-term efficacy and safety - What happened this year? *Curr Opin Neurol.* Dec 2005;18(6):623–630.

50. Tang JK, Moro E, Lozano AM, et al. Firing rates of pallidal neurons are similar in Huntington's and Parkinson's disease patients. *Exp Brain Res.* Oct 2005;166(2):230–236.

51. Tang JK, Moro E, Mahant N, et al. Neuronal firing rates and patterns in the globus pallidus internus of patients with cervical dystonia differ from those with Parkinson's disease. *J Neurophysiol.* Aug 2007;98(2):720–729.

52. Kuncel AM, Cooper SE, Wolgamuth BR, Grill WM. Amplitude- and frequency-dependent changes in neuronal regularity parallel changes in tremor With thalamic deep brain stimulation. *IEEE Trans Neural Syst Rehabil Eng.* Jun 2007;15(2):190–197.

53. Glenn WW, Holcomb WG, Hogan J, et al. Diaphragm pacing by radiofrequency transmission in the treatment of chronic ventilatory insufficiency. Present status. *J Thorac Cardiovasc Surg.* 1973;66(4):505–520.

54. Elefteriades JA, Quin JA. Diaphragm pacing. *Chest Surg Clin North Am.* 1998;8:331–357.

55. Bradley WE, Chou SN, and French LA. Further experience with radio transmitter receiver unit for the neurogenic bladder. *Neurosurg.* 1963;20:953–960.

56. Stenberg CC, Burnett WH, and Bunts RC. Electrical stimulation of human neurogenic bladders: experience with four patients. *J Urol.* 97: 79–84, 1967.

56a. www.medtronic.com/your-health/overactive_bladder/ device.index.htm [accessed 12/20/2008].

57. Kessler DK. The CLARION Multi-Strategy Cochlear Implant. *Ann Otol Rhinol Laryngol Suppl* 1999;177:8–16.

57a. www.cochlear.com/corp/Investor.2403.asp [accessed 12/20/ 2008].

58. Jeglic A, Vanken E, Benedik M. Implantable muscle/nerve stimulator as part of an electronic brace. Paper presented at: 3rd International Symposium on external control of human extremities, 1970; Nauka.

59. Waters RL, McNeal D, Perry J. Experimental correction of footdrop by electrical stimulation of the peroneal nerve. *J Bone Joint Surg.* 1975;57A:1047–1054.

60. Strojnik P, Acimovic R, Vavken E, Simic V, Stanic U. Treatment of drop foot using an implantable peroneal underknee stimulator. *Scand J Rehabil Med.* 1987;19:37–43.

61. Kenney L, Bultstra G, Buschman R, Taylor P, Mann G, Hermens H. An implantable two channel drop foot stimulator: initial clinical results. *Artif Organs.* 2002;26: 267–270.

62. Burridge JH, Haugland M, Larsen B, et al. Phase II trial to evaluate the ActiGait implanted drop-foot stimulator in established hemiplegia. *J Rehabil Med.* Apr 2007;39(3): 212–218.

63. Hoffer JA, Sinkjaer T. A natural 'force sensor' suitable for closed-loop control of functional neuromuscular stimulation. Paper presented at: Proc. 2nd Vienna International Workshop on Functional Electrostimulation, 1986.

64. Haugland M, Sinkjaer T, Haugland M, Sinkjaer T, Haugland M, Sinkjaer Ts. Method and implantable systems for neural sensing and nerve stimulation. US patent 0144710 A1, 2003.

65. Sharma M, Marsolais EB, Polando G, et al. Implantation of a 16-channel functional electrical stimulation walking system. *Clin Orthop Relat Res.* Feb 1998(347):236–242.

66. Davis JA, Jr., Triolo RJ, Uhlir JP, et al. Surgical technique for installing an eight-channel neuroprosthesis for standing. *Clin Orthop Relat Res.* Apr 2001(385):237–252.

67. Agarwal S, Kobetic R, Nandurkar S, Marsolais EB. Functional electrical stimulation for walking in paraplegia: 17-year follow-up of 2 cases. *J Spinal Cord Med.* Spring 2003;26(1):86–91.

68. Heilman BP, Audu ML, Kirsch RF, Triolo RJ. Selection of an optimal muscle set for a 16-channel standing neuroprosthesis using a human musculoskeletal model. *J Rehabil Res Dev.* Mar–Apr 2006;43(2):273–286.

69. Liu LQ, Nicholson GP, Knight SL, et al. Interface pressure and cutaneous hemoglobin and oxygenation changes under ischial tuberosities during sacral nerve root stimulation in spinal cord injury. *J Rehabil Res Dev.* Jul–Aug 2006;43(4): 553–564.

70. Liu LQ, Nicholson GP, Knight SL, et al. Pressure changes under the ischial tuberosities of seated individuals during sacral nerve root stimulation. *J Rehabil Res Dev.* Mar–Apr 2006;43(2):209–218.

71. Bogie KM, Wang X, Triolo RJ. Long-term prevention of pressure ulcers in high-risk patients: a single case study of the use of gluteal neuromuscular electric stimulation. *Arch Phys Med Rehabil.* Apr 2006;87(4):585–591.

72. Wilkenfeld AJ, Audu ML, Triolo RJ. Feasibility of functional electrical stimulation for control of seated posture after spinal cord injury: A simulation study. *J Rehabil Res Dev.* Mar–Apr 2006;43(2):139–152.

73. Forrest GP, Smith TC, Triolo RJ, et al. Energy cost of the case Western reserve standing neuroprosthesis. *Arch Phys Med Rehabil.* Aug 2007;88(8):1074–1076.

74. Mushahwar VK, Aoyagi Y, Stein RB, Prochazka A. Movements generated by intraspinal microstimulation in the intermediate gray matter of the anesthetized, decerebrate, and spinal cat. *Can J Phys Pharmacol.* Aug-Sep 2004; 82(8–9):702–714.

75. Mushahwar VK, Collins DF, Prochazka A. Spinal cord microstimulation generates functional limb movements in chronically implanted cats. *Exp Neurol.* 2000;163(2): 422–429.

76. Saigal R, Renzi C, Mushahwar VK. Intraspinal microstimulation generates functional movements after spinal-cord injury. *IEEE Trans Neural Syst Rehabil Eng.* Dec 2004;12(4): 430–440.

77. Guevremont L. [Ph.D.]. Edmonton: Biomedical Engineering, University of Alberta; 2006.

78. Moritz CT, Lucas TH, Perlmutter SI, Fetz EE. Forelimb movements and muscle responses evoked by microstimulation of cervical spinal cord in sedated monkeys. *J Neurophysiol.* Jan 2007;97(1):110–120.

79. Peckham PH, Creasey GH. Neural prostheses: clinical applications of functional electrical stimulation in spinal cord injury. *Paraplegia*. 1992;30(2):96–101.

80. Peckham PH, Keith MW, Kilgore KL, et al. Efficacy of an implanted neuroprosthesis for restoring hand grasp in tetraplegia: a multicenter study. *Arch Phys Med Rehabil*. 2001;82(10):1380–1388.

81. Hall SW. *Commercializing Neuroprostheses: The Business of Putting the Brain Back in Business* [B.A. Molecular Biology]. New Jersey: Princeton University; 2003.

82. Kilgore KL, Hart RL, Montague FW, et al. An implanted myoelectrically-controlled neuroprosthesis for upper extremity function in spinal cord injury. *Conf Proc IEEE Eng Med Biol Soc*. 2006;1:1630–1633.

83. Spensley J. STIMuGRIP(R); a new Hand Control Implant. *Conf Proc IEEE Eng Med Biol Soc*. 2007;1:513.

84. Gan LS, Prochazka A, Bornes TD, Denington AA, Chan KM. A new means of transcutaneous coupling for neural prostheses. *IEEE Trans Biomed Eng*. Mar 2007;54(3): 509–517.

85. Anderson KD. Targeting recovery: priorities of the spinal cord-injured population. *J Neurotrauma*. Oct 2004;21(10): 1371–1383.

86. Frankel HL, Coll JR, Charlifue SW, et al. Long-term survival in spinal cord injury: a fifty year investigation. *Spinal Cord*. 1998;36:266–274.

87. Prochazka A, Gan LS, Olson J, and Mohart M. The stimulus router system (SRS): first human intra-operative testing of a novel neural prosthesis. In: *Neural Interfaces Conference*. Cleveland: 2008.

88. Gaunt RA, Prochazka A. Control of urinary bladder function with devices: successes and failures. *Prog Brain Res*. 2006;152:163–194.

89. Brindley GS. An implant to empty the bladder or close the urethra. *J Neurol, Neurosurg Psychiatry*. 1977;40:358–369.

90. Tanagho EA, Schmidt RA, Orvis BR. Neural stimulation for control of voiding dysfunction: A preliminary report in 22 patients with serious neuropathic voiding disorders. *J Urol*. 1989;142:340–345.

91. Heine JP, Schmidt RA, Tanagho EA. Intraspinal sacral root stimulation for controlled micturition. *Invest Urol*. 1977;15: 78–82.

92. Brindley GS, Polkey CE, Rushton DN. Sacral anterior root stimulators for bladder control in paraplegia. *Paraplegia*. 1982;20:365–381.

93. Rijkhoff NJ. Neuroprostheses to treat neurogenic bladder dysfunction: current status and future perspectives. *Childs Nerv Syst*. Feb 2004;20(2):75–86.

94. Bhadra N, Grunewald V, Creasey GH, Mortimer JT. Selective activation of the sacral anterior roots for induction of bladder voiding. *Neurourol Urodyn*. 2006;25(2): 185–193.

95. Weil EH, Ruiz-Cerda JL, Eerdmans PH, Janknegt RA, Bemelmans BL, van Kerrebroeck PE. Sacral root neuromodulation in the treatment of refractory urinary urge incontinence: a prospective randomized clinical trial. *Eur Urol*. 2000;37(2):161–171.

96. Nashold BS, Friedman H, Glenn JF, Grimes JH, Barry WF, Avery R. Electromicturition in paraplegia: implantation of a spinal neuroprosthesis. *Proc Veterans Adm Spinal Cord Injury Conference*. 1971;18:161–165.

97. Nashold BS. Electromicturition in paraplegia. *Nursing Times*. 1974;70(1):22–23.

98. Prochazka A, Mushahwar VK, McCreery DB. Neural prostheses. *J Physiol*. 2001;533(Pt 1):99–109.

99. McCreery DB, Lossinsky A, Agnew WF, Bullara LA. *Functional microstimulation of the lumbosacral spinal cord. Quarterly Progress Report #4*. NIH-NINDS contract # 1-NS-2-2340; 2002.

100. Buss RR, Shefchyk SJ. Sacral dorsal horn neurone activity during micturition in the cat. *J Physiol*. Aug 15 2003;551 (Pt 1):387–396.

101. Shefchyk SJ. Spinal mechanisms contributing to urethral striated sphincter control during continence and micturition: "how good things might go bad". *Prog Brain Res*. 2006;152:85–95.

102. Pikov V, Bullara L, McCreery DB. Intraspinal stimulation for bladder voiding in cats before and after chronic spinal cord injury. *J Neural Eng*. 2007;4:356–368.

103. Matsuura S, Downie JW. Effect of anesthetics on reflex micturition in the chronic cannula-implanted rat. *Neurourol Urodyn*. 2000;19(1):87–99.

104. Gaunt R, Prochazka A. *Functional microstimulation of the lumbosacral spinal cord. Quarterly Progress Report #23*: NIH-NINDS; 2007. contract # 1-NS-2-2342.

105. Sawan M, Elhilali MM, Sawan M, Elhilali MMSawan M, Elhilali MMs; Victhom, assignee. Electronic stimulator implant for modulating and synchronizing bladder and sphincter function. U.S. patent 6,393,323, 2002.

106. Abdel-Gawad M, Boyer S, Sawan M, Elhilali MM. Reduction of bladder outlet resistance by selective stimulation of the ventral sacral root using high frequency blockade: a chronic study in spinal cord transected dogs. *J Urol*. 2001;166(2):728–733.

107. Lee YH, Creasey GH. Self-controlled dorsal penile nerve stimulation to inhibit bladder hyperreflexia in incomplete spinal cord injury: a case report. *Arch Phys Med Rehabil*. Feb 2002;83(2):273–277.

108. Boggs JW, Wenzel BJ, Gustafson KJ, Grill WM. Frequency-dependent selection of reflexes by pudendal afferents in the cat. *J Physiol*. Nov 15 2006;577(Pt 1): 115–126.

109. Boggs JW, Wenzel BJ, Gustafson KJ, Grill WM. Bladder emptying by intermittent electrical stimulation of the pudendal nerve. *J Neural Eng*. Mar 2006;3(1): 43–51.

110. Yoo PB, Klein SM, Grafstein NH, et al. Pudendal nerve stimulation evokes reflex bladder contractions in persons with chronic spinal cord injury. *Neurourol Urodyn*. 2007;26(7):1020–1023.

111. Yoo PB, Grill WM. Minimally-invasive electrical stimulation of the pudendal nerve: a pre-clinical study for neural control of the lower urinary tract. *Neurourol Urodyn*. 2007;26(4):562–569.

112. Kilgore KL, Bhadra N. Nerve conduction block utilising high-frequency alternating current. *Med Biol Eng Comput*. May 2004;42(3):394–406.

113. Bhadra N, Kilgore K, Gustafson KJ. High frequency electrical conduction block of the pudendal nerve. *J Neural Eng*. Jun 2006;3(2):180–187.

114. Tai C, Wang J, Wang X, de Groat WC, Roppolo JR. Bladder inhibition or voiding induced by pudendal nerve stimulation in chronic spinal cord injured cats. *Neurourol Urodyn*. 2007;26(4):570–577.

115. Tai C, Wang J, Wang X, Roppolo JR, de Groat WC. Voiding reflex in chronic spinal cord injured cats induced

by stimulating and blocking pudendal nerves. *Neurourol Urodyn.* 2007;26(6):879–886.

116. Boger A, Bhadra N, Gustafson KJ. Bladder voiding by combined high frequency electrical pudendal nerve block and sacral root stimulation. *Neurourol Urodyn.* Nov 27 2007.

117. Gaunt RA, Prochazka A. Activation and blockade of the pudendal nerve using transcutaneously coupled electrical stimulation. Paper presented at: Society for Neuroscience Online., 2007; San Diego, CA.

118. Gaunt RA, Prochazka A. High-frequency blockade of the pudendal nerve using a transcutaneously coupled stimulator in a chronically implanted cat. Paper presented at: Proceedings of the 12th Annual Meeting of the International Functional Electrical Stimulation Society; Nov. 10–14, 2007; Philadelphia, PA.

119. Ashley EA, Laskin JJ, Olenik LM, et al. Evidence of autonomic dysreflexia during functional electrical stimulation in individuals with spinal cord injuries. *Paraplegia.* 1993;31(9):593–605.

120. Matthews JM, Wheeler GD, Burnham RS, Malone LA, Steadward RD. The effects of surface anaesthesia on the autonomic dysreflexia response during functional electrical stimulation. *Spinal Cord.* 1997;35(10):647–651.

121. Aggarwal RK, Connelly DT, Ray SG, Ball J, Charles RG. Early complications of permanent pacemaker implantation: no difference between dual and single chamber systems. *Br Heart J.* Jun 1995;73(6):571–575.

122. Kowalczewski JA, Chong S, Prochazka A. Home-based upper extremity rehabilitation in spinal cord injured patients. Paper presented at: Society for Neuroscience, 2007; San Diego, CA.

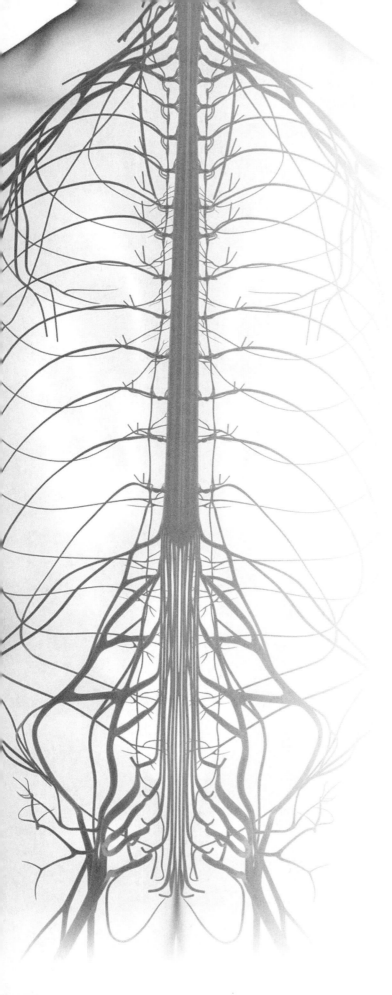

Promoting Maximal Restoration of Function

Assessment of Function   **6**

Sarah A. Morrison, PT

After reading this chapter, you will be able to:

OBJECTIVES

- Identify the justification for standardizing assessment measures for individuals with spinal cord injury (SCI)
- Describe various measurement tools used to assess altered body structures and functions for individuals with SCI
- Identify measurement tools used to assess the performance of activities for individuals with SCI
- Describe various assessment tools used to measure the level of participation for individuals with SCI

OUTLINE

Introduction

Assessing function for individuals with spinal cord injury (SCI) can be challenging, yet it is imperative that clinicians working with researchers standardize the measures by which they assess function. As medical and rehabilitation researchers and/or clinicians discover methods to restore function and quality of life to individuals with a SCI, it is important to develop easily replicated measures for demonstrating the efficiency and effectiveness of services provided in order to facilitate comparisons of outcomes among different clinical trials.[1] In addition to validating neurological or functional recovery, standardized measurements of function can also:

1. Justify cost reimbursement for medical and rehabilitative services.[2,3]
2. Predict long-term caregiver needs and estimate the amount of assistance necessary.[3,4,5]
3. Facilitate communication among health-care professionals by comparing the efficacy of different rehabilitation treatments.[2,3,4,6]
4. Guide management to initiate improvements within the rehabilitative continuum of care.[4]

This chapter will describe and discuss various assessments that have been used in SCI treatment to measure an individual's level of function. The International Classification of Functioning, Disability and Health (ICF) provides a conceptual framework for consequences of disease and injury.[7] In keeping within this framework, functional assessments will be reviewed in the *body functions and structures*, *activity*, and *participation* domains as described by the ICF.[7] These three domains address disturbances in terms of functional changes associated with the body, person, and society.[7]

The first domain of *body functions and structures* is the loss or abnormality of body structure or of a physiological or psychological function.[7] For individuals with SCI, the loss or abnormality of body structure applies to altered activity of neural structures, such as those measured by muscle weakness and sensory loss.[7,8] The second domain of *activity* is "the execution of a task or action."[7] Limitations in activities relate to an individual's difficulty in performing an activity or set of activities such as self care or mobility.[7,8] The third domain of *participation* addresses a person's involvement in life situations.[7] This third domain identifies changes in social roles, including vocational, marital, and avocational roles.[7]

The assessments of function described in this chapter will be organized using the above ICF domains. The procedures for the administration of each assessment will be reviewed along with a discussion of how they are to be scored and interpreted. In addition, the results of investigations regarding each specific assessment of function will be discussed. An overview of measures and their associated strengths and limitations are given in Table 6-1.

Table 6-1
Summary of Outcome Measures for Assessing Body Functions and Structures, Activities, and Participation in Individuals with SCI

Body Functions and Structures	Measures	Strengths	Limitations
International Standards for Neurological Classification of Spinal Cord Injury (ASIA) Examination	Sensory and motor assessment to determine neurological level, extent of injury, and level of impairment	Well-established international standards for evaluation of persons with SCI Motor scores collected early have predictive validity in functional outcomes.[12] Offers training videos, Internet-based training and manuals	Lower reliability for individuals with incomplete SCIs[9] Motor scores obtained in the supine position only
University of Miami Neuro-Spinal Index (UMNI)	Sensory and motor assessment used as a quantitative scale for spinal cord function	May be more sensitive than the ASIA Examination in detecting change due to the increased number of muscles and dermatomes tested	Used less frequently than the ASIA Examination The full assessment takes longer than the ASIA Examination due to the increased number of muscles and dermatomes tested

Table 6-1

Summary of Outcome Measures for Assessing Body Functions and Structures, Activities, and Participation in Individuals with SCI—cont'd

Body Functions and Structures	Measures	Strengths	Limitations
Yale Scale	Assesses severity of SCI[28]	Uses percentage of recovery ratio to compare various treatment modalities	More general results due to the averaging of motor and sensory scores Limits the dermatomes for assessing position sense and deep pain
National Acute Spinal Cord Injury Scale	Assesses motor and sensory function	An objective measure for neurological recovery	Not used widely. Has been replaced as the research standard by the ASIA Examination
Manual muscle test (MMT)	Determines the strength of individual muscles or muscle groups	Assessment is helpful for predicting functional potential as well as level of injury from a myotomal perspective	Decreased sensitivity for the higher levels of strength or for detection of the small changes in increased strength[30]
Myometry	Objective method for muscle strength assessment using a handheld dynomometer	Can detect changes in muscle strength not detected by traditional manual muscle tests[37,38]	Cannot detect trace muscles as it takes away the examiner's ability to palpate muscle contractions

Activities	Measures	Strengths	Limitations
Functional Independence Measure (FIM)	Measures level of independence and predicts the burden of care	Internationally recognized Offers a telephone version Has an assessment tool for children (WEEFIM)	Assessment is not SCI specific. Ceiling and floor effect for some levels of injury Cognitive subscale ceiling effect for most individuals with SCI
Modified Barthel Index (MBI)	Measures level of independence and reflects the burden of care	One of the most highly researched tools	Assessment is not SCI specific Ceiling and floor effects for some levels of injury
Spinal Cord Independence Measurement (SCIM)	Measures the functional independence of individuals with SCI	Designed specifically for individuals with SCI More sensitive than the FIM to detect functional change in individuals with SCI[62]	Not as widely used as the FIM Ceiling and floor effects for individuals with very high or very low levels of injury
Spinal Cord Injury Ability Realization Measurement Index (SCI-ARMI)	Measures the component of activity that is likely to be affected by rehabilitation	Designed specifically for individuals with SCI Enables objective and quantitative evaluation of functional changes	Not well published

Continued

Table 6-1
Summary of Outcome Measures for Assessing Body Functions and Structures, Activities, and Participation in Individuals with SCI—cont'd

Activities	Measures	Strengths	Limitations
Quadriplegia Index of Function (QIF)	Assesses function for individuals with tetraplegia	Designed specifically for individuals with SCI More sensitive than the MBI and the FIM[39]	Difficult to score due to the weighted scale Assessment for individuals with tetraplegia only
Capabilities of Upper Extremity Instrument (CUE)	Measures the action of grasp, release, and reaching in individuals with tetraplegia	Designed specifically for individuals with SCI	Assessment for individuals with tetraplegia only
Spinal Cord Injury Functional Ambulation Inventory (SCI-FAI)	Assesses deviation in various gait parameters	Designed specifically for individuals with SCI Measures the level of independence in the home and community, quality of gait, and the use of assistive devices	Does not take into consideration the amount of assistance required
Walking Index for Spinal Cord Injury (WISCI-II)	An ordinal scale describing amount of assistance needed for walking function	Designed specifically for individuals with SCI Includes assistance required as well as assistive devices used	Does not consider walking speed or endurance Does not measure quality of walking
6-Minute Walk Test (6MWT)	Measures walking endurance	Measures gait endurance Easy to administer	Does not measure the quality of gait or describe assistance or assistive devices required Requires more space to complete the assessment
10-Meter Walk Test (10MWT)	Measures walking speed	Easy to administer Minimal equipment/space requirement	Does not measure the quality of gait or describe assistance or assistive devices required Does not measure walking function in the community
Timed Up and Go (TUG)	Assesses sitting, standing, and walking function	Easy to administer Incorporates mobility and balance	Distance walked is only 3 meters Does not measure endurance of walking
Ambulatory Motor Index (AMI)	Measures the sum of hip and knee strength grades as a percentage of normal	Can predict requirements for LE orthoses, upper extremity assistive devices[71]	Does not measure the function of walking

Table 6-1

Summary of Outcome Measures for Assessing Body Functions and Structures, Activities, and Participation in Individuals with SCI—cont'd

Activities	Measures	Strengths	Limitations
Wheelchair Circuit	Assesses the performance of various wheelchair propulsion skills	Developed specifically for the SCI population	Tasks performed are only relevant to manual wheelchair users
Wheelchair Assessment Tool	Measures the ability and time to perform wheelchair skills for individuals with paraplegia	Developed specifically for the SCI population	Tasks performed are only relevant to manual wheelchair users who are diagnosed with paraplegia
Wheelchair Skills Test (WST)	Assesses the ability to perform 50 separate skills	Tasks cover a wide range of difficulty and is made up of many functional skills	Less than half of the items tested are directly concerned with wheelchair mobility Limited testing on the SCI population
Obstacle Course Assessment of Wheelchair User Performance (OCAWUP)	Evaluates the wheelchair user's performance in difficult environmental situations	Measures the degree of ease as well as the level of performance Considers environmental barriers for individuals who propel a wheelchair in the community	Not well published for use in individuals who have a SCI
Wheelchair Users Functional Assessment (WUFA)	Assesses wheelchair skills in individuals who use a manual wheelchair for 80% of their mobility	Considers environmental barriers for individuals who propel a wheelchair in the home and community environment	Requires particular equipment/environments to complete the assessment
Wheelchair Physical Functional Performance (WC-PFP)	Assesses the ability to complete various tasks from the wheelchair	Includes skills for maneuvering the wheelchair as well as completing various tasks from the wheelchair level	Further investigation is indicated to assess reliability within the SCI population Duplicates skills required of other functional performance assessments
Functional Evaluation in a Wheelchair (FEW)	Assesses functional performance from a manual and/or power wheelchair	Includes the assessment of power wheelchair skills as well as manual wheelchair skills	Completed by questionnaire

Continued

Table 6-1

Summary of Outcome Measures for Assessing Body Functions and Structures, Activities, and Participation in Individuals with SCI—cont'd

Participation	Measures	Strengths	Limitations
Craig Handicap Assessment and Reporting Technique (CHART)	Measures handicap among individuals living in a community	Establishes norms of handicap Easy to complete Has been widely published	Ceiling effect for the lower levels of SCI Total score can be misleading
Canadian Occupational Performance Measure (COPM)	A client-centered outcome measurement tool	Areas covered are individually relevant	No published norms for different levels of injury Not appropriate for persons that lack insight
Assessment of Life Habits (Life-H)	Assesses the quality of social participation of individuals with disability	Incorporates interaction of the individual and the environment	No normative data for individuals with SCI
Impact on Participation and Autonomy (IPA)	A generic questionnaire that addresses perceived participation and autonomy	Relatively short questionnaire that can be used across diagnoses	Limited information for individuals with SCI

Body Functions and Structures

Standard examination and classification procedures are necessary for clinicians and researchers to accurately communicate the extent of injury and the degree of recovery for individuals with SCI.[9] This section will review specific assessments in the "body functions and structures" domain that address altered activity of neural structures as measured by tests of sensory and motor function.

International Standards for Neurological Classification of SCI

In 1982, the American Spinal Injury Association (ASIA) developed standards for the neurological testing of individuals with SCI.[10] The neurological examination is a standardized clinical examination that assesses the degree of functional disability as well as the prognosis for recovery (Appendix 6-A on page 131).[11] The ASIA standards for neurological classification of SCI has two main components, sensory and motor, which together determine the neurological level of the injury, the extent of the injury, and the level of impairment.

Sensory Examination

The sensory examination is completed by testing 28 key sensory points along the dermatomes on the right and left sides of the body. Each of these points are tested and scored separately for the light touch and the pinprick sensory modalities. A 3-point scale is used to score each modality of sensation (0, absent; 1, impaired; 2, normal).[10] Sensory scores are calculated by adding the scores for each dermatome for a total possible score of 112 each for pinprick and light touch (56 for each side of the body). Changes in sensation over the acute, subacute, and chronic phases of injury are identified by comparing sensory scores. A higher score indicates the individual perceives more sensation. The sensory level is defined as the most caudal dermatome to have intact sensation for both pinprick and light touch on both sides of the body.[10] In addition to the key sensory points, the external anal sphincter is tested, and perceived sensation is recorded as present or absent.[10]

Overall light touch and pinprick assessments have high intra-rater and inter-rater reliability; however, the reliability of sensory scores is greater for individuals with a complete injury compared to those with an incomplete injury.[9] Interclass correlation coefficients (ICC) for sensory and motor scores by neurological category are given in Table 6-2.

Motor Examination

The motor examination is completed by testing 10 key muscles for the left and right sides of the body (5 for the

Table 6-2

ICC for Pinprick, Light Touch and Motor Index Scores by Neurological Category

	Para Complete	Para Incomplete	Tetra Complete	Tetra Incomplete
Pinprick				
UE	0.15	–0.06	0.94	0.62
Trunk	0.97	0.74	0.94	0.84
LE	0.71	0.89	1.00	0.89
Light Touch				
UE	1.00	–0.06	0.93	0.89
Trunk	0.94	0.65	0.94	0.32
LE	0.93	0.06	0.99	0.73
Motor Index				
UE Muscles	1.00	0.95	0.99	0.76
LE Muscles	1.00	0.95	1.0	0.97

Reprinted with permission from *Topics in Spinal Cord Injury Rehabilitation.* 1996;1(4): 24–26. Thomas Land Publishers. Available at: http://www.thomasland.com

upper body and 5 for the lower body).[10] Each of the key muscles represents a neurological segment between C5–T1 and L2–S1 and are listed below:

C5 – elbow flexors
C6 – wrist extensors
C7 – elbow extensors
C8 – long finger flexors
T1 – small finger abductors
L2 – hip flexors
L3 – knee extensors
L4 – ankle dorsiflexors
L5 – long toe extensors
S1 – ankle plantarflexors

The above muscles are examined in the supine position, beginning with the most rostral muscles and proceeding in a caudal direction.[10] The strength of each muscle is graded using a 6-point grading scale:

0 – total paralysis
1 (trace) – palpable contraction
2 (poor) – active movement with full range of motion (ROM) with gravity eliminated
3 (fair) – active movement with full ROM against gravity
4 (good) – active movement with full ROM against moderate resistance
5 (normal) – active movement with full ROM against full resistance

In addition to testing the key muscles, the external anal sphincter is tested and recorded as present or absent. The grade of each key muscle is added together, and the total is referred to as the *motor index score.* The motor index score can range from 0 to 100 (0 to 50 for each side of the body) and provides a means of numerically documenting changes in motor function. To provide the clinician with additional information regarding muscle strength and level of injury, ASIA recommends evaluating additional muscles such as the diaphragm (via fluoroscopy), abdominals (via the Beevor's sign), medial hamstrings, and hip adductors. However, the strength of these muscles are not used in determining the motor score or motor level.[10] Muscle testing for the ASIA standards differs from those of more traditional muscle testing and will be discussed later in this chapter.

Once motor scores are obtained, a motor level is determined for the left and right sides of the body by determining the most caudal segment of the spinal cord with a motor function score of at least a 3/5, provided that the next most rostral key muscle scores a 5/5. For the spinal levels that are not clinically tested for motor function (T2–L1), the motor level is recorded as the same as the sensory level.

The reliability of the motor index score that results from the muscle test has excellent inter- and intra-rater scoring (ICC ranging from 0.91 to 0.99).[9] Table 6-2 shows the ICC for motor index scores by neurological category.

A standard time interval after the initial injury for completing the motor and sensory assessment is recommended. Brown and colleagues[12] showed that a 72-hour muscle test score is a better predictor of recovery at 3 months post-injury than an examination performed within 24 hours of injury.[12] The authors described several reasons for the superiority of the 72-hour test, including (1) an improvement of the individual's ability to cooperate with the testing procedure, (2) the inherent progression of neurological damage, and (3) early surgical or medical interventions that may have altered the scores.[12]

ASIA Impairment Scale

The results of the motor and sensory examination give the necessary information to determine the ASIA Impairment Scale (AIS). The AIS was modified from the Frankel classification,[13] and the AIS describes the degree of impairment as listed below. Reliability for the AIS shows excellent overall agreement between raters (kappa = 0.72).[14]

A – Complete: No sensory or motor function preserved in the sacral segments S4–S5.
B – Incomplete: Sensory but not motor function is preserved below the neurological level including the sacral segments S4–S5.
C – Incomplete: Motor function is preserved below the neurological level, and more than half of the key muscles below the neurological level have a muscle grade less than 3 (grades 0–2).
D – Incomplete: Motor function is preserved below the neurological level, and at least half of the key muscles below the neurological level have a muscle grade of 3 or more.
E – Normal: Sensory and motor function is normal.

The AIS has been shown to predict recovery patterns for various impairment levels. For example, Marino et al.[15] reported that individuals with a violent etiology of injury are significantly more likely than those with a nonviolent etiology to have a complete injury (65% versus 46%, $p < 0.001$). Individuals with a violent etiology are also more likely to remain complete from discharge from inpatient rehabilitation (94% vs 86%; $p < 0.001$).[15] It has been shown that one-third of individuals classified as an AIS B remain motor complete while one-third of these individuals convert to AIS C and one-third convert to AIS D or E.[15]

Other authors such as Burn et al[16] showed that 105 individuals classified as AIS C or D tetraplegia upon admission ambulate 200 feet by the time of discharge from inpatient rehabilitation.[16] In addition, 90% of individuals under the age of 50 years old who are classified as AIS C and 40% of the individuals older than

50 years old who are classified as AIS C are able to ambulate 200 feet.[16] It appears that AIS B subgroups with preserved pinprick sensation at 72 hours post-injury have a better chance of regaining walking function compared to those without pinprick sensation.[16–18] The more favorable prognosis for individuals with pinprick sensation may be explained by the close anatomical relationship of the corticospinal tract to the lateral spinal thalamic tract.[17]

Motor recovery following SCI has been well researched. Ditunno et al.[19] found that roughly 70% to 80% of acutely injured individuals who score a muscle grade of 1/5 or 2/5 at 1 week post-injury recover to the next neurological level within 3 to 6 months; however, those with no motor strength show less recovery during this same time period. Other authors have noted that individuals with SCI having an initial muscle grade of 1/5 (trace) recover to muscle grade of 3/5 (fair) within 3 months of the initial injury.[20] Wu and colleagues[21] showed that subjects with no initial motor function have a better chance of muscle recovery to a grade of 3/5 (fair) strength by 1 year post-injury if they have acquired a 2/5 (poor) strength grade by 3 months post-injury. In addition, 68% to 82% individuals with muscle strength scores of 1 to 2.5/5 at admission improve to a grade of 3/5 or better between 3 and 6 months and 90% within 9 to 12 months. Conversely, only 14% to 36% of individuals who have no motor power recover during the same period of time.[22]

Studies have also found a positive correlation between function and strength.[23] For example, AIS motor scores can predict the level of ambulatory capacity following SCI.[11] Individuals with AIS lower extremity motor scores equal to or less than 20/50 show decreased outcomes compared to those individuals whose lower extremity motor scores are 30 or more.[6] Individuals with a lower extremity motor score of 20 or less use a wheelchair as their primary mode of locomotion: if they achieve ambulation, it is, at best, at a household level, using bilateral knee ankle foot orthoses.[6] In addition, they walk at a slower pace (3.5 meters/minute) with a higher heart rate (130 beats/minute) and exert more pressure through their upper extremities onto an assistive device.[6] On the other hand, individuals with lower extremity scores of 30 or more are likely to become community ambulators, with physiological parameters comparable to that of able-bodied individuals.[6] Individuals who have a lower extremity score more than 30 have an increased walking speed (57.5 meters/minute), a lower heart rate (108 beats/minute), and exert less pressure on their assistive device compared to their counterparts who had a lower extremity score of 20 or less.[6]

Authors have also shown that motor scores can predict the level of independence an individual with SCI achieves while performing activities of daily living.[24–26] There is increased independence noted in individuals whose injuries have a more caudal neurological level.[25] This observation is not surprising when one considers that injuries with a more caudal neurological level have more intact musculature and that the functional activities of daily living require muscle function to perform. When predicting self-care function in individuals with SCI, the motor level appears to be superior to the neurological or sensory level in determining the relationship with functional tasks.[26]

University of Miami Neuro-Spinal Index

The University of Miami Neuro-Spinal Index (UMNI) is a quantitative scale for assessing spinal cord function.[27] The UMNI is composed of two subscales: sensory and motor. The sensory and motor scale scores are indicators of overall spinal cord functional capacity. The total scores (sum of motor and sensory scores) range from 0 to 460, where 0 represents no detectable function and the score of 460 indicates normal function. The motor score is obtained by muscle testing 44 muscle groups on a 6-point (0 to 5) scale. Motor scores range from 0 to 220. Sensory scores range from 0 to 240 and are obtained by assessing pain and vibratory sensation. Each stimulus is tested on 30 dermatomes for each side of the body and scored as 0, absent; 1, impaired, or 2, normal. The UMNI is used less frequently than the AIS assessment; however, the UMNI may be a more sensitive assessment tool to detect change in spinal cord function due to the increased number of muscles and dermatomes tested.

The UMNI has a high inter-rater reliability for both the motor scale score ($r = 0.85$) and the sensory scale score ($r = 0.93$).[27]

Yale Scale

The Yale Scale assesses the severity of SCI and is used as a measure of prognosis for individuals with SCI.[28] The scale is based on a neurological examination that numerically grades selected spinal cord functions below the level of injury. The scale combines motor and sensory function in selected muscle groups and dermatomes. The motor severity scale assesses the strength of 10 selected muscle groups from each side of the body using a 0 to 5 grading scale. An average is obtained by dividing the sum of the graded muscles by the number of muscles tested.

Sensory scores are obtained by assessing pinprick, position sense, and deep pain, independently of each other. Pinprick is graded on a scale of 0 to 2 (0, no sensation; 1, abnormal sensation; 2, intact sensation).[28] A score is obtained by dividing the sum of the responses in the dermatomes below the level of injury by the number of dermatomes tested. Position sense is tested for the fifth finger and the first toe and is scored using the same 3-point scale used for the pinprick assessment. The scores for each are averaged and rounded off to the nearest tenth. Deep pain is tested by compressing the Achilles tendon or by squeezing the first toe and is scored on a 2-point scale (0, no sensation; 1, sensation detected).

The motor score and the three sensory scores are added and referred to as the *Yale Scale score*. The Yale Scale scores range from 0 (complete absence of motor/sensory function below the level of the injury) to 10 (intact function).[28] Relative recovery of the initial deficit measured as a percentage recovery ratio is presented as an analytical tool for comparison of effectiveness of different methods of therapy.[28]

National Acute Spinal Cord Injury Scale

The National Acute Spinal Cord Injury Scale (NASCIS) was used in assessing the effectiveness of methylprednisolone in the 1980s and 1990s. In this assessment, motor function is evaluated in 14 muscle groups on both sides of the body and is graded from 0 to 5, with a total motor score between 0 and 70.[29] Sensory function is divided into pinprick and light touch for 29 dermatomal levels from C2 through S5. Each dermatome is scored on a 3-point scale (1, absent; 2, decreased; 3, normal).[29] A total score for sensation ranges from 29 to 87. Again, this assessment is not used as widely as the AIS exam, but it was an important measurement used in the NASCIS studies.

Assessment of Muscular Strength

The manual muscle test (MMT) remains one of the most commonly used tools in the assessment of individuals with SCI. The MMT is universally accepted as a clinical tool to determine strength of individual muscles or muscle groups, as well as for assessments of neurological classification (as with AIS). MMT scores provide clinicians with the necessary information to guide them during therapeutic planning and outcome evaluation.[30] The MMT grades strength according to the ability of a muscle to move a joint against gravity and/or resistance applied by an examiner. The grading scale described by Daniels and Worthingham[31] is as follows:

0 (zero)—No muscle contraction
1 (trace)—Trace muscle contraction
2 (poor minus)—Muscle can perform partial ROM with gravity eliminated
2 (poor)—Muscle can perform full ROM with gravity eliminated
3 (fair)—Muscle can perform full range of motion against gravity
3+ (fair plus)—Muscle can perform full ROM against gravity and added minimal resistance
4 (good)—Muscle can perform full ROM against gravity and added moderate resistance
5 (normal)—Muscle can perform full ROM against gravity and added normal resistance

Other MMT scales have additional + and − grades; however, the use of additional gradations are discouraged as they have been shown to be unreliable.[31] Test–retest reliability coefficients for MMT ranged from moderate to excellent ($r = 0.63$ to 0.98).[32,31] Inter-rater reliability in individuals with SCI has shown to be excellent ($r = 0.94$).[33]

The MMT described here is different from the one described by the International Standards for Neurological classification of SCI.[10] First, the grading scale is different. International Standards[10] do not permit the use of + or − modifiers in the grading of muscle strength. Second, the individual is positioned based on the muscles being tested and whether the muscle is tested in the gravity-eliminated position or the antigravity position. The International Standards[10] dictate that the individual must be in the supine position when grading all muscles regardless of the strength of the muscle.

Muscle strength scores correlate with functional abilities for individuals with SCI. Welch[34] explored the importance of 3+ muscle scores in wrist extension and elbow extension and compared these scores to the ability to become independent in a variety of activities. Other authors have found that muscle strength in the elbow flexors, shoulder flexors, and wrist extensors correlates with the ability to perform bladder management, toileting, dressing, and transfers.[35] Fujiwara[36] found a very strong correlation (Spearman correlation 0.93, $p < 0.001$) between scapular/shoulder muscle scores and the ability to perform bed-to-wheelchair transfers.

Some authors have shown that the MMT does not have sufficient sensitivity to distinguish between increments of higher levels of strength or to detect the small or moderate increases in strength observed in individuals with SCI.[30] This lack of sensitivity has resulted in the investigation of other methods for determining strength, such as myometry.

Myometry is a quantitative and objective method for muscle strength assessment using a handheld dynomometer. This device (of which there are many types) measures the maximal isometric strength of the muscle using a continuous scale that reflects the force exerted against the device (usually measured in pounds or kilograms). An increase of mean myometry values was found to correspond to a proportional increase of MMT scores.[30] Schwartz[33] found a moderate to excellent association between MMT and myometry ($r = 0.59$ to 0.94) for elbow flexors and wrist extensors in 122 individuals with tetraplegia. The stronger associations between MMT and myometry were noted for muscles whose strengths scored less than a 4 (good).[33] Results suggest that a handheld myometer is capable of detecting change in muscle strength that is not detected by MMT.[37,38]

The test–retest reliability coefficients for the myometer ranged from 0.69 to 0.90.[32] The MMT was less discriminating than the myometer in identifying small differences in muscle strength.[32] Disadvantages of using the myometer are that the device comes between the hands of the examiner and the muscle being tested and can be difficult to stabilize when testing stronger individuals.[32]

Activities

As stated earlier, *activity* is defined as the execution of a task or action.[7] Activity differs from body functions as it is more at the "person level" rather than the "system level." Most of the assessments performed in a rehabilitation setting fall into the activities domain, as they define a level of independence. Noting improvements in level of independence is necessary for rehabilitation reimbursement, but one must note that these improvements do not necessarily reflect neurological recovery and could be due to the results of compensatory training. The goals of inpatient rehabilitation are to reduce disability by increasing an individual's independence in performing activities and to minimize the limitations of impairments.[39,40] Rating scales to measure the ability to perform mobility and activities of daily living have been developed to provide objective measures of functional status and change during and after acute rehabilitation for individuals with SCI.[4]

An assessment of activities should meet certain basic criteria. The assessment should be reliable and valid, feasible for use in clinical investigations, and sufficiently sensitive to the magnitude of change that one can reasonably expect to achieve with the treatment(s) under study.[41] A scale that is not sensitive will miss real changes in the individual's functional status. Many assessment tools exist to measure the ability of an individual to perform functional skills; however, only a few will be described.

Functional Independence Measure

The Functional Independence Measure (FIM) is the predominant measure to assess activities of daily living for all types of disabilities. The FIM is the most commonly used measure to evaluate the functional ability of individuals with SCI.[3,42–44] The FIM was added to the National SCI Database in 1988 because of the need to have a way to measure disability.[45] The FIM is also used by the Model Spinal Cord Injury System supported by the National Institute on Disability and Rehabilitation Research (NIDRR)[39] and the NASCIS.[29] The FIM is also a major component of the functional related groups (a classification system used to determine payment for rehabilitation).[46]

The FIM consists of 18 items (13 motor and 5 cognitive). Each item is scored on a 1 to 7 ordinal scale, with 1 representing total dependence and 7 representing total independence without the use of equipment.[39] A total FIM score ranges from 13 (total dependence) to 126 (totally independent). In addition to a total score, the FIM provides two domain scores (motor and cognitive), 6 subscale scores (self care, sphincter control, transfers, locomotion, communication, and social cognition), and 18 individual item scores.[47] Motor scores range from 13 to 91, and the cognitive scores range from 5 to 35.

The main objective of this assessment tool is to predict the burden of care.[48] Higher scores indicated fewer care hours required. The time to administer the FIM is roughly 20 to 30 minutes.[39]

The FIM demonstrates excellent inter-rater reliability as well as high internal consistency.[47,49,50] For assessment of individuals with SCI, the FIM shows good reliability, validity, sensitivity, and practicality.[64] The ICC for the total FIM, motor FIM, and cognitive FIM is 0.96, 0.96, and 0.91, respectively.[64] The ICC for each subscale score is high and ranges from 0.89 to 0.94.[64] There are statistically significant differences in FIM scores between individuals with SCI who have differing levels of impairment severity ($p < 0.005$).[49] The more severe the SCI, the lower the FIM scores: incomplete paraplegia scores (FIM = 105) > complete paraplegia (FIM = 97) > incomplete tetraplegia (FIM = 95) > complete tetraplegia (FIM = 72).[49]

Stineman et al.[51] used the FIM instrument to generate functional outcome benchmarks among inpatients with traumatic SCI. The majority of individuals whose motor FIM scores were above 30 at the time of admission were able to groom, dress the upper body, manage bladder function, use a wheelchair, and transfer to/from the bed and chair at the level of supervision or higher (FIM scores 5 to 7) by the time of discharge from inpatient rehabilitation. Most individuals whose admission scores were above 52 achieved independence in all but the most difficult FIM tasks (stairs and tub/shower transfers).[51]

The total FIM also has predictive value in relation to the percentage of individuals with SCI who return home following discharge from inpatient hospitalization. A study by New[40] showed that individuals with a lower total FIM score are less likely to return home following discharge. Individuals with a FIM admission score of 44 returned home whereas individuals with a score of 29 did not return home ($p < 0.001$).[40]

Personal care assistance services are among the most costly aspects of daily living following a SCI. Personal care assistance services account for as much as 44% of the recurring costs for individuals with SCI.[52] When looking at predictors for the need of personal care assistance, the total FIM has a greater predictive value than length of stay, days in a nursing home, neurologic category, employment, living environment, insurance, gender ethnicity, age, and years post-injury.[53] In a sample of 2154 individuals with SCI, the average number of hours for personal care services was 8.63 hours per day (3.39 hours per day of paid services and 4.86 hours of unpaid services).[53] There appeared to be a relation with total FIM scores, number of years post-injury, and the amount of personal care assistance required. Each additional point of motor FIM corresponded to reductions of 8.0, 10.0, and 18.4 minutes in paid, unpaid, and total hours of personal care assistance, respectively.[53] In addition, each subsequent year following the SCI was associated with 6.6 fewer minutes of total assistance.[53]

There are some identified limitations of the FIM when using it to assess function for individuals with SCI. First, the FIM was designed for evaluation of individuals with all types of impairment, and consequently, it fails to measure specific functional skills that are important in the rehabilitation of individuals with SCI. Second, the FIM's main purpose is to determine "burden of care" rather than measure the ability to perform complex tasks. Third, individuals with SCI have a notable ceiling effect on the FIM cognition subscale scores, with roughly 65% to 93% obtaining the maximum scores for the cognitive categories.[40] Last, some studies have shown a lack of sensitivity of scores between individuals with C8 tetraplegia, high-level paraplegia, and low-level paraplegia.[54,55]

Modified Barthel Index

The Barthel Index was originally developed by Mahoney and Barthel[56] and was later revised by Granger et al.[1] to the Modified Barthel Index (MBI). The MBI was created for individuals with neuromuscular or musculoskeletal disorders and used to measure their level of independence.[56] The MBI has 15 activities that are scored based on the level of independence achieved (Table 6-3).[1]

The total score ranges from 0 to 100 and reflects the burden of care. A score of 60 to 100 indicates independence. A score of 40 or below suggests severe dependence, while a score of 20 or below suggests total dependence.[56] However, the MBI measures basic activities of daily living, and an individual may score 60 to 100, but still need assistance with more complex skills that are not represented in the MBI assessment. This assessment tool is easily understood and can be scored quickly by anyone who adheres to the item definitions.[56] The MBI assessment tool has high internal consistency (alpha = 0.92), high test–retest reliability (0.89), and high inter-rater reliability (>0.95).[1,57]

The MBI has been shown to be a sensitive and reliable assessment scale to record change in function over time among individuals with SCI. For individuals who have a complete SCI, a strong and statistically significant relationship is found between MBI scores and the severity of the spinal cord lesion. Individuals with a higher level of lesion will have significantly lower MBI scores than the individuals with a lower-level SCI lesion.[58]

A study of 708 individuals with SCI showed that the MBI was sensitive to functional changes over the course of rehabilitation. There was a significant ($p < 0.001$) change in the scores at admission to rehabilitation (mean score = 24.6) compared to discharge from rehabilitation (mean score = 58.9).[59] Results from the analysis of covariance showed that total discharge MBI scores relate to injury level ($p < 0.001$), completeness of injury ($p < 0.001$), and admission MBI score ($p < 0.001$), but not to age.[59] In addition, a significant interaction between level and completeness of injury exists ($p < 0.001$) such that the difference in discharge MBI scores between individuals

Table 6-3
Modified Barthel Index[1]

Item	Independence	Assistance	Dependence
Self-Care Tasks			
Drinking from cup	4	2	0
Eating	6	3	0
Upper body dressing	5	3	0
Lower body dressing	7	4	0
Brace donning	0	-2	0
Grooming	5	3	0
Bathing	6	3	0
Bladder continence	10	5	0
Bowel continence	10	5	0
Mobility Tasks			
Chair transfer	15	7	0
Toilet transfer	6	3	0
Tub transfer	1	0	0
Walk on level, 50 yards	15	10	0
Up and down stairs, 1 flight	10	5	0
Wheelchair 50 yards	5	0	0

with complete and incomplete tetraplegia is significantly greater than the difference between individuals with complete and incomplete paraplegia.[59]

Spinal Cord Independence Measure

The Spinal Cord Independence Measure (SCIM) was specifically designed for the functional assessment of individuals with SCI. The SCIM consists of 18 tasks, which are divided into three subscales of function (self care, respiratory and sphincter management, and mobility (Appendix 6-B on page 133).[18] Items and scoring for each subscale are listed below. A final score ranges from 0 to 100. The SCIM takes about 30 to 45 minutes to administer.[42,60,61]

- Self care includes feeding, bathing, dressing, and grooming. Scores range from 0 to 20.[60]
- Respiration and sphincter management includes respiration, bladder management, bowel management, and use of a toilet. Scores range from 0 to 40.[60]

- Mobility is divided into two parts: tasks performed in the bedroom and bathroom and tasks performed all over the house and outdoors. Mobility in the bedroom and bathroom includes mobility in the bed and transfers to and from the bed, wheelchair, and toilet/tub. Mobility in other parts of the house and outdoors includes mobility for short, moderate, and long distances, stair management, and transfers to and from the wheelchair and car. Scores for this subscale range from 0 to 40.[60]

The SCIM has been shown to be a more precise assessment than the FIM when tested on individuals with SCI.[60–63] Inter-rater reliability studies indicate excellent consistency of the SCIM measurements ($r = 0.91$ to 0.99; $p < 0.0001$).[60] The SCIM shows an 80% frequency of identical scoring by two independent raters for 13 of 18 individual functions listed (64% to 100% range for all tasks).[61] In the self-care subscale, frequency of identical scoring was 80% to 99%.[61] There was a relationship noted between the scores of both the SCIM and FIM scales ($r = 0.85$, $p < 0.01$); however, the SCIM was more sensitive than the FIM to changes in function for individuals with SCI. The SCIM detected all the functional changes detected by the FIM total scoring, but the FIM missed 26% of the changes detected by the SCIM total scoring.[62] All functional fluctuations detected by the FIM total score were also detected by the SCIM total score in the subgroups of tetraplegia, paraplegia, complete lesions, and incomplete lesions.[62] The FIM, however, missed 25% to 27% of the functional changes detected by the SCIM.[62] The mean difference between consecutive scores was significantly higher for the SCIM ($p < 0.01$). These results indicate that the SCIM is a reliable disability scale that is more sensitive to changes in function than the FIM for individuals with SCI.[60]

The SCIM has the following advantages: (1) it includes functional skills relevant to individuals with SCI; (2) scores are more sensitive for those achievements considered more important for individuals with SCI; (3) each area of function is assessed according to its weight relative to the overall activity; and (4) scoring criteria are precisely defined and presented in the evaluation sheet.[60] The disadvantage is that the SCIM is not as widely used as the FIM assessment.

Spinal Cord Injury Ability Realization Measurement Index

The Spinal Cord Injury Ability Realization Measurement Index (SCI-ARMI) uses the combined scores of the International Standards for Neurological Classification of SCI and the SCIM to create the SCI ARMI.[64] It is an assessment of disability that is weighted for the neurological deficit. The weighted disability is represented by the ratio of the actual functional performance score to the potential performance score given a certain neurological status. The SCI-ARMI (score range 0 to 100) is intended to replace intuitive estimation of the chances and possible effect of rehabilitation, which are independent of neurological status. The new instrument is designed to measure the component of activity that is likely to be affected by rehabilitation in individuals with SCI lesions and thus help predict and evaluate the outcome and efficiency of rehabilitation. The SCI-ARMI enables objective and quantitative evaluation of functional changes in individuals with SCI, isolating them from the effect of neurological changes. Further exploration of this assessment tool is indicated.

Quadriplegia Index of Function

Of individuals who have sustained a SCI, 52.9% are diagnosed as having tetraplegia.[65] The Quadriplegia Index of Function (QIF) (Table 6-4) was developed in 1980 because the Barthel Index was deemed too insensitive to document the small but significant functional gains made by individuals with tetraplegia.[66]

The QIF consists of two parts. The first part assesses nine categories: transfers, grooming, bathing, feeding, dressing, wheelchair mobility, bed activities, bowel program, and bladder program. The second part is a supplemental questionnaire that assesses the individual's understanding of personal care. Understanding personal care is assessed via multiple choice questions covering 10 content areas such as skin care, nutrition, equipment, medication, and infections.[63,67]

Each category in the QIF contains individual items that are scored from 0 to 4 in order of increasing independence (0, total dependence: 1, assistance needed; 2, supervision; 3, independent with devices; and 4, independent). Category scores are obtained by summing the item scores in a particular category. The category and questionnaire scores are then weighted by multiplying the score of each category by the assigned relative weight (percentage) of each category. A final score ranges from 0 to 100, and subscores for each variable are available if needed. The estimated time to administer the QIF is 15 to 20 minutes.[39,66]

The QIF is more sensitive than other popular assessment tools, such as the MBI.[39] Scores by different raters, working independently, were found to be significantly positively correlated for all subscores ($p < 0.001$). Pearson coefficient correlation values for the ratings by different observers showed statistical significance ($p < 0.001$).[39] The QIF shows a high correlation with the FIM ($r = 0.97$, $p < 0.001$)[61] and shows a good to high correlation with motor ($r = 0.91$, $p < 0.001$), pinprick ($r = 0.65$, $p < 0.01$), and light touch scores ($r = 0.64$, $p < 0.001$) of the International Standards for Neurological Classification of SCI.[23] The improvement indicated by the ASIA motor scores shows a good correlation with the gain in QIF scores ($r = 0.68$, $p < 0.001$) but shows a poor correlation with FIM gain scores ($r = 0.38$, $p > 0.05$).[23] The average gain in QIF and FIM scores are 30.12 out of 180 points and 14.20 out of 126 points, respectively.[23] The QIF scoring is able to identify improvements in functional abilities for persons with tetraplegia, whereas the FIM score may not reflect a change in ability.[39]

A short-form QIF has been developed due to previous work suggesting that the items within self-care and mobility categories of the QIF can be reduced to 6 items without losing discriminatory information.[67] Regression analysis identified the following items to be the best predictors of the total 37-item QIF score: (1) wash/dry hair, (2) turn supine to side in bed, (3) put on lower body clothing, (4) open carton/jar (feeding), (5) transfer from bed to chair, and (6) lock wheelchair.[67] Scores for the short QIF range from 0 to 24. The short form retains good internal consistency characteristics with less redundancy.[67] The Spearman correlation coefficient between the short-form QIF and 37-item QIF score is shown to be 0.978.[67] Further research is indicated to assess if the short from QIF is as sensitive to change as the 37-item QIF.

Table 6-4
Quadriplegia Index of Function

Category	Component Activities (Scored separately)	Relative Weights of Category (%)
Transfers	1. Bed–Chair 2. Chair–Bed 3. Chair–Toilet/Commode 4. Toilet/Commode–Chair 5. Chair–Vehicle 6. Vehicle–Chair 7. Chair–Shower/Tub 8. Shower/Tub–Chair	8
Grooming	1. Brushing Teeth/Managing Dentures 2. Brushing/Combing Hair 3. Shaving (men) 4. Managing tampon (women)	6
Bathing	1. Wash/Dry upper body 2. Wash/Dry lower body 3. Wash/Dry feet 4. Wash/Dry hair	4
Feeding	1. Drink from cup/glass 2. Use spoon/fork 3. Cut food (meat) 4. Pour liquids out 5. Open carton/jar 6. Apply spreads to bread 7. Prepare simple meals 8. Apply adaptive equipment	12
Dressing	1. Upper indoor clothes on/off 2. Lower indoor clothes on/off 3. Upper outdoor (heavy) clothes on/off 4. Socks on/off 5. Shoes on/off 6. Fasteners	10
Wheelchair Mobility	1. Turn corners 2. Reverse direction 3. Lock wheelchair brakes 4. Propel wheelchair on rough/uneven surface 5. Propel wheelchair on an incline 6. Move and position in chair 7. Maintain sitting balance	14

Table 6-4
Quadriplegia Index of Function—cont'd

Category	Component Activities (Scored separately)	Relative Weights of Category (%)
Bed Activities	1. Supine–prone 2. Supine–long sitting 3. Supine–side 4. Side–side 5. Maintain long sitting balance	10

Bladder Program	Separate sets of scoring criteria for:
	A. Voluntary voiding
	  1. Toilet
	  2. Commode
	B. Intermittent catheterization program
	C. Autonomic bladder program
	D. Indwelling catheter
	E. Ileal diversion
	F. Crede
		14

Bowel Program	Separate sets of scoring criteria for:
	A. Complete control
	  1. Toilet
	  2. Commode
	B. Suppository
	  1. Toilet
	  2. Commode/Bed/Chux pad
	C. Digital disimpaction
	  1. Toilet disimpaction
	  2. Commode/Bed disimpaction
	D. Digital or mechanical stimulation
	  1. Toilet
	  2. Commode/Bed
		12

Understanding Personal Care	1. Skin Care 2. Diet/Nutrition 3. Medication 4. Equipment 5. Range of motion 6. Autonomic dysreflexia 7. Upper respiratory infection 8. Urinary tract infection 9. Deep vein thrombosis 10. Obtaining human services	10

From Gresham GE, Labi MLC, Dittmar SS et al. *Paraplegia* 1993;31:225–233.

Capabilities of Upper Extremity Instrument

The Capabilities of Upper Extremity Instrument (CUE) is a 32-item questionnaire that measures the actions of grasp, release, and reaching in individuals with tetraplegia.[8] The CUE measures reaching and lifting, pulling and pushing, wrist actions, hand and finger actions, and bilateral actions. The first four categories are examined separately for the right and the left sides of the upper body.[8] The individual is then asked to rate each skill on the amount of limitation they experience (*limitation* is defined by either not doing or having trouble performing the action in order to complete everyday activities). The limitations are scored using the following scale:

7—Not at all limited
6—A little limited
5—Some limitation
4—Moderately limited
3—Very limited
2—Extremely limited
1—Totally limited, can't do at all

The CUE exhibits good validity and high test–retest reliability (ICC = 0.94).[8] Pearson and Spearman rank correlations display a high correlation with the upper extremity motor scores and the FIM for the total sample of individuals diagnosed with motor-complete SCI. The CUE has also shown to have a good correlation for those diagnosed with motor-incomplete SCI. When examined by motor levels, CUE scores increase with motor level and can discriminate between individuals who are at least two motor levels apart.[8]

Walking Assessments

Factors that influence walking potential include the individual's level of conditioning, motivation, and severity of paralysis.[68] It is estimated that between one-quarter and one-third of individuals with SCI in rehabilitation regain some ability to walk by the time of discharge from inpatient hospitalization.[69] The potential for an individual with SCI to become a community ambulator by 1 year post-injury has been reported to be 100% for individuals with tetraplegia with lower extremity scores of 20 or more and for individuals with paraplegia with lower extremity scores of 10 or more on the motor portion of the International Standards for Neurological Classification of SCI. In contrast, only 45% of individuals with complete paraplegia become community ambulators.[70] When compared with an able-bodied population, individuals with SCI who are ambulatory have a 52% slower velocity (41 m/min vs 80 m/min), a 23% greater rate of oxygen consumption (14.9 mL/kg/min vs 12.1 mL/kg/min), and a 240% higher oxygen cost per meter (0.52 mL/kg/m vs 0.15 mL/kg/m).[71]

Many of the previously mentioned assessment scales are for an overall assessment of function and are not specific to walking function. Since individuals with SCI can become ambulatory, assessment tools are important to measure change in those who have some ambulatory function, and there are a number of such tools available for this purpose.

Spinal Cord Injury Functional Ambulation Inventory

The Spinal Cord Injury Functional Ambulation Inventory (SCI-FAI) is an observational gait assessment.[72] The SCI-FAI addresses three separate domains: gait, assistive device use, and walking mobility (Table 6-5).

The range of composite scores for each of the three domains is 0 to 20, 0 to 14, and 0 to 5, respectively. Because these scores measure different domains of function, it is not recommended to combine these scores into a total score. The advantage of the SCI-FAI over other gait assessment tools is that it not only measures the level of independence in the home and community but also the quality of the gait and the use of assistive devices.

The SCI-FAI has been shown to be a reliable, valid, and sensitive measure of walking ability in individuals with SCI.[72] There is a moderate to good negative correlation ($r = -0.742$ and -0.700) found between the gait score and time required to walk a specified path. Inter-rater reliability is moderate to good for the live score and the videotaped records (ICC = 0.703, 0.800, 08.40, respectively). Intra-rater reliability is high (ICC = 0.903, 0.960, and 0.942, and 0.850 for raters 1 to 4). Moderate correlation is found between the change in gait score and the change in lower extremity strength ($r = 0.58$). In addition, there is complete agreement (100%) among raters for the objective domains of inventory (assistive device use and walking mobility score).[72]

Walking Index for Spinal Cord Injury

Developed in 2000 and revised in 2001, the Walking Index for Spinal Cord Injury (WISCI-II) is an ordinal scale describing walking function on a 21-level scale (0 to 20) (Table 6-6).

The WISCI-II also integrates assistive devices such as walkers/canes and lower-limb extremity orthotics. This scale is based on the premise that there is a hierarchical improvement in the ability to ambulate that can be captured in terms of bracing, assistive device use, and amount of assistance required.[73]

The WISCI-II has face validity, criterion validity, and shows responsiveness to change.[19,47,73,74] Inter-rater reliability scoring of 40 video clips showed 100% agreement.[19] In addition, data suggests agreement among the experts in rank ordering of original items ($W = 0.843$, $p < 0.001$).[19] The WISCI-II scale is more sensitive to incremental change than the Barthel Index, FIM, or the SCIM.[75] There is a significant positive correlation between WISCI-II and other scales: Barthel Index ($r = 0.67$), SCIM ($r = 0.97$), and FIM ($r = 0.70$) with $p < 0.001$ for each.[74] Lower extremity

Table 6-5
The Spinal Cord Injury Functional Ambulation Inventory (SCI-FAI)

Name: Parameter	Session: Criterion	Date: L	R
Weight Shift	Shifts weight to stance limb	1	1
	Weight shift absent or only onto assistive device	0	0
Step Width	Swing foot clears stance foot on limb advancement	1	1
	Stance foot obstructs swing foot on limb advancement	0	0
	Final foot placement does not obstruct swing limb	1	1
	Final foot placement obstructs swing limb	0	0
Step Rhythm (relative time needed to advance swing limb)	At heel strike of stance limb, the swing limb begins to advance in <1 second or requires 1–3 seconds to begin advancing or requires >3 seconds to begin advancing	2 1 0	2 1 0
Step Height	Toe clears floor throughout swing phase or toe drags at initiation of swing phase only or toe drags throughout swing phase	2 1 0	2 1 0
Foot Contact	Heel contacts floor before forefoot or forefoot or foot flat first contact with floor	1 0	1 0
Step Length	Swing heel placed forward of stance toe or swing toe placed forward of stance toe or swing toe placed rearward of stance toe	2 1 0	2 1 0
	Parameter Total		Sum __/20

Assistive Devices		L	R
Balance/Weight-bearing devices	None	4	4
	Cane(s)	3	3
	Quad cane(s), crutch(es) (forearm/axillary)	2	2
	Walker	2	
	Parallel bars	0	
Assistive devices	None	3	3
	AFO	2	2
	KAFO	1	1
	RGO	0	0
	Assistive Device Total		Sum __/14

CE Measures			
Typical walking practice as opposed to W/C use	Walks:		
	Regularly in community (rarely/never use W/C)	5	
	Regularly in home/occasionally in community	4	
	Occasionally in home/rarely in community	3	
	Rarely in home/never in community	2	
	For exercise only	1	
	Does not walk	0	
	Walking Mobility Score		Sum __/5

(distance walked in 2 minutes) Distance walked in 2 minutes = _____

Table 6-6
Walking Index for Spinal Cord Injury (WISCI-II)

00	Patient is unable to stand and/or participate in assisted walking
01	Ambulates in parallel bars, with braces and physical assistance of two people, less than 10 m
02	Ambulates in parallel bars, with braces and physical assistance of two persons, 10 m
03	Ambulates in parallel bars, with braces and physical assistance of one person, 10 m
04	Ambulates in parallel bars, no braces, and physical assistance of one person, 10 m
05	Ambulates in parallel bars, no braces, and no physical assistance, 10 m
06	Ambulates with walker, with braces and physical assistance of one person, 10 m
07	Ambulates with two crutches, with braces and physical assistance of one person, 10 m
08	Ambulates with walker, no braces, and physical assistance of one person, 10 m
09	Ambulates with walker, with braces and no physical assistance, 10 m
10	Ambulates with one cane/crutch, with braces and physical assistance of one person, 10 m
11	Ambulates with two crutches, no braces and physical assistance of one person, 10 m
12	Ambulates with two crutches, with braces and no physical assistance, 10 m
13	Ambulates with walker, no braces, and no physical assistance, 10 m
14	Ambulates with one cane/crutch, no braces, and physical assistance of one person, 10 m
15	Ambulates with one cane/crutch, with braces and no physical assistance, 10 m
16	Ambulates with two crutches, no braces, and no physical assistance, 10 m
17	Ambulates with no devices, no braces, and physical assistance of one person, 10 m
18	Ambulates with no devices, with braces and no physical assistance, 10 m
19	Ambulates with one cane/crutch, no braces, and no physical assistance, 10 m
20	Ambulates with no devices, no braces and physical assistance, 10 m

Reprinted with permission from Macmillan Publishers Ltd: *Spinal Cord.* 2005;43:655.

muscle strength correlates with the WISCI-II levels, and the progression of the individuals recovering from SCI follows the hierarchical ranking of the WISCI-II.[75]

Initial AIS classification may be predictive of mobility outcome on the WISCI-II. Morganti et al.[74] showed that 6.4% (5 of 78) of individuals with a classification of ASIA A attained independent walking during inpatient rehabilitation, versus 23.5% (4 of 17) of individuals with AIS B, 51.4% (56 of 109) of individuals with AIS C, and 88.6% (39 of 44) of individuals with AIS D. AIS grades and WISCI-II exhibit a strong correlation, which further supports the construct validity of the scale. The highest correlation is shown for individuals who are AIS C and D.[74] Correlation of AIS grades with WISCI-II levels were significant at initial ambulation ($p < 0.03$) and at maximum recovery of walking function ($p < 0.001$).[73]

6-Minute Walk Test

The 6-Minute Walk Test (6MWT) was originally developed as a measure of gait endurance for individuals with respiratory disease.[76] The assessment consists of asking the individual to walk as far as possible for a duration of 6 minutes. There are standard phrases used to encourage the individual during the walking test, as altering the method of encouragement can affect the individual's pace by up to 30%.[77] The measurement recorded is the distance walked. It is not known whether it is best to express change in the 6MWT by an absolute value, a percent change, or a change in percentage of predicted values.[77] Secondary measures can include fatigue and dyspnea.[78]

In 6 minutes, healthy individuals walk between 400 and 700 meters.[78] Factors that decrease the distance walked in 6 minutes include shorter height, older age, higher body weight, being female , impaired cognition, and shorter corridor. Factors that increase the distance walked in 6 minutes include taller height, being male, high motivation, and having previously performed the test.[77]

The 6MWT has been shown to be a valid and reliable measure for assessing walking function for individuals with SCI.[79] Individuals with chronic incomplete SCI have shown improvement in the 6MWT post-locomotor training.[80] Intra-rater reliability and inter-rater reliability are high ($r > 0.95$; $p < 0.001$ for each).[79] A statistically significant mean increase in 6MWT in a group of participants is often much less than a clinically significant increase in a single individual.[77]

10-Meter Walk Test

The 10-Meter Walk Test (10MWT) was developed as a measure for walking speed in individuals with stroke.[81] The clinician instructs the individual to "walk as fast as you can." The equipment used to measure the 10MWT is a straight walkway (a minimum of 14 meters long) and a stopwatch. The individuals accelerate for the first 2 meters and decelerate the last 2 meters. The final time is recorded as the number of seconds it takes the individual to walk the middle 10 meters of the walking path.[79]

The 10MWT has been shown to be a valid and reliable measure for assessing walking function in individuals with SCI.[79] Intra-rater and inter-rater reliability are high ($r > 0.05$; $p < 0.001$ for each).[79] The 10MWT shows significant increase in mean gait speed (0.11 ± 0.10 m/s; $p < 0.001$) after locomotor training in chronic incomplete SCI.[80] However, for individuals with poor walking ability (0 to 10 WISCI), the results of the 10MWT must be interpreted with caution.[80]

Timed Up and Go

The Timed Up and Go (TUG) measures the time (in seconds) required for an individual to stand up, walk 3 meters, return to a chair, and sit down. The TUG has been shown to be a valid and reliable measure for assessing walking function in individuals with SCI.[79] Intra-rater and inter-rater reliability is high ($r = 0.979$ and $r = 0.973$; $p < 0.001$, respectively).[79] As with the 10MWT, the results of the TUG should be interpreted with caution for individuals with poor walking ability (0 to 10 WISCI-II).[80]

Van Hedel et al.[79] compared the three timed walking tests (6MWT, TUG, and 10MWT) and an excellent correlation among tests ($r > 0.88$) was demonstrated. A moderate correlation with the WISCI-II ($r > 0.60$) was also shown. The correlation between the timed tests for individuals with poor walking ability remains high ($r > 0.70$), but the correlation between the timed tests and the WISCI-II was low ($r < 0.35$). High correlation coefficients ($r < 0.97$) were found for intra- and inter-rater reliability in use of the TUG. The TUG and 10MWT reliability measures were negatively influenced by poor walking function. When individuals have a WISCI-II score of 0 to10, the correlation coefficients are $r = 0.92$, -0.70, and -0.96 between the TUG and 10MWT, the 6MWT and the TUG, and the 6MWT and the 10MWT, respectively. When the WISCI score is within the range of 11 to 20, the correlation coefficients were 0.79, -0.78 and -0.93 for each of the timed tests.[79]

Ambulatory Motor Index

The Ambulatory Motor Index (AMI) is a sum of the hip- and knee-strength grades expressed as a percentage of normal. The muscles tested are hip flexion, abduction, extension, and knee extension and flexion using a modified scale. Instead of a traditional 6-point scale for grading the muscle strength, a 4-point scale is used: 0, absent; 1, trace/poor; 2, fair; 3, good or normal.[68,71] The maximum possible score is 30 (15 for each side of the body).[68,71]

The AMI can predict requirements for lower extremity orthoses, upper extremity assistive devices, and the amount of arm work necessary to support oneself as measured by peak axial load on an upper extremity assistive device.[68] An AMI of less than 40% is associated with the need for two knee-ankle-foot orthoses (KAFO) to ambulate, while an AMI of 58% indicates that the individual does not require KAFOs.[68] Also, AMI seems to parallel the need for upper extremity assistive devices.[71] On average, if the AMI is 79% or greater, no assistive devices are needed, whereas scores of 68%, 44%, and 34% indicate the need for one cane/crutch, two crutches, or a walker, respectively.[71] It is not surprising that the peak axial loads of the upper extremities on the assistive device correlate with the AMI scores as individuals with greater lower extremity paralysis need to rely more on their arm strength to ambulate with assistive devices. The peak axial load ranges from 0% for individuals who do not require an assistive device to 39.2% for individuals who require the use of a walker.[68] Lastly, the AMI correlates with gait velocity and cadence ($r > 0.7$; $p < 0.001$ for each), oxygen cost per minute ($r = 0.77$; $p < 0.001$), and peak axial load ($r = 0.91$, $p < 0.001$).[68]

Wheelchair Mobility Assessments

Among individuals with SCI, 82% depend on wheelchairs as their primary means of mobility.[82] To function independently in the community, wheelchair users must achieve independence in a variety of wheelchair skills to allow them to negotiate physical barriers within the home and community environments.[83] Wheelchair mobility assessment tools should make it possible to identify difficult environmental situations and the extent of the difficulties encountered by wheelchair users.[43] Assessment of wheelchair skills is not only important for documentation of rehabilitation outcomes, but also to assist engineers in the development and assessment of new wheelchair technologies. Many of the tasks essential for independence in wheelchair mobility are not appropriately reflected on the FIM, MBI, QIF, or SCIM. Therefore, other assessment tools have been developed to more accurately reflect the activities necessary to accomplish independence in wheelchair mobility. Several of these measurement tools will be discussed.

Wheelchair Circuit

The Wheelchair Circuit consists of eight standardized tasks related to activities of daily living. Test scores are reported for ability, performance time, and physical strain.[84–86] The ability score is the main score. All items that can be performed adequately and independently are scored between 0.5 and 1.0. All points are summed to give an overall score. The ability score ranges from 0 to 8. The performance time score is the sum of the performance times for completing a figure eight and the 15-meter sprint. The addition of the timed score makes it possible to detect changes in wheelchair skill performance in subjects who have achieved the maximum ability score.[86] Physical strain is calculated using the peak heart rates achieved during the performance of the 3% and 6% slope items on the treadmill.

Tasks are to be performed in fixed sequence as described below:

1. Figure eight: The individual is to propel a wheelchair in a figure eight shape around three markers placed 1.5 meters apart. A maximum time of 1 minute is allowed for completion of this task.
2. Crossing a doorstep: The individual propels the wheelchair up and over a wooden doorstep that measures 0.4 meters high, 0.15 meters wide, and 1.2 meters long. A maximum time of 2 minutes is allowed.
3. Mounting a platform: The individual propels the wheelchair up a wooden platform that is 0.1 meters high, 1.2 meters wide, and 1.2 meters long. A maximum time of 2 minutes is allowed.
4. Sprint: The individual is asked to propel the wheelchair as fast as possible for 15 meters. A maximum time of 1 minute is allowed.
5. 3% slope: This skill is performed while on a treadmill at a starting speed of 0.56 meters per second with 0% slope. After 10 seconds, the slope is raised to 3% for 10 seconds before the incline returns to 0%.
6. 6% slope: This activity mirrors the 3% slope described above, but the maximum incline is 6%.
7. Wheelchair driving: The individual is asked to propel the wheelchair for 3 minutes at a speed of 0.83 meters/second.
8. Transfer: The individual transfers between the wheelchair and a table set at the same height as the top of the wheelchair cushion.

The Wheelchair Circuit has shown to be a valid test to assess wheelchair skill performance during inpatient rehabilitation.[84] The intra-rater reliability of the sum of tasks that each subject is able to perform is high (ICC = 0.98), as is the inter-rater reliability (ICC = 0.97).[84] Figure eight, sprint, and transfers also show a high inter- and intra-rater reliability (ICC ≥ 0.94).[84]

For individuals with SCI, ability scores are significantly different between levels of injury.[84] Individuals with paraplegia score significantly higher than those with tetraplegia. The ability score is positively correlated with the FIM mobility scores, peak power output, and peak oxygen consumption.[84] Individuals with higher values of peak power output and/or stronger muscle test scores have better scores on the Wheelchair Circuit than individuals with lower values. When an individual improves his/her peak power output and/or manual muscle test sum score, it is associated with better wheelchair skill scores.[85]

Wheelchair Assessment Tool

A Wheelchair Assessment Tool was developed by Harvey et al.[87] and was designed to assess mobility in wheelchair-dependent individuals with paraplegia. The scoring system is a 6-point scale (1, dependent; 6, independent) and is similar to the scale used for the FIM. The wheelchair assessment tool scores the level of assistance as well as the time required to complete each of the tasks. The six tasks include the following: supine to long sit; horizontal transfer 20 centimeters from a plinth; vertical transfer from the floor back into the wheelchair; propelling a wheelchair around 2 markers placed 25 meters apart; pushing a wheelchair around two markers placed 15 meters apart on a 1:12 graded ramp; and negotiating curbs ranging from 15 to 25 centimeters high.[87] The assessment can be administered in 15 minutes and does not require special equipment.[86] It has been shown to have high inter-rater reliability for each task (r = 0.82 to 0.96) for individuals with paraplegia who were wheelchair dependent.[86]

Wheelchair Skills Test

The Wheelchair Skills Test (WST) includes the performance of 50 separately scored skills. The skills address handling of the wheelchair, transfers to and from the wheelchair, maneuvering the wheelchair, and negotiating obstacles.[88] All skills are scored on a 2-point scale (0, failure; 1, pass). The order of the skills being tested begins with the easier skills and progresses to the more difficult tasks. A total goal attainment score is calculated as follows:

$$\text{Goal attainment score} = \frac{(\text{total raw score}) - (\text{\# of skills scored})}{(\text{total raw score possible}) - (\text{\# skills scored})} \times 100\%$$

The mean time taken to administer the WST is 27.0 minutes, with a range of 12 to 70 minutes.[88] Test–retest and intra-rater, inter-rater reliability have ICCs for total scores that are 0.904, 0.959, and 0.968, respectively.[88]

There appears to be a negative correlation with WST scores and age. The older the individual, the lower the WST score (r = –0.434, p < 0.001).[88] Regression analysis identifies sex as a significant factor (p < 0.001), with men scoring significantly higher than women.[88] The amount of experience an individual has propelling a wheelchair significantly effects the total WST scores as well.[88] Individuals who have used a wheelchair for 21 days or less have a 59.6% lower score than those who have wheelchair use experience for more than 21 days ($p < 0.006$).[88] In addition, individuals using a conventional weight wheelchair have lower total WST scores than those using a lightweight wheelchair, with mean values of 6.4% and 75.1%, respectively ($p < 0.001$).[88]

A disadvantage to this wheelchair assessment tool is that less than half (15 of the 33) items are directly concerned with actual wheelchair mobility.[86] In addition, there is a low correlation between WST scores and FIM scores, which is attributable to the fact that the FIM measures many different skills in addition to wheelchair mobility.[88]

Obstacle Course Assessment of Wheelchair User Performance

The purpose of the Obstacle Course Assessment of Wheelchair User Performance (OCAWUP) is to evaluate the wheelchair user's performance in potentially difficult environmental situations.[44] The wheelchair assessment tool consists of 10 obstacles divided into four environmental categories (negotiating in tight spaces, getting over obstacles of varying height, negotiating different types of terrain, and negotiating different levels of inclines). Execution time (measured in seconds) and degree of ease are used to evaluate the wheelchair user's performance in negotiating each obstacle.[44] The degree of ease is measured on a 4-point scale: 3, total success; 2, success with difficulty; 1, partial failure; and 0, complete failure. The global score of ease ranges from 0 to 30.[44] Test–retest reliability varies from good to excellent ($r = 0.74$ to 0.99). The analyses show a strong positive association between the global score of ease and FIM partial score ($r = 0.84$, $p \leq 0.05$).[44]

Wheelchair Users Functional Assessment

The Wheelchair Users Functional Assessment (WUFA) is designed to assess wheelchair skills in individuals who use a manual wheelchair for at least 80% of their home and community mobility. The WUFA includes a 13-item test scored similar to that of the FIM (ranging from 1, total dependence to 7, completely independent). The total score obtained ranges between 13 and 91. Unlike the FIM, a score of 7 can be given for individuals using a manual wheelchair if the user meets a certain time requirement.[89] The skills include maneuvering in tight spaces, negotiation over uneven terrain, door management, crossing the street, ascending ramps and curbs, a bed transfer, a toilet transfer, a floor transfer, bathing; upper and lower body dressing, and reaching and picking up objects from the floor.[89] The time to administer this assessment is roughly 1.0 to 1.5 hours.

Equipment needed to complete the WUFA includes a thick carpet, a doorway, an area for straight propulsion, a curb cut, portable ramps and curbs, a bed or low plinth, a toilet with grab bars, a floor mat, a tub with bath bench, specific clothing items, an adjustable shelf, a water jug and cup, a broom with dustpan, kitty litter, a waste basket, two quarters, and an 8-pound sandbag. Inter-rater reliability and stability of the WUFA are high (ICC = 0.96 and 0.78, respectively).[89] The Cronbach's alpha measure of reliability resulted in high internal consistency (0.96) between the 13 items on the WUFA.[89]

Wheelchair Physical Functional Performance

The Wheelchair Physical Functional Performance (WC-PFP) assessment is an adaptation of the Continuous Scale for Physical Functional Performance Measure.[90] The score includes measures of upper body strength, upper body flexibility, balance and coordination, and endurance.[91] Scores range from 0 (inability to perform task) to 100 (highest performance). A WC-PFP total score is derived from averaging all tasks. The tasks measured include lifting and transferring a pan of specified weight, transferring and pouring water from a jug into a cup, donning and doffing a jacket, putting Velcro-closed straps over a shoe, picking up scarves from the floor, transferring laundry from a washer to a dryer, placing and removing a sponge from an adjustable shelf, carrying groceries, pulling open and passing through a door, transferring to a standard chair, and a undergoing a 6-minute wheel test.[91] The advantage of this assessment is that it includes skills for maneuvering the wheelchair as well as completing various tasks from the wheelchair level. Further investigation is indicated to assess reliability within the SCI population.

Functional Evaluation in a Wheelchair

All wheelchair functional measures discussed to this point have been assessments specific for manual wheelchair users. One instrument, the Functional Evaluation in a Wheelchair (FEW), investigates functional performance of both manual and power wheelchair users.[92] The FEW is designed as a self-administered questionnaire. It serves as a dynamic indicator or profile of perceived user functions related to wheelchair use. The FEW consists of 10 categories: transfer, reach, accessing task surfaces, transportation/portability, human–machine interface, architectural barriers, transportation/accessibility, transportation/securement, natural barriers, and accessories. This instrument requires further refinement, but it nonetheless shows potential for the inclusion of power wheelchair mobility assessments.

Participation

The literature contains for fewer published assessments to evaluate *participation* compared to the assessments for *activities*. However, it appears that there is a growing interest in defining and objectively measuring participation for individuals with various disabilities, including SCI. The goal of assessing participation for individuals with SCI is to measure the return of an individual to pre-injury societal roles.[93] By identifying various behaviors that prevent the individual from obtaining pre-injury societal roles/functions, treatment interventions can focus on improving the specific activities associated with a lack of participation.

Craig Handicap Assessment and Reporting Technique

The Craig Handicap Assessment and Reporting Technique (CHART) was developed in the late 1980s and measures handicap among individuals undergoing rehabilitation living in a community setting.[94] The CHART is administered by interview or self-report and contains 32 questions within six domains. Its objective is to quantify the extent to which individuals fulfill various social roles.[95] The domains, as described by Whitneck et al.,[93,96] are as follows:

1. *Occupation:* Hours per week spent working, schooling, homemaking, maintaining one's home, doing volunteer work, recreating and other self-improvement activities. The occupation domain score is calculated by the formula:

   2 × (hours/week in working, schooling, homemaking or performing home maintenance) + (hours/week volunteering and performing recreation and/or other improvement activities)

   One hundred points indicates a person with no occupational handicap.[94]

2. *Physical independence:* The ability to sustain a customary effective independent existence. The physical independence domain score is calculated by the following formula:

   100 − (4 × (hours/day that care [paid and unpaid] is provided)

   If the individual takes primary responsibility for instructing or directing caregivers, the number of hours is multiplied by a factor of 3 instead of 4 as indicated above.[94]

3. *Mobility:* The ability to move about effectively in one's surroundings. The mobility domain score is calculated by the formula:

   2 × (hours/day out of bed) + 5 × (days/week out of the house)

   In addition, a maximum of 10 points is awarded for questions pertaining to home accessibility, and up to 20 points each are awarded to individuals for spending nights away form home and for independence in transportation.[94]

4. *Social integration:* The ability to participate and maintain customary social relationships. The social integration domain score assesses household composition and romantic involvement. Up to 30 points can be earned. Additional points are given for the number of individuals with whom regular contact is maintained

and for the frequency of initiating conversations with strangers and acquaintances.[94]

5. *Economic self-sufficiency:* The ability to sustain customary socioeconomic activities and independence. This domain is measured by the total household family income from all sources not used for medical care. Net resources are then compared with governmental poverty scales. A score of 100 is given if the figure is two times the poverty level.[94]

6. *Orientation:* The ability to orient oneself to his/her surroundings. Measured by performance in other dimensions, such as successful employment, mobility, and social integration.[94]

A total CHART score is produced by adding the scores of the physical independence, mobility, occupation, social integration, and economic self-sufficiency dimensions. A maximum of 100 points may be scored for each for the subscales of Occupation, Physical independence, Mobility, Social integration, and Economic self-sufficiency. The maximum score for the CHART is 500 points, which is indicative of absence of handicap.[94] However, it is recommended that users do not calculate CHART total scores, but base analyses on the individual subscores so that important inter-group differences are not obscured.[96]

The CHART has been shown to be a valid and reliable assessment tool.[94,97] Rasch analyses demonstrates that CHART is a well-calibrated linear scale with a good fit of both items and individuals to its data.[94] The CHART shows high test–retest reliability for the total score ($r = 0.93$) and for each of the subscales ($r = 0.80$ to 0.95).[96]

The CHART has been shown to be a sensitive measure for individuals with SCI.[95,97] The CHART scores showed the expected trends in terms of level and completeness of injury, age, time since injury, and other correlations.[96] The more severe impairments show a more significant handicap across all of the five domains.[94] Individuals with AIS D reach the maximum scores most often, while individuals with high tetraplegia (AIS A, B, C) obtain maximum subscale scores least often.[96] It is evident that completeness and level of injury have a significant influence on physical independence, mobility, and occupation subscale scores and, consequently, on the total score. It is noted that the lower the level of injury, the greater the community integration and the less important completeness of injury becomes. On the other hand, the scores of social integration and economic self-sufficiency are not significantly different among different levels of injury. Table 6-7 shows anticipated CHART scores for the different levels and severity of SCI.

Canadian Occupational Performance Measure

The Canadian Occupational Performance Measure (COPM) is a client-centered, individualized outcome

Table 6-7
CHART Scores for Different Level of Injuries and Impairments

| Subscale | ASIA A, B or C | | | | | | ASIA D | | | | | |
| | High Tetraplegia | | | Low Tetraplegia | | | Paraplegia | | | All | | |
	Mn	SD	n	Mn	SD	n	Mn	SD	n	Mn	SD	n
Physical Independence	49.9	30.4	253	71.8	28.3	498	90.3	19.8	787	90.7	20.6	340
Mobility	58.5	28.0	267	76.0	25.6	513	85.5	21.0	804	86.2	22.4	346
Occupational Status	34.5	32.9	270	51.0	36.9	512	61.8	35.5	793	62.1	36.5	347
Social Integration	78.7	25.6	261	83.5	23.1	493	85.6	20.4	760	86.7	20.2	331
Economic Self-Sufficiency	59.6	40.7	128	62.0	36.7	274	66.0	37.6	460	77.6	32.0	201
Total score	294.1	101.4	116	369.2	89.9	259	404.1	87.5	419	420.5	85.3	186

Reprinted with permission from *Topics in Spinal Cord Injury Rehabilitation.* 1998; 4(1): p20, Thomas Land Publishers.
Available at: http://www.thomasland.com.

measure administered using a semistructured interview to allow the individual to identify areas of difficulty in the three domains of self care, productivity, and leisure.[98] The COPM was developed to detect change in an individual's self-perception of occupational performance in the context of his or her environment.[98]

Once the areas of difficulty are identified, the individual rates the importance of each issue. From this list, individuals choose up to five problems they wish to focus on during their treatment sessions. Individuals rate their current level of performance and satisfaction with their performance in each of these five identified areas. A scale from 1 to 10 is used, with 10 being the most important (1, great difficulty or not satisfied, and 10, no difficulties or completely satisfied). The performance and satisfaction scores of the selected activities are summed and averaged over the number of problems identified. Upon reassessment, the COPM guidelines recommend that the individual review the same areas they identified on the initial assessment. A change score is obtained by subtracting the post-treatment score from the initial score. A change score of 2 or more is considered clinically significant; however, this has not been confirmed for the SCI population.[99] The COPM, is not appropriate for individuals who lack insight, have dementia, or cannot make decisions for themselves.[99]

The COPM has been shown to be a valid measure of occupational performance.[100] The COPM has demonstrated excellent test–retest reliability for both the performance and satisfaction scores when tested 1 week apart (ICC ≥ 0.88).[101] Studies have also reported that the COPM has been responsive to changes in

client outcomes over time and when compared to other measures such as the Short Form-36.[102]

The COPM provides a unique glimpse into the personal issues faced by those who have sustained a SCI. These measures are more sensitive to change than standard measures of function and are often the foundation for goal-based, individualized treatment programs.[98] The most common goals identified by individuals with SCI were self care (79%), productivity (12%), and leisure (9%), while the most frequently reported problems were functional mobility, dressing, and grooming/hygiene issues.[98]

Assessment of Life Habits

Life habits are defined as "those habits that ensure the survival and development of a person in society throughout his or her life."[103] The Assessment of Life Habits (LIFE-H) questionnaire was developed to assess the quality of social participation of individuals with disability regardless of the impairment.[103,104] The LIFE-H assessment documents two domains of function: performance of daily activities and participation in various social roles.[104] The LIFE-H assessment includes a total of 12 categories (6 in each domain) of life habits. Activities of daily living items include nutrition, fitness, personal care, communication, residence and mobility. Social role items include responsibility, interpersonal relations, community, education, employment, and recreation. A 10-point scale (0 to 9) is used to describe the level of difficulty in performing each task, as well as the type of assistance required for each task.[103] If a specific life habit is not part of one's lifestyle, the item is scored as "not applicable." A raw score is obtained for each life habit category by adding the accomplishment scores of each applicable item. A higher score indicates an easier accomplishment of life habits.

The LIFE-H has a long form consisting of 240 items and a short form consisting of 69 items, both of which cover all 12 categories of life habits. Whether the long or short form is used, the questionnaire is completed based on the person's judgment as to how well he or she accomplishes the various activities and social roles. The short form takes roughly 30 to 60 minutes to complete; the long form takes roughly 50 to 180 minutes.[104]

The LIFE-H has been shown to have construct validity.[105] Intra-class coefficients for total LIFE-H scores suggest a good level of reliability (ICC = 0.74) for an adult sample of individuals with SCI.[103] The inter-rater reliability for the total scores and daily activities subscores are highly reliable (ICC ≤ 0.89), and the social role subscore is moderately reliable (ICC = 0.64).[106] The life habits score that showed the highest level of reliability in adult individuals with SCI was personal care (ICC = 0.91) and the lowest was nutrition (ICC = 0.13) and interpersonal relations (ICC = 0.21)[103]

In a study of 482 individuals with SCI, individuals identified significant disruptions in the accomplishment scores of 58% of all life habits (a *disruption* was defined as an accomplishment score of ≤6 for 25% of the subjects).[107] Within the activities of daily living, all life habits related to personal care and mobility were disrupted. These habits included activities that generally require a higher level of motor function, such as indoor and outdoor home maintenance, taking part in physical fitness, meal preparation, and transportation.[107] Within the social role items, the life habits that were most frequently disrupted were in the categories of education, recreation, employment, job hunting, attending cultural events, and having sexual relations. The least disrupted life habits were associated with social roles that require maintaining an emotional relationship with others or the creation of friendships.[107] Interestingly, the disruptions of the social role life habits were not associated with the severity of the individual's injury.[107]

The disruptions in life habits appeared to be associated with age and severity of injury.[107] More than 60% of life habits showed significant differences of accomplishment scores between individuals with complete versus incomplete injuries and individuals with tetraplegia versus paraplegia. In most life habits, there was an increase of accomplishment scores with a lesser severity of injury. This finding is not surprising as many of the life habits require motor function and cannot be achieved without assistance from others.

The LIFE-H measures the quantity and the quality of social participation.[103] It allows collection of information in several areas related to rehabilitation and social integration. Rehabilitation teams can benefit from the results of the LIFE-H questionnaire as it will allow them to identify the areas of handicap within each person's environment, allowing the rehabilitation teams to intervene accordingly.

Impact on Participation and Autonomy

The Impact on Participation and Autonomy (IPA) is a generic questionnaire that addresses perceived participation and autonomy.[108] This assessment focuses on life role performance and the control an individual feels over everyday life.[108] The IPA reflects five domains: autonomy indoors, autonomy outdoors, family role, social relationships, and work/education. There are 31 items that are scored on a 5-point scale (very good, good, fair, poor, very poor) that describe the individual's perceived participation and autonomy. A second rating for eight items (mobility, self care, family role, financial situation, leisure, social relations, work, and education) is scored to reflect the perceived problems that restrict participation. This second rating is scored using a 3-point scale describing the problems experienced in each item (no problem, minor problems, and severe problems).[109] Perceived participation and problems are reflected in two separate scores with higher scores representing greater restrictions in participation.[110]

The IPA has been shown to have good homogeneity and construct validity.[108] Cronbach's alpha was considered good, ranging between 0.84 (family role) and 0.87 (self care and appearance). Test–retest reliability of the IPA showed that there was no significant difference between the mean scores of the measurements. ICCs ranged from 0.83 (family role) and 0.91 (autonomy outdoors).[111]

A study by Lund et al.[109] assessed 161 individuals with SCI to identify how they perceived their participation in life situations. This study also evaluated the influence of age, sex, level of injury, time since injury, marital status, and access to social support on perceived problems with participation. Results indicated that the majority of individuals with SCI perceived their participation as sufficient (score of very good, good, or fair) in most activities. For example, in the domain of social relations, more than 90% of the participants reported sufficient participation, and 80% or more reported that their autonomy indoors was sufficient.[109]

Reports of insufficient (poor or very poor) participation were perceived in the domains of family role and autonomy outdoors, work, and education.[109] Further analysis showed that access to social support was the most important variable in predicting perceived severe problems with participation on all items.[109] Access to social support appeared to have a greater impact on perceived problems with participation than the level of injury, time since injury, age, sex, and marital status.[109] The results of the this study reinforce the importance of focusing on the influence of social support.

The IPA can be used to describe the impact of disease on daily functioning, to quantify the needs for adaptations and care, and to evaluate the possible effects of rehabilitation interventions.[108] For individuals with SCI, the IPA is an important assessment for rehabilitation teams, as it can assist in identifying areas of perceived difficulties that can then become the main focus of treatment interventions.

Summary

The advancement of science in the areas of medical and rehabilitative treatment for individuals with SCI has been actively increasing in recent years, which has led to an increasing need for standardized measurement of impairment, ability, and rehabilitation. To determine the effectiveness of therapeutic trials and/or various rehabilitative treatments for individuals with SCI, assessments must include valid, reliable, and sensitive measurements. The ultimate goal for SCI assessments is to have internationally standardized methods for assessing the level of an individual's impairment and the individual's ability to perform various activities, then to transition these activities into participation in life situations for individuals with SCI. If researchers and clinicians can agree on various standardized measurements of function, it will be a much less daunting task to identify the efficacy of different treatment methodologies.

REVIEW QUESTIONS

1. What are the justifications for using standardized functional assessment tools?
   a. To demonstrate effectiveness of services provided
   b. To justify cost reimbursement
   c. To facilitate communication between health-care professionals
   d. To guide management decisions regarding program development
   e. All of the above.
2. Which functional assessment does not measure the domain of *activity*?
   a. Functional Independence Measure
   b. Spinal Cord Injury Measurement
   c. Walking Index for Spinal Cord Injury
   d. Wheelchair Skills Test
   e. International Standards for Neurological Classification of Spinal Cord Injury
3. Which of the following assessments of walking function do *not* take into consideration the assistive devices used for ambulation?
   a. Spinal Cord Injury Functional Ambulation Inventory
   b. Walking Index for Spinal Cord Injury
   c. Ambulatory Motor Index
   d. None of the above

4. Which of the following wheelchair assessments can be used to assess individuals who use either a manual or power wheelchair?
   a. The Wheelchair Circuit
   b. The Obstacle Course Assessment of Wheelchair Use Performance
   c. Wheelchair Users Functional Assessment
   d. Functional Evaluation in a Wheelchair
5. Which domains are measured by the CHART?
   a. Occupation
   b. Physical Independence
   c. Mobility
   d. Social Interaction
   e. Economic Self Sufficiency
   f. Orientation
   g. All the above
6. Which group of individuals with SCI implies a more significant handicap as measured by the CHART?
   a. High tetraplegia
   b. Low-level tetraplegia
   c. Paraplegia
   d. AIS D
7. The higher LIFE-H score indicates the individual has more difficulty accomplishing life habit activities.
   a. True
   b. False
8. The IPA shows that the most important variable in predicting severe problems with participation was which variable?
   a. Access to social support
   b. Level of injury
   c. Time since injury
   d. Marital status

REFERENCES

1. Granger CV, Albrecht GL, Hamilton BB. Outcome of Comprehensive Medical rehabilitation: Measurement by PULSES profile and the Barthel Index. *Arch Phys Med Rehabil.* 1979;60:145–154.
2. Cole B, Finch E, Gowland C et al. *Physical Rehabilitation Outcomes Measures.* Toronto, Ontario: Canadian Physiotherapy Association; 1994.
3. Watson AH, Kanny EM, White DM et al. Use of standardized activities of daily living rating scales in spinal cord injury and disease services. *Am J Occup Ther.* 1995;49(3): 229–234.
4. Roth E, Davidoff G, Haughton J et al. Functional assessment in spinal cord injury: A comparison of the modified Barthel Index and the "adapted" functional independence measure. *Clin Rehabil.* 1990;4:277–285.
5. Grey N, Kennedy P. The Functional Independence Measure: A comparative study of clinician and self ratings. *Paraplegia.* 1993;31:457–461.
6. Waters RL, Adkins R, Yakura J et al. Prediction of ambulatory performance based on motor scores derived from standards of the American spinal injury associations. *Arch Phys Med Rehabil.* 1994;75:756–760.

7. World Health Organization. International Classification of Functioning, Disability and Health: ICF. Geneva, Switzerland: World Health Organization; 2001.

8. Marino RJ, Shea JA, Stineman MG. The capabilities of upper extremity instrument: Reliability and validity of a measure of functional limitation in tetraplegia. *Arch Phys Med Rehabil.* 1998;79(12):1512–1521.

9. Cohen ME, Sheehan TP, Herbison GJ. Content validity and reliability of the international standards for neurological classification of spinal cord injury. *Top Spinal Cord Inj Rehabil.* 1996;1(4):15–31.

10. International Standards for Neurological Classification of Spinal Cord Injury. 2002; Chicago, IL, American Spinal Injury Association.

11. Curt A, Dietz V. Ambulatory capacity in spinal cord injury: Significance of somatosensory evoked potentials and ASIA protocol in predicting outcome. *Arch Phys Med Rehabil.* 1197;78(1):39–43.

12. Brown PJ, Marino RJ, Herbison GJ et al.. The 72-hour examination as a predictor of recovery in motor complete quadriplegia. *Arch Phys Med Rehabil.* 1991;72(7):546–548.

13. Waters, RL, Adkins, RH, Yakura, JS. Definition of complete spinal cord injury. *Paraplegia.* 1991;9:573–581.

14. Cohen ME, Bartko JJ. Reliability of ISCSCI-92 for neurological classification of spinal cord injury. In: Ditunno JF, Donovan WH, Maynard FM, editors. *Reference Manual for the International Standards for Neurological and Functional Classification of Spinal Cord Injury.* Chicago IL: American Spinal Injury Association; 1994.

15. Marino RJ, Ditunno JF, Donovan WH et al. Neurological recovery after traumatic spinal cord injury: Data from the model spinal cord injury systems. *Arch Phys Med Rehabil.* 1999;80:1391–1396.

16. Burns SP, Golding DG et al. Recovery of ambulation in motor incomplete tetraplegia. *Arch Phys Med Rehabil.* 1997;78:1169–1172.

17. Crozier KS, Graziani V, Ditunno JF Jr et al. Spinal Cord injury: Prognosis for ambulation based on sensory examination in patients who are initially motor complete. *Arch Phys Med Rehabil.* 1991;72:119–121.

18. Waters RL, Adkins RH, Yakura JS et al. Motor and sensory recovery following incomplete tetraplegia. *Arch Phys Med Rehabil.* 1994;75:306–311.

19. Ditunno JFJr, Ditunno PL et al. Walking Index for Spinal Cord Injury (WISCI): An international multicenter validity and reliability study. *Spinal Cord.* 2000;38:234–243.

20. Mange KC, Marino RJ, Gregory PC et al. Course of motor recovery at the zone of injury in complete spinal cord injury. *Arch Phys Med Rehabil.* 1990;71:796.

21. Wu L, Marino RJ, Herbison GJ et al. Recovery of zero-grade muscles in the zone of partial preservation in motor complete quadriplegia. *Arch Phys Med Rehabil.* 1992;73:40–43.

22. Ditunno JF, Stover SL, Freed MM et al. Motor recovery of the upper extremities in traumatic quadriplegia: A multicenter study. *Arch Phys Med Rehabil.* 1992;73:431–436.

23. Yavuz N, Tezyurek M, Akyuz M. A comparison of two functional tests in quadriplegia: The quadriplegia index of function and the functional independence measure. *Spinal Cord.* 1998;36:832–837.

24. Lazar RB, Yarkony GM, Ortolano D et al. Prediction of functional outcome by motor capability after spinal cord injury. *Arch Phys Med Rehabil.* 1989;70:819–822.

25. Middleton JW, Truman G, Geraghty TJ. Neurological level effect on the discharge functional status of spinal cord injured persons after rehabilitation. *Arch Phys Med Rehabil.* 1998;79:1428–1432.

26. Marino RJ, Rider-Foster D, Maissel G et al. Superiority of motor level over single neurological level in categorizing tetraplegia. *Paraplegia.* 1995;33:510–513.

27. Klose KJ, Green BA, Smith RS et al. University of Miami Neuro-spinal Index (UMNI): A quantitative method for determining spinal cord function. *Paraplegia.* 1980;18:331–336.

28. Chehrazi B, Wagner FC, Collins WF et al. A scale for evaluation of spinal cord injury. *J Neurosurg.* 1981;54:320–315.

29. Bracken MB, Shepard MJ, Collins WF, et al. Methylprednisolone or naloxone treatment after acute spinal cord injury: 1 year follow-up data. *J Neurosurg.* 1992;76: 23–31.

30. Noreau L, Vachon J. Comparison of three methods to assess muscular strength in individuals with spinal cord injury. *Spinal Cord.* 1998;36:716–723.

31. Daniels L, Worthingham C. *Muscle Testing Techniques of Manual Examinations.* 5th edition. Philadelphia: W. B. Saunders; 1986.

32. Wadsworth CT, Krishnan R, Sear M et al. Intrarater reliability of manual muscle testing and hand-held dynametric muscle testing. *Phys Ther.* 1987;7(9):1342–1347.

33. Schwartz S, Cohen ME, Herbison GJ et al. Relationship between two measures of upper extremity strength: Manual muscle test compared to hand-held myometry. *Arch Phys Med Rehabil.* 1992;73:1063–1068.

34. Welch RD, Lobley SJ, O'Sullivan SB et al. Functional independence in quadriplegia: Critical levels. *Arch Phys Med Rehabil.* 1986;67:235–240.

35. Velozo CA, Magahaes LC, Pan AW et al. Functional scale discrimination at admission and discharge: Rasch analysis of the level of rehabilitation scale-III. *Arch Phys Med Rehabil.* 1995;76(8):705–712.

36. Fujiwara T, Hara Y, Akaboshi K et al. Relationship between shoulder muscle strength and functional independence measure (FIM) score among C6 tetraplegics. *Spinal Cord.* 1999;37:58–61.

37. Herbison GJ, Isaac Z, Cohen ME et al. Strength post-spinal cord injury myometer vs manual muscle test. *Spinal Cord.* 1996;34(9):543–548.

38. Jacquemin GL, Burns SP, Little JW. Measuring hand intrinsic muscle strength: Normal values and interrater reliability. *J Spinal Cord Med.* 2004;27:460–467.

39. Marino RJ, Huang M, Knight P et al. Assessing self-care status in quadriplegia: Comparison of the quadriplegia index of function (QIF) and the functional independence measure (FIM). *Paraplegia.* 1993;31:225–233.

40. New PW. Functional outcomes and disability after non traumatic spinal cord injury rehabilitation: Results form a retrospective study. *Arch Phys Med Rehabil.* 2005;8:250–261.

41. Jette AM. Functional status index: Reliability of a chronic disease evaluation instrument. *Arch Phys Med Rehabil.* 1980;61(9):395–401.

42. Itzkovich M, Tamir A, Philo O et al. Reliability of the Catz-Itzkovich spinal cord independence measure assessment by interview and comparison with observation. *Am J Phys Med Rehabil.* 2003;82:267–272.

43. Hall KM, Cohen ME, Wright J et al. Characteristics of the functional independence measure in traumatic spinal cord injury. *Arch Phys Med Rehabil.* 1999;80:1471–1476.

44. Routhier F, Desrosiers J, Vincent C et al. Reliability and construct validity studies of an obstacle course assessment of wheelchair user performance. *Int J Rehabil Res.* 2005;28(1): 49–56.

45. Stover SL, DeLisa IA, Whiteneck GG. *Spinal cord injury: Clinical outcomes from the model systems.* Gaithersburg, MD; Aspen; 1995. p. 170.

46. Stineman MG et al. A Prototype Classification System for Medical Rehabilitation. Washington DC: American Rehabilitation Association; 1994.

47. Hamilton BB, Laughlin JA, Fiedler RC et al. Interrater reliability of the 7-level functional independence measure (FIM). *Scand J Rehabil Med.* 1994;26:115–119.

48. Granger CV, Hamilton BB, Keith RA et al. Advances in functional assessment for medical rehabilitation. *Top Geriatr Rehabil.* 1986;1(3):59–74.

49. Dodds TA, Martin DP, Stolov WC et al. A validation of the functional independence measurement and its performance among rehabilitation inpatients. *Arch Phys Med Rehabil.* 1993;74(5):531–536.

50. Ottenbacher KJ, Mann WC, Granger CV et al. Interrater agreement and stability of functional assessment in the community-based elderly. *Arch Phys Med Rehabil.* 1994;75: 1297–1301.

51. Stineman MG, Marino RJ, Deutsch A et al. A functional strategy for classifying patients after traumatic spinal cord injury. *Spinal Cord.* 1999;37(10):717–725.

52. Harvey C, Wilson SE, Greene CG et al. New estimates of the direct costs of traumatic spinal cord injuries: Results of a nationwide survey. *Paraplegia.* 1992;30:834–850.

53. Weitzenkamp DA, Whiteneck GG, Lammertse DP. Predictors of personal care assistance for people with spinal cord injury. *Arch Phys Med Rehabil.* 2002;83:1399–1405.

54. Menter RR, Whiteneck GG, Charlifue SW et al. Impairment, disability, handicap and medical expenses of persons aging with spinal cord injury. *Paraplegia.* 1991;29(9):613–619.

55. Ota T, Akaboshi K, Nagota M et al. Functional assessment of patients with spinal cord injury: Measured by the motor score and the functional independence measure. *Spinal Cord.* 1996;34:531–535.

56. Mahoney FI, Barthel DW. Functional evaluation: The Barthel Index. *MD State Med J.* 1965;14:61–65.

57. Yarkony GM, Roth EJ, Heinemann AW et al. Functional skills after spinal cord injury rehabilitation: Three-year longitudinal follow-up. *Arch Phys Med Rehabil.* 1988;69(2): 111–114.

58. Post MW, Van Asbeck FW, Van Dijk AJ et al. Dutch interview of the Barthel index evaluated in patients with spinal cord injuries. *Ned Tijdschr Geneeskd.* 1995;139(27): 1376–1380.

59. Yarkony GM, Roth EJ, Heinemann AW et al. Spinal cord injury rehabilitation outcome: The impact of age. *J Clin Epidemiol.* 1988;41(2):173–177.

60. Catz A, Itzkovich M, Agranov E et al . SCIM-Spinal Cord Independence Measure: A new disability scale for patients with spinal cord lesions. *Spinal Cord.* 1997;35:850–856.

61. Catz A, Itzkovich M, Steinberg F et al. The Catz-Izkovich SCIM: A revised version of the Spinal Cord Independence Measure. *Disabil Rehabil.* 2001;23(6):263–268.

62. Catz A, Itzkovich M, Agranov E et al. The Spinal Cord Independence Measure (SCIM): Sensitivity to functional changes in subgroups of spinal cord lesion patients. *Spinal Cord.* 2001;39:97–100.

63. Itzkovich M, Tripolski M, Zeileg G et al. Rasch analysis of the Catz-Itzkovich Spinal Cord Independence Measure. *Spinal Cord.* 2002;40(8):396–407.

64. Catz A, Greenberg E, Itkovich M et al. A new instrument for outcome assessment in rehabilitation medicine: Spinal Cord Injury Ability Realization Measurement Index. *Arch Phys Med and Rehabil.* 2004;85:399–404.

65. National Spinal Cord Injury Statistical Center. Spinal Cord Injury: Facts and Figures at a Glance. Birmingham, AL: University of Alabama; 2005.

66. Gresham GE, Labi MLC, Dittmar SS MAP et al. The Quadriplegia Index of Function (QIF): Sensitivity and reliability demonstrated in a study of thirty quadriplegic patients. *Paraplegia.* 1986;24:38–44.

67. Marino RJ, Goin JE. Development of a short form quadriplegia index of function scale. *Spinal Cord.* 1999;37: 289–296.

68. Waters RL, Yakura JS, Adkins R et al. Determinants of gait performance following spinal cord injury. *Arch Phys Med Rehabil.* 1989;70(11):811–818.

69. Barbeau H, Ladouceur M, Norman KE et al. Walking after spinal cord injury: Evaluation, treatment, and functional recovery. *Arch Phys Med Rehabil.* 1999;80:225–235.

70. Gittler MS, McKinley WO, Steins SA et al. Spinal cord injury medicine. 3. Rehabilitation outcomes. *Arch Phys Med Rehabil.* 2002;83 3 Suppl 1:S66–71, S90–8.

71. Waters RL;Yakura JS, Adkins RH. Gait performance after spinal cord injury. *Clinical Orthopaedics and Related Research.* 1993;288:87–96.

72. Field-Fote EC, Fluet GG, Schafer SD et al. The Spinal Cord Injury Functional Ambulation Inventory (SCI-FAI). *J Rehabil Med.* 2001;33:177–181.

73. Ditunno PL, Ditunno JF Jr. Walking Index for Spinal Cord Injury (WISCI II: Scale revision). *Spinal Cord.* 2001;39(12):654–656.

74. Morganti B, Scivoletto G, Ditunno P et al. Walking Index for Spinal Cord Injury (WISCI): Criterion validity. *Spinal Cord.* 2005;43:27–33.

75. Ditunno JF Jr, West C, Schmidt M. et al. Validation and refinement of the Walking Index for Spinal Cord Injury (WISCI) in a clinical setting. *J Spinal Cord Med.* 2004;27:160.

76. Butland RJA, Pang J, Gross ER et al. Two-six, and 12-minute walking tests in respiratory disease. *BMJ.* 1982;284:1607–1608.

77. American Thoracic Society. ATS statement: Guidelines for the six-minute walk test. *Am J Respir Crit Care Med.* 2002;166:111–117.

78. Enright PL. The six-minute walk test. *Respir Care.* 2003;48(8):783–785.

79. Van Hedel HJ, Wirzam, Dietz V. Assessing walking ability in subjects with spinal cord injury: Validity and reliability of 3 walking tests. *Arch Phys Med Rehabil.* 2005;86(2):190–196.

80. Wirz M, Zemon DH, Rupp R et al. Effectiveness of auto-mated locomotor training in patients with chronic incomplete spinal cord injury: A multicenter trial. *Arch Phys Med Rehabil.* 2005;86:672–680.

81. Collen FM, Wade DT, Bradshaw CM. Mobility after stroke: Reliability measures of impairment and disability. *Int Disabil Stud.* 1991;12:6–9.

82. Post MW, van Asbeck FW, van Dijk AJ et al. Services for spinal cord injured: Availability and satisfaction. *Spinal Cord.* 1997;35:109–115.

83. Kilkens OJ, Post MW. Wheelchair skills tests: A systematic review. *Clin Rehabil.* 2003;17:418–430.

84. Kilkens OJ, Post MW, van der Woude LH et al. The wheelchair circuit: Reliability of a test to assess mobility in persons with spinal cord injury. *Arch Phys Med Rehabil.* 2002;83(12):1783–1788.

85. Kilkens OJ, Dallmeijer AJ, Nene AV et al. The longitudinal relation between physical capacity and wheelchair skill performance during inpatient rehabilitation of people with spinal cord injury. *Arch Phys Med Rehabil.* 2005;86:1575–1581.

86. Kilkens OJ, Dallmeijer AJ, de Witte LP et al. The wheelchair circuit: Construct validity and responsiveness of a test to assess manual wheelchair mobility in persons with spinal cord injury. *Arch Phys Med Rehabil.* 2004;85:424–431.

87. Harvey LA, Batty J, Fahey A. Reliability of a tool for assessing mobility in wheelchair dependent paraplegics. *Spinal Cord.* 1998;36:427–431.

88. Kirby RL, Dupuis DJ, MacPhee AH et al. The Wheelchair Skills Test (version 2.4): Measurement properties. *Arch Phys Med Rehabil.* 2004;85:794–804.

89. Stanley RK, Stafford DJ, Rasch E et al. Development of a functional assessment measure for manual wheelchair users. *J Rehabil Res Dev.* 2003;40(4):301–307.

90. Cress ME, Buchner DM, Questad KA et al. Continuous-scale physical functional performance in healthy older adults: A validation study. *Arch Phys Med Rehabil.* 1996;77:1243–1250.

91. Cress ME, Kinne S, Patrick DL et al. Physical functional performance in persons using a manual wheelchair. *J Orthop Sports Phys Ther.* 2002;32:104–113.

92. Mills T, Holm MB, Trefler E, et al. Development and consumer validation of the Functional Evaluation in a Wheelchair (FEW) instrument. *Disabil. Rehabil.* 2002;24:38–46.

93. Whiteneck G, Tate D, Charlifue S. Predicting community reintegration after spinal cord injury from demographic and injury characteristics. *Arch Phys Med Rehabil.* 1999;80:1485–1491.

94. Whiteneck GG, Charlifue SW, Gerhart KA et al. Qualifying handicap: A new measure of long-term rehabilitation outcomes. *Arch Phys Med Rehabil.* 1992;73(6): 519–526.

95. Walker N, Mellick D, Brooks CA et al. Measuring participation across impairment groups using the Craig hospital handicap assessment reporting technique. *Am J Phys Med Rehabil.* 2003;82:936–941.

96. Hall KM, Dijkers M, Whiteneck G et al. The Craig handicap assessment and reporting technique (CHART): Metric properties and scoring. *Top Spinal Cord Inj Rehabil.* 1998;4(1):16–30.

97. Dijkers M. Scoring CHART: Survey and sensitivity analysis. *J Amer Paraplegia Soc.* 1991;14:85–86.

98. Donnelly C, Eng JJ, Hall J et al. Client–centered assessment and the identification of meaningful treatment goals for individuals with a spinal cord injury. *Spinal Cord.* 2004;42:302–307.

99. Donnelly C, Carswell A. Individualized outcome measures: A review of the literature. *Can J Occup Ther.* 2002;69:84–94.

100. McColl MA, Paterson M, Davies D et al.. Validity and community utility of the Canadian occupational performance measure. *Can J Occup Ther.* 2000:67:22–23.

101. Cup EH, Sholte op Reimer WJ, Thijssen MC et al. Reliability and validity of the Canadian occupational performance measure in stroke patients. *Clin Rehabil.* 2003;17:402–409.

102. Lewis J, Jones P. Measuring handicap in rheumatic disease: Evaluation of the Canadian occupational performance measure. *ARHP Annual Meeting.* 2001;45(6):S90.

103. Fougeyrollas P, Noreau L, Bergeron H et al. Social consequences of long term impairments and disabilities: Conceptual approach and assessment of handicap. *Int J Rehabil Res.* 1998;21:127–141.

104. Noreau L, Fougeyrollas P, Vincent C. The LIFE-H: Assessment of the quality of social participation. *Technol Disabil.* 2002;14:113–118.

105. Desrosiers J, Noreau L, Robichaud L et al. Validity of the assessment of life habits in older adults. *J Rehabil Med.* 2004;36:177–182.

106. Noreau L, Desrossiers J, Robichaud L et al. Measuring social participation: Reliability of the LIFE-H in older adults with disabilities. *Disabil Rehabil.* 2005;26(6):346–352.

107. Noreau L, Fougeyrollas P. Long-term consequences of spinal cord injury on social participation: The occurrence of handicap situations. *Disabil Rehabil.* 2002;22(4):170–180.

108. Cardol M, de Haan RJ, de Jong BA et al. The development of a handicap assessment questionnaire: The impact on participation and autonomy (IPA). *Clin Rehabil.* 1999;13:411–419.

109. Lund ML, Nordlund A, Nygard L et al. Perceptions of participation and predictors of perceived problems with participation in persons with spinal cord injury. *J Rehabil Med.* 2005;27:3–8.

110. Cardol M, de Jong BA, van den Bos GAM et al. Beyond disability: Perceived participation in people with a chronic disabling condition. *Clin Rehabil.* 2002;16:27–35.

111. Cardol M, de Haan RJ, de Jong BA et al. Psychometric properties of the impact on participation and autonomy questionnaire. *Arch Phys Med Rehabil.* 2001;82:210–216.

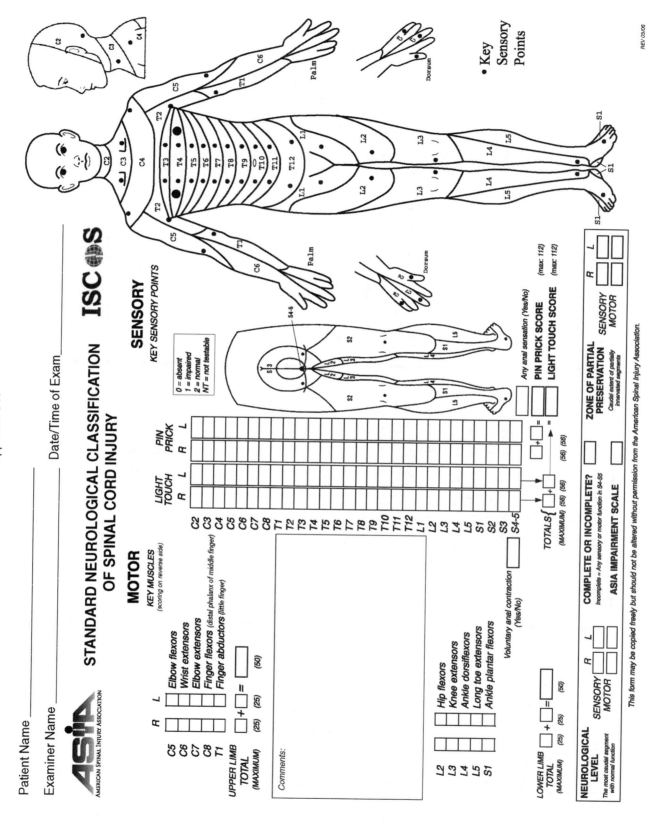

MUSCLE GRADING

0   total paralysis

1   palpable or visible contraction

2   active movement, full range of motion, gravity eliminated

3   active movement, full range of motion, against gravity

4   active movement, full range of motion, against gravity and provides some resistance

5   active movement, full range of motion, against gravity and provides normal resistance

5*   muscle able to exert, in examiner's judgement, sufficient resistance to be considered normal if identifiable inhibiting factors were not present

NT not testable. Patient unable to reliably exert effort or muscle unavailable for testing due to factors such as immobilization, pain on effort or contracture.

ASIA IMPAIRMENT SCALE

☐   **A = Complete:** No motor or sensory function is preserved in the sacral segments S4-S5.

☐   **B = Incomplete:** Sensory but not motor function is preserved below the neurological level and includes the sacral segments S4-S5.

☐   **C = Incomplete:** Motor function is preserved below the neurological level, and more than half of key muscles below the neurological level have a muscle grade less than 3.

☐   **D = Incomplete:** Motor function is preserved below the neurological level, and at least half of key muscles below the neurological level have a muscle grade of 3 or more.

☐   **E = Normal:** Motor and sensory function are normal.

CLINICAL SYNDROMES (OPTIONAL)

☐   Central Cord
☐   Brown-Sequard
☐   Anterior Cord
☐   Conus Medullaris
☐   Cauda Equina

STEPS IN CLASSIFICATION

The following order is recommended in determining the classification of individuals with SCI.

1. Determine sensory levels for right and left sides.

2. Determine motor levels for right and left sides.
   Note: in regions where there is no myotome to test, the motor level is presumed to be the same as the sensory level.

3. Determine the single neurological level.
   This is the lowest segment where motor and sensory function is normal on both sides, and is the most cephalad of the sensory and motor levels determined in steps 1 and 2.

4. Determine whether the injury is Complete or Incomplete (sacral sparing).
   If voluntary anal contraction = No AND all S4-5 sensory scores = 0 AND any anal sensation = No, then injury is COMPLETE. Otherwise injury is incomplete.

5. Determine ASIA Impairment Scale (AIS) Grade:

   Is injury Complete?   If YES, AIS=A Record ZPP
       NO   (For ZPP record lowest dermatome or myotome on each side with some (non-zero score) preservation)

   Is injury motor incomplete?   If NO, AIS=B
       YES   (Yes=voluntary anal contraction OR motor function more than three levels below the motor level on a given side.)

   Are at least half of the key muscles below the (single) neurological level graded 3 or better?
       NO   YES
      AIS=C   AIS=D

   If sensation and motor function is normal in all segments, AIS=E
   Note: AIS E is used in follow up testing when an individual with a documented SCI has recovered normal function. If at initial testing no deficits are found, the individual is neurologically intact; the ASIA Impairment Scale does not apply.

Appendix 6-B

Spinal Cord Independence Measure (SCIM)

LOEWENSTEIN HOPSITAL REHABILITATION CENTER
Affiliated with the Sackler Faculty of Medicine, Tel-Aviv University

Department IV, Medical Director: Dr. Amiram Catz

Patient Name: _____ **ID:** _____   **Examiner Name:** _____

(Enter the score for each function in the adjacent square, below the date. The form may be used for up to 6 examinations.)

SCIM–SPINAL CORD INDEPENDENCE MEASURE   Version III, Sept 14, 2002

Self-Care   DATE

Exam 1 2 3 4 5 6

1. Feeding (cutting, opening containers, pouring, bringing food to mouth, holding cup with fluid)
- 0. Needs parenteral, gastrostomy, or fully assisted oral feeding
- 1. Needs partial assistance for eating and/or drinking, or for wearing adaptive devices
- 2. Eats independently; needs adaptive devices or assistance only for cutting food and/or pouring and/or opening containers
- 3. Eats and drinks independently; does not require assistance or adaptive devices

2. Bathing (soaping, washing, drying body and head, manipulating water tap.) **A–upper body; B–lower body**
- A. 0. Requires total assistance
- 1. Requires partial assistance
- 2. Washes independently with adaptive devices or in a specific setting (e.g., bars, chair)
- 3. Washes independently; does not require adaptive devices or specific setting (not customary for healthy people) (adss)
- B. 0. Requires total assistance
- 1. Requires partial assistance
- 2. Washes independently with adaptive devices or in a specific setting (adss)
- 3. Washes independently; does not require adaptive devices (adss) or specific setting

3. Dressing (clothes, shoes, permanent orthoses: dressing, wearing, undressing). **A–upper body; B–lower body**
- A. 0. Requires total assistance
- 1. Requires partial assistance with clothes without buttons, zippers or laces (cwobzl)
- 2. Independent with cwobzl; requires adaptive devices or in a specific setting (adss)
- 3. Independent with cwobzl; does not require adss; needs assistance or adss only for bzl
- 4. Desses (any cloth) independently; does not require adaptive devices or specific setting
- B. 0. Requires total assistance
- 1. Requires partial assistance with clothes without buttons, zippers or laces (cwobzl)
- 2. Independent with cwobzl; requires adaptive devices or in a specific setting (adss)
- 3. Independent with cwobzl; does not require adss; needs assistance or adss only for bzl
- 4. Desses (any cloth) independently; does not require adaptive devices or specific setting

4. Grooming (washing hands and face, brushing teeth, combing hair, shaving, applying makeup)
- 0. Requires total assistance
- 1. Requires partial assistance
- 2. Grooms independently with adaptive devices
- 3. Grooms independently without adaptive devices

SUBTOTAL (0–20)

Respiration and Sphincter Management

5. Respiration
- 0. Requires tracheal tube (IT) and permanent or intermittent assisted ventilation (IAV)
- 2. Breathes indpendently with TT; requires oxygen, much assistance in coughing or TT management
- 4. Breathes independently with TT; requires little assistance in coughing or TT management
- 6. Breathes independently without TT; requires oxygen, much assistance in coughing, a mask (e.g., peep) or IAV (bipap)
- 8. Breathes independently without TT; requires little assistance or stimulation for coughing
- 10. Breathes independently without assistance or device

6. Sphincter Management—Bladder
- 0. Indwelling catheter
- 3. Residual urine volume (RUV) >100cc; no regular catheterization or assisted intermittent catheterization
- 6. RUV <100cc or intermittent self-catheterization; needs assistance for applying drainage instrument
- 9. Intermittent self-catheterization; uses external drainage instrument; does not need assistance for applying
- 11. Intermittent self-catheterization; continent between catheterizations; does not use external drainage instrument
- 13. RUV <100cc; needs only external urine drainage; no assistance is reqeuired for drainage
- 15. RUV <100cc; continent; does not use external drainage instrument

7. Sphincter Management—Bowel
- 0. Irregular timing or very low frequency (less than once on 3 days) of bowel movements
- 5. Regular timing, but requires assistance (e.g., for applying suppository); rare accidents (less than twice a month)
- 8. Regular bowel movements, without assistance; rare accidents (less than twice a month)
- 10. Regular bowel movements, without assistance; no accidents

8. Use of Toilet (perineal hygiene, adjustment of clothes before/after, use of napkins or diapers).
- 0. Requires total assistance
- 1. Requires partial assistance; does not clean self
- 2. Requires partial assistance; cleans self independently
- 4. Uses toilet independently in all tasks but needs adaptive devices or special setting (e.g., bars)
- 5. Uses toilet independently; does not require adaptive devices or special setting

SUBTOTAL (0–40)

DATE   Exam 1 2 3 4 5 6

Mobility (room and toilet)

9. Mobility in Bed and Action to Prevent Pressure Sores

   0. Needs assistance in all activities: turning upper body in bed, turning lower body in bed, sitting up in bed, doing push-ups in wheelchair, with or without adaptive devices, but not with electric aids

   2. Performs one of the activities without assistance

   4. Performs two or three of the activities without assistance

   6. Performs all the bed mobility and pressure release activities independently

10. Transfers: bed-wheelchair (locking wheelchair, lifting footrests, removing and adjusting arm rests, transferring, lifting feet).

   0. Requires total assistance

   1. Needs partial assistance and/or supervision, and/or adaptive devices (e.g., sliding board)

   2. Independent (or does not require wheelchair)

11. Transfers: wheelchair-toilet-tub (if uses toilet wheelchair: transfers to and from; if uses regular wheelchair: locking wheelchair, lifting footrests, removing and adjusting armrests, transferring, lifting feet)

   0. Requires total assistance

   1. Needs partial assistance and/or supervision, and/or adaptive devices (e.g., grab-bars)

   2. Independent (or does not require wheelchair)

Mobility (indoors and outdoors, on even surface)

12. Mobility indoors

   0. Requires total assistance

   1. Needs electric wheelchair or partial assistance to operate manual wheelchair

   2. Moves independently in manual wheelchair

   3. Requires supervision while walking (with or without devices)

   4. Walks with a walking frame or crutches (swing)

   5. Walks with crutches or two canes (reciprocal walking)

   6. Walks with one cane

   7. Needs leg orthosis only

   8. Walks without walking aids

13. Mobility for Moderate Distances (10–100 meters)

   0. Requires total assistance

   1. Needs electric wheelchair or partial assistance to operate manual wheelchair

   2. Moves independently in manual wheelchair

   3. Requires supervision while walking (with or without devices)

   4. Walks with a walking frame or crutches (swing)

   5. Walks with crutches or two canes (reciprocal walking)

   6. Walks with one cane

   7. Needs leg orthosis only

   8. Walks without walking aids

14. Mobility Outdoors (more than 100 meters)

   0. Requires total assistance

   1. Needs electric wheelchair or partial assistance to operate manual wheelchair

   2. Moves independently in manual wheelchair

   3. Requires supervision while walking (with or without devices)

   4. Walks with a walking frame or crutches (swing)

   5. Walks with crutches or two canes (reciprocal walking)

   6. Walks with one cane

   7. Needs leg orthosis only

   8. Walks without walking aids

15. Stair Management

   0. Unable to ascend or descend stairs

   1. Ascends and descends at least 3 steps with support or supervision of another person

   2. Ascends and descends at least 3 steps with support of handrail and/or crutch or cane

   3. Ascends and descends at least 3 steps without any support or supervision

16. Transfers: wheelchair-car (approaching car, locking wheelchair, removing arm and footrests, transferring to and from car, bringing wheelchair into and out of car)

   0. Requires total assistance

   1. Needs partial assistance and/or supervision and/or adaptive devices

   2. Transfers independent; does not require adaptive devices (or does not require wheelchair)

17. Transfers: ground-wheelchair

   0. Requires assistance

   1. Transfers independent with or without adaptive devices (or does not require wheelchair)

SUBTOTAL (0–40)

TOTAL SCIM SCORE (0–100)

Reprinted with permission from *Topics in Spinal Cord Injury Rehabilitation.* 1998; 4(1): p20, Thomas Land Publishers. Available at: http://www.thomasland.com.

Maximizing Mobility

7

Jennifer D. Hastings, PT, PhD, NCS

Edelle C. Field-Fote, PT, PhD

After reading this chapter, the reader will be able to:

OBJECTIVES

- Understand mechanical leverage and its application to functional mobility
- Describe how the principles of motor learning can be applied to mobility skills
- Understand the fundamental elements of joint protection for the preservation of joint integrity in both the paralyzed and the intact limbs
- Describe the strategy for teaching balance to a newly spinal cord-injured individual
- Understand the basic mechanism of an efficient short-sitting transfer
- Discuss factors that contribute to optimal wheelchair push mechanics

Introduction

Mobility after spinal cord injury (SCI) requires the acquisition of new movement strategies and skills. The individual with a recent SCI is has altered voluntary control over his or her body and must learn to use it to acquire an entirely new set of mobility skills. These skills include the ability to move within a wheelchair, to move forward and back on the seat, to move from side to side, and to pick up a leg and cross the foot over the opposite knee. Mobility also includes the ability to move on a bed, to roll to either side or from prone to supine position and back to prone, to get up from supine to sitting position, to move over in the bed or off the bed, and to lift the lower extremities up onto the bed or off the bed, among other abilities. All of these functional tasks require relearning after SCI. Mobility is important as it represents the ability to get around in the environment, but it is important for other reasons as well. Immobility can cause pain, discomfort, and skin breakdown. Immobility can also lead to frustration, hopelessness, and even depression. Through mobility training, the therapist empowers the individual with SCI by providing opportunities for early and successful movement, while attending to issues such as passive range of motion, joint integrity, skin health, and optimal postural alignment.

For individuals who will not return to walking as the primary means of over-ground mobility, skilled wheelchair use is the key to independence. An understanding of body mobility is a prerequisite to skilled wheelchair use and to the ability to transfer (i.e., to move from one seated position to another seated position). In addition, the ability to maintain balance during movement (i.e., dynamic balance ability) and the ability to stop or change direction of a movement are essential to mastering independent mobility. These skills become intuitive with repeated practice and allow the individual to capitalize on the mechanical assistance provided by leverage and body (or body part) alignment in order to move the body fluidly into and out of the desired positions. The experienced therapist has an understanding of the fundamental concepts and essential elements of successful movement and is able to identify the optimal strategies and approaches to use to train the individual for independence in these skills.

There are few studies that directly address the issue of wheelchair mobility. Available studies primarily address wheelchair propulsion and related skills. While the individual with SCI must learn many aspects of wheelchair propulsion, skillful wheelchair use requires far more than simply the ability to propel the wheelchair. The individual must also acquire the ability to safely and efficiently negotiate through the environment in a wheelchair. Studies of wheelchair skill[1–5] tend to focus on the effect of training or quantification of skill acquisition, while studies of wheelchair propulsion typically consist of biomechanical analyses that assess the influence of position,[6,7] speed,[8] and level of injury,[9] or compare manual versus power-assisted wheels.[10,11] In general, these studies show that wheelchair skills improve with training, including the training of the propulsive stroke.

Beyond the ability to propel the wheelchair and negotiate through the environment, the independent wheelchair user must be able to safely transfer into and out of the wheelchair. As with wheelchair mobility, there is little available literature regarding teaching and learning transfer skills. There have been descriptive studies assessing the frequency of transfers and correlative studies assessing pain associated with transfers,[12–15] but these studies do not compare the relative advantages or disadvantages of various transfer techniques. Studies related to transfer skills have investigated movement strategies employed,[16–19] as well as a transfer-related upper extremity joint forces[20,21] and muscle demand.[19] However, these studies have been small, laboratory-based, descriptive studies addressing a specific, defined type of transfer; furthermore, in two of these studies, the subjects were able-bodied indi-viduals.[17,20] In a published review of research related to transfer skills, the authors concluded that "existing studies of transfers among individuals with SCI have relied on small groups of either asymptomatic or nonimpairedsubjects, with minimal integration of kinematic, kinetic, and electromyographic data."[22] To date, there have been no published studies describing and/or comparing transfer techniques that are intended to increase efficiency or decrease mechanical load.

The dearth of literature related to mobility after SCI exists for other aspects of post-SCI activity and function as well. A state-of-the-science review of SCI rehabilitation published in 2006 suggested that therapies should include muscle strengthening, range of motion, and training in transfers, gait, activities of daily living (ADLs), and use of equipment. But the authors found few evidence-based analyses of specific exercise therapies.[23] There is no current literature that directly investigates the therapeutic interventions that are used for functional training after SCI.

Functional Potential

The therapist evaluates both what an individual with SCI *can* do and what the individual has the *potential* to do, even if the limits of length of stay in a rehabilitation facility are not likely to allow the individual to attain the ultimate level of function during that time. Recognition of functional potential is critical because everything the newly-injured person knows about SCI is learned during this initial rehabilitation stay. The acute rehabilitation team has a tremendous influence on what a person knows and believes about his or her future function and life.

In his autobiography, Wayne Rainey, a world champion motorcycle racer at the time of his SCI (T4 paraplegia secondary to a crash during a race), wrote, "In the hospital they said 'there's no way you can get in the chair from the ground by yourself,' but I was determined to do it. But it's a real struggle if I fall. I've only done it twice with no help."[24] However, in truth, with appropriate training an individual with T4 level of injury *should* be able to transfer from the floor into the chair, as full innervation of the upper extremities is preserved in a T4 injury. The ability to transfer from the floor to the chair is an essential skill, not only in the event of a fall, but also for whenever there is a need or desire to get on the floor. If this individual's recollection is accurate, it represents a striking example of how a knowledge deficit can limit the functional outcome of an individual with SCI. The knowledge and attitude of the therapist can empower the individual to achieve optimal functional outcomes. To this end, it is the responsibility of the therapist to know the functional potential of the individual based on his or her motor capabilities, train the individual in skills that will serve as a foundation for optimal function, and educate the individual to prevent the development of poor movement habits.

Learning a new motor skill requires problem-solving skills and practice, therefore, choosing interventions and selecting equipment that encourage activity will promote the development of new skills. While learning new motor skills, the individual will become independent earlier if taught to attend to available sensory cues to provide information about what strategies are successful. Information from the preserved proprioceptive and equilibrium systems can often compensate for impairment in other sensory systems, but learning to use this information will occur only with experience and practice. An excellent resource for principles of motor learning is provided by Schmidt and Wrisberg.[25]

Motor-Complete Injuries

In terms of ADLs and transfers, individuals with motor-complete C6 SCI have the same potential for independence in self care as do individuals with motor-complete L2 SCI; the difference is in *how* the activities are accomplished and *how long* it takes to obtain the skills. Table 7-1 describes the expected functional outcomes for individuals

Table 7-1
Expected Functional Outcomes for Motor Compete SCI Based on Neurologic Level

C4	Dependent in self care and independent in mobility using a power wheelchair. Should be able to direct others in all care needs.
C5	Unlikely to be independent in transfers, (with rare exceptions). Pressure relief ability is also limited, although the individual is able to perform an adequate pressure change. With this level of injury, an individual will generally be independent in community mobility from a power wheelchair and require attendant assistance for all ADLs.
C6	Potential to reach independent transfers without a board, but mastery of this level of function requires the individual to have a high level of motivation, good pre-morbid fitness, and minimal secondary complications. Will use adaptive equipment for self care, able to dress with some difficulty, and often may use attendant care for efficiency. Manual wheelchair independence is possible, as is driving in a lift- or ramp-equipped van with transfer to the vehicle seat. Depending on environment and lifestyle, power mobility may be selected.
C7	Independence in all self care (may require adaptive equipment) from a manual wheelchair. Independent transfers without a board, including off the floor and over height. Independent stowing a wheelchair into a car. Wheelie skills, including curbs up and down (may be limited to jumping up 4-inch curbs due to lack of grip strength).
C8–L2	Independence in all self care from a manual wheelchair. Independent transfers without a board, including off the floor and over height. Independent stowing a wheelchair into a car. Wheelie skills, including curbs up and down.
L3	Potential for functional community ambulation. Will need wheelchair for sports, distance, parenting, and maybe work. Independent in all self care. Requires bilateral AFO and UE assistive devices for gait (arch supports in the AFOs).

with motor-complete SCI (while it is understood that individuals are classified as motor-incomplete if they retain voluntary anal contraction, for the purpose of clarity, the term *motor-complete* will be defined in this chapter as lacking voluntary limb or trunk motor function below the stated neurologic level).

In a subsequent section of this chapter, entitled "Transitions," the specific strategies for accomplishing these outcomes will be described in detail.

Motor-Incomplete Injuries

Incomplete spinal injuries are more common than complete injuries,[26] and working with an individual with a motor-incomplete injury can be a challenging and rewarding experience for the therapist. Because functional potential in individuals with incomplete injuries depends on the preserved motor and sensory capabilities (as well as comorbidities), the training approach and functional outcome are highly individualized. In addition to a systematic examination of remaining function to determine abilities, the training approach requires the capacity to teach the individual to maximize function by using these abilities in a creative way. For example, if function in the lower extremities and trunk is preserved to a greater extent than function in the upper extremities, successful strategies for movement will capitalize on these assets.

The Ability to Move

Functional training is directed at providing the experiences the individual needs in order to acquire the ability to move and accomplish meaningful activities. The therapist's knowledge of musculoskeletal anatomy related to the origin, insertion, and action of residual musculature contributes to understanding the mobility potential of the individual. Analyzing how to best teach an individual to perform a motor task also uses the therapist's knowledge of the mechanics of movement and the optimal use of gravity. Biomechanical factors such as length of the lever arm, location of the axis of rotation, size of the base of support, and height of the center of gravity are all considered when analyzing a task.

Spinal cord injury rehabilitation, and particularly functional skill training in individuals with SCI, has much in common with coaching an athlete. Critical observation skills and movement analyses are required. The therapist determines what the individual needs to do to accomplish the task, analyzes the individual's performance, determines how to improve the technique, and devises ways to coax out just a little more function. The motivation and encouragement the therapist provides are also important. Ultimately, the goal is for the individual to learn concepts rather than a particular pattern of movement so that he or she will be able to apply these concepts regardless of the context of the movement.

Working with Gravity

Learning to work with gravity is one of the keys to optimizing functional mobility. The optimal use of gravity will aid in the accomplishment of any motor tasks, while working directly against gravity will always be the hardest way to accomplish a task. Gravity may be thought of as being directed downward toward the floor. Individuals with paresis or paralysis can maximize movement by using gravity and substituting leverage for muscle power. Levers are classified according the positions of the fulcrum and the load relative to the force required to lift the load (Fig. 7-1 illustrates the three classes of levers). The position of the fulcrum relative to the lever arm and the load determines the length of the lever arm and the amount of effort that will be required to lift the load. In some situations, the position of the fulcrum (and therefore the length of the lever arm) can be modified; in these situations, applying force with the longest lever arm and decreasing the length of the lever arm on the side of the load will give the best mechanical advantage.

The following examples demonstrate how gravity, levers, and fulcrums can be applied to mobility tasks in an individual with SCI. For clarification, in the discussions of mobility activities, the side toward which the individual is moving is termed the *leading* side, while the side opposite the direction of the movement in termed the *trailing* side.

Example 1: Pushing open a heavy door. The individual reaches across the body to push on the handle of the door, using the hand on the opposite side of the body to maximize the leverage of the pushing force and minimize the resistance of the door. The individual propels the wheelchair with hand on the side nearest the door handle

Example 2: Lifting the trailing leg onto a bed. The individual holds the leg securely under the knee and leans back to lift the leg onto the bed, the pelvis acts as a fulcrum about which the legs and the trunk pivot. Flexing the hip and knee will shorten the lever arm of the load to be lifted.

Example 3: Surface-to-surface transfers. The individual uses the upper body and gravity to lift the lower body around the fulcrum of the fixed upper extremities (especially on the side of the trailing arm). The head moves in the direction opposite the direction of movement of the pelvis.

The concepts of stability and instability are related to gravity and leverage. Support surfaces that are larger offer more stability than those that are smaller. Likewise, body positions with a larger base of support are inherently more stable than those with a smaller base of support. Therefore, if the goal is to create stability, then a wide base of support is best, but if the goal is to facilitate movement, then a narrower base of support creates instability and increases the ease of movement. The lower

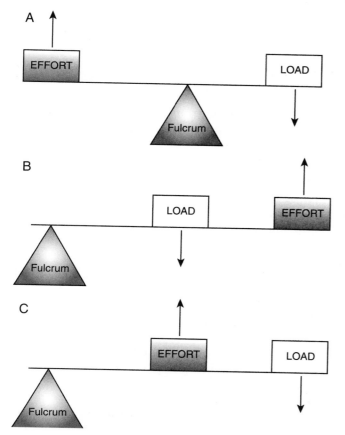

Figure 7-1. Classes of levers. The relative position of load, effort, and fulcrum in lever systems. (A) Class 1 lever. The fulcrum is between the load and the effort. A biomechanical example of a Class 1 lever is an individual reaching overhead while lying supine. The elbow joint is the fulcrum about which the forearm moves as a result of the force (effort) produced by the triceps muscle on the opposite side of the fulcrum. (B) Class 2 lever. The load is between the fulcrum and the effort. A biomechanical example of a Class 2 lever is rising up onto the toes in the standing position. The weight of the body (load) falls between the fulcrum (the ball of the foot) and the source of effort (forces generated by the plantar flexor muscles). (C) Class 3 lever. The effort is between the fulcrum and the load. Elbow flexion activities are biomechanical examples of a Class 3 lever. The elbow is the fulcrum about which the load in the hand is lifted by the force (effort) produced by the biceps muscle that inserts in the forearm between the elbow and the hand.

extremities can provide a critical biomechanical lever and base of support. They can assist movement or, if placed in the wrong position, become an obstacle to movement. In mobility training, the therapist also assesses the position of body parts to ensure that the movement is attempted in a manner that maximizes leverage by positioning the limbs in such a way as to increase or decrease the base of support and take advantage of gravity. For example, in early mobility training, moving from sitting to supine position is easier than the reverse, because moving from sitting to supine position takes advantage of the assistance of gravity and involves moving from a less stable position, with a smaller base of support, to

a position that is more stable, with a larger base of support.

Using momentum is another way to take advantage of gravity as an aid in the mobility training program, but momentum is used with discretion. In rolling from supine to prone position, the individual may use momentum by "winding up" and throwing the arm in the direction of the roll. To optimally use momentum in this task, the individual must continue to reach in the direction of the roll after throwing the arm, protracting at the shoulder, and continuing to reach after the arm motion has stopped. If the roll is not accomplished with the first throw, then the therapist evaluates the technique or setup to determine what should be changed to make the next attempt successful, perhaps by altering the direction of the throw or the leverage. Unless something about the task is altered, repeating the same technique is unlikely to be any more successful on subsequent attempts than it was on the first attempt. Another way that momentum frequently is incorporated into mobility activities is through the use of rocking (accompanied by counting "1, 2, 3") prior to transfer. When using this technique, the rocking is most effective if it is in the diagonal direction, opposite the direction of the transfer (rather than in the anterior-posterior plane). Rocking in the diagonal plane opposite the direction of the transfer sets up the individual to rotate the trunk away from, and the pelvis toward, the direction of the support surface.

Capitalizing on Biomechanics

The body is an interconnected system in which the structural biomechanics impart inherent patterns of coordination. In the presence of paralysis, capitalizing on this inherent coordination provides an advantage for movement. In muscles that are under voluntary control, the origins and insertions of the muscles will dictate the direction of movement of the bone segments when the muscle is activated. But movement can also arise from passive mechanics of the bones, joints, and soft tissues. For example, in an individual with high thoracic or cervical injury in whom voluntary control of the trunk musculature is lost, it is nevertheless possible for the individual to rotate the trunk via the passive interaction among body segments. By moving the upper limbs to their end-range position, movement can be created at the shoulder girdle that is, in turn, transmitted to the trunk. The individual can employ this strategy in rolling over from the supine position. Reaching up and across the body in a diagonal direction places the latissimus dorsi muscle near its end range, and if the shoulder girdle is then protracted forward, the latissimus dorsi muscle will pull at its distal origin on the pelvis, drawing the pelvis over to complete the roll.

Using the above example of rolling over, the same result could be accomplished by active contraction of an innervated upper extremity muscle. If the individual grasps a bar after reaching across the body, the roll can be completed by shortening contraction of the latissimus dorsi muscle, actively pulling the trunk attachment toward the fixed arm. Alternatively, rather than assisting movement, the same mechanics can also resist movement and make mobility activities more difficult. For instance, the passive force created by the hamstrings in a long-sitting position (when the hamstrings are lengthened over both the hip and the knee joints) poses a resistive force such that the individual would have difficulty lifting or moving their lower extremities in this position. This type of resistance to movement will be discussed in greater detail in the section entitled "Identifying Obstacles to Movement."

An individual's residual muscle function is an important consideration when planning a movement or motor task. This plan should effectively harness knowledge of relevant musculoskeletal anatomy and biomechanics in an effort to devise the most efficient and effective strategy possible. The goal is to select the strategy with optimal biomechanical efficiency, moving the body in a manner that takes the least muscular work by capturing the biomechanical properties of the muscles, joints, and limb segments and using leverage and gravity to their optimum advantage. In mobility after SCI, technique is critical in optimizing the efficiency and effectiveness of mobility skills.

Fundamentals of Mobility Training

The therapist works to build success into the mobility program while challenging the individual to achieve new levels of skill. Some tasks are easier for the individual to accomplish than others, and these tasks are the logical place to begin so that the individual builds confidence in his or her abilities. Some tasks are simply not possible for individuals with certain impairments to perform. For example, the individual with acute C5 level tetraplegia is not able to roll over on initial evaluation. The therapist first considers what skills the individual must acquire and what components of the task are difficult for the individual due to his or her specific functional capacity and physical attributes.

Incorporating Principles of Motor Learning

In structuring the learning activity, the therapist takes into account factors related to the task (e.g., how much precision is required, whether speed of performance will affect the outcome, whether gravity will assist or resist the movement task) and the environment (e.g., the size/ firmness/ stability of the support surface) and how these will affect the success of the individual's efforts. After analyzing the task, the therapist designs a therapeutic environment that maximizes the ability of the individual and minimizes the difficulty of the problem components. In many cases, a therapist can break down an activity into its component

parts to allow the individual to focus on the components that are most difficult (i.e., part-task training). In other cases, tasks are best performed in their entirety (i.e., whole-task training) in order to take advantage of factors such as momentum or in cases when the parts of the task are highly interrelated. Applying this knowledge and creating the appropriate learning experiences contributes to the development of movement strategies that optimize the individual's capabilities. Examples of this include the following:

- If an individual has difficulty with balance in the short-sitting position, the therapist may select a large, soft surface.
- If the individual has mastered balance on a large soft surface, progressing to a narrower firm surface increases the difficulty of the task.
- If the goal is moving across a surface, then a firmer surface may be selected
- If the task is dressing/undressing, training may begin with the task of undressing, as this is (in most cases) the easier task.
- If the task is getting into out of bed, the therapist may choose to begin with getting into/out bed as the assistance of gravity makes this an easier task than getting out of bed.
- If the task is maneuvering over curbs in a wheelchair, both ascending and descending require skill, but because gravity will assist the descent, it is the easier task and therefore represents the better starting place.

Careful observation of the individual during execution of new skills provides the therapist with opportunities to identify the characteristics of successful attempts and point these characteristics out to the individual. The therapist also assesses whether the instructions being given to the individual are effective in furthering skill development. The motor learning literature (for review, see Winstein[27]) indicates that external feedback (e.g., verbal cues from the therapist) are useful in the early stages of learning when the individual is developing an understanding of the task and conceptualizing what must be done to accomplish the task. Extrinsic feedback about performance (i.e., knowledge of performance) such as, "your hands are too close to your body on the transfer board," provides information that contributes to the individual's understanding of the essential components of the task. Because practicing tasks on a random schedule is most effective for promoting motor learning (compared to repeatedly practicing the activity within a block of time), the opportunity to practice activities in varied environments at various periods throughout the day is most favorable for skill acquisition.

As skill develops, allowing the individual to rely to a greater extent on intrinsic feedback (i.e., information the individual acquires on his or her own from visual, kinesthetic, tactile, and vestibular senses) promotes the development of problem-solving skills that will be required when the individual is alone and faced with a challenging tasks or environmental obstacle. In the later stages of learning, if extrinsic feedback is provided, giving the individual information about the results of the attempt (i.e., knowledge of results) such as, "your balance would be better if you ended your transfer further back on the mat," is more useful for skill development than is knowledge of performance, as the individual is able to find their own solutions that will change the result in subsequent attempts. The therapist progressively restructures the task and the environment to allow the individual to practice under a variety of conditions. Ideally, the goal is that the individual will able to transfer skills to similar tasks (e.g., balance skills learned in short-sitting position on the mat will transfer to improved balance while propelling the wheelchair) and that skills gained with the practice of one task will generalize to other tasks (e.g., awareness of the influence of body position developed in transfer training is generalized to adjusting position while maneuvering curbs).

The therapist designs a mobility training program that will allow the individual to build confidence by challenging the individual within the realm of his or her capability for success. There are likely to be mobility skills that are difficult for a particular individual, for whatever reason. Often, it is best to postpone efforts on that task for a while, encouraging efforts on alternate tasks with component skills similar to those for the task with which the individual is experiencing difficulty. Not surprisingly, when the individual returns to the original task, he or she will often be able to accomplish it with greater ease.

Identifying Obstacles to Movement

Often, body position or position of a limb segment becomes an obstacle to movement and a hindrance to successful performance of a mobility task. As part of the movement analysis that accompanies mobility training, the therapist identifies obstacles to movement and assists the individual in learning to identify and correct these obstacles. If obstacles to movement are not identified, the individual may expend excessive effort to accomplish the task and may ultimately be unsuccessful. A simple example is in rolling from supine to prone position, wherein if the arm (or leg) on the side the individual is rolling toward is not aligned with the trunk, then the limb becomes an obstacle to completion of the roll. The individual may think that performing the task is not possible, when without the obstacle the efforts would have been successful.

In transfers, the most common obstacle to movement is lack of clearance to permit leg rotation. The individual may expend great effort to push and rotate the body to perform a transfer, but if the posterior aspect of the trailing leg is firmly against the edge of the seating surface, then the transfer will not be possible. Because the individual is unlikely to be able to feel the contact with the seating surface, he or she is unable to identify the problem. Analyzing the setup, the therapist identifies the obstacle, draws the individual's attention to the issue, and assists the individual in identifying a solution (i.e., moving forward in the seat prior to initiating the transfer). Occasionally, the individual's leading leg will be an obstacle to execution of a transfer, but this is more obvious and therefore easier for the individual to identify because the leading leg will strike the mat or become stuck inside the wheelchair frame.

Posture that creates a biomechanical disadvantage is another obstacle to movement. For instance, attempting to lift the leg while seated in an anterior pelvic tilt posture creates a biomechanical disadvantage that increases the required effort and may result in inability to perform the task. The movement may also be blocked by the pelvis/femur interaction. Simply changing the posture to one of posterior pelvic tilt decreases the required effort. The task is made easier still if the individual is taught to move the pelvis in the opposite direction while lifting the legs. Similarly, if the individual attempts to lift the body with hands positioned in the same plane as the hip joints, he or she is at a biomechanical disadvantage and will find it difficult or impossible to lift the body. By placing the hands slightly forward of the hip joints and flexing at the hips, leaning the trunk forward of the hands, the individual is able to lift, using the hands as a fulcrum. This strategy is especially effective for an individual who is wearing a thoracolumbosacral orthosis (TLSO), as the orthosis elongates the trunk, increasing the relative distance the individual must reach to contact the support surface. Prior to attempting mobility training with an individual in a TLSO, the therapist inspects the orthosis to ensure that it is well-fitted, with snug contours under the ribs, proximal trim lines allowing for pectoral girdle movement, and distal trim lines that allow hip flexion while maintaining appropriate position of the pelvis.

Weight bearing or lack thereof can also be an obstacle to movement. If the task requires a limb to be lifted, it will be almost impossible to perform if the individual is leaning on the limb, or if the limb is bearing weight or providing support. Conversely, if the goal is to use the limb as a support, then the limb should bear weight. In early transfer training, the problem of having the hand slide on the support surface is not uncommon. While some therapists may place nonskid material under the hands or encourage the individual to lick the hand for increased friction, what is actually required is increased weight bearing on the upper extremity. Often, increased weight bearing on an upper extremity is achieved simply by having the individual place the hand in closer proximity to the body.

In some individuals, spasticity and muscle spasms can be obstacles to movement. Unanticipated spasms can throw a person off balance or interfere with an intended motion. Typically, however, the individual can learn to anticipate spasms. Moreover, it is not unusual for individuals to learn to "trigger" a muscle spasm to assist with transfers and/or mobility. The potential functional mobility of an individual should not be hindered by the belief that spasticity limits function. The therapist and the person with SCI should attend to positional or movement triggers in an effort to anticipate this potential obstacle.

Other obstacles to movement include lack of passive range of motion or the attempt to move beyond the normal anatomical end range of a joint. When promoting functional mobility in individuals with SCI, considering the way an able-bodied individual would accomplish the task often provides a helpful reminder of the most efficient and effective approach. For example, to reach to put on a shoe, the nondisabled individual usually bends at the hip and the knee rather than attempting to put the shoe on with the knee extended. Some of the more frequently encountered obstacles to the successful performance of mobility tasks are given in Table 7-2.

Sequence and Integration

The acquisition of mobility skills follows a specific sequence that is much like the motor developmental sequence described by Rood:[28] mobility, stability, controlled mobility, and skill. In the mobility stage, the individual is able to move the limbs if external postural stabilization is provided (e.g., reaching up while lying on a mat). At the stability stage, the individual is able to hold himself in a stable posture (e.g., sitting in a long-sitting posture). When controlled mobility has been achieved, the individual is able to move the proximal segments while the distal segments are fixed (e.g., rocking forward and back while in the quadripedal position). Finally, at the stage of skill, the individual is able to move the distal extremities while maintaining a stable posture (e.g., reaching out while sitting to grasp an object) and is able to move between postures (e.g., transfer from the wheelchair to the mat).

Using the sequence of balance training as an example, the individual must first be able to balance statically within a posture, then move within a posture, then move into and out of a posture. Balance training also requires practicing transitions, moving between postures or positions with control. Good balance is reflected in the ability to move smoothly and comfortably between postures without landing abruptly on or bearing excessive weight on the upper extremity. A good foundation in balance training alleviates the fear of falling.

Mobility skills are best acquired through practice in different environments. If an individual can transfer independently between level surfaces in the clinic, then

Table 7-2
Common Obstacles to Movement

Mobility Problem	Potential Obstacle	Solution
Difficulty lifting leg	Pelvis in anterior tilt	Place pelvis in poster tilt
	Individual is leaning on the leg	Lean away from leg
	Obstruction blocking leg	Remove obstruction
Loss of balance during a transfer	Hands positioned in same plane as the hip joint	Position hands anterior or posterior to hip joint (depending on direction of movement)
	Feet positioned too far back	Position feet forward of knees
Inability to complete transfer	Lack of clearance for rotation of trailing leg	Move forward in seat
	Leading leg collides with mat	Rotate legs away from mat
	Trunk/shoulders rotated toward direction of transfer	Rotate trunk/shoulders away from direction of transfer
Inability to roll over	Leading arm blocking movement	Position arm under body or over head
	Leading side leg blocking roll	Position leg in plane of body
	Poor use of leverage	with triceps control, reach up and extend neck (look up) *or* without triceps control, flex neck, reach down and across body

the next goal would be to master level transfers from the wheelchair to a bed. In addition to transfers, other skills that are incorporated into the early mobility training program include bed mobility, with training in leg management skills (i.e., getting the legs on and off the bed), and advanced balance skills. Bed mobility skills and balance in short- and long-sitting positions are prerequisites to other skills such as dressing. If these mobility skills are learned early, then the individual has the foundation to be successful when attempting tasks related to ADLs.

When working on the development of balance and wheelchair mobility activities, prescription of the most appropriate wheelchair is essential. A wheelchair that is not optimal has the potential to impede development of key skills. While it might seem that a power wheelchair with power tilt would be appropriate for a newly injured individual with motor-incomplete SCI who is not yet independent in propelling the chair or in performing pressure relief, such a wheelchair would hinder the individual's ability to acquire skill in these activities. By providing excessive stabilization and protecting the individual from balance challenges, such a chair provides over-ground mobility at the expense of skill acquisition. To acquire balance and motor control, the individual must be able to experience instability. Through mobility training, the therapist provides a safe environment wherein the individual is able to challenge the limits of his or her stability.

The individual will be in different stages of skill development for each skill that must be acquired. Progress through the various stages depends on the difficulty of the task relative to the individual's capabilities. Factors such as the amount of force required, the impact of gravity, the height of the center of gravity, the size of the base of support, the advantage or disadvantage of the levers, and the environment all contribute to the level of difficulty of the task.

Therapeutic Assistance

The individual with SCI is learning new movement strategies and new motor skills using a body that is moving in new ways after the SCI. In some cases, especially in the early stages of mobility training, the individual may be completely unfamiliar with the strategy that will be required to accomplish a task. In this period, it is often helpful for the therapist demonstrate the activity and then to assist the individual to move through the whole pattern or task so that the individual can conceptualize the mobility task and acquire a kinesthetic and/or visual sense of what is required to accomplish the task. The therapist provides assistance for components of a task for which the individual is unable to overcome the resistance of gravity or where grip is poor. For example, the trunk rotation component of a transfer is often difficult for many individuals in the early period of training; the therapist can assist with the transfer with manual contact.

The therapist promotes success and guides the appropriate movement pattern so that the individual can acquire a kinesthetic sense of the motion. As the individual progresses toward independence, the amount of assistance is reduced and may be replaced with manual cues. The therapist is vigilant for faulty movement patterns and offers assistance to correct them so that the individual does not practice and acquire a poor movement habit.

The use of equipment for assisting with mobility can be enabling, but overreliance on equipment can limit independence. An individual who is only able to accomplish rolling independently when using specific stationary equipment such as a hospital bed, bed rails, or grab bars will be limited in his ability to accomplish ADLs in different environments. Furthermore, this deficit will also limit the individual's capacity for full participation in social roles. The ability to stay independently in a hotel and to travel for business or pleasure is compromised by overreliance on specialized equipment. If business travel is limited, so then may be job opportunities. Maximized ability with minimized equipment is the goal whenever possible. The therapist encourages creative solutions to mobility issues. For example, the wheelchair is always positioned at bedside for ease of access, but it may also assist with bed mobility. For some individuals, the wheelchair handrim will provide sufficient assistance for independence in rolling over, or for pushing up onto an elbow to sit up. The goal is for the individual to achieve maximum independence and flexibility by using the environment in creative ways and avoiding reliance on rigid methods that are restrictive and limiting.

Joint Protection

Protection of joint integrity in paralyzed limbs is an essential part of therapeutic intervention. During mobility training, the therapist evaluates the individual's movement strategies to ensure protection of joint integrity. The therapist is attentive to limb positions and postures (e.g., hyperextension of the shoulder) that have the potential to injure a joint. The therapist also teaches the individual to be attentive to these postures and positions. Particular attention/education is directed to lower extremity positions and areas below the level of normal sensation. In individuals with spastic paresis or spastic paralysis, spasticity or muscle contracture may pull on one side of a joint. In the lower extremity, hip flexion contractures have the potential to create posterior instability of the hip joint that may result in subluxation or dislocation. The therapist emphasizes that prevention of joint instability is one of many reasons that it is important to preserve normal joint range of motion, but that care must also be taken not to overstretch the soft tissues that provide the joint with structural stability.

Preserving the Structural Stability of Joints

It is a common misconception that the individual with SCI needs to increase the length of the hamstring or the shoulder musculature beyond the length that would be considered "normal," in order to have functional mobility for tasks such as dressing. Consequently, individuals with SCI have historically been encouraged to aggressively stretch the hamstrings.[29–31] In truth, overly aggressive stretching creates laxity in the passive structures in the posterior aspect of the lower limb, resulting in hypermobility and joint instability. In the absence of muscle activity, passive structures are necessary to maintain the joint alignment. Once elongated, these structures will not return to their original length. Education is the key to protecting joints over a lifetime of use.

Hip dislocation is a recognized problem in the pediatric SCI population,[32–35] and there are also reports in the adult population.[36,37] Joint malalignment changes the platform for sitting and therefore changes the postural alignment of body parts above the pelvis. This altered postural alignment can have a negative influence on many systems (respiratory, skin, and upper limb musculoskeletal health). Measures to reduce the risk of hip dislocation include maintaining hip extension range of motion and not overstretching the posterior structures of the hip. Moving in a manner that keeps the femoral head seated in the acetabulum protects the soft tissue structures that surround the hip and assists in maintaining integrity of the hip joint. To this end, when teaching an individual with SCI to maneuver the lower extremities, the individual practices keeping the hips in external rotation and abduction whenever possible. A tip for remembering this pattern is that when moving, the knee leads on the leading limb while the foot leads on the trailing limb, such that the feet are kept close to each other and the knees are kept apart from each other. Figure 7-2 illustrates the difference between a potentially damaging pattern and the recommended positioning for the trailing leg during transfers.

The therapist evaluates movement patterns for combinations of motion that could potentially damage a joint. If a repetitive movement pattern is used that could threaten the integrity of a joint, then the therapist instructs the individual in an alternative movement strategy.

In the SCI literature, much as been written about the association between upper limb pain and wheelchair propulsion or the performance of transfers,[14,21,38–41] as well as discussions of the upper limbs "wearing out" and "overuse" pain. Musculoskeletal pain associated with overuse is the most common cause of shoulder pain in individuals with SCI.[42] However, no studies have established a causal link between long-term wheelchair use and upper extremity pain, and there is evidence that the experience of pain is not well correlated with activity level.[43] Nonetheless, individuals with SCI use their upper

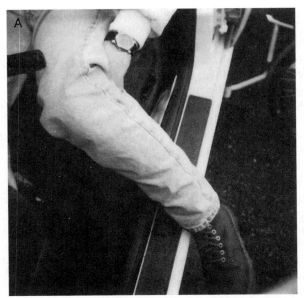

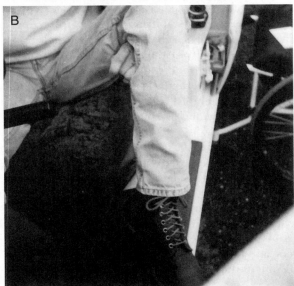

Figure 7-2. A potentially damaging hip position (A) with hip internal rotation, adduction, and flexion versus a hip protective pattern (B) with hip external rotation, abduction, and flexion.

extremities for all ADLs, including transfers, pressure relief lifts, and wheelchair propulsion, so intuitively it seems wise to protect these joints.

Joint Protection During Transfers

Transfers and pressure relief lifts involve high joint forces in which each upper extremity must bear a substantial portion of the individual's body weight for a prolonged period of time; therefore, transfers are a potential threat to upper limb musculoskeletal health. Mastery of biomechanically sound transfer techniques contributes to the protection of joint (and skin) integrity, as such skills make the individual less likely to sustain injury compared to an individual with poor or marginal skills. In addition to attending to the forces generated with upper extremity mobility activities, attending to joint position also contributes to preservation of joint integrity. Joints operate best at mid range wherein articular surfaces are optimally aligned. Therefore, the therapist teaches the individual to avoid loading a joint when it is in its end-range position whenever possible. Accordingly, because muscle imbalance around a joint creates the potential for joint incongruence, maintaining range of motion is also important. In cases of asymmetrical motor involvement, care must be taken to minimize malalignment that may result from imbalance in the forces around a joint.

In the shoulder, the relative positions of the scapula and the humerus are important in determining the stability of the joint. The shoulder is stable for weight bearing when the scapula is rotated and protracted to maintain congruence between the articular surfaces of the glenoid fossa and the humeral head; this is achieved with the trunk flexed over the hips in sitting when the hands are resting on the seating surface. If an individual is transferring between surfaces of different heights, then the low arm should bear the larger proportion of the load as it is in the more advantaged position in terms of the biomechanics of the shoulder. If the individual is going to transfer by pulling on an overhead bar, the shoulder should be externally rotated and in a scaption plane with pull from the latissimus dorsi (elbow moving in the posterior direction), pectoralis major, and the biceps.

While much attention is focused on protection of the shoulder joints, it is also important to consider other upper extremity joints. Mechanically locking the elbow joint during transfers should be avoided; passive extension of the elbow in the midrange of joint motion is possible if gravity and the biomechanical properties of the limbs are used to advantage (this is discussed further in the section entitled "Transitions"). The wrist is best positioned in neutral when performing transfers; positioning the hand so that the metacarpalphalangeal joints are off the edge of the transfer surface or grabbing around the wheelchair frame are examples of ways that a neutral wrist position can be achieved.

Reducing Joint Forces During Wheelchair Propulsion

While in the typical wheelchair user, propulsion does not use the same high levels of prolonged force that are required for transfers, the repetitive nature of propulsion also has the potential to threaten the musculoskeletal health of the upper limb. One important aim of wheelchair selection and training in propulsion techniques is to minimize upper extremity forces while maximizing efficiency. The use of ultralight manual wheelchairs, with customization for optimal postural support and training in proper push mechanics, aids in upper limb protection.[44] The wrist is subject to stress from excessive finger extrinsic activity during wheelchair propulsion if the individual develops the improper habit of gripping and releasing the handrim with every stroke. Excessive finger extrinsic activity in poor wrist positions can contribute to the development of carpal tunnel syndrome and lateral epicondylitis. In addition to the stress on the wrist and hand, the habit of repetitively gripping and releasing the handrim is counterproductive; the increased resistance at the terminal phase of the stroke does not allow full advantage to be made of the forward momentum and actually causes the wheelchair to slow. Instead of gripping the handrim, the individual can smoothly propel the wheelchair with a relaxed and slightly open hand contact on the rim. This technique will eliminate the need for the individual to grip and release the handrim, except during the forceful propulsion required for maneuvering inclines or curbs. Proper wheelchair propulsion techniques are discussed in detail in the section entitled "Propelling a Wheelchair."

Balance and Postural Stability

Optimal balance has two essential components: (1) the ability to anticipate and prepare for postural conditions that will perturb balance and (2) the ability to respond quickly and appropriately to perturbations that are not anticipated. Poor balance and postural stability can also contribute to upper extremity musculoskeletal problems. Individuals with poor postural stability or poor balance will often use the upper extremity to hold the trunk upright. For example, individuals who stabilize their posture by propping on their hands while doing computer work will use positions of hyperextension of the wrist with excessive lengthening of the flexor tendons. Propping for inadequate stability creates stress at the wrist and hand and may contribute to the development of carpal tunnel syndrome. Balance training can make an important contribution to preserving upper extremity joint integrity, but balance is also important for a multitude of other reasons.

In individuals with SCI, there is likely to be impairment or loss of the sensorimotor contributions to balance below the level of the SCI. Despite this, postural control can be achieved if the individual learns how to anticipate threats to balance. Through balance training, the individual gains an understanding of the point of balance as well as the boundaries around this point (within which he or she can move without exceeding the limits of stability). The individual also learns how best to use gravity, passive positioning, and residual motor control to maximize dynamic balance. The individual learns what challenges can be overcome with subtle postural corrections, what situations require more substantial strategies, and when it will be necessary to increase the base of support (i.e., protective extension). To facilitate this knowledge, the therapist structures a program that fosters recognition of internal feedback associated with balance challenges, both challenges generated internally by the individual's own movement and those imposed from external sources. The acquisition of skill in balance typically begins with the ability to respond to internally generated balance challenges prior to acquiring the ability to respond to externally generated challenges.

Training in short-sitting balance begins by assisting the individual into a position of balance, providing the opportunity for the individual to experience this balanced posture. The size of the base of support is maximized, with full contact of the posterior thigh against the support surface, thighs parallel to floor (or knees slightly higher than hips), and feet flat on the floor. The true balance position is often anterior of the position the individual perceives as being balanced, and he or she will tend to push back into extension. With a paralyzed trunk, when the trunk is extended and shoulders positioned posterior to the hip joint, there is no support against the pull of gravity. Conversely, with slight trunk flexion and positioning of the shoulders slightly forward of the hip joint, the individual will be able to balance with support afforded by intra-abdominal pressure and tension in the posterior longitudinal ligament.

While in the absence of voluntary trunk control the short-sitting posture will not be erect, an individual with upper extremity function and trunk paralysis can be quite stable in this position. For individuals in a TLSO, balance is harder to achieve, and the boundary around the balance point is smaller because the orthosis places the individual in a more erect posture, thereby eliminating the availability of passive support from intra-abdominal pressure and tension in the posterior longitudinal ligament. On the other hand, individuals with cervical immobilization have an easier time learning short-sitting balance, but they are discouraged from spending extended periods of time in this position as it imposes cervical strain.

It is important for individuals with SCI to learn that there is a limit to their balance and to experience what those limits are in a safe environment. This is particularly true when seated in the wheelchair with good postural alignment. If an individual has impaired or absent voluntary control of the trunk muscles, this seated position has a small boundary of control. These boundaries must be considered when performing tasks with the upper extremities. While there may be sufficient balance control in short-sitting position to allow the individual to perform two-handed activities close to body (and therefore close to the balance point), it may be necessary to change to a more stable position (e.g., scooting the buttocks forward and assuming a posterior pelvic tilt) when performing two-handed tasks farther away from the body. While the poorly aligned postures that provide stability for two-handed tasks farther away from the body can be tolerated infrequently for short periods, using such postures habitually puts the musculoskeletal system at risk for injury. Balance while reaching is best achieved by performing the reach as a two-armed activity; one arm reaches forward to manipulate the environment while the other arm provides stability for balance. Lifting items from the floor is also a two-armed activity, wherein one hand grasps the item while the other hand holds onto some aspect of the wheelchair and pulls the trunk back to the upright position.

Transitions

Earlier in the chapter, Table 7-1 described the expected functional outcomes for individuals with motor-complete SCI based on neurologic level. The following section discusses these concepts in detail, focusing on the sequential addition of contributions from muscles innervated by progressively more caudal levels of the spinal cord between the segmental levels of C5 and C8 and the impact these muscles have on available movement strategies.

The Functional Impact of Neurological Level

Innervation at C5

At the C5 segmental level, the biceps muscle is the key muscle that becomes available. This muscle provides elbow flexion, forearm supination, and a weak ability to flex the shoulder. The biceps is only partially innervated by C5 because additional innervation to this muscle is provided by the C6 segmental level. The clavicular head of the pectoralis muscle also is partially innervated at C5, as are the three heads of the deltoid (anterior, middle, and posterior). In the posterior aspect of the shoulder girdle, the rhomboid muscle is fully innervated at C5, and the rotator cuff muscles of external rotation are partially innervated. The individual with C5 motor innervation has good movement of the shoulder and elbow, but the shoulder is not fully innervated and not inherently stable. The lack of strong shoulder internal rotator and adductor muscles is a limitation to functional mobility. The individual with C5 SCI has no innervation of the major muscles that attach to the trunk, with the exception of the trapezius muscle, therefore the limb muscles must be used to move the trunk. For this reason, it is unusual for an individual with the C5 level of motor function to be able to independently transfer or perform bed mobility.

Innervation at C6

With innervation at the C6 segmental level there is a significant enhancement in functional potential. From the perspective of mobility, the pivotal functional advantage afforded with C6 innervation is stability and power of the shoulder muscles. Innervation at C6 provides internal rotation with strong subscapularis, weak latissimus dorsi, and moderately strong teres major muscles. The teres major and the latissimus dorsi muscles also provide adduction. The serratus anterior muscle has two levels of innervation for functional protraction. The posterior rotator cuff muscles and the deltoid muscle are fully innervated, as is the biceps muscle. The individual with a C6 motor level has the ability to reach across the front of the body, active shoulder protraction, a stable shoulder, and has the muscular capacity to move the trunk over a fixed arm. Therefore, the individual with C6 motor function has full capabilities for transfers, assuming full joint range of motion and reasonable body weight (i.e., not overweight). The C6 segment also affords the ability to extend the wrist, providing the capacity for a tenodesis grip. This distal function is important for the ability to manipulate small objects, for oral and facial hygiene, and for eating.

Innervation at C7

Segmental level C7 provides innervation to the triceps for active elbow extension; this segment also strengthens many of the larger muscles that attach the upper limb to the thoracic wall (e.g., the serratus anterior, pectoralis major, and latissimus dorsi muscles), which significantly improves the ability to move the body over a fixed hand for transfers. Active triceps muscles increase the ease of transferring from a low to a high surface by adding some lift with the leading side (high) arm. Seated push-ups for pressure change or repositioning in the wheelchair are also easier. In addition, this muscle increases the ease of pushing up from supine to sitting position and provides the capacity for reaching overhead and for extending the arm against gravity or resistance. This capacity improves the ease of bed mobility and self-care tasks. Innervation at C7 also increases the stability and strength at the wrist, adding wrist flexion and strengthening active pronation.

Innervation at C8

Innervation at C8 contributes additional power and stability to the shoulder girdle and, in particular, to the large muscles attached to the thoracic wall. Innervation at C8 also provides active grip and release in the hand.

Thoracic Innervation

Innervation at successively more caudal thoracic levels is associated with increased control of the postural muscles and therefore increasing balance and postural stability. Active rotation is available as the oblique muscles are innervated.

Rolling

Rolling is a mobility skill that is necessary for moving in bed and for pressure relief to maintain skin health. It also is an important component of other functional activities such as stretching and dressing (for individuals who dress in bed). The ability to roll also contributes to sleeping comfort and sexual intimacy. As with training any mobility task, instruction in rolling begins with components of the skill that the individual is likely to be successful at performing. Starting in the side-lying position, the individual works on the ability to push back into the supine position or roll forward into the three-quarter prone position. As an early mobility activity, gaining proficiency in rolling is empowering because individuals with SCI are regularly positioned in side-lying position during the acute inpatient period. Ability to move into and out of side-lying provides the individual with options for positioning. Rolling is a task in which the passive mechanics of the upper extremities can be used to achieve trunk movement. Rather than reaching for a rail to pull on, the individual is encouraged to learn to use gravity and body mechanics to accomplish the roll.

Practice activities begin with the individual reaching forward and making small excursions from the side-lying position toward the prone position, then progressing to larger excursions. The individual also practices moving from the side-lying position to the supine position by retracting the scapula and pulling the arm back behind the body, leading with the elbow. If more leverage is needed, the motion may be performed with the elbow extended. This technique uses the concept of moving to the end range of motion of the more proximal component and then reaching farther to draw the distal attachment along in the same direction of movement. If the support surface is soft, then it will be necessary to overcome inertia, and roll may not begin immediately. The individual learns to continue to reach, using leverage to its fullest advantage, and wait for the motion to begin. If the roll is not accomplished, the therapist and the individual reevaluate the setup and the motion to determine what must be changed to successfully complete the roll.

Reflecting on stable and unstable body positions offers insights about how the rolling task can be made easier. Lying on the side with the trunk and lower extremities aligned in extension provides a narrow and unstable base of support for the body, therefore attempting a roll from this starting position will minimize the necessary effort. The leverage that arises from moving the arms forward or backward is all that is required to cause the body to roll in the same direction. Conversely, an individual positioned on the side with flexed lower extremities provides a comparatively larger base of support, making it more difficult to roll from this flexed starting position. Indeed, the flexed legs present an obstacle to rolling toward prone.

Once the individual has acquired an understanding of what is required for rolling, the concepts learned in rolling from the side-lying position can also be applied when the individual is rolling from a prone or a supine starting position. As with training for any mobility task, the therapist selects the technique that will best achieve the desired outcome for the individual based on physical attributes and the particular circumstances. An individual with paraplegia who is in a TLSO will roll most easily using an extension pattern with upper extremities lifting up and across the body, extending the neck, and reaching overhead. Conversely, an individual with a cervical injury and cervical immobilization but a free trunk will roll best using trunk flexion and reaching down and across to pull the body over.

Pushing Up from Weight Bearing on an Elbow

Pushing up from the position of weight bearing on an elbow is an essential skill that is easily learned with proper instruction. This is a component skill of many other mobility tasks and should be taught first to facilitate skill acquisition in other tasks. This technique is particularly important for individuals who have no active triceps function. As with many skills, this skill is best learned in reverse (described below in the discussion of part-task training). The therapist can assist the individual to drop down onto one elbow in a supported long-sitting position and then provide the individual with verbal and tactile cues for the maneuver. The motion should be done with the powerful shoulder girdle muscles and does not require active elbow extension. The key elements for successful execution of this mobility task are the angle of push relative to the line of gravity and the leverage established by positioning (*see* Fig. 7-3A and B). While bearing weight on the elbow, the hand is positioned away from the trunk (shoulder external rotation and slight abduction) with the palm down; the resultant position is with the angle between the forearm and the upper arm greater than 90 degrees. The individual then presses firmly on the hand and "flips" the elbow upward off the mat, using forceful shoulder internal rotation. The weight shift off the elbow and over the hand is necessary, and the therapist may need to facilitate this weight shift during early training. Manual cues at the hand for downward pressure, at the posterior distal humerus for lift (rotation upward), and assistance to support the weight of the trunk will facilitate this acquisition of this skill.

Supine to Sit

When moving from the supine position to the short-sitting position, the individual with motor-complete SCI should move through the long-sitting position. This strategy provides the most protection to the lower limb joints and is the safest. Once in long-sitting position, the individual can maneuver the legs off the bed in a sequential manner. Moving the leading leg is most easily accomplished by placing the contralateral hand under the leg just below the knee and pushing the leg laterally. The ipsilateral arm can then pull the trailing leg over toward the leading leg and repeat the actions. Movement of the pelvis away from the side of the bed will assist in achieving a stable short-sitting position perpendicular to the long axis of the bed. When practicing this maneuver, the therapist alerts the individual to the fact that he will have less forward balance as the legs move off the mat; this allows the individual to anticipate the imbalance.

The move from supine to a long-sitting position can be achieved in two different ways. The first approach is most often employed by individuals with thoracic level injury and is the method required during the use of a

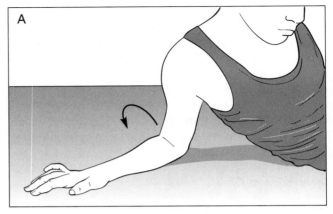

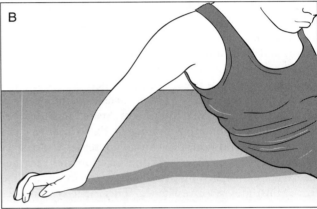

Figure 7-3. Pushing up from prone on elbows. The starting position (A) is with hand away from body in shoulder external rotation, with internal rotation of the shoulder (B) the elbow is lifted off the surface and extended.

TLSO; it requires moving up from supine in two stages. Rather than moving straight up against gravity, the individual uses two lateral/upward moves (this is akin to the difference between climbing a mountain by hiking straight up versus traversing the switchbacks). The first stage is to push up into weight bearing on one elbow; the second stage is pushing off the elbow, using the technique described above to achieve sitting. To move onto one elbow, those with full hand function may grab the side of the mat or bed to facilitate pulling up onto the elbow (persons without hand function may find hooking the wheelchair handrim provides a sufficient anchor). The contralateral hand is placed palm down close to the trunk between the waist and hip with the elbow not in contact with the surface (shoulder internal rotation, slight abduction, and forearm pronation). The motion is to push the trunk laterally over the elbow while also pulling the trunk up using the elbow flexors of the weight-bearing arm. The key elements to success with this mobility skill are leverage and body part alignment. It is important not to start this maneuver while positioned too close to the edge of the mat as room is required to align the forearm away from the trunk in order to accommodate the move off the elbow.

The second approach for moving from supine to long-sitting position is often used by individuals with tretraplegia, as less arm function is required compared with the first approach. In the second approach, moving to long-sitting position is accomplished by moving from supine to prone on elbows. Then, from the prone on elbows position, the individual "walks" on elbows around toward the knees while bending at the waist (*see* Figs. 7-4A–C).

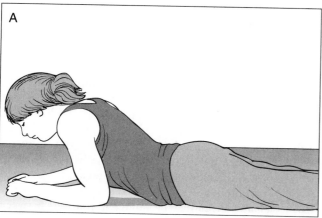

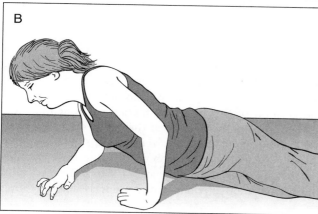

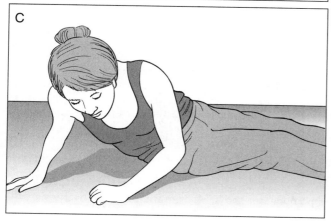

Figure 7-4. Initial steps of the prone to long-sitting transition. First from prone on elbows (A), the individual "walks" with the arms toward long-sitting position, flexing at the waist while maintaining trunk extension (B and C)

The trunk stays elongated, such that the individual does not bend too close to the knees with the trunk. Moving around to hook the outside knee with the leading hand and using the lower extremities to stabilize, the individual pushes up off the trailing elbow (using the technique described above for pushing up from weight bearing on an elbow). The individual then pulls the hooked knee out to the side (hip abduction), allowing the pelvis to drop over and pull the trunk into the upright position.

Part-task Training for Transitions

Transitioning from supine to long-sitting position is a stepwise progression. It is sometimes helpful to practice this progression by starting in reverse. From the long-sitting position, the individual drops down onto one elbow (with the therapist supporting most of the body weight from behind and not allowing the person to drop completely into the supine position). The individual is then instructed to come immediately back up to the long-sitting position. As noted previously, the hand is positioned away from the body, with the elbow in toward the side (shoulder external rotation), and then the elbow flips upward off the support surface. The session includes several practice trials in both directions. Thereafter, the individual practices trials in which he is closer to being completely supine, but with the trunk slightly elevated and supported (by the therapist who is kneel-sitting behind the individual). From this position, the individual works on the component of pushing onto one elbow. Once the individual is able to perform the component skills, the components may be added together progressively to achieve the whole task. The same concept of part-task training can be applied to training for transition from supine to prone to long-sitting position. As with developing any new motor skill, the individual may require hands-on assistance and manual cues to learn the proper pattern. Once the individual is able to conceptualize what is required to accomplish the movement, the skill will be readily mastered. If the individual appears to have a concept of what is required to accomplish the movement, but continues to have difficulty mastering the task, the therapist seeks obstacles to movement and modifies the approach accordingly. For example, if the individual has tight hamstrings, it will be necessary to work with knees flexed and hips externally rotated and slightly abducted. Alternatively, the individual can be positioned with the feet hanging over the end of the bed.

Transfers

Fundamentals of Wheelchair Transfers

The fundamentals of a mechanically efficient transfer are the same for all individuals regardless of body type, height, arm length, or level of injury. Body position and setup greatly influence the ease with which a transfer is performed. Leg and foot position also play a role in proper transfers, as they contribute stability to the base of support. Even if the lower extremities are paralyzed, they contribute to the transfer and have the potential to make the transfer easier or more difficult. To provide mechanical assistance and to prevent the legs from becoming an obstacle to the movement, the feet are placed midway between the mat and the wheelchair. Both lower extremities must have space for movement. The legs can create an obstacle to movement if the leading leg has insufficient clearance to pivot forward or if the trailing leg has insufficient clearance behind the knee to allow it to rotate.

In preparation for the transfer, the individual moves forward on the seat. In the early stages of transfer training, moving forward in the seat is often difficult for the individual, and the therapist may assist with this component at that stage of learning. The three-pronged support configuration of a tripod serves as a good analogy for a mechanically efficient transfer with a large base of support. A tripod is created by the two hands positioned forward of the pelvis. The proper positioning of the individual's hands for a mat-to-wheelchair transfer is described in Table 7-3.

The transfer begins with the individual pushing into the hands using shoulder protraction, taking weight off the leading hip by leaning over the trailing hand, and rotating the trunk so that the chest is directed away from the direction of transfer and the pelvis moves in the direction of transfer. The motion of the transfer swings the body approximately 90 degrees around the axis of the knees on the fulcrum of the hands. With the distal aspect of the leading arm fixed, adduction of the shoulder draws the body toward the mat. The transfer is completed with protraction of the trailing shoulder to push the body into the final position (*see* Figs. 7-5A–D). This technique uses momentum to its greatest advantage,

as the head and upper trunk counterbalance the pelvis, propelling the pelvis in the direction of the transfer; conversely, attempting the transfer by leaning forward over the legs would create undesired momentum in the forward direction rather than in the direction of the transfer.

The individual with SCI learns that all transfers make use of the same general skills and the same general components of movement. The therapist is consistent but not rigid. For example, the individual's hand positions may differ slightly depending on what seems to work best for the individual. In general, in individuals with cervical injury, a more anterior hand position (near the upper one-third of the thigh) may be favorable, but if the hand is too far forward, there will be no power for a lift. Individuals with full innervation of the upper limb have the serratus anterior, pectoralis major, and the latisimus dorsi muscles to provide the lift and will have better ability to lift with the hands placed more widely apart (i.e., with greater shoulder abduction). Conversely, for individuals with tetraplegia, who have less muscle power, it may be necessary to place the hands closer in to the body and to move in incremental steps.

The techniques described above for the mat-to-wheelchair transfer may be applied to transfers between a myriad of other support surfaces. Some advanced transfers may require alternative leg positioning. For instance, in a wheelchair-to-tub transfer the leading leg (or both legs) are placed inside the tub wall. For transfers in confined spaces, the therapist determines the best leg placement by analyzing the pivot-swing trajectory of the intended transfer, the wheelchair setup angle, and the position of the legs. The therapist is watchful for a nose-in angle of the wheelchair that is too tight to accommodate the pivot clearance required by the legs, such that they would create an obstacle to the transfer. This may be especially problematic with a shorter-framed, rigid wheelchair. Another potential obstacle is created by leaving

Table 7-3
Hand Placements for Wheelchair Transfers

Leading Hand Position	Trailing Hand Position
Forward of the hips	Slightly forward of the hips but posterior to the position of the leading hand
Away from the body (gripping wheelchair frame or placed on front of cushion)	Close to the body
Knuckles directed forward and slightly inward toward the body	Fingers pointing out and away from the direction of transfer
Wrist in neutral	Wrist begins in extension but moves toward a neutral position as transfer proceeds

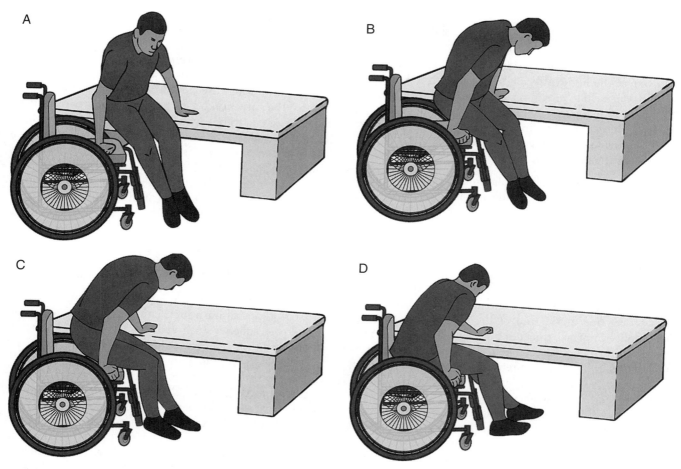

Figure 7-5. The wheelchair transfer. The setup of the transfer forms a tripod configuration, with the two hands forward of the pelvis. The feet are positioned midway between the start and end surfaces with clear pivot space. The individual moves his buttocks forward toward the edge of the mat (A). The individual lowers the head and protracts the shoulders pushing into the hands to take weight off the hips (B). Rotating the trunk away from the direction of the transfer and moving the head over the trailing limb moves the hips and the direction of the wheelchair (C). Finally, the individual pushes back into the wheelchair seat (D).

the feet on the footrest; at a tight angle, the feet will tangle in the footrest.

Some individuals with long-standing SCI have developed a compensatory habit of transferring with the lower extremities extended at the knee and resting on the surface to which they are transferring. This habit is often observed in individuals with poor dynamic balance (e.g., secondary to inadequate rehabilitation or overstretched hamstrings). This transfer setup position can provide a sense of stability and a large base of support, and elevating the feet prevents the legs from dragging at the end of the transfer. However, transferring with the feet elevated on the support surface results in significant upper limb strain as it moves the center of gravity posteriorly and pushes the pelvis downward into the seat, thereby creating a mechanical disadvantage for the transfer. There are occasional situations, however, in which foot elevation can be advantageous; for instance, positioning the feet on the strap above the footrest can aid a transfer to a higher surface.

Additionally, for transfers to a higher surface, the wheelchair should be angled with the footrest directed outward to provide more stability because there is no issue related to rear wheel clearance since the individual is moving over the wheel.

Transfer Training

During transfer training activities, the therapist uses body positioning and manual assistance/cuing to assist the individual in the activity. The therapist is positioned seated or half kneeling in front of the individual and slightly toward the side of the direction of transfer. This position offers security to the individual who is learning to transfer, as the therapist is in a position to prevent a fall forward onto the floor. In addition, from this position the therapist is available to assist the individual with the transfer activity. To assist the transfer during the early stages of transfer training, the therapist assumes the following hand/leg placements:

- The therapist's leading side hand is at the posterior lateral scapula (hooking the posterior acromion) of the individual's leading shoulder.
- The therapist's trailing side hand reaches across the front of the body, offering security from forward loss of balance while providing assistance at the individual's trailing side hip.
- The therapist's trailing side leg blocks (assists) the individual's trailing side knee, using this block to prevent the body from sliding too far forward.

These positions and hand placements allow the therapist to lead the movement and to assist the individual in rotating the upper trunk and head in the direction away from the transfer while the hips are moving in the direction of the transfer.

Transfer training may begin with a transfer board, but the components of the transfer are the same. The "lift" is more of an "unweighting" early on, and at this stage there is more emphasis on the trunk rotation and shoulder protraction at the end of the transfer. As skill and confidence improve, the cues can begin to emphasize the need to lift, then rotate. When beginning to train without a transfer board, it is often easier to transfer toward a surface that is slightly lower in height. For uneven height transfers (and any transfer that is awkward), it is a good habit to learn to land on, or at least near, the leading hand. With the head down and away from the transfer, it is not possible for the individual to see if he or she has safely landed. However, if the individual sits on the leading hand, it offers a cue about the position, and he or she can then finish sliding onto the surface before lifting the head and moving the hand. In uneven transfers, the arm on the lower side is the primary worker, actively protracting for lift and controlling the descent through eccentric muscle activity. When transferring to a surface that is significantly lower, the speed of impact with the support surface is controlled by the speed at which the individual lifts the head. The head and upper trunk counterbalance the lower body around the fulcrum of the upper extremities. Rapidly lifting the head will result in abrupt contact with the support surface and has the potential to damage the skin. Slowly raising the head controls the rate of descent of the pelvis. The therapist may offer cues for head/trunk position through manual contact at the posterior lateral scapula.

Once the basic mechanics of a transfer are mastered, the skills may be generalized to other contexts. Whenever possible, the goal of transfer training is skill in both directions of movement, that is, the ability to transfer into the wheelchair toward the right or toward the left. However, if one arm is significantly more impaired than the other (either in terms of greater weakness or pain), then whenever possible the individual should lead with the impaired side, as the trailing arm performs more muscular work during a transfer.[45] In some situations, the direction of the transfer will be determined by the environment. In particular, toilet and tub transfers will likely have only one possible direction of approach; in such cases, early training should be specific to the required direction of movement.

Mastery of transfer skills includes the ability to stop at any point during the transfer task, to reposition, to reverse the direction, or to move between two unstable surfaces (e.g., from a wheelchair to wheelchair without locks). To achieve this level of mastery, the individual must understand and use the concepts of head–hips counterbalance and adduction of the leading arm as essential to the transfer. It is this skill that allows the individual to maintain the stability of an ultralight wheelchair during transfers.

Wheelchair Skills

Propelling a Wheelchair

Basic wheelchair mobility involves pushing on level surfaces. Optimal push mechanics on a level surface call for a low-frequency push with the hand dropping below the pushrim on recovery. This stroke pattern decreases the workload on the joints of the upper extremity.[46] Contact with the rim is made during the forward swing of the arm. All joints of the upper extremity should be moving in the midrange of their available motion. Shoulder or wrist hyperextension or excessive elbow flexion are indications that the wheelchair seating and axle position require evaluation. In a well-tuned ultralight wheelchair, there is a period of glide between push strokes, allowing the wheelchair to roll unencumbered by hand contact with the rim. Light friction contact may be used to correct the direction of motion of the wheelchair.

As described in the section on joint protection, gripping the handrim for each propulsive stroke is neither necessary nor recommended. Repetitive forceful gripping is considered a significant risk factor for carpal tunnel syndrome.[47] The individual is instructed to push with a relaxed open hand, using a neutral wrist position and open fingers on the handrim. This hand posture results in a distribution of the push forces with most force centered on the thenar eminence on the wheel. While it has the disadvantage of putting the hands at risk of infection and being chronically dirty, the use of gloves, especially when outdoors, alleviates this problem.

Alternative handrims are available that attempt to provide optimal push mechanics without the need for the hand on the tire. The basic modification is that the space between the wheel and the handrim has a surface designed for thumb push, and the handrim has a more oblong shape to promote open fingers. However, these handrims result in a slightly more abducted and internally rotated shoulder position because they place the hand in a more lateral position during propulsion. Care must be taken to avoid compromising the shoulder while improving the wrist mechanics. Mounting the handrims close to the wheel can provide improved push mechanics for individuals with tetraplegia or others who do not want the thumb to slide into the space between the rim and wheel. Handrims can be fitted with a plastic or foam coating that can aid individuals with decreased hand function. Rim projections (previously called "quad knobs") can potentially overstretch the tendons of the hand and impair a tenodesis grip; these projections can make slowing a wheelchair difficult and dangerous. Rim projections are not a necessary feature on ultralight wheelchairs and should be avoided.

The placement of the wheel axle relative to the seat frame is critical for facilitating optimal push mechanics. The rear axle should be mounted forward of the shoulder when measured with the individual sitting upright.[48] However, in an individual whose balance and wheelchair skills will not tolerate the resultant rearward instability of the chair, the axle is positioned farther rearward. The axle height relative to the seat position should be such that the axle falls between the fingertips and the base of the fingers when the arm is hanging at the side with the individual sitting upright. An alternative method of determining the correct axle position is to have the individual place a hand on the top of the handrim; when seated in this position, the individual's elbow and shoulder should each be in a comfortable position with no greater than 90 degrees flexion at the elbow and with no hyperextension at the shoulder. If the elbow has less than 60 degrees of flexion, then the individual is seated too high relative to the wheels, and it is advisable to decrease the vertical distance between the shoulder and the axle.[49,50]

Individuals with tetraplegia who have absent or impaired triceps function and who use a manual wheelchair will benefit from a more forward position of the rear wheel. Such a position allows the arc of propulsion to be concentrated on the back upper quadrant of the wheel, allowing the biceps and anterior deltoid to provide the propulsive stroke. However, because the forward axle placement makes the wheelchair more unstable to the rear, care must be taken in the frame selection and setup to increase the weight distribution to the front end. Squeeze frames with an anterior hinge allow a more forward rear wheel, while maintaining stability via weight distribution characteristics.

Pushing up inclines requires a change in push technique, with a forward inclination of the trunk and a shorter, higher frequency stroke at the top/forward portion of the wheel. Prior to ascent, the rider may benefit from performing a lift and reseating the buttocks farther back in seat than usual; this promotes greater hip flexion for pushing up the incline. At the top of the incline, the individual should reposition himself or herself to the proper seated position. During ascent, care must be taken not to push on the back half of the wheels as this will cause the casters to lift off the ground. Rough terrain requires a similar higher frequency push stroke; however,

a more upright trunk posture is required because leaning forward will increase the weight on the front of the chair and drive the casters into the terrain. If wheelchair skills permit, rough terrain can be maneuvered in a low wheelie.

Wheelies

The ability to master balancing in a wheelie is an important skill for the wheelchair user as wheelies permit access to areas and environments that would otherwise be inaccessible. Wheelie mastery means more than being able to balance in a wheelie. It requires understanding the dynamic balance of the chair such that the individual is able to use the wheelie automatically and without excessive effort as necessitated by the circumstances or the environment. Wheelies are used in numerous circumstances. Examples of circumstances in which wheelie skills aid mobility are given in Box 7-1.

Skilled wheelie technique reflects an intimate connection with the wheelchair. The wheelchair and the body are highly integrated and coordinated for optimally efficient mobility. The wheelchair configuration and the user position in the wheelchair have a direct impact on the ability to perform wheelies. Teaching wheelie balance skills employs a process similar to that of teaching postural balance. The individual gains a greater understanding of the dynamics of balance and of their ability to control it through the wheelie skills training.

Training in wheelie skills begins by placing the individual in a balanced wheelie position while the therapist guards against a rearward fall. The individual is encouraged to experiment with the effect of trunk positions on the balance of the wheelchair. The lowest wheelie is achieved with the trunk relaxed on the backrest. Leaning forward moves the center of gravity forward so that balance is achieved by raising the casters into a high wheelie. The individual then experiments with the effect of moving the wheels and is instructed to grip the wheels firmly and move the wheels forward and back (rather than allowing the hands to slide over the wheels). Through this exercise, the individual learns that the effect of wheel position on wheelie balance is predictable: pull back on the wheels and the casters will drop, push forward on the wheels and the casters will rise. The ability to lift into a wheelie should

---

BOX 7–1
Situations Requiring Use of Wheelies
- Ascending over a curb
- Descending a curb or steps, which can be done balanced on the rear wheel while rolling off the step
- Descending a steep incline
- Maneuvering over obstacles
- Maneuvering rough and uneven terrain
- Turning in tight spaces
- Dancing

not require rolling backward, as this technique limits the situations in which the individual is able to use a wheelie. Wheelies need to be available while moving forward. After training in the initial concepts of balance in a wheelie, the therapist can begin to teach its functional uses.

Wheelie training is often not offered to individuals who are elderly or overweight. However, most individuals with sufficient upper extremity function can be taught to perform wheelies and to maneuver 2-inch curbs. The intuitive understanding of personal balance (which must include the wheelchair in individuals who are full-time wheelchair users) is a fundamental underpinning to confident mobility and mastery of the wheelchair. Anti-tip devices are often prescribed for the safety of individuals who lack wheelie skills. However, for numerous reasons, anti-tip devices can be problematic. They typically increase the overall length of the wheelchair (and therefore the turn radius), increase the frame length for stowing the wheelchair into a vehicle, and for a van user the anti-tip device can create difficulty with lift and ramp use. Anti-tip devices can make it difficult to maneuver even minor terrain obstacles such as doorway thresholds. For this reason, they are often adjusted to an elevated height, in which case, the device will not prevent a rearward flip of the wheelchair. Thus, anti-tip devices tend to be a nuisance in real life and are frequently removed by individuals with SCI or their families. Mastery of wheelie skills eliminates the need for such devices and alleviates the potential for rearward falls. However, individuals who use a wheelchair with anti-tip devices in place also benefit from wheelie skills training because of the limitations of the anti-tip devices. A detailed guide for wheelie training is offered in the Appendix of this chapter.

Jumping Curbs

Mastery of basic wheelie skills, while not required for success at jumping curbs, makes it easier to perform curb jumping and makes the individual more expert in doing so. However, if the individual is unable to perform a static wheelie, then the dynamic rolling wheelie or controlling a wheelie down a gentle incline are good preliminary skills from which to begin training in jumping curbs. The critical element for successfully jumping a curb is that the front casters are lifted up onto the curb and placed down *before* the rear wheels hit the curb. As the rear wheels hit the curb, the individual shifts the body weight forward to assist the rear wheels over the curb. However, the body weight must not be too far forward or the rear wheels will lose traction. A quick follow-through push stroke on the rear wheels drives the wheels forward after they contact the edge of the curb and pushes them over the top. The follow-through stroke should start with the hands placed approximately 20 degrees forward of the highest point of the wheel, and the push force is directed downward, with the hand position finishing low on the front of the wheel.

While it might seem that momentum would assist the jump to a greater degree if the wheelchair approaches the curb at a higher speed, in truth, the difficulty of the jump increases the faster the wheelchair travels. The reason is that the faster the wheelchair approaches the curb, the less time will be available to execute the maneuver; therefore, greater skill and timing will be required. Consequently, moving way back to "get a run" at the curb (or "running curbs") is not encouraged. Ideally, the curb should be approached at a normal wheeling speed, with a wheelie lift and follow-through on the subsequent stroke.

If the individual is not successful on the first attempt, he or she will have the opportunity to attempt the task again. The available options to setup for a repeat attempt at the task are: (1) rolling back to the point where the casters are on the edge of the curb, leaning forward while pushing forcefully with the hands placed at the highest point of the wheel, and performing a follow-through stroke to the ground; (2) pulling the chair up onto the curb using a fixed object such as a parking meter or tree; (3) pushing up using a parked car (requires more power); (4) having an assistant give a push at the lower aspect of the backrest while the rider pushes; or (5) backing off to bring the casters off the curb and trying again. Descending a single curb does not require balancing in a wheelie as descent can be achieved with a slight lift of the casters while leaving the curb and landing on all four wheels simultaneously. However, a wheelie is an option for descending a curb and is necessary for forward descent of steps, which can be done balanced on the rear wheel while rolling off the step. A detailed guide for curb training is offered in the Appendix of this chapter.

Odd skills

Hopping a wheelchair

Hopping a wheelchair can be a very empowering skill for which there are many uses. The task requires hopping the chair straight up. The actual mechanics of performing this skill are not easily articulated, therefore it is best taught by simply asking the individual to try to hop the chair and, if possible, demonstrating the skill for the individual. This skill taught early in the rehabilitation stay builds confidence in the individual with a recent SCI, because it is a skill that is perceived as difficult, but is actually fairly easy to perform. It can be done by anyone with full hand function, and many individuals with tenodesis grip will also be able to achieve it. Hopping a wheelchair can (and initially should) be done with the anti-tip devices in place. This technique may be used for maneuvering on a landing to open an outward-swinging door, maneuvering in a bus or other vehicle to position for transfer or tie downs, negotiating tight hallways, etc. This skill is most useful when the individual can hop and also rotate the wheelchair to the left or right about the vertical axis. It is also useful for the individual to be able to hop sideways.

Removing a wheel

Rigid frame wheelchairs can be pulled up onto one wheel to remove the opposite wheel. The individual may remove the wheel while holding onto a grab bar, pole, or other stable object. This is a skill that might be used, for example, when the individual notices the axle wasn't locked when last getting out of the car. Removal of one wheel can offer a method for accessing small doorways (e.g., most European bathrooms and many European hotel elevators). Learning this skill early in mobility training helps increase the user's connection to the wheelchair and the understanding of its dynamics. It also increases the individual's confidence in his or her abilities. At the very least, this skill should be demonstrated and practiced with a one-person assist. The more agile and able individual with lower level paraplegia will be able to master it independently.

CASE STUDY 7:1 Component Skill Training and Transfer of Training

Tim is having difficulty mastering a lateral transfer without a transfer board. His therapist observes that he is not leaning sufficiently over his trailing arm to achieve unweighting of his hips. The therapist reasons that Tim is insecure about sitting balance and fearful of falling. The therapist structures different learning activities that will incorporate the component skills of leaning forward and balancing. The selected activities include

- opening heavy doors,
- pushing a shopping cart, and
- ascending curbs.

The therapist also elects to work on transfers in a different environment. Instead of working on the level transfer without a board in the clinic, Tim is given the opportunity to work on car transfers with a board. While the component skills are the same as the level transfer without a board, the longer excursion and the different seat heights of the car transfer require Tim to lean more toward the trailing hand. Once the car transfer was mastered, Tim had no difficulty performing the level transfer in the clinic without a sliding board.

Summary

Learning to move one's body and to maneuver in the environment in a wheelchair are essential skills after SCI. Functional mobility skills required to move in bed, get into and out of the wheelchair, and maneuver the wheelchair can be acquired by individuals with complete SCI at neurological levels C6 and below, although

there will be differences in the approach used by individuals with different levels of injury. All of the mobility skills discussed in this chapter can be taught during the acute rehabilitation time frame, while the injured individual is wearing post-operative immobilization devices and is under spinal precautions. Therapists provide the opportunity for early mobility training and work to empower individuals with successful movement strategies that challenge them to develop their maximum potential for skilled mobility.

Movement after SCI can be dexterous and fluid with proper training and the maintenance of normal range of motion. Persons with skillful mobility will not need to think about how to do the specific tasks but rather will be able to concentrate on the functional outcome. An intrinsic awareness of balance and automatic use of leverage and mechanical advantage allow mastery of mobility skills. This awareness and skill are acquired with proper guidance, practice, and experience. Individuals who learn to balance without upper extremity support, who maintain anatomical range of motion in the lower extremities, and who have patterns of movement that are mechanically advantageous will have positive outcomes with self care and can avoid the negative sequelae from falls or skin breakdown; they will also have more opportunities to participate in society.

REVIEW QUESTIONS

1. Describe an example of how a therapist might use leverage and gravity to the advantage of an individual with SCI during a functional task.
2. List three instructions a therapist might offer an individual regarding joint protection during a functional task.
3. Discuss the critical aspects of balance training in the individual with a new SCI.
4. Describe the technique employed by an individual with SCI when moving from supine to long-sitting.
5. List the essential components of a successful short-sitting transfer.
6. Discuss how optimal manual wheelchair push mechanics are accomplished.

REFERENCES

1. De Groot V, Hollander. Wheelchair propulsion technique and mechanical efficiency after 3 weeks of practice. *Med Sci Sport Exer.* 2001;756–766.
2. May LA, Butt C, Minor L et al. Measurement reliability of functional tasks for persons who self-propel a manual wheelchair. *Arch Phys Med Rehabil.* 2003;84(4):578–583.

3. Kirby RL, Swuste J, Dupuis DJ et al. The Wheelchair Skills Test: A pilot study of a new outcome measure. *Arch Phys Med Rehabil.* 2002;83(1):10–18.

4. Kirby RL, Lugar JA, Breckenridge C. New wheelie aid for wheelchairs: Controlled trial of safety and efficacy. *Arch Phys Med Rehabil.* 2001;82(3):380–390.

5. Rodgers MM, Keyser RE, Rasch EK et al. Influence of training on biomechanics of wheelchair propulsion. *J Rehabil Res Dev.* 2001;38(5):505–511.

6. Rodgers MM, Keyser RE, Gardner ER et al. Influence of trunk flexion on biomechanics of wheelchair propulsion. *J Rehabil Res Dev.* 2000;37(3):283–295.

7. Boninger M, Baldwin M, Cooper R et al. Manual wheelchair pushrim biomechanics and axle position. *Arch of Phys Med Rehabil.* 2000;81:608–613.

8. Boninger M, Cooper R, Shimada S et al. Shoulder and elbow motion during two speeds of wheelchair propulsion: A description using a local coordinate system. *Spinal Cord.* 1998;36:418–426.

9. Kulig K, Newsam CJ, Mulroy SJ et al. The effect of level of spinal cord injury on shoulder joint kinetics during manual wheelchair propulsion. *Clin Biomech (Bristol, Avon).* 2001;16(9):744–751.

10. Somers M, Wlodarczyk S. Use of a pushrim-activated, power-assisted wheelchair enhanced mobility for an individual with cervical 5/6 tetraplegia. *Neurology Report.* 2003;Vol 27(1):22–28.

11. Corfman TA, Cooper R, Boninger M et al. Range of motion and stroke frequency differences between manual wheelchair propulsion and pushrim-activated power-assisted wheelchair propulsion. *J Spinal Cord Med.* 2003;26:135–140.

12. Curtis KA, Roach KE, Applegate EB et al. Development of the Wheelchair User's Shoulder Pain Index (WUSPI). *Paraplegia.* 1995;33:290–293.

13. Pentland WE, Twomey LT. The weight-bearing upper extremity in women with long term paraplegia. *Paraplegia.* 1991;29(8):521–530.

14. Subbarao JV, Klopfstein J, Turpin R. Prevalence and impact of wrist and shoulder pain in patients with spinal cord injury. *J Spinal Cord Med.* 1995;18(1):9–13.

15. Dalyan M, Cardenas DD, Gerard B. Upper extremity pain after spinal cord injury. *Spinal Cord.* 1999;37(3):191–195.

16. Allison GT, Singer KP, Marshall RN. Transfer movement strategies of individuals with spinal cord injuries. *Disabil Rehabil.* 1996;18(1):35–41.

17. Nawoczenski DA, Clobes SM, Gore SL et al. Three-dimensional shoulder kinematics during a pressure relief technique and wheelchair transfer. *Arch Phys Med Rehabil.* 2003;84(9):1293–1300.

18. Gagnon D, Nadeau S, Gravel D et al. Biomechanical analysis of a posterior transfer maneuver on a level surface in individuals with high- and low-level spinal cord injuries. *Clin Biomech (Bristol, Avon).* 2003;18(4):319–331.

19. Gagnon D, Nadeau S, Gravel D et al. Movement patterns and muscular demands during posterior transfers toward an elevated surface in individuals with spinal cord injury. *Spinal Cord.* 2005;43(2):74–84.

20. Wang YT, Kim CK, Ford HT, 3rd et al. Reaction force and EMG analyses of wheelchair transfers. *Percept Motor Skill.* 1994;79(2):763–766.

21. Bayley JC, Cochran TP, Sledge CB. The weight-bearing shoulder. The impingement syndrome in paraplegics. *J Bone Joint Surg Am.* 1987;69(5):676–678.

22. Nyland J, Quigley P, Huang C et al. Preserving transfer independence among individuals with spinal cord injury. *Spinal Cord.* 2000;38(11):649–657.

23. Sipski ML, Richards JS. Spinal cord injury rehabilitation state of the science. *Am J Phys Med Rehabil.* 2006;85(4):310–342.

24. Scott M. *Wayne Rainey His Own Story.* Newbury Park: Haynes Publications Inc.; 1997.

25. Schmidt RA, Wrisberg CA. *Motor Learning and Performance.* 3rd edition. Champaign, IL: Human Kinetics; 2004.

26. National Spinal Cord Injury Statistical Center. Spinal Cord Injury Facts and Figures at a Glance. Available at: www.spinalcord.uab.edu. Accessed February 20, 2006.

27. Winstein C. Knowledge of results and motor learning—implications for physical therapy. *Phys Ther.* 1991;71(2):140–149.

28. Stockmeyer SA. An interpretation of the approach of Rood to the treatment of neuromuscular dysfunction. *Am J Phys Med.* 1967;46(1):900–961.

29. O'Sullivan S, Schmitz T. *Physical Rehabilitation Assessment and Treatment.* 4th edition. Philadelphia: F. A. Davis; 2001.

30. Somers M. *Spinal Cord Injury Functional Rehabilitation.* 2nd edition. Upper Saddle River, NJ: Prentice-Hall Inc.; 2001.

31. Nixon V. *Rehabilitation Institute of Chicago Procedure Manual. Spinal Cord Injury: A Guide to Functional Outcomes in Physical Therapy Management.* Rockville, MD: Aspen; 1985.

32. Vogel LC, Krajci KA, Anderson CJ. Adults with pediatric-onset spinal cord injury. Part 2. Musculoskeletal and neurological complications. *J Spinal Cord Med.* 2002;25(2): 117–123.

33. Rink P, Miller F. Hip instability in spinal cord injury patients. *J Pediatr Orthoped.*1990;10(5):583–587.

34. Betz RR, Mulcahey MJ, Smith BT et al. Implications of hip subluxation for FES-assisted mobility in patients with spinal cord injury. *Orthopedics.* 2001;24(2):181–184.

35. McCarthy JJ, Chafetz RS, Betz RR et al. Incidence and degree of hip subluxation/dislocation in children with spinal cord injury. *J Spinal Cord Med.* 2004;27 Suppl 1:S80–83.

36. Young J, Giertz K, Goldstein B. Hip subluxation and scoliosis in individual with paraplegia. Paper presented at: American Spinal Injury Association Annual Scientific Meeting, 1998; Cleveland, OH.

37. Baird RA, DeBenedetti MJ, Eltorai I. Non-septic hip instability in the chronic spinal cord injury patient. *Paraplegia.* 1986;24(5):293–300.

38. Curtis KA, Drysdale GA, Lanza RD et al. Shoulder pain in wheelchair users with tetraplegia and paraplegia. *Arch Phys Med Rehabil.* 1999;80(4):453–457.

39. Nichols PJ, Norman PA, Ennis JR. Wheelchair user's shoulder? Shoulder pain in patients with spinal cord lesions. *Scand J Rehabil Med.* 1979;11(1):29–32.

40. Sie IH, Waters RL, Adkins RH et al. Upper extremity pain in the postrehabilitation spinal cord injured patient. *Arch Phys Med Rehabil.* 1992;73(1):44–48.

41. Gellman H, Sie I, Waters RL. Late complications of the weight-bearing upper extremity in the paraplegic patient. *Clin Orthop Relat R.* 1988;233:132–135.

42. Dyson-Hudson TA, Kirshblum SC. Shoulder pain in chronic spinal cord injury. Part I. Epidemiology, etiology, and pathomechanics. *J Spinal Cord Med.* 2004;27(1):4–17.

43. Finley MA, Rodgers MM. Prevalence and identification of shoulder pathology in athletic and nonathletic wheelchair users with shoulder pain: A pilot study. *J Rehabil Res Dev.* 2004;41(3B):395–402.

44. Boninger M, Waters RL, Chase T et al. *Preservation of Upper Limb Function Following Spinal Cord Injury: A Clinical Practice Guideline for Health-Care Professionals.* Washington DC: Paralyzed Veterans of America Consortium for Spinal Cord Medicine; 2005.

45. Tharakeshwarappa N. *Biomechanical Analysis of Independent Transfers: Reliability of Measures and Pilot Study Involving Persons with Paraplegia.* Pittsburgh, PA: Department of Rehabilitation Science and Technology, University of Pittsburgh; 2005.

46. Boninger ML, Souza AL, Cooper RA et al. Propulsion patterns and pushrim biomechanics in manual wheelchair propulsion. *Arch Phys Med Rehabil.* 2002;83(5):718–723.

47. Smith MB. The Peripheral Nervous System. In: Goodman C, Boissonnault WG, editors. *Pathology: Implications for the Physical Therapist.* 1st edition. Philadelphia: W. B. Saunders Co.; 1998. pp. 811–837.

48. Boninger ML, Baldwin M, Cooper RA et al. Manual wheelchair pushrim biomechanics and axle position. *Arch Phys Med Rehabil.* 2000;81(5):608–613.

49. Richter WM. The effect of seat position on manual wheelchair propulsion biomechanics: A quasi-static model-based approach. *Med Eng Phys.* 2001;23(10):707–712.

50. van der Woude LH, Veeger DJ, Rozendal RH et al. Seat height in handrim wheelchair propulsion. *J Rehabil Res Dev.* 1989;26(4):31–50.

APPENDIX 7-1

WHEELIE PROGRESSION, FALLING, AND CURB TRAINING GUIDELINES

KEY POINTS

1. The therapist stands behind the chair, with one foot forward of the other; this position allows the therapist to use a leg under chair to catch a tip backward. One hand is placed under the push handle, the other hand is poised over shoulder of the individual in the wheelchair (contact is made only if necessary). For rigid frame wheelchairs without push handles, a strap on the rigidizer bar may be used. The strap should be loose so it does not affect balance.
2. The individual with SCI may practice with a therapist only and is strongly advised not to practice with anti-tip devices in place and not to begin a habit of resting tipped back on the anti-tip devices.

STATIC AND DYNAMIC WHEELIE SKILLS

Static balance in wheelie
1. The therapist guards from behind, and places the individual into the wheelie position.
2. The individual is instructed that proper hand placement is on top of wheel, with shoulders and elbows in slight flexion to allow pushing/pulling of the wheel to correct for balance.
3. The individual works on maintaining balance in the wheelie position.

Hand control
1. The individual is placed in wheelie position and directed to pull the wheels back sharply (casters will fall to ground).
2. The individual is placed in a wheelie position and directed to push wheels forward sharply (wheelchair will tip backward).
3. The individual's hands should remain on the wheels and should not move on/off the wheel to "chase" the balance point.

Pop up front casters
1. The individual grips the wheel posterior to the axle and pushes forward sharply.
2. The individual pops up the front casters to achieve a balanced wheelie position.
3. Encourage the individual to experiment with the wheelie height; for example, when resting against the backrest, the balance point is achieved with the casters closer to the ground, and when leaning forward off backrest, the balance point is achieved with the casters farther from the ground
4. Once the individual is able to pop up to balance position, emphasis is on maintaining this position.

GOAL: Maintain static balance for 10 minutes in a 2-square foot space.

Note: The individual is encouraged to work on dynamic wheelie skills (below) prior to achieving mastery of the 10-minute static wheelie.

Dynamic balance within wheelie
1. Wheeling forward
2. Wheeling backward
3. Balancing in a wheelie position using one hand only
4. Turning 360 degrees
5. Wheeling around corners
6. Wheeling down inclines (the rims are allowed to slide through the hands for control of speed)

GOAL: Maintain dynamic balance for 10 minutes without loss of wheelie.

Note: The individual is encouraged to begin curb training (below) prior to achieving mastery of the 10-minute dynamic wheelie.

CATCHING A FALL AND RETURNING TO UPRIGHT

Catching a Fall

The individual must be out of thoraco-lumbar-sacral orthosis (TLSO) or medically cleared for this activity before learning to catch a fall.

1. The individual practices with an 8-inch mat behind the wheelchair.
2. The therapist assists/guards from behind to provide a slow descent (simulating a fall).
3. The individual is instructed to hold the head up and forward (away from the direction of the fall) and to keep elbows flexed in preparation for the catch impact.
4. The individual may catch the fall by reaching in the direction of the fall with one or both hands. If using a single hand to catch the fall, the other hand holds the frame at the front of the seat.

Returning to upright after a fall

In the early stages of wheelchair training, the individual is taught to get out of the chair, right the chair, and use a floor-to-wheelchair transfer to get back into the chair. However, the more advanced wheelchair user can learn to return to the chair to upright while seated in the chair. There are three common methods for accomplishing this, are described below.

Method 1: Return to upright from the ground
The individual

1. lowers back of the chair to the ground;
2. locks the brakes;
3. reaches across the lap to hold on to the front of frame at the front of the seat with a pronated grip, allowing the trunk to pull up and away from the backrest;
4. pushes the backrest up from the ground with the free hand while pushing down on front of the frame with the other hand;
5. leans the trunk over the wheel and walks the support hand around side of the chair as the backrest rises;
6. leans forward toward the feet to right the wheelchair.

Method 2: Return to upright from a support arm
The individual

1. never drops the backrest all the way to the floor, but supports weight with one arm;
2. reaches across the body with the free arm to grasp the opposite wheel;
3. pulls the wheel sharply toward the backrest;
4. rights the chair.

Method 3: Return to upright with the help of an assistant
The individual

1. lies on the backrest and grasps wheels to pull the buttocks into the seat;
2. instructs an assistant to grasp the footrests (rigid wheelchair);
3. instructs the assistant to place one foot on the axle bar on the lowest cross frame;
4. instructs the assistant to pull down on the footrest, then leans back and lowers the body as the chair rights;
5. holds buttocks firmly in seat and leans forward toward the thighs to assist righting of the wheelchair.

Progression of training in catching a fall and returning to upright after a fall

1. The individual practices with sequentially lower mat heights.
2. The individual practices without mat(s) and with decreased guarding by therapist.
3. The individual, once independent in safely catching a fall and able to perform floor-to-wheelchair transfer **or** a walk around push up, may discontinue use of anti-tip devices in daily activities

Note: It is important that the individual be instructed that wheelies are to be performed only under the supervision of the therapist until such time as the anti-tip devices are disconnected. Once the individual is independent in these skills, the therapist documents that the individual is cleared for independent wheelies and the anti-tip devices may be removed.

Individuals in TLSOs

Special consideration must be given to the individual in a TLSO. Those in a TLSO must be at least 2 months post-surgery before wheelchair skills training is undertaken. If the individual in a TLSO has mastered all wheelie skills (static and dynamic wheelies), it is appropriate to learn how to catch a fall. *Only* the two-hand catch should be used in this case, and the wheelchair should not be lowered all the way to the floor (practice is performed with mats stacked behind the wheelchair). The individual is taught an assisted return (method 3) to upright or an off-the-floor transfer. Independent pull up (methods 1 and 2) is practiced only after discontinuation of the TLSO.

CURB TRAINING

While the following training progression is recommended because it builds on sequential skills, alternative progression sequences may be effective for some individuals.

Aluminum handrims are strongly recommended for curb training in all individuals who have good hand function. Individuals with other types of handrims may experience limited success with wheelies for descending curbs or ramps.

Safely descending curbs

Method 1: Assisted rear approach
1. The therapist guards/assists while standing off the curb. The individual in the wheelchair leans forward, grasping and controlling the wheels.
2. The individual wheels to the edge of curb and is cued to align wheels evenly with the edge of the curb.
3. The therapist leans into the back of the wheelchair, using the legs to slow the wheelchair's descent as the individual backs off the curb.

Method 2: Independent rear approach
1. The individual wheels to the edge of curb and is cued to align the wheels evenly with the edge of the curb.
2. The individual leans forward onto the thighs, pulling the wheels back and immediately grabbing the front frame.
3. The individual is instructed not to stop the wheels until the wheelchair is completely off the curb and on level ground (as the wheelchair can flip backward with momentum of the descent).

Method 3: Descend and turn
1. The individual leans forward, keeping the hands on the wheels, and slowly lowers the rear wheels off the curb.
2. The individual then turns sharply to the side to get casters off the curb.

Safely ascending ("popping") curbs
The proper technique for ascending curbs evokes images of skateboards or bikes jumping up curbs. The technique relies heavily on timing rather than power or speed; greater speed requires more perfect timing for successful performance.

Note: Training in curb-ascent skills should not be attempted in wheelchairs equipped with high-mount wheel locks. Remove the wheel locks for training or install low-mount or scissor wheel locks. This precaution is necessary to protect the thumbs from trauma.

1. Training begins on 2-inch curbs and progresses to increased heights as skill is mastered (typically an individual will have mastered descending curbs in a wheelie prior to attempting ascent of a 4-inch curb).
2. The individual approaches the curb in a wheelie and strives to set the casters down on top of the curb before the rear wheels hit the curb.
3. Once the casters are down, the individual shifts the body weight forward and pulls the rear wheels up over the edge of the curb.
4. If the wheelie is too early, the footrest will hit the curb (forward guard is necessary).
5. If the wheelie too high or too late, the rear wheels will hit the curb and the chair will tip rearward.

Practice drills for descending and ascending curbs
Rolling Wheelie
1. With the wheelchair gliding freely (i.e., no hand contact after push), the individual pops up into a low wheelie on cue. There is no attempt to balance in the wheelie, just a low caster lift and an immediate push on to the front half of the rear wheel for follow-through.
2. Once the glide to wheelie to follow-through has been mastered, the individual practices the same approach over a 2-inch curb, striving for glide to wheelie to follow-through over the curb.

Ascending 2-inch curbs from a static wheelie position
1. From a stationary position facing a curb, the individual performs a low wheelie to lift casters onto the curb.
2. The individual then rolls back so that the casters are close to the edge of the curb (to gain as much distance as possible for the pop up) and sits as erectly as possible.
3. With hands on top of the wheel, the individual simultaneously leans forward with momentum (to shift the body weight forward) and pushes down (to propel the wheelchair forward).
4. The individual must follow through on the push, taking the hands as low as possible to bring the wheels up and over the curb.

Progressing to higher curbs
Working on the ascent of 2-inch curbs from the static position will promote skill in dynamic ascent of 4-inch curbs from a rolling wheelie because the individual gains skill in weight-shifting techniques.
     The sequence for training ascent of 4-inch and 6-inch curbs is similar to that of 2-inch curbs; begin with dynamic curbs, then static, then increase the height and return to dynamic, etc.

Note: Individuals wearing a TLSO will be unable to ascend a 6-inch curb from the static wheelie position due to inability to fully flex the trunk and achieve adequate forward lean/weight shift, but these individuals may achieve a dynamic 6-inch curb.

DESCENDING CURBS IN A WHEELIE
Descending a curb in a wheelie creates momentum and forces that cause the chair to tilt back. The individual must correct for these forces either before or after the descent. The most dangerous possibility in descending a curb occurs with the casters dropping first off the curb. The therapist guards from behind, but with a hand poised over the individual's shoulder to protect against the possibility of a forward fall. There are two methods for descending curbs in a wheelie.

Method 1: Four-wheeled landing
The individual

1. approaches the curb on a gliding roll;
2. lifts into a low wheelie;
3. drops off the curb, landing on all four wheels (or with casters dropping immediately after the rear wheels touch).

Method 2: Rear wheel landing
The individual
1. approaches the curb in a balanced wheelie;
2. drops off the curb, landing on the rear wheels only.

The latter technique is necessary for higher drops and for learning to descend stairs forward.
     If the individual *pushes* on the rear wheels to propel off the curb in a wheelie, the result is that the casters will lift and the chair will tip rearward. To counter this, the individual needs to pull back (or brake) as he or she goes off the curb to stabilize the chair (this is the technique required for stair descent in a wheelie).

ADVANCED WHEELCHAIR SKILLS
Mastery of the following indicates advanced achievement in wheelchair skills.
Independent in using wheelies for curbs 6 inches and lower
Independent going up curbs 6 inches and lower
Independent going down and incline in a wheelie
Independent going downstairs (backward) with a railing
Independent performing a pullover return from a wheelie catch
Optional: Independent going down up to four steps in wheelie (forward)
Wheelchair skills training is discontinued when skills are maximized, when the individual has plateaued in skill progression, or when the individual desires to discontinue training.

8

Seating and Wheelchair Prescription

Jennifer D. Hastings, PT, PhD, NCS
Kendra L. Betz, MS, PT, ATP

After reading this chapter, the reader will be able to:

OBJECTIVES

- List the fundamental components of "seating"
- Recognize the features of an ultralight manual wheelchair, compare frame styles, and understand configuration options
- Understand the different power mobility options for base and seat selections
- Discuss the benefits and challenges for use of power mobility
- Discuss common theories of cushion design for skin protection and postural support
- Discuss the interaction between components of the seating system
- Describe the required components of a postural examination for seating purposes
- Discuss the influence of seated posture on dynamic function
- Justify the need for selected/prescribed seating system components
- Be able to defend time spent in seating planning and intervention as therapeutic time for the client

OUTLINE

Introduction

Seating is the foundation for optimal outcomes in the spinal cord-injured population, especially for those who use wheelchairs for full-time mobility. There is an intimate and obligatory relationship between the posture of a paralyzed body and the support provided from the seating system. Postural alignment directly impacts respiration, swallowing, speech, skin, and musculoskeletal health and function. Posture may also affect the body image of an individual and feelings of self-worth and therefore participation in the community after spinal cord injury (SCI). The multi-factorial influence of posture on health outcomes makes seating a premier concern for early intervention and constant vigilant monitoring throughout the injured person's lifetime.

Understanding the interactions of the seating system and the resulting postural alignment requires careful integration of information from the physical therapy examination and an understanding of the potential, as well as the constraints, of the equipment. Specifying an orthotic seating system is a specialty skill. It provides therapeutic benefits for the client. The therapist must evaluate the impact of selected parameters of a seating system and any adjustments made and must understand the effect on the client/user. Seating requires critical thinking, analysis, and integration of knowledge by the therapist. The actual mechanics of seating system configuration changes may be delegated to qualified support personnel, but the evaluation, specification, and fitting should never be relegated to anyone other than a skilled seating therapist (i.e., physical or occupational therapist).

In this chapter, the concepts of the evaluation for and prescription of a therapeutic system will be described, and a strategy for defining the specifications will be developed for a client. However, an exhaustive review of all available products is beyond the scope of this text and the fact is that specific device-related information would soon be outdated. More importantly, seating for the client with SCI needs to be individualized based on examinations, assessments, and interventions. There is no such thing as the "best wheelchair" or the "best cushion," although there may well be an optimal wheelchair configuration or cushion for the *individual* in question. Upon completion of this chapter, the reader will understand seating system selection and configuration for the client with SCI in order to optimize seated posture: The goal of optimal seated posture is to promote maximum independence via the achievement of functional skills, comfort, and skin health.

An explicit overarching message in this chapter is that seating *is* therapy. For the population of individuals with SCI, seating is a vital therapy, and the process of thoughtful seating should begin even before the new rehabilitation client gets out of the intensive care unit bed. A properly selected and set up wheelchair as the *first* wheelchair experience can set the stage for a successful rehabilitation. Early use of an appropriate system promotes overall health, mobility skill achievement, and the early success of the patient. An appropriate seating system is also important as a preventive strategy. Appropriate wheelchair setup and optimized posture will decrease the musculoskeletal stresses associated with prolonged sitting and wheelchair propulsion as well as protect against skin breakdown. Quality equipment, which optimizes functional ability, improves overall health and protects against systemic pathologies such as cardiovascular impairment and obesity. Self-efficacy in community mobility skills is also likely to improve a wheelchair user's mental health status.

The following is an overview of current evidence relative to seating and wheelchairs for the client with SCI. Research relative to postural alignment is limited, especially studies specifically addressing seated posture in individuals with SCI. Evidence is available to support the hypothesis that posterior pelvic tilt and spinal flexion posture correlates with negative sequelae.[1-5] Research concerning manual wheelchairs has been targeted toward durability, configuration for stability, and configuration for propulsion. In general, the literature supports the use of high-strength, lightweight materials for manual wheelchairs and a forward position of the rear wheel to improve the propulsion mechanics.[6] Published research pertaining to power wheelchairs is extremely limited. While high-end power bases have been shown to be most durable, there is no published research to indicate a preferred drive wheel position. Some research has been completed to define optimal power seat functions and configuration relative to skin integrity at the sitting surface. With the many variables associated with cushion materials, design, and properties, published research supports individualized cushion selection for the client with SCI.

Fundamentally, there are three primary components of a seating prescription for the client with SCI: (1) the mobility base (the wheelchair, either power or manual); (2) the seating interface (the cushion and backrest); and (3) the size and configuration of the equipment. The final component is perhaps the most important. The actual *size and configuration of the equipment* is the feature that will provide the optimal stability and mobility for the spinal cord-injured person. The correct size and configuration of the equipment is derived from a systematic evaluation of the client with particular attention to anatomical measurements. The seating system is literally built upon the foundation of the size and configuration of the wheelchair. If the seat depth is longer than the anatomical thigh length, then the individual will not be able to sit erect. Similarly, if the available hip range of motion does not match the angle between the seat and backrest, then optimal pelvic positioning will not be achieved. There are also three distinct but interrelated goals for a seating system: postural goals, mobility goals, and functional goals. To a large extent, the overall health outcomes of the individual, including musculoskeletal health, respiratory function, and skin integrity, will depend on how well these goals are addressed.

Alignment and Musculoskeletal Pain

In the general population, normal standing alignment is a "plumb-line posture," such that a plumb line will align the ear lobe, shoulder, hip, and knee. This alignment establishes the normal spinal curves. The plumb line posture is known to take the least muscular work to maintain.[7] Essentially, this posture capitalizes on gravity to assist in the maintenance of posture, with the line of gravity passing just posterior to the hip and just anterior to the knee. Any deviation from this posture will increase the work of standing. Postural abnormalities are also known to be associated with pain. For instance, Greenfield[8] found that forward head position is associated with shoulder pain. In a seminal manuscript, Keegan[9] illustrated that optimal health of the lumbar spine is promoted with sitting postures as closely approximating those in standing as possible. Optimal posture, whether standing or sitting, is achieved when

the center of gravity is over the base of support. This posture requires the least amount of muscular work to maintain, and it is the posture from which it is the easiest to move.

Muscles function to support or move a joint. In general, if passive stability is insufficient, muscles will work harder to provide contractile support to maintain a joint in a given postural position. If postural support is lacking, the residual trunk and upper extremity muscles (superficial back muscles) work excessively in an attempt to stabilize. Muscles generally have a length at which they operate most efficiently. Muscles can be physiologically too short (active insufficient) or too long (passive insufficient). Muscles working outside of their optimal length are disadvantaged and tend to fatigue. Muscles also fall into physiologic categories: phasic muscles are best suited for short bursts of activity requiring high speed or force, while tonic muscles are best suited for prolonged, low-forces activities. Postural muscles are typically tonic muscles that work best in midrange or shortened length. In the condition of kyphosis, posterior postural muscles become over-lengthened and ineffective.

Chronic poor posture negatively impacts the strength and balance of forces around the shoulder joint. A depleted muscle is one that is tapped of all glucose supply or working beyond its vascular capacity for refueling and waste removal; pain can arise from a depleted muscle. A muscle working excessively, beyond its capacity for force generation or at a frequency beyond its tolerance, can also be a source of pain. Mechanical pain in the musculoskeletal system can also be articular in origin. Alignment is critical for appropriate articular function; malalignment created by muscle imbalance can contribute to the creation of articular pain by not maintaining appropriate articular surface congruency. In the upper extremity, postural malalignment will create altered glenohumeral joint mechanics.

Alignment and Function

Appropriate seating is the platform for upper limb function. The shoulder and upper limb are designed for optimal mobility to facilitate hand placement in all dimensions. The upper limb articulates with the axial skeleton via the pectoral girdle. Muscles and ligaments largely suspend the pectoral girdle in order to allow maximal movement and flexibility. The only bony articulation between the trunk and upper limb is at the sternoclavicular joint. The glenohumeral joint (true shoulder) lacks bony constraint throughout the normal range of motion. This design is essential for upper limb mobility; however, stability through bony factors is minimal. Stability is established by the soft tissues (e.g., ligaments, capsule, labrum, muscles) and by alignment. End range stability is achieved when soft tissues, particularly the ligaments and capsule, are stretched to their physiologic limit. Dynamic stability is achieved by concavity compression and glenohumeral balance in midranges of motion.[10] Concavity compression is a mechanism in which the humeral head is compressed into the glenoid fossa by muscles (particularly the rotator cuff musculature), thereby resisting translational forces. Glenohumeral balance is a stabilizing mechanism in which the glenoid fossa (therefore the scapula) is positioned in the most stable position (i.e., so that the net humeral joint reaction force passes through the glenoid fossa). Because of the articulation to the axial skeleton via the sternoclavicular joint, the shoulder girdle is obligatory in its relationship to the spine. Spinal posture determines alignment and positioning of the scapula. Therefore, the resting lengths of the shoulder girdle musculature and the resulting biomechanical stability of the shoulder are dependent on spinal posture.

The spinal cord-injured population is unique not only in that they use their upper extremities for mobility and weight bearing, but that they are also paralyzed, significantly in the trunk and gluteal muscles, and they are seated. Individuals with significant truncal paralysis do not have normal trunk control against gravity. Compensatory strategies for absent trunk innervation include stabilization with the upper extremities and a C-sitting spinal posture.[11] A C-sitting posture is characterized by a posterior pelvic tilt and flexion of the lumbar and thoracic spine. C-sitting creates an overall shorter sitting posture and a tendency for a forward head posture. In a study assessing sitting stability with reaching task, Seelen and Vuurman[12] noted that persons with SCI had significantly more electromyographic (EMG) activity in the latisimus dorsi and trapezius muscles compared to able-bodied control subjects. The authors suggest that this is a compensatory mechanism to substitute for the absence of erector spinalis muscle activity. Similarly, Janssen-Potten and colleagues[13] showed that posterior pelvic tilt was associated with more EMG activity in the thoracic postural muscles. In an intact able-bodied individual, full range of overhead reach is achieved only with spinal extension. In individuals who sit full time, there is likely to be more frequent and maintained overhead reaching. If the habitual seated posture is one of posterior pelvic tilt, spinal flexion, forward head, and rounded shoulders, and the individual has no active spinal extension, reaching will be impaired. Furthermore, reaching may even be potentially damaging to the joint structures due to increased impingement. However, this same individual may be provided with the external support of an orthotic seating system and gain significantly improved reach.[14]

Normal trunk innervation allows unilateral or bilateral upper extremity tasks with synergistic stabilization by the trunk muscles. In this regard, the movement strategies of the individual with truncal paralysis differ significantly from the biomechanics used in the able-bodied population. The impact of the difference in trunk stabilization is illustrated in a study that assessed the relationship between motor lesion level and rotator cuff disorders. The authors found a significantly higher prevalence of rotator cuff disorder in the subjects with high-level paraplegia (defined as T2–T7).[15] The therapeutic goal of seating is to avoid the negative sequelae of compensations for instability. Therefore, the seating system must make use of gravity to assist with attaining stability, promote optimal pelvic alignment, and allow positioning of the normal spinal curves on top of the pelvis.

The obligatory interaction between the spine and the shoulder girdle makes it imperative to recognize spinal posture as the platform for upper extremity function. Therefore, the joint angles of the upper extremity (for instance with wheelchair propulsion) cannot be ascertained without knowing the position of the trunk. In the same wheelchair with the hand at the top of the pushrim (at the 12 o'clock position), the shoulder and elbow positions and angles will differ if the buttocks are at the rear of the seat or at the front, or if the trunk leans forward. Push mechanics cannot be analyzed without considering posture. Posture impacts the range of motion of all the upper extremity joints.

When an individual uses a manual wheelchair, the propulsion of the wheelchair must be considered a potential source of stress for the shoulder. Intuitively, push mechanics appear to be important. At issue are the positions in which the joints of the upper extremity are working. Evidence supports the idea that the joint positions are a significant factor for forces across the joint.[16–19] It is important to assess whether the wheelchair configuration is dictating movement at the extremes of joint range of motion or in positions of instability. Extremes of joint range force muscles to work at a mechanical disadvantage, usually overlengthened or overshortened, causing physiologic insufficiency. For the shoulder, hyperextension or the combination of abduction with internal rotation are positions of the joint that are not optimal for joint function; they are believed to be impinging positions for the rotator cuff muscles as they decrease the subacromial space.

Alignment, Respiration, and Skin Health

Kyphotic postures will reduce the individual's respiratory function by decreasing lung volume.[4,20] Combined with the absent abdominal wall function, kyphosis can severely decrease the ability for forceful expulsion through coughing. In extreme cases of postural malalignment, there is difficulty with swallowing and even with management of saliva. Mechanical swallowing problems can lead to aspiration pneumonia. Decreased tidal volume can also lead to decreased phonation. Fatigue and decreased systemic ability due to decreased oxygenation are also sequelae.

Pressure sores are the most frequent secondary medical complication in individuals with SCI[21] and are a leading cause for rehospitalization following traumatic SCI.[22] Individuals with SCI are at risk of skin compromise due to limited mobility, impaired circulation, altered sensation, abnormal muscle control, loss of tissue, and altered postural alignment. If not properly addressed, limited range of motion due to spasticity, contractures, heterotopic ossification (abnormal bone formation in the soft tissues), and spinal stabilization often lead to postural deformity that may result in increased pressures when sitting. Asymmetrical sitting postures increase the risk of skin breakdown in load-bearing areas.

Orthotic Seating

Very little information exists in the literature regarding the impact of wheelchair configuration on posture. Early work by Zacharkow[23] addressed the issue of posture and the wheelchair. He recommended a number of modifications to a standard wheelchair that would optimize spinal posture while allowing balance and function. Harms[24] did similar work comparing three standard wheelchair configurations used in England at the time of the study and concluded that the sling upholstery backrest created the most kyphosis and was the most uncomfortable for users. In a series of four case studies in persons with tetraplegia, Bolin and colleagues[25] showed that wheelchair configuration modifications did change posture and outcome measures related to pain and function. A series of lab-based studies assessing the effects of a chair configuration on balance in a bimanual reaching task concluded that a posterior pelvic tilt was a stable position,[26] that a forward inclination (wedging up the back of the seat) would not create an anterior pelvic tilt,[13] and that the footrest did not appear to contribute to balance for reaching.[27] Tomlinson performed mathematical modeling and computer simulation to determine the impact of the manual wheelchair configuration on roll resistance, maneuverability, and stability.[28] However, none of these simulations brought the backrest forward to vertical, which is a key component of a pelvic-stabilizing configuration and is believed to significantly impact seated stability and balance. In personal communication, the author (Hastings) asked Tomlinson to plot the characteristics of an individual with T6 paraplegia into his simulated equation and then bring the backrest to vertical. In the model, this change resulted in an erect spinal posture with improved stability at least equivalent to the slump kyphotic sitting assumed with buttocks forward.[29] More recently, a therapist in Europe has developed the ergonomic seating system, which is a frame design of a wheelchair that the designer calls a "wheeled orthosis,"[30] and that contains the key parameters of a pelvic-stabilizing system. A study by Maurer and Sprigle[31] assessed the seated pressure distribution of a seating configuration with various seat slopes and found that there are no significant differences in peak pressures with different seat slope inclinations. This study is significant because it refutes one of the concerns levied by therapists against pelvic-stabilizing wheelchair configurations, that of increased ischial pressure.

Orthotic seating and the design of a pelvic-stabilizing system through wheelchair configuration are concepts that have been advanced in the literature.[14,32,33] This approach is founded in the work of Keegan[9] and based on the interactions of the anatomy of the pelvis and lumbar spine, the length of the muscles of the thigh, and the principles of orthotic fabrication. The pelvic stabilizing configuration uses three points of control to stabilize the pelvis in neutral alignment. The seat slope is positive (front higher than rear) and the seat-to-backrest angle is acute (generally, with the backrest being perpendicular to the floor or forward of this position). The backrest is either low or contoured to allow the normal spinal curves above a neutral pelvis. This orthotic wheelchair configuration was shown to decrease forward head posture and shoulder protraction and increase humeral elevation when compared to the standard factory setup of a lightweight wheelchair.[14] Because wheelchair configuration can provide orthotic support to maintain proper spinal alignment, the wheelchair configuration can directly impact the articular function and biomechanics of the shoulder in tasks such as wheelchair propulsion, reaching, and transfers.

Prevention

Prevention science models suggest that the crux of prevention is to identify and reduce known risk factors while enhancing protective factors.[34] Postural malalignment is a known risk factor for musculoskeletal pain, and optimal spinal alignment is a protective factor. The support of optimal spinal posture is the key to prevention of potential musculoskeletal pain, as well as a treatment for existing pain secondary to malignment and muscle imbalance. In a study assessing the spinal deformities in adults who were acutely spinal cord-injured prior to the age of 16 years, Bergstrom[35] found a high prevalence of scoliosis and kyphosis. The author suggested that habitual positioning in poor alignment was a contributing cause and that maintenance of seated posture that most closely mirrors the alignment of the spine in a standing position may prevent or reduce spinal deformity.

Identification of modifiable factors is essential to the development of an optimal treatment program. In the presence of trunk paralysis, the immediate environment of the wheelchair and the extent to which it provides postural support is a modifiable factor and the target of a seating intervention. The intervention is *postural change*; the mechanism of obtaining this intervention in a population with truncal paralysis secondary to SCI is the configuration of a customized seating system.

Theoretically, upper-quadrant musculoskeletal pain after SCI has two main and interrelated causes: postural pain and pain from aberrant upper limb joint biomechanics.

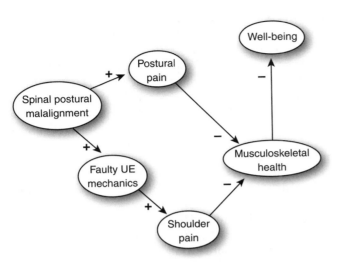

Figure 8-1. Poor postural alignment has negative sequelae. Failure to achieve proper spinal postural alignment with optimal wheelchair seating results in poor push mechanics and pain. These factors in turn degrade musculoskeletal health and ultimately have a negative impact on quality of life and overall well-being.

The posture of the individual is a direct predictor of pain and also indirectly contributes to pain through upper extremity biomechanics (Fig. 8-1). Further spinal postural malalignment can negatively impact health even in the absence of pain. Postural malalignment contributes to skin breakdown, impaired respiratory function, and poor self-image. Physical health impairments, to the extent that they interfere with social engagement and social participation, are known to be linked to decreased quality of life.[36]

The Mobility Base

Functions of a Wheelchair

A well-prescribed wheelchair is a mobile seating orthosis and, as such, can stabilize, support, enhance, or substitute for function. As with any orthosis, the design and configuration of the wheeled orthosis is dependent upon the impairments and functional needs of the individual. Likewise, to determine the specifications of the orthosis, a careful physical examination (including testing of motor and sensory integrity and passive range of motion) is performed in complement with a movement evaluation and an assessment of the environmental needs.

Much of the remainder of this chapter will discuss the components of the evaluation that lead to the determination of the postural support needs that must be provided by the system. The functional assessment addresses the question, "What does the wheelchair need to do for the individual with SCI?" On the face of it, that may seem to be a foolish question. Obviously, the wheelchair allows mobility in the place of walking. For the most able individual with SCI having mastery of diverse wheelchair skills and functional mobility, that is indeed the sole function of the wheelchair. However, there are many variations in the functions of wheelchairs. A poorly prescribed wheelchair can actually *limit* function. This section of the chapter will illustrate how the optimal functional tasks of the wheelchair for a given individual can be predicted based on an assessment of the environment, the lifestyle, and the individual's current (and potential) functional skills.

There are three basic roles the mobility base can provide. These are mobility, a seated position, and a platform for function. There is a wide range of function within each of these categories, and it is necessary to define the specific needs of the individual. There are factors to be considered regarding mobility. Is this the all-day and exclusive form of mobility? Does the individual have any walking ability, even for short distances? If the individual stands or partially stands for any functional activity, the front frame length and the footrest configuration is a consideration. Does the individual drive? If not, then the wheelchair provides much more mobility. What kinds of distances or terrain are likely to be traveled? For what duration of time is the individual away from home? If the individual does not drive, access to public transportation and maneuverability within its confines must be considered, as well as weight limits for lift equipment (i.e., for power wheelchairs). Additionally, portability of the wheelchair for transportation in the vehicles of friends or caregivers must be considered. How easy is the wheelchair to transport? In the case of a power wheelchair that will provide the primary source of community mobility, consideration of ground clearance, battery life, and durability is important. If the individual does drive, what kind of vehicle will be used? If it is a lift- or ramp-equipped vehicle, then weight limits, head clearance, and maneuverability in the vehicle, and wheelchair handling skills, must all be considered. If the individual will stow the wheelchair into the vehicle, the therapist must consider where and how it will be stowed. The vehicle may dictate some features of the wheelchair. For the individual who is newly spinal cord-injured and who is purchasing new equipment, vehicle suggestions can be made to allow optimal wheelchair selection. However, a vehicle is a larger investment than a wheelchair, and existing vehicles may dictate wheelchair parameters.

Body Weight

The body weight of the wheelchair user is a factor that must be considered in wheelchair prescription. Individuals over 250 pounds are over the weight limit for many manufacturers' light and ultralight wheelchairs, requiring wheelchairs to be reinforced to accommodate the body weight. Many companies will not warranty folding wheelchairs at the higher rider weight, yet rigid wheelchairs can be a problem for these individuals. The larger user and the larger wheelchair strain the clearance behind a steering wheel when attempting to stow the wheelchair in a car. Some manufacturers are producing newer-technology folding ultralight wheelchairs that handle higher body weight; this may be a better option for driving independence. Body weight is also a factor for the power wheelchair user as the combined weight of the user and the wheelchair cannot exceed the load capacity of lift equipment for transportation.

Self Care

If the individual dresses in his or her wheelchair, this places certain requirements on the configuration of the wheelchair. Some flexibility may be required in the back-rest to allow for the trunk extension to lift the hips for pants clearance. Also, for this technique, there will be an increased need for rearward stability of the wheelchair. Alternatively, if the technique is to scoot forward and lift hips with flexion and hip hiking, then a slightly longer front frame may be beneficial. In power equipment, the ability to open the seat-to-backrest angle may facilitate caregiver ability to manage clothing.

Individuals who use wheelchairs full time will be required to perform bladder management from their wheelchair; therefore, consideration must be given to how the individual voids. Leg bag management requires the ability to maneuver the wheelchair closer to a toilet for spill-free drainage. The individual who self-catheterizes may need more seat depth or front frame length to maneuver into a posterior pelvic-tilted position within the wheelchair, while a seat depth that is too long will interfere with voiding into a urinal. Those requiring caregiver support may have specific equipment needs to allow efficient and safe assistance.

Seated Position

Assessment of lifestyle and abilities are key factors in determining the functions of the wheelchair in this category. At one extreme, for the individual with high tetraplegia who is dependent for all mobility needs, the wheelchair provides the all-day seated environment. The wheelchair functions must therefore include the ability to change positions for pressure relief and to support the performance of functional activities to the client's fullest capabilities. Power seat functions such as tilt, recline, and elevators, or a combination of all three, may be required to meet the individual's needs. At the other extreme, if the individual has mastery of a wide variety of transfers, alternative positional functions in the wheelchair are typically not required. This individual will transfer out of the wheelchair to drive, to relax, to watch a movie, to exercise, etc. For this individual, the wheelchair can be setup for a single-seated position that optimizes posture and wheelchair propulsion ability.

Somewhere between the extremes illustrated by these two cases is the individual with marginal transfer skills, or who requires assistance, who may not get out of the wheelchair with any frequency during the day. If this individual drives a vehicle from the wheelchair, they will require a higher backrest on the wheelchair, and a head-rest is recommended. They may also desire armrests or other accessories to optimize seated stability.

Wheelchair Skills

Wheelchair skills, and especially wheelie mastery, heavily influence the functions the wheelchair must provide. If an individual has minimal wheelchair skills and/or poor ability in wheelchair propulsion, then the wheelchair must provide for the biomechanics of an assistant. Push handles and higher backrests may be needed. Larger caster diameter will traverse terrain obstacles easier and may be needed if the individual cannot lift casters to clear these obstacles.

Transfers

The individual's method of transferring to and from the wheelchair must be considered to encourage optimal techniques and efficiency. For the individual who transfers independently with either one or both feet on the floor, front frame design is important in order to allow appropriate foot placement. Swing-away leg rests or flip-up footplates are preferred by some to allow a firm contact of both feet on the ground while minimizing the influence of the front frame. When the individual maintains the feet on the footrest during an independent transfer, the orientation of the front frame relative to the caster placement should provide forward and lateral stability of the wheelchair. Individuals who require a positive seat angle (front seat height greater than rear seat height) often require specific transfer training to support independence. For those who transfer with assistance or by dependent methods, swing-away and removable leg rests are beneficial. When the individual performs assisted transfers with feet on the ground, seat-to-floor heights must be considered.

Foot Propulsion

If the individual propels the wheelchair with the feet, then the configuration will be distinctly different from an arm-propelled wheelchair. There are obvious needs for lower seat-to-floor height and having either remov-able footrests or omitting them altogether; however, it is also necessary to think about upper extremity sup-port and increasing the anterior space for improved foot maneuverability. The functional demands on the wheelchair are more limited in terms of the usual ter-rain it will cover, but they are also more varied as it is likely that it will be necessary to set up the wheelchair for the independent foot-propelled function as well as the dependent propulsion over long distances or rough terrain.

Social Roles

Individuals who work or travel have equipment preferences to allow them to be optimally functional in varied environments. Wheelchair users with young children may also express specific needs for their seating system. A thorough assessment of the individual's social roles, lifestyle, environment, functional abilities, and limitations will help the therapist derive a list of wheelchair requirements to meet the function-specific demands. Now, the therapist is ready to guide the selection of specific wheelchair components. Table 8-1 provides information on the basic manual wheelchair components.

Table 8-1
Basic Manual Wheel Chair Components

Component	Usual Options	Considerations
Casters	Diameter ranging from 3 to 8 inches. *Material options:* Polyurethane Pneumatic Semi-pneumatic/soft roll	Larger diameter traverses obstacles more easily. Smaller diameter casters have less roll resistance and turn with greater ease. Foot clearance: Larger diameter casters usually require more forward foot position for clearance. Wider contact will increase roll resistance, especially for turning. Narrower contact decreases roll resistance and increases vibration from terrain obstacles. Pneumatic casters lose air quickly (increase maintenance) and low pressures will increase roll resistance.
Rear wheel	Diameter	Rear wheel diameter (22 to 26 inch) should be considered along with axle position to ensure good arc of push without excessive joint motions. In general, larger diameter wheels offer less resistance. Larger wheel size traverses terrain more easily.
	Wheel Options: Spoked with high or low flange	Aluminum spokes are lightweight and provide some shock absorption, but require maintenance.
	"Mag" High-end composites *Tire options:*	"Mag" wheels are heavy, but require no maintenance. Composites purport a smoother ride and are lighter than aluminum spokes.
	Pneumatic: Range of pressures from high to low (110 lbs/inch^2 to 45 lbs/inch^2) Airless inserts *Tread options:*	Air is a shock absorber, therefore more air at lower pressure provides more shock absorption. Higher pressure provides less roll resistance. Airless inserts add a significant amount of weight.
	Range from smooth to mountain bike tire	Tread selected is determined by the environment of use. Higher tread provides more traction and increased roll resistance.
	Composite tires	Generally, these tires have smooth to low tread features and offer an alternative to airless inserts. They are heavier than pneumatic tires, with less shock absorption.
Armrests		The amount and frequency of weight bearing on the armrest should be considered.
	T-shaped single post	T-shaped armrests are better for weight bearing, although no armrests are designed to support full body weight.

Table 8-1
Basic Manual Wheel Chair Components—cont'd

Component	Usual Options	Considerations
	L-shaped swing away	Swing-away armrests generally have a separate side guard and allow the rear wheel to be positioned closer to the frame.
	Flip back	Flip-back armrests are less stable laterally.
Push handles	Bolted on to rigidizer bar (rigid frame wheelchair)	Consider ease of reach if the rider uses hooking for functional stability.
	Integrated in back cane	If the backrest is low, with acute seat-to-backrest angle to provide lumbar support, then the integral push handles may interfere with push or cause rubbing on the lateral trunk.
	Some manufacturers offer fold-down integrated push handles, quick-release, or height-adjustable push handles.	If push handles are for occasional assistance, then consider removable and higher placement for improved mechanics.

Manual Wheelchairs

The ideal manual wheelchair is lightweight, durable for long-term use, and custom-configured to meet the specific needs of the intended user. While many manual wheelchair options exist, the ultralight class of wheelchairs is the best choice for the consumer with SCI due to its inherent features. The ultralight offers a number of adjustable features and configurations for individualized customization and is the lightest-weight option available. The ultralights are the easiest to manage. Because decreased weight is directly related to decreased roll resistance, a lighter-weight chair requires less force to propel. Lower force propulsion is important for minimizing the risk of upper extremity pathology in wheelchair users as high forces are correlated with shoulder pathology,[37,38] pain, and injury at the wrist.[39] Additionally, an ultralight is the easiest to manage when the wheelchair user is not in the wheelchair, as in the case of stowing the chair in a vehicle. In addition to the lightweight nature of the wheelchair frame, ultralights typically have a rear wheel quick-release feature that disengages the rear wheels when the axle pin is manually depressed. This allows the wheels and frame to be lifted independently, which requires less upper extremity work than managing the entire assembled system. When compared to the other classes of manual wheelchairs, the ultralights are the most durable, as higher-quality materials are used for the frames, components, and accessories. Superior durability means that ultralights are more cost effective despite a higher initial purchase price, and they may also be a more reliable and safer selection.[40]

The ultralights are the only class of manual wheelchairs that allow customized configuration. In addition to selection of seat sizes, frame designs, and accessories, ultralights can be configured and adjusted to optimize performance and functional independence while minimizing injury risk. Whether by adjustment or custom build, the ultralight can be specifically fit to the consumer in a manner that allows for comfort,[41] postural support,[14] skin protection,[42] and efficient wheelchair propulsion.[43,44] One key feature unique to the ultralights is adjustability of the rear wheel in multiple planes. The rear wheel is adjustable forward in the horizontal plane, which has been demonstrated to improve push mechanics[17,43,45,46] and therefore potentially reduce the risk of upper extremity injuries. The rear wheel should be positioned as far forward as possible without causing the wheelchair to be unstable rearward ("tippy").[6] Orientation of the rear wheel in the vertical dimension can be fixed or adjusted in the ultralight chairs. Once posture is optimized, the rear wheel should be positioned such that the distance between the shoulder and wheel hub is minimized[47] and the elbow angle (with the hand at top dead center of the handrim) is between 100 and 120 degrees.[17,48]

Products vary widely within the class of ultralight wheelchairs. Generally, frames are available in either folding or rigid form, with a wide range of configuration and component options available. Selection of the appropriate ultralight is based on findings from the comprehensive evaluation, therapist knowledge of available options, and client preferences.

Folding ultralight wheelchairs range in design from highly adjustable to completely custom. Most clients who prefer folding chairs are long-term wheelchair users whose habitual technique for stowing their wheelchair into their vehicles is to fold it, usually without removal of the rear wheels. The collapse of the folding wheelchair for stowage in a vehicle is a primary benefit of this frame style. One concern with most folding wheelchairs is that postural support is compromised when the back angle is at a fixed position of a 90-degree backrest-to-seat angle. In effect, this will result in the backrest being reclined when there is a positive slope (front seat height higher than rear seat height). To preserve optimal postural alignment, a folding chair with either an adjustable or custom-specified back angle is recommended. A second concern with folding ultralights is lost push efficiency due to the inherent flex in the frame. Folding ultralights with either a locking center frame or articulated rigid footplate may reduce folding frame inefficiencies.

Nonfolding, rigid ultralights can be specifically adjusted or custom ordered to optimize postural support. They are efficient to push because upper extremity forces applied to the wheel are not diminished by flex in the frame. The rigid wheelchairs vary not only in degree of adjustability but also in the style or design of the frame. In general, adjustments for seat-to-backrest angle, backrest height, and footrest length are available, while degree of adjustability of other features depends on the style of the frame.

One style of rigid ultralights is the box frame. The rigid box frame wheelchairs have a top frame tube and a bottom frame tube with at least one cross tube welded to both sides (Fig. 8-2). With the most adjustable box-style welded frame, the rear wheels and front casters are mounted to the frame tubing by plate interfaces. On these frames, most of the components and accessories can be moved on the frame in multiple dimensions to customize the fit to the user. As an example, the rear wheel can be moved horizontally, vertically, and laterally without additional parts. Another option in the box-style

wheelchair is the welded frame with an axle tube spanning the width of the chair to interface with the rear wheels. The frame is built to specified dimensions. Typically, only adjustment of the rear wheel in the horizontal plane is available. The minimization of moving parts and adjustments typically provides improved comfort, efficiency, and performance.

Another option in rigid ultralight manual wheelchairs is the squeeze frame. This frame design has a hinge at the front of the frame to allow rear seat height adjustment by moving the rear seat position up or down. The rear wheel position is fixed in the vertical dimension. Since the rear wheel does not move up or down, the front caster housing is fixed. Rear wheel adjustment in the horizontal plane is preserved.

A popular low-profile frame is the cantilever or monotube design, also referred to as a *minimalist* frame (Fig. 8-3). With one style of cantilever wheelchair, the rear wheels are mounted by brackets suspended from, and extending below, the rear frame. When the rear wheels are removed, the cantilever style typically has the lowest profile frame of all the chairs, making it easier to maneuver the wheelchair when stowing into a vehicle. With the adjustable cantilever models, there are many options available for seat angle configuration and rear wheel position. However, along with adjustability comes more moving parts. In some cases, this adds increased weight despite the appearance of low weight with a minimal frame design. Additionally, it is important to remember that the more adjustable parts there are on a wheelchair, the more potential for breakage or maladjustment.

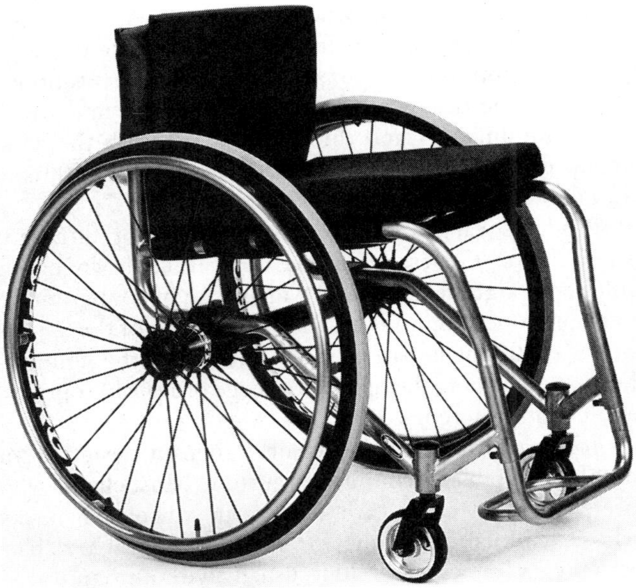

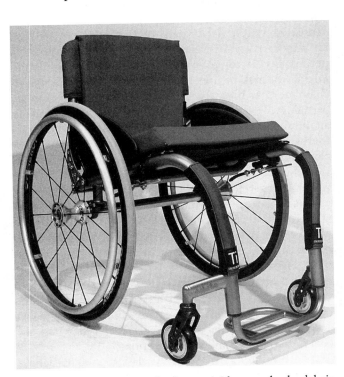

Figure 8-3. Cantilever-style frame rigid manual wheelchair. (Photo courtesy of TiLite, Kennewick, WA.)

Figure 8-2. Box-style frame rigid manual wheelchair. (Photo courtesy of Invacare Top End.)

On frames where there are both adjustable components and fixed components, it is important to recognize the secondary impact of purposeful adjustment. For instance, with the front hinge-style frame, the result of increasing the seat slope (lowering the rear seat height) is that the user sits deeper in the wheels (i.e., closer to the axles), thereby increasing the joint excursion of all upper extremity joints during propulsion. Additionally, this change causes the knee position to be more flexed. In contrast, with a cantilever frame design, increasing the seat slope will not change the knee angle, but will position the footrest at a more forward angle relative to the floor and increase the overall length of the wheelchair. For all chairs that allow adjustment as an inherent feature, it is important to confirm that desired chair alignment is preserved when extremes of adjustments are used. For example, when the rear seat height is adjusted to the lowest setting, the backrest should still achieve a vertical position and the front caster housing perpendicular orientation must be maintained.

The most advanced style of ultralight manual wheelchairs is the custom-configured welded frames. Available in a number of different designs from several manufacturers, the welded chairs are manufactured based on specific prescribed dimensions for all aspects of the chair. In addition to seat width and depth, the chair is built to specific dimensions relative to front and rear seat heights, frame lengths, backrest orientation, caster position, and footrest design. Depending on the manufacturer and the specific model, adjustability in rear wheel horizontal position and backrest angle can be preserved to fine-tune the fit of an otherwise fixed frame. Generally, some adjustment of backrest height and footrest length is maintained to accommodate different cushion heights. Because the welded chairs are custom designed for the specific consumer and are constructed with few moving parts, they are the lightest-weight, most durable, most highly maneuverable, and most energy-efficient chairs available. However, because there is minimal adjustability, the skills of a highly experienced and confident therapist are required to design and fit a fixed wheelchair that best meets the complex needs of the user with SCI.

Many ultralights are also available with suspension. The function of suspension is to absorb shock that is transmitted through the wheelchair. Suspension frames are available in both adjustable and highly customized models. The location of the suspension on the frame and the type of system used varies by manufacturer. Several chairs have the suspension located directly under the seat, with attachment to both the frame and underside of the seat. When the system is "loaded" by the individual sitting in the chair, the hydraulic system under the seat will compress. In a center-mount suspension design, the seat sinks between the two wheels when the suspension device is loaded. By contrast, other suspension chairs use independent rear wheel suspension. Either a spring or elastic polymer is incorporated into the mounting hardware for each rear wheel. When the seat is loaded, the suspension device at each wheel compresses independently. The independent rear wheels will respond to an asymmetric load, as occurs when traversing uneven terrain. With either suspension design, the rear seat height will be lowered when the suspension device is loaded; therefore, it is critical to evaluate the implications for seat slope, backrest position, and rider orientation to the rear wheels for propulsion. Suspension for front casters is also available as an accessory that can interface with most manual wheelchairs. Potential clinical indications for rear and/or front suspension include improved ease and comfort when negotiating uneven terrain and decreased jarring and vibration during wheeling. Cooper and Wolf[49] evaluated shock and vibration at the seat and footrest in wheelchairs with and without suspension. They found that shock and vibration is reduced with caster fork suspension more than with rear frame suspension. While there are identified benefits to the use of suspension with manual wheelchairs, the choice must be balanced with consideration of increased weight to the system, maintenance needs, and potential impaired efficiency of propulsion on varied surfaces.

Regardless of the style of chair selected for an individual, the dimensions and configuration of the wheelchair deserve critical attention in order to maximize mobility, support, and comfort. Additionally, the prescribing therapist must clearly understand the reference points for all chair dimensions, which will ultimately dictate the configuration of the final wheelchair. Unfortunately, reference dimensions vary from one manufacturer to another, so for each manufacturer there is only one correct way to measure. The therapist is urged to *read the directions* on the order form with care.

Manual Wheelchair Propulsion Assistance

Add-on rear wheel options that provide assistance during propulsion are available for certain models of wheelchairs. These rear wheel propulsion-assist technologies are typically accessory devices that are mounted and interfaced with a new or existing manual wheelchair and are targeted toward improved mobility as well as decreased pain and risk of upper extremity injury for individuals who propel manual wheelchairs.

One available option is the pushrim-activated power-assist wheelchair (PAPAW). The wheelchair is accessorized with battery-powered wheels that provide supplemental power output when the handrim is engaged during propulsion. Depending on the manufacturer, the power wheels may interface with just one type of wheelchair or may be retrofitted to a wide range of wheelchairs by alternative mounting hardware. Arva and colleagues[50] found that metabolic energy and user power were lower, and mechanical efficiency higher, during propulsion with the PAPAW. Laboratory findings associated with the PAPAW include decreased energy demands,[51-54] decreased stroke frequency,[52] decreased upper extremity range of motion during propulsion,[55] and decreased surface EMG of upper extremity muscles.[56] Alsgood and colleagues[54] found that individuals with tetraplegia traversing a four-obstacle course in both standard manual wheelchairs and with PAPAW rated the obstacles as significantly easier with PAPAW. Functional wheelchair skills do not appear to be significantly influenced by the use of PAPAW. In a study comparing acquisition of wheelchair skills in a wheelchair with standard rear wheels versus power-assist wheels, there was no significant difference in skill achievement as measured by the total score on a wheelchair skills test.[57] However, the authors noted that the added torque appeared to offer an advantage for skills for which power was required (such as inclines), but disadvantaged skills requiring control (such as wheelie-based skills). This study was done in able-bodied subjects, so the results may not be generalized to clients with SCI who have limited hand function. Evidence supports the metabolic benefit and the increased torque provided by PAPAW; however, it is not clear whether there is an overall improvement at the community participation level. A community-based study[58] found no difference in distance traveled in a 2-week period in manual wheelchairs versus PAPAW.

Another rear wheel accessory specifically designed to aid wheelchair propulsion is a geared wheel that allows the individual to switch between standard pushing and a lower gear. Similar to riding a geared bicycle, the low gear provides decreased resistance to propulsion. With decreased resistance over a given terrain, the wheel is easier to propel, but it requires increased push frequency to traverse the same distance. Preliminary reports suggest that the geared wheel may decrease upper limb pain[59] but more research investigation of the geared rear wheel is needed.

Accessory rear wheel options appear to offer some benefit to individuals who prefer to continue pushing a manual wheelchair versus transitioning to a power wheelchair. When considering prescription of add-on wheels, the ability of the users to operate the wheels must be evaluated, in such areas as turning the assistance on and off, installing and removing the wheels, and ease of charging the battery. These considerations are especially important for the individual with tetraplegia with upper extremity weakness and impaired hand function. Evaluation of management of the wheelchair with power wheels must also take into consideration tasks such as stowing the wheelchair in a vehicle. The significant weight of each wheel creates an increased risk for injury when attempting independent stowing of the wheels. It is recommended that an individual using add-on wheels use a van with a lift or ramp or, if traveling in a car, seek assistance for stowing the wheels. Battery life and how it is affected by the terrain the individual typically traverses are important factors to consider when assessing for power-assist wheels. For the currently available power-assist systems, there is significant added weight and roll resistance if propelling the wheelchair without the power-assist feature engaged. Other considerations for the rear wheel propulsion-assist accessories include maintenance needs, cost, and the need for additional wheelchair skills training.

Power Wheelchairs

Power wheelchairs are the appropriate equipment choice for many individuals with SCI. Like manual wheelchairs, there are a multitude of power wheelchair options with variable features and functions. The ideal power system is one that best meets the comprehensive needs of the client, with decisions guided by a thorough assessment combined with simulation and trials of appropriate options. The power system must provide maximal mobility while also meeting the fundamental seating goals for postural support, comfort, skin protection, and optimized function. Because the needs of individuals with SCI who require power mobility are typically complex, most are best served by a power base with an adjustable "rehab-style" seat that is designed to meet the dimensional, postural, comfort, and functional needs of a person and can also accommodate dynamic power seat functions such as tilt in space, reclining backrests, and seat elevation. Scooters and basic power wheelchairs with integral seats (i.e., captain's seating) usually do not adequately address mobility and seating requirements for the client with SCI. For aggressive, full-time wheelchair users functioning in both indoor and varied outdoor environments, wheelchairs must be highly maneuverable, durable, and reliable, both in known and unpredictable circumstances. Fass and colleagues[60] found the most advanced, high-end, custom wheelchair bases to be the most durable. Individuals with higher-level cervical injuries require a power system that will meet mobility and support needs and also interface with alternative specialty controls to allow them to operate their power system and to control their environment. The following overview of power bases, power seat options, and input devices will guide clinical reasoning for power system recommendations for the client with SCI.

Power wheelchair bases are available with a variety of features, including control processor capabilities (i.e., programmability of control parameters including speed, acceleration, braking, and tremor dampening), suspensions, and motor packages. A common method of comparing bases involves position of the drive wheels, such as rear wheel drive (RWD), front wheel drive (FWD), and midwheel drive (MWD). Within these three general categories, there are significant variations of the drive wheel position with different manufacturers and models. The drive wheel position relative to the power base and relative to the seat orientation over the base carries significant implications for wheelchair performance.

Factors influenced by drive wheel position include turning radius, overall wheelchair length, maneuverability, speed, stability, traction, and the ability to negotiate obstacles. There are inherent benefits and concerns for each of the power base options. The appropriate power base selection for the individual requires that the pros and cons of product options be carefully weighed and integrated with the client's specific needs and preferences. Fass and colleagues[60] identified no differences in durability between RWD, FWD, and MWD power wheelchairs. There is currently no published research to support that one drive wheel position is superior to another.

A RWD power base has the large drive wheels positioned posteriorly, relative to the center of the base, with smaller casters at the anterior aspect of the base. The seat is positioned such that the driver's center of gravity (COG) is forward of the drive wheels. With this posterior placement of the drive wheels, power to the wheels functions to "push" the wheelchair forward when it is activated by the driver. A low-ratio RWD configuration allows for a smaller percentage of driver body weight (~65%) over the drive wheels, while a high-ratio RWD allows for a greater percentage of driver body weight over the drive wheels (~85%); these are factors that impact drive performance.[61] Traction is improved with increased weight over the drive wheels. Relative to other power bases, RWD performance is most consistent with increased stability at high speeds and predictable reaction on uneven surfaces. The RWD power wheelchairs typically have a longer wheelbase, with an associated increase in turning radius. RWD wheelchairs are most stable while descending inclines, but may be unstable on steep ascents (rearward instability). Additionally, the rear-positioned drive wheels are challenged for uphill climbing because of increased power demands. When traversing a side slope, the inherent configuration of RWD will cause the front of the wheelchair to turn downward, the extent of which is highly dependent on the weight over the casters. The RWD wheelchairs are less maneuverable over thresholds, obstacles, and in soft terrain because the front casters must first overcome the environmental challenge. A key consideration relative to the front casters is lower leg and foot position. To allow clearance for caster swivel without contacting the driver's foot, the front rigging (i.e., leg rest and foot support) typically needs to extend forward from the seat, which may result in an increased overall wheelchair length.

The FWD power base is configured with the large drive wheels most forward on the base and the smaller casters trailing behind (Fig. 8-4). The driver's COG while seated is behind the drive wheels. Because the seat is positioned over the base, the footrest is the most forward aspect of a FWD power wheelchair and therefore must be considered relative to obstacle negotiation. Having the footrest positioned forward of the anterior drive wheels allows for many options in lower leg and foot position. Similar to RWD, there are low-ratio and

high-ratio wheel configurations in FWD systems.[61] With the drive wheels located anteriorly, input to the wheels functions to "pull" the wheelchair in the desired direction. FWD wheelchairs have a wheelbase similar to that of RWD wheelchairs; however, the maneuvering configuration is quite different. Driving a FWD wheelchair has been described as similar to driving a forklift, because the major part of the wheelchair is posterior to the drive wheels. FWD wheelchairs are known to be less stable at higher speeds and are more difficult to control over uneven terrain. However, recent improvements in technology have improved tracking and overcome instability concerns with most FWD wheelchairs, which are especially beneficial to those driving with switch-activated controls. FWD wheelchairs likely represent the most effective wheelchair for negotiating thresholds and obstacles and also for ascending small curbs. This is because the large drive wheels encounter the challenge first and function to pull the wheelchair up and over obstacles. FWD wheelchairs are highly effective for climbing hills, but are less stable than other bases for descending inclines. On a side slope, the rear aspect of a FWD wheelchair turns downward, forcing the front of the wheelchair to turn upward and requiring the user to compensate with driving skill.

The MWD power wheelchair bases have the large drive wheel positioned centrally on the base under the driver's center of mass. Depending on the specific model

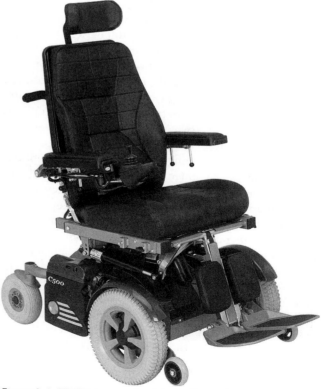

Figure 8-4. FWD power wheelchair. (Permobil C500, courtesy of Permobil, Inc.)

and configuration, the drive wheel may be biased forward or rearward, which impacts wheelchair performance in varied conditions. The MWD wheelchairs typically have the shortest wheel base and smallest turning radius, which may make them easiest to manage for sharp turns and tight spaces. MWD wheelchairs have the most weight over the drive wheels, which improves traction, but compromises forward and rearward stability. To compensate for instability, front and rear casters or "stabilizers" are necessary, such that MWD wheelchairs function with six wheels. With static stabilizers (those that do not change position), the wheelchair may high-center or get stuck over grade transitions, such as when driving from a flat surface to a ramp. Dynamic stabilizers, or independent suspensions on the front and rear stabilizer wheels, prevent high-centering and allow for improved obstacle negotiation and control in unpredictable terrains. Technological developments for MWD wheelchairs are targeted toward increased stability in all environments. The impact of increased speed on stability depends on the bias of the center wheel backward or forward, which correlates with identified tendencies of the RWD and FWD wheelchairs, respectively. MWD wheelchairs tend to be the least predictable for straight line driving on a side slope, because the pull of the wheelchair upward or downward is influenced both by the actual position of the drive wheel and by the specific side slope. MWD wheelchairs have more footrest options than RWD, but the orientation of the lower legs and feet must be considered relative to the front stabilizers.

A power seat with dynamic functions mounted to the selected power base provides necessary body movement that is typically compromised as a result of SCI. While the power base allows the individual to move from one place to another and to maneuver in varied environments, the power seat provides for specific changes in body position, which promotes physiologic health, comfort, postural support, and energy conservation. Power seat options include recline, tilt (two dimensions), seat elevation, standing, and leg rest elevation (Fig. 8-5).

The selection and configuration of power seat options are based on assessment of client needs balanced with consideration of the specific benefits and concerns associated with a given feature. Interaction between components must also be considered. While power seats offer a number of inherent advantages, installation of a power seat can result in increased seat-to-floor height and increased overall wheelchair length as compared to standard nonpowered seats. Actuators, which mechanically control the power seat functions, must be stacked to allow for multiple seat functions (i.e., tilt combined with elevation), which will increase seat-to-floor height.

Power recline pivots the backrest posteriorly, increasing the seat-to-backrest angle and allowing the user to assume a more recumbent position. Power recline is used as a pressure-relief technique; improved pressure distribution is provided and high pressures are shifted away from the

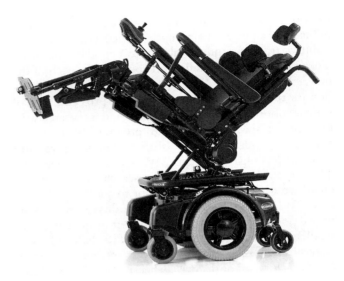

Figure 8-5. Tilt power seat function.

sitting surface when a much greater surface area is available. Published research relative to the extent of recline necessary to achieve adequate pressure relief is limited. Two studies have indicated that there is a significant decrease in seated pressures with recline but also found increased shear forces.[62,63] In a study of 63 healthy subjects, Stinson and colleagues found that average pressures were reduced with recline at 120 degrees; however, maximum pressures were not significantly altered.[64] There is no published research evaluating the seated pressure associated with varying degrees of recline greater than 120 degrees, independent of other seat functions. Recline may be indicated when the seated individual cannot achieve upright sitting, such as when available hip flexion range of motion is less than 90 degrees or in the case of a fixed thoracic kyphosis wherein recline restores vertical head position. Recline can be used to allow a position of rest, away from upright sitting. Power recline allows for an increased hip angle, which may be beneficial for dynamic passive joint motion, comfort, improved access for bladder management, and increased ease of clothing adjustment. There are several concerns relative to recline systems used by the Client with SCI. As the backrest moves through recline and the return to neutral, shear forces at the buttocks and posterior trunk increase the risk of skin breakdown. Recline creates a challenge for maintaining postural support. As the backrest comes forward to return to an upright position, the user may be pushed forward in the seat, compromising postural alignment and support. Most people who require a power-reclining backrest lack the functional mobility to correct their seated position. Highly contoured cushions and backrests are not typically compatible with recline systems due to the potential shift in body alignment. Additionally, for those with upper motor neuron injuries, such as SCI, movement into a supine position may elicit a spastic reflex that may further compromise position in the wheelchair.

Power tilt allows the entire seat to pivot while maintaining the seat-to-backrest angle. While rearward tilt is most commonly prescribed, power tilt is also available in the forward and lateral directions. Rearward tilt is another mechanism used for pressure relief as weight is shifted from the seated surface to the posterior trunk in the tilted position. Henderson and colleagues[65] demonstrated that there is a significant decrease in seated pressures with 65 degrees of tilt, but only minimal change in pressure with 35 degrees of tilt. The distribution of pressure while tilted is likely not as good as that achieved with a fully reclined position as less surface area is available, although this has not been reported in the scientific literature. However, because the pressure relief provided by tilt lacks the shear effects inherent with full recline, tilt is the preferred method for preserving skin integrity. Like recline, the tilted position is beneficial for shifting body orientation in space and as a position of relative rest. The benefits to tilt are that body position is maintained through the excursion into tilt and back to upright, thereby eliminating shear and allowing the individual to maintain postural alignment and support. Tilt systems do not allow for passive joint motion as there is no change in seat angles; therefore, access for bladder management may be a challenge for some users. Because the flexed body posture is consistently maintained, extensor spasticity is better controlled in a tilt system. While not commonly prescribed for the SCI population, forward tilt may have a specific benefit related to transfers for the client with partial lower limb innervation whose feet are supported on the ground for assisted or independent transfers. Lateral tilt may be effective for providing vertical upper body and head alignment for the individual who sits with severe pelvic obliquity and excessive trunk curvature.

A combination power tilt and recline seat may be an appropriate choice for the client with SCI who will benefit from the advantages of each system. In a tilt/recline combination system, the driver first tilts the wheelchair, then reclines the backrest. The reverse maneuver (return from recline, then return from tilt) is used to achieve the upright seated posture. The major negative aspects of recline—shear forces on the skin and a shift in body position—are negated when the seat is in the tilted position, as the impact of gravity on the body is minimized. The concern for fixed hip position with tilt is addressed as recline following tilt allows partial extension of the hip joint without facilitating extension reflexes. The goal of the combination of power tilt and power recline is to reduce pressure and minimize shear. Hobson[62] demonstrated that maximum pressure and shear reduction was achieved with 120 degrees of recline and 25 degrees of tilt. Pellow,[66] in a case series on two subjects with C5 tetraplegia, found the greatest pressure relief with a combination of 150 degrees of recline and 45 degrees of tilt. Vaisbuch and colleagues[63] studied five seated positions for 15 children with complete paraplegia due to myelomeningocele and 15 nondisabled children. While tilt alone and recline alone were found to significantly decrease seated pressures, the combination of tilt with recline reduced pressures to the greatest degree. Aissaoui and colleagues[67] evaluated multiple combinations of tilt and recline in 10 able-bodied subjects in a simulation chair. The greatest pressure relief was demonstrated with 45 degrees of tilt and 120 degrees of recline. Compliance with use of powered tilt and recline systems was evaluated in a study reporting the results of 40 client interviews.[68] Ninety seven and a half percent of subjects used their power tilt/recline systems daily, predominantly to provide comfort and a rest position. Further research is necessary to specify clinical indications and optimum tilt and recline angles for individuals with SCI.

Power seat elevation allows the entire seat to translate upward in space while all seat angles and system configurations are preserved. Seat elevation allows improved environmental access in home, work, and community environments by providing a vertical upward transition that allows the individual to interact above the standard seated level.[69] Personal interactions at eye level may provide improved psychosocial adjustment for wheelchair users. Eye level communication reduces the need for chronic cervical hyperextension and may thereby decrease musculoskeletal pain in persons with limited ability to adjust position. Kirby[70] reported that sustained cervical extension and rotation resulted in increased neck discomfort in wheelchair users. Power seat elevation facilitates maximal functional mobility when moving from the wheelchair. An increased seat-to-floor height allows level or downhill lateral transfers, which have been shown to decrease upper extremity muscle effort.[71] Sit-to-stand transfers are also improved with seat elevation as lower extremity muscles have a biomechanical advantage from a raised seat height. A literature review[72] confirmed that performance of sit-to-stand transfers is strongly influenced by the seat height. Seat elevation also plays a role in minimizing the risk of upper quadrant musculoskeletal injury and discomfort for wheelchair users. Increased height in space minimizes the frequency of overhead reaching, which has been implicated as a contributing factor in shoulder pain[73] and shoulder muscle load.[74–76]

Wheelchairs that allow passive standing have some similar advantages to seat elevation. However, when considering standing for the client with SCI, potential risk for lower extremity fractures, skin compromise, and hypotension must be carefully evaluated. In general, wheelchairs that allow alternative positioning do not preserve optimal seated postural support.

Power-elevating leg rests (ELRs) are another feature that can be beneficial to the client with SCI. ELRs can be operated either simultaneously with or independent of power tilt and/or recline. When used in conjunction with recline, additional increased surface area is provided for pressure distribution, but increased shear forces result unless tilt in space is also incorporated. Specific attention to lower extremity range of motion is critical when using ELRs in any wheelchair system. If the leg rest is elevated beyond the user's available hamstring length, the individual will shift into a posterior pelvic tilt to relieve excessive muscle tension. When using ELRs for management of lower extremity edema, they should be interfaced with the power tilt function so that the legs can be positioned above the heart to facilitate fluid management.[77] Use of power ELRs should be judicious as they are heavy, may increase overall wheelchair length, and may create additional maintenance requirements.

Prescription of a power system includes critical attention to the drive control, in addition to power base and seat selections. The comprehensive client evaluation will provide key information relative to best options for drive control selection. While it is beyond the scope of this chapter to review the multitude of joystick and alternative specialty control options, the correlation between power wheelchair operation and seated posture must be emphasized. In order for the individual with SCI to be successful using any potential drive control—whether by upper extremity, head, oral, or other physical function—postural alignment and support must be addressed first. Providing the individual with an appropriate seating system with posture optimized will allow optimal functional performance for using power controls. Additionally, proper seating is likely to decrease the risk of musculoskeletal discomfort and injury that is linked to repetitive, sustained activity such as that required for operating a power wheelchair.

Overview of Wheelchair Configuration Recommendations and Considerations

The final configuration for both power and manual wheelchairs is determined by selecting the features of the wheelchair and specifying the measurements and angular setup. Table 8-2 provides some recommendations and considerations for the wheelchair configuration for the client with SCI.

Power Versus Manual Decision

The decision to prescribe power mobility for the acutely injured individual with SCI should be made very thoughtfully, and the use of power should be judicious in any case of incomplete SCI. In the case where the use of power is obviously required, the selection of drive control (e.g., selecting sip and puff versus facilitated hand driving) should be made with just as much care. Because there is always the potential for improved function due to neuroplasticity, the individual should be given every opportunity to move functionally in biomechanically appropriate ways. Decreased use promotes learned nonuse[78] and, more importantly, the establishment of the habit of compensatory patterns of movement. Sometimes

the compensatory function is actual dependence on assistance from another, and this can be a vicious cycle if the caregiver enables dependency.

Motor learning literature suggests the idea that new motor skills are acquired through a process of practice, with error and internal correction, with mastery after generalization to varied environments.[79–81] Balance after SCI is a new motor skill because there is a new neurologic platform. It is very important not to oversupport or over-immobilize an individual in the early period post-SCI. Minimal equipment with dynamic challenge will optimize facilitory situations. Of course, care must be taken to avoid fatigue and deterioration of function. A progressive seated activity schedule or alternative positioning can help avoid this issue.

The case of the individual with newly acquired incomplete tetraplegia, especially with central cord syndrome, is an example of a circumstance in which power mobility should be avoided. Facilitation of lower extremity activity with foot propulsion mobility will increase endurance and strength of the lower extremities and set up better potential for independent transfer, functional standing, and perhaps walking. Foot propelling a manual wheelchair creates dynamic balance challenge. Trunk control is especially crucial to those with limited or no upper extremity function. Dynamic manual wheelchair activity facilitates trunk stability.

There is no evidence to support the idea that power wheelchairs will prevent musculoskeletal pain after SCI. While there is evidence that there is a high prevalence of pain in wheelchair users,[82–85] many studies have shown that there is no identifiable association between pain and the type of wheelchair used (power versus manual). Indeed, studies suggest that among persons with SCI there is a higher prevalence of pain in persons with tetraplegia,[82,86,87] who are more likely to use power mobility. Evidence supports the belief that optimized postural support in an ultralight manual wheelchair and attention to biomechanics of wheelchair propulsion, in terms of both wheelchair setup and propulsive stroke training, is protective to the upper extremities.[6] Body weight is also a key issue. Lack of basic low-level maintenance exercise will promote weight gain, and increased body weight is associated with more musculoskeletal pain and functional compromise.[82]

The decision to use power mobility should be made based on functional need. If the individual in question has the ability to transfer independently and can drive a vehicle, he or she will likely be better served with manual mobility. In the situation where the individual is dependent in transfers or cannot drive, he or she may be better served with power mobility. Most persons with C6 level injury without comorbidity can successfully master both transfers and driving; therefore, manual mobility is recommended for acutely injured individuals with injury at this level and below. The functional ability of those persons discharged in manual mobility is often increased

Table 8-2

Seating the Client with SCI: Wheelchair Configuration Recommendations and Considerations

Frame Parameter Key Issues	General Recommendations	Considerations
Seat and Back Widths Too wide → inadequate postural control Too narrow→ may create skin compromise, provide inadequate support, or cause a postural shift	Snug fit without causing adverse pressure at trochanters or posterolateral ribs. Body measurements at pelvis, hips, knees, and trunk must be considered. Frontal plane alignment and flexibility must be incorporated in width selection. Armrests with panel or rigid clothing guards (manual wheelchairs) can assist with postural control and protection of soft tissue at hips. Consider clothing bulk relative to seasonal differences, but avoid excessive widths: provide education for clothing selections. If aftermarket backrest is specified, ensure that the backrest frame width is sufficiently wide to accommodate it.	Excessive seat and/or back widths contribute to postural deformity as the body may shift to fill extra space. If a discrepancy exists between body measurements for seat and trunk widths, prescribe separate/independent seat and back widths. Seat width correlates to overall chair width, which must be considered relative to environmental access. Some manual chairs are available with a tapered seat (front more narrow than rear). Tapered seats may allow improved leg positioning and increase environmental access. For some power chairs, the space available between the armrests is greater than the actual seat width measurement. Consider actual space available between armrests when selecting seat width.
Seat Depth Too long → posterior pelvic tilt Too short → inadequate support	Appropriate seat depth should provide support for the pelvis and posterior thighs, with adequate space remaining between seat upholstery and the posterior knee. "Adequate" depends on functional ability: the dependent person can have less space, an independent person with full hand function requires ~2 inches, and an independent person with impaired hand function needs more space. Specific attention to upper leg lengths, lower extremity range of motion measures, and sagittal plane posture and flexibility is necessary. Seat depth selection must be considered relative to the front frame or footrest angle. Knee flexion position on front frame or footrest is important. Increased knee flexion typically requires a shorter seat depth.	A common mistake is seat depth that is too long. Excessive seat depth is a direct cause of postural compromise, with facilitation of a posterior pelvic tilt. Excessive seat depths also increase overall frame lengths, which negatively impacts accessibility. Seat depths that are too short provide inadequate support under posterior thighs, which may increase pressure under the pelvis. Short seat depths may interfere with transfers secondary to a decreased support platform. Seat depth (upholstery or solid seat) may be prescribed independent of the frame length (i.e., shorter seat on longer frame). Backrest selection and orientation impacts actual seat depth. Installation of aftermarket backrest may increase or decrease the available seat depth, which impacts support, posture, and chair performance.

Continued

Table 8-2
Seating the Client with SCI: Wheelchair Configuration Recommendations and Considerations—cont'd

Frame Parameter Key Issues	General Recommendations	Considerations
		An asymmetric seat depth should be prescribed for true upper leg length discrepancies or apparent asymmetric upper leg lengths that are related to fixed deformities, such as pelvic rotation or a dislocated hip.
Seat Slope Determined by the difference between front and rear seat-to-floor heights divided by the frame depth	Information from the mat evaluation and empirical trials is *critical* for determining optimal seat slope for postural support. As a general rule, the greater the degree of trunk muscle paralysis, the greater the degree of seat slope to substitute for trunk instability (i.e., with a 16-inch seat depth and extensive trunk paralysis best with 3 to 4 inch front to rear difference vs. intact trunk 1 to 2 inch difference) although highly variable. Seat slope has significant impact on postural alignment.[14]	Seat slope and backrest configuration must be addressed in concert. Transfers may be impacted by increased seat slope. Therapists must be competent in teaching transfer techniques from sloped seats. Increased seat slope does not increase interface pressures at the sitting surface.[31]
Front Seat Height Front seat height must be considered relative to rear seat height to achieve desired seat slope for postural support.	Must allow appropriate clearance under tables and desks while also allowing adequate clearance under footplate for ground clearance. Consider seat height relative to transfers and vertical position in space. Lower leg lengths, range of motion, footrest position, and cushion heights must be incorporated when determining ideal seat-to-floor height.	Must consider front seat heights relative to driving a vehicle from the wheelchair as clearance under steering column is critical. Front seat height configuration requires attention to frame design, caster diameter, caster fork length, and caster stem length.
Rear Seat Height Must be considered relative to front seat height to achieve desired seat slope for postural control.	Rear seat height determines the actual sitting height of the individual. For manual wheelchairs, consider rear seat height relative to rear wheel position. With optimized posture and hand at top dead center of handrim, recommended elbow flexion angle is 100 to 120 degrees[17,48]	For manual chairs with suspension, consider the impact of suspension on rear seat height when the suspension is loaded. Is rear seat height altered when the suspension system is loaded? Is rear seat height compromised as suspension system ages? Rider body weight changes may result in compromised positioning.
Backrest Angle Backrest angle must be considered relative to seat slope as the interaction between the seat and back significantly impacts postural support.	Findings from evaluation and empirical trials indicate optimal back angle position. The available range of motion at the hip must be considered when determining back-to-seat angle. Back angle must also be considered in conjunction with backrest height	Backrest angle can either be adjustable posterior (recline) and anterior or may be a fixed welded angle. Backrest position posterior to vertical may facilitate a posterior pelvic tilt. Adequate lumbar support must be incorporated to support a neutral pelvic position.

Table 8-2
Seating the Client with SCI: Wheelchair Configuration Recommendations and Considerations—cont'd

Frame Parameter Key Issues	General Recommendations	Considerations
		The reclined (posterior to vertical) backrest position is overprescribed in individuals with SCI. Individuals with low cervical injuries and those with paraplegia with neutral postural alignment often do well with a vertical backrest that provides lumbar and midtrunk support and allows full scapular and shoulder motion.

In manual wheelchairs, a reclined backrest requires that the rear wheel be in a more rearward position, which negatively impacts UE propulsion mechanics.

Consider the influence of rear suspension on back angle. When the suspension is loaded, does the back angle shift toward posterior? If so, the backrest angle should be anterior prior to loading. |
| *Backrest Height* Backrest height must be considered in conjunction with backrest angle. | Height of backrest is determined based on prioritization of postural support needs and upper extremity function.

Should be high enough that pelvis and trunk are well supported, and low enough to allow normal thoracic extension over the backrest. Back height should not inhibit trunk motion (unless desired) or upper extremity function.

Backrests in power-tilt and recline systems must be high enough to provide adequate trunk support when reclined. Central support is the most critical so that the individual is not resting solely on the headrest; contoured relief for scapulae can be incorporated when elbow blocks are provided to support arms when seat is tilted. | Available in adjustable or fixed heights.

A common mistake is positioning the backrest too high. A high backrest contributes to increased thoracic kyphosis, which consequently contributes to a posterior pelvic position, protracted scapulae with the humerus forward in the glenoid, and cervical hyperextension.

Avoid positioning the back height immediately above or below spinal stabilization rods as hypermobility at that segment may be facilitated and/or discomfort may result.

High backrests must have appropriate contours to allow normal spinal curvature. |
| *Front Frame or Footrest Drop Angle* Impacts leg position and overall frame length | Configuration or selection of the front frame or footrests must be considered relative to seat slope and front seat-to-floor height.

Postural presentation, knee, and ankle range of motion and spasticity must be considered.

Consider angle selection relative to overall chair length, which impacts environmental access and chair maneuverability. | In chairs with adjustable seat slope by the rear axle position, alteration of the seat slope alters front frame or footrest angle relative to the floor.

A front frame or footrest angle that is closer to vertical requires increased knee flexion. This may be beneficial for inhibition of extensor spasticity if adequate range of motion is available.

Front frame or footrest angle also must be considered relative to stability of the |

Continued

Table 8-2
Seating the Client with SCI: Wheelchair Configuration Recommendations and Considerations—cont'd

Frame Parameter Key Issues	General Recommendations	Considerations
		front of the chair. With feet positioned farther in front of the frame or base, a longer lever arm creates forward instability. Caster position relative to the front frame or footrest is also important for addressing forward stability.
Footplate Height	Determine appropriate vertical position relative to the front seat height and ground clearance needs. Lower leg lengths as well as ankle position and range of motion must be considered. Cushion height must be incorporated when determining footplate height. Footplate height is directly related to front frame or footrest angle. For the same lower leg length, a more vertical front frame or footrest angle decreases footplate distance from the floor.	The angle of the actual footplate must be considered relative to the height off the floor. Often, footplates positioned to accommodate plantar flexion contractures increase the actual length required to support the foot, thereby decreasing distance for ground clearance. Footplate position is based on individual needs and personal preferences. However, lower ground clearance requires wheelie mastery in a manual wheelchair and may inhibit rough terrain clearance in a power wheelchair.
Armrest Height	Posture in the sagittal plane must be optimized prior to determining armrest height. Armrests should be positioned such that the elbow and forearm are supported while facilitating a neutral position of the humerus in the glenoid fossa.	Armrests that are too low will allow shoulder subluxation in individuals without a fully innervated or weak rotator cuff. Armrests that are too low facilitate trunk flexion with kyphosis, scapular protraction, forward humerus and cervical hyperextension. Armrests that are too high may cause subacromial impingement or undue pressure on elbow. A manual wheelchair configured as an orthotic device provides appropriate postural support. The armrests are not needed for balance or support and can be eliminated.

at 1 year post-injury, whereas the functional ability of those discharged in power mobility will often decline.

The decision to *change* to power mobility at some point during the life of an individual with SCI should be based on individual medical and functional reasons. Functional limitations tend to accrue with aging and health decline; this is true in the general population and may be magnified in the SCI population. It is important to assess how the current functional ability is impacting participation. If limitations begin to interfere with social roles, then there may be a domino effect of increased social isolation and declining physical function. However, it is important to recognize that many people will see the move to power as symbolic of their decline in ability or an increase in disability, a "giving in." For some long-term manual wheelchair users there is a certain pride in their ability to be independent in their mobility without power.

The decision to transition to a power wheelchair is multifaceted, and a thorough assessment with empirical trials should be performed. The change to power may require a change of vehicle, changes in the home environment, and changes in some functional movement strategies. However, if the functional benefits of power mobility outweigh these detriments, then the changes can be successfully made. An example of a functional benefit is propulsion speed, or velocity. The average minimum speed necessary to safely cross a street intersection is 1.06 m/s.[88] If the individual cannot consistently propel a manual wheelchair at this minimal threshold despite the provision of appropriate equipment and optimal propulsion techniques, power mobility may be indicated.

New power wheelchair designs are smaller in overall width and turn radius, so often there are fewer environmental differences than might be expected. If the individual is well seated and comfortable in the manual wheelchair, then attempts should be made to replicate the sitting position in the new power equipment. Because of the multifaceted nature of this change to powered mobility and the potential for an emotional resistance to it, the process may take 6 months to a year. Generally, a slower, sequential approach will create the more positive outcome.

The Seating Interface

The selection of the cushion and backrest plays a significant role in contributing to the success of a mobility system for the individual with SCI. The cushion and backrest provide the direct interface between the individual and the mobility base. For this reason, the cushion and backrest combination are referred to as the seating interface. When the seating interface is appropriately selected and configured, the individual's ability to function from a wheelchair is optimized. While there are a myriad of seating interface products available, the components to be tested in empirical trials can be narrowed and final selection optimized when the individual's needs and the goals of the overall seating system are carefully considered. Impaired function as a result of paralysis, postural deformity, impaired sensation, altered skin integrity, and issues with pain and discomfort create challenges for long-term successful seating interventions. Results from a comprehensive evaluation will guide determination of appropriate seating interface products to be included in trials. Typically, the key goals for the seating interface for an individual with SCI are to (1) provide necessary postural support for proximal stability, (2) promote skin protection, (3) provide comfort, and (4) encourage optimal function. The relative priority for each of these goals is specific to each individual and must be considered when determining which seating products may be most appropriate. Skin protection is always a high priority for the wheelchair user with SCI because of the high risk of skin compromise due to the nature of the disability. However, when providing products that promote skin protection, it is essential to consider needs for postural support, comfort, and function. An understanding of the key features and considerations for different types of cushions and backrests and the necessary interaction between the two will assist the therapist in matching equipment to the client's individual needs and priorities.

Wheelchair cushions and backrests are commercially available in a broad range of materials, shapes, sizes, and configurations. They vary in degree of support and skin protection provided and span a wide spectrum of shapes and contour, from standard to highly customized. Without an attempt to individually review specific equipment, a discussion of the unique aspects of different types of products will guide the therapist's thought process for determining seating interface solutions to best meet the needs of an individual with SCI. In all cases, selection of the seating interface is unique and specific for each person.

Two key factors to consider when evaluating various seating interface products are materials and shape. The materials from which the product is constructed, combined with the shape of a given product, will guide determinations for postural support, stability for function, comfort, pressure and shear management, airflow and temperature characteristics, weight, and durability. Materials and shape also dictate how the interface product will function for the individual. The adjustability of cushions and backrests will differ depending on the materials used. It is also necessary to clearly understand and address the interface of the cushion with the backrest and the interaction of both with the mobility base. Selection of appropriate products combined with the proper orientation on the wheelchair is necessary for optimal outcomes when seating the individual with SCI.

Cushions

There are two primary approaches to cushion design for skin protection: the distribution of pressure across the sitting surface and the off-loading of high-risk bony prominences. Pressure distribution requires that the cushion materials and shape deform under load, which allows pressures to disperse across the entire sitting surface. A cushion designed for off-loading requires a firm material and specific shape that does not change under load in order to achieve the desired redirection of sitting forces.

A third, less common, design approach is the dynamic cushion. Alternating inflation cushions use a battery-powered motor that provides intermittent inflation to a series of air bladders. The air bladders are inflated and deflated sequentially, with the aim of decreasing the duration of sitting pressures to allow improved blood flow to the tissues of the sitting surface. While pressures on dynamic cushions have been measured to be very low during the deflation cycle, pressures during the inflation cycle increase significantly.[89] The benefit of dynamic cushions is intermittent reduction of pressure at different regions of the sitting surface. The significant concerns with the dynamic cushions are lack of seated stability, difficulty providing necessary postural supports, maintenance of the cushion, maintenance of the motor and battery, and increased weight added to the overall seating system. Koo et al. found that pressure management characteristics of an alternating inflation cushion were not as good as those of either air inflation or polyurethane foam cushions.[90]

Cushion selection should be highly individualized for each wheelchair user. A fundamental understanding of cushion materials and properties is necessary to guide clinical recommendations for cushion prescription. A wide variety of material is used in cushion construction. While some cushions are constructed of a single type of material, as in the case of single-density foam cushion or an air inflation cushion, many products use a combination of materials to achieve the desired outcome. Materials commonly used either alone or in combination include open cell foam, closed cell foam, viscoelastic foam, elastomer gels, viscous fluids, air, and flexible matrix thermoplastics.

Foam is a lightweight cellular material is characterized by density (weight per unit volume) and stiffness (resistance to deformation). Different types of foams are used for different applications based on the density and stiffness characteristics. For example, foams that are very stiff are typically used for base materials and for specific applications where the foam must hold its shape under load. Viscoelastic foam has both elastic and viscous properties that dictate that the foam will deform under load, and to the original shape when unloaded. The time required for the foam to return to the original shape is dependent upon properties of the foam (which change as the cushion ages), the amount of load, and the amount of time the load was in place. The benefits to foam cushions are that they are typically lightweight, are available in a wide range of thickness and contour, and require little maintenance. However, some foam cushions are difficult to keep clean, will retain odors, lose contoured shape under load, and require frequent replacement due to deterioration of materials. Foam cushions have been found to produce higher temperatures[91] as well as increased relative humidity associated with increased temperature.[92] Cushions constructed of a flexible honeycomb matrix formed by a fusion bonding process function in a manner similar to foam cushions. The thermoplastic cushions are lightweight, allow airflow for temperature and moisture management, require little maintenance, and are easy to clean. The flexible honeycomb matrix provides increased shear management. Incorporation of fluids in cushion fabrication is common.

A wide variety of viscous fluids, gels, and pastes, as well as water, are incorporated into cushion construction. While these fluids vary significantly from cushion to cushion, the general aim is to use the fluid as a means of distributing pressure around and away from bony prominences. Cushions that incorporate gels, pastes, or water typically provide elements of both postural support via a firm base and skin protection via load distribution. However, fluid cushions are typically heavier than foam or air cushions and have been shown to significantly increase humidity at the sitting surface due to perspiration.[92] The specific heat of a given fluid will influence skin temperature at the sitting surface.[93] Water has a high specific heat and is likely to increase skin temperature, whereas air has a low specific heat and therefore is not likely to increase skin temperature.

Air has characteristics similar to fluid and is used in cushions that are commonly prescribed for the client with SCI. Immersion of the buttocks into an air inflation cushion usually provides good distribution of pressures due to envelopment of the sitting surface. When compared to other cushions, air flotation cushions have demonstrated improved distribution of seated pressures.[94,95] Air inflation cushions typically control shear forces as the individual air cells move with the body. An element of shock absorption is another benefit to the air cushion. The primary concerns with the air inflation cushions are the required maintenance, with risk for puncture or valve dysfunction, difficulty determining and maintaining ideal inflation parameters, and inherent sitting instability. Most air inflation cushions now offer multichamber adjustments to improve postural support for deformity and to offer increased stability.

In addition to the materials used to construct the cushion, cushion shape must also be given critical consideration. When viewing the superior aspect of the cushion (top), cushions range from flat to highly contoured, with most falling somewhere in between. A number of studies have demonstrated that, compared to flat cushions, contoured cushions distribute pressure better[96–98] and allow improved functional skills such as reach.[99] The specific materials used play a key role in the shape as well as the function of a specific cushion. An understanding of what happens to the original shape when loaded by the individual is important. Is the original shape preserved? Does it remain rigid and maintain shape for stability? Or is it compressed to match individual contours (immersion)? Or compressed to the point that protection of bony prominences is compromised? The combination of materials and shape gives the overall specific characteristics of any given cushion. For example, the Jay 2 cushion is constructed with firm, nondeforming closed-cell foam, with specific contours for the pelvis and thighs used as a base support. A fluid and foam overlay over the firm base is used to provide skin protection properties when the client is immersed in the fluid, while preserving the base shape for stability. Understanding the interaction of materials with shape guides clinical reasoning for cushion trials and selection.

Immersion of the buttocks into the cushion defines the shape that the cushion will assume under load and therefore impacts the function of the cushion. One way to understand the concept of immersion is to think about how far the pelvis and legs will sink into the cushion when the cushion is loaded by body weight and how the cushion reacts to that load. Depending on the cushion construction, the amount of immersion varies widely. An air inflation cushion is designed to allow the body to sink into the cushion, this allows the cushion shape to conform to the body thereby increasing the area over which seating pressures are distributed. A firm cushion with contours is designed to preserve its shape under load, providing postural support. A cushion that has an initial flat shape is typically expected to conform to the body under load, while a firm cushion with highly specific contours is expected to maintain its shape under load so that the body conforms to the shape of the cushion.

When evaluating shapes of cushions, the orientation and degree of cushion contours must be considered relative to the individual client. The findings from a comprehensive client evaluation must be the basis for determining potential appropriate cushions for that individual. Based on the client evaluation, goals for the cushion are determined that will guide trials and selection. In general, an individual who sits with neutral alignment and symmetric orientation in all planes is most appropriately fitted with a cushion that will match that symmetry, whether by existing symmetric contours in the cushion or by immersion of the symmetric body into the cushion. Conversely, postural correction or accommodation requires a supportive material that will not deform under load. An individual who sits asymmetrically and has flexibility to tolerate correction toward neutral alignment requires a cushion that will provide the supportive correction and will maintain its shape under load so that the individual does not shift toward asymmetry. At the other end of the spectrum is the individual who sits asymmetrically and who does not have flexibility available to assume a more neutral orientation. In this case, the individual is usually best served with a cushion that accommodates the existing postural asymmetry, yet provides support to prevent further progression of the deformity. It is the composite angle of the wheelchair frame configuration and the cushion contours that dictate the posture and seated stability; therefore, care must be taken when prescribing new equipment. Trials are critical for integrating a new cushion with existing equipment.

Backrests

Backrest selection and configuration requires the same critical thought as that required for cushions. Based on the client evaluation and assessment, goals for the overall seating system will be identified and will guide clinical problem solving for the wheelchair backrest as well. Like cushions, backrests vary widely in materials, shape, and degree of adjustability and customization. Selection and orientation of the cushion and backrest must be coordinated in every seating system. The backrest must interface appropriately with the cushion and the mobility base in a specific orientation to provide support, comfort, and skin protection while promoting maximal function in the wheelchair. If the backrest is not addressed as an integral interaction with the cushion, the specific qualities of the chosen cushion may be lost. If the backrest is not optimally orientated relative to wheelchair, the performance of the entire system may be compromised.

Like cushions, the materials, construction, design, and functionality of backrests vary significantly for both manual and power wheelchairs. The broad categories for backrests are soft sling, planar, contoured, and custom. Backrest materials and shape will determine ability to provide postural support, stability for function, comfort, pressure and shear management, airflow and temperature characteristics, weight, and durability. Backrests have not been studied extensively in research settings.

Sling upholstery is the standard default backrest for most manual wheelchairs and some power wheelchairs. The advantages to sling upholstery are that it is low maintenance, low cost, and readily available. These backrests are also lightweight and add no bulk to the wheelchair, so that the chair is easier to transport. The greatest disadvantage to standard sling upholstery is that the material has a tendency to stretch over time, which can result in the compromise of postural support. An excellent upgrade from the standard sling upholstery, now available from most manufacturers, is the padded nylon sling that is tension adjustable by straps positioned posterior to the backrest. The series of tension-adjustable straps allow a fine-tuned fit to provide positional support for the pelvis, lumbar spine, and trunk. Additionally, maintenance of the strap tension preserves orientation of the backrest between the back posts and negates the effect of material stretch over time. It is critical that the adjustable tension backrest be appropriately padded with quality materials to avoid skin irritation and bruising from the straps. Several sling-style backrests also offer subtle lateral supports as well, which can assist with pelvis and trunk support. When properly configured, the adjustable-tension sling upholstery can be an appropriate device for the wheelchair user with SCI.

Linear backrests are commonly used in wheelchair configurations, particularly power wheelchairs. Linear backrests are either flat or curved, with a minimal lateral contour. They are typically constructed of a solid, strong base material such as plywood, metal, or a plastic composite and covered by a foam overlay. Subtle customization of the backrest shape is possible with the addition of lumbar padding and articulated lateral supports. Linear backrests are durable, and the provided strength is reliable for high-load situations such as that needed with a power tilt pressure relief. The linear backrests typically allow mounting of headrests and lateral positional supports. Installation of a linear backrest will usually result in a loss of effective seat depth. Because of the fixed configuration of the solid base, the linear backrest is most appropriate for those with neutral, symmetric sitting postures when appropriate trunk contours are provided, such as a lumbar support. Because human anatomical alignment is curved, not linear, most clients with SCI will be better served with a contoured backrest.

Contoured backrests are available in a wide range of material, size, shape, and adjustability. Contoured backrests are mounted to the back canes with a hardware interface. Some contoured backrests are lightweight, such as those constructed of carbon fiber, aluminum, or plastic composites. Others are quite heavy, especially when higher weight metals are used or articulation is incorporated in the backrest. When evaluating the weight of the backrest, it is imperative to consider the weight of the mounting hardware as well. Most contoured backrests have a symmetric lateral shape, with the degree of lateral contours highly variable in both height and depth. Most offer some degree of customization, such as addition of lumbar and trunk contouring by foam supports or additional mounted hardware. Many contoured backrests offer a great degree of adjustability in height, angle, and fore-aft positioning on the wheelchair, which is an advantageous feature for this type of backrest. Because the contoured backrests inherently have a firm, symmetric shape, they are appropriate for those individuals with good flexibility who can achieve and maintain trunk symmetry while sitting. Individuals who sit with trunk asymmetry in multiple planes may require a custom-molded backrest.

Custom-molded backrests are effective for providing specific postural support by strategic and precise contact with the trunk. Most custom backrests are constructed from an impression or mold of the individual in optimal orientation. When fit properly, the custom backrest provides the necessary support for posture and function. The increased contact area inherent to a custom backrest preserves skin integrity by improved pressure distribution and decreased shear forces. Because of the individualized support provided, the molded backrest functions most like a stabilizing orthosis, such as a TLSO (thoraco-lumbar-sacral orthosis, or "body jacket") used to stabilize the spine following acute SCI. A stabilizing orthosis is specifically intended to restrict or control movement. While the restrictive control is desirable in some seating cases where a molded system is indicated, it is imperative that the control provided does not impair function. Custom-molded backrests are most appropriate for individuals who require precise postural control to either correct a significant postural asymmetry or to prevent progression toward further deformity. Key considerations when evaluating custom-seating products are weight, materials used, interface with the cushion and mobility base, availability of adjustments and modifications, and relative cost.

Integration of the Cushion and Backrest

When evaluating seating interface products (cushions and backrests) for an individual with SCI, the availability of various sizes, adjustments, and modifications of a given product is important. Because the fit of the overall seating system is highly individualized and customized for each client, the seating interface products must allow for that individualized fit. Relative to cushion sizes, it is important to know that it is standard in the rehabilitation industry to refer to cushion dimensions as width first, followed by depth. For example, an 18 inch by 16 inch cushion is 18 inches wide and 16 inches deep, which is completely different from a cushion that is 16 inches by 18 inches. Backrest measurements are referenced first by width, then by height. Thus, a backrest that is 16 inches by 14 inches is 16 inches wide and 14 inches high. Some products are available in a selection of standard sizes only, while others are available in a wide range of combination sizes or can be modified by the manufacturer, or in the clinic, for a specific size. In most cases, it is not acceptable to compromise by using a standard dimension cushion as a default. For example, if the client evaluation reveals that the individual is best served with a 15-inch seat depth, the cushion should also be 15 inches deep. Compromise with a 16-inch-deep cushion may have a negative effect on seated position or function while compromise with a 14-inch-deep cushion may compromise positional support and skin protection. Similarly, if it is determined that an individual is best served with a 14-inch backrest height, compromise with use of a 16-inch backrest height is likely to result in impaired support and function.

The interaction of the cushion and backrest requires that the two components be addressed, both together and individually. The cushion selection and the backrest selection must complement each other. The cushion offers the platform for inferior aspect of the pelvis and posterior legs. The backrest is the support for the posterior pelvis and trunk. The cushion and backrest must be selected and oriented in such a way that there is an appropriate transition between the posterior aspect of the cushion and the inferior aspect of the backrest such that the seated individual is supported in the desired anatomical position. A compromised backrest orientation will negate the supportive qualities of the cushion.

Conversely, the backrest and cushion selections should also be addressed individually as there may be differences in needs between the two. Consider a woman with SCI to illustrate the need for different width in cushion and backrest support. Because of the natural female shape and distribution of body weight, a woman may require a backrest that is significantly more narrow than the cushion and wheelchair width. When indicated, the more narrow backrest must be provided. If not, she is likely to develop a postural asymmetry as a result of sitting with inadequate trunk support from a backrest that is too wide. Similarly, an individual with a pelvis narrower than his trunk must have a cushion that fits the pelvis, not the width of the backrest. In the case of an individual with flexible postural asymmetry, the process is to first address the pelvic obliquity. The individual may require a cushion that is adjustable, modified, or even customized in order to provide the necessary support under the pelvis. After the pelvis is addressed with an appropriate cushion, trunk symmetry is often achieved, which allows the individual to use a standard symmetric backrest. Only if more support is required would a modified or custom backrest be considered.

With contoured products, it is imperative to understand that the dimensions of the product must be fit to the client first, then to the wheelchair. Consider an obese individual with SCI to illustrate this point. With increased adipose tissue, the actual size of the skeleton does not change, but the overall body width does. Therefore, a man with a pelvis that is 16 inches wide using a contoured cushion requires a 16-inch-wide cushion so that the anatomical contours of the cushion match the body dimensions. However, since the adipose tissue exceeds the 16-inch width, the necessary wheelchair width may be 18 inches and the adipose tissue will exceed the 16-inch-wide cushion. In this case, the best solution is to prescribe a 16-inch-wide cushion custom modified to extend laterally for support of adipose tissue and to fill the space for the 18-inch wheelchair width. If an 18-inch-wide contoured cushion is used for a 16-inch-wide pelvis, the pelvis will be unsupported by the lateral cushion contours, which may result in skin compromise and lack of postural stability. This approach is also appropriate for an individual who sits with extreme pelvic obliquity and associated lateral trunk curvature. Positioning of a cushion under the pelvis may require a lateral extension on the side of the obliquity to fill the space for the required wheelchair width. With the challenges associated with the seated client with SCI, it is often necessary to adjust, modify, or customize a product to best meet the individual's needs. The availability and ease of customization, whether by the manufacturer or in the clinic, is a key consideration for equipment selection.

The selection as well as the orientation of interface products relative to the mobility base carries significant implications when seating the client with SCI. Each product must be considered not only relative to the interface with the client, but also how one product impacts the outcome of the overall system for the individual. For example, the height or thickness of the cushion plays a key role in wheelchair seat-to-floor height, footrest height, armrest height, clearance under tables, and transfers to varied surfaces. The orientation of the backrest must be considered relative to several aspects of the overall seating system. The angle and height of the backrest has implications for stability in a manual wheelchair. A backrest that is reclined causes a manual wheelchair to be unstable to the rear. A reclined backrest also allows the pelvis to rotate posteriorly, which shifts the pelvis forward on the cushion and creates an increased midthoracic kyphosis with cervical hyperextension. Ideally, the backrest must be high enough to provide adequate pelvic and lumbar support, yet low enough to allow normal thoracic curvature over the top of the backrest. This backrest orientation will maximize upper extremity function for propulsion and daily living tasks. A backrest that is too high compromises both posture and function. In a power wheelchair with a power tilt system, the backrest height must be high enough to support the individual when tilted. For power tilt users with shoulder function, the backrest should be shaped such that the center provides support for tilt while the lateral shape allows appropriate space for scapular mobility.

Pressure Mapping

Interface pressure mapping (IPM) is a clinical tool that, when used correctly, adds valuable information for seating interventions. IPM provides objective measurement with visual representation of the pressure between two objects or surfaces. In wheelchair-seating assessment, IPM measures the force applied by the client's sitting surface to the cushion and/or by the client's trunk against the backrest support.

The use of IPM has gained attention for seating the client with SCI due to the prevalence of pressure sores in this population. One goal of an appropriately configured seating system is to provide skin protection. For the client with SCI, evaluation and management of seated pressures is a mandatory consideration when addressing comprehensive seating system needs. A correlation between increased seated interface pressures and incidence of pressure ulcers has been demonstrated in published studies.[96,100]

An IPM system consists of a computer and monitor, the pressure-mapping software, the data collection sensor pad(s), an electronics unit, and a power source. The sensor pad is placed between the seated individual and corresponding surface. A digital color representation of interface pressures across the contact surface is displayed on the monitor. Software display options exist for viewing the pressure data, such as 2-dimensional with color isobar, 3-dimensional pressure contour, or with a numeric grid that reports the numeric pressure reading for each sensor cell. Additionally, pressure distribution histograms and pressure-versus-time graphs are available. The center of gravity can be displayed, as well as statistical information regarding average pressures across the sensor pad, peak pressure, and total contact area. The sensitivity of the sensor pad can be adjusted for more discerning evaluation. Some IPM systems allow wireless programmed recording of IPM data that is downloaded for evaluation once the recording session is complete. Ideally, pressure mapping in dynamic conditions should be incorporated into clinical practice as investigations have shown that seated pressures increase during wheelchair propulsion.[101,102]

IPM is commonly used for relative comparison of seating interventions and equipment assessment. Following a comprehensive client evaluation, changes in wheelchair configuration and/or cushion trials are attempted, with the goal of improving postural alignment and/or distribution of pressure. Since neutral, symmetric sitting posture typically best distributes pressure, seating interventions to optimize posture should precede pressure management strategies. Published research has demonstrated that interface pressures are influenced by seated postures.[62,90] Typically, a baseline IPM measurement is taken and compared to measurements following adjustment of the seating system (an *intervention*) by an experienced therapist. In most cases, the desired result is to decrease pressure at a region of concern or to ensure that pressures have not been increased. IPM is beneficial for measuring the presence, location, and distribution of pressure, and it is also valuable for demonstrating the absence of contact or complete off-loading of a body surface. IPM is useful for evaluating the influence of specific wheelchair configuration adjustments, as well as the client's pressure picture on different cushions and backrests. When combined with other essential assessment factors such as comfort, postural support, functional skills, and skin inspection, IPM data is helpful in assisting with equipment selection and configuration. It is recommended that a clinical IPM protocol be adopted for the collection and interpretation of data. A standard international protocol for IPM would assist with identifying reliable practices for collecting and interpreting IPM data, but this is not currently available.

IPM is also a powerful education tool. It is particularly useful when used as a component of client training for effective pressure relief. With the client seated on the sensor pad, he or she can watch the pressure map display on the monitor for visual feedback to determine the effectiveness of a pressure relief effort. IPM is valuable for therapist education as well. When used properly, IPM is used to confirm or deny a clinical hypothesis. For example, when the hands-on evaluation reveals that a client sits with a pelvic obliquity, higher pressures are expected under the lower ischial tuberosity, which can be confirmed with pressure mapping. The therapist can use IPM in conjunction with palpation to confirm postural alignment and the location of bony prominences.

IPM can also be used to guide modifications to existing equipment. When the IPM display indicates a high-pressure area for a seated individual, palpation of the sensing mat at its outside margins allows a grid to be determined, with markings on the cushion to specifically locate the high-pressure area under the seated person.

This allows the cushion to be modified at the precise problem area, as determined by coordinate markings, once the individual transfers out of the wheelchair.

IPM has several valuable clinical uses; however, the limitations of this technology must be considered as well. Understanding how *not* to use the technology guides the therapist in using pressure mapping as one appropriate "tool."

Pressure Mapping Does Not Stand Alone. IPM serves as an adjunct to the comprehensive evaluation with hands-on assessment, including skin inspection. IPM alone does not provide adequate information to guide clinical decision making.

Pressure Mapping Measures Interface Pressures Only. The sensors measure force applied, in a vertical dimension, by the client to the sitting surface. Key factors that are not measured by IPM are capillary pressure, tissue perfusion, and shear forces.

Pressure Mapping Cannot Substitute for Skin Inspection. Skin inspection is mandatory for all seating evaluations and interventions. If there is an area of high pressure, the skin will redden or have evidence of breakdown at that site. If the pressures are well distributed and there are no areas of excess pressure, the skin will not be discolored. Skin inspection reveals areas of scars from previous skin compromise and surgeries. Palpation of the skin and underlying tissue will reveal alteration of normal tissue integrity that may indicate pressure-related problems beneath the skin.

Pressure Mapping Does Not Substitute for Knowledge of Equipment Options. IPM should not be used to "guess" at a potential seating intervention. Professionals providing seating intervention must possess comprehensive knowledge of equipment options and available adjustments. Identification of specific client needs narrows the field of equipment choices that are then appropriate to be "mapped" for supplemental information.

Pressure Maps Cannot Be Generalized. While IPM adds important information about a specific individual sitting on a particular surface, the information cannot be generalized to other people. The same cushion usually maps very differently under different people because each individual has unique sitting positions, anatomical orientation, and tissue integrity.

Pressure Maps Never Negate the Need for Pressure Relief. Even with the best possible pressure map, individuals with SCI must continue to perform consistent pressure relief with complete off-load of the sitting surface.

Pressure mapping is a valuable tool for measuring interface pressures for the client with SCI. When used judiciously as an adjunct tool in the evaluation and intervention process for wheelchair seating interventions, IPM provides objective information that is useful for decreasing the risk of debilitating pressure ulcers.

Pulling it Together: Evaluation for Seating Systems

Evaluation

Successful seating system prescription requires that a qualified therapist or team of professionals complete a comprehensive evaluation of the wheelchair user. Individuals who may be involved in the evaluation or sharing of information include the client, the family and/or caregivers, the physician, physical therapist, occupational therapist, recreation therapists, and/or other members of the health-care team. Regardless of length of time since SCI, the following information is critical for prescribing a seating system that will result in optimal outcomes.

Medical Background

Pertinent information regarding medical issues can be obtained from medical record review combined with a client interview. Age, length of time since SCI, and American Spinal Injury Association (ASIA) scores with indication of upper motor neuron (UMN) versus lower motor neuron (LMN) damage provide important information. ASIA scores combined with a documented course of rehabilitation and time since injury indicate prognosis for recovery of function. Body morphology—height, weight, and body type—should be investigated relative to preinjury body build and course of weight fluctuation since injury. Individuals typically lose significant weight following the initial injury and often gain weight back to baseline or beyond their "walking weight" following initial rehabilitation. Those with LMN injuries will typically atrophy significantly in their lower bodies in the first several years with SCI. Those who gain weight will often carry the weight in the trunk and upper body, with loss of tissue mass in the buttocks and legs. Current and past medical history should be reviewed with attention to respiratory issues, cardiac function (with review of circulation and blood pressure management), and metabolic disorders. Critical attention must be paid to secondary issues associated with SCI, including spasticity, pain, skin compromise, and orthopedic complications such as heterotopic ossification and hip subluxation or dislocation. The review of past surgical history includes investigation of the extent and nature of spinal stabilization and history of surgical interventions for wound management.

Physical Assessment

A thorough physical examination is mandatory when evaluating for the seating system. The basic clinical evaluation skills learned in entry-level professional programs are invaluable for adding critical information to comprehensive assessment. Passive range of motion (PROM) measures and flexibility testing identify limitations in body motion that can have significant implications for postural alignment and support in the seating system. Strength evaluation determines which muscles are innervated and available for functional use and which are in need of strengthening. Evaluation of muscle tone and reflexes provides information about optimal orientation in the seating system to inhibit undesired involuntary responses. Assessment of sensation is critical for determining needs for skin protection and tolerance of external supports. Examination of the skin at the sitting surface and trunk details current issues with compromised skin and past issues indicated by scar tissue. Respiratory functional assessment in various positions indicates potential positions for optimal ventilation. Measurements of body dimensions and leg lengths are also specifically considered relative to seating system prescription.

A comprehensive postural evaluation is a key component of the physical assessment. When combined with the physical measurements above, postural presentation indicating the body's reactions to gravity guides the therapist's approach for configuring the seating system as an orthotic device. Observation of the individual in three circumstances is recommended: sitting in existing mobility system, short-sitting on a firm mat with minimized external support, and supine on a firm mat. Transitioning the individual from sitting in the wheelchair to sitting on the mat indicates how the current wheelchair impacts the client's postural presentation. Sitting on the firm mat without support provides information on the body's natural reaction to gravity. While sitting on the mat, we expect an individual with full or partial trunk paralysis to assume a position of posterior pelvic tilt with lumbar and thoracic flexion to achieve stability against gravity. In this position, key information about trunk flexibility into flexion and extension can be assessed with manual contacts and passive movement into available ranges of motion. After sagittal plane current and potential alignment is understood, the extent of frontal plane asymmetry, such as a pelvic obliquity, can be assessed. Observation of the individual's alignment in the supine position eliminates the influence of gravity. Trunk and lumbopelvic flexibility testing in three planes, combined with the passive range-of-motion (PROM) evaluation, indicates the body's ability to assume a neutral postural presentation with manual facilitation. This information is then used to guide initial simulation of seating system configuration to provide control that is needed and can be tolerated in the upright sitting position.

When documenting the postural evaluation, a simple sketch is an efficient way to represent the information gathered from palpation and observation as a supplement to written text. Figure 8-6a–c illustrates schematic examples of how a postural evaluation may be documented. Figure 8-6a illustrates neutral alignment in the frontal plane, which is the desired seating goal; Figures 8b and 8c show pelvic obliquity and a "windswept posture," respectively, common deviations from neutral postures.

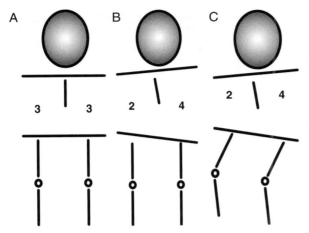

Figure 8-6. Schematic documentation of postural evaluation. In the simple diagram, the circle represents the head, the superior horizontal line represents the shoulders, and the lower horizontal line represents the pelvis. The short vertical line below the shoulder line represents the orientation of the sternum. The numbers indicate the space between the top of the iliac crest and the lowest rib. The actual number references how many of the therapist's fingers fit in that space. The vertical lines below the pelvis line show the alignment of the upper and lower legs. (A) The desired neutral posture, wherein the individual is well aligned. (B) Pelvic obliquity, wherein one hemipelvis is elevated with respect to the other. (C) Windswept posture, wherein pelvic rotation results in malalignment of the legs, trunk, and shoulders.

In general, *correction* is attempted for postural deviations found to be flexible, while *accommodation* is the approach for fixed alignments. There is also an important sequence to postural correction. The sagittal plane must be corrected first. The architecture of the spinal column is such that in a more flexed position there is more medial-lateral play, as well as more play in frontal plane rotation; therefore, improper sequence can result in overcorrection of a frontal plane deviation. It is also critical to understand that there are few postural deformities that are truly fixed, as most will progress with time toward further deformity unless appropriate stabilizing supports are incorporated in the seating system. Whether an individual has had a recent SCI or is a longstanding wheelchair user, the information from the physical examination, including the postural evaluation, is critical for determining ideal seating system parameters. Table 8-3 shows critical physical measures that influence seating configuration.

Equipment Evaluation

Examination of equipment currently being used provides important information relative to the individual's physical presentation. Attention should be directed toward the mobility system configuration, specifically to the seat dimension, seat slope, backrest configuration, and frame design (including front frame or footrest orientation). The cushion and backrest are evaluated for supportive and protective qualities. The presence of additional external supports provides insight into prior attempts to provide postural stability. The accessories on the existing wheelchair, such as friction-coated handrims or anti-tip bars on a manual wheelchair, may indicate functional limitations. Patterns of wear on wheelchair components and cushions provides key information for the client's typical postural alignment in the wheelchair, functional habits, and mobility strategies. Pressure mapping, described earlier in this chapter, provides objective information regarding body contact with the existing system that can be useful during the evaluation process.

Psychosocial Profile

The wheelchair user's cultural background, cognition, education level, behaviors, preferences, and social support systems (friends, family, caregivers) may carry significant implications for the seating system prescription. Some individuals may have strong preferences for equipment configuration or may have specific requirements based on priorities for appearance or functional needs in specific environments. Others, especially those with more recent SCI or with cognitive impairment, may rely heavily on the therapists recommendations for equipment selections. In all cases, the therapist must respectfully communicate with the individual, allowing the client to participate in the process to his or her comfort level. A thorough psychosocial review will assist with determining appropriate seating system configuration.

Functional Assessment

Discussion and observation of the client's movement strategies indicates the extent of impaired mobility and associated compensations that allow optimal function. Relative to seating needs, the functional exam includes observation of balance strategies and coordination relative to wheelchair propulsion or driving patterns, transfer techniques, pressure relief methods, and self-care strategies such as dressing and bladder management. It is important to investigate functional performance beyond the clinical setting, which gives a more realistic view of the client's situation. For example, frequent transfers to varied heights may impact selection of wheelchair seat heights. Asymmetric repetitive actions, such as consistently reaching toward one side, may have implications for postural presentations such as pelvic obliquity with scoliosis. Observation of movement skills and habits, combined with expectations for functional outcomes based on level of injury and ASIA Impairment Scale (AIS) scores, guides determination of wheelchair needs to encourage optimized function. Additionally, areas for needed education and training can be identified to encourage maximized functional potential while preventing injuries associated with long-term disability.

Table 8-3
Critical Measures that Influence Seating Configuration

Passive Range of Motion Limitation	Component Affected
Hip flexion without posterior pelvic tilt (measure hip only not allowing spine motion)	Need to accommodate range if less than that needed for seat-to-back inside angle (drop the front of seat toward floor whenever possible instead of reclining backrest).
	Unilateral hip flexion limitation will create a low contralateral pelvis; accommodate the flexion limitation to correct the obliquity.
Hip extension without anterior pelvic tilt (measure hip only, not allowing spine motion).	Accommodate hip flexor contracture to decrease lordotic pull (steep seat slope).
Inside hamstring length with hip flexed at 90 degrees (or intended seat-to-back inside angle).	Front frame or footrest drop angle should be tighter and placement of pivot point closer (accommodates the hamstring tightness to avoid posterior pelvic tilt).

Environmental Profile

The anticipated various environments in which the mobility system will be used must be thoroughly explored. The climate in which the individual lives may impact the selection and configuration of seating system components. Most individuals with SCI will use their wheelchair both indoors and outdoors. The transitions must be evaluated, as many ramped doorways will have a significant sill or threshold, and landings may have limited space with an outward swinging door. Indoor settings almost always include carpet and tight spaces for wheelchair negotiation. Outdoor terrain includes slopes in all directions, uneven surfaces, and architectural barriers. When prescribing a new wheelchair, it is important to address dimensions and limitations in the home and work settings as well as other places frequented. It is important to ask the individual where he or she spends time in a given week or month.

Transportation

Methods of transportation must also be critically assessed relative to wheelchair recommendations. Functional skills and exploration of whether the individual will use a personally owned vehicle or public transportation must be carefully considered. With personally owned vehicles, some manual wheelchair users will transfer to the driver's seat, independently stow the wheelchair, and drive independently with adaptive driving controls. In some instances the wheelchair will be stowed in a trunk or rear compartment of a vehicle.

Power wheelchair users will require either a ramp or lift to enter and exit the vehicle. Some manual wheelchair users also choose this option. Thus, compatibility between the individual's wheelchair and the vehicle to be used must be considered. Some power wheelchair users will transfer to the vehicle driver's seat, some will drive the vehicle from their wheelchair, and others will stay in their wheelchair to be transported as a nondriving passenger. Most who use public transportation will stay in their wheelchair and access the vehicle via a lift or ramp. Regardless of the vehicle, when an individual is transported in a wheelchair, proper support in the wheelchair must be provided and an appropriate occupant restraint (vehicle mounted) and wheelchair tie-down system must be used.

Seating system prescription necessitates a comprehensive evaluation for all clients, whether a first-time or long-standing wheelchair user. Those with long-standing SCI typically will provide more comprehensive information and often have firm preferences. While the newly injured individual without significant medical complications typically presents as symmetric and flexible, it is nonetheless important to document the comprehensive evaluation to have a baseline for future follow-up. The first-time wheelchair user can greatly benefit from the education gained during the evaluation process. Discussion of findings, review of available equipment options, and mobility techniques education will empower individuals to understand their body and take responsibility for their choices and actions.

Equipment Selection

Proper selection of a wheelchair requires consideration of the needs of the user, both the postural and functional needs, was well as the demands on the functions of the wheelchair. The postural evaluation provides the information on the orthotic requirements of the equipment. Through the postural evaluation, the therapist can establish the parameters needed for the wheelchair set up.

Clinical decision making about equipment should follow a systematic pathway as represented in the schematic in Figure 8-7. Specifically, the requirements for seat slope, inside seat-to-backrest angle, and the height of the backrest should be determined. This resembles the process of determining what features a lower extremity orthosis must provide to the individual after the examination and gait evaluation. The therapist creates a list of requirements and client-specific needs that must be met by the wheelchair design.

Once the therapist has determined the orthotic requirements of the equipment, this information is combined with the functional demands of the equipment in terms of both mobility and lifestyle function requirements for the individual. At this point, the therapist is ready to select equipment for empirical trials.

The client should only try equipment that is appropriate. This means that a list of equipment should be generated based on the clinical judgment of the therapist. This list should not include any equipment that will not meet the client's needs, nor should it include equipment that is not needed. The therapist must be certain that the need for all components of equipment that are offered for trial can be justified. The therapist must determine the equipment that will meet the *needs* of the individual and select only from this subset of equipment for a trial. A trial in an ultralight manual wheelchair with a suspension shock system and off-road mountain bike tires for a user who requires friction-coated handrims and anti-tip devices is a misfit. Similarly, consideration of a power wheelchair with a large wheelbase and maximum torque settings for an individual who is expected to drive only indoors and on paved surfaces is inappropriate.

Equipment trials are very important and often not done due to time constraints or lack of access. Every attempt should be made to provide trials. If the trials are done after the stepwise assessment, there should be only a limited number of options. A client should have the opportunity to try different makes and models of equipment (from the subset of those appropriate for his or her

needs) and select the one that best meets his or her tastes or preferences.

It is imperative to do trials correctly. The trials must be a comparison of "apples to apples." Therefore, each wheelchair must be appropriately configured for the postural support needs and best push mechanics or drive mechanics of the individual, and all the wheelchairs used in the trial should be set up the same. The more specific the postural needs of the individual, the more important it will be to set up the wheelchairs in the *same* configuration so that a true comparison can be made. If the therapist simply does not have access to the specific equipment the client wishes to purchase, the therapist should attempt to simulate the features of the target equipment with the equipment that is available.

Trials should be guided by the therapist and therefore limited to the wheelchairs that meet the medical/postural and environmental/functional needs of the client. When there is no difference in the performance of the equipment, personal preference should be considered, as well as cost. When there is no difference in the cost of the equipment, considerations such as service record or time-to-delivery may be made. A particular make and model should be selected prior to measuring for the wheelchair. If equipment selection follows this careful algorithm, with documentation accompanying all decisions, then it will be easy to medically justify the final equipment (Fig. 8-8).

The properly prescribed and fitted seating system (wheelchair and interface) will support optimal posture and function. For the first seating system, this prescription should be completed with knowledge of the individual's potential function. There is no justification for compromise on the first wheelchair. The therapist is encouraged not to prescribe a more stable or less dynamic wheelchair just because it is a first wheelchair. Such a wheelchair will limit, and perhaps block, the acquisition of functional skills. Regardless of length of time since onset of SCI, manual wheelchair users should be provided with a wheelchair that may be customized to

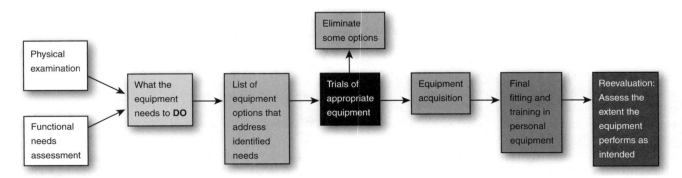

Figure 8-7. Flow diagram of clinical decision making in wheelchair prescription. Selection of equipment, wheelchair components, and configuration follows a systematic pathway. In each step, the therapist documents the requirements and the specifications required to meet these requirements.

Date:
Patient:
Physician:
Therapist:
Vendor:

Letter of Justification

To Whom It May Concern:

Client is a 63-year-old woman who has been a full-time manual wheelchair user since 1980 when she sustained a T9 incomplete SCI. Client has nonfunctional lower extremity motor control with some sensory sparing. She cannot ambulate for any distance; she cannot stand. She independently uses an ultralight manual wheelchair for all mobility when out of bed; she transfers to and from this wheelchair independently with a lateral lift transfer with full weight bearing on her upper extremity. Client complains of fatigue with excessive distance pushing and difficulty with stowing her current wheelchair into her car.

Client is currently using a manual wheelchair that is not appropriate for her postural or functional needs. Additionally, her current wheelchair is approximately eight years old making acquisition of parts impossible. The current equipment: Kuschall 3000 ST (rated K0005) manual wheelchair and a ~2-inch foam cushion (very compressed).

Client reports shoulder pain with stowing this wheelchair into her car (into passenger front seat of 2-door car). She also has difficulty with independent propulsion up steeper inclines and controlling steep descent. These difficulties are due to the weight of the current wheelchair and the lack of postural stability, which will be corrected by customized postural support incorporated into the frame parameters of a new wheelchair. Client is unable to functionally propel a lightweight or standard manual wheelchair due to the weight of the chairs and the limited positioning options.

Home environment: Primary residence is on rural 40 acres. Secondary (new) residence is a condominium in city—not an ADA accessible unit with some limitations in bathroom access. The primary residence is rural requiring daily transfers into the car to access any enterainment or essentials such as groceries.

With the current equipment, Client presents with the following postural problems: pelvic obliquity and frontal plane scoliosis, mild forward head and thoracic kyphosis, poorly controlled lower extremities. She reports some postural pain with prolonged sitting in the wheelchair. Client is 5'3" and ~135 pounds. She reports a history of multiple tendon releases secondary to siginificant spasticity and muscle shortening.

Client requires a new custom ultralight manual wheelchair. The specific equipment requested is a [*Name the exact make and model*] custom-specified titanium wheelchair with the following custom specifications:

• Custom-sized seat with tapering to accommodate the disparate hip to distal thigh width
• 14-inch seat depth to accommodate her short stature and lower extremity contractures
These features are not available in a K0004 chair.
• Custom backrest with tapering, rotation, and adjustable tension upholstery to accommodate disparate hip to back width and thoracic scoliosis
This feature is not available in a K0004 chair.
• Reinforced backrest rigidizer bar to support use as a handhold for physical assistance up and down stairs **for emergency egress from nonaccessible venues** (engineered to support body weight rather than just provide rigidity to back)
• Custom rear axle placement and frame parameters including seat to floor at front and rear and footrest drop angle to optimize postural support and provide for functional stability
4-inch difference front to rear with a 14-inch seat depth is not available on a K004 chair.
• Angle adjustable footplate to provide for accommodation of plantarflexion contractures and significant lower extremity spasticity
• Scissor wheel locks to provide safety for transfers while having no lock parts obstructing wheelchair propulsion or interfering with transfer providing skin safety for hands, posterior thigh, and buttocks
• Rigid side guards to augment the pelvic control by centering cushion and rider in the wheelchair

This wheelchair is significantly lighter than her current wheelchair (~30%); a lighter wheelchair will benefit Client in terms of maintaining the ability to independently stow the wheelchair into the car. Client has been a manual wheelchair user for more than 20 years and there is evidence to support an increase in shoulder pain and degeneration in spinal cord–injured persons greater than 15 years post-injury, therefore protecting the shoulder joint from biomechanical stress is a focus of preventative health care.

The dampening inherent in a titanium wheelchair should help decrease her current lower extremity spasticity especially the ankle clonus as well as decrease her low-back pain. If spasticity is a hyperactive stretch response; the innate reflexive contration that is caused by a quick stretch to the muscle spindle is hyper-responsive due to the motor neuron condition created by the client's spinal cord injury at the level of T9. Spasiticity is elevated by noxious stimulus anywhere in the body, thus a urinary tract infection or an ingrown toenail can elevate spasticity. Any physiologic pain, even if unperceived by the individual secondary to the interruption of spinal pathways, can elevate spasticity in an individual with an upper motor neuron syndrome. Titanium is a metal with natural shock-dampening characteristics, thus decreasing the stimulus to the muscle spindle and decreasing the expression of spasticity. The general increased ride comfort created by the characteristics of the material decrease stress to the body including weight-bearing seated surfaces and the lower back. The ultralight feature of the overall chair decreases the biomechanical stress of wheelchair propulsion. Any or all of the above can combine to decrease the expression of hypertonicity.

Her primary postural needs are for a custom wheelchair to fit her small stature and disparate hip-to-trunk measurements and scoliosis. Seat slope characteristics will accommodate hip flexion contractures while custom frame features will ensure lower extremity control and stability on inclines. Frontal plane corrections/accommodations are needed after sagittal plane is established and will likely be achieved through a modified cushion but will be augmented with the control from the custom backrest.

The patient has had successful trials in a wheelchair mocked up to meet most of the custom specifications.

I will be happy to answer any questions you have regarding this request. Thank you for your timely attention to this matter. I can be reached by phone at [*contact #*] or email: wherever@some.com

Sincerely,
Jennifer Hastings PT, PhD, NCS

Attachments: Wheelchair specifications, Drawings of specified wheelchair

Figure 8-8. Sample letter of justification. The letter details the specific requirement of the client to substantiate the need for the various components identified by the therapist.

the individual and that is constructed with high-strength, lightweight materials as supported by accepted clinical practice guidelines.[6] In most cases, a rigid manual wheelchair is the appropriate selection for the SCI person who will independently propel the chair. The wheelchair should be custom configured to support posture through pelvic stabilization, which is built into the frame parameters and enhanced by the selected cushion and backrest interface. The options on the wheelchair should be selected based on functional needs as determine by lifestyle and abilities (current and potential). The power wheelchair system should likewise be optimized to provide the best possible postural support and the overground mobility necessary to meet the requirements of the individual's lifestyle with only the required power and seat functions. The clinical tendency in power is to overprescribe. The pressures of believing that there is "one shot" with third-party payers have led to too many functions being provided in a first wheelchair. The therapist should remember to prescribe based on needs, both postural and functional. When the individuals are "overstabilized" or "overprovided" with function, their potential for functional and neurological recovery is truncated. New equipment for the long-term user should never decrease function. The desired outcome is that the new equipment enhances abilities. In the delivery of new equipment, the individual should be assessed for just that. Functional skills should be checked out as a component of the final fitting. All habitual transfers should be evaluated; the ability to independently maneuver in a usual manner, including the use of wheelies and jumping curbs, etc., should be checked during delivery of the final system. Both vehicle access for power mobility systems and stowing the wheelchair into the vehicle for manual systems need to be specifically evaluated. It is likely that some fine-tuning of the setup may be needed to optimize posture and function.

Fitting and Education

Issue and Fit Process

Clearly, a significant investment of time, money, and brainpower is associated with determining the appropriate seating system for an individual with SCI. Perhaps the most important component in providing a seating system takes place when the final products are delivered to the client. The bottom line is that seating system products will not work optimally in the form in which they arrive from the manufacturer. It is the configuration, adjustment, and customized fitting to the individual that allows prescribed products to work for the client. The following is a proposed framework for fitting a seating system once prescribed products have been received:

- Review the products received: check measurements, orientation, and configuration to ensure that what was prescribed is what was actually received. The therapist should not settle for anything less than what was

ordered. An inaccurate dimension or configuration typically carries significant negative implications for the client and must be rectified prior to scheduling the client for equipment fitting.
- Arrange for the complete seating system to be assembled and operational before the client arrives for the fitting and adjustment process.
- Get in the wheelchair and push it or drive it to rule out any problems (such as tracking or instability issues) before the client arrives.
- Following general assembly, adjustments and a fine-tuned fit to the individual make all the difference in the world. A general guideline for a sequence of adjustments once the client has been positioned in the seating system follows:

1. Check basic fit, with cushion, backrest, and accessories in place.
2. Adjust the backrest angle.
3. Adjust backrest height.
4. Adjust footrest height.
5. Adjust accessory supports.
6. Adjust rear wheel position (manual wheelchair skills).
7. Set up the drive control; install switches, and program parameters to maximize control in all settings (power wheelchairs).
8. Check wheelchair skills and maneuverability in varied environments and terrain.
9. Further adjust seating system as needed.
10. Perform pressure mapping and skin inspection to identify concerns.
11. Further adjust seating system as needed.
12. Provide comprehensive education.

Client Education

Throughout the process of evaluation and provision of seating system interventions, client education must be an integrated theme. The amount, extent, and content of the actual education provided varies depending on the length of time the individual has been a wheelchair user, the strength of his or her preferences, and the willingness to consider new concepts and technology.

With the issuance of definitive seating system equipment, the following education topics should be addressed with the client.

- Review of proper seating system configuration (e.g., cushion orientation)
- Basic equipment operation and safety
- Maintenance recommendations
- Push mechanics (manual) or driving strategies (power) for efficiency and injury prevention
- Review of transfers to and from the wheelchair to varied surfaces
- Recommendations for pressure relief and skin protection
- Stow techniques into a vehicle (manual) or driving strategies to access a van or public transportation (manual or power)

In addition to education specific to equipment management and mobility, several topics should be addressed with all wheelchair users. Activity of daily living (ADL) techniques must be emphasized to minimize the risk of upper extremity injury while performing functions from a wheelchair. Fitness, weight management, and general wellness strategies should be encouraged to promote lifelong health. Appropriate stretching, strengthening, and conditioning exercises can be prescribed to encourage optimal function while preventing injury. It is typically appropriate to stretch the anterior chest and shoulder musculature and strengthen the posterior shoulder, trunk, and intrascapular muscles as needed, depending on the client's presentation. Comprehensive client education empowers individuals to take responsibility for their own body, to make informed decisions, and to live a healthy and balanced life despite reliance on a wheelchair for mobility.

Outcomes

Seating interventions must be documented with outcome measures. Objective goals for the seating system will help determine the appropriate outcome measure. If the goal is to improve functional endurance with a lighter wheelchair that has less roll resistance, then the therapist should document the current ability. Timing the ability to maneuver an obstacle course or a 6-minute push test (the wheeled mobility equivalent of the 6-minute walk test) are appropriate assessments. Include a perceived exertion score[103] after completing the mobility test. Vital signs may also be helpful for documenting the heart rate or respiratory rate after propulsion in persons with SCI below T6.

Document the same measure in the ultralight wheelchair. If the therapist can do this during trials, the information provides the evidence to support the letter of justification. The therapist must be sure to document these measures as an outcome in the definitive equipment chosen.

First wheelchairs are prescribed based on the evidence in the literature. For instance, the current evidence supports the fact that the individual with SCI is best served in an ultralight manual wheelchair made from high-strength, lightweight material with customized configuration for optimal posture and push mechanics.[6] New equipment for seating, whether it be a complete system, a mobility base, or an interface component (backrest or cushion), must also have goals and outcome measures.

If the goal of the intervention is postural support, then the therapist should objectively document current posture. Photographs and anatomical measures such as rib-to-iliac clearance, sternal angle off vertical, and seated height are recommended for preintervention and postintervention documentation. These measures will show that posture was indeed changed with the new seating configuration.

Whether or not the postural change matters to the individual is best documented with a subjective or patient-reported outcome scale. The Posture Scale for Wheelchair Users was developed to assess the wheelchair users perception of seated posture (see Appendix). In a pilot study, this measure showed good face validity, concurrent validity, and good internal consistency (reliability).[104]

If the client's complaint was musculoskeletal pain and the postural intervention was directed at the postural contribution to mechanical pain, then the therapist will want to use a measure such as the Wheelchair User's Shoulder Pain Index[105,106] to document change in pain.

If the seating intervention was directed at skin issues, the therapist will need objective measures such as pressure mapping, as well as frequency, severity, and location of skin concerns. These measures should be documented preintervention and postintervention.

Functional ability in a wheelchair can be affected by seating. If the seating intervention is directed at functional improvement, an outcome measure of function may be appropriate. One such measure is the Functioning Evaluation in a Wheelchair (FEW) measure.[107] Additional outcome measures specific to wheelchair skills are the Wheelchair Circuit[108,109] and the Wheelchair Skills Test.[110,111]

Seating for SCI as Lifelong Disability

One of the goals of early proper postural support through appropriate seating prescription is to avoid negative sequelae. Many of the common secondary complications associated with SCI are preventable, and proper postural support is critical to prevention.

However, even with the best initial prescription based on the thorough postural and functional evaluation delineated earlier in this chapter, it is necessary to monitor posture and seating throughout the client's lifetime. The reasons are many. One aspect is the growing knowledge of rehabilitation science and evolving technology in equipment. With time, rehabilitation science pertaining to seating is getting better. We have increased our knowledge of postural interaction with the upper limb mechanics, and we will continue to investigate postural interactions with other health outcomes. Equipment will continue to evolve, offering more possibilities with design features and perhaps more advantages in new materials. Another reason is that people are dynamic. They are not static in their life interests, social roles, or functional needs. These changes may therefore change the requirements of their equipment. Physically, people are not static either. With aging, all people will change physiologically. There is a change in tissue structure with aging. Bones tend to decrease in density, muscles tend to atrophy, fat distribution changes, and skin loses its elasticity. With SCI, all of these changes continue to occur and some at an accelerated pace.[112] There are physiologic changes in organ function with aging as well. Generally, there is a decrease in systematic circulation, loss of vital capacity in lung function, and a slowing of gastrointestinal and urologic functions. Again, all of these changes occur with SCI as well, and most at an accelerated rate.

For seating, these changes may be reflected most in the requirements for skin protection. The loss of muscle tissue and subcutaneous fat combined with a decrease in skin elasticity and decreased circulation increases the risk of skin breakdown. The physiologic changes with aging often drive functional and lifestyle changes in the general population, and this is no different for individuals with SCI. Again, this may occur at a more rapid rate, and thus the functional needs and the abilities must be frequently monitored to determine whether they indicate a change in equipment. Unfortunately, not every individual with SCI was afforded the best postural support early after injury and therefore may have acquired postural deformities that need to be corrected (if possible) or accommodated through seating prescription. Because many of these deformities have developed progressively over years, it is common that individuals slowly and progressively accommodate their functional techniques to their physical capacities. It is imperative that a seating therapist who is evaluating an individual with long-standing SCI be very careful and thorough in the evaluation of the functional strategies and how the current equipment interfaces with the individual's functional movement strategies. Habits are hard to break, and function is a very strong motivator. The therapist evaluates function as a component of seating intervention to ensure that the chair supports function and the particular movement habits that work best for the individual. The intervention may be needed for skin health or postural alignment, but if function is lost, it will not be successful (and if the individual has the option they will discard the new system). Pain is the only motivator stronger than function, so unless the individual has pain that goes away after a seating intervention, the intervention will be declined if function is threatened.

Some examples of well-intended but failed interventions:

Prescription: A new ultralight titanium folding manual wheelchair to an individual with paraplegia who is 20 years post-injury.
Goals: Increased mobility with better push mechanics in lighter adjustable equipment
Justification: Shoulder pain and aging.

Reason for Failure:

1. The transfer technique was to put the feet up on the surface being transferred to; the new wheelchair would tip rearward with this activity.
2. The wheelchair stow habit was behind the front passenger seat. The new wheelchair did not fold to be narrow enough and required the rear wheels to be removed.

In this example both of the functional habits had the potential to be changed in order to successfully use the new wheelchair. The client should have been evaluated for the potential for, and interest in, learning new techniques for both transfer and wheelchair stowing. It is important to remember that functional techniques often evolve out of progressive physical impairments. In this case, the individual had significantly overstretched hamstrings, resulting in loss of ability to perform short-sitting without a backrest. Changing his transfer technique was not a viable option. If wheelchair stowing had been evaluated, then the client would have been very clear that he was not open to removing the rear wheels nor acquiring a new vehicle.

Marginal function should be considered sacred. Some individuals can just barely move, but most relish this movement. Some individuals have adopted sitting postures that allow this limited mobility, and it works for them in their movement strategies. The therapist must be very wary of taking this away.

An individual with C6 tetraplegia who is a manual wheelchair user for 25 years. Posture is kyphotic with posterior pelvic tilt. He has had skin breakdown, which is now healed. The individual uses a 2-inch open cell foam cushion with nylon upholstery. Referral is for a new cushion with increased skin protection and postural correction.
Prescription: Hybrid technology cushion with an anterior wedged base and an immersion overlay.
Goals: Increased postural support to decrease posterior tilt with the anterior wedge feature and improved skin protection with pressure distribution via immersion.
Justification: History of recent skin breakdown with postural deviation.

Reason for Failure:

1. Postural correction interferes with function. This individual's ability to transfer depends on his ability to move forward in the seat, which is lost on the contoured base; additionally, the immersion surface is less stable and decreases his ability to move.
2. The increased skin protection is gained by the immersion feature of the cushion but this feature decreases this individual's function. Due to the instability, his transfer and his pressure relief method are lost.

Negotiated Solution: the same thing he has been successfully using (open cell foam with nylon cover) but new and one inch thicker with replacement at six months.

Table 8-4 provides examples of typical postural presentations that can occur in individuals with long-standing SCI. The postural deviation is defined, and potential causes of the deviations are given, along with recommended seating interventions for each deviation.

Table 8-4
Common Postural Deviations in Individuals with SCI

Typical Presentation	Postural Deviation	Potential Causes	Recommended Seating Interventions
Forward head position: Collapsing forward, propping with upper extremities Anterior thoracic fold at base of sternum Lumbar flexion Increased thoracic kyphosis Scapular protraction with humeral head forward in glenoid fossa High cervical hyperextension *Skin:* Bilateral ischial skin breakdown, perineal skin breakdown, may present with sacrum and coccyx pressure, and at spinous process at apex of thoracic kyphotic curve. May have anterior moisture breakdown in skin folds *Pain:* May complain of head ache, upper back pain, discomfort with prolonged sitting in wheelchair, shoulder pain with propulsion	*Posterior pelvic tilt:* Pelvis is rotated backward from neutral sagittal plane alignment	*Anatomical:* Limited hamstring length Fixed kyphosis Limited lumbar extension Anterior chest tightness *Equipment:* Seat depth too long Lack of posterior pelvic and lumbar support Backrest reclined Backrest too high Footrests too low	*Flexible spine:* Provide support for neutral pelvic position and lumbar extension. Likely corrections are seat slope, backrest angle and backrest height (or backrest contours where height is required) *Inflexible spine:* Address seating system configuration to accommodate posterior pelvic position and resultant kyphosis. Rotate system in space to provide horizontal line of sight and prevent musculoskeletal pain. Provide support to prevent progression of deformity. *Education:* As appropriate, stretching for hamstrings, thoracic extension, anterior chest and shoulder muscles. Strengthening posterior shoulder and intrascapular muscles. Stretch for posterior neck muscles and sternocleidomastoid.
Asymmetrical shoulders- Shoulder elevated same side as low pelvis Neck musculature shortening same side as low pelvis Asymmetrical stomach with abdominal bulge laterally same side as low pelvis Asymmetrical pelvis Spinal scoliosis with rotation Pelvic rotation may exist.	Pelvic obliquity One side of the pelvis is lower, creating frontal plane asymmetry. Compensatory curve away from low side.	*Anatomical:* Limited hip flexion contralateral to obliquity Unilateral hip flexion contracture Asymmetric spinal fusion Asymmetric lateral abdominal or hip flexor spasticity contralateral to obliquity Asymmetric flexibility due to habitual function: reach to one side, rotate to one side for access, one side only transfers	*Flexible spine:* Provide support to lift low side of pelvis; provide associated trunk support if needed *Limited hip range:* Accommodate to allow neutral pelvis *Inflexible spine:* Accommodate and provide support at pelvis at high side to increase pressure distribution and support trunk to prevent progression of deformity.

Continued

Table 8-4
Common Postural Deviations in Individuals with SCI—cont'd

Typical Presentation	Postural Deviation	Potential Causes	Recommended Seating Interventions
Skin: Breakdown at the ischial tuberosity, greater trochanter or posterior-lateral ribs on same side as low pelvis *Pain:* Cervical pain on same side as low pelvis; may present with shoulder pain either side		Head righting, seeking a head vertical; eyes horizontal and forward line of sight will exacerbate compensatory deformity created by an asymmetric pelvic platform *Equipment:* Trunk shift due to lack of adequate support or equipment that is too wide. Joystick drive control with lateral placement	*Education:* Stretching for lateral trunk and neck musculature. Avoid repetitive functional activities that elongate or shorten in the pattern of the deformity
Arching over the top of the backrest Excessive lumbar lordosis May sit with pelvis forward to reverse curve Flat thorax Unstable sitting balance. Pelvis sits posterior on cushion with ischii at most posterior aspect of cushion *Skin:* Issues at perineum or coccygeal breakdown (from backrest or bed surface) *Pain:* Upper back and neck pain, may present with upper limb pain	*Hyper-anterior pelvic tilt:* Pelvis is rotated forward from neutral sagittal plane alignment	*Anatomical:* Hip flexion contractures Spinal fusion in extension Premorbid lumbar hyper-extension Hypermobile lordosis below spinal fusion *Equipment:* Horizontal seat plane in the presence of truncal paralysis and hip flexion contractures Overstretched backrest upholstery Inadequate backrest support Backrest too low	*Flexible spine:* Configure seating system to facilitate neutral pelvic and trunk alignment. This requires a significantly steep slope or a combination of seat slope and cushion contour to decrease pull of the hip flexor contractures on the lumbar spine. *Inflexible spine:* Ensure appropriate cushion support under pelvis. Adjust back support for lumbar extension. Rotate the system in space to provide horizontal line of sight. Configure for stability. Configure seating system to prevent progression of deformity. *Education:* Stretching for hip flexors and spinal extensors.
Asymmetrical lap Trunk rotation Uneven pelvis One knee forward of the other, creating transverse plane asymmetry	Upper leg length discrepancy (LLD) Short limb internally rotated	*Anatomical:* A true pre-SCI leg length discrepancy Subluxed or dislocated hip on short side History of femur fracture with resultant shortening	*Flexible:* (i.e. pelvic rotation) Provide support and stabilization to neutralize pelvic position.

Table 8-4

Common Postural Deviations in Individuals with SCI—cont'd

Typical Presentation	Postural Deviation	Potential Causes	Recommended Seating Interventions
		Equipment: If equipment angles or dimensions do not accommodate anatomical limitations, the equipment will create or increase deformity	*Fixed:* Provide seat depth and cushion modifications to accommodate LLD. Accommodate fixed pelvic and trunk positions. *Education:* With fixed LLD, allow asymmetric lower extremity (LE) alignment vs. attempting to correct with pelvic rotation. Educate about the interaction of the pelvis with spine and the curvature with rotation need to compromise LE positioning to preserve upper body alignment and biomechanics
Windswept posture One upper leg abducted with external rotation while opposite leg is adducted with internal rotation May present with skin issues at feet, knees, or greater trochanter	Pelvic rotation Pelvic obliquity Scoliosis Unilateral cervical contracture	*Anatomical:* Pelvic rotation Trunk rotation Unilateral or asymmetric hip adductor spasticity Limited hip flexion (adducted leg) Limited hip abduction (adducted leg) Limited hip adduction (adducted leg) *Equipment:* If equipment angles or dimensions do not accommodate anatomical limitations, the equipment will create or increase deformity.	*Flexible:* Provide support for pelvis, trunk, and lower extremities to position at neutral alignment *Fixed:* Accommodate with cushion and backrest modifications. Provide supports to prevent progression of deformity. *Education:* LE, trunk, and cervical stretching.

When SCI Occurs in the Young

There is considerable literature to support the belief that postural deformities are more prevalent in persons for whom SCI occurred as a child.[35,113] There are high rates of dislocated hips and scoliosis, and many children with SCI are prescribed long-term spinal orthoses use or have surgical stabilization against progressive spinal deformity. It is hypothesized that the immature skeletal system plays a part in the development of these deformities. These concepts will be explored in greater detail in Chapter 25.

If a paralyzed trunk is unsupported, then it will align to a position of stability, which is spinal flexion. If a pelvis is not contained with medial and lateral support, then it may shift to one side, setting up a pattern of scoliosis from lack of a stable platform. A seating system that is too large is *much* more dangerous than one that is too small when the outcome of concern is postural alignment. Too often, children are seated in equipment that is too large. Even if the seat itself has been properly downsized to fit the child, the wheelchair base is often heavy and cumbersome. What is known from the body of research on upper limb musculoskeletal pain in individuals with SCI is that posture and proper upper limb biomechanics are essential. Furthermore, wheelchair roll resistance should be minimized through engineering to protect the individual who will push a wheelchair for full-time mobility. The person who suffers SCI earlier in life is the *most* in need of this protection, as they have the longest life remaining. As soon as a child is mature enough to safely maneuver his or her own equipment the child should be granted all of the same considerations discussed throughout this chapter. Nearly all of the high-end ultralight wheelchair manufacturers have some version of a trade up or discounted rate to rebuild for growth. Nearly all of the power mobility manufacturers have seating components that can grow over the mobility base. It is imperative that seating professionals do the best possible job of prescribing seating systems for children with SCI and of advocating for the best available equipment.

Wheelchairs for Sport and Recreation

Wheelchairs designed for sports and recreation are often used by individuals with SCI. While it is beyond the scope of this chapter to discuss in detail the appropriate prescription of wheelchairs for various adaptive sports and recreation activities, we will outline some important considerations.

- It is imperative that the same issues be addressed as those for everyday seating systems: postural support, skin protection, comfort, and function.
- A clear understanding of the client's interests, experience, goals for the specific equipment, intentions for use (whether recreational or competitive), and available support for pursuing a sports or recreational goal is necessary for appropriate prescription.
- Sports wheelchairs vary greatly; therefore, a thorough understanding of the sport activity is necessary for appropriate wheelchair prescription. In a team sport, it is important to consider the position played.
- The experience and skill level of the athlete also guides equipment decisions.

Sports wheelchair prescription requires a number of specific considerations in order to prescribe an appropriate athletic device. Therapists who lack competence in prescribing sports and recreation equipment are encouraged to seek guidance and mentorship from colleagues with this specific skill set.

Case Studies

The following two cases illustrate key concepts related to the wheelchair prescription that have been discussed in this chapter.

CASE STUDY 8-1   Individual with C5 Tetraplegia Seated in a Power Wheelchair

The client is a 22-year-old woman with C5 tetraplegia with partial motor preservation in C6 on the right, who is seen in an outpatient seating clinic. She breathes independently and uses a joystick-controlled power wheelchair. A car accident 4 years ago resulted in SCI. The client lives at home with her parents and attends community college. She hopes to transfer to an out-of-state university next fall. For school, she uses a note taker in class and a dictation system at home. The family owns a ramped minivan in which she travels as a passenger while seated in her power wheelchair. She does not drive and has no intention to return to driving.

Client is 5 foot 5 inches tall, with a reported weight of 125 prior to SCI. She believes she now weighs approximately 135. She reports she is in a wheelchair from about 8 a.m. to 10 p.m. She reports she does not use the elevating leg rests and cannot use them independently. The client states she does not use the tilt for pressure relief but she does use it once a day, as a rest position.

Client reports she has had no skin health issues. Her mother reports one area in high sacrum that gets red.

Key Concerns

1. Client: "It feels like I am tipping more forward since my injury, and through the day, my neck is pulling me down. I also tip to the left. It does not seem like spasms." Client also does not like the fact that her legs are spread apart.
2. Mother: She is concerned that her daughter is leaning over to the left, developing scoliosis that seems to be worsening.
3. Regular PT states: The wheelchair is contributing to the kyphosis and rounded shoulder and poor lateral control.

The interview will help determine the functions this client requires in a wheelchair. From what is already known, a list of the functions of her wheelchair can be created.

For mobility:

Must provide all-day mobility
Must provide for 12 to 14 hours of battery life in community mobility
Must be able to access family minivan

CASE STUDY 8-1   Individual with C5 Tetraplegia Seated in a Power Wheelchair—cont'd

Platform for function:

Must provide all day sitting position
Must provide pressure relief
Must provide positional change for functional tasks
Must provide comfort
Must provide postural stability

Considering this list, the therapist determines whether the current power base and interface equipment is appropriate.

Current System Information

Make/model of wheelchair/base: Permobil Chairman tilt in space with elevating leg rests and elevator (a FWD power base, with rehab seating and power functions).

Make/model of backrest: Jay 2 Deep Contour (adult large, 18-inch shell height) backrest is bolted on to backrest (a contoured backrest with lateral contours). Pan not mounted with hardware.

Make/model of cushion: High Profile Roho 10 × 9 (an air-filled cushion).

A review of the client's needs and the characteristics of the power base and seating interface reveal that the equipment is appropriate. The Permobil is a high-end power base with adequate range and ground clearance for community mobility. The power tilt offers pressure relief ability and the elevator allows ease of dependent function as well as positional changes required for varied tasks. The fact that the elevating leg rests are not under power control and not used means that they are likely an unnecessary component. Physical examination results will determine whether they are also potentially detrimental to postural support. The Jay 2 Deep Contour backrest also appears to have the potential to meet the needs of this client; the size may be an issue due to the small stature of the client. The high-profile Roho cushion is at the high end of skin protection, but may provide less-than-needed postural stability.

Physical Examination

Client and range of motion measurements are as follows:

PROM:	Left	Right
Hip flexion without post pelvic tilt	100	100
Hip extension without anterior pelvic tilt	−25	−15
Knee extension with hip at 90 (inside <)	135	135
Rule out hip limitations (abduction/ adduction, or rotation)		
Problem? No		
Thigh length (mat to popliteal)	15.5	15.5
Dorsiflexion ROM	20	20
Foot/ankle deformity? No		
Upper extremity deficits? Yes		

Scapulae bilaterally are excessively elevated with inferior angle approximation. Limited extension on the right glenohumeral joint. Right upper extremity is stronger than left

Current equipment measures and angles are as follows:

Seat depth: 18 inches
Seat width: 17 inches
Backrest height: 24 inches
Footrest length: 15 inches
Front seat-to-floor height: 20 inches
Rear seat-to-floor height: 18.5 inches
Inside angle seat to backrest: 100 degrees
Seat to footrest angle: 95 degrees

Postural Evaluation

(Schematic representation of the shoulder and pelvis by lines; rib-to-iliac space indicated in number of fingers.)

Short-sitting evaluation:
    (Fig. 8-9 illustrates initial   3   2
    seated posture)
Some rotation of the pelvis, transverse plane
Supine: (hip flexor tightness
    with hyperlordosis)

                              2   2

The physical examination will help the therapist determine the postural needs.

Postural Issues

Truncal paralysis suggests a need for orthotic support in the sagittal plane
Client is wider at hips than the back, which suggests she may need narrower backrest to fit appropriately
Significant hamstring and hip flexor contractures require accommodation with seat slope via frame configuration or interface
Sits with scoliosis with a rotatory deformity; however, this may be partially functional, as she can straighten in supine. It may also be partially due to oversized equipment providing less-than-adequate support

Reviewing the findings will give the therapist a general impression and some hypotheses as to the problems in the configuration of the current equipment.

Impression:

- Seat depth is too long (it is longer than her thigh measurement).
- Backrest is too high (laterals impinging on axilla).
- Reclined backrest is facilitating posterior pelvic tilt.
- Leg control is poor with down-sloped thighs and abduction.
- There is apparent pelvic obliquity with right side low— the pelvic obliquity appears to be a somewhat flexible deformity as lifting appeared to improve alignment and aid stability.

Continued

CASE STUDY 8-1   Individual with C5 Tetraplegia Seated in a Power Wheelchair—cont'd

The most critical component of successful seating is for the equipment to *fit* the individual. Equipment that is *too large* is detrimental to posture, especially in the condition of truncal paralysis. Because the client's seat depth measures 2.5 inches *longer* than her thigh length, she absolutely cannot sit without a significant posterior pelvic tilt. Until this is neutralized, it is not possible to have a true assessment of the rest of her postural deformity. Because her pelvis is being pulled forward by the lower leg, the asymmetrical hip flexion contracture may explain the postural deviations above the pelvis.

At this point, empirical trials are required to determine the affect of a shorter seat depth. The sagittal plane orthotic support can be created using a base wedge (or the tilt function) to create a positive seat slope, decreasing the seat-to-backrest angle, and lowering the backrest. Because the backrest is mounted without the adjustable hardware, the initial position will need to be more reclined than ideal, and the lower backrest will not allow

optimal pelvic positioning (Fig. 8-10 illustrates interim seated posture).

The adjustment of the current equipment is sufficient to verify that these changes are on the right track. To finalize the changes, it will be necessary to order different equipment, in particular a kit to shorten the seat depth and a tubular backrest to allow optimal mounting of aftermarket backrests with appropriate angle adjustment.

With final equipment, the seating is significantly improved (Fig. 8-11 illustrates final seated posture). This case primarily illustrated a change in configuration of the equipment. The power base and the interface equipment remained the same. The size and configuration of the equipment changed. The seat depth was shortened, the seat-to-backrest angle was closed (but the top of the backrest reclined), and a positive seat slope was added.

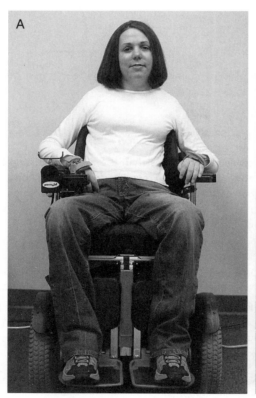 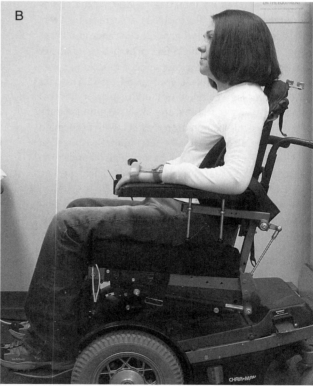

Figure 8-9. Initial posture of subject in Case Study 8-1. (A) Frontal view. Note apparent pelvic obliquity and abduction/external rotation of the hips. (B) Sagittal view. Note reclined backrest, posterior tilt of the pelvis, and downsloped thighs.

CASE STUDY 8-1   Individual with C5 Tetraplegia Seated in a Power Wheelchair—cont'd

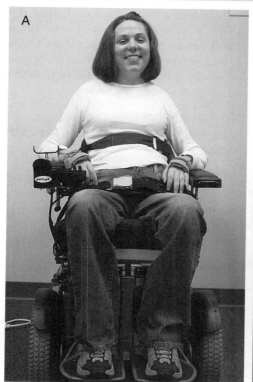
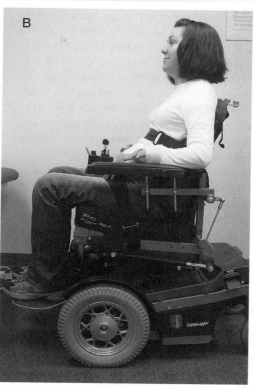

Figure 8-10. Interim posture of subject in Case Study 8-1 with original equipment. While some desired adjustments were not possible with the original equipment, reconfiguration resulted in improved postural positioning. (A) Frontal view. Note improved positioning of the legs. (B) Sagittal view. Note improved thigh-trunk angle created using the tilt function on the wheelchair, decreasing the seat-to-backrest angle and lowering the backrest.

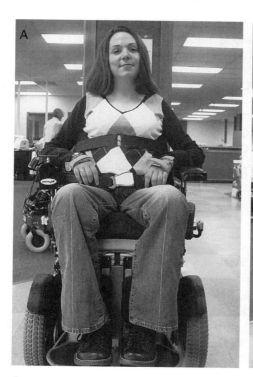
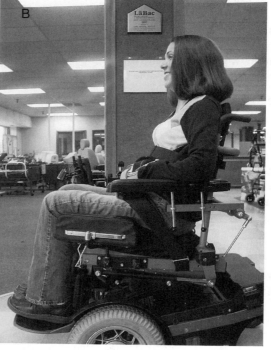

Figure 8-11. Post-intervention posture of subject in Case Study 8-1 with new equipment. (A) Frontal view. Note improved alignment of the trunk and pelvis that places even the shoulders in a more natural position. (B) Sagittal view. Note more optimal position of legs and trunk with shorter seat depth and positive seat slope.

CASE STUDY 8-2   Individual with T9 Paraplegia Seated in a Manual Wheelchair

The client is a 63-year-old woman who has been a full-time manual wheelchair user since age 40 when she sustained a T9 incomplete SCI. Client reports incomplete, but nonfunctional, lower extremity motor function. Client is self-referred for seating evaluation in an outpatient clinic with the goal of acquiring a new manual wheelchair. Client reports her current wheelchair is approximately 8 years old.

Client reports that she has some postural problems with some associated pain in upper back and neck. She reports shoulder pain, especially with stowing wheelchair into car (into passenger front seat of two-door car).

Client reports no history of skin problems. She reports low lumbar scoliosis without correction and a history of releases in hip flexors, knees (hamstring), and adductor tendons approximately 18 years ago. Client reports lower extremity spasticity, especially into plantarflexion. Client is 5 feet 3 inches tall and weighs approximately 135 pounds.

Client reports some wheelie skills, but no curbs and few sidewalks in her environment.

Client reports dressing in the wheelchair as well as self-catheterization.

Client is independent in lateral transfers to level surfaces with marginal skills. She requires a firmly locked wheelchair. She reports she does not often transfer out of the wheelchair except to bed.

The client's primary residence is on a rural island property of 40 acres. She has a secondary (new) residence in a condominium in urban locality. The unit offers limited accessibility to the wheelchair including some limitations in bathroom access (requires turning radius limited to that of current wheelchair).

Her husband will assist up steeper inclines and down steeper descents for control. Additionally, client has local family with stairs to access the home; husband pulls her up backward in the wheelchair, which requires a push handle assembly. Client requests a removable push handle system.

Key Concerns

1. Client is hoping for the lightest wheelchair possible to maintain her independence.

The information from the interview will assist the therapist in determining the functions the client requires in a new wheelchair. From what is known, a list of the functions of her wheelchair can be created.

For Mobility

Must cover rough terrain with limited skills
Must be set up for dependent assist
Must be lightweight (for stow and removal from car)
Must provide all-day sitting position

Platform for function

Requires rearward stability (for dressing in wheelchair)
Requires adequate seat/frame depth (for self-catheterization)
Requires stable platform for transfers
Requires compact wheelchair for accessibility

Summarizing what has been learned, it is possible to predict what wheelchair components are appropriate. The client's mobility habits and skills and her environment suggest an ultralight manual wheelchair set up for good forward and rearward stability, with treaded tires, moderate-sized soft roll casters, push handles, and, perhaps, armrests.

Physical Examination

Client and range of motion measurements are as follows:

PROM:	Left	Right
Hip flexion:	120	130
Hip Extension	−30	−−35
Hamstring length	120	130
(inside angle with hip at 90)		
DF	−5	−10
Thigh length	15 inches	15 inches

LE contractures with firm end feels

Trunk with some flexibility but limited in lateral flexion to left

Current equipment measures and angles are as follows:
Kuschall 3000 ST (an ultralight cantilever frame wheelchair) and an ~2-inch foam cushion (very compressed)

Seat depth: 16 inches
Seat width: 16.5 inches
Backrest height: 16 inches
Footrest length: 16.5 inches
Front seat-to-floor: 19.25 inches
Rear seat-to-floor: 16 inches
Inside seat-to-backrest angle: 90 degrees
Seat to footrest angle: 80 degrees
Inside footrest: 11 inches
Camber: ~3 degrees
Wheel clearance: .75 inch
Center of gravity (measure of rear axle forward of rear frame): 2.5 inches
Rear frame to caster tube: 15 inches
Overall width: 25.5 inches
Overall length (including toes): 33 inches

Postural Evaluation

Short-sitting evaluation findings are as follows (Fig. 8-12 illustrates initial seated posture):

Left pelvis is low, right shoulder is low
Right hip is externally rotated and slightly abducted
Left hip is slightly internally rotated and adducted
Sagittal plane appears highly unstable to the rear
Down-sloped thighs
Posterior pelvic tilt
Mild forward head
Thoracic kyphosis

CASE STUDY 8-2   Individual with T9 Paraplegia Seated in a Manual Wheelchair—cont'd

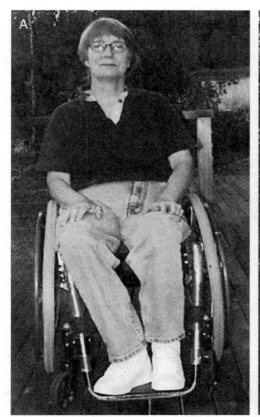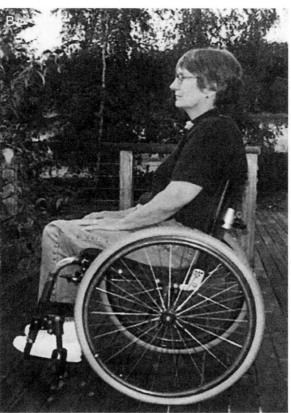

Figure 8-12. Initial posture of subject in Case Study 8-2. (A) Frontal view. Note curvature of trunk and rotation of pelvis. (B) Sagittal view. Note reclined position of backrest imposes forward head posture.

The physical examination will help the therapist determine the postural needs.

Postural Issues

Truncal paralysis requires orthotic support in sagittal plane
Scoliosis with rotatory deformity, which suggests some
   accommodation for appropriate contour and support
Significant hamstring and hip flexor contractures
   (requires accommodation in frame configuration)

Reviewing the findings of the physical examination and the measurements of the current equipment will give the therapist a general impression of problems with the current equipment and indications of the best directions for configuration of the new equipment.

Impression:

Her postural support needs suggest a wheelchair that can be highly customized.
Frame features will include

- a fairly steep seat slope with the front of seat higher than the rear of seat at approximately 14 degrees above horizontal. This feature will accommodate her hip flexion contractures and provide orthotic sagittal plane support.

- a tight front frame drop angle (approaching vertical); this feature will accommodate the hamstring contractures.

However, this configuration can be quite unstable and she requires stability, therefore

- caster position should be forward with the foot support between the casters.
- axle position can be adjusted to improve rearward stability
- the backrest angle will be either vertical or forward of vertical.
- inside seat-to-backrest angle will be acute (<90).
- her frontal plane asymmetry may require correction, but this will be evaluated after sagittal plane correction with proper wheelchair frame configuration.
- rotatory deformity is a fixed deformity and must be accommodated with asymmetry built into backrest.

At this point, some configuration changes to her existing equipment are warranted in order to prepare the client for the recommended changes that will be incorporated in new equipment. Trials in appropriate wheelchairs should be arranged.

The final selection for this client was a custom titanium rigid wheelchair with the following frame parameters:

Continued

CASE STUDY 8-2   Individual with T9 Paraplegia Seated in a Manual Wheelchair—cont'd

Front STF: 19 inches
Rear STF: 15 inches
Seat depth: 14 inches
Footrest: 14 inches
Width: 16 inches rear, 14 inches front
Inside seat-to-backrest angle (right cane 2 degrees
     forward of left): 75 inches
Backrest height: 14 inches
Inside footrest: 10 inches
Footrest angle: 80 (to floor)
Camber: 4 degrees
Wheel clearance: .75 inches
Center of gravity: 3 inches
Rear frame to caster tube: 17 inches
Overall width: 25 inches
Overall length: 31.5 inches

Note the following changes to the wheelchair configuration:

- A shorter seat depth and footrest length: These measures now match her anatomy. (Fig. 8-13 illustrates final seated posture.)

- A steeper seat slope, shorter backrest, and more acute seat-to-backrest inside angle: These features accommodate hip flexion contractures and provide sagittal plane orthotic support to spinal alignment.
- Shorter seat depth and decreased footrest drop angle: These features accommodate her hamstring contractures.
- Longer frame measure between the rear frame and caster housing: This feature improves the stability of the wheelchair.

A letter of justification to the third-party payer (Refer to Fig. 8-8 for sample letter) was written to facilitate acquisition of this wheelchair. The therapist justified the need for the wheelchair in general, the need for the category of wheelchair being requested, and the need for each specific specialized component, which will include charges for customization as well as any equipment beyond standard.

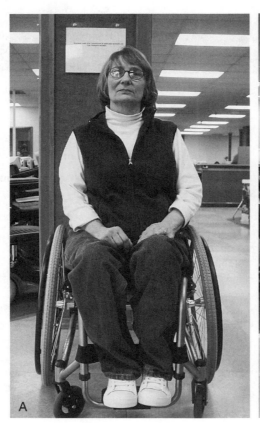 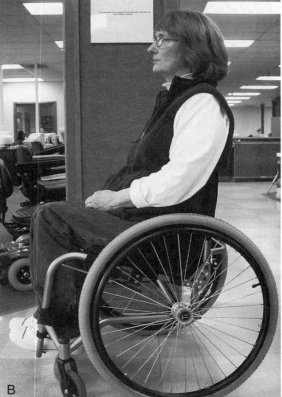

Figure 8-13. Post-intervention posture of subject in Case Study 8-2 with new equipment. (A) Frontal view. Note improved trunk, pelvis, and leg alignment. (B) Sagittal view. Note more acute seat-to-backrest angle to accommodate hip flexion contractures and decreased footrest angle to accommodate hamstring contractures.

Summary

The ideal seating system for the individual with SCI maximizes mobility and activity, minimizes injury risk, is comfortable, and provides an optimal platform for both physical and physiologic function. Optimal seating outcomes are the result of a comprehensive client evaluation, equipment trials with appropriate products, and provision of a final system that matches the unique needs and preferences of the individual. A thorough client evaluation includes assessment of physical, functional and social needs. Once the client's requirements are identified, the broad field of equipment choices may be narrowed to coordinate appropriate trials with products that are likely to meet specific objectives. Seating prescription must begin with postural support, which requires that equipment is first *sized* correctly and then *configured* appropriately to provide optimal musculoskeletal alignment and support. When postural support is provided with strategic selection and configuration of all seating system components, subsequent outcomes include optimized function, comfort, and skin protection, all of which are critical considerations for any wheelchair user. A successful seating system for the individual with SCI meets identified needs and preferences and, as a result, contributes to improved quality of life.

REVIEW QUESTIONS

1. List three common problems encountered by individuals with SCI who rely on wheelchairs for primary mobility.
2. List 10 key components that should be included in a seating evaluation for an individual with SCI.
3. Explain why it is important to examine the current equipment used by a client during a seating evaluation.
4. Describe the appropriate sequence in a seating intervention.
5. What are the advantages of a fully customized ultra-light manual wheelchair?
6. What is the primary feature that differentiates the power bases? How does this affect chair maneuverability and performance?
7. Describe (three) beneficial features of power seat functions. For each of the independent power seat functions, name one relative concern.
8. What are two key considerations when determining if an individual is best served with a manual or power wheelchair?
9. How does a therapist determine the "best" cushion to prescribe to a particular client?
10. Outline (three) critical elements to include when providing justification for a seating system.

REFERENCES

1. Hobson DA, Tooms RE. Seated lumbar/pelvic alignment. A comparison between spinal cord-injured and noninjured groups. *Spine.* 1992;17(3):293–298.
2. Alm M, Gutierrez E, Hultling C et al. Clinical evaluation of seating in persons with complete thoracic spinal cord injury. *Spinal Cord.* 2003;41(10):563–571.
3. Finley MA, Lee RY. Effect of sitting posture on 3-dimensional scapular kinematics measured by skin-mounted electromagnetic tracking sensors. *Arch Phys Med Rehabil.* 2003;84(4):563–568.
4. Massery M. What's positioning got to do with it? *Neurol. Rep.* 1994;18(3).
5. Samuelsson KA, Larsson H, Thyberg M et al. Back pain and spinal deformity—Common among wheelchair users with spinal cord injuries. *Scand J Occup Ther.* 1996;3:28–32.
6. Boninger M, Waters RL, Chase T et al. *Preservation of Upper Limb Function Following Spinal Cord Injury: A Clinical Practice Guideline for Health-Care Professionals.* Washington DC: Paralyzed Veterans of America Consortium for Spinal Cord Medicine; 2005.
7. Norkin C, Levangie P. *Joint Structure and Function a Comprehensive Analysis.* 2nd edition. Philadelphia: F. A. Davis; 1992.
8. Greenfield B, Catlin PA, Coats PW et al. Posture in patients with shoulder overuse injuries and healthy individuals. *J Orthop Sports Phys Ther.* 1995;21(5):287–295.
9. Keegan JJ. Alterations of the lumbar curve related to posture and seating. *J Bone Joint Surg.* 1953;35A(3):589–605.
10. Matsen FA, Lippitt SB, Sidles JA et al. *Practical Evaluation and Management of the Shoulder.* Philadelphia: W. B. Saunders; 1994.
11. Minkel JL. Seating and mobility considerations for people with spinal cord injury. *Phys Ther.* 2000;80(7):701–709.
12. Seelen HA, Vuurman EF. Compensatory muscle activity for sitting posture during upper extremity task performance in paraplegic persons. *Scand J Rehabil Med.* 1991;23:89–96.
13. Janssen-Potten YJ, Seelen HA, Drukker J et al. The effect of seat tilting on pelvic position, balance control, and compensatory postural muscle use in paraplegic subjects. *Arch Phys Med Rehabil.* 2001;82(10):1393–1402.
14. Hastings JD, Fanucchi ER, Burns SP. Wheelchair configuration and postural alignment in persons with spinal cord injury. *Arch Phys Med Rehabil.* 2003;84:528–534.
15. Sinnott KA, Milburn P, McNaughton H. Factors associated with thoracic spinal cord injury, lesion level and rotator cuff disorders. *Spinal Cord.* 2000;38:748–753.
16. Boninger ML, Cooper RA, Shimada SD et al. Shoulder and elbow motion during two speeds of wheelchair propulsion: A description using a local coordinate system. *Spinal Cord.* 1998;36(6):418–426.

17. Boninger M, Baldwin M, Cooper R et al. Manual wheelchair pushrim biomechanics and axle position. *Arch Physl Med Rehabil.* 2000;81:608–613.

18. Boninger ML, Souza AL, Cooper RA et al. Propulsion patterns and pushrim biomechanics in manual wheelchair propulsion. *Arch Phys Med Rehabil.* 2002;83(5):718–723.

19. Rodgers MM, McQuade KJ, Rasch EK et al. Upper-limb fatigue-related joint power shifts in experienced wheelchair users and nonwheelchair users. *J Rehabil Res Dev.* 2003;40(1):27–37.

20. Massery M. Musculoskeletal and neuromuscular interventions: A physical approach to cystic fibrosis. *J R Soc Med.* 2005;98 Suppl 45:55–66.

21. McKinley WO, Jackson AB, Cardenas DD et al. Long-term medical complications after traumatic spinal cord injury: A regional model systems analysis. *Arch Phys Med Rehabil.* 1999;80(11):1402–1410.

22. Cardenas DD, Hoffman JM, Kirshblum S et al. Etiology and incidence of rehospitalization after traumatic spinal cord injury: A multicenter analysis. *Arch Phys Med Rehabil.* 2004;85(11):1757–1763.

23. Zacharkow D. Essential wheelchair modifications for proper sitting posture. *Wheelchair Posture and Pressure Sores.* Springfield, IL: CC Thomas; 1984. pp. 18–38.

24. Harms M. Effect of wheelchair design on posture and comfort of users. *Physiotherapy.* 1990;76:266–271.

25. Bolin I, Bodin P, Kreuter M. Sitting position—posture and performance in C5–C6 tetraplegia. *Spinal Cord.* 2000;38(7):425–434.

26. Janssen-Potten YJ, Seelen HA, Drukker J et al. Chair configuration and balance control in persons wtih spinal cord injury. *Arch Phys Med Rehabil.* 2000;81:401–408.

27. Janssen-Potten YJ, Seelen HA, Drukker J et al. The effect of footrests on sitting balance in paraplegic subjects. *Arch Phys Med Rehabil.* 2002;83(5):642–648.

28. Tomlinson JD. Managing maneuverability and rear stability of adjustable manual wheelchairs: An update. *Phys Ther.* 2000;80(9):904–911.

29. Tomlinson JD. Personal communication. Tacoma, WA; 2000.

30. Van Breukelen K. The ergonomic seating system. Paper presented at: 3rd International Congress on Restoration of (Wheeled) Mobility in Spinal Cord Injury, April 4, 2004; Amsterdam, The Netherlands.

31. Maurer CL, Sprigle S. Effect of seat inclination on seated pressures of individuals with spinal cord injury. *Phys Ther.* 2004;84(3):255–261.

32. Hastings JD. Seating assessment and planning.*Phys Med Rehabil Clin North Am.* 2000;11(1):183–207.

33. Hastings JD, Goldstein B. Paraplegia and the shoulder. *Phys Med Rehabil Clin North Am: Shoulder Rehabilitation, Part II.* 2004;15(3):699–718.

34. Kraemer H, Kraemer K. Designing, conducting, and analyzing programs within the prevention intervention research cycle. In: Mrazek PJ, Haggerty RJ, eds. *Reducing Risks for Mental Disorders, Frontiers for Preventive Intervention Research.* Washington DC: National Academy Press; 1994. pp. 359–414.

35. Bergstrom EMK. The effect of childhood spinal cord injury on skeletal development. *Spinal Cord.* 1999;37:838–846.

36. Putzke JD, Richards JS, Hicken BL et al. Interference due to pain following spinal cord injury: Important predictors and impact on quality of life. *Pain.* 2002;100(3):231–242.

37. Andersen JH, Kaergaard A, Frost P et al. Physical, psychosocial, and individual risk factors for neck/shoulder pain with pressure tenderness in the muscles among workers performing monotonous, repetitive work. *Spine.* 2002;27(6):660–667.

38. Frost P, Bonde JP, Mikkelsen S et al. Risk of shoulder tendonitis in relation to shoulder loads in monotonous repetitive work. *Am J Ind Med.* 2002;41(1):11–18.

39. Roquelaure Y, Mechali S, Dano C et al. Occupational and personal risk factors for carpal tunnel syndrome in industrial workers. *Scand J Work Environ Health.* 1997;23(5):364–369.

40. Fitzgerald SG, Cooper RA, Boninger ML et al. Comparison of fatigue life for 3 types of manual wheelchairs. *Arch Phys Med Rehabil.* 2001;82(10):1484–1488.

41. DiGiovine MM, Cooper RA, Boninger ML et al. User assessment of manual wheelchair ride comfort and ergonomics. *Arch Phys Med Rehabil.* 2000;81(4):490–494.

42. Cook AM, Hussey AM. Seating systems as extrinsic enablers for assistive technologies. *Assistive Technologies Principles and Practice.* 2nd ed. St. Louis, MO: Mosby; 2002.

43. Brubaker CE. Wheelchair prescription: An analysis of factors that affect mobility and performance. *J Rehabil Res Dev.* 1986;23(4):19–26.

44. Beekman CE, Miller-Porter L, Schoneberger M. Energy cost of propulsion in standard and ultralight wheelchairs in people with spinal cord injuries. *Phys Ther.* 1999;79(2):146–158.

45. Hughes CJ, Weimar WH, Sheth PN et al. Biomechanics of wheelchair propulsion as a function of seat position and user-to-chair interface. *Arch Phys Med Rehabil.* 1992;73(3):263–269.

46. Masse LC, Lamontagne M, O'Riain MD. Biomechanical analysis of wheelchair propulsion for various seating positions. *J Rehabil Res Dev.* 1992;29(3):12–28.

47. Richter WM. The effect of seat position on manual wheelchair propulsion biomechanics: A quasi-static model-based approach. *Med Eng Phys.* 2001;23(10):707–712.

48. van der Woude LH, Veeger DJ, Rozendal RH et al. Seat height in handrim wheelchair propulsion. *J Rehabil Res Dev.* 1989;26(4):31–50.

49. Cooper RA, Wolf E, Fitzgerald SG et al. Seat and footrest shocks and vibrations in manual wheelchairs with and without suspension. *Arch Phys Med Rehabil.* 2003;84(1):96–102.

50. Arva J, Fitzgerald SG, Cooper RA et al. Mechanical efficiency and user power requirement with a pushrim activated power assisted wheelchair. *Med Eng Phys.* 2001;23:699–705.

51. Cooper RA, Fitzgerald SG, Boninger ML et al. Evaluation of a pushrim-activated, power-assisted wheelchair. *Arch Phys Med Rehabil.* 2001;82(5):702–708.

52. Algood SD, Cooper RA, Fitzgerald SG et al. Impact of a pushrim-activated power-assisted wheelchair on the metabolic demands, stroke frequency, and range of motion among subjects with tetraplegia. *Arch Phys Med Rehab.* 2004;85(11):1865–1871.

53. Levy CE, Chow JW. Pushrim-activated power-assist wheelchairs: Elegance in motion. *Am J Phys Med Rehabil.* 2004;83(2):166–167.

54. Algood SD, Cooper RA, Fitzgerald SG et al. Effect of a pushrim-activated power-assist wheelchair on the functional capabilities of persons with tetraplegia. *Arch Phys Med Rehabil.* 86;2005:380–386.

55. Corfman TA, Cooper RA, Boninger ML et al. Range of motion and stroke frequency differences between manual wheelchair propulsion and pushrim-activated power-assisted wheelchair propulsion. *J Spinal Cord Med.* 26;2003: 135–140.

56. Levy CE, Chow JW, Tillman MD et al. Variable-ratio pushrim-activated power-assist wheelchair eases wheeling over a variety of terrains for elders. *Arch Phys Med Rehabil.* 85;2004:104–112.

57. Best KL, Kirby RL, Smith C et al. Comparison between performance with a pushrim-activated power-assisted wheelchair and a manual wheelchair on the Wheelchair Skills Test. *Disabil Rehabil.* 2006;28(4):213–220.

58. Fitzgerald SG, Arva J, Cooper RA et al. A pilot study on community usage of a pushrim-activated, power-assisted wheelchair. *Assist Technol.* 2003;15:113–119.

59. Gordes KL, Finley MA, Meginniss S et al. Effect of two-speed manual wheel on shoulder pain in wheelchair users: Preliminary findings. Paper presented at: International Seating Symposium; 2006; Vancouver, BC.

60. Fass MV, Cooper RA, Fitzgerald SG et al. Durability, value, and reliability of selected electric powered wheelchairs. *Arch Phys Med Rehabil.* 2004;85(5):805–814.

61. Dennison I, Guyton D. Power wheelchairs—A new definition. Paper presented at: International Seating Symposium, 2002; Vancouver, BC.

62. Hobson DA. Comparative effects of posture on pressure and shear at the body-seat interface. *J Rehabil Res Dev.* 1992;29(4):21–31.

63. Vaisbuch N, Meyer S, Weiss PL. Effect of seated posture on interface pressure in children who are able-bodied and who have myelomeningocele. *Disabil Rehabil.* 2000;22(17): 749–755.

64. Stinson MD, Porter-Armstrong A, Eakin P. Seat-interface pressure: A pilot study of the relationship to gender, body mass index, and seating position. *Arch Phys Med Rehabil.* 2003;84(3):405–409.

65. Henderson JL, Price SH, Brandstater ME et al. Efficacy of three measures to relieve pressure in seated persons with spinal cord injury. *Arch Phys Med Rehabil.* 1994;75(5): 535–539.

66. Pellow TR. A comparison of interface pressure readings to wheelchair cushions and positioning: a pilot study. *Can J Occup Ther.* 1999;66(3):140–149.

67. Aissaoui R, Lacoste M, Dansereau J. Analysis of sliding and pressure distribution during a repositioning of persons in a simulator chair. *IEEE Trans Neural Syst Rehabil Eng.* 2001;9(2):215–224.

68. Lacoste M, Weiss-Lambrou R, Allard M et al. Powered tilt/recline systems: Why and how are they used? *Assist Technol.* 2003;15(1):58–68.

69. Arva J, Schmeler M, Lange M et al. RESNA position on the application of seat-elevating devices for wheelchair users. Rehabilitation Engineering Society of America. 2005. Available at: http://www.rstce.pitt.edu.

70. Kirby RL, Fahie CL, Smith C et al. Neck discomfort of wheelchair users: Effect of neck position. *Disabil Rehabil.* 2004;26(1):9–15.

71. Wang YT, Kim CK, Ford HT, 3rd et al. Reaction force and EMG analyses of wheelchair transfers. *Percept Motor Skill.* 1994;79(2):763–766.

72. Janssen WG, Bussmann HB, Stam HJ. Determinants of the sit-to-stand movement: A review. *Phys Ther.* 2002;82(9): 866–879.

73. Herberts P, Kadefors R, Hogfors C et al. Shoulder pain and heavy manual labor. *Clin Orthop Relat Res.* 1984(191): 166–178.

74. Sigholm G, Herberts P, Almstrom C et al. Electromyographic analysis of shoulder muscle load. *J Orthop Res.* 1984;1(4): 379–386.

75. Palmerud G, Forsman M, Sporrong H et al. Intramuscular pressure of the infra- and supraspinatus muscles in relation to hand load and arm posture. *Eur J Appl Physiol.* 2000;83(2–3):223–230.

76. Jarvholm U, Palmerud G, Karlsson D et al. Intramuscular pressure and electromyography in four shoulder muscles. *J Orthop Res.* 1991;9(4):609–619.

77. Sprigle S, Spasato B. Physiologic effects and design considerations of tilt and recline wheelchairs. *Orthop Phys Ther Clin North Am.* 1997;6(1):99–122.

78. Taub E. Somatosensory deafferentation in research with monkeys: Implications for rehabilitation medicine. In: Ince L, ed. Behavioural Psychology and Rehabilitation Medicine. Baltimore, MD: Williams & Wilkins; 1980. pp. 371–401.

79. Schmidt RA, Young DE. Methodology for motor learning: A paradigm for kinematic feedback. *J Motor Behav.* 1991;23(1):13–24.

80. Schmidt RA, Wrisberg CA. Motor Learning and Performance. 3rd ed. Champaign, IL: Human Kinetics; 2004.

81. Lotze M, Braun C, Birbaumer N et al. Motor learning elicited by voluntary drive. *Brain.* 2003;126(4):866–872.

82. Dyson-Hudson TA, Kirshblum SC. Shoulder pain in chronic spinal cord injury, Part1: Epidemiology, etiology and pathomechanics. *J Spinal Cord Med.* 2004;27:4–17.

83. Finley MA, Rodgers MM. Prevalence and identification of shoulder pathology in athletic and nonathletic wheelchair users with shoulder pain: A pilot study. *J Rehabil Res Dev.* 2004;41(3B):395–402.

84. Dalyan M, Cardenas DD, Gerard B. Upper extremity pain after spinal cord injury. *Spinal Cord.* 1999;37(3):191–195.

85. Samuelsson KA, Tropp H, Gerdle B. Shoulder pain and its consequences in paraplegic spinal cord-injured, wheelchair users. *Spinal Cord.* 2004;42(1):41–46.

86. Curtis KA, Tyner TM, Zachary L et al. Effect of a standard exercise protocol on shoulder pain in long-term wheelchair users. *Spinal Cord.* 1999;37(6):421–429.

87. Boninger ML, Cooper RA, Fitzgerald SG et al. Investigating neck pain in wheelchair users. *Am J Phys Med Rehabil.* 2003;82(3):197–202.

88. Hoxie R, Rubenstein L. Are older pedestrians allowed enough time to cross intersections safely? *J Am Geriatr Soc.* 1994;42(3):241–244.

89. Burns SP, Betz KL. Seating pressures with conventional and dynamic wheelchair cushions in tetraplegia. *Arch Phys Med Rehabil.* 1999;80(5):566–571.

90. Koo TK, Mak AF, Lee YL. Evaluation of an active seating system for pressure relief. *Assist Technol.* 1995;7(2):119–128.

91. Seymour RJ, Lacefield WE. Wheelchair cushion effect on pressure and skin temperature. *Arch Phys Med Rehabil.* 1985;66(2):103–108.

92. Stewart SF, Palmieri V, Cochran GV. Wheelchair cushion effect on skin temperature, heat flux, and relative humidity. *Arch Phys Med Rehabil.* 1980;61(5):229–233.

93. Brienza DM, Geyer MJ. Understanding support surface technologies. *Adv Skin Wound Care.* 2000;13(5):237–244.

94. Aissaoui R, Kauffmann C, Dansereau J et al. Analysis of pressure distribution at the body-seat interface in able-bodied and paraplegic subjects using a deformable active contour algorithm. *Med Eng Phys.* 2001;23(6):359–367.

95. Yuen HK, Garrett D. Comparison of three wheelchair cushions for effectiveness of pressure relief. *Am J Occup Ther.* 2001;55(4):470–475.

96. Brienza DM, Karg PE, Geyer MJ et al. The relationship between pressure ulcer incidence and buttock-seat cushion interface pressure in at-risk elderly wheelchair users. *Arch Phys Med Rehabil.* 2001;82(4):529–533.

97. Sprigle S, Chung KC, Brubaker CE. Reduction of sitting pressures with custom contoured cushions. *J Rehabil Res Dev.* 1990;27(2):135–140.

98. Brienza DM, Karg PE, Brubaker CE. Seat cushion design for elderly wheelchair users based on minimization of soft tissue deformation using stiffness and pressure measurements. *IEEE Trans Rehabil Eng.* 1996;4(4):320–327.

99. Aissaoui R, Boucher C, Bourbonnais D et al. Effect of seat cushion on dynamic stability in sitting during a reaching task in wheelchair users with paraplegia. *Arch Phys Med Rehabil.* 2001;82(2):274–281.

100. Geyer MJ, Brienza DM, Karg P et al. A randomized control trial to evaluate pressure-reducing seat cushions for elderly wheelchair users. *Adv Skin Wound Care.* 2001;14(3):120–129, 131–122.

101. Dabnichki P, Taktak D. Pressure variation under the ischial tuberosity during a push cycle. *Med Eng Phys.* 1998;20(4):242–256.

102. Kernozek TW, Lewin JE. Seat interface pressures of individuals with paraplegia: Influence of dynamic wheelchair locomotion compared with static seated measurements. *Arch Phys Med Rehabil.* 1998;79(3):313–316.

103. Borg GA. Psychophysical bases of perceived exertion. *Med Sci Sports Exerc.* 1982;14(5):377–381.

104. Hastings JD. Instrument development: A postural scale for wheelchair users. *J Spinal Cord Med.* 2005;28(2):163.

105. Curtis KA, Roach KE, Applegate EB et al. Reliability and validity of the Wheelchair User's Shoulder Pain Index (WUSPI). *Paraplegia.* 1995;33(10):595–601.

106. Curtis KA, Roach KE, Applegate EB et al. Development of the Wheelchair User's Shoulder Pain Index (WUSPI). *Paraplegia.* 1995;33:290–293.

107. Mills T, Holm MB, Trefler E et al. Development and consumer validation of the Functional Evaluation in a Wheelchair (FEW) instrument. *Disabil Rehabil.* 2002;24(1–3):38–46.

108. Kilkens O, Post M, van der Woude LH et al. The wheelchair circuit: Reliability of a test to assess mobility in persons with spinal cord injuries. *Arch Phys Med Rehabil.* 2002;83(12):1783–1788.

109. Kilkens O, Dallmiejer A, De Witte L et al. The wheelchair circuit: Construct validity and responsiveness of a test to assess manual wheelchair mobility in persons with spinal cord injury. *Arch Phys Med Rehabil.* 2004;85(3):424–431.

110. Kirby RL, Swuste J, Dupuis DJ et al. The Wheelchair Skills Test: A pilot study of a new outcome measure. *Arch Phys Med Rehabil.* 2002;83(1):10–18.

111. Kirby RL, Dupuis DJ, Macphee AH et al. The Wheelchair Skills Test (version 2.4): Measurement properties. *Arch Phys Med Rehabil.* 2004;85(5):794–804.

112. Mentor R, Hudson L. Effects of age at injury and the aging process. In: Stover S, DeLisa J, Whiteneck G, editors. Spinal Cord Injury: Clinical Outcomes from the Model Systems. Gaithersburg, MD: Aspen; 1995. pp. 277–288.

113. Vogel LC, Krajci KA, Anderson CJ. Adults with pediatric-onset spinal cord injury: Part 2: Musculoskeletal and neurological complications. *J Spinal Cord Med.* 2002;25(2):117–123.

Appendix 8-1

Postural Scale for Wheelchair Users: Scoring and Metric Properties

The Postural Scale for Wheelchair Users provides a rating of the wheelchair user's perception of seating problems and concerns. The scale includes the domains of pain (P), aesthetics (A), health (H), and function (F).

Scoring Instructions

For each item, a box is checked to indicate agreement with the associated descriptor. The numerical values assigned to each checked box are transcribed in the associated triangle (on the right side). Vertical columns are added to obtain a summed score for each of the subscales. The subscale scores are summed for a total score.

The scale range is 0-48; subscale range is 0-12. A higher score indicates a perception of more problematic posture associated with seating.

A total score of 24 (50%) or greater, or a subscale score of 9 (75%) or greater, indicates that referral for seating evaluation and intervention would be of benefit to the wheelchair user.

Scale Metrics

Statistical testing of the Postural Scale for Wheelchair Users indicates high internal consistency (Cronbach's alpha = 0.86; subscale to scale: all significant [range = 0.76 − 0.86]; subscale to subscale: all significant [range = 0.40 − 0.72]; and item to subscale: all significant [range = 0.42 - 0.88]), and high test-retest reliability = 0.73.

Scale developed by Jennifer Hastings, PT, PhD, NCS

Postural Scale for Wheelchair Users

This is a questionnaire to assess how you feel about your posture. Please read each statement below and then determine how strongly you agree or disagree with the statement. Please check the box that matches the strength of your agreement/disagreement.

Type of wheelchair? Power _____, Manual _____

If you use both, select one for the purpose of the questionnaire.

	Completely Disagree	Somewhat Disagree	Somewhat Agree	Completely Agree	For administrative use only			
					P	A	H	F
1. Whenever I see a mirror I tend to correct my posture in my wheelchair	☐ 0	☐ 1	☐ 2	☐ 3		☐		
2. I feel sitting upright in my wheelchair is 'work'	☐ 0	☐ 1	☐ 2	☐ 3	☐			
3. I worry that how I sit may lead to skin breakdown	☐ 0	☐ 1	☐ 2	☐ 3			☐	
4. My wheelchair was custom-designed to meet my needs	☐ 3	☐ 2	☐ 1	☐ 0				☐
5. I limit how long I sit in my wheelchair due to discomfort	☐ 0	☐ 1	☐ 2	☐ 3				☐
6. I think I could breathe easier if I sat differently	☐ 0	☐ 1	☐ 2	☐ 3			☐	
7. I have pain, or discomfort, that I think is related to how I sit in my wheelchair	☐ 0	☐ 1	☐ 2	☐ 3	☐			
8. I get tired during the day and I believe it is related to how I sit	☐ 0	☐ 1	☐ 2	☐ 3	☐			
9. I sit with my hips forward to improve my balance	☐ 0	☐ 1	☐ 2	☐ 3				☐
10. I think my posture may lead to some problems down the line	☐ 0	☐ 1	☐ 2	☐ 3			☐	
11. My chair is not supportive enough	☐ 0	☐ 1	☐ 2	☐ 3				☐
12. I think my muscular fatigue is due to how I sit in my wheelchair	☐ 0	☐ 1	☐ 2	☐ 3	☐			
13. I believe I have poor posture	☐ 0	☐ 1	☐ 2	☐ 3		☐		
14. I believe the way I sit makes my spasticity worse	☐ 0	☐ 1	☐ 2	☐ 3			☐	
15. I think I would look better if I could sit up taller	☐ 0	☐ 1	☐ 2	☐ 3		☐		
16. I feel good about how I look in my wheelchair	☐ 3	☐ 2	☐ 1	☐ 0		☐		
Sums								
Totals =					+	+	+	
Overall Total =								

Please fill out the following information:

Age _____ Neurological condition that requires use of a wheelchair _____ .
                                                                    (include level of injury if SCI)

Do you use your wheelchair full-time? ___Y ___ N

Year of beginning wheelchair use _____ .

Male _____ Female _____

Psychological Aspects of Living With Spinal Cord Injury: Emotional Health, Quality of Life, and Participation

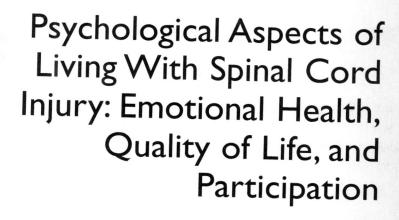

Susan Magasi, PhD, OTR

Allen W. Heinemann, PhD, ABPP (Rp)

Catherine S. Wilson Psy D, ABPP (Rp)

OBJECTIVES

After reading this chapter, the reader will be able to:

- Explain key models of psychological adjustment to disability and the implications for clinical interventions for people with spinal cord injuries (SCIs)
- Differentiate the concept of quality of life/life satisfaction from health-related quality of life and describe the relevance to SCI rehabilitation
- Identify the key factors that contribute to quality of life during different times in the life course of people with SCIs
- Define participation and discuss barriers to participation in employment, marriage and parenting, and access to health care experienced by people with spinal cord injuries and identify solutions to these barriers
- Describe how barriers to participation affect emotional adjustment and quality of life

OUTLINE

Introduction

The person with a newly acquired spinal cord injury (SCI) is confronted not only with the loss of mobility and physical function but also with a tremendous amount of uncertainty about what the future holds. Most people do not have personal or immediate experience with disability and often have negative preconceptions about disability and its impact on quality of life and social participation. The media often portrays people with disabilities in stereotypical ways—as objects of pity, objects of terror, or, in rare cases, as inspirational overcomers. The lives of real people with SCI, however, defy these stereotypes. They hold jobs, go to school, fall in and out of love, raise families. In short they are capable of engaging in a broad array of social roles. Their lives ought not to be objects of pity, fear, or inspiration. Each of these portrayals is detrimental because it obscures the complexity of the lives of people with disabilities; yet, in the absence of complete information, stereotypes are what many people use when trying to understand what a newly acquired SCI means for them. Disability research and much of clinical practice perpetuates negative conceptualizations of SCI by approaching research from a deficits-based approach. While relying on empirical research that highlights the negative impact of SCIs, this chapter seeks to debunk some of the myths of life with a SCI by providing a realistic picture of psychosocial adaptation, quality of life, and community participation for people with SCIs.

This chapter will describe the dominant perspectives on psychosocial adjustment to SCIs and the implications for therapeutic interventions. Psychosocial adjustment is closely related to quality of life and community participation outcomes. Each of these topics will be discussed, concluding with a discussion of participation that is influenced by SCI. Practical suggestions that rehabilitation professionals may integrate into their clinical work with people who have SCIs are offered. This chapter strives to integrate a traditional psychological rehabilitation focus with a disability studies perspective, so as to provide a balanced and nuanced view of the lived experience of life following SCI.

The purpose of this chapter is to provide a comprehensive guide to the most current thinking regarding the psychological aspects of living with SCI for rehabilitation practioners. This chapter is designed to provide the autonomous practitioner with the scientific evidence to determine effective rehabilitation interventions for individuals with SCI. The target readership for this chapter is rehabilitation specialists, both in practice and those in training. In keeping with the current focus on "evidence-based practice," the aim of this chapter to is to demonstrate how state-of-the-art research may be applied to rehabilitation practices. The goal for this chapter is to complement other contributions in this text so as to demystify cutting edge lines of scientific investigation, thus allowing the reader to develop into a more savvy consumer of the research literature related to SCI.

Psychosocial Reactions and the Process of Adjustment Following SCI

Psychosocial reactions to SCI and the onset of permanent impairments have been discussed extensively in the rehabilitation literature (*see* Vash and Crewe[1]). The incidence of SCI remains relatively low in the general population, and as a result, there are no models of psychosocial adjustment that were developed exclusively in this population. Researchers and clinicians working in the area of SCI rehabilitation tend to apply more general models of adjustment to disability to this group.

Model of Values Change

One of the early models of disability acceptance was described by Dembo, Leviton, and Wright[2] and later elaborated by Wright.[3,4] Based on extensive interviews with veterans who sustained amputations, they developed a model of value changes to define the concept of disability acceptance. This model focuses on intrapsychic processes that influence self-perception and one's value in the world by focusing on personal assets (rather than deriving self-worth from comparisons with other people) and by de-emphasizing the importance of the physical body. This disability acceptance framework has been applied to people with SCI and serves as the basis for adjustment processes. For example, Hernandez[5] found that men with violently acquired SCI came to see their injuries as positive life events that allowed them to reassess their lives and make positive changes and choices.

Stage Models of Adjustment to Disability

Early research on adjustment to SCI was dominated by stage models. Similar to Kubler-Ross[6] stages of death and dying, stage models of adjustment to disability posit a predictable and sequential series of reactions. Stage models have been criticized as an explanatory framework for understanding the process of psychosocial adjustment to disability in general and SCI in particular; yet they have an enduring allure for some rehabilitation professionals because they offer a predictable road map for explaining the dynamic process of psychosocial adjustment.

In her seminal work on the impact of SCI, Trieschmann[7] contends that the myth of stages of adjustment pathologize people with SCIs by demanding that all people experience psychological problems such as denial or depression in response to the injury. If the client states that no such psychological problems exist, then this is judged as denial and the client is diagnosed as having a psychological problem. Stage theories both pathologize and normalize reactions to disability. By labeling depression as a stage in the adjustment process, the experience of depression is normalized as a phase that one must pass through. This is problematic because research indicates that depression in people with SCIs is often undiagnosed and untreated. While depression is not a universal reaction to SCI, estimates of prevalence of depressive symptoms in people with SCI range from 16–60%[8] The high prevalence of depression and anxiety reinforces the need for health-care professionals to attend to issues of psychosocial adaptation to SCI[9] Depression can have a significant negative impact on people living with SCIs as it is associated with decreased quality of life and community participation. Depression also creates a risk for substance abuse and suicide (both of which are experienced at much higher rates among people with SCI). Suicide rates in particular are five times higher among people with SCI than among the general population,[10] with the highest rates of suicide found in the first 5 years post-injury (a time when the person is still adjusting to his or her life with a SCI). Depression can also be a barrier to participation in the rehabilitation and the long-term health maintenance processes.

In addition to conceptual limitations of stage theories, there is little empirical evidence to support these models. Trieschmann[7] characterized stage models as based on the "clinical impressions of the particular author and no data have been presented in any of the studies to demonstrate reliably and validly the existence, sequence or duration of these stages."

A paradox inherent in the use of stage models is related to the determination of an end point of the process.[11] If adjustment consists of a series of sequential stages, when the person reaches the final stage, the process ought to be complete. But even if an individual has successfully adapted to impairments, they are still judged by outsiders (including rehabilitation professionals, family, friends, and strangers) on the basis of their impairments. Like all people, individuals with SCI must adjust and readjust to changes in their physical and social environment, and consequently, no end point is ever achieved. Individuals with SCI can come to see themselves "like everyone else, they adapt to the full array of possibilities and limitations afforded by the complete panorama of their biological states and their social and physical environments . . . The question [for psychology] is how they come to satisfactory and satisfying terms with the same world in which everyone lives."

Shontz[11] proposes that psychological adjustment is no different for people with disabilities than it is for anyone else, and no special psychology of disability is needed. Trieschmann[7] echoes this perspective in her model of SCI adjustment. Her model is based on the assumption that adjustment to disability is not a finite process with a specific end point but rather is a dynamic, life-long process. The individual with a SCI strives for a balance in life by constantly adjusting and adapting to body systems issues (such as paralysis, pain, and fatigue), psychological resources (such as coping strategies, locus of control, and sense of coherence), and environment factors (such as the availability of social support, physical access, and societal attitudes). Within this model, rehabilitation is defined as "the process of teaching people to live with their disabilities in their own environment." This model is true to the principles of the biopsychosocial model of disability[12] that dominates rehabilitation theory, research, and policy and that serves as the basis for the World Health Organization's International Classification of Functioning, Disability and Health (ICF).[13]

In response to the criticisms of traditional stage models of adjustment to disability, Antonak and Livneh[14] developed a model of reactions to disability. Using a cross-disability sample, including people with SCI, they found evidence of a hierarchical, but nonlinear, multidimensional process of adaptation to disability. Using a sample of 118 people who sustained disability an average of 8 years earlier, they documented adaptation to disability as a developmental process in which the gradual acceptance of changes to body, self, and social interactions occur. They describe eight reactions (*see Box 9-1*) to disability, which they categorized as *nonadaptive* or *adaptive*.

Although considerable variations were noted in the sequence of these reactions, they observed a pattern in which nonadaptive reactions of anxiety, depression, internalized anger, and externalized hostility were prerequisites for adaptive responses of acknowledgment and adjustment. Shock was observed to be a prerequisite for depression and internalized anger, which are in turn are prerequisites for acknowledgment and adjustment. Only denial was independent of the other reactions.

Antonak and Livneh's[14] hierarchical model of reactions to disability has been used as the basis for exploring other factors that influence the rehabilitation process. For example, Martz[15] explored the relationship between adaptation to disability and future time orientation. Future time orientation is the degree of general concern, engagement, and involvement in the future. It is an important construct for rehabilitation professionals because the client-centered rehabilitation process demands that the client be able to participate in long-term planning and focus on future goal setting.[16,17] Traumatic injury such as an SCI can disrupt future time orientation and make it difficult to conceive of oneself as having a career, family, or normal life span. In a study of 317 people with SCI, Martz[15] found that shock, depression, and adjustment were related to future time orientation. Because of their negative association with the ability to conceive of a plan for a future, shock and depression may indicate the need for psychosocial interventions.

While empirical evidence for a developmental perspective may provide a useful framework for understanding the process of adjustment, Kendall and Buys[18] contend that all "stage models are largely descriptive and provide little information about the factors that contribute to individual difference in the adjustment process, even though an understanding of these factors will provide the key to maximizing the effectiveness of rehabilitation."

Psychological Reactions to SCI

- Stage models are of limited clinical utility in treatment planning because they fail to account for how adjustment occurs.
- Stage models have been criticized for promoting a recipe book for treatment and forcing all individuals to adhere to a narrowly defined set of responses.
- Rehabilitation professionals should not assume they know what the client is experiencing. They must ask and provide opportunities for engagement.
- The rehabilitation specialist must meet clients where they are and not where they are expected to be.
- Issues of depression, anxiety, and shock have important long-term consequences and must be assessed, diagnosed, and treated appropriately with pharmacological and/or psychosocial interventions as appropriate for the individual client. All members of the interdisciplinary team must be vigilant for signs of psychological distress and make referrals to the appropriate team member.

BOX 9–1
Model of Reactions to Disability[14]

Nonadaptive Reactions

1. Shock: A reaction of psychological numbness, depersonalization, disorganization, and decreased speech and mobility.
2. Anxiety: Involves panic, confused thinking, cognitive flooding, physical responses, and purposeless activity.
3. Denial: The tendency to negate or downplay the long-term consequences of injury because of inability to deal with the psychological consequences.
4. Depression: Feelings of helplessness, hopelessness, despair, isolation, self-deprecation, and distress.
5. Internalized anger: Self-directed reaction associated with blaming oneself and feeling guilty regarding the onset of the disability
6. Externalized hostility: May include aggression, antagonism, criticisms, accusations, and abusive verbalizations against others, or passive aggressive behaviors that may obstruct treatment.

Adaptive Reactions

7. Acknowledgement of disability: Cognitive acceptance of the disability
8. Adjustment to disability: Emotional and behavioral adjustment to the disability and integration of the disability into one's life.

Stress Appraisal Coping Model

Research in the area of adjustment following SCI has moved away from static models to focus on the dynamic interaction between effective problem-solving, coping, and social support. Livneh and Martz's[19] review on the relationship between coping and adjustment to disability reported that successful adjustment is linked to coping styles exemplified by self-confidence, cooperation, and sociability;[20] purpose in life;[21] perceived self-efficacy;[22,23] and increased sense of coherence post-injury[24] Similarly, Elfström and associates'[25] study of 255 people with SCI found that coping factors accounted for most of the variability in psychological outcome reactions. Sociodemographic variables (with the exception of education) and disability-related variables were weak predictors of psychological outcomes.

Lazarus and Folkman[26] described a stress appraisal and coping model that has been applied extensively to SCI research. They describe a dynamic process in which the individual perceives a stressor in the environment, appraises its potential impact on his or her life, and mobilizes coping strategies and coping resources to mediate the effect of the stressor. Each of the core concepts of this model are discussed in turn, along with empirical evidence to supporting its inclusion in the model.

Stressors

Stressors represent a particular relationship between the person and the environment that is seen by the individual as taxing or exceeding the resources that are available to deal with it, thereby endangering well-being. SCI can reasonably be considered a stressful event for most people. Other potential stressors experienced by people who have sustained a SCI include sudden functional status loss; altered social relationships; and decreased access to work, health care, and housing. Negative stress responses can include depression, anxiety, and emotional distress. While depression is not a universal outcome of SCI, people with SCI report significantly higher rates of depression than the general population.[8,9] Similarly, anxiety has been viewed as a normal early reaction following the onset of severe bodily injury and sudden functional loss.[27,28] Anxiety levels are higher among people with SCIs than in community samples, with a prevalence level of about 30%.[29] Anxiety is not, however, a universal reaction to SCI, but represents psychosocial distress. Anxiety is associated with poorer psychosocial adjustment following SCI.[20] Acute anxiety reactions in the form of posttraumatic stress disorders have been reported in people following SCI.[30,31]

Longitudinal studies of people with SCIs indicate that anxiety levels remain high up to 2 years post-injury.[29,32] For example, Holicky and Charlifue[33] reported the findings of a longitudinal study of the impact of stress and psychological outcomes in people with SCI who were at least 20 years post-injury. They reported three significant findings: (1) the nonrelationship between stress and severity of impairments among long-term SCI survivors; (2) strong relationships between stress and other psychological outcomes, especially increased depression and decreased life satisfaction and quality of life; and (3) a lack of strong relationships between stress and medical outcomes. Clearly, stress and one's reaction to it has important implications for the long-term adjustment to SCI.

Mediators

In response to stressors, people appraise the level of threat and their ability to deal with the threat. Lazarus and Folkman's[26] stress-appraisal coping model describes a primary and secondary appraisal process.

Primary Appraisal

Primary appraisal is an inference about a life situation determined by factors such as individual psychological characteristics, past experience, and expectations for the future. It is not an objective analysis of the stressors and resources, but a scan of the situation to determine its potential harm. Situations may be deemed irrelevant, benign/positive, or stressful. The stress appraisals after SCI include the degree of harm or threat to the individual. For example, someone who sees SCI as a catastrophic event that will exclude them from active engagement in valued life roles such as worker, athlete, and lover will appraise the situation as more threatening than someone who can envision adapted means of participation and role fulfillment. The threat of the SCI is therefore mediated by both the importance of the issues being threatened and the individual's belief about his or her ability to control the situation.

Secondary Appraisal

Secondary appraisal is a more calculated process by which the individual decides what can be done to decrease the stressful situation. It is a complex evaluative process that takes into account available coping resources, the adequacy of these resources, and the feasibility of putting them into action. Secondary appraisal can occur at an unconscious level or as a metastrategy whereby the person actively assesses the demands of a situation to select appropriate coping strategies and resources to deal with the stressor.

Empirical Support

A great deal of research has been focused on the psychological impact of a person's appraisal of the attribution of blame for SCI. Research on the relationship between appraisal and emotional adjustment has been contradictory. For example, Bulman and Wortman[34] found that people with SCI who perceived their injuries as avoidable and thus controllable demonstrated better adjustment than those who blamed external factors. While self-blame and specific attributions may be adaptive in the acute phase, they do not appear to serve that function as time passes. The passage of time allows people to reframe their experience of injury and impairment in ways that promote positive self-evaluations. While questions of "why me?" may be important to psychosocial well-being in the immediate aftermath of injury, their resolution allows energy to be refocused to the social world, relationships, and the pursuit of short- and long-term goals.

Coping

Lazarus and Folkman[26] define coping as the "constantly changing cognitive and behavioral efforts to manage specific external and/or internal demands that are appraised as taxing or exceeding the resources of the person." Two main types of coping strategies have been proposed: emotion-focused and problem-focused coping.

Emotion-focused coping involves changing or regulating emotional responses. These strategies are used when individuals believe that a situation is beyond their control and includes strategies such as wish-fulfilling fantasy, emotional expression, and substance use.

Problem-focused coping is aimed at managing the stressful situation itself. These strategies tend to be used when people believe that the situation is controllable and that they have the skills needed to control it. Problem-focused strategies include asking questions, considering alternative courses of action, and evaluating consequences of coping efforts.

Empirical Support

Coping is an extensively studied aspect of the stress appraisal model; empirical evidence suggests a strong relationship between coping and emotional adjustment.

People who use emotion-focused coping report higher rates of depression, anxiety, and life stress[35,36] and poorer emotional adjustment than those using problem-focused strategies.[37] Furthermore, people's belief in their ability to effectively solve problems was predictive of depression and emotional distress.[38] Coping strategies were more strongly associated with greater psychological adjustment than were age, time since injury, level of injury, locus of control,[39] marital status, or functional independence.[40] The types of coping strategies used remained fairly consistent over time, but the tendency to seek emotional and instrumental social support decreased with time. Most people with SCIs used adaptive strategies such as acceptance regardless of time since injury.[36]

In summary, coping strategies have a greater mediating effect on psychosocial adjustment than do sociodemographic variables such as age, time since injury, marital status, and functional independence. Coping is a dynamic process, with some strategies being more adaptive at some times than others, and may be influenced by individual needs and circumstances.[41]

Coping Resources

The final modifier in the stress appraisal coping model is coping resources. Unmodifiable coping resources are traits inherent in an individual (e.g., age, gender). They cannot be changed by rehabilitation or intervention. Modifiable coping resources are amenable to change and may be an appropriate therapeutic target. Social support is an example of a modifiable resource." Modifiable and unmodifiable coping resources are discussed next.

Unmodifiable Resources

Age Younger individuals demonstrate greater emotional adjustment. Galvin and Godfrey[42] hypothesize that younger individuals may have greater flexibility in the path their lives will follow and therefore may be more adaptable to change.

Gender Women tend to be more accepting of SCI-associated loss than men. Differential role expectations may allow women to move more freely in and out of the job market. Higher rates of sexual difficulties may contribute to poorer adjustment for men.

Modifiable Resources

Social Support Social support is the most important and extensively studied coping resource and mediator of emotional adjustment. For example, in a study of 179 people with SCI, Elliott and associates[38] found that support characterized by reassurance of worth and independence is associated with good emotional adjustment, while relationships characterized by nurturing support was associated with poor adjustment. Given its importance to psychosocial adjustment, social support will be discussed in detail in later in this chapter.

Evidence-Based Interventions to Promote Psychological Adjustment

In spite of our growing understanding about the process of adjustment, there are few evidence-based interventions reported in the literature.[42,43] One potentially valuable intervention is cognitive behavioral therapy (CBT). CBT is increasingly recognized as an effective technique for managing psychosocial disorders, especially depression and anxiety.[44,45] It provides a structured and effective therapeutic approach to changing behavioral and cognitive patterns by implementing behavioral contingencies, isolating negative or maladaptive thought patterns, and teaching adaptive coping strategies. CBT has been used to prepare people for community reentry. Group CBT provides rehabilitation practitioners with an efficient means of treating people with similar concerns in a group setting while providing opportunities for peer support and social learning.

Craig and associates[46] used a nonrandomized, controlled trial to assess the long-term efficacy of an inpatient CBT group. Treatment consisted of a 10-week program that addressed anxiety, depression, self-esteem, assertiveness, sexuality, and family relationships. This skills-based approach included realization training techniques, cognitive restructuring, opportunities to improve social skills and assertiveness, sexual education sessions, and participation in increasingly pleasant events. Due to a relative low incidence of psychological problems in either the control or the intervention group, no significant differences in depression or anxiety were found. However, a subsample of people with high levels of depression and anxiety demonstrated significant improvements in depression immediately after treatment and at 1 year post-injury. These findings suggest that not all people with SCI need psychosocial and CBT interventions, but that those experiencing psychological distress can benefit from CBT. Craig and associates[32] reassessed the participants 2 years post-injury and found that the treatment group had fewer hospital readmissions, reported less drug use, and had better emotional adjustment than the control group, indicating that CBT may have long-term benefits for emotional adjustment.

Kennedy and associates reported similar benefits with coping effectiveness training (CET) on psychological adjustment, self-perception, and adaptive coping.[47-49] CET is a group-based CBT intervention based on Lazarus and Folkman's[26] stress appraisal coping theory.

CET aims to teach appraisal skills, a range of standard cognitive behavioral skills along with a metastrategy to flexibly guide the choice of coping strategies and their application.[47-49] Since the effectiveness of coping strategies fluctuates with situational demands, the ability to accurately appraise a situation and apply an appropriate strategy is a critical element.

CET consists of seven 60- to 75-minute sessions twice a week. Box 9-2 outlines the organization and content areas of each session. Participants in these studies reported that they valued the opportunities for shared discussion and problem solving that the group format afforded them.

In summary, preliminary evidence suggests that individual and group CBT are effective in promoting emotional adjustment after SCI.

Social Support

Social support is an important coping resource and has been extensively studied among people with SCIs. High levels of social support and satisfaction with social contacts have been associated with increased levels of well-being when controlling for health and income,[50] increased life satisfaction, better self-assessed physical health, and reduction of secondary health conditions.[51] Spousal support in particular has been associated with decreased depression, increased life satisfaction, and psychological well-being,[33] while social support from friends was the best indicator of acceptance and was positively correlated with adaptive coping strategies.

McColl, Lei, and Skinner[41] examined the relationship between social support and coping in people returning to community living after SCI. They found that patterns of social support changed over time. At 1 month after discharge, there was a higher concentration of informational support, whereas emotional support took precedence at 4 and 12 months post-discharge. The changing levels and types of support may reflect patterns of need in the community reintegration process. In the initial phases of community integration, emphasis is on learning how the service systems work and how to negotiate society as a person with a disability. With time, emphasis may shift to taking care of emotional health and well-being.

Not only has the amount of support been shown to be important, the manner in which support is provided also impacts long-term outcomes. For example, Elliott and associates[38] found people whose social support relationships afforded opportunities for assertiveness reported lower levels of depression than people who received primarily nurturance and caretaking. People with SCIs whose social relationships were characterized by assertiveness also reported higher levels of social integration and a reassurance of their self-worth. These findings highlight the importance of allowing people to assert choice and control over how they live their lives and how support is provided and received. Cardol and associates[52] stressed the importance of decisional autonomy (the ability to make one's own decisions) even when independent function (executional autonomy) is compromised. The right to exert choice and control over one's life is a core value within the disability rights and independent living movements as well.[53]

In spite of the positive benefits of social support, people with SCI report support levels approximately 10% lower than their nondisabled peers.[54] Social support is conventionally characterized as a temporary need, which may not correspond with the ongoing needs of people with SCIs.[55] Norris and Kaniasty[56] described a social support deterioration model based on evidence of a fading effect of social support over time for people with ongoing support needs. Erosion of perceived support has been linked to depression, distress, and decreased life satisfaction among people with disabilities.[51,56,57] Using a strength-based qualitative approach, Devereux and associates[58] sought to understand how people maintain high levels of support. Participants highlighted the importance of maintaining autonomy, reciprocity, and a positive outlook. These responses demonstrate that social support is an interaction between two people, both of whom have needs and desires. Social support is best understood as a multidirectional flow between parties. The person with SCI is not a passive recipient, but has strengths and contributions to offer.

Support Providers

A unique situation occurs when members of a social network assume the role of informal and usually untrained support provider. While disability scholars, such as Jenny Morris,[59,60] contend that the emphasis on care partners and caregiver burden casts the person with a disability in the role of passive recipient of care and detracts from discussions about the right to adequate community resources, the impact of support provision is an important consideration in the lifelong care of people with SCIs.

Informal support providers such as family and friends provide a tremendous amount of physical and emotional

---

BOX 9–2
CET Sessions[47-49]

Session 1: Introduction to the concept of stress and attempts to normalize stress reactions.
Session 2: Stress appraisal skills.
Session 3: Problem solving, including SCI-specific role plays.
Session 4: Examination of connection and distinction between thoughts, feelings, and behaviors. Also includes pleasant activity scheduling and relaxation training.
Session 5: Awareness of negative assumptions, thoughts, and expectations and how to change them.
Session 6 and 7: Metastrategy training.

support to community-dwelling individuals with SCI.[61–63] These arrangements can have unintended and detrimental consequences, such as increased stress and depression and decreases in the support-provider's health and life satisfaction. Reliance on a single informal support provider also creates risks if the support provider is no longer willing or able to provide support.[64–67] Using a mixed methods design, Boschen, Tonack, and Gargaro[68] found that being a support provider was a major life change, and many people felt inadequately prepared, both cognitively and emotionally. Support providers felt that their productivity suffered and that they were invisible within the rehabilitation and social service systems. Similarly, Post, Bloeman, and de Witte[69] found that support providers experienced a greater burden. Factors that contributed to caregiver burden included amount of assistance provided, poor psychological adjustment by the person with the SCI, partner age and gender, functional independence, and time since injury.

Social Support

- Training and support of informal support providers can help prepare them for this unanticipated role.
- Monitoring support providers' needs and functioning for signs of burnout or deterioration is critical.
- Adequate community-based resources, such as personal attendant services, can help promote the autonomy of both members of the support dyad.
- Peer networks and social support groups for sharing strategies and struggles can help support providers.
- Support providers can benefit from knowledge-building activities to enhance their effectiveness.

Peer Mentoring

While social support from family and friends is clearly an important determinant of psychosocial adjustment, the beneficial impact of support from disabled peers and mentors is gaining increased recognition. For example, a 2-year mixed method study by Boschem, Tonack, and Gargaro[70] found that while substantial adjustments are required after SCI, both social support and peer mentoring are valuable parts of the process. By providing opportunities to learn from people with similar experiences, peer mentoring helped to compensate for perceived gaps in the rehabilitation process related to the real life experience of living with a SCI. Similarly, Sherman, Sperling, and DeVinney[71] examined the impact of past mentoring experiences on adjustment. Although the majority of peer-mentoring relationships are short lived (87% last less than 1 year) and informal (79%), participants who reported prior peer-mentoring experiences showed greater satisfaction with life and mean

occupational activity. The relationship between peer mentoring and work outcomes is intriguing because of the significant relationship between employment, psychosocial adjustment, and quality of life.[70,71]

Peer Mentoring

- Peer mentoring programs and opportunities should be integrated into clinical practice.
- Formal and informal peer mentoring programs allow sharing of advice, insider perspectives on disability, and community integration experiences. Facilitate opportunities for patients to network and interact with other people with SCIs.

Quality of Life

As medical management of SCI has improved and life expectancy has increased, there has been a shift in the focus of rehabilitation efforts from issues of physical and functional improvements to quality of life. While a SCI does represent a major lifestyle and functional change, it does not necessarily diminish quality of life. Quality of life for people with SCI can be very similar to that of their nondisabled peers. In what they labeled the "disability paradox," Albrecht and Devlieger[72] found that most people with disabilities rate their quality of life as good to excellent despite outsiders' impressions that their existence is "undesirable." This disjuncture between insider and outside perspectives on quality of life is well documented and persists even among experienced professionals.[73,74] People with disabilities report that quality of life depends on finding a balance between body, mind, and spirit and on establishing and maintaining harmonious relationships within one's social environment.[72] While such ideas resonate ideologically, they are difficult to integrate into clinical practice. To ensure that the values and experiences of people with SCIs are integrated into practice, researchers and clinicians must define and operationalize quality of life.

Definitions of Quality of Life

There is no single agreed-upon definition of *quality of life*. In fact, two separate but related constructs of quality of life are represented in the research literature. These are subjective quality of life/life satisfaction and health-related quality of life (HRQOL). Both are relevant for clinicians working with people with SCIs.

Quality of Life/Life Satisfaction

The World Health Organization defines quality of life as individuals' "perception of their position in life in the context of the culture and value systems in which they live, and in relation to their goals, expectations, standards and concerns."[75] Quality of life, also called *life satisfaction*, is the broader of the two quality of life constructs and encompasses all the things that a person values.[76] It reflects a person's overall perception of and satisfaction with how things are in their life.[77–79] Issues such as material, physical, and emotional well-being; functional capacity; social relationships; personal freedom; respect from others; and opportunity for work and leisure may all be included, depending on the individual's values.[77]

Health-Related Quality of Life

Stemming in part from recognition that not all areas of value to people have a realistic potential of being addressed by health-care systems and interventions, researchers sought to focus the definition of *quality of life*.[80] The concept of health-related quality of life is the result of these efforts. Experts have yet to agree on a single definition of HRQOL, yet there is a general consensus that it takes into account individuals' perceptions of their physical, mental, social, and role functioning, as well as their perceptions of health and well-being.[81–84] HRQOL is more related to functional performance than is quality of life/life satisfaction.

Definitions of Quality of Life

- It is important for clinicians to be aware of the differences between HRQOL and quality of life/life satisfaction. Both are important constructs, but to optimize interventions, treatment goals will address different phenomena of interest.
- HRQOL is likely to be more influenced by interventions that address activities of daily living and instrumental activities of daily living.
- Quality of life/life satisfaction may be more appropriately addressed at the level of community participation by addressing barriers in the physical and social environment.

Factors Influencing Quality of Life

Although once deemed elusive and too individualized to study, there is a growing body of evidence about factors that affect quality of life. These factors fall into two broad categories.

1. Individual demographic and impairment characteristics that often are not amenable to change or clinical intervention.
2. Medical, functional, social, and participation variables that may be improved by rehabilitative interventions.

Both categories provide important information that the clinician can use to enhance the quality of life of the clients they serve. Individual demographic characteristics such as age, level of injury, length of time since onset, gender, and race can be used to identify people who are at high risk for decreased quality of life and who may benefit from targeted interventions. The second group of medical, functional, social, and participation issues provides important information on what issues to target and address with clients. True to the principles of client-centered practice, intervention decisions ought to be made in collaboration and consultation with the person with SCI. An understanding and knowledge of the issues that affect quality of life can provide clinicians with a solid grounding from which they can facilitate the process of learning to live with SCI. For example, demographic characteristics that have been associated with reduced quality of life, include:

- Male gender
- Racial minority status, especially African American and Hispanic
- Recent onset of SCI
- Lower levels of community participation
- Lower educational attainment, especially for those with less than a high school diploma
- Unemployment
- Living in an institution

Quality of life issues and client-rated quality of life change over time as different issues take primacy during different stages of the adjustment process. In the first 2 years after SCI, self-rated quality of life tends to reach low levels as people work to adjust to the physical, functional, and lifestyle changes that accompany their injuries.[85] Lower quality of life is associated with greater pain, spasticity, incontinence, less physical independence and mobility, and the ability to return to work.[86–89] Higher quality of life is associated with satisfying relationships, maximizing function, meaningful activities, and access to the environment.[90] Understanding and addressing quality of life in the early phases is important because reduced quality of life predicts later stress, depression, and impaired psychological well-being.[91]

Quality of life tends to improve gradually over time.[85] Perceived quality of life in people with SCIs is relatively high and stable over time. Charlifue and Gerhart[91] reported that only 22% of people rate their quality of life as fair or poor, indicating that quality of life is not dramatically lower for people with SCI than for the general population.[92] Based on survey data from 2183 people with SCI, Dijkers[93] found that gender, time since injury, and social participation outcomes are major determinants of quality of life during the period of 1 to 20 years post-injury. Health status as measured by rehospitalization also had a direct effect on quality of life. The effects of impairment (such as level and completeness of injury) and disability (functional status) are experienced indirectly by how they affect social participation. Race, ethnicity, and education also are related to quality of life through their influence on participation. Cushman and Hasset[94] found that the ability to live in a preferred situation, a private home versus a nursing home, was strongly related to quality of life. Qualitative research on subjective quality of life identified four factors that are not typically assessed by most instruments but that were found to be associated with quality of life. These factors include environmental accessibility, disability stigma, spontaneity, and health-promoting behaviors.[95] These issues are closely related to social participation and are important areas to explore collaboratively with clients.

Quality of life and life satisfaction reflect developmental processes. Quality of life starts to decrease around 30 years post-injury and between the ages of 45 and 55.[96,97] Research on aging with a disability indicates that people with disabilities tend to experience the effects of aging at earlier ages than their nondisabled peers. People with SCI express greater anxiety about aging in general and express specific concerns related to their overall health, their ability to remain independent, and their ability to sustain a satisfying lifestyle.[98]

The quality of life literature makes it clear that access and opportunity for meaningful community participation and social engagement are key determinants of quality of life. The following section provides an overview of community participation and explores key aspects of participation that are important to people with SCIs.

Participation

Since 2001, the concept of participation has become increasingly important in rehabilitation, research, and policy. At that time, the World Health Organization brought forth a revised classification system for health and disability. The ICF[13] significantly revised the framing of disability and impairment by replacing the concept of handicap with that of participation. The ICF defines participation as "involvement in life situations" and outlines nine areas of participation (see Box 9-3 for areas of participation defined by the ICF).

The ICF represents a shift from the negative terminology of *handicap* to the more active concept of participation and reframing research and practice rehabilitation focus away from deficits to a greater focus on active engagement. The ICF provides a taxonomy to facilitate interdisciplinary communication for goal setting and treatment planning by providing clinicians common language that is not discipline specific.[106] As described earlier, participation is both an important goal for people with SCI and a significant contributor to quality of life and emotional adjustment. In the following section, key areas of participation that have been shown to influence quality of life and emotional adjustment in people with SCI are examined, including employment and education, martial status and parenting, and access to health care.

Measuring Quality of Life

- The selection of assessment tools to measure quality of life should reflect the salience of issues at different points in time. A working group of SCI and quality of life researchers developed assessment guidelines for use at different times post-SCI.[77] During the acute phase when issues of pain, physical mobility, functional status, and emotional adjustment are of primary importance, they recommend the Functional Independence Measure,[99] the Hospital Anxiety and Depression Scale,[100,101] and a Visual Analogue Scale for Pain. After discharge, they recommend use of the SF-36,[102] the Craig Handicap Assessment and Reporting Technique (CHART),[103] and the Quality of Well-Being Scale[104] or the Life Satisfaction Questionnaire.[105]
- For people whose motor and functional status is unlikely to improve, it is important to use measures of quality of life that allow the individual to evaluate the importance of physical function.
- Quality of life measures ought to be completed by the person with a SCI. Surrogates such as health professionals and support providers tend to underestimate quality of life.
- Clinicians should consider age-related changes. The ability to age in place and maintain meaningful community participation is of particular importance to older adults. Since these individuals are well past the acute and rehabilitative phases, they may not have access to the information, education, and interventions that can help them adapt to their changing needs. Health professionals can facilitate information acquisition.

BOX 9–3
Areas of participation defined by the International Classification of Functioning, Disability, and Health

- Learning and applying knowledge
- General tasks and demands
- Communication
- Mobility
- Self care
- Domestic life
- Interpersonal interactions and relationships
- Major life areas (such as work and education)
- Community, social, and civic life

Employment and Education

Employment rates and the closely aligned issue of economic self-sufficiency are of primary importance to people with SCIs. Employment affects more than just financial security—it is related to self-esteem, self-worth, and personal identity.[107] People with SCI who are employed tend to be more active, have fewer medical treatments, perceive themselves with fewer problems, are more satisfied with their lives, and rate their overall adjustment higher.[108,109] People with SCI are chronically underemployed, with employment rates ranging from 16% at first anniversary[64] and peaking at 33% at the tenth anniversary.[110] The rate of employment varies widely depending on how employment is defined and the time after injury.[111] For example, some studies include home-making and student roles as part of employment, while others include only paid employment. Employment rates increase with number of years post-injury.[110,111]

A variety of sociodemographic and impairment-related factors predict (re)employment. These are

- age at onset,
- length of time since onset,
- race,
- level of injury, and
- education.

Level of education is associated with return to work. For example, 65% to 89% of people with 16 or more years of education return to some form of work, compared with only 22% of people with a high school diploma.[112] Education not only reflects a higher socioeconomic status but increases the range of jobs available. People with SCI are much more likely to be employed in clerical, office, administrative, professional, and technical jobs than is the general population. Not only are these jobs better suited to the functional capacity of people with SCI, they are also more likely to have health insurance benefits that may offset the financial disincentives to work. Employment rates are roughly equal for men and women, although men are more likely to be engaged in paid work while women are more likely to be in unpaid roles, such as homemakers, volunteers, and students. Although the evidence regarding the relationship between level of injury and return to work is inconclusive, it does suggest that people with paraplegia and/or incomplete injuries are more likely to be employed than people with tetraplegia and complete injuries. People of color are less likely to be employed, even when controlling for age, education, gender, and neurological category.

Nearly three-quarters of people with SCI require product and worksite modification to maintain or improve productivity.[113] Access to and effective use of assistive technology is a major influence on employment success.[114] Participation in vocational rehabilitation program has been shown to increase (re)employment rates,

although some people with SCI note that occupational and educational choices are sometimes restricted by vocational counselors' perceptions about individuals' potential.[115] Despite the passage of the Americans with Disabilities Act[116] in 1990, which prohibits employment discrimination, the barriers of discrimination and lack of reasonable accommodations persist. These barriers include a lack of worksite and community accessibility, inadequate medical benefits, inadequate public transportation, employer bias, inflexible work schedules, and unreliable personal attendant services.[117,118]

Employment and Education

- Rehabilitation professionals in work preparedness programs must not only examine the person's ability to perform the job demands, but also evaluate environmental factors such as transportation, flexible scheduling, and availability of attendant care on the job.
- Employers' concerns about costs and difficulties of providing accommodations may be reduced if they learn from peers about the value of adapting the work environment and equipment to meet the needs of employees with SCIs. Most worksite modifications are relatively inexpensive.

Marital Status and Parenting

Marital status is related to quality of life and social support in people with SCIs. Unfortunately, after the first 3 years post-injury, divorce rates for people with SCIs are two to three times higher that that of the general population.[64] Divorce rates are higher for people who are younger,[119] African-American,[119,120] have previously been divorced,[121] are childless, and have more severe injuries.[122] People who are unmarried at the time of their injuries are also less likely to marry than their peers.[123]

As discussed in the section on social support, many spouses take on the role of support providers to their partners with SCI, either by choice or by a lack of adequate personal attendant care services. The emphasis on support provision, especially assistance for activities of daily life (ADLs), risks disrupting the spousal relationship and places a strain upon it. Other stressors can include financial instability due to disrupted employment, both parties' adjustment to altered functional status, and social role functioning.[124]

Parenting is another major life role that may be strained for people with SCIs. Parents with mobility impairments, including SCI, report that they experience attitudinal barriers about their fitness to parent. For example, David Lykken created a controversy with his award address published in the *American Psychologist* when he proposed that society license couples to become parents.[125] He included people "incapacitated by physical and mental disorders," along with people with violent criminal records and histories of substance abuse, among the category of people requiring special dispensations to have children. This speech drew strong criticism from many within the disability and rehabilitation communities, including the American Association of Spinal Injury Psychologists and the National Resource Center for Parents with Disabilities. This type of public statement perpetuates negative stereotypes about parents with disabilities, prejudices that are especially pronounced for mothers. Outsiders tend to emphasize the performance of specific childcare activities rather than the complete set of tasks, skills, and values that encompass parenting.[17,127–129] Evaluations of parental incapacity are often made without providing parents with disabilities the appropriate adaptive equipment, and so what gets evaluated is not parenting but disability obstacles.[130] Concerns have also been raised that children of disabled parents are robbed of their childhoods by being forced to act as "young caregivers." A recent nationwide study conducted through seven model system SCI centers indicated that there are no significant differences in family and child adjustment between families with mothers with and without a SCI.[131] Prejudice about parental capacity and fitness may create fear among parents with SCIs and prevent them from disclosing their need for assistance.[129] There is nothing inherent in a SCI that prevents a parent from creating a nurturing, caring, and safe environment that facilitates a child's physical and emotional growth.

Access to Health Care

Health status has been demonstrated to be an important predictor of quality of life for people with SCI. However, people with disabilities often face systematic barriers when trying to access services. For example, the National Organization on Disability[132] found in a nationwide survey that 28% of people with disabilities reported that they needed therapies, equipment, or medications that were not covered by their health plans, compared with only 7% of people without disabilities. Similarly, 19% of people with disabilities reported that they needed medical care within the previous year that they did not receive, compared with 6% of nondisabled people.

Unequal access to health care is in part a funding issue, but it has also been found that misconceptions about people with disabilities contribute to disparities in services. Medical providers tend to focus on disability-specific issues, creating an "underemphasis on health promotion and disease prevention activities."[133,134] For example, people with severe mobility impairments such as SCIs receive significantly fewer screening and preventative services, such as mammograms, Pap smears, and tobacco queries.[135] Stereotypes and stigma about living with a disability also create barriers to comprehensive care, such as limiting discussion of mental health and sexuality.[136] The neglect of mental health needs of people with SCIs is important because people with these injuries have a risk five times greater risk than the general population for depression, anxiety, and suicide.

Finally, access issues such as inaccessible doctor's offices[137] and reliance on overbooked and financially strapped paratransit services create barriers to entering a physician's office. Issues of access to health care are important because people with SCIs often have a "thinner margin of health" than their nondisabled peers due to functional limitations; risk of secondary conditions and functional loss, such as pressure ulcers and urinary track infections; fewer opportunities for health maintenance and preventative health care; and the earlier onset of chronic health conditions.[138]

Martial Status and Parenting

- Given the strain that a SCI may place on a relationship, the needs of both parties in a couple ought to be considered. This consideration includes addressing and assessing their needs, both as individuals and as part of a dyad.
- Access to supportive community-based resources and personal attendant services can help disentangle support provision from the spousal relationship.
- Parents with SCIs can benefit from the support of therapists to help strategize adaptive and alternative methods to perform child-care tasks.
- Clinicians should be aware that fear may prevent parents from raising issues related to child care in a clinical setting. Clinicians should work to create a safe and supportive environment in which these issues may be discussed and addressed.

Access to Health Care

- All medical and psychological service offices should comply with the Americans with Disability Act accessibility guidelines.
- All rehabilitation professionals must consider the entire person with a SCI, and not just the diagnosis, in order to provide the most comprehensive care possible.

CASE STUDY 9-1: Assessment, Intervention and Consultation Issues

Background Information

Violet, a 32-year-old married woman, sustained complete tetraplegia at the C6–C7 level as the result of a motor vehicle accident. She experienced hallucinations at the acute care hospital and told her husband that she could not live paralyzed.

At rehabilitation admission, Violet was dependent for all her ADLs, locomotion, and transfers. A complete rehabilitation program was recommended, including psychological assistance for patient and family. After 4 weeks, Violet was discharged because her Halo brace limited participation in rehabilitation. After the Halo brace was removed 2 months later, Violet was readmitted and resumed inpatient rehabilitation.

Pre-Injury Social History

Violet had a stable 6-year marriage with her husband, Chuck. They were childless by choice. Violet was college educated and worked full-time at the time of her injury. Her hobbies included "working in my massive garden, which has two water gardens, raising three dogs, and my koi fish." Violet came from a close-knit family who lived nearby. She was a practicing Roman Catholic and attended Mass weekly, even during rehabilitation.

Initial Interview

Upon initial interview, Violet appeared somewhat dysphoric, anxious, and frustrated. She reported that she worried about "being a burden for my family and husband . . . I don't want to be cared for the rest of my life." She brought up the fear that she would no longer be attractive to her husband and he might abandon her. She reported awakening at night fearing that she may stop breathing. Her parents stayed with her around the clock to alleviate her anxiety. She feared being dropped during transfers.

Violet described her pre-accident personality as competent, independent, and fun loving. She had always "directed others with ease . . . [but] now I worry about confronting staff, not wanting to be seen as demanding." She was timid with staff, preferring to direct her family to help when staff were unresponsive. She reported that she was irritable with her family, felt periodically overwhelmed, and was frustrated with her disability. Her strengths included her strong spiritual beliefs, her self-confidence, and a good social support network.

Psychosocial Interventions

Violet's psychologist recommended individual and group psychotherapy, which she willingly accepted. Early in her rehabilitative stay, Violet expressed the following thoughts: "I can't imagine living like this the rest of my life . . . I don't want to live this way . . . my parents are always with me . . . I feel like a child . . . I worry my husband will leave me . . . I'm no longer attractive . . . I will never accept this . . . I am sad when I think about my future." Violet also reported, "I lost my body and my way of life."

It is not unusual for a person to experience a mourning process immediately following a SCI. It is therefore important to differentiate normal grieving from clinical depression. In grieving, one does not usually experience helplessness, hopelessness, low self esteem, psychomotor agitation, and anhedonia. Violet was able to clearly state realistic goals and looked forward to her future, including regaining arm and hand function and returning to work. These statements were corroborated by the results of the Zung Self-Rating Depression Scale[139] and used to rule out depression. The Zung was chosen because it does not contain somatic items that can be confused with the physical symptomatology of SCI. Her psychologist focused on helping Violet cope with multiple losses, including self-identity, independence, and mobility.

Violet's good pre-morbid problem-solving skills, her goal-directed strategies, and her current hope were indicators of her resiliency and were targeted for therapeutic interventions. During her first hospitalization, the primary therapeutic concerns focused on her anxiety, helplessness, and suicidal ideation. Violet was taught to identify her specific fears and clarify their realistic and irrational components. She learned to use relaxation techniques to deal with the anxiety they provoked. Given Violet's fear of being dropped during transfers, the therapy and nursing staff developed consistent transfer techniques to help her feel more secure. Violet attributed her suicidal ideation to the shock of the injury and did not truly want to end her life.

The 2-month interruption of rehabilitation helped Violet to clarify her goals and identify her strengths and priorities. Violet stated, "After being home, I realized I can still plan my garden and direct the plantings . . . I know I will regain more function. . . . I love my life, and with time I want to go back to work. . . . I am still connected with my dogs, and they need me . . . I will never give up." She also gained insight into emotional and psychological needs to participate in outside activities.

During her second rehabilitation stay, Violet's psychologist used behavioral and psychodynamic techniques in addition to support and education. Violet had the capacity to identify catastrophizing "what if" statements, fortune-telling, and other self thoughts, images, and statements that anticipated negative outcomes. As time progressed, Violet started to regain control of her environment. She became more assertive in interaction with patients, staff, and family, indicating a more constructive psychological state. In light of Violet's strong connection to her religious community, the rehabilitation psychologist (with Violet's permission) contacted her local parish and requested their presence in the hospital, including having the priest say Mass at the hospital. These efforts provided solace to both Violet and her family.

Continued

CASE STUDY 9-1:   Assessment, Intervention and Consultation Issues—cont'd

Spousal Psychotherapeutic Contacts

SCI can affect an entire family system. With Violet's consent, psychotherapeutic contacts were initiated with her husband. He reported feeling that "her parents had come in and taken over Violet's complete care . . . I feel like I am her boyfriend not her husband . . . I know she thinks I'm no longer physically attracted to her . . . I feel that I have let her down." Chuck was profoundly overwhelmed. He wanted to support his wife but did not know how to do it. Psychotherapeutic interventions included support, educa-

tion, insight, and behavioral strategies. Chuck was supported in finding ways to reestablish his husband role and spend time alone with Violet without hurting or distancing his in-laws. Toward the end of his sessions, Chuck said, "I feel more connected."

This case study highlights issues of assessment, intervention, and consultation in SCI rehabilitation. It demonstrates some of the ways that rehabilitation psychologists can address psychosocial concerns to help facilitate the process of community reintegration.

Summary

Most people with SCIs report having satisfying lives with good emotional health and quality of life. There is an important association between meaningful participation in valued life roles, quality of life, and emotional adjustment. There is, however, a significant minority who experience psychosocial problems such as depression, anxiety, suicidal ideation and attempts, decreased quality of life, and barriers to participation. These problems are associated with both demographic (e.g., age) and injury-specific (e.g., neurological level, pain) factors, as well as with barriers in the physical and social environment. It is vital that health professionals who work with people with SCIs not only be aware of, but also address, personal and societal factors to maximize social and emotional functioning. By adopting a holistic, interdisciplinary, and client-centered approach, rehabilitation professionals can help people with SCIs achieve the satisfying lives that they deserve and desire.

REVIEW QUESTIONS

1. Identify two limitations of hierarchical stage models of adjustment to SCI.
2. List and define the eight types of emotional reactions to disability described by Antonak and Livneh. Differentiate adaptive and nonadaptive reactions.
3. Name and define the three main components of the stress appraisal coping model and discuss their relevance to SCI rehabilitation.
4. List four factors that contribute to quality of life for people with SCIs.
5. Identify two core areas of participation that can be negatively impacted by a SCI.

REFERENCES

1. Vash CL, Crewe NM. *Psychology of Disability.* 2nd edition. New York: Springer Publishing; 2004.
2. Dembo T, Leviton G, Wright BA. Adjustment to misfortune: A problem in social-psychological rehabilitation. *Artificial Limbs.* 1956;3:4–62.
3. Wright BA. *Physical Disability: A Psychological Approach.* New York: Harper and Row; 1960.
4. Wright BA. *Physical Disability: A Psychosocial Approach.* 2nd edition. New York: Harper and Row; 1983.
5. Hernandez B. A voice in the chorus: Perspectives of young men of color on their disabilities, identities, and peer-mentors. *Disabil Soc.* 2005;20(2):117–133.
6. Kubler-Ross E. *On Death and Dying.* New York: Macmillan; 1969.
7. Treischmann RB. *Spinal Cord Injuries: Psychological, Social, and Vocational Rehabilitation.* 2nd edition. New York: Demos Medical Publishing; 1988.
8. Elliott TB, Frank RG. Depression following spinal cord injury. *Arch Phys Med Rehabil.* 1996;77:816–823.
9. Kennedy P, Rogers BA. Anxiety and depression after spinal cord injury. *Arch Phys Med Rehabil.* 2000;81(7): 932–937.
10. DeVivo MJ, Black KJ, Stover SL. Causes of death during the first 12 years after spinal cord injury. *Arch Phys Med Rehabil.* 1993;74:248–254.
11. Shontz FC. Adaptation to chronic illness and disability. In: Millon T, Green C, Meagher R, editors. *Handbook of Clinical Health Psychology.* New York: Plenum Publishing; 1982: pp. 153–172.
12. Engel GL. The need for a new medical model: A challenge for biomedicine. *Science.* 1977;196:129–136.
13. World Health Organization. *International Classification of Functioning, Disability, and Health: ICF.* 2001. Geneva, Switzerland: World Health Organization.
14. Antonak RF, Livneh H. A hierarchy of reactions to disability. *Int J Rehabil Res.* 1991;14:13–24.
15. Martz E. Do reactions of adaptation to disability influence the fluctuation of future time orientation among individuals with spinal cord injuries? *Rehabil Couns Bull.* 2004;47(2):86–95.

16. Rumrill P, Roessler R. New directions in vocational rehabilitation: A career development perspective on closure. *J Rehabil.* 1999;65(1):26–30.

17. Szymanski EM, Hershenson DB. Career development of people with disabilities: An ecological model. In: Parker RM, and Szymanski EM, editors. *Rehabilitation Counseling: Basics and Beyond.* 3rd edition. Austin, TX: ProEd; 1998. pp. 327–378.

18. Kendall E, Buys N. An integrated model of psychosocial adjustment following acquired disability. *J Rehabil.* 1998;64(3):16–20.

19. Livneh H, Martz E. Psychosocial adaptation to spinal cord injury: A dimensional perspective. *Psychol Rep.* 2005;97: 577–586.

20. Alfano DP, Neilson PM, Fink MP. Long-term psychosocial adjustment following head or spinal cord injury. *Neuropsychiatry Neuropsychol Behav.* 1993;6:117–125.

21. Thompson NJ, Coker J, Krause JS et al. Purpose in life as a mediator for adjustment after spinal cord injury. *Rehabil Psychol.* 2003;48:100–108.

22. Hampton NZ. Self-efficacy and quality of life in China. *Rehabil Couns Bull.* 2000;43:66–74.

23. Middleton JW, Tate RL, Geraghty TJ. Self-efficacy and spinal cord injury: Psychometric properties of a new scale. *Rehabil Psychol.* 2003;48:281–288.

24. Lustig DC. The adjustment process for individuals with spinal cord injury: The effect of perceived premorbid sense of coherence. *Rehabil Couns Bull.* 2005;48:146–156.

25. Elfström ML, Rydén A, Kreuter M et al. Linkages between coping and psychological outcome in the spinal cord lesioned: Development of SCL-related measures. *Spinal Cord.* 2002;40:23–29.

26. Lazarus RS, Folkman S. *Stress, Appraisal, and Coping.* New York: Springer Publishing; 1984.

27. Livneh H, Antonak RF. *Psychosocial Adaptation to Chronic Illness and Disability.* Gaithersburg, MD: Aspen Publishers; 1997.

28. Vash CL, Crewe NM. *Psychology of Disability.* 2nd edition. New York: Springer Publishing; 2004.

29. Hancock KM, Craig AR, Dickson HG et al. Anxiety and depression over the first year of spinal cord injury: A longitudinal study. *Paraplegia.* 1993;3:349–357.

30. Radnitz CL, Schlein IS, Walczak S et al. The prevalence of post-traumatic stress disorder in veteran with spinal cord injury. *Spinal Cord Injury Psychosocial Process.* 1995;8: 145–149.

31. Martz E, Cook DW. Physical impairments as risk factors for the development of posttraumatic stress disorder. *Rehabilitation Counseling Bulletin.* 2001;44(4):217–221.

32. Craig AR, Hancock K, Dickson H. Improving the long term adjustment of spinal cord injured persons. *Spinal Cord.* 1999;37:345–350.

33. Holicky R, Charlifue S. Aging with spinal cord injury: The impact of spousal support. *Disabil Rehabil.* 1999;21(5/6): 250–257.

34. Bulman RJ, Wortman CB. Attributions of blame and coping in the 'real world': Severe accident victims react to their lot. *J Pers Soc Psychol.* 1977;35:351–363.

35. Frank RG. Differences in coping styles among persons with spinal cord injury: A cluster-analytic approach. *J Consult Clin Psych.* 1987;55:727–731.

36. Kennedy P, Marsh N, Lowe R et al. A longitudinal analysis of psychological impact and coping strategies following spinal cord injury. *Brit J Health Psychol.* 2000;5:157–172.

37. Moore AD, Bombardier CH, Brown PB et al. Coping and emotional attributions following spinal cord injury. *Inter J Rehabil Res.* 1994;17:39–48.

38. Elliott TR, Godshall FJ, Herrick SM et al. Problem solving appraisal and psychological adjustment following spinal cord injury. *Cogn Ther Res.* 1991;15:387–398.

39. Buckelew SP, Baumstark KE, Frank RG et al. Adjustment following spinal cord injury. *Rehabil Psychol.* 1980;35:101–109.

40. Kennedy P, Lowe R, Grey N et al. Traumatic spinal cord injury and psychological impact: A cross sectional analysis of coping strategies. *Br J Clin Psychol.* 1995;34:627–639.

41. McColl MA, Lei H, Skinner H. Structural relationships between social support and coping. *Soc Sci Med.* 1995;41(3):395–407.

42. Galvin LR, Godfrey HPD. The impact of coping on emotional adjustment to spinal cord injury (SCI): Review of the literature and application of a stress appraisal and coping formulation. *Spinal Cord.* 2001;39:615–627.

43. McAweeney M, Tate D, McAweeney W. Psychosocial intervention in the rehabilitation of people with spinal cord injury: A comprehensive review. *Spinal Cord Injury Psychosocial Process.* 1997;10:58–63.

44. Andrews G. The evaluation of psychotherapy. *Curr Opin Psychiatry.* 1991;4:379–83.

45. Andrews G. The essential psychotherapies. *Br J Psychol.* 1993;162:447–451.

46. Craig AR, Hancock KM, Dickson H et al. Long term psychological outcomes in spinal injured persons: Results of a controlled trial using cognitive behaviour therapy. *Arch Phys Med Rehabil.* 1997;78:330–338.

47. King C, Kennedy P. Coping effectiveness training for people with spinal cord injury: Preliminary results of a controlled trial. *Brit J Clin Psychol.* 1997;38:5–14.

48. Kennedy P, Duff J, Avare M et al. Coping effectiveness training reduces depression and anxiety following traumatic spinal cord injuries. *Br J Clin Psychol.* 2003;42:41–52.

49. Kennedy P, Taylor NM, Duff J. Characteristics predicting effective outcomes after coping effectiveness training for patients with spinal cord injuries. *J Clin Psychol Med Settings.* 2005;12(1):93–98.

50. Schulz R, Decker, S. Long-term adjustment to physical disability: The role of social support, perceived control, and self-blame. *J Pers Soc Psychol.* 1985;48:1162–1172.

51. Rintala DH, Young ME, Hart KA et al. Social support and the well-being of persons with spinal cord injury living in the community. *Rehabil Psychol.* 1992;37:155–164.

52. Cardol M, DeJong BA, Ward CD. On autonomy and participation in rehabilitation. *Disabil Rehabil.* 2002;24(18): 970–974.

53. Barnes C, Mercer G, Shakespeare T. *Exploring Disability: A Sociological Introduction.* Cambridge, England: Polity Press; 2000.

54. White GW, Branstetter AD, Seekins T, editors. *Secondary Conditions among People with Disabilities from Minority Cultures: Proceedings and Recommendations of a Working Conference.* University of Kansas: Research and Training Center on Independent Living; 2000.

55. Braithewaite DO, Eckstein NJ. How people with disabilities communicatively manage assistance: Helping as instrumental social support. *J Appl Commun Res.* 2003;1(1):1–26.

56. Norris FH, Kaniasty K. Received and perceived social support in times of stress: A test of the social support deterioration deterrence model. *J Pers Soc Psychol.* 1998;71(3): 498–511.

57. Fontana A, Kerns R, Violetnberg R et al. Support, stress, and recovery from coronary heart disease: A longitudinal causal model. *Health Psychol.* 1989;8:175–193.

58. Devereux PG, Bullock CC, Bargmann-Losche J et al. Maintaining supporting in people with paralysis: What works? *Qual Health Res.* 2005;15(10):1360–1376.

59. Morris J. Impairment and disability: Constructing an ethics of care that promotes human rights. *Hypatia.* 2001;16(4): 1–16.

60. Morris J. Independent living and community care: A disempowering framework. *Disabil Soc.* 2004;19(5): 427–442.

61. Elliott TR, Shewchuk RM. Recognizing the family caregiver: Integral and formal members of the rehabilitation process. *J Vocat Rehabil.* 1998;10:123–132.

62. Mintz S. Caregiving counts. *Paraplegia News.* 1997;51(3): 14–15.

63. Mintz S. Share the caring. *Paraplegia News.* 1999;53(9): 12–14.

64. Dijkers MP, Abela MB, Gans BM et al. The aftermath of spinal cord injury. In: Stover SL, DeLisa JA, and Whiteneck GG, editors. *Spinal Cord Injury: Clinical Outcomes from the Model Systems.* Gaithersburg, MD: Aspen Publishers; 1995. pp. 185–209.

65. Grant JS, Elliott TR, Giger JN et al. Social problem-solving abilities, social support, and adjustment among family caregivers of individuals with a stroke. *Rehabil Psychol.* 2001;46:44–57.

66. Kolakowsky-Hayner SA, Miner KD, Kreutz JS. Long-term quality of life and family needs after traumatic brain injury. *J Head Trauma Rehabil.* 2001;16:374–384.

67. Meade MA, Taylor L, Kreutzer JS et al. A preliminary study of acute family needs after spinal cord injury: Analysis and implications. *Rehabil Psychol.* 2004;49:150–155.

68. Boschen KA, Tonack M, Gargaro J. The impact of being a support provider to a person living in the community with a spinal cord injury. *Rehabil Psychol.* 2005;50(4): 397–407.

69. Post MWM, Bloeman J, de Witte LP. Burden of support for partners of persons with spinal cord injuries. *Spinal Cord.* 2005;43:311–319.

70. Boschen KA, Tonack M, Gargaro J. Long-term adjustment and community reintegration following spinal cord injury. *Int J Rehabil Res.* 2003;26:157–162.

71. Sherman JE, Sperling KB, DeVinney DJ. Social support and adjustment after spinal cord injury: Influence of past peer-mentoring experiences and current live-in partner. *Rehabil Psychol.* 2004;49(2):140–149.

72. Albrecht GL, Devlieger PJ. The disability paradox: High quality of life against all odds. *Soc Sci Med.* 1999;48: 977–988.

73. Bach JR, Tilton MC. Life satisfaction and well being measures in ventilator assisted individuals with traumatic tetraplegia. *Arch Phys Med Rehabil.* 1994;75:626–632.

74. Gerhart KA, Koziol-McLain J, Lowenstein SR et al. Quality of life following spinal cord injury. Knowledge and attitudes of emergency care providers. *Ann Emerg Med.* 1994;23:807–812.

75. World Health Organization. *The World Health Organization Quality of Life Assessment. Field Trial Version for Adults. Administration Manual.* 1995; Geneva, Switzerland, World Health Organization.

76. Scheer L. Experiences with quality of life comparisons. In: Szalai A, Anderson FM, editors. *The Quality of Life: Comparative Studies.* Newbury Park, CA: Sage Publications;1980.

77. Wood-Dauphinee S, Exner G, Bostanci B et al. Quality of life in patients with spinal cord injury—basic issues, assessment, and recommendations. *Restor Neurol Neurosci.* 2002;20:135–149.

78. Hornquist JO. The concept of quality of life. *Scand J Soc Med.* 1982;10:57–61.

79. Whiteneck GG. Measuring what matters: Key rehabilitation outcomes. *Arch Phys Med Rehabil.* 1994;75:1433–1439.

80. Ware JE. Standards for validating health measures: Definitions and content. *J. Chron Dis.* 1987;40:473–480.

81. Berzo RA, Hays RD, Shumaker SA. International use, application, and performance of health-related quality of life instruments. *Qual Life Res.* 1993;2:367–368.

82. Bowling A. *Measuring Disease: A Review of Disease-Specific Quality of Life Measurement Scales.* Buckingham, England: Open University Press;1995.

83. Fitzpatrick R, Fletcher A, Gore S et al. Quality of life measures in health care. 1: Application and issues of assessment. *Br Med J.* 1992;305:1074–1077.

84. Pope A, Tarlov A. *Disability in America: Toward a National Agenda for Prevention.* Washington, DC: National Academy Press; 1991.

85. Krause JS, Crewe NM. Long-term prediction of self reported problems following spinal cord injury. *Paraplegia.* 1990;28:186–202.

86. Siösteen BA, Lundqvist C, Blomstrand C et al. The quality of life of three functional spinal cord injury subgroups in a Swedish community. *Paraplegia.* 1990;28:476–488.

87. Anke AGW, Stenehjem AE, Stanghelle JK. Pain and life quality within 2 years of spinal cord injury. *Paraplegia.* 1995;33:555–559.

88. Lundqvist C, Siösteen A, Blomstrand C et al. Spinal cord injuries: Clinical, functional, and emotional status. *Spine.* 1991;16:78–83.

89. Putze JD, Elliot TR, Scott RJ. Marital status and adjustment 1 year post-spinal cord injury. *J Clin Psychol Med Settings.* 2001;8(2):101–107.

90. Kennedy P, Rogers B. Reported quality of life of people with spinal cord injuries: A longitudinal analysis of the first 6 months post-discharge. *Spinal Cord.* 2000;38:4 98–503.

91. Charlifue S, Gerhart K. Changing psychosocial morbidity in people aging with spinal cord injury. *NeuroRehabilitation.* 2004;19:15–23.

92. Dijkers M. Quality of life after spinal cord injury: A meta analysis of the effects of disablement components. *Spinal Cord.* 1997;35:829–840.

93. Dijkers M. Correlates of life satisfaction among persons with spinal cord injury. *Arch Phys Med Rehabil.* 1999;80:867–876.

94. Cushman LA, Hassett J. Spinal cord injury: 10 and 15 years after. *Paraplegia.* 1992;30:690–696.

95. Manns PJ, Chad KE. Components of quality of life for persons with a quadriplegic and paraplegic spinal cord injury. *Qual Health Res.* 2001;11(6):795–811.

96. McColl MA, Stirling P, Walker J et al. Expectations of independence and life satisfaction among aging spinal cord injured adults. *Disabil Rehabil.* 1999;21(5/6):231–240.

97. Krause JS, Broderick L. Outcomes after spinal cord injury: Comparisons as a function of gender and race and ethnicity. *Arch Phys Med Rehabil.* 2005;85:355–362.

98. McColl MA, Violetnthal C. A model of resource needs of aging spinal cord injured men. *Paraplegia.* 1994;32: 261–270.

99. Uniform Data System for Medical Rehabilitation. *Inpatient Rehabilitation Facility Patient Assessment Instrument (IRF-PAI) Training Manual.* Buffalo, NY: Uniform Data System for Medical Rehabilitation; 2004.

100. Zigmond AS, Snaith RP. The Hospital Anxiety and Depression Scale (HADS). *Acta Psychiatr Scand.* 1983;67:361–370.

101. Woolrich RA, Kenndy P, Tasiemski T. A preliminary psychometric evaluation of the Hospital Anxiety and Depression Scale (HADS) in 963 people living with a spinal cord injury. *Psychol Health Med.* 2006;11(1):80–90.

102. McHorney CA, Ware JE, Raczek AE. The MOS 36-Item Short-Form Health Survey (SF-36). II. Psychometric and clinical trials of validity measuring physical and mental health constructs. *Med Care.* 1993;31(3):247–263.

103. Whiteneck GG, Charifue SW, Gerhart KA et al. Quantifying handicap: A new measure of long-term rehabilitation outcomes. *Arch Phys Med Rehab.* 1992;73:519–526.

104. Kaplan RM, Anderson JP. The general health policy model: An integrated approach. In: Spilker B, editor. *Quality of Life and Pharmacoeconomics in Clinical Trials.* New York: Raven Publishing;1996. p. 309.

105. Fugl-Meyer AR, Bränholm I-B, Fugl-Meyer KS. Happiness and domain-specific life satisfaction in adult Northern Swedes. *Clin Rehabil.* 1991;5:23–35.

106. Jette A. Toward a common language for function, disability, and health. *Phys Ther.* 2006;86(5):726–734.

107. Rice RW, Near JP, Hunt RG. The job satisfaction-life satisfaction relationship. A review of empirical research. *Basic Appl Soc Psychol.* 1980;1:37–64.

108. Krause JS. The relationship between productivity and adjustment following spinal cord injury. *Rehab Couns Bull.* 1990;33:188–199.

109. Krause JS. Employment after spinal cord injury. *Arch Phys Med Rehabil.* 1992;73:163–169.

110. Krause JS, Anson CA. Employment after spinal cord injury: Relation to selected participant characteristics. *Arch Phys Med Rehabil.* 1997;77:737–743.

111. Yasuda S, Wehman P, Targett D et al. Return to work after spinal cord injury: A recent review of the literature. *Neurorehabilitation.* 2002;17:177–186.

112. Krause JS, Kewman D, DeVivo MJ et al. Employment after spinal cord injury: An analysis of cases from the Model Spinal Cord Injury Systems. *Arch Phys Med Rehabil.* 1999;80:1492–1500.

113. Dowler D, Batiste L, Whidden E. Accommodating workers with spinal cord injuries. *J Vocat Rehabil.* 1998; 10:1998.

114. Inge K, Strobel W, Wehman P et al. Vocational outcomes for persons with severe physical disabilities: Design and implementation of workplace supports. *NeuroRehabilitation.* 2000;15(2):175–187.

115. Shapiro JP. *No Pity: People with Disabilities Forging a New Civil Rights Movement.* New York: Crown Publishing Group; 1994.

116. Americans with Disabilities Act of 1990, Title I, Pub. L. No. 101–336, 42nd United States Congress, 12101 note.

117. Anderson CJ, Vogel LC. Domain-specific satisfaction in adults with pediatric spinal cord injuries. *Spinal Cord.* 2002;41:684–691.

118. Targett P, Wehman P. Successful work supports for persons with spinal cord injuries. *Psychosocial Process.* 2003;(Spring):6–11.

119. Brown JS, Giesy B. Marital status of persons with spinal cord injury. *Soc Sci Med.* 1986;66:313–322.

120. Crewe NM, Athelson GT, Krumberger BA. Spinal cord injury: A comparison of pre-injury and post-injury marriages. *Arch Phys Med Rehabil.* 1979;60:252–256.

121. El Ghahtit AZ, Hanson RW. Outcomes of marriages existing at time of a male's spinal cord injury. *J Chronic Dis.* 1975;28:383–388.

122. Crewe NM, Krause JS. Marital status and adjustment to spinal cord injury. *J Am Paraplegia Soc.* 1992;15:14–18.

123. DeVivo MJ, Fine PR. Spinal cord injury: Its short term impact on marital status. *Arch Phys Med Rehabil.* 1985;66(8):501–504.

124. Chan RK. How does spinal cord injury affect marital relationship? A story from both sides of the couple. *Disabil Rehabil.* 2000;22(17):764–775.

125. Lykken DT. Parental licensure. *Am Psychol.* 2001;56: 885–894.

126. Kocher M. Mothers with disabilities. *Sex Disabil.* 1994: 12(2):127–133.

127. Wates M. *Disabled Parents: Dispelling the Myths.* Cambridge, England: National Childbirth Trust Publishing; 1997.

128. Wates M, Jade R. *Bigger than the Sky: Disabled Women on Parenting.* London: Women's Press; 1999.

129. Prilletensky O. My child is not my career: Mothers with physical disabilities and the well-being of children. *Disabil Soc.* 2004;19(3):210–223.

130. Tuleja C, DeMoss A. Babycare assistive technology. *Technol Disabil.* 1999;10:1–8.

131. Alexander CJ, Hwang K, Sipski ML. Mothers with spinal cord injuries: Impact on martial, family, and children's adjustment. *Arch Phys Med Rehabil.* 2002;83: 24–30.

132. National Organization on Disability. *2000 N.O.D./Harris Survey of Americans with Disabilities.* Washington, DC: National Organization on Disability; 2000.

133. Iezzoni LI, O'Day BL. *More Than Ramps: A Guide to Improving Health Care Quality and Access for People with Disabilities.* New York: Oxford University Press; 2006.

134. Iezonni L, McCarthy EP, Davis RB et al. Mobility impairments and use of screening and preventative services. *Am J of Public Health.* 2000;90(6): 955–961.

135. U.S. Department of Health and Human Services. *Healthy People 2010*. Washington, DC; U.S. Department of Health and Human Services; 2000.

136. Panko Reis J, Breslin ML, Iezzoni LI et al. *It Takes More than Ramps to Solve the Crisis of Healthcare for People with Disabilities*. Chicago: Rehabilitation Institute of Chicago; 2004.

137. Kirschner KL, Breslin ML, Iezzoni LI. Structural impairments that limit access to health care for patients with disabilities. *JAMA*. 2007;297:1121–1125.

138. DeJong G. Primary care for persons with disabilities: An overview of the problem. *Am J Phys Med Rehabil*. 1997;76 Suppl:S2–S8.

139. Zung WWK. A self-rating depression scale. *Arch Gen Psychiatry*. 1965;12:63–70.

Upper Extremity Orthotic and Postsurgical Management

10

Amy S. Bohn, OTR/L

Allan E. Peljovich, MD, MPH

OBJECTIVES

After reading this chapter, the reader will be able to:

- Discuss the reasons why rehabilitation of the hand and upper extremity should commence as soon as medically possible in the individual with tetraplegia
- Discuss the goals of upper extremity management in the acute, subacute, and chronic phases of spinal cord injury and the role of splinting
- Describe the tenodesis grasp, what is required for tenodesis grasp to be effective, and the motions that should be avoided in order to preserve tenodesis grasp
- Describe the general process by which tendon transfer procedures are undertaken to provide power to a paralyzed muscle and identify the most important grip pattern to restore with tendon transfer procedures
- Describe the fundamental elements of the postsurgical rehabilitation protocol for an individual who has undergone a tendon transplant procedure

Introduction

For individuals with tetraplegia due to spinal cord injury (SCI), upper extremity impairment is among the most disabling aspects of this injury. The loss of hand and arm function severely limits an individual's independence and quality of life. Several studies support the importance of focusing on upper extremity rehabilitation as part of the comprehensive management program. As early as 1976, Hanson and Franklin[1] documented the importance of restoring hand function, both for the individual with SCI and the individual's caregiver. Early in the collective experience treating individuals with tetraplegia, Waters[2] noted, ". . . the greatest potential for improvement in the quality of life lies in the rehabilitation and maximal restoration of upper extremity function." More recent studies continue to reaffirm the value that upper extremity rehabilitation has in this population of individuals.[3–5]

Since the 1940s, the body of knowledge related to rehabilitation of the hand and arm in individuals with tetraplegia has expanded considerably. Proper management of the upper extremity throughout the individual's continuum of care is essential for optimizing functional outcomes. The main goals of upper extremity management include restoring as much function as possible, maintaining normal appearance, and preserving joint integrity so that the hands remain supple and flexible. Achieving these goals requires a coordinated, interdisciplinary team approach that incorporates the expertise of therapists, physiatrists, and surgeons, as well as the supportive care provided by case managers, nurses, and all ancillary staff. In this chapter, options for the nonsurgical and surgical management of the upper extremity following cervical SCIs will be reviewed for all phases of rehabilitation, from the acute phase to chronic phase of injury.

Acute Phase of Injury

Rehabilitation of the upper extremity begins as soon as medically permissible. While the immediate care of the individual with SCI is rightly devoted to life-saving measures and to preserving neurological function, failure to attend to the limbs, especially the arms and hands, can have devastating consequences on the subsequent potential to restore function. Left unattended in the early stages of injury, the upper limbs will quickly become contracted, stiff, swollen, and painful. This sequence of events, once begun, can take an inordinate amount of time and effort to reverse in order to regain upper limb health.[6] Too many individuals have their ultimate potential compromised as a direct result of delayed attention to the upper extremities. For this reason, planning and forethought are critical during the early stages of injury recovery.

The primary goals of upper extremity management in the acute phase following cervical SCI are to maintain joint suppleness, prevent contractures, treat edema, control pain, and control spasticity. Moberg,[7] long considered one of the "fathers" of restorative surgery for individuals with tetraplegia, noted that most individuals desire supple hands, not stiff and rigid hands. It is this principle upon which acute care management of the upper extremity is modeled. In order to accomplish these goals, therapy is focused on edema management, positioning, splinting, pain management, tone and spasticity management, exercise (range of motion), and education.

Edema Management

Edema in the acute stage of SCI is most commonly the result of neurogenic shock that affects both the somatic and autonomic nervous systems. Loss of sympathetic drive leads to abnormalities in vasomotor control characterized by increases in arteriovenous shunting, an increase in capillary and venous pressures, and venous dilatation. Proteins leak across endothelial basement membranes, inducing similar migration of plasma fluids. This fluid cannot be readily returned into the vascular system because the normal pumping action of the skeletal muscles is absent in the paralyzed limb.[6] Edema is one of the primary causes of limited range of motion, but it can be minimized thorough daily active and passive range of motion, retrograde massage, and proper positioning of the upper extremity, both when the individual is in bed and in the wheelchair.

Positioning

One of the primary strategies for the control of edema in the upper limbs is to position the hands such that they are elevated above the level of the heart. In addition, proper positioning of the wrist will allow the venous and lymphatic drainage from the digits and hand via veins and lymphatic ducts that pass across the dorsum of the hand. In a paralyzed hand, edema in the dorsal aspect of the hand is the area that is most problematic. Left unsupported, gravity will cause the wrist to fall into flexion, resulting in the shortening of the extensor tendons and hyperextension of the metacarpophalangeal (MCP) joint. However, if the wrist is positioned in extension, then the viscoelastic properties of the flexor muscles of the fingers will flex the fingers at the MCP joint, resulting in a compressive force on the dorsal soft tissues. This compressive force increases interstitial pressure sufficiently to reduce edema. Thus, the appropriate position of the hand is one of wrist extension with MCP flexion; this position may be achieved with the support of pillows or splints.

Positioning of the upper limbs is also intended to counter the tendency of the limbs to assume abnormal postures, which if left untreated, may interfere with attainment of functional goals in addition to being undesirable for reasons of cosmesis. For example, when the individual is positioned in the supine position, a soft pillow or wedge is used to support the upper trunk (rather than just the head), thereby placing the pectoral muscles in a relatively stretched position and preventing the shoulders from rolling forward. When addressing the issues of positioning for an individual with SCI in the acute phase, it is helpful to consider the specific patterns of positioning associated with the different levels of injury; these patterns are described in Table 10-1.[6]

If proper positioning is not attended to, these patterns will result in characteristic restrictions. For example, for an individual with a C5 level of injury, the typical posturing can lead to protracted shoulders, resulting in shoulder pain, and shortened upper chest muscles, resulting in upper rib tightness that restricts the upper chest expansion necessary for optimal respiration. In the individual with a C6 level injury, the typical posture results from unopposed activity of the shoulder elevators (trapezius, levator scapulae), external rotators, abductors (supraspinatus, deltoids), and the flexors of the elbow. This posturing places the individual at risk for development of abduction contractures of the shoulder and flexion contractures of the elbow.

An individual with a C7 level of injury has some sparing of shoulder depressor and elbow extensor muscles that give rise to the typical pattern of posturing. Therefore, while the shoulders may still tend toward an abducted posture and the elbows tend to a flexed posture, it does not occur to the extent observed in the individual with C6 injury. The wrist extensors are strong and unopposed. The intrinsic-plus position is considered the safe position, as it can be maintained for extended periods without the development of stiffness. Positioning of the hand in this position with an intrinsic-plus splint will be considered in the following section. In an individual with a C8 level of injury, the presence of innervation for most of the arm muscles means that abnormal arm posturing is uncommon; however, the finger extensors are unopposed

Table 10-1
Positioning the Upper Extremity in the Acute Phase of Injury

Level of Injury	Postural Tendencies	Optimal Positioning
C5	Shoulder adduction, forearms pronation, arms held across the chest	Shoulder abduction, forearms supination, elbow extension, appropriate wrist support
C6	Shoulder elevation and abduction, elbow flexion, may have some wrist extension posturing	Shoulder adduction with arms extended by the side, adequate wrist and hand support
C7	Shoulders may be abducted, elbow may be flexed (although not to the extent observed with a C6 injury), wrist and fingers extended or hyperextended in claw-hand posture	Shoulder and elbow positioning as for C6 injury (if required). Early splinting with wrist and fingers in intrinsic-plus position. MP blocking splint may be fabricated for functional activities.
C8	Abnormal posturing of the arm is rare; however, claw-hand posture is common.	Early splinting (intrinsic-plus splint) is required for positioning. MP blocking splint may be fabricated for functional activities.

by the intrinsic muscles, which may result in the development of a claw-hand posture (or "clawing" of the hand) wherein the MCP joints are extended and the interphalangeal (IP) joints are flexed.

Splinting

Splinting is important for the prevention of deformity, promotion of function, and preservation of a normal hand appearance. Two different approaches have emerged regarding the management of the upper extremities with splinting. One approach emphasizes the goal of maintaining a supple hand. By keeping the fingers supple, there are more available options for management, including universal cuff orthoses and adaptive equipment with large handles or universal cuff handles. In addition, the individual with active wrist extension can use a tenodesis grasp. This grasp takes advantage of the natural biomechanics of the hand such that the fingers are flexed when the wrist is extended (providing grasp), and the fingers are extended when the wrist is flexed (providing release). While the tenodesis grasp does not provide as strong a grasp as would be afforded by an orthotic, it may allow for easier acquiring and releasing of an object and precludes the need for assistance that may be required to don and doff an orthotic device. This functional hand position is often achieved using an *intrinsic-plus splint*, which positions the wrist at 20 degrees of extension, the MCP joints at 80 to 90 degrees of flexion, the IP joints fully extended or in minimal flexion, and the thumb in the natural position of opposition (Fig. 10-1). A night splint is often provided to maintain the hand in the intrinsic-plus position. This position allows for reduction of edema, preservation of modified tenodesis, and prevention of fixed contractures.

The therapist determines whether the individual would benefit from a day splint, a splint applied to the forearm (depending on wrist motion and level of awareness of limbs, the splint may be short or long), for initiation of functional activities in the acute phase (Fig. 10-2). Supple digits are the goal of this approach, while avoiding thumb instability and MCP joint hyperextension. Impaired sensation may dictate that the initial splints require frequent adjustments to prevent pressure points that can result in skin breakdown.

The alternative approach to maintaining a supple hand is to maximize function by intentionally allowing the development of contractures that will position the hand in a tenodesis posture. This posture may provide sufficient tip pinch to pick up light objects, as, in effect, the fingers and thumb become akin to anatomical tools that imitate the tongs of pliers. These "tongs" are controlled by the wrist through stiffening the IP and MCP joints. Proponents of this philosophy include Nickel and colleagues,[8] who believe that the primary goal of splinting is to stabilize the hand in one selected position and then use all residual muscle power to provide active grasp and release. Their approach is to use the three radial digits to accomplish this. Based on this philosophy, the flexor hinge splint was developed. Few individuals accepted the flexor hinge splint for long-term use because of associated discomfort and inconvenience, especially when another individual was required to assist with donning the device. Despite the fact that most individuals with SCI discontinue use of this device at some point, the flexor hinge splint continues to be used in the initial phases of rehabilitation for early functional training. The issue of rejection of an orthotic device is true of many orthotics; they are far from being universally accepted by individuals, and their usage rates decline with time.[9,10] Ultimately, most individuals strongly desire to be brace free.[7]

Aside from the issue of poor acceptance of orthotics by users, another problem with the intentional development of contractures is that these contractures are almost impossible to overcome by conservative methods within

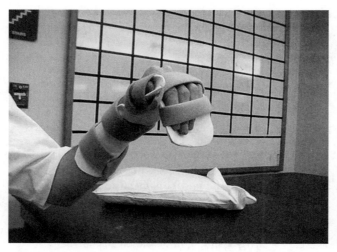

Figure 10-1. Volar intrinsic-plus splint. This splint maintains the alignment of the wrist and fingers that promote tenodesis grasp.

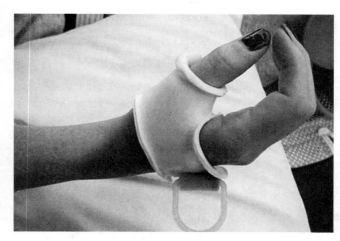

Figure 10-2. Short opponens splint for use during functional training.

a reasonable time frame. Severe contractures can present problems with skin breakdown in the palm of the hand or in the finger joints. These contractures must be surgically released, both delaying other procedures and limiting surgical alternatives for restoration in the future. A supple hand without contractures is more pleasant and acceptable to the individual.[7]

Pain Management

Upper extremity pain following spinal cord trauma arises from injury to hard and soft tissues (i.e., nociceptive pain from fractures and muscle and tendon trauma) and to neural tissue (i.e., neuropathic pain from injury to nerve roots and damage to the spinal cord).[11] In the early post-injury phase, if pain interferes with positioning, splinting, or exercise, then a comprehensive approach to care for the pain is ideal. Careful examination and identification of the source of pain is essential. In addition to pharmacological options, nonpharmacological treatments such as transcutaneous nerve stimulation, traction, acupuncture, massage, and mobilization techniques may be incorporated into a pain management program.[6] Persistent or worsening pain is a sign that there may be occult injury or progression of a known injury. The expertise of a pain specialist is required if pain cannot be managed using pharmacological or physical therapeutic interventions. The issue of pain will be discussed in greater detail in Chapter 17.

Tone and Spasticity

Uncontrolled upper limb spasticity that develops in the acute period must be treated aggressively. Nonpharmacological treatments may include heat, cold, massage, manipulation, and electrical stimulation. Pharmacological intervention and/or serial casting provide other options. For example, botulinum toxin injection along with serial casting is an alternative means of controlling spasticity. It has been especially successful in C5–C6 level of injuries to block spasticity of forearm muscles.[12,13] The issue of spasticity will be discussed in greater detail in Chapter 18.

Range-of-Motion Exercise

Passive range-of-motion and stretching exercises should be performed twice each day. Stretching is performed slowly, and joints are never forced. The individual is encouraged to assist with the movement activities as much as possible. Aggressive range-of-motion exercises along with pillow splints (Fig. 10-3) to maintain the limb and joint in the desired position are often the first line of defense in maintaining muscle length and joint range of motion. Often, more aggressive splinting is needed, such as a static elbow extension splint or even a dynamic elbow extension splint.[14]

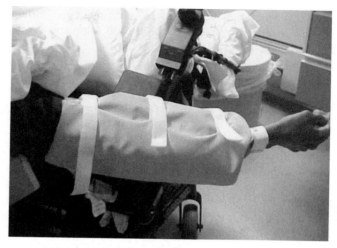

Figure 10-3. Pillow splint for elbow extension.

Maintaining shoulder range of motion is important at all levels of injury as proximal range of motion and stability are required for distal function. It is important to bear in mind that positioning as well as stretching are essential in preventing shoulder tightness. Particular attention is given to internal and external rotators to prevent capsular tightness. Elbow range of motion is an issue especially for individuals with an injury at the C5–C6 level. Due to the lack of triceps innervation, these individuals often position themselves with elbows flexed and arms crossed over the chest.

In an individual with tetraplegia, the wrist and fingers should be stretched in the natural tenodesis pattern to take advantage of the functional nature of this synergistic movement pattern. The fingers should be extended when the wrist is flexed and the fingers flexed when the wrist is extended to avoid overstretching the structures that support tenodesis. MCP joint hyperextension should be avoided to prevent claw-hand posture as well as loss of the important palmar supports needed in grasp. If this posture is present, a metacarpophalangeal (MP) blocking splint (Fig. 10-4) should be fabricated for use during the

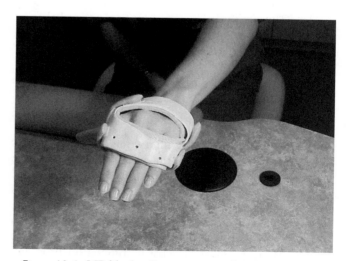

Figure 10-4. MP block splint to prevent claw-hand posture.

day for functional activities. In addition, care should be taken not to overstretch the thumb joint and create carpometacarpal (CMC) joint instability.

Education

Early education for the individual, family, and caregiver focuses on teaching passive range of motion, donning and doffing of splints, proper positioning in bed to prevent contractures, and checking for pressure areas. Once these skills have been acquired, the individual with SCI is encouraged to direct his or her own care, and families and caregivers are encouraged to participate in the program. The therapist ensures that the patient and family members all understand the purpose and goals of any therapeutic intervention and provides a home program of activities to ensure continuation of therapy.

Surgical Intervention in the Acute Phase

In this acute phase, surgery is only considered with regards to preserving joint and anatomic integrity. In particular, upper extremity injuries should be treated to the extent permitted by the individual's medical status, and treatment should be as aggressive as it would be for a nondisabled individual. The treatment of fractures, tendon injuries, nerve injuries, joint dislocations, or ligament injuries is the same as would be provided to nondisabled individuals.

In the absence of appropriate acute management, the ensuing stiffness or instability may limit future function and may render a restorative surgical plan ineffective. For example, distal radius fractures are often undertreated by physicians who presume that paralysis serves as a relative contraindication to aggressive surgical management. The problem with this philosophy is that by withholding surgical management of the fracture, stiffness is likely to develop. This stiffness precludes an effective finger tenodesis effect that many individuals rely upon for function and upon which many plans for restorative surgery are based. As such, it is strongly recommended that, at the very least, management of upper extremity injuries be directed toward maximizing passive function and joint integrity.

Subacute/Rehabilitation Phase of Injury

In the first weeks following injury, the individual begins the process of adapting to the injury. In this subacute stage of injury, the basic rehabilitation strategies initiated in the acute stage are continued. There may be changes in tone and spasticity that require adjustments to the splinting and positioning approaches. In addition to maintaining the therapeutic protocol, an aggressive strengthening program, electrical stimulation program, and splinting for functional use should be incorporated.

Maintaining Range of Motion

In the subacute phase, assuming the individual received appropriate care in the acute phase, it is likely that the limbs will be supple and pain free, allowing the individual to begin moving forward toward the goal of greater independence. However, if the upper limbs were neglected in the acute phase, the limbs may be painful and have restricted range of motion. In general, slow, static stretching is likely to be the safest immediate treatment. The initial goal is to achieve gains in range of motion at each therapy session, maintain the gains with splinting, and then turn the focus to strengthening for functional abilities. Spasticity may become a growing problem at this time. The following section describes areas that require special attention during the subacute phase of injury.

Management of the Shoulder Joint

Shoulder problems are all too common in the SCI population. Silfverskiold and colleagues[15] studied a small sample of individuals with SCI and determined that, of individuals with tetraplegia, 78% experienced some shoulder symptoms during the first 6 months following injury. Overuse problems are a very common source of reduced function. Campbell and Koris[16] identified capsular contracture and/or capsulitis, rotator cuff pathology and instability, osteonecrosis, and osteoarthritis as common causes of shoulder pain in the early stages of recovery in individuals with tetraplegia. These problems may be prevented or mitigated with appropriate upper extremity management.

In the absence of proper positioning and vigorous range-of-motion exercises in the acute stage of injury, range of motion in the glenohumeral joint rapidly becomes restricted, resulting in contracture in a posture of internal rotation. Frequently, this contracture becomes associated with shoulder pain that interferes with therapy and becomes problematic for the rehabilitation team. At the subacute stage, aggressive treatment, including pain control through modalities (e.g., ultrasound, thermal agents, transcutaneous electrical nerve stimulation [TENS]); anti-inflammatory, antispastic, and antiadrenergic pharmacology; and persistent aggressive range-of-motion exercises are essential.[6] Intra-articular corticosteroid injection may help reduce pain and stiffness in the joint and render therapy more effective.

With loss of function in the muscles that stabilize the glenohumeral and scapulothoracic joints, shoulder instability may be another problem and source of pain for individuals with tetraplegia. This condition is often associated with pain as the muscles and ligaments become overstretched. Any preexisting injury to the rotator cuff further complicates this issue. Aggressive range of motion, along with strengthening of both the anterior and posterior musculature, is important to prevent the development of stiffness. Shoulder taping may be useful when scapular winging is noted to aid in posterior stabilization.

Management of the Elbow Joint

In individuals with tetraplegia, the elbow assumes a considerable weight-bearing function in mobility activities such as transitions, transfers, and pressure relief lifts; therefore, maintaining elbow range of motion is essential for optimal function. In the presence of severe spasticity of the elbow flexors, effective splinting is necessary to prevent the development of contractures. In addition to aggressive range-of-motion exercises, other aids to prevent contractures include spasmolytic medication, heat, and stretching to the elbow flexor muscles (biceps brachii, brachialis, and brachioradialis) and electrical stimulation of the triceps (assuming muscle contraction can be elicited with stimulation of this muscle). If these techniques are not effective in maintaining elbow range of motion, then more aggressive procedures such as botulinum toxin and/or phenol injection, serial casting (or a combination of injection and serial casting), rubber band traction from the wrist cuff to the foot of the bed, or dynamic elbow extension orthosis (Fig. 10-5) may be required.

All individuals with C5 and C6 level of tetraplegia, as well as some individuals with C7 level injuries, experience muscle imbalance in the forearm. This may result in a supination contracture or pronation contractures. Supination contractures are a particular problem faced by some individuals who are classified as American Spinal Injury Association (ASIA) classification C5 or high C6. These individuals typically retain voluntary biceps brachii and supinator muscle function, but in the case of motor complete injuries, they lack an innervated pronator teres (innervated at C6–C7) or pronator quadratus (innervated at C7–C8–T1) muscle. The result is a chronic imbalance between active and potentially spastic

forearm supinator and flaccid forearm pronator muscles. The brachioradialis (innervated at C5–C6) may act as a secondary pronator muscle in these individuals; however, this muscle is unlikely to be strong enough to be an effective antagonist in the face of a particularly strong or spastic supination moment.[17] In some individuals, whether because of poor upper extremity management in early rehabilitation, spasticity, or the particular neural damage, a persistent supinated posture develops. This posture can eventually become fixed if the interosseous membrane and proximal and distal radioulnar joints become contracted.[18,19] This deformity is detrimental to function because most hand activities require pronation. Furthermore, the deformity is aesthetically unacceptable to the individuals.[18–20] For this reason and others, early control of bicep muscle spasticity is important in order to prevent forearm muscle contractures. When performing range-of-motion exercises, it is important to fully extend the elbow and pronate the forearm so that the bicep, the brachioradialis, and extensor carpi radialis longus (ECRL) muscles are stretched. The therapist may also use pronation and supination straps during times when the individual is not actively participating in therapy. If range-of-motion issues remain unresolved, surgical intervention may be necessary. The surgical solutions to the paralytic supination deformity include a biceps rerouting transfer or a radial osteotomy.[19,21]

Management of the Wrist Joint

The wrist joint is another common area where problems may develop due to inadequate upper extremity management. Individuals with tetraplegia who have higher levels of spasticity in the upper extremities in general, and the wrist flexor muscles in particular, may develop a flexed wrist posture. This posturing may also occur in individuals with low or no spasticity if wrist support is not provided or when the wrist support does not place the joint in a sufficiently extended posture. In such cases, the wrist will be in a flexed position, and wrist drop will result. Early identification of wrist-positioning issues is needed so that the wrist joint can be managed early and aggressively with proper positioning, range-of-motion exercises, and splinting.

Management of the Hand

In individuals with cervical injury, the goal of hand range-of-motion exercises and stretching is to achieve a hand that is supple but that will provide the structural support needed for a tenodesis grip for grasp and release function. This grip is achieved via the passive biomechanics of the hand wherein the fingers are flexed when the wrist is extended (grasp) and the fingers are extended when the wrist is flexed (release). The effective grip may be between the fingers and the palm or between the thumb and fingers. Passive range-of-motion exercises are performed while taking care not to stretch the fingers

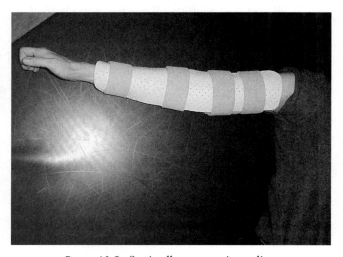

Figure 10-5. Static elbow extension splint.

and wrist simultaneously into full extension. Excessive stretching of the wrist extensor muscles is also avoided when splinting and, in individuals who have some voluntary wrist/hand function, during strengthening exercises as well. If contractures begin to develop in any of the joints of the fingers, additional stretching and splinting is implemented to maximize a functional tenodesis grasp and to prevent skin breakdown.

Strengthening

In individuals with tetraplegia, strengthening exercises directed at improving the force-generating capacity of the remaining muscles contributes to the functional capacity of the arm and hand. While distal muscle is likely to be more impaired than proximal muscle function, strengthening of proximal muscles provides the required stability that allows meaningful distal function to be possible. Likewise, strengthening of both anterior and posterior musculature contributes to balanced posture. The goals of the strengthening program include consideration for future options such as tendon transfers and other surgical interventions that might be performed to increase functional independence. Muscles that may be targeted for transfers include the posterior deltoid and biceps (elbow extension transfers), brachioradialis (wrist extension, thumb extension, finger extension transfers), and the ECRL (finger flexion transfer).

The principles of strengthening are the same as those for nondisabled individuals; progressive increases in resistance are key to increasing muscle strength. Progressive resistance training and endurance training are both effective in strengthening muscles, and the strength of a muscle contraction increases as more motor units are recruited. Care must be taken to isolate the muscle of interest so that habitual use of a detrimental compensatory pattern of movement is not encouraged. In individuals with motor incomplete SCI, because the pattern of residual muscle function is different from one individual to another, the therapist is instrumental in designing a strengthening program tailored to the unique requirements of each individual.

Massed Practice Training

Early after SCI, individuals often learn to use compensatory strategies to accomplish upper extremity functional tasks. In the subacute phase of injury, there is likely to be some recovery of functional capacity. However, the habitual use of well-learned compensatory strategies may mask the individual's ability to perform activities in more "typical" manner. Massed practice training, with the goal of acquiring more typical movement strategies for hand-related activities, may allow the individual to use the hand in more functional ways. These concepts are explored in detail in Chapter 11.

Electrical Stimulation

Provided that the motor neuron and nerve that innervate the muscle are intact, electrical stimulation to the motor nerve will evoke a muscle contraction in muscles innervated by spinal levels caudal to the injury. Muscles below the level of injury undergo disuse atrophy that can be reversed to some extent using electrical stimulation as part of an exercise program. Electrical stimulation using surface electrodes to elicit muscle contraction may improve muscle strength and endurance.[22-25] Stimulation may also be used to assist in moving joints through their range of motion, thereby preventing the development of contractures. Additionally, the changes in muscle contractile properties that result in conversion of slow twitch (fatigue-resistant) muscles to a fast twitch (fatigable) fiber type in individuals with SCI can be reversed with a program of electrical stimulation[22,23] (this concept is discussed in detail in Chapter 3).

Splinting

During the subacute phase of injury, splinting continues to focus on preventing deformity as it did during the acute phase of injury; however, there is an increased emphasis the use of splints for performing functional tasks and on the incorporation of these splints into the daily routine. The goals of therapy in the subacute phase is to maximize functional performance. During the day, static and dynamic splints are used for functional activities, and night splints are used for positioning at night.

Static orthoses are prescribed in the acute and subacute phases of rehabilitation to

- prevent overstretching of ligaments (e.g., as for maintaining a tenodesis grasp),
- maintain functional positions,
- prevent deformity, and
- protect and stabilize flail joints.[26]

It is important to establish clear goals with the individual regarding splinting and orthoses. Early incorporation of splints into functional retraining provides the individual with a demonstration of the functional advantage they offer before less-functional compensatory strategies are developed, making it more likely the individual will use the splint.

An example of a functional splint is a universal cuff (Fig. 10-6), which can be adapted for use with many different types of utensils and handles. Different splints provide different functional advantages; therefore, understanding the individual's needs is critical in providing them with the most effective splints. Table 10-2 describes the recommended hand-splinting approaches that are used based upon level of injury.

Although splinting is an important strategy for improving limb function and one that should be emphasized,

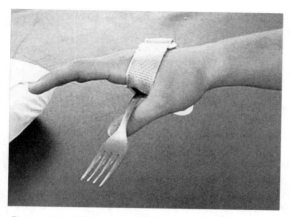

Figure 10-6. Universal cuff for functional retraining.

studies have shown that despite a carefully chosen program, the rate of splint use among individuals with tetraplegia varies from as low as 39% to as high as 89%.[10] The majority of the individuals who desire surgical reconstruction usually reject the orthoses because they want to be less reliant on orthoses and have a more typical appearance.

Surgical Intervention in the Subacute Phase

In the subacute phase of rehabilitation, the maintenance or achievement of supple joints remains a priority. The development or persistence of joint contractures despite application of appropriate and aggressive nonsurgical treatment is a possible indication for surgery in this

Table 10-2
Hand Splints Based Upon Level of Injury

Level of Injury	Splint	Purpose	Wearing Schedule
C1–C4	Resting hand splint	Maintains the hand in a functional position, prevents deformity, maintains aesthetic hand appearance	When in bed, complete passive range-of-motion exercises daily
C5	Long opponens splint	Provides a stable post against which index finger can prehend; positions thumb in functional key pinch position	As needed to increase function
	Dorsal wrist support	Protects integrity of wrist joint; acts as a universal cuff for functional activities	As needed to increase function
	Intrinsic-plus splint (Fig. 10-1)	Protects integrity of wrist and fingers; aligns thumb for lateral pinch	In bed
	Elbow extension splint (Fig. 10-5)	Prevents biceps contracture	In bed
C6	Short opponens splint (Fig. 10-2)	Supports use of the tenodesis grasp in individuals who have some ability to extend the wrist	As needed to increase function
	Wrist drive flexor hinge splint	Augments natural tenodesis and alignment of fingers	As needed to increase function
	Universal cuff (Fig. 10-6)	Assists in holding objects for functional tasks	As needed to augment function
	Elbow extension splint	Prevents biceps contracture	In bed
	Intrinsic-plus splint	Protect integrity of wrist and fingers; aligns thumb for lateral pinch	In bed

Continued

Table 10-2

Hand Splints Based Upon Level of Injury—cont'd

Level of Injury	Splint	Purpose	Wearing Schedule
C7	MP block splint (Fig. 10-4)	Prevents hyperextension deformity of the MCP joints	As needed to increase function and decrease deformity
	Universal cuff	Assist in holding objects for functional tasks	As needed to increase function
	Intrinsic-plus splint	Protect integrity of wrist and fingers; aligns thumb for lateral pinch	In bed
C8	MP block splint (Fig. 10-4)	Prevents hyperextension deformity of the MCP joints	As needed to increase function and decrease deformity
	Intrinsic-plus splint	Protect integrity of wrist and fingers; aligns thumb for lateral pinch	In bed

phase. The importance of nonsurgical management as the initial course of treatment cannot be overemphasized. Surgery is reserved for when nonsurgical interventions fail to achieve meaningful goals.

Among those individuals in whom it is deemed appropriate to perform surgical intervention in the subacute phase of injury, joint manipulation under anesthesia is the most commonly performed surgical procedure. Presurgical radiographs are important to ensure that the stiffness is not the result of heterotopic ossification or occult injury. Joints that respond well to joint manipulation include the shoulder and the digital IP joints. Elbow joints may also be manipulated in cases in which stiffness is not resolved by splinting and casting. Arthroscopic surgical releases or open surgical releases may be indicated in cases where joint manipulation under anesthesia fails to achieve the desired outcome; the hand surgeon and the individual should be prepared for this possibility. In the case of the elbow, significant contractures usually require an open surgical release in order to avoid injury to the ulnar nerve.[27,28] Fixed forearm contractures may also be corrected in the subacute phase. A rotational osteotomy may be the best option in this circumstance.[21] Alternatively, biceps rerouting tendon transfers have been reported, but this procedure is only effective if the contracture is not fixed; as such, it should be reserved until it is certain that maximal neurological recovery from the injury is complete.[20]

Chronic Phase of Injury

Rehabilitation during the chronic phase of injury (beginning approximately 1 year post-injury) continues with the strengthening, positioning, and splinting interventions for both positional and functional purposes. The individual should have a daily regimen that may be performed at home independently or in which a caregiver may assist. This daily exercise regimen may include a scheduled period for practicing fine motor tasks such as those employed with massed practice training (for details *see* Chapter 11), as this intervention has been shown to improve hand and arm use even in individuals with chronic tetraplegia. By this time, with good rehabilitation care, the individual will have achieved the highest possible level of function, using upper extremities as possible either with or without assistive devices. Surgical restorations are offered in this stage with the goals of restoring functional independence without the use of braces.

History of Tendon Transfers

Surgical restoration of hand function in individuals with tetraplegia has evolved significantly in recent decades; new techniques have been developed to meet the social, functional, and cosmetic needs of individuals with SCI.[29–32] In individuals with tetraplegia, tendon transfers are the most common surgical intervention for restoring hand function. The early conceptualization of tendon transfers to augment upper extremity function in SCI was largely influenced by experiences with individuals with residual deficits from poliomyelitis.[32,33] Using the tendon transfer approach, the function of a paralyzed muscle is restored by substituting a muscle (the "donor muscle") over which the individual has voluntary control. The tendon of a nearby donor muscle is detached from its normal insertion and sewn into the muscle that the intervention is meant to restore. An effective donor muscle must have sufficient voluntary strength (typically at least active movement against gravity with resistance or the equivalent of a manual muscle test grade of 4–5), and the loss of the contribution of this muscle to its typical action must not impair the function of the individual. The ideal donor muscles are redundant. For example, the biceps brachii muscle makes a suitable donor muscle for a paralyzed triceps muscle provided the brachialis muscle is still under voluntary control.

An alternative surgical technique incorporates an implanted electrical stimulation (neuroprosthetic) system. The function of the paralyzed muscle is restored by inducing muscle contraction via electrical stimulation. This technology is a promising advancement for individuals with tetraplegia who have lack voluntary control of the desired muscle but in whom the motor neuron and motor nerve are intact. This technology offers the potential for restoring multiple muscles[34] and was discussed in detail in Chapter 5.

In the following sections, surgical interventions for improving upper extremity function using the tendon transfer approach will be described. Essential elements of the presurgical evaluation for selection of candidates, principles of tendon transfers, surgical interventions, and postsurgical rehabilitation will be discussed.

Timing of Surgery

The chronic phase of SCI is when neurological recovery is considered complete, and this is the earliest that surgical restoration should be performed.[6,35] It is commonly accepted that by 1 year post-injury, those with complete SCI are likely to make no significant additional neurologic improvement. In those individuals with incomplete injury, however, recovery may continue longer than 1 year; indeed, interventions such as massed practice training have been shown to improve hand and arm function in individuals with chronic incomplete tetraplegia. When serial assessments confirm that the individual has reached a plateau, and the individual is motivated to undergo the procedure, then surgical intervention may be appropriate. We postulate that the dogmatic one-year minimum from injury prior to surgery may not be scientifically accurate, but continue with this practice until medical research alters our understanding of neurological recovery.

Criteria for Surgical Restoration

The decision to undertake surgical restoration should be a deliberate and structured process. Some surgeons are of the opinion that all individuals with traumatic tetraplegia who are in the acute and subacute phases of recovery should be considered potential candidates for surgery, regardless of whether the individual believes at that time that he or she will undergo surgery in the future. This optimizes the rehabilitative process, including the beneficial outcomes of joint stability and suppleness, splinting, and functional rehabilitation. The fact is that not all individuals are good candidates for surgery. Studies indicate that between 50% and 60% of all individuals with tetraplegia will meet criteria for tendon transfer-based surgical restoration,[36,37] and 13% of individuals will meet criteria for surgical restoration using implantable functional electrical stimulation (FES) systems.[9] Individuals with tetraplegia have impairments and conditions that are specific to the individual that must be considered in the process of surgical decision making. The surgical plan is primarily based upon the individual's physical examination (discussed in the next section), but is often modified by other factors.

The evidence suggests that desirable postsurgical outcomes are achieved when the individual is able to meet strict psychosocial and physical criteria.[6,21] For example, individual must have reasonable, achievable goals for undergoing surgery. The individual who is hoping for independent digital function sufficient to play piano will be disappointed in the outcome; on the other hand, the individual who hopes to become more independent and less reliant on orthotics and attendants for activities of daily living (ADLs) such as eating, grooming, and self-care will be satisfied.

Then, too, the individual must be motivated and dedicated to the process. For a period of 1 to 3 months post-surgery, the individual will be more dependent on others for care as the arm recuperates. The arm will be casted or splinted for a period of time and will be temporarily less useful than it was prior to the surgery. This is often a stressful time for the individual as he or she is likely to be reminded of the immediate post-injury condition. The individual may be fearful of losing the function he or she has spent a great deal of effort and time to gain, regardless of how little function that may be. Unmotivated and undedicated individuals are likely to become noncompliant with therapy and lose the potential benefits of the surgery.

The individual should additionally have a strong system of social support. Family, friends, and caregivers become especially important for the individual during this initial phase of recuperation. The stress of surgery is not only greater in individuals who have poor support, but the logistics of their greater dependency and greater therapy requirements after surgery may preclude the attainment of desirable outcomes. Sound case management is also important to ensure that appropriate adaptive equipment or nursing care is available for a period of time after surgery. For example, an individual who has only a manual wheelchair will require a motorized chair until the limb is no longer immobilized and is sufficiently strong to propel the chair.

The individual's ability to adhere to the required postsurgical plan is yet another requirement. An individual who has a demonstrated a history of nonadherence to the prescribed plan of care, for whatever reason, will not make a good candidate for surgery, as postsurgical care, including therapy, is likely to be even more intense than that which was previously experienced. Analogously, the individual with cognitive problems related to previous head trauma or other condition may not make good a candidate for tendon transfer if he or she cannot participate actively in the required postsurgical retraining program. Other requirements for a good candidate are more general. The individual must be in good general health; those who have chronic hospitalizations, problems with infections, nephrolithiasis, or pressure ulcers are not good candidates. Perhaps most importantly, the individual must motivated to achieve the best outcomes after surgery.

Presurgical Evaluation

Maximal neurological recovery and the psychosocial criteria described above must be met for an individual to be considered a reasonable candidate for surgical reconstruction. Once met, physical capability of the individual then becomes the basis for the surgical plan, as well as the achievable goals of restoration. A good assessment of the individual begins with a directed medical history. The implications of any prior upper extremity trauma, such as dislocations, fractures, and brachial plexus injuries, sustained at time of injury or prior to injury must be considered. Likewise, any history of conditions that affect joints, such as inflammatory or degenerative arthritis, must be considered.

Examination begins with inspection. Previous scars, surgical incisions, or indications of difficulty with scarring or wound healing are noted. Any evidence of dystrophic changes or abnormal neurovascular or sudomotor findings are also noted. A thorough sensory examination of the arm and hand is important. Good sensibility in the digits is not a prerequisite for surgery, but individuals who have good thumb and index finger sensibility will be more functional after surgery. Individuals who do not have good sensibility of the thumb and index are still candidates, but they must understand that they will require visual feedback to control the hand, and therapy must emphasize the importance of using visual feedback. Hypersensitive skin presents a particularly worrisome situation. The hypersensitivity must be cared for via desensitization techniques so that it does not interfere with postsurgical rehabilitation.

Baseline assessments of the upper extremity mobility include active and passive motion of all upper extremity joints. Assessment of scapular and glenohumeral stability is important for all candidates to ensure that there is adequate proximal control for distal function. All muscles are graded for strength using a scale[37] that is equivalent to the standard muscle test scores employed by physical therapists. Using this convention, muscle strength is graded as: 0 = no contraction; 1 = flicker or trace of contraction; 2 = active movement with gravity eliminated; 3 = active movement against gravity; 4 = active movement against gravity and resistance; 5 = normal power.

Muscles with strength grades of 4 to 5 or higher are well suited for tendon transfer. Grade 3 to 5 muscles may occasionally be useful for transfer. Tendon transfer success relies on voluntary donor muscle control, strength of the donor muscle, and suppleness of the joint to be mobilized via transfer. Therefore, particular attention is paid to whether spasticity is present, as a spastic muscle is a poor donor muscle. Attention is also paid to joint suppleness, as a stiff joint will remain stiff after transfer. Full passive mobility is ideal, but functional passive motion is sufficient. For example, a 20-degree elbow flexion contracture would not preclude the success of an elbow extension transfer; however, a 60-degree contracture would preclude success.

Any limitations that can be resolved should be addressed prior to proceeding with surgical interventions. In addition, assessment of current level of performance of ADLs is performed in establishing goals for surgery. The therapist educates the individual about the expected outcomes and postsurgical plan and provides him or her with information that will give insight into personal goals and desires. Education regarding the procedure and commitment to the process are important to the postsurgical rehabilitation. In the process of educating the individual and family/caregiver, evaluation of resources in terms of equipment and assistance available is essential, as tendon transfer surgery requires temporary immobilization and a course of aggressive rehabilitation. Important required equipment includes a power wheelchair with power tilt and a Hoyer lift for transfers. It is also important to discuss resources available to perform bowel and bladder routines, skin checks, and turns during immobilization periods in order to prevent secondary complications.

There are numerous classification schemes available to characterize the injury/impairment in individuals with tetraplegia. The American Spinal Cord Injury Association (ASIA) Impairment Scale (AIS) is probably the most widely used classification scheme, and it facilitates communication about functional status based on injury level. For example, it is understood that an individual with AIS C7 injury will be fairly independent, because the functional abilities of an individual with C7 injury have been well characterized.[31] Despite the simplicity and general usefulness of the system, the ASIA classification does not provide sufficient information when considering surgical restoration in tetraplegia. This was the impetus for the development of the International Classification of Tetraplegia (IC) motor-scoring system created in 1984 by a group of hand surgeons devoted to the care of individuals with tetraplegia.[31,38] This classification system is based upon the normal progressive segmental innervation of the forearm and hand musculature,[6] and scores are based on the results of manual muscle testing and testing of two-point discrimination. Each grade is determined by the most distally innervated muscle with grade 4 strength; this aids the surgeon in determining the presence and number of potential suitable donor muscles for transfer. The classification system in its present form is given in Box 10-1.

Principles of Surgical Restoration via Tendon Transfers

The great difficulty in executing a surgical plan is that it is not possible with currently available techniques to completely restore upper extremity function to the pre-injury capacity. Surgical strategies rely primarily on tendon transfer-based restoration and/or FES neuroprosthesis-based restoration. For tendon transfer-based restoration, the number of functions and joints that can be restored is directly proportional to the level of injury. In the case of FES neuroprosthesis-based restoration, the number of muscles that can be activated is limited by available technology and the fact that some muscles remain permanently denervated from injury.[39] Upper extremity function must be distilled into its most fundamental elements to maximize gains from limited options. Compromise and creativity form the basis of planning surgery for a particular individual. That said, there are traditional compromises and priorities that exist based upon experience gained in treating individuals with paralysis of all forms.

Surgical Planning for Tendon Transfers

The upper extremity performs the act of physically manipulating our environment. In a sense, the hand is the universal "tool" for manipulation, and the shoulder, elbow, and forearm provide the mode of transporting the hand in space and positioning it for function. The complex combination of muscle strength, digital mobility, and sensory perception within the hand itself creates the dexterity necessary for functional use of the upper extremity. Therefore, two primary functions of the upper extremity are critical: transport of the hand in space and the various forms of manipulation or grasp/release modes. Transport of the hand in space and the work space available for the hand relies on active shoulder, elbow, and forearm motion. Manipulation of the hand is dependent upon the functional capacity of the hand and wrist. For the individual with traumatic tetraplegia, both the transport function and the manipulation function are severely compromised.

In order to maximize the work space available for the hand, elbow, and shoulder, maintaining full range of motion of all joints must be a priority in good rehabilitation care. Injury to the C5/6 spine is the most common level of tetraplegia, the typical individual with this level of injury retains voluntary control of shoulder mobility and elbow flexion, but elbow extension is deficient. In cases of motor-complete SCI, only those people with injuries at or below the level of the C7 nerve roots will retain elbow extension. Elbow extension is among the most important contributors to functional independence[40] as it makes an important contribution to the individual's ability to reach into and engage his or her work space. For this reason restoration of elbow extensor function is often a priority for surgical intervention.

When it comes to manipulation of objects, it is necessary to make some compromises in regard to desired outcomes. The basis for hand function in most individuals is the wrist tenodesis effect, the key to which is strong wrist extension. Surgical restoration of hand

---

Box 10–1

IC Motor-Scoring Scale

		AIS Equivalent
0	No grade 4 muscle below elbow	C4, 5
1	Brachioradialis (BR)	C5
2	BR + Extensor carpi radialis longus (ECRL)	C6
3	Above + Extensor carpi radialis brevis (ECRB)	
4	Above + Pronator teres (PT)	
5	Above + Flexor carpi radialis (FCR)	C7
6	Above + Finger extensors	
7	Above + Thumb extensor	
8	Above + Partial digital flexors	C8
9	Lacks only intrinsics	

SENSORY

Cu (cutaneous) if 2 Point Discrimination in thumb/index < 10 mm
O (ocular) if 2 Point Discrimination in thumb/index > 10 mm

function seeks to prioritize wrist extension first and then, when possible, build upon that by creating strong and precise grasp and release patterns. Previous studies have documented that most ADLs are accomplished with two grasp patterns, namely lateral pinch (key pinch) and palmar grasp.[41] Lateral pinch, being even more critical to accomplishing ADLs than palmar grasp, is prioritized in situations wherein it is not possible to restore both forms of pinch. One important concept that cannot be overlooked in restoring grasp patterns is the release phase of the activity. Reliable and useful grasp and pinch requires the individual to be able to release an object. A limitation to surgical restoration is that to date, sensation cannot be restored.[42]

The most common level of injury in tetraplegia is C5–C6 injury. With this level of injury, the typical individual retains shoulder function, elbow flexion, and possibly strong wrist extension. In such an individual, the priority in tendon transfer-based restoration would be restoration of elbow extension, lateral pinch (if brachioradialis is available for transfer), and possibly palmar grasp (if ECRL is available for transfer). If the individual had C4 level tetraplegia, then tendon transfer-based restoration of the upper extremity would be impossible. At the same time, if the individual has a C7 level of injury, elbow extension usually does not require restoration, and other procedures, for restoration of lateral pinch and grasp, can be applied.

Other Important Considerations for Tendon Transfer Surgery

There are a number of other important issues that must be considered in planning for tendon transfer surgery. First, each muscle is uniquely organized to perform its specific task. The properties of muscles that are considered in transfers are its excursion (the distance through which it contracts) and the force (or tension) that it can develop, a property understood as the work capacity of the muscle. A suitable donor muscle mimics the properties of the muscle that it will replace in the transfer. For example, the muscles that flex the fingers typically have an excursion of 7 centimeters. The flexor carpi ulnaris (FCU), a muscle whose work capacity is similar to the finger flexors, has a potential excursion of only 4.2 centimeters.[43] The FCU would thus be a poor donor muscle for finger flexion since its contraction would not be sufficient to make a fist. The ECRL, on the other hand, has a slightly greater work capacity and excursion than the finger flexors and serves as an excellent potential donor muscle. Surgeons must be familiar with these properties.[44]

Second, the ideal donor muscle must be expendable and have strength that is (at least) sufficient to actively move the limb segment against gravity with resistance (i.e., the equivalent of a manual muscle test grade of 4 to 5) in order to be considered a potential donor. Using the

ECRL as a donor muscle when there are no other strong wrist extensors present will result in the loss of wrist extension—clearly not a beneficial tendon transfer. In addition, the minimum strength requirement is needed because donor muscles lose strength following tendon transfer for a variety of reasons, and the general expectation is that the transferred muscle will lose a grade of strength. Third, the joint that is to gain mobility must be supple. Full range of motion is not required, but passive motion must at least be functional in order for the tendon transfer to be useful. Stiff joints are not reversed with a tendon transfer.[42]

Fourth, in order to minimize adhesions that can reduce excursion, and reduce angles that can diminish the strength of a transfer, it is preferable to have a straight line of pull from the donor motor to the recipient whenever possible. If this is not possible, the surgeon must be certain that the biomechanics of the donor motor are suitable accounting for the lost strength from angular pulls. Ideally, each donor muscle restores one function. It is not always possible to create this condition, and this must be accounted for and understood in order for the tendon transfer to be successful. In the example of an individual with C5 tetraplegia, the brachioradialis is commonly used to replace the flexor pollicis longus (FPL), a function for which it is biomechanically well suited. The problem is that the brachioradialis originates proximal to the elbow and is then used to power a muscle that crosses multiple joints in the hand. The power of the tendon transfer is thus enhanced by stabilizing several hand joints, in particular, the CMC and IP joints, to maximize the force of contraction at the MCP joint. The power of the tendon transfer is further enhanced by stabilizing the elbow with an elbow extension transfer.[45] *Synergism* in tendon transfers aids in rehabilitation and is used when possible. This concept refers to the combination of movements that create function. In the case of grasping an object, the wrist typically goes into slight extension as the fingers flex to acquire and grip. A wrist extensor would then be a synergistic donor muscle to restore finger flexion and ease tendon transfer retraining. This is not a strict feature of tendon transfers, as illustrated by the success of using the biceps as a donor muscle for elbow extension.[46,47]

Finally, there are numerous challenges when it comes to tendon transfer restoration in individuals with tetraplegia. As previously discussed, the functions to be restored must be prioritized based upon the number of donor muscles available, and individuals with tetraplegia have only a limited number of suitable donor muscles. As such, the usefulness of each donor must be maximized to achieve as much function as possible considering that it will cross multiple joints to flex or extend a finger. In these cases, tendon transfers are often combined with joint stabilization procedures such as arthrodeses or tenodeses to minimize the number of joints a donor muscle activates. For example, and as illustrated below in the discussion of lateral pinch, the pinch is distilled into flexion of the thumb metacarpophalangeal joint so that all the power of the transfer is not dissipated across the carpometacarpal joint. In other cases, passive tendon transfers, or *tenodeses*, are used in place of tendon transfers. An example is "powering" finger extension by surgically attaching the extensor tendons proximal to the wrist so that wrist flexion produces greater finger extension than would be provided by the static properties of the more elastic muscle. Principles are occasionally disregarded and expectations adjusted. For example, a grade 3 ECRL may be used to restore a relatively weak pinch because, in these individuals, restoring a weak pinch is better than having no pinch.[48] Such concepts will be apparent as the techniques of restoration are discussed below.

General Principles of Postsurgical Care

Immediately after surgery, the upper extremity is placed in a bulky but durable plastersplint and then coverted to a cast as necessary over the next 3-4 weeks to protect the transfers while they heal. During the period of immobilization, it is essential to maintain range of motion of the joints that are not casted, as well as that of the extremity that did not undergo surgery. Education for individuals and the families and caregivers should focus on signs of infection, proper positioning, and precautions. The individual should be instructed on how to perform transitions and transfer for mobility and adaptations that need to be made for ADLs, wheelchair mobility, and weight shifts.

Cast removal occurs approximately 3 to 4 weeks after surgery. General rehabilitation considerations at time of cast removal are as follows:

- Identify what muscles are involved in tendon transfer and understand functional purpose.
- Position the individual's hand and arm to protect tendon transfer.
- Explain to the individual the procedure for cast removal and what to expect in appearance when cast is removed.
- Explain to the individual what motions are to be avoided and demonstrate how to position or hold the extremity while out of cast or splint.
- Remove bulky dressing and observe wounds, sutures, dressing, and incision.
- Note any signs of drainage, infection, or pressure from the cast.
- Cleanse arm with clean, warm soapy water and saline/water over incision.
- If areas are open, dress wounds with nonstick gauze and a stockinette.

Therapy after cast removal emphasizes protective splinting, scar mobilization, retrograde massage, and active range of motion (re-education activities). To protect the tendon transfer and to prevent the development or reoccurrence of deformity, protective splints are fabricated to position the extremity in the appropriate position. Splints are lined with thin foam to protect insensate areas.

Retrograde massage and scar mobilization are performed prior to active range-of-motion exercises. Retrograde massage may be used for edema reduction.[49] Scar mobilization is initially performed along the perimeter of the incision, and when the incision is well healed, it is performed over the surgical site. Scar mobilization with firm pressure should be performed at least twice daily.[50] Active range-of-motion exercises and muscle re-education focuses on retraining the individual how to use the muscle in its new function. There are many alternative techniques available to assist with training for individuals who may have difficulty learning how to perform the new function. Techniques such as biofeedback or surface electrical stimulation may be incorporated into the training program.[51,52] Early practice of functional skills will aid in the retraining process.

Specifics of Surgical Reconstruction and Rehabilitation

The various types of tendon transfer procedures are discussed in the following section in order of priority. Each surgical procedure has unique features, both surgically and in terms of rehabilitation, which will be discussed in below. While projected time frames are given for postsurgical rehabilitation, it is important to bear in mind that unexpected issues may arise that may require the schedule to be revised.

Restoration of Elbow Extension

Moberg has stressed the importance of restoring active elbow extension for the individual with tetraplegia. Without elbow extension, the individual with tetraplegia cannot reliably reach for overhead objects. The individual must propel a manual wheelchair using the shoulder muscles for propulsion, which means that the individual does not have the ability to "push through" with a full motion, making propulsion less efficient and more energy consuming. Elbow extension is important for a variety of other functional activities, such as reaching, accurately positioning the arm in space, pressure relief techniques, transfers, and locomotion.

Active elbow extension also improves the outcomes of more distal tendon transfers to restore hand function.[37] Moberg[53] emphasizes the beneficial effect of restoring elbow stability on the functional outcome of procedures that use either the brachioradialis or ECRL for muscle transfers. Brys and Waters[45] found that pinch strength following brachioradialis-to-FPL tendon transfer increased by 150% when the elbow could be stabilized. Today, two surgical procedures are advocated to restore active elbow extension: these are the posterior deltoid-to-triceps transfer and the bicep-to-triceps transfer.

Surgical Technique: Posterior Deltoid-to-Triceps Transfer

Surgical Description

Restoring elbow extension using the deltoid as a donor muscle has been the traditional procedure used since it was first described by Moberg in 1975.[7] In this procedure, the function of the triceps is restored by using the posterior one-third to one-half of the posterior deltoid as a donor muscle. In terms of biomechanical properties of the tendon transfer, the deltoid has more than sufficient excursion, but it can generate only 20% to 50% of the force of the triceps.[54] This is consistent with the observed outcomes of the tendon transfer surgery in that it is sufficient to provide antigravity strength, but not to generate the large forces required for performing mobility transfers.[55–57] There are two aspects of the posterior deltoid-to-triceps procedure that merit mentioning. The first is that the deltoid tendon does not have the length to be directly inserted into the triceps tendon, and thus the distance must be made up by some form of graft. The tensor fascia lata, extrinsic toe extensors, tibialis anterior, and triceps tendon turn-up flap have all been used to bridge this gap without any study evaluating their relative merits.[37,58–60] Second, this tendon transfer is particularly prone to stretching in the postsurgical period, which may seriously weaken the tendon transfer; thus a demanding and precise postsurgical rehabilitation program is necessary to maximize results.[61]

Specific Guidelines for Postsurgical Rehabilitation

Following surgery, the upper extremity is placed in a long arm cast with the elbow in no more than 20 degrees of flexion and with the wrist and hand mobile.[7,62] While the individual is in bed, the arm is elevated to prevent edema, and the shoulder is positioned in 30 degrees of abduction. Passive range of motion of the shoulder should begin after surgery, with shoulder flexion and shoulder abduction limited to 90 degrees and horizontal adduction to midline. No lifting under the axilla area should occur. All these restrictions are intended to avoid shoulder positions that could stretch the graft during the early postsurgical period.

The cast is removed 3 to 4 weeks after surgery. A dial-hinge elbow orthosis (Fig. 10-7) is used to further protect the tendon transfer and to prevent overstretching or rupture of the tendon transfer. Initially, the orthosis is locked in 0 degrees of extension for the first week and is worn at all times, except during therapy and skin checks. The hinged orthosis is progressed 15 degrees of flexion per week, provided that active motion to full elbow extension is present.[7,63,64] The therapist increases flexion only when it is certain that full range of elbow extension is present. If the individual demonstrates a restriction in the extension range of motion, then it is better to maintain the brace position and increase strength prior to increasing allowable flexion. When the hinged orthosis is advanced to 15 degrees of flexion (during day wear), a static elbow extension brace is fabricated for nighttime wear. When the dial-hinge elbow orthosis reaches 90 degrees of flexion for 1 week, the brace is discontinued.[63]

Therapy initially focuses on successful activation of the tendon transfer. In order to achieve elbow extension successfully via the tendon transfer, the shoulder is positioned in 90 degrees of abduction, and the individual is cued to pull the shoulder back (horizontal abduction). It is important to ensure that the individual is not substituting with external rotation and the use of gravity to complete elbow extension. The active range of motion of elbow extension continues in this gravity-eliminated plane. A powder board may be used to assist the individual at the beginning of the retraining. As the individual progresses, strengthening activities in all planes of motion are added to the therapy. Active elbow flexion beyond the limits of the orthosis is avoided until 12 weeks after surgery, at which time retraining in performing transitions, transfers, and wheelchair propulsion may be considered. A soft splint to avoid elongation of the tendon is worn at night for a total of 6 months. The tendon transfer will continue to strengthen and become more useful for a year or more after surgery.

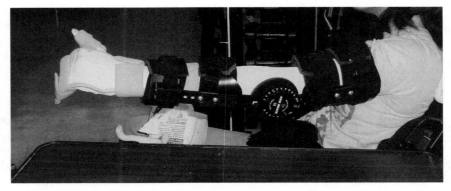

Figure 10-7. Postsurgical active lateral pinch and biceps-to-triceps transfer showing dorsal intrinsic-plus splint and dial-hinge elbow orthosis.

Surgical Technique: Biceps-to-Triceps Transfer

Surgical Description

The first published description of using a biceps tendon transfer to provide elbow extension appeared in 1954.[65] This procedure has gained momentum as a useful alternative to the deltoid-to-triceps transfer, and in some clinics, it has become the primary mode of surgically restoring elbow extension.[46,47,66] The literature indicates that the biceps proves as strong if not stronger than the deltoid as a donor for elbow extension.[47,66] Multiple authors have noted a loss of elbow flexion strength on the order of 50%, and a smaller reduction is also noted with the deltoid tendon transfer; however, the functional gains associated with having elbow extension more than compensate for the reduction in elbow flexion strength.[46,66] Zancolli and colleagues[67] advocated this type of tendon transfer early on, but noted problems when the biceps was routed laterally around the elbow as it could produce radial nerve compression. For this reason, Revol and colleagues[46] advocated a medial routing of the biceps. The advantage of this approach is that the biceps tendon can be directly inserted on the triceps and the triceps tendon without the need for graft, it tends to allow for earlier movement than the deltoid tendon transfer, and it is performed in less time than the deltoid tendon transfer. Some have argued that the biceps donor is particularly indicated in the presence of an elbow flexion contracture, since correcting this contracture often requires a lengthening of the biceps.[40,47,68] In this example, there is not a straight line of pull, and the tendon transfer is not synergistic, yet there is a gain in function. This transfer demonstrates how compromises between tendon transfer principles are sometimes required in individuals with tetraplegia, and desirable outcomes are still obtained.

Specific Guidelines for Postsurgical Rehabilitation

After surgery, the upper extremity is placed in a long-arm cast, with the elbow fixed in no more than 20 degrees of flexion and the wrist and hand mobile. While the individual is in bed, the arm is elevated to prevent edema, and the shoulder is positioned in 30 degrees of abduction. Passive range-of-motion exercises for the shoulder should begin after surgery and is limited to 90 degrees of shoulder flexion and shoulder abduction.

The cast is removed 3 to 4 weeks after surgery. A dial-hinge elbow orthosis is used to further protect the tendon transfer and prevent overstretching or rupture of the tendon transfer. Initially, the orthosis is locked 0 degrees of extension for the first week and worn at all times except for therapy and skin checks. The hinged orthosis is progressed 15 degrees of flexion per week provided that active motion to full elbow extension is present without substitution. When the hinged orthosis is advanced to 15 degrees of flexion (day wear), a static elbow extension brace is fabricated for nighttime wear.

When the dial-hinge elbow orthosis reaches 90 degrees of flexion for 1 week, the brace is discontinued.

Therapy initially focuses on successful activation of the tendon transfer. In order to achieve elbow extension successfully by the tendon transfer, the shoulder is positioned in 90 degrees of abduction and the individual is cued to supinate the forearm. It is important to ensure that the individual is not substituting external rotation and the use of gravity to complete elbow extension. The active range of motion of elbow extension continues in this gravity-eliminated plane. A powder board may be used to assist the individual at the beginning of the retraining. As the individual progresses, strengthening should take place in all planes of motion. Active elbow flexion beyond the limits of the orthosis is avoided until 12 weeks after surgery, at which time mobility transfers and wheelchair propulsion may be considered. A soft splint to avoid elongation of the tendon is worn at night for a total of 6 months. The tendon transfer will continue to strengthen and become more useful for a year or more after surgery (Fig. 10-8).

Restoration of Passive Lateral Pinch

Moberg[7] pointed out that in individuals with higher levels of injury (e.g., those who have IC motor scores of 0 or 1) voluntary wrist extension is either absent or weak; therefore, the goal of surgical restoration must be restoration of an automatic lateral tenodesis pinch (also termed passive lateral pinch). A tendon transfer is utilized to provide or augment wrist extension. A series of secondary procedures are then created to augment the strength of natural tenodesis pinch. The passive lateral pinch provides the ability to securely grasp lightweight objects. It may help with self-catheterization, writing, feeding, and other fine motor activities involving grasping lightweight or small objects.

Surgical Technique: Brachioradialis for Restoration of Passive Tenodesis Grip and Pinch

Grasp restoration hinges upon successful performance of four phases of the activity: (1) object acquisition, (2) grasp, (3) hold/manipulation, (4) object release.[42] The functional outcome of the surgical restoration procedure requires the coordination of precise digital motions so that all phases of the pattern can be accomplished. In the case of lateral pinch, object acquisition depends upon the thumb extending sufficiently (extensor pollicis longus [EPL], extensor pollicis brevis [EPB], abductor pollicis longus [APL]) with wrist flexion. Secure grasp is best achieved as the thumb moves into opposition (abductor pollicis brevis [APB]) and firmly rests against the index finger with force (FPL, adductor pollicis [AdP], index flexors, index intrinsics). The grasp must be secure enough so that the individual can maintain it with minimal fatigue while an object is handled, and then he/she must be able to easily release the object. In most individuals with C5–C6

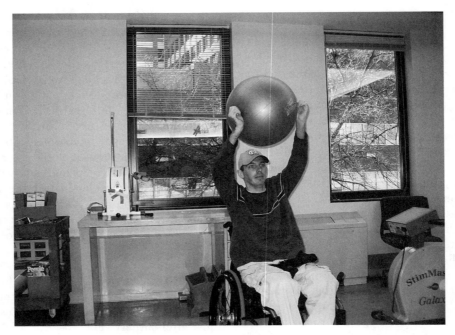

Figure 10-8. An individual with C5 ASIA A SCI 12 weeks after biceps-to-triceps transfer.

tetraplegia, the number of muscles remaining under voluntary control is insufficient to replace the many paralyzed hand and forearm muscles. Therefore, the challenges of this procedure are to recreate a meaningful pinch, as well as achieve precise digital positioning.

This procedure illustrates the need for *secondary* procedures that compliment tendon transfers in order to achieve the positioning and strength required for effective pinch. As each digital ray is a series of intercalated joints, stabilizing one or some concentrates the effect of a tendon transfer on a specific desired joint instead of allowing the force to be dissipated over several joints. Joint stabilizing procedures can also be used to set the position of the joint so as to create the best angle of motion. For example, by stabilizing the thumb IP and positioning the CMC joint, the powered FPL will concentrate its tension on the MCP joint in a pre-set opposition attitude. Tenodesis, another type of secondary procedure creates muscle tension through the action of joint motion; for example, wrist flexion can power thumb extension if a thumb extensor is surgically anchored proximal to the wrist. These synergistic strategies are employed when there are more functions to be restored than there are donor muscles to restore them. For passive lateral pinch, the focus is on opposition position, thumb flexion against the flexed index finger, and thumb extension for release. Careful attention to physical examination forms the basis of the surgical plan. The following questions are asked:

- Does the thumb extend well with the individual's own gravity-induced wrist flexion?
- In wrist extension, does the thumb naturally come into opposition and flexion?

- Is the MCP joint stable?
- Is the CMC joint of the thumb stable or loose?
- Does the index finger flex sufficiently in wrist extension to rest against the thumb?
- Does the index finger extend sufficiently with wrist flexion?

In some individuals, voluntary wrist extension is insufficient to produce a meaningful tenodesis grasp. In these individuals, the brachioradialis may be required to power or augment wrist extension, especially if the strength of extension is insufficient to hold against gravity (i.e., manual muscle test grade of less than 3 to 5). Digital positioning in these individuals is usually achieved through natural tenodesis, but if necessary, the thumb CMC joint, when fused in opposition, ensures that the thumb will approximate the side of the index finger.[69,70] A variety of surgical techniques have been devised to avoid fusing the CMC joint of the thumb.[6,71,72] and improve tenodesis for maximization of pinch strength and opposition. Powered pinch is achieved via passive FPL tenodesis.[73,74] To both avoid a hyperflexed IP joint that will miss the index finger and to focus tension on the MCP joint, the IP is stabilized by a "bridle transfer," in which the radial half of the FPL is detached from its insertion on the distal phalange of the thumb volarly and secured into the EPL dorsally.[75,76] The result, in part, is that it creates a resting IP position of neutral to slight flexion. When the FPL 'pulls' the thumb into flexion against the side of the finger this advantageous position is maintained because half of the FPL inserts dorsally into the EPL thereby preventing the IP joint from hyperflexing while simultaneously concentrating the flexion moment of the tenodesis to the

MCP and maximizing force of pinch. If thumb extension is insufficient with the individual's natural wrist tenodesis, extension can be augmented via a passive tenodesis. House[69] confirmed that all the components of lateral pinch reconstruction can be achieved with a single surgical procedure. This combination of procedures and its recent modifications form the original "key-pinch" procedure devised by Moberg, which is the currently favored intervention.[6,37,72,77]

As the IC motor scores improve, lateral pinch reconstruction is more effective.[6,21,78] In fact, as the IC motor scores improve, and more than two donor muscles are available without sacrificing wrist extension (i.e., muscles with IC motor scores of 3 and, in some cases, IC motor scores of 2), both lateral pinch and palmar grasp can be reconstructed. Tendon transfer procedures are typically prioritized to create power, that is, flexion for pinch and grasp, with extension provided by passive tenodesis if necessary. As the IC motor score improves to a score of 4 or greater and more donor muscles become available, both flexion and extension can be powered. Reconstructions that will involve providing both flexion and extension are best performed in two separate surgical procedures. This is due to the postsurgical therapy regimens, which require focus on either flexion or extension to the exclusion of the other. The efficacy of the flexor or extensor procedure would compromise the other if both were performed simultaneously. The topic of two-stage reconstructions is discussed later in this chapter.

Specific Guidelines for Postsurgical Rehabilitation

Following the surgical procedure for restoration of passive lateral pinch, the arm is immobilized for 3 to 4 weeks in 90-degrees elbow flexion, 20-degrees wrist extension, and flexion of the thumb and index MCP joints. The arm is elevated to limit edema while the individual is in bed. Shoulder range-of-motion exercises continue on the surgical side, with no limitations. Following cast removal, a dorsal splint is fabricated to position the wrist in 20 degrees of extension, with the thumb and index MCP joints in flexion. It is not necessary to splint the elbow; however, to protect the brachioradialis tendon transfer, activities involving high stress (hooking of the arm around wheelchair) should be avoided. The first 2 weeks of rehabilitation should concentrate on scar mobilization and on successful voluntary activation of the tendon transfer. In order to activate the passive pinch, the forearm is positioned in a neutral position and the individual is instructed to bend the elbow.

When the individual is consistently activating the tendon transfer, practice is continued with the elbow positioned at different angles of flexion. In addition, functional activities are initiated when the individual is consistently able to activate the tendon transfer. When practicing grasp activities, the objects to be grasped should be of small diameter so as not to stretch out the

FPL tenodesis pattern. The thumb should be positioned between the index and middle finger during functional tasks to avoid resistive pinch until 8 to 10 weeks after surgery. Wrist flexion angle should not exceed the angle that is passively available, nor should thumb extension exceed what is passively available. At 8 weeks postsurgery, wrist extension should be approaching presurgical range. At this time, strengthening of the transfer may occur by adding resistance to wrist extension exercises. A daytime splint is worn until the individual demonstrates consistent activation of the tendon transfer, good control of wrist extension, and sufficient range of motion to allow placement of the thumb pad against the fingers. This is usually occurs 3 to 4 weeks after cast removal. Nighttime splinting is continued indefinitely to ensure optimal posture of the hand.

Restoration of Active Lateral Pinch and Active Grip

In individuals with lower levels of cervical injury (i.e., those who have IC motor scores ≥ 2), the presence of suitable donor muscles results in the ability to convert a passive procedure as previously described into active and voluntary transfers. Instead of relying upon wrist tenodesis to generate the power of a tenodesis pinch, a donor muscle can be used to create active pinch, and if enough donor muscles are available, active palmar grasp. The lower the level of injury, and hence the more donor muscles available, the more elegant and functional the restorative plan can become.

The active lateral pinch provides the ability to secure small objects. The active lateral pinch will enhance ADL function, including self-catheterization, writing, feeding, and other fine motor grasping activities. When there are sufficient donor muscles available, an active grip procedure is often performed at the same time as the active lateral pinch procedure. The combination of both pinching and grasping will enhance ADL function, including grasping for propulsion of manual wheelchair, opening doorknobs, and grasping various-sized objects. The combination of both pinch and grip will enhance many fine motor-grasping activities.

Surgical Technique: Brachioradialis to Flexor Pollicis Longus; Extensor Carpi Radialis Longus to Flexor Digitorum Profundus

When wrist extension is sufficiently strong, that is, with an IC motor score greater than 2, a donor muscle is typically available to power pinch. For individuals with IC motor scores of 2 or 3, the brachioradialis is transferred into the FPL with the thumb stabilized and positioned as described in the section on passive lateral pinch.[69,70,79,80] In individuals having IC motor scores of 4 or greater, there are even more options. In these individuals, the BR, ECRL and pronator teres (PT) are, at a minimum, available as donor muscles. The ECRL is typically reserved to power finger flexion; therefore, the BR and PT are the available donor muscles that could be used to create active lateral pinch. House[69] devised methods of reconstructing thumb pinch: one method used FPL activation via tendon transfer and thumb CMC fusion for strength, the other used FPL activation via tendon transfer and another tendon transfer creating opposition for precision/dexterity. The former method is as described above. In the latter technique, the BR powers opposition using the ring finger flexor digitorum superficialis (FDS) tendon attached to the APB as a graft, and the PT powers the FPL. It is most common to apply the adduction-opponensplasty (i.e., surgical restoration of the adduction-opposition function of the thumb) when the surgeon is performing a bilateral reconstruction in which one thumb is reconstructed for strength, the other for dexterity.[69] Other reports have described various methods of achieving thumb position without the need for CMC fusion.[81] Thumb extension, if needed, is achieved either with a tenodesis procedure or by using brachioradialis to power digital extension. Thumb IP stabilization remains an important part of the procedure in order to create an effective pinch platform on the flexed index finger.

As with the lateral pinch, palmar grasp requires the coordinated motions of a variety of joints that are synchronized with wrist motion. Also, like lateral pinch, compromises are made, since donor muscles are likely to be insufficient in number. The typical coordination between the extrinsic forearm muscles and the intrinsic hand muscles must be considered in restoration of palmar grasp. Both of these muscle groups work in concert to create normal digital flexion and extension, with the intrinsic muscles being largely responsible for MCP flexion and IP extension.[82] Many individuals with tetraplegia have a hand posture of MCP extension, with partial flexion of the IP joints of the fingers and thumb (i.e., an intrinsic-minus hand position), therefore some capacity for MCP flexion during grasp improves strength.[83] The palmar grasp procedure is not typically performed unless lateral pinch can be restored (IC motor score greater than 2), and results may be better in individuals with lower levels of injury (IC motor score 4 or greater).[6]

Finger flexion is achieved by powering the action of the flexor digitorum profundus (FDP), which will flex all the joints. Finger extension is achieved by powering the extensor digitorum communis (EDC) and occasionally the EIP and EDM. Because the goal is a strong grasp, powering the FDP via a tendon transfer is prioritized over activating the extensors. In individuals in whom natural tenodesis fails to produce adequate finger extension to allow grasp function, the extensors are grafted to the dorsal surface of the distal radius using a variety of techniques. Finger extension is powered only if there are sufficient donor muscles. In addition, if finger extension tenodesis or active tendon transfer is to be performed, then it is preferable to perform the finger extension procedure as part of a two-stage reconstruction.

Powering the FDP via tendon transfer is usually achieved with the ECRL as the donor muscle. It requires an individual with an IC motor score of 3 or greater. Since one muscle cannot recreate independent digital motion, the ECRL is weaved into all four tendons of the FDP. In order to create an effective palmar grasp, the tendon transfer is first performed whereby all four tendons are sewn to each other such that, with active wrist extension, all four fingers flex level to each other (referred to as reverse cascade FDP synchronization). The ECRL is then weaved into the FDP mass proximal to the synchronization sutures. All this can be accomplished via the same radial forearm incision used for the lateral pinch procedure.

Restoration of intrinsic muscle function may also be considered in a select group of individuals. Careful presurgical examination helps identify the individual's specific tenodesis grasp pattern. If the MCP joint remains extended during flexion, the surgeon may consider performing a simultaneous *intrinsicplasty* (i.e., surgical restoration of the function of the intrinsics) designed to create MCP flexion passively with wrist extension.[67] This method involves using the FDS tendons. If the individual exhibits a significant limitation in the proximal interphalangeal (PIP) extension with wrist flexion, then another method that restores PIP extension is performed.[69]

Specific Guidelines for Postsurgical Rehabilitation

After the surgical procedure for restoration of active lateral pinch and active grip, the arm is casted for 3 to 4 weeks with the elbow fixed at a flexion of 90 degrees. The arm is elevated to limit edema while the individual is in bed. Shoulder range-of-motion exercises should continue with no limitations while in the arm is in the cast. If the active grip procedure was performed, then the volar surface of the fingers should not be casted, but supported with a strap. Beginning the day after surgery, the strap is removed at least two times per day, and the individual should gently activate the grip transfer. This is done in an effort to decrease the risk of adhesions.

After cast removal, a dorsal-based splint is fabricated to position the wrist in 20 degrees of extension, with the thumb aligned for lateral pinch, and MCP joints of digits are fixed at 90 degrees of flexion

The splint is worn at all times during the first week after cast removal, except for therapy and skin checks. The splint may be discontinued during light ADLs (i.e., eating, grooming, writing, etc.) when individual is able to do the following: verbalize an understanding of postsurgical precautions, demonstrate awareness of restrictions (see below) during therapy activities, and demonstrate the ability to consistently activate all transferred muscles. The splint can be used for night wear only when the individual demonstrates consistent control/activation of the tendon transfer without substitution, demonstrates functional range in the restored joint, and demonstrates an understanding of postsurgical precautions. As a general guideline, splints are changed to a night wear-only schedule approximately 2 to 3 weeks after cast removal. The K-wire for IP is removed 3 to 4 weeks post-surgery. However, if a CMC fusion was performed, then the individual will wear a protective thumb splint until the CMC K-wire is removed (wrist support during day may be discontinued if the above guidelines are met). The CMC fusion is x-rayed at week 8 post-surgery, and if healed, the K-wire is removed at that time.

General precautions following the surgical procedure are as follows: no forced wrist extension beyond the available passive range, no forced thumb extension beyond the available passive range, no forced thumb flexion beyond the available passive range, no heavy weight bearing for at least 6 to 8 weeks after surgery. After that time, the surgeon's evaluation may determine that heavy weight bearing may be initiated. Manual wheelchair propulsion and transferring should be added when the surgeon discerns that criteria have been met.

Therapy initially focuses on scar management and successful activation of the tendon transfer. In order to achieve active pinch and grip, the positioning will depend on which muscles have been transferred. Activation of pinch function will be the initial focus. If the brachioradialis was transferred to the FPL, in order to activate pinch function, the wrist is positioned in neutral and the forearm in a pronated position. The individual is then cued to activate the brachioradialis by bending the elbow toward the mouth. If the pronator teres was transferred to the FPL, the wrist and forearm are positioned in neutral (Fig. 10-9) and the individual is cued to pronate the forearm. In either case, the therapist will want to be certain that the appropriate muscles are being activated and that the individual is not substituting wrist extension to perform or enhance the motion. Once the individual is successful in activating the lateral pinch, training for activation of grip in initiated.

In order to activate the grip, the forearm is positioned in neutral and the individual is cued to extend the wrist in the radial direction. Training the active range of motion of both the pinch and grip continues in the gravity-eliminated plane until the individual is able to perform each consistently. Once the activation of the pinch and grip is consistent, the individual must learn to activate the tendon transfer in multiple planes as well as coactivate these functions with other procedures that may have been done at the same time. Early incorporation of light functional activities should be stressed. The activities should be of interest to the individual and should include different elbow and wrist motions and levels of resistance to increase strength. As general guideline, light ADLs should begin 2 to 3 weeks after cast removal. Functional activities that generate high forces and resistance, such as manual wheelchair propulsion and transfers, should be added when the surgeon has determined that criteria have been met.

Restoration of Active Grip and Release as a Two-Staged Procedure

The provision of active pinch and grasp is considered when sufficient donor muscles are available. Typically, the donor muscle must have an IC motor score of 3 or greater and preferably when IC motor score is 4 or greater. The potential problem with restoration of active grip is that creating active flexion moments can ultimately lead to digital imbalance and the consequent development of either positional or fixed flexion contractures over time. If contractures develop, the release phase of grasp weakens and becomes inefficient. For these reasons, reconstruction of extension is often performed when the surgical plan calls for restoring both active pinch and grasp. Such restorations, unlike others, are performed in two stages, one procedure to restore flexion and one procedure to restore extension. This is because the rehabilitative protocols for extensor reconstruction contradict those for flexion. Advantages of restoring both flexion and extension are greater durability and, perhaps, more dexterity. The main disadvantage is that two procedures are required per hand.

Surgical Technique: Passive Extensor Activation of Extensor Digitorum Communis and Extensor Pollicis Longus; Flexor Phase with Extensor Carpi Radialis Longus to Flexor Digitorum Profundus and Pronator Teres or Brachioradialis to Flexor Pollicis Longus

The surgical procedures for restoration of the flexion and extension are performed 2 to 6 months apart, depending on how the wounds heal and how supple the tendon transfers are at the time of second stage. There are two original descriptions for this sequence, one in which the flexors are reconstructed first and the other in which the extensors are reconstructed first.[67,69] Extensor reconstruction results in extensor activation (EDC and EPL) passively by tenodesis or by tendon transfer to the EPL, APL, and EDC (IC motor score 4 or greater) using a

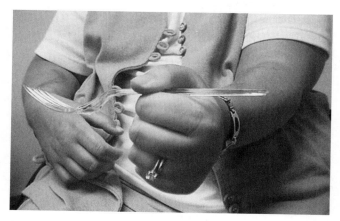

Figure 10-9. Individual with C6 ASIA B SCI, 8 weeks after active lateral pinch and grip.

number of donor muscles.[6,67,84-86] An intrinsicplasty is typically performed during the extensor phase. The thumb is treated by a CMC arthrodesis (if opponensplasty not performed) or APL tenodesis (if opponensplasty is performed). The flexor phase consists of transferring the ECRL tendon to power the FDP muscle and transferring the pronator teres tendon or brachioradialis tendon to power the FPL muscle (depending upon what is done during the extensor phase and how the thumb is to be reconstructed). The IP is stabilized by a FPL split tendon transfer. Variations using alternative tendon transfers and alternative ordering of the surgical procedures have been described and illustrate the importance of individualizing the surgical plan to fit the candidate's needs.[6,21,67,84-86]

Specific Guidelines for Postsurgical Rehabilitation

STAGE 1 (Extensor Stage). The individual is casted for 3 to 4 weeks. After cast removal, during the first 2 weeks of therapy, the focus is on active range of motion of the wrist flexors to facilitate passive tenodesis opening or to initiate passive motion of the brachioradialis. In addition, passive range-of-motion exercises of the proximal and distal IP joint is performed.[29-33] These exercises are performed with the wrist positioned in extension to avoid stretching the tendon transfers. Muscle re-education of the brachioradialis muscle and active range-of-motion exercises for the ECRL are initiated during the 6th week after surgery, and by week 8, strengthening activities are performed.

STAGE II (Flexor Stage). When full wrist flexion is obtained, typically between 7 to 10 weeks after surgery for the extensor stage, the flexor stage reconstruction is performed. The rehabilitation for this stage is the same as the active pinch and grip section.

It is inevitable that there will be situations when the outcome of the surgical procedure is not typical. Problem-solving strategies for common issues that may arise during the course of postsurgical rehabilitation are summarized in Table 10-3.

Table 10-3
Problem Solving for Common Issues in Rehabilitation of Tendon Transfer

Problem	Suggested Solutions
The individual is unable to activate the transferred muscle and/or the therapist does not palpate a contraction along the entire length of the transferred muscle.	• Reposition the individual's arm. • Provide an alternative form of cueing to elicit the restored movement. • Consult another therapist for opinion. • Call the surgeon to assess for disruption or adhesions.
The individual is having difficulty activating and isolating the transferred muscle(s).	• Be certain that the individual is attempting to activate the intended muscle and not a synergistic muscle to achieve the restored motion. • Provide an alternative form of cueing to elicit the restored movement. • Maintain the individual's arm in a position that blocks compensatory strategies. • Consider biofeedback if medically cleared by the surgeon. • Consider electrical stimulation if medically cleared by the surgeon.
The individual is gaining motion in direction of the antagonist too slowly (per protocols).	• Cue the individual to actively pull the joint in the direction of the antagonist. • Palpate the muscles that should be working to be certain that the patient is activating the correct muscle(s) to achieve the restored movement. • Incorporate pain management strategies if necessary. • Consult the surgeon to evaluate and advise.

Table 10-3

Problem Solving for Common Issues in Rehabilitation of Tendon Transfer—cont'd

Problem	Suggested Solutions
The individual is gaining motion in the direction of the antagonist too quickly.	• Emphasize terminal end range of the restored motion. • Exercise within the range desired versus the individual's full range. • Extend the immobilization time with splints according to surgeon's orders. • Consult the surgeon to evaluate and advise
The individual has a weak motor response.	• Ensure adequate trunk support. • Be sure that arm is positioned to move in a gravity-eliminated plane. • Provide an alternative form of cuing to elicit the restored movement. • Try alternate upper extremity position(s). • Try isometric resistance if cleared by the surgeon. • Try electrical stimulation if cleared by the surgeon.
The individual has pain.	• Decrease resistance during exercise. • Decrease number of repetitions. • Arrange treatment sessions/home program sessions to allow more rest between exercise sets. • Incorporate stretching while adhering to postsurgical precautions.
Know when to begin coactivation of transplants in the individual who has had simultaneous tendon transfers.	• Training c-activation begins when the individual can activate each muscle in isolation.

CASE STUDY 10-1   Upper Extremity Management in an Individual with Acute Tetraplegia

Assessment

Morgan is a 38-year-old woman who sustained a C5 SCI who sustained 4 days ago. Morgan underwent a posterior spinal fusion from C5–C7. There were no other significant injuries sustained. On bedside assessment, the therapist finds the individual lying supine in bed with shoulders held in adduction, forearm pronated, elbows flexed 90 degrees, and arms held tightly across chest. Her wrist has fallen into full flexion and hands are in a fisted posture. Morgan has pillows positioned to prevent skin breakdown. Assessment of passive range of motion reveals that full passive range is attainable at all joints. Morgan has active deltoids and biceps. No tone/spasticity is present at this time.

Intervention

The therapist positions Morgan with pillows in the following pattern: shoulders abducted, forearms neutral with elbows out to side. At this point, therapist notes that elbows do not comfortably remain in this position. Therefore, pillow splints are used; these will help prevent elbow flexion contracture. Therapist fabricates intrinsic-plus splints to hold the wrist in slight extension, MP joints at 90 degrees, and IP in minimal flexion. The thumb is in lateral abduction. All of above measures will assist in edema management, contracture prevention, and pain management from poor positioning. The therapist educates the team (including the family) about positioning when supine and lying on the side. In addition, the family is instructed in range-of-motion exercises, with precautions not to overstretch the muscles or force the joints. Basic spinal cord education is initiated.

CASE STUDY 10-2   Upper Extremity Management in an Individual with Chronic Tetraplegia

Mario is a 27-year-old man who sustained a C6 SCI in a diving accident 15 months previously. He reports that he completed an aggressive inpatient rehabilitation and day treatment program. He is participating in outpatient therapy and is interested in what he can do to improve his function.

History and Assessment of Activities

Mario reports the following: After his injury, he had skin breakdown on his sacrum, which has completely healed. He has urinary tract infections occasionally. He experiences autonomic dysreflexia due to bladder and bowel conditions, but has never had autonomic dysreflexia related to casting or splinting devices. Mario has spasticity that is controlled with spasmolytic medication (oral baclofen). Mario lives with his mother in disabled-accessible apartment. His mother is his primary caregiver, and he also has a sister and brother-in-law who live nearby and assist with his care. He has a power wheelchair with power tilt, roll-in shower chair, and Hoyer lift. Mario's ability to use his upper extremities for function are as follows:

- is independent in feeding with universal cuff (after setup)
- brushes teeth with universal cuff after setup
- washes face with minimal assistance
- shaves with universal cuff minimal assistance
- bathes upper extremity with minimal assistance
- bathes lower extremity with maximal assistance
- zips zippers and buttons buttons with moderate assistance
- use ATM card with maximal assist
- removes money from wallet with moderate assistance
- writes with universal cuff with modified independence
- turns pages in a book with pencil in universal cuff with modified independence
- types on computer with pencil in universal cuff with modified independence
- completes lateral transfers with moderate assistance
- propels manual wheelchair 100 feet before tiring
- is dependent in emptying leg bag.
- wears intrinsic-plus night splints for positioning

Assessment of Body Functions

Mario reports no pain or hypersensitivity in either upper extremity. He has good shoulder stability, good stability in the wheelchair, full passive range of motion, and a good tenodesis alignment with fair CMC stability. Mario's muscle test scores are listed in the following table.

Upper Manual Muscle Test Scores for the Upper Extremities (from Maximum Score of 5)

Muscle	Right Upper Extremity Score	Left Upper Extremity Score
Deltoids	5	5
External rotation	4+	4−
Internal rotation	4+	4−
Biceps	5	5
Brachioradialis	5	5
Supinator	5	5
Triceps	0	0
Pronator teres	2	0
Pronator quadratus	2	0
Extensor carpi radialis longus	4−	4−
Extensor carpi radialis brevis	4−	4−
Extensor carpi ulnaris	0	0
Wrist flexors	0	0
Finger flexion	0	0
Finger extension	0	0
Thumb movement	0	0

This assessment warrants C6 ASIA A classification and International Classification (IC), right upper extremity: O(Cu) 3; left upper extremity: O(Cu) 3. O, ocular; Cu, cutaneous.

Goals

Mario indicates that he would like to be able to straighten his elbows and have a better pinch in order to complete functional skills. He would like to be able to complete activities without needing adaptive equipment and splints. Mario's functional goals included the following: feeding, brushing teeth, washing face, managing money, painting, self-catheterization, writing, transferring, pulling covers down in bed, transferring self, and propelling manual wheelchair, all with modified independence (including no equipment or splints). Mario wishes to proceed with his right upper extremity first because it is his dominant side pre-injury.

Surgical Planning

From a functional perspective, the restoration of elbow extension would be the first priority among the planned tendon transfer procedures. The surgeon opted to use the biceps-to-triceps reconstruction procedure. The second

CASE STUDY 10-2   Upper Extremity Management in an Individual with Chronic Tetraplegia—cont'd

priority was restoration of lateral pinch. Based on available donor muscles, the surgeon selected to perform the brachioradialis-to-flexor pollicis longus tendon transfer with a split procedure to prevent hyperflexion at the thumb IP joint. The CMC joint was fused due to instability.

The surgeon and the therapist discussed the anticipated course of postsurgical rehabilitation with Mario. The case manager worked with the family to schedule assistance in the postsurgical period because Mario will be in a long arm cast for 3 weeks and then require continued assistance for up to 12 weeks after surgery. Discussions resolved issues related to the need for transfers via Hoyer lift, showering, bowel/bladder routine, daily tasks, and weight shifts. Mario and the family showed good motivation, dedication, and planning for surgical procedures.

Surgical Procedure

The planned surgical procedures were completed on the right upper extremity. Mario was placed in a long arm cast for 3 weeks post-surgery. While he was in bed, the arm was elevated to prevent edema, and the shoulder was positioned in 30 degrees of abduction. Passive range of motion of the shoulder began after surgery, with the limitation of 90 degrees of shoulder flexion and shoulder abduction.

Postsurgical Rehabilitation

When Mario came to the clinic for cast removal, he was informed about what he should expect. Upon removal of the cast, all incision sites were closed and appeared to be healing well. The first step in learning to make functional use of the tendon transfer was to begin activation of the active lateral pinch transfer. Mario was positioned with the elbow fully extended and the wrist in neutral. Mario was cued to think of bending his elbow, and he was successful in activating lateral pinch. The training then moved to activation of elbow extension. Mario was position with his shoulder in 90 degrees of abduction, and he was cued to supinate the forearm. Mario was successful in activating elbow extension.

When it was evident that Mario was able to activate the tendon transfers, he was placed in a dorsal intrinsic-plus splint and a dial-hinge elbow orthosis set at 0 degrees of extension. During the first week of therapy, focus remained on activation of both tendon transfers and scar management. Mario and his family were instructed in a home program consisting of activating the tendon transfer and scar massage.

At the beginning of week 2, Mario began activating the elbow extension transfer in the range of 15 degrees of flexion to 0 degrees of extension in the gravity-eliminated plane. Therefore, the angle of the dial-hinge elbow orthosis was increased to 15 degrees of flexion during the day, and a

static night elbow extension splint set at 0 degrees of extension was fabricated for nighttime wear, along with the dorsal intrinsic-plus splint. Lateral pinch strength was 1 pound. In week 2, light functional activities were initiated, such as holding a piece of paper, holding a pen, and holding a catheter in light pinch. In addition, Mario practiced grasping and releasing objects that had been placed in locations that required him to bend his elbow and then activate elbow extension in order to acquire the objects. The home program continued with activation of tendon transfers and scar management.

At the beginning of week 3, Mario was activating the elbow extension transfer in the range of 30 degrees of flexion to 0 degrees of extension in the gravity-eliminated plane. When moving against gravity, Mario was activating the transfer in the range of 10 degrees of flexion to 0 degrees of extension. Lateral pinch strength was 2 pounds. At this time, the angle of the dial-hinge elbow orthosis was increased to 30 degrees of flexion during the day. Mario began activating the pinch and elbow extension in multiple planes, as well as continuing to increase functional activities. At night, use of the static night elbow extension splint set at 0 degrees of extension was continued, along with the dorsal intrinsic-plus splint. Mario demonstrated consistent control/activation of the tendon transfer without substitution, functional range in the restored joint, and an understanding of postsurgical precautions; therefore, the dorsal intrinsic-plus splint schedule changed to night wear only. The IP K-wire was removed at this time. Because the CMC K-wires had not yet been removed, a thumb spica splint was fabricated for day wear.

At the beginning of week 4, Mario was activating the elbow extension transfer in the range of 45 degrees of flexion to 0 degrees of extension in the gravity-eliminated plane. When moving against gravity, Mario was activating the transfer in the range of 20 degrees of flexion to 0 degrees of extension. Therefore, the angle of the dial-hinge elbow orthosis was increased to 45 degrees of flexion during the day. Lateral pinch strength was 3 pounds. At night, use of the static night elbow extension splint set at 0 degrees of extension was continued, along with dorsal intrinsic-plus splint. Therapy focused on increasing the ability to activate the tendon transfers in multiple planes and increasing functional activities.

At the beginning of week 5, Mario was activating the elbow extension transfer in the range of 60 degrees of flexion to 0 degrees of extension in the gravity-eliminated plane. When moving against gravity, Mario was activating the elbow extension transfer in the range of 35 degrees of flexion to 0 degrees of extension. Therefore, the angle of the dial-hinge elbow orthosis was increased to 60 degrees of flexion during the day. Lateral pinch strength was

Continued

CASE STUDY 10-2   Upper Extremity Management in an Individual with Chronic Tetraplegia—cont'd

3.5 pounds. At night, use of the static night elbow extension splint set at 0 degrees of extension was continued, along with dorsal intrinsic-plus splint. Focus of therapy continued to be on activating the tendon transfers in multiple planes and increasing functional activities. The CMC K-wires were removed, allowing discontinuation of the thumb spica splint.

At beginning of week 6, Mario was activating the tendon transfer in the range of 75 degrees of flexion to 0 degrees of extension in the gravity-eliminated plane. When moving against gravity, Mario was activating the tendon transfer in the range of 50 degrees of flexion to 0 degrees of extension. Therefore, the dial-hinge elbow orthosis is increased to 75 degrees of flexion during the day. Lateral pinch strength was 4 pounds. At night, use of the static night elbow extension splint set at 0 degrees of extension was continued, along with dorsal intrinsic-plus splint. Therapy continued to focus on activating tendon transfers in multiple planes and increasing functional activities. In therapy, Mario began working on activating pinch and elbow extension at same time (coactivation) and separately. Training for pinch tasks progressed to activities requiring increased force and larger circumferences since the CMC K-wires had been removed.

At beginning of week 7, Mario was activating the tendon transfer in the range of 90 degrees of flexion to 0 degrees of extension in a gravity-eliminated plane. When moving against gravity, Mario was activating the tendon transfer in the range of 70 degrees of flexion to 0 degrees of extension. Therefore, the angle of the dial-hinge elbow orthosis was increased to 90 degrees of flexion during the day. At night, use of the static night elbow extension splint set at 0 degrees of extension was continued, along with dorsal intrinsic-plus splint. Therapy continued to focus on activating tendon transfers in multiple planes, coactivating the pinch and elbow extension transfers, and increasing functional activities. During this week, the same procedure was performed on the left arm.

At beginning of week 8, Mario was activating the tendon transfer in the range of 100 degrees of flexion to 0 degrees of extension in a gravity-eliminated plane. When moving against gravity, Mario activated the tendon transfer in the range of 90 degrees of flexion to 0 degrees of extension. Therefore, the angle of the dial-hinge elbow orthosis was increased to 90 degrees of flexion during the day. At night,

use of the static night elbow extension splint set at 0 degrees of extension was continued, along with a dorsal intrinsic-plus splint. Therapy continued to focus on activating tendon transfers in multiple planes, coactivating the transfers, and increasing functional activities. With the surgeon's clearance, weight-bearing activities on the right upper extremity were initiated.

Weeks 9 thorough 12 focused on continued high-resistance activities in the right upper extremity. During week 10, the cast was removed from the left upper extremity, and rehabilitation began on left side.

At the end of 12 weeks of rehabilitation on the left upper extremity, Mario's functional capacity was as follows:

- right lateral pinch 6.5 pounds
- left lateral pinch 5.5 pounds
- full elbow extension overhead with manual muscle strength scores of 4 to 5 strength bilaterally

Mario was independent in the following activities with no assistive devices:

- feeding
- brushing teeth
- washing face independently
- shaving
- bathing upper extremity
- zipping zippers and buttoning buttons
- removing money from wallet
- writing with regular pen
- turning pages in a book
- typing on computer keyboard
- propelling manual wheelchair (all day)
- bladder care, including emptying leg bag and self-catheterization

In addition, Mario could perform the following activities independently with the appropriate assistive device (i.e., modified independent):

- bathing lower extremities with pinch-holding handle of long-handled sponge
- performing lateral transfers with transfer board
- using ATM card with adaptation to card modified independent

Mario and his family expressed satisfaction with the outcome of his surgery and rehabilitation.

Summary

A well-planned and comprehensive program for management of the hand and upper extremity will result in increased functional independence and improved quality of life for the individual with tetraplegia. Early management of the upper extremity is essential and should begin in the acute phase of injury. Strategies to preserve joint range of motion and retain suppleness of the hand and arm provide the basis for interventions that may be planned in the future. In the subacute phase of injury, upper extremity management continues to be important, and functional training is emphasized with or without the aid of assistive devices to maximize the individual's ability to use the upper extremity to the best of his or her ability. Proximal muscle and joint function and range of motion are essential both for performing weight-bearing and propulsive activities and for transporting the hand to its destination in reaching tasks. Wrist and hand functions allow the pinch and grasp functions required for many activities of daily living. In the chronic phase of injury, upper extremity management is aimed at increasing functional gains by restoring the ability to actively extend the elbow, pinch, grasp, and release (depending on the individual's level of injury). Many different surgical approaches are available to assist in the restoration of upper extremity function; the selection of the approach depends on the unique characteristics of the individual and the function that is desired. Each surgical approach has associated time frames and established rehabilitation protocols, but it is important to bear in mind that issues may arise that require adjustment of the schedule and protocol. Perhaps the greatest benefit of aggressive upper extremity management may be upon the individual's psyche, with dramatic improvements in self-image, confidence, and overall quality of life. In the words of Sterling Bunnell from many years ago, "if you have nothing, a little is a lot."[7]

REVIEW QUESTIONS

1. What are the reasons why rehabilitation of the hand and upper extremity should commence as soon as medically possible in the individual with tetraplegia?
2. What are the goals of upper extremity management in the acute, subacute, and chronic phases of SCI?
3. What is the tenodesis grasp, what is required for tenodesis grasp to be effective, and what are the motions that should be avoided in order to preserve tenodesis grasp?
4. What is the general process by which tendon transfer procedures are undertaken to provide power to a paralyzed muscle? What is the most important upper extremity motion to restore and the most important grip pattern to restore with tendon transfer procedures?
5. What are the fundamental elements of the postsurgical rehabilitation protocol for an individual who has undergone a tendon transplant procedure?

REFERENCES

1. Hanson RW, Franklin MR. Sexual loss in relation to other functional losses for spinal cord injured males. *Arch Phys Med Rehabil*. 1976;57:291–293.
2. Waters RL, Sie IH, Gellman H et al. Functional hand surgery following tetraplegia. *Arch Phys Med Rehabil*. 1996; 77(1):86–94.
3. Anderson KD. Targeting recovery: Priorities of the spinal cord-injured population. *J Neurotrauma*. 2004;21(10): 1371–1383.
4. Snoek GJ, IJzerman MJ, Hermens HJ et al. Survey of the needs of patients with spinal cord injury: Impact and priority for improvement in hand function in tetraplegics. *Spinal Cord*. 2004;42(9):526–532.
5. Snoek GJ, IJzerman MJ, Post MW et al. Choice-based evaluation for the improvement of upper-extremity function compared with other impairments in tetraplegia. *Arch Phys Med Rehabil*. 2005;86(8):1623–1630.
6. Hentz VR, Leclercq C. *Surgical Rehabilitation of the Upper Limb in Tetraplegia*. London: W.B. Saunders; 2002.
7. Moberg E. Surgical treatment for absent single-hand grip and elbow extension in quadriplegia. Principles and preliminary experience. *J Bone Joint Surg-Am*. 1975;57(2):196–206.
8. Nickel V, Perry J, Garret AL. Development of useful function in the severely paralyzed hand. *J Bone Joint Surg-Am*. 1963;45:933.
9. Gorman PH, Wuolle KS, Peckham PH et al. Patient selection for an upper extremity neuroprosthesis in tetraplegic individuals. *Spinal Cord*. 1997;35(9):569–573.
10. Wuolle KS, Doren CLV, Bryden AM et al. Satisfaction with and usage of a hand neuroprosthesis. *Arch Phys Med and Rehabil*. 1999;80:206–213.
11. Sie IH, Waters RL, Adkins RH et al. Upper extremity pain in the postrehabilitation spinal cord injured patient. *Arch Phys Med Rehabil*. 1992;73(1):44–48.
12. Cromwell SJ, Paquette VL. The effect of botulinum toxin A on the function of a person with poststroke quadriplegia. *Physical Therapy*. 1996;76(4):395–402.
13. Richardson D, Edwards S, Sheean GL et al. The effect of botulinum toxin on hand function after incomplete spinal cord injury at the level of C5/6: A case report. *Clin Rehabil*. 1997;11(4):288–292.
14. Grover J, Gellman H, Waters R. The effect of a flexion contracture of the elbow on the ability to transfer in patients who have quadriplegia at the sixth cervical level. *J Bone Joint SurgAm*. 1996;78(A):1397–1400.
15. Silfverskiold J, Waters RL. Shoulder pain and functional disability in spinal cord injury patients. *Clin Orthop Relat Res*. 1991(272):141–145.
16. Campbell CC, Koris MJ. Etiologies of shoulder pain in cervical spinal cord injury. *Clin Orthop Relat Res*. 1996(322):140–145.
17. Lemay MA, Crago PE, Keith MW. Restoration of pronosupination control by FNS in tetraplegia—Experimental and biomechanical evaluation of feasibility. *J Biomech*. 1996;29(4):435–442.
18. Freehafer A. Flexion and supination deformities of the elbow in tetraplegics. *Paraplegia*. 1977;15:221–225.
19. Zancolli E. Paralytic supination contracture of the forearm. *J Bone Joint SurgAm*. 1967;49(A):1275–1284.
20. Gellman H, Kan D, Waters RL et al. Rerouting of the biceps brachii for paralytic supination contracture of the forearm in tetraplegia due to trauma. *J Bone Joint Surg-Am*. 1994;76(3):398–402.
21. Peljovich AE, Kucera K, Gonzalez E et al. Rehabilitation of the hand and upper extremity in tetraplegia. In: Mackin EJ, Callahan AD, Osterman AL et al., editors. *Rehabilitation of the Hand and Upper Extremity*. 5th edition. St. Louis: Mosby; 2002.
22. Keith MW, Kilgore KL, Peckham PH et al. Tendon transfers and functional electrical stimulation for restoration of hand function in spinal cord injury. *J Hand Surg-Am*. 1996;21(1):89–99.

23. Peckham P, Mortimer J, Marsolais E. Alteration in the force and fatigability of skeletal muscle in quadriplegic humans following exercise induced by chronic electrical stimulation. *Clin Orthop Relat R*. 1976;114:326–334.

24. Keith MW. Restoration of tetraplegic hand function using an FES neuroprosthesis. In: Hunter J, Schneider L, Mackin E, editors. *Tendon and Nerve Surgery in the Hand: A Third Decade*. St. Louis: Mosby; 1997.

25. Kilgore KL, Peckham PH, Keith MW et al. An implanted upper-extremity neuroprosthesis. Follow-up of five patients. *J Bone Joint Surg-Am*. 1997;79(4):533–541.

26. Krajnik SR, Bridle MJ. Hand splinting in quadriplegia: Current practice. *Am J Occup Ther*. 1992;46(2):149–156.

27. Ring D, Adey L, Zurakowski D et al. Elbow capsulectomy for posttraumatic elbow stiffness. *J Hand Surg-Am*. 2006;31(8):1264–1271.

28. Ring D, Jupiter JB. Operative release of complete ankylosis of the elbow due to heterotopic bone in patients without severe injury of the central nervous system. *J Bone Joint Surg-Am*. 2003;85-A(5):849–857.

29. Hentz V, House J, McDowell C et al. Rehabilitation and surgical reconstruction of the upper limb in tetraplegia: An update. *J Hand Surg-Am*. 1992;17(A):964–967.

30. McDowell C, Moberg E, House J. The second international conference on surgical rehabilitation of the upper limb in tetraplegia (quadriplegia). *J Hand Surg-Am*. 1986;11(A): 604–608.

31. Moberg E. Surgical rehabilitation of the upper limb in tetraplegia. *Paraplegia*. 1990;28(5):330–334.

32. Moberg EA, Lamb DW. Surgical rehabilitation of the upper limb in tetraplegia. *Hand*. 1980;12(2):209–213.

33. Moberg E. The new surgical rehabilitation of arm-hand function in the tetraplegic patient. *Scand J Rehabil Med*. 1988;17 Suppl:131–132.

34. Keith MW, Peckham PH, Thrope GB et al. Functional neuromuscular stimulation neuroprostheses for the tetraplegic hand. *Clin Orthop*. 1988(233):25–33.

35. Keith M, Lacey S. Surgical rehabilitation of the tetraplegic upper extremity. *J Neuro Rehabil*. 1991;5:75–87.

36. Curtin CM, Gater DR, Chung KC. Upper extremity reconstruction in the tetraplegic population, a national epidemiologic study. *J Hand Surg-Am*. 2005;30(1):94–99.

37. Moberg E. *The Upper Limb in Tetraplegia: A New Approach to Surgical Rehabilitation*. Stuttgart, Germany: Georg Thieme Publishers; 1978.

38. Landi A, Mulcahey MJ, Caserta G et al. Tetraplegia: Update on assessment. *Hand Clin*. 2002;18(3):377–389.

39. Mulcahey M-J, Smith B, Betz R. Evaluation of the lower motor neuron integrity of upper extremity muscles in high level spinal cord injury. *Spinal Cord*. 1999;37: 585–591.

40. Hoyen H, Gonzalez E, Williams P et al. Management of the paralyzed elbow in tetraplegia. *Hand Clin*. 2002;18(1): 113–133.

41. Boelter L, Keller A, Taylor C et al. Studies to determine the functional requirements for hand and arm prosthesis. Final report to the National Academy of Sciences. University of California, Los Angeles: National Academy of Sciences; 1947. Report nr Contract VA M-212223AU.

42. Peljovich AE. Tendon transfers for restoration of active grasp. In: Kozin SH, editor. *Atlas of the Hand Clinics*. Philadelphia: W.B. Saunders; 2002. pp. 79–96.

43. Brand P, Beach R, Thompson D. Relative tension and potential excursion of the muscles in the forearm and the hand. *J Hand Surg-Am*. 1981;6(A):209–219.

44. Brand P. *Clinical Mechanics of the Hand*. St. Louis: Mosby; 1985.

45. Brys D, Waters RL. Effect of triceps function on the brachioradialis transfer in quadriplegia. *J Hand Surg-Am*. 1987;12(2):237–239.

46. Revol M, Briand E, Servant J. Biceps-to-triceps transfer in tetraplegia: The medial route. *J Hand Surg-Am*. 1999;24B(2):235–237.

47. Kuz J, Van Heest A, House J. Biceps-to-triceps transfer in tetraplegic patients: Report of the medial routing technique and follow-up of three cases. *J Hand Surg-Am*. 1999;24(A):161–172.

48. Haque M, Keith M, Bednar M et al. Clinical results of ECRB to FDP transfer through the interosseous membrane to restore finger flexion. Presented at: 8th International Conference on Surgery of the Upper Limb in Tetraplegia; 1998; Cleveland, Ohio.

49. Knapp ME. Massage. In: Krusen FH, Kotke FJ, Ellwood PM, editors. *Handbook of Physical Medicine and Rehabilitation*. 2nd edition. Philadelphia: W.B. Saunders; 2003. pp. 381–384.

50. Totten PA. Therapist's management of de'Quervain's disease. In: Hunter JM, Schneider LH, Mackin EJ, editors. *Rehabilitation of the Hand: Surgery and Therapy*. 3rd edition. St. Louis: Mosby; 1990. pp. 308–317.

51. Kolumban SL. Preoperative and postoperative management of tendon transfers. In: Hunter JM, Schneider LH, Mackin EJ, editors. *Rehabilitation of the Hand*. 2nd edition. St. Louis: Mosby; 1984. pp. 476–478.

52. Stanley BG. Preoperative and postoperative management of tendon transfers after median nerve injury. In: Hunter JM, Schneider LH, Mackin EJ, editors. *Rehabilitation of the Hand: Surgery and Therapy*. 3rd edition. St. Louis: Mosby; 1990. pp. 705–713.

53. Moberg E. Helpful upper limb surgery in tetraplegia. In: Hunter J, Schneider L, Mackin E et al., editors. *Rehabilitation of the Hand*. St. Louis: Mosby; 1978.

54. Friden J, Lieber RL. Quantitative evaluation of the posterior deltoid-to-triceps tendon transfer based on muscle architectural properties. *J Hand Surg-Am*. 2001;26(1): 147–155.

55. Dunkerley AL, Ashburn A, Stack EL. Deltoid triceps transfer and functional independence of people with tetraplegia. *Spinal Cord*. 2000;38(7):435–441.

56. Mennen V, Boonzaier A. An improved technique of posterior deltoid-to-triceps transfer in tetraplegia. *J Hand Surg-Br Eur*. 1991;16(B):197–201.

57. Paul SD, Gellman H, Waters R et al. Single-stage reconstruction of key pinch and extension of the elbow in tetraplegic patients [comments]. *J Bone Joint Surg-Am* 1994;76(10):1451–1456.

58. Castro-Sierra A, Lopez-Pita A. A new surgical technique to correct triceps paralysis. *Hand*. 1983;15(1):42–46.

59. Lacey S, Wilber R, Peckham P et al. The posterior deltoid-to-triceps transfer, a clinical and biomechanical assessment. *J Hand Surg-Am*. 1986;11(A):542–547.

60. Rabischong E, Benoit P, Benichou M et al. Length-tension relationship of the posterior deltoid-to-triceps transfer in C6 tetraplegic patients. *Paraplegia*. 1993;31: 33–39.

61. Friden J, Ejeskar A, Dahlgren A et al. Protection of the deltoid-to-triceps tendon transfer repair sites. *J Hand Surg-Am.* 2000;25(1):144–149.

62. Freehafer A, Kelly C, Peckham H. Planning tendon transfers in tetraplegia: "Cleveland Technique." In: Hunter J, Schneider L, Mackin E, editors. *Tendon Surgery in The Hand.* St. Louis: Mosby; 1987. pp. 506–515.

63. Bryden A, Wuolle K, Frost F. Training of tetraplegic persons with new upper extremity tendon transfers: A cost-sensitive program. *J Am Paraplegia Soc.* 1994;17:230.

64. Freehafer AA, Peckham PH, Keith MW. New concepts in the treatment of the upper limb in tetraplegia: Surgical restoration and functional neuromuscular stimulation. In: Tubiana AR, editor. *The Hand.* Vol. 4. Philadelphia: W.B. Saunders; 1991. pp. 564–574.

65. Friedenberg Z. Transposition of the biceps brachii for triceps weakness. *J Bone Joint Surg.* 1954;36(A):656–658.

66. Mulcahey MJ, Lutz C, Kozin SH et al. Prospective evaluation of biceps-to-triceps and deltoid-to-triceps for elbow extension in tetraplegia. *J Hand Surg-Am.* 2003;28(6):964–971.

67. Zancolli E, Zancolli E. Tetraplegies traumatiques. In: Tubiana R, editor. *Traite' de Chirurgie de la Main.* Paris: Masson; 1991.

68. Ejeskar A. Elbow extension. *Hand Clin.* 2002;18(3):449–459.

69. House JH. Reconstruction of the thumb in tetraplegia following spinal cord injury. *Clin Orthop.* 1985(195):117–128.

70. House JH, Shannon MA. Restoration of strong grasp and lateral pinch in tetraplegia: A comparison of two methods of thumb control in each patient. *J Hand Surg-Am.* 1985;10(1):22–29.

71. Colyer RA, Kappelman B. Flexor pollicis longus tenodesis in tetraplegia at the sixth cervical level. A prospective evaluation of functional gain. *J Bone Joint Surg-Am.* 1981;63(3):376–379.

72. Garber SL, Gregorio TL. Upper extremity assistive devices: Assessment of use by spinal cord-injured patients with quadriplegia. *Am J Occup Ther.* 1990;44(2):126–131.

73. Hentz VR, Brown M, Keoshian LA. Upper limb reconstruction in quadriplegia: Functional assessment and proposed treatment modifications. *J Hand Surg-Am.* 1983;8(2):119–131.

74. Hentz VR, Hamlin C, Keoshian LA. Surgical reconstruction in tetraplegia. *Hand Clin.* 1988;4(4):601–607.

75. Mohammed K, Rothwell A, Sinclair S et al. Upper limb surgery for tetraplegia. *J Bone Joint Surg.* 1992;74B:873–879.

76. Van Heest A, Hanson D, Lee J et al. Split flexor pollicus longus tendon transfer for stabilization of the thumb interphalangeal joint: A cadaveric study. *J Hand Surg-Am.* 1999;24(6):1303–1310.

77. Rieser TV, Waters RL. Long-term follow-up of the Moberg key grip procedure. *J Hand Surg-Am.* 1986;11(5):724–728.

78. Allieu Y. General indications for functional surgery of the hand in tetraplegic patients. *Hand Clin.* 2002;18(3):413–421.

79. Waters R, Moore KR, Graboff SR et al. Brachioradialis to flexor pollicis longus tendon transfer for active lateral pinch in the tetraplegic. *J Hand Surg-Am.* 1985;10(3):385–391.

80. Waters R, Stark L, Gubernick I et al. Electromyographis analysis of brachioradialis to flexor pollicis longus tendon transfer in quadriplegia. *J Hand Surg-Am.* 1990;15A:335–339.

81. Kelly CM, Freehafer AA, Peckham PH et al. Postoperative results of opponensplasty and flexor tendon transfer in patients with spinal cord injuries. Part 1. *J Hand Surg-Am.* 1985;10(6):890–894.

82. Smith R. Intrinsic muscles of the finger: Function, dysfunction and surgical reconstruction. *AAOS Intructional Course Lectures.* Vol. 24. St. Louis: Mosby; 1975. pp. 200–220.

83. McCarthy CK, House JH, Van Heest A et al. Intrinsic balancing in reconstruction of the tetraplegic hand. *J Hand Surg-Am.* 1997;22(4):596–604.

84. Zancolli E. Surgery for the quadriplegic hand with active, strong wrist extension preserved. A study of 97 cases. *Clin Orthop.* 1975(112):101–113.

85. Zancolli E. Functional restoration of the upper limb in traumatic quadriplegia. Structural and dynamic bases of hand surgery. 2nd edition. Baltimore, MD: Lippincott; 1979. pp. 229–262.

86. Zancolli E, Zancolli EJ. Surgical reconstruction of the upper limb in middle-level tetraplegia. In: Tubiana R, editor. *The Hand.* Vol. 4. Philadelphia: W.B. Saunders; 1993. pp. 548–563.

Upper Extremity Training for Individuals With Cervical Spinal Cord Injury: Functional Recovery and Neuroplasticity

Larisa R. Hoffman, PT, PhD

Edelle C. Field-Fote, PT, PhD

OBJECTIVES

After reading this chapter the reader will be able to:

- Discuss the neural plastic changes that occur following cervical spinal cord injury (SCI) that impact upper limb function
- Describe the impact of level of injury and chronicity on arm and hand function, cortical plasticity, and spinal plasticity in individuals with cervical SCI
- Compare and contrast the prognosis for recovery of arm and hand function in individuals with motor-complete and motor-incomplete cervical SCI
- Describe non-surgical interventions for improvement of hand function in individuals with cervical SCI
- Describe the cortical and spinal mechanism for recovery of function following non-surgical rehabilitation interventions for arm and hand function

Introduction

The most common form of spinal cord injury (SCI) is to the cervical spinal cord. Injury to the cervical spinal cord frequently results in impaired arm and hand function, which impacts an individual's ability to participate in self-care, work, and recreational activities. Many individuals with tetraplegia cite recovery of arm and hand function as the most important goal during rehabilitation.[1,2] In a survey of 681 individuals with chronic SCI, 48.7% of the individuals with tetraplegia stated that regaining arm and hand function would be the single factor that would most improve their quality of life.[1] In another report, 77% of individuals with tetraplegia stated they expected a significant change in their quality of life if they regained hand function.[2] Therefore, improving arm and hand function should be a compelling goal for rehabilitation specialists working with individuals with cervical SCI.

The activity limitations that an individual experiences is dependent on the chronicity, severity, and level of the injury. Here, we will discuss the etiology of upper extremity dysfunction in individuals with cervical SCI and how the chronicity of the injury, severity of the injury, and level of the injury influences upper limb function. We will conclude with a comparison of interventions that are designed to optimize upper extremity function in individuals with cervical SCI.

Etiology of Upper Extremity Dysfunction in Individuals With Cervical SCI

On the surface, the mechanisms underlying upper extremity dysfunction following SCI seem unambiguous. Information from the cortex is essential for functional hand and arm movement, and damage to the spinal tracts limits the amount and rate of transmission of information from the cortex to the muscle.[3] This leads to impaired activation of intrinsic and extrinsic hand muscles, impaired sensory perception of the hand and arm, and disrupted modulation of muscle tone.[4] However, beyond damage to the spinal tracts, evidence suggests that additional mechanisms contribute to upper extremity dysfunction in individuals with cervical SCI by decreasing effectiveness of the remaining corticospinal tract connections. Detrimental plastic reorganization in the cortical motor areas and spinal cord may create further loss of function. Fortunately, preliminary evidence suggests that these plastic changes may be reversible through interventions provided by rehabilitation specialists, thereby improving upper extremity function, independence, and participation.

Cortical Reorganization in Individuals With Cervical SCI

Learned Non-use

Learned non-use is a phenomenon most commonly associate with stroke. It is the result of failed attempts to use the more affected arm early after stroke when there is hypotonicity of the extremities. Later, when the nervous system begins to recover from the insult and some upper extremity function might be possible, the individual does not attempt to use the arm since prior attempts were unsuccessful. This decreased use is associated with cortical reorganization wherein the hand region of the motor cortex is invaded by areas representing more proximal arm control.[5,6] This reorganization is detrimental to function. Thus, there is a persistent cycle of decreased use leading to detrimental cortical reorganization leading to decreased use. There is much evidence now available to indicate that this detrimental cortical reorganization is reversible through mechanisms of activity-dependent plasticity.

Decreased Cortical Motor Representation

Investigations with functional magnetic resonance imaging (fMRI), transcranial magnetic stimulation (TMS), positron emission testing (PET), and electroencephalography (EEG) have identified profound cortical reorganization in individuals with SCI.[3,4,7–18] Neuroimaging techniques have demonstrated that individuals with tetraplegia have significantly less activation of cortical motor areas than either individuals with paraplegia or nondisabled individuals.[12] Furthermore, individuals with greater upper extremity deficits have less activation of supplementary motor area, sensorimotor area, and ipsilateral cerebellum.[11] Not only is there less total cortical motor activity, but muscles distal to the lesion also have decreased cortical motor representation,[15] and the more proximal musculature expands into the areas that typically control more distal muscles.[7] Thus, individuals with tetraplegia have smaller cortical motor hand and arm representation relative to both nondisabled individuals (Fig. 11-1 compares a cortical motor map of an individual with SCI and a nondisabled individual[19]) and individuals with paraplegia.[12]

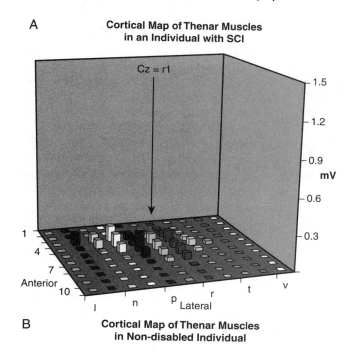

A   Cortical Map of Thenar Muscles in an Individual with SCI

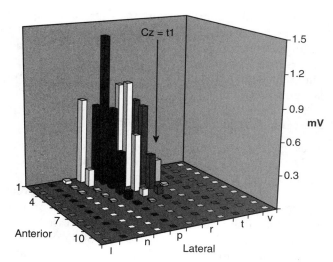

B   Cortical Map of Thenar Muscles in Non-disabled Individual

Figure 11-1. Cortical motor maps elicited through transcranial magnetic stimulation in an individual with cervical SCI and a nondisabled individual. Note in the individual with SCI the responses are much smaller and there are fewer responses relative to the responses in the nondisabled individual.

Posterior Shift of Cortical Motor Representation

In addition to the reduction in size of the hand region of the motor cortex, there is evidence to suggest that in individuals with SCI, the cortical area that controls hand function is shifted posteriorly compared to nondisabled individuals.[13,14] It has been suggested that individuals with SCI may rely less on the motor cortex and more heavily on other cortical areas that contribute to the corticospinal tract, such as the sensory cortex[13] (Fig. 11-2). In intact animals, the sensory cortex makes

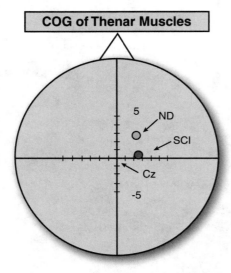

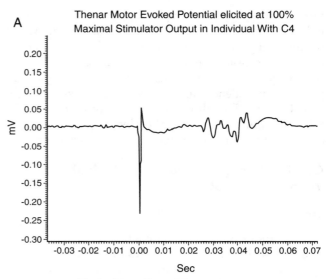

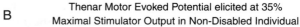

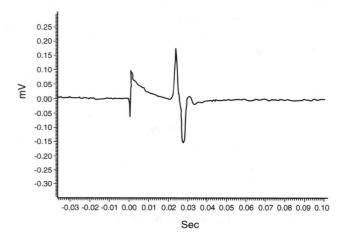

Figure 11-2. Mean center of gravity of cortical motor maps of the thenar muscles in five individuals with cervical SCI and five nondisabled individuals. Note that the center of gravity is posteriorly shifted in individuals with SCI.

Figure 11-3. Motor evoked potential (MEP) of the thenar muscles in response to TMS to the motor cortex in a nondisabled individual and an individual with incomplete cervical SCI. Note in the individual with SCI, the high intensity of the stimulation required to achieve a minimal motor response and the distortion of the shape of the response.

a considerable contribution to the corticospinal tract.[20,21] Furthermore, in humans, stimulation of the sensory cortex can induce movement.[22] For individuals who recover hand function after the acute injury, the hand representation shifts back to its more typical anterior position.[14]

Decreased Cortical Motor Excitability

Investigations using neurophysiological techniques have established that in individuals with SCI, muscles affected by the injury have lesser levels of cortical motor excitability.[23] Studies investigating the impact of blocking afferent input or limiting voluntary movement of the arm in nondisabled individuals suggest that the decreased cortical motor excitability in individuals with SCI may be due to the combination of deafferentation and deefferentation. Blocking afferent input through either local anesthetic block[24] or ischemic nerve block[25] decreases the cortical motor excitability of the muscles associated with that segment.[24,25] Likewise, immobilization of the wrist due to an orthopedic injury results in decreased excitability of the affected segment.[26] It may be that one of the consequences of decreased movement is decreased movement-related afferent input to the sensory cortex, which thereby decreases cortical motor excitability. Hence, the relative impact of either decreased sensory input or motor output on cortical motor excitability cannot be distinguished. Individuals with cervical SCI have varying degrees of deafferentation due to the damage of ascending pathways, decreased voluntary movement due to the damage of the descending pathways, as well as loss of movement-related afferent information, all of which are associated with decreased cortical motor excitability (Fig. 11-3).

Impaired Cortical Drive

The cortical motor reorganization also negatively affects muscle recruitment patterns, specifically in the hand musculature. In nondisabled individuals, low levels of muscle contraction (10% maximum voluntary contraction) of hand musculature create a facilitory effect at the level of the motor cortex, but further increases in muscle contraction do not increase cortical motor excitability.[23] In individuals with cervical SCI, this facilitation is not observed until much greater muscle activation is produced (50% maximum voluntary contraction).[23] It's possible that those muscles with less voluntary drive are not able to recruit all motoneurons available for that muscle such that it requires more voluntary effort to produce the same muscle response.[27] This requires individuals with tetraplegia to use greater effort over a similar force range compared to nondisabled individuals.

Decreased Intracortical Inhibition

While the role of intracortical inhibition is not known, it has been hypothesized that this inhibitory network is involved in the plastic changes of muscle representation that occur within the motor cortex.[28] As a consequence of their injury, individuals with motor-incomplete cervical SCI American Spinal Cord Injury (ASIA) Impairment Scale (AIS)[29] classification C and D) have impaired cortical drive,[23] which may lead to adaptive changes in inhibitory cortical circuits.[30,31] Compared to nondisabled individuals, individuals with incomplete cervical SCI have less intracortical inhibition to the corticospinal tract, specifically to intrinsic hand muscles.[31] It has been suggested that this decrease in inhibition is an adaptive mechanism at the level of the cortex to increase the descending cortical drive.[32] Support for this concept is provided from individuals with stroke who also exhibit loss of intracortical inhibition in both the affected and nonaffected cortex,[33,34] with greater loss of intracortical inhibition observed in the affected hemisphere.[33]

Impaired Somatosensory System

Disrupted sensory input and decreased movement-related afferent information also induces cortical reorganization within the sensory cortex, specifically in the S1 region.[35] Individuals with cervical SCI have significantly less gray matter in the hand and leg region within S1 compared to nondisabled individuals.[36] It is thought that the atrophy of this region is a secondary plastic change due to the decrease in afferent input and not a direct result of the injury.[36,37] In addition to the atrophy of S1, the sensory cortex (S1, S2, and S3) also undergoes plastic reorganization such that the more proximal sensory regions of the sensory cortex (such as the face) invade the more distal regions (such as the arm and hand).[38] This reorganization is similar to that which is seen in the cortical motor system and, like the motor system, may be modifiable with rehabilitation interventions.

Spinal and Peripheral Nerve Reorganization in Individuals With Cervical SCI

Impaired Modulation of Spinal Reflexes

Following cervical SCI, hyperreflexia or spasticity in the upper extremities is detrimental to upper limb function, both limiting performance of activities and causing pain (Fig. 11-4 depicts extensor spasm of thumb muscles). In an investigation including 354 individuals with SCI, problematic spasticity was correlated with incomplete cervical SCI; of these individuals, 60% experienced spasticity in their upper extremities.[39] The mechanisms behind spasticity are thought to be partially related to the

loss or disruption of normal supraspinal influence over multiple spinal reflexes, including reciprocal inhibition, presynaptic inhibition, and recurrent inhibition.[40,41] It is important to recognize that it is likely that a similar mechanism underlies hyperreflexia in both the upper and lower limb in individuals with SCI.

Lower Motoneuron Damage

In addition to the disruption of the modulation of spinal reflex circuits, there may be damage to the spinal motor neurons, as well as the peripheral motor nerve.[42] This change in excitability at the spinal level in individuals with cervical SCI may contribute to upper extremity weakness and thereby decrease arm and hand function. In a study investigating the integrity of the peripheral motor nerve in individuals with cervical SCI, more than 50% had a reduced or absent muscle response to maximal stimulation to the peripheral nerve (M-wave).[42] The reduced motor response is likely related to damage to the motoneuron or spinal nerve root.[42]

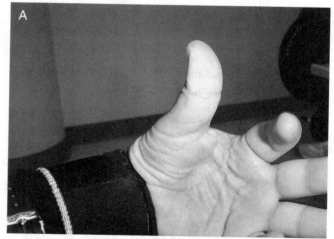

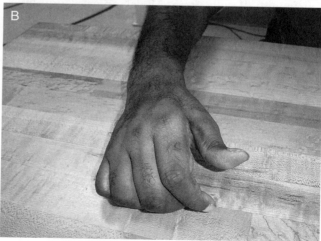

Figure 11-4. Hyperreflexia in thumb extensors in two different individuals with cervical SCI. (A) C7 motor-complete SCI and (B) C5 motor-complete SCI.

With recovery of injury, residual motoneurons may sprout new connections to compensate for the loss.[27] However, this results in the creation of large motor units and decreases the ratio of number of motoneurons per muscle fiber.[43,44] Maintaining a high ratio of motoneurons to muscle fibers is vital for grading muscle force[45], and altering this ratio such that the motor neuron must innervate a larger number of muscle fibers results in the inability to precisely control force.[46]

Influence of Chronicity on Arm and Hand Function in Individuals With Cervical SCI

Acute Stage of Recovery of Arm and Hand Function

Sensorimotor Function in the Acute Stage

Individuals with cervical SCI frequently experience notable improvements in sensorimotor function and grasping function during the first post-injury year. The greatest improvement in sensorimotor scores occurs within the first 50 to 100 days post-injury.[32] However, recovery of sensorimotor function continues throughout the first 300 post-injury days.[32] During this time, there are greater changes in recovery of motor function than recovery of sensory function.[10] Upper extremity motor scores are useful during the acute phase of recovery, as they can be used to predict future grasping function; upper extremity motor scores are highly correlated with future grasping function.[10]

Some individuals (10% to 15%) with an initial diagnosis of complete (AIS A) tetraplegia upon reevaluation (6 to 12 months post-injury) were reclassified as having an incomplete injury (AIS B or C).[47] Likewise, 66% of individuals with motor-complete (AIS B) tetraplegia were reclassified as motor-incomplete (AIS C or D) at 1 year follow-up.[47] Results from Model Spinal Cord Injury System indicates that 16% of individuals initially assigned a diagnosis of neurologically complete injury improve at least one AIS grade within the first post-injury year.[47] Sensorimotor function typically plateaus between 300 and 400 days post-injury.[32]

Cortical Neurophysiology in the Acute Stage

Plastic cortical reorganization, described in the previous section, occurs rapidly after injury. Investigations of the cortical motor map of upper limb muscles suggest that cortical reorganization occurs in individuals with cervical SCI as early as 6 days post-injury.[48] However, within the first post-injury year, the motor responses to cortical stimulation are highly variable and become stable only after 1 year of injury.[32]

In individuals with cervical SCI, neurophysiological signals from the upper limb early after injury can be used to predict future hand motor function. Specifically, prognosis of grasping function can be identified through the presence or absence of motor responses (motor evoked potentials [MEPs]) in response to stimulation of the corticospinal tract in the motor cortex (via TMS).[10] During the acute stage of recovery, a motor response in the abductor digiti minimi in response to stimulation of the corticospinal tract (via TMS) is correlated with recovery of grasping function, whereas the absence of a muscle response in the abductor digiti minimi is correlated with poorer recovery. Furthermore, those individuals who do not have a motor response to a cortical stimulus in either biceps brachii or digiti minimi typically do not recover functional hand use.[10] The ability to voluntarily activate muscles is positively correlated with the presence of an MEP in that muscle.[8] Thus, the presence of voluntary activity in intrinsic hand muscles early after injury is a positive indicator of ultimate recovery of grasping function.[10]

Just as muscle responses elicited from the motor cortex are indicative of future hand function, responses in the sensory cortex in the acute phase also predict hand function in the chronic phase.[49] The presence of a response in the sensory cortex to an electrical stimulus of the median or ulnar nerve (somatosensory evoked potentials [SSEPs]) is correlated with recovery of grasping function.[49] Likewise, a diminished or absent response in the sensory cortex to a median or ulnar nerve stimulus (SSEPs) is correlated with impaired grasping and sensory function.[4] Clinicians may not have access to neurophysiological equipment to access SSEPs, however vibratory perception threshold moderately correlates with presence of SSEPs[4] and therefore may be useful in predicting future hand function. Thus, the sparing of sensory pathways is indicative of future hand function, where greater sensory responses are associated with greater recovery of grasp and sensory function.[4]

Spinal Neurophysiology in the Acute Stage

Shortly after injury, many individuals with cervical SCI experience "spinal shock," a period of hypotonicity in which the individual does not have voluntary motor control, sensation, or spinal reflexes below the level of injury.[50] During this period, the excitability of the spinal motoneuron is significantly depressed compared to individuals with chronic SCI and nondisabled individuals.[42,51] For individuals in whom the motoneurons and peripheral nerves remain intact, resolution of spinal shock coincides with resolution of spinal depression and an increase in the excitability of spinal motoneurons (as measured by the motor response, or F-wave, in response to a supramaximal stimulus to the peripheral motor nerve).[42] In those individuals who have damage to the motoneurons or peripheral nerves, denervation results in persistent depression of motoneuron excitability. The extent of motoneuron damage impacts the recovery of spinal motoneuron excitability, where the greater the motoneuron injury, the less spinal motoneuron excitability recovers.[42]

A denervating injury can be identified by a lack of motor response to an electrical stimulus to the peripheral nerve (also called a compound motor action potential or M-wave) and does not change between the acute and chronic stage.[42] Thus, early after injury, decreased motor function and hypotonicity may be related to either depressed spinal excitability or denervated muscle, and further investigation to the origin of hypotonicity may provide prognostic information for recovery of motor function.

Chronic Stage of Recovery of Arm and Hand Function

Sensorimotor Function and Neurophysiology in the Chronic Stage

Motor scores obtained during the chronic stage of recovery are more highly correlated with grasping function than those obtained in the acute stage.[10] This is likely due to the fact that motor scores are relatively stable after 1 year of injury.[32] Thus, investigations of rehabilitation interventions that induce changes in sensori-motor function in individuals with chronic injury can be attributable to the intervention rather than spontaneous recovery. While the rate of improvement in function is much less than that which occurs in the acute stage, improvements in sensorimotor function may occur up to 5 years post-injury.[52] The severity of injury is much less likely to change following the first post-injury year; however, a small proportion (5.5%) of individuals convert between AIS classifications in the chronic stage.[52] Of those individuals that transition between AIS classifications, those with cervical SCI have a greater likelihood of converting compared to individuals with thoracic or lumbar injuries.[52] In addition, individuals with more incomplete injuries are more likely to improve in sensorimotor scores over time.[52] Thus, individuals with incomplete cervical SCI appear to have good potential for some recovery with the appropriate rehabilitation intervention. Similar to the sensorimotor scores, cortically evoked responses become stable around 1 year post-injury,[32] and therefore a similar deduction can be made that changes in cortical organization that occur in individuals with chronic injury can be attributed to the intervention.

Influence of Severity on Arm and Hand Function in Individuals With Cervical SCI

For individuals with cervical SCI, factors used to identify prognosis of recovery of arm and hand function include severity of injury and the neurological level of injury.[53,54] As would be expected, individuals with incomplete cervical SCI (AIS B, C, and D) demonstrate greater motor recovery than do individuals with complete SCI (AIS A).[10,53] Recovery of upper limb function is almost two times greater in individuals with incomplete SCI (AIS B, C, and D) compared to individuals with complete SCI (AIS A).[53]

Motor-Incomplete Cervical SCI (AIS C and D)

Functional Recovery in Individuals With Motor-Incomplete Cervical SCI

Of individuals who have tetraplegia, individuals with motor-incomplete cervical SCI (AIS C and D) have the greatest potential for recovery of upper extremity function,[53-56] and recovery of function at the next caudal level occurs much faster in individuals with motor-incomplete SCI.[57] Waters et al.[58] found in individuals with motor-incomplete cervical SCI (AIS C and D), 100% of muscles that had an initial score of 2 out of 5 were able to move against gravity at 1 year post-injury. Furthermore, 73% of muscles that had an initial score of 1 out of 5 were able to move against gravity at 1 year post-injury, and 20% of muscles that had an initial score of 0 out of 5 were able to move against gravity at 1 year post-injury.[58] In these individuals, functional recovery of the upper extremities begins to plateau around 9 to 12 months.[56,59]

Incomplete Spinal Cord Syndromes

Individuals with incomplete cervical SCI (AIS B, C, and D) can be further characterized according to the distribution of their sensorimotor scores and classified into syndromes: central cord, Brown-Sequard, and anterior cord.[29,60] Earlier versions of the International Classification System for Individuals with Spinal Cord Injury also included posterior cord syndrome and mixed syndrome, but these were eliminated due to the low incidence of posterior cord syndrome and indefinable nature of mixed syndrome.[60] Among individuals with incomplete SCI, those individuals classified as having either central cord syndrome or Brown-Sequard syndrome have the best prognosis for recovery.[61]

Central cord syndrome is characterized by greater upper extremity than lower extremity dysfunction.[29,60] Many individuals that fall into this classification make dramatic improvements in their sensorimotor scores.[62] An investigation of 112 individuals with central cord syndrome found that at 2 years post-injury the average motor score was 92 out of a total 100.[62] While the prognosis for functional recovery is good for individuals with central cord syndrome, the pattern is such that intrinsic hand function is the last to recover and is most likely to display residual deficits.[63,64] Many individuals with only minor impairment in sensorimotor scores demonstrate moderate to severe limitations in the performance of functional activities.[62] In individuals with central cord syndrome, many factors influence the amount of motor recovery, return of functional skills, and perceived health quality of life. Factors that predict recovery in individuals with central cord syndrome include level of education, presence of spasticity, and age, where a higher level of education, absence of spasticity, and younger age was positively correlated with improved functional outcome.[62]

Brown-Sequard syndrome is frequently caused by a penetrating injury and characterized by ipsilateral hemiplegia, ipsilateral hypoesthesia, and contralateral hemianalgesia.[60] These clinical findings can be explained by the organization of the spinal pathways within the spinal column, where the descending cortical spinal tract and the ascending dorsal column medial lemniscus decussate at the level of the brainstem, whereas the descending spinal thalamic pathway decussates at or within one to two segments of the root level where the nerves exit. Thus, for an individual who has Brown-Sequard syndrome, the pathways that carry light touch, deep pressure, and proprioceptive information, as well as motor information, will be disrupted on the same side as the injury; the pathways that carry pain and temperature will be disrupted on the opposite side of the injury. Most individuals classified under this syndrome have a relative asymmetry of symptoms and not a pure form of Brown-Sequard syndrome.[60] One of the most important factors impacting functional recovery in individuals with Brown-Sequard syndrome is the preservation of motor function in the dominant hand.[53]

Anterior cord syndrome is characterized by loss of function of anterior pathways (including motor function and sensation of pain and temperature), but relative preservation of the dorsal columns (including proprioception, light touch, and deep pressure).[60] Among individuals who are classified with an incomplete cervical SCI syndrome, those with anterior cord syndrome demonstrate less functional recovery than other incomplete syndrome classifications due to the damage to the motor pathways and or motoneurons.[61]

Motor-Complete Cervical SCI

Functional Recovery in Individuals With Sensory-Incomplete Cervical SCI (AIS B)

The presence of sensation at any spinal level increases the probability of motor return at that level, especially if perception of pinprick (pain) is intact.[55] It is thought that the close proximity of the lateral spinal thalamic tract to the lateral corticospinal tract may indicate that if one is preserved, the other pathway may also be preserved. Thus, preservation of the perception of pain that would be relayed through the lateral spinal thalamic pathway may indicate that other pathways that travel in the lateral columns may also be preserved.[53]

Functional Recovery in Individuals With Complete Cervical SCI (AIS A)

Individuals with complete cervical SCI (AIS A) frequently recover at least one level of sensory or motor function, with the greatest rate of recovery occurring within the first 3 months.[53] The level of injury may determine the relative amount of sensory or motor recovery in individuals with complete tetraplegia. Individuals with complete C4 injury (AIS A) have less likelihood of regaining sensorimotor function at the C5 level than do individuals with a complete C5 injury (AIS A), who have a greater likelihood of regaining sensorimotor function at C6.[65] The presence of initial voluntary muscle activation indicates the probability of achieving antigravity muscle strength for that muscle.[53] Only 27% of individuals with complete cervical SCI (AIS A), who initially had a motor score of 0 at the next caudal level, regained antigravity muscle activation at 1 year post-injury, whereas 97% of individuals with complete cervical SCI (AIS A), who initially had a motor score of 1 at the next caudal level, regained antigravity muscle strength.[58] In individuals with complete cervical SCI (AIS A), functional recovery of upper limb function begins to plateau around 12 to 18 months after injury.[58,59,65]

Compensatory Strategies

It is important to recognize that while some individuals may not have all of the necessary sensorimotor functions required to perform a particular task in the typical manner, many individuals can learn compensatory strategies that allow them to perform the task successfully and independently. There are many different compensatory strategies, but the most common may include the use of a supinated hand, the use of the hand as a hook, and tenodesis. All three of these strategies rely on the passive forces of the extrinsic finger flexors. This occurs when the extrinsic finger flexors that cross the wrist joint and insert into the phalanges are allowed to shorten; thus, when the wrist is actively or passively extended, the shortened finger flexor tendons passively close the hand. A supinated hand held against gravity falls passively into wrist extension; thus, the long finger flexors are passively shortened and the individual can hold objects that are placed in the hand (Fig. 11-5). Individuals with tetraplegia can use their hands passively to hook onto an object that has a handle, such as bag, mug, or pitcher (Fig. 11-6). Tenodesis grasp is the use of active wrist extension to passively shorten the long finger flexors and tendons to grasp objects. Objects can be released by eccentrically controlling wrist extension, elongating the finger flexors (Fig. 11-7).

While compensatory strategies may be useful for the individual with more severe sensorimotor impairments, they have several limitations. They are inefficient, in that these strategies take greater amount of time to perform

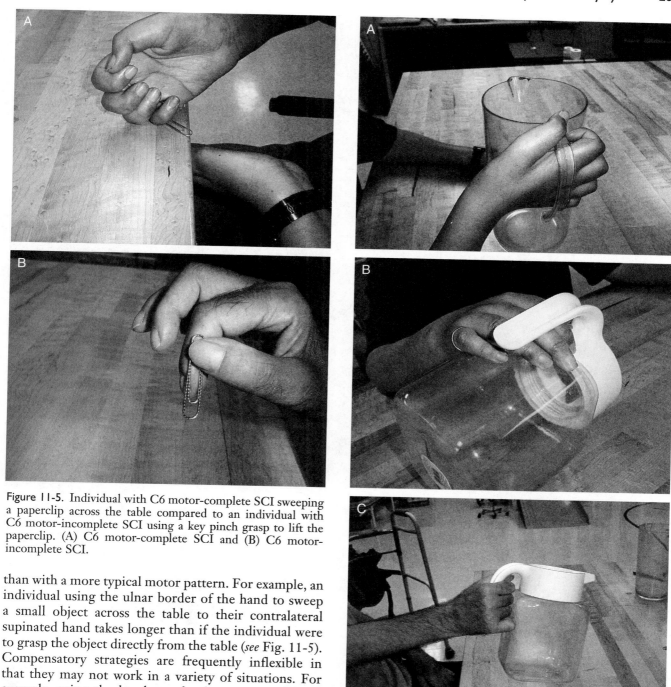

Figure 11-5. Individual with C6 motor-complete SCI sweeping a paperclip across the table compared to an individual with C6 motor-incomplete SCI using a key pinch grasp to lift the paperclip. (A) C6 motor-complete SCI and (B) C6 motor-incomplete SCI.

than with a more typical motor pattern. For example, an individual using the ulnar border of the hand to sweep a small object across the table to their contralateral supinated hand takes longer than if the individual were to grasp the object directly from the table (*see* Fig. 11-5). Compensatory strategies are frequently inflexible in that they may not work in a variety of situations. For example, using the hand as a hook to grasp a handle works well if the handle of the object is closed, but if the handle of the object is not connected on both sides, this grasping pattern will fail (*see* Fig. 11-6). Compensatory strategies may require more energy than using a more typical movement pattern and therefore may be more fatiguing than a typical movement pattern. For example, the use of a tenodesis grasp to pick up heavier objects frequently requires multiple trials to achieve the required alignment such that the object does not slip

Figure 11-6. Individual with C6 motor-complete SCI using the hand as a hook to grasp two pitchers, one with a handle that is closed and one with the handle open. Note that the hook strategy becomes ineffective with the open handle, whereas the individual with C6 motor-incomplete SCI is able to use finger flexors and thumb opposition to grasp a handle. (A) C6 motor-complete SCI, (B) C6 motor-complete SCI, and (C) C6 motor-incomplete SCI.

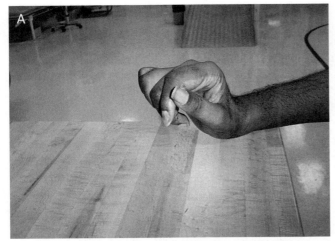

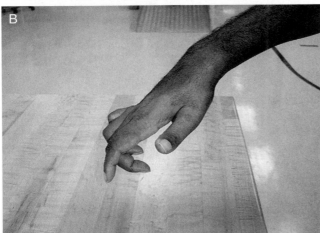

Figure 11-7. Individual with cervical SCI using tenodesis to increase grasping power. This individual does not have active finger flexors or thenar muscles in the right hand. (A) Grasp and (B) release.

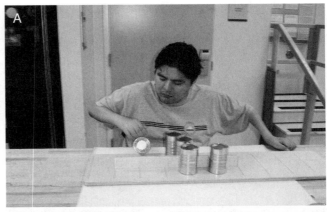

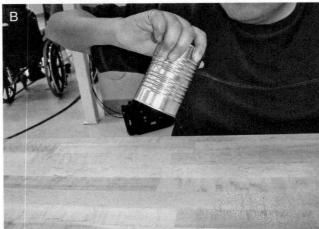

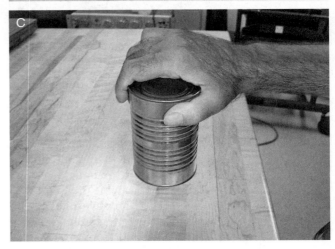

out of the hand (Fig. 11-8). After multiple tries to lift a heavy object, individuals with hand and arm weakness may easily become fatigued. Finally, compensatory strategies increase risk of overuse injuries in joints that are used more frequently. For example, to increase the power of a tenodesis grip, many individuals must further extend their wrist. To increase wrist extension and keep the hand and fingers on the object, the individual may internally rotate and abduct their shoulder, thereby elevating the elbow and increasing wrist extension (Fig. 11-9). This puts the individual at increased risk of shoulder impingement and tendonitis, a frequent injury in individuals with cervical SCI. Therefore, if it is possible to relearn a more typical pattern of movement, it may be more beneficial for the individual to work toward independence using the more typical and flexible strategy; however, there are cases in which compensatory strategies are the only option and provide a useful tool.

Figure 11-8. Individual with C6 motor-complete SCI using tenodesis to grasp a soup can. Note that the individual is able to grasp the can using tenodesis, but requires several tries to complete the task; an individual with C6 motor incomplete SCI using finger flexors to grasp a soup can is much more consistently able to grasp the object. (A) C6 motor-complete SCI, (B) C6 motor-complete SCI, and (C) C6 motor-incomplete SCI.

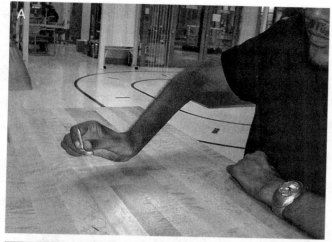

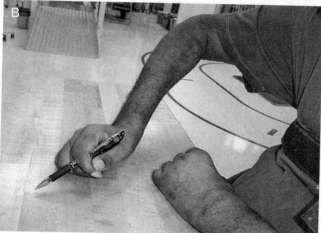

Figure 11-9. Two individuals with cervical SCI using excessive shoulder abduction and medial rotation to increase wrist extension for two different tasks, placing them at increased risk of shoulder overuse injuries.

Influence of Level of Injury on Arm and Hand Function in Individuals with Cervical SCI

Individuals with cervical SCI with similar levels of injury have a variety of patterns of sensorimotor return and arm and hand function. This is especially true of individuals with more incomplete injuries. Therefore, describing the functional capabilities expected for individuals with specific levels of injury may not prove to be useful, as individuals will demonstrate unique capabilities and activity limitations based on their individual pattern of sensorimotor recovery. It may be more useful for the rehabilitation specialist to learn the process of evaluating the sensorimotor functions and impairments unique to the individual, identify the sensory and motor requirements for a particular task, and plan the best intervention strategy to address the activity limitations.

Evaluation of Arm and Hand Function

There are a variety of ways in which one could perform an evaluation of upper limb dysfunction in an individual with cervical SCI. In this section, we will identify the components of an examination that may be important for the rehabilitation specialist in identifying the impairments of individuals with different levels of injury, as well as the motor requirements for four different activities frequently performed by individuals with cervical SCI. The purpose of this section is to provide a logical way to identify the relationship between impairments and activity limitations for individuals with different levels of injury.

Motor Examination for Upper Extremity Function

The most widely used component of an upper extremity examination in an individual with cervical SCI is the International Standards for Neurological Classification of Spinal Cord Injury of the American Spinal Cord Injury Association (ASIA),[29] also referred to as the ASIA Motor and Sensory Scores. The motor portion of the examination provides information regarding both the level of injury and the severity of injury.[29] During this examination, the rehabilitation specialist can gain information regarding the individual's ability to isolate movement at a single joint (or selective activation of a single muscle) and grade the level of force the individual is able to generate about that joint. In areas of weakness, the rehabilitation specialist may need to further explore the strength of other muscles beyond the key muscles identified by the ASIA Motor and Sensory Scores. Table 11-1 describes the level of innervation of different muscles. Finally, the fatigability of upper limb muscles weakened by injury should be assessed,[66] which may be accomplished by analyzing the effect of multiple muscle contractions on the ability to produce muscle force.

Sensory Examination for Upper Extremity Function

The sensory portion of the examination includes assessment of perception of pinprick and light touch. These scores define the sensory level, with the most caudal level having sufficient innervation to achieve a score of 2 out of 2 points (normal). As discussed in the section on influence of severity of injury, these pathways provide information regarding the integrity of the lateral and dorsal columns that may afford prognostic information regarding return of motor function. Additional sensory information that will be useful includes assessments of proprioception, vibration, and thermal sense.[67] These measures of sensory function may identify areas of sensory dysfunction in regions where sensory scores are unable to detect them.[68] Furthermore, vibratory perception threshold is moderately correlated with presence of SSEPs.[69]

Table 11-1
Level of Innervation of Upper Extremity Muscles

Level of Innervation	Key Muscle	Upper Extremity Muscles
C5	Biceps brachii and brachialis	Levator scapulae, rhomboid major, rhomboid minor, serratus anterior, pectoralis major, latissimus dorsi, deltoid, supraspinatus, infraspinatus, teres minor, teres major, biceps brachii, brachialis, brachioradialis, supinator.
C6	Extensor Carpi radialis longus and extensor carpi radialis brevis	Serratus anterior, pectoralis major, latissimus dorsi, deltoid, supraspinatus, infraspinatus, teres minor, teres major, coracobrachialis, biceps brachii, brachialis, brachioradialis, supinator, pronator teres, extensor carpi radialis longus, extensor carpi radialis brevis, extensor carpi ulnaris, flexor carpi radialis, palmaris longus, extensor digitorum, extensor indicis, extensor digiti minimi, abductor pollicis longus, extensor pollicis brevis.
C7	Triceps brachii	Serratus anterior, pectoralis major, latissimus dorsi, coracobrachialis, triceps brachii, anconeus, pronator teres, extensor carpi radialis brevis, extensor carpi ulnaris, flexor carpi radialis, palmaris longus, extensor digitorum, extensor indicis, flexor digitorum superficialis, extensor digiti minimi, abductor pollicis longus, extensor extensor pollicis brevis.
C8	Flexor digitorum profundus	Pectoralis minor, pectoralis major, latissimus dorsi, triceps brachii, anconeus, pronator quadratus, extensor carpi ulnaris, flexor carpi ulnaris, extensor digitorum, flexor digitorum superficialis, flexor digitorum profundus, extensor digiti minimi, abductor digiti minimi, flexor digiti minimi brevis, opponens digiti minimi, palmaris brevis, lumbricals, dorsal interossei, palmar interossei, abductor pollicis longus, flexor pollicis longus, flexor pollicis brevis, abductor pollicis brevis, opponens pollicis, adductor pollicis.
T1	Abductor digiti minimi	Pectoralis minor, pectoralis major, latissimus dorsi, pronator quadratus, flexor carpi ulnaris, flexor digitorum profundus, abductor digiti minimi, flexor digiti minimi brevis, opponens digiti minimi, palmaris brevis, lumbricals, dorsal interossei, palmar interossei, flexor pollicis longus, flexor pollicis brevis, abductor pollicis brevis, opponens pollicis, adductor pollicis.

Additional Factors That Influence Upper Extremity Function

In addition to sensorimotor testing, other factors that impact upper limb function and should be formally evaluated include upper extremity passive range of motion, muscle tone in upper limb musculature, strength of trunk musculature, and static and dynamic sitting balance. Limited range of motion in hands and fingers may lead to impairments in grasping function, whereas limited range of motion of the shoulders may limit reaching function. Measures of muscle tone that may be useful include spasticity (measured by Ashworth scale), influence of co-contraction on movement, and severity and frequency of muscle spasms. In addition, the pattern of movement synergies that impair functional movement should be described. Weakness in trunk musculature and impaired sitting balance may negatively impact bilateral hand function. If an individual requires the use of one arm for sitting balance, then only one hand remains free to perform the task. Thus, when evaluating hand function and potential for recovery, a very thorough examination of the individual's impairments and activity limitations must be completed, as many different factors may contribute to hand and arm use.

Functional Examination for Upper Extremity Function

A functional assessment of arm and hand use provides the rehabilitation specialist with information about how the individual is able to use his or her sensorimotor function effectively to perform a task. The ability to use the upper extremities to perform gross motor tasks such as bed mobility skills, transfers, and wheelchair mobility skills should be evaluated. The ability to perform fine motor skills such as reaching, performing unimanual tasks (each hand individually), and bimanual tasks (use of the hands together) should also be evaluated. Different grasping patterns to be assessed may include lateral pinch, tip-to-tip pinch, three jaw chuck, tripod grasp, and power grip.

Effect of Level of Injury on Function

During the evaluation, the rehabilitation specialist must determine the prognosis for arm and hand function. In order to identify the functional activities the individual will most likely be able to perform successfully (after intervention), careful analysis of different tasks must be completed. The rehabilitation specialist should identify the muscles required to perform the task. It is important to recognize that nondisabled individuals and individuals with tetraplegia may use different muscles or strategies to perform the same task. The important sensory components of the task should be considered. A fine motor activity may require greater haptic information than a gross motor upper-extremity task. Finally, the relative amount of range of motion, trunk strength, and sitting balance requirements to complete the task should be identified. In the next section, the muscles used by individuals with different levels of cervical SCI in the performance of four different activities will be identified.

Reaching

The ability to reach allows individuals to use their hands or assistive devices for activities of daily living as well as direct the attention of others by pointing. For individuals with cervical SCI, the primary muscle used for forward reaching is the pectoralis major; for directions other than forward reaching, different combinations of pectoralis major and posterior deltoid are used.[70] The innervation to the pectoralis major comes from many different spinal levels, thus the ability to activate this muscle must be evaluated on an individual basis. However, in order to use the distal extremity during a reach, flexors of the elbow (such as biceps brachialis and brachioradialis) are required.[71] Elbow flexors are intact in individuals with a C5 level injury, and individuals with incomplete injuries at higher levels may have varying amounts of biceps function. In order to reach and grasp an object without using an assistive device, an individual must have either intact wrist extension, extrinsic finger flexors, or other intrinsic hand muscles.

Wheelchair Propulsion

Individuals with cervical SCI frequently use a wheelchair as their primary means of locomotion, and therefore propelling a wheelchair becomes an important skill. Propelling a wheelchair may be divided into two phases: push and recovery.[72] The push phase is the phase in which the individual propels the rims forward. The recovery phase is the period in which the individual repositions his or her hands on the rims. Muscles important for the push phase of wheelchair propulsion include anterior deltoid, pectoralis major, serratus anterior, biceps brachii, and the muscles of the rotator cuff. During the recovery phase, the middle and posterior deltoid, supraspinatus, subscapularis, middle trapezius, and triceps brachii are used.[72] Individuals with C6 SCI have weakness in their pectoralis major, triceps, and wrist and finger flexors and therefore propel their wheelchairs at significantly slower velocity than do either individuals with C7–C8 SCI or individuals with paraplegia.[72]

Wheelchair Transfers and Pressure Relief

The ability to weight shift and transfer weight to upper limbs is a necessary skill for activities such as relieving pressure from weight-bearing surfaces and transferring to and from different surfaces. Not surprisingly, individuals without upper extremity weakness (individuals with paraplegia and nondisabled individuals) primarily use their triceps brachii to transfer weight to their upper limbs.[71] However, individuals who lack active elbow extension (such as individuals with motor-complete injuries, AIS A and B, at C6 or higher) and individuals with weak elbow extensors are able to transfer weight to their upper extremities using an alternative strategy. Individuals with tetraplegia are able to compensate for triceps weakness by using gravity to assist in elbow extension (through hyperextension of the elbow) and using more proximal shoulder muscles, such as pectoralis major, latissimus dorsi, and deltoid, for pressure relief.[71] Transfers require greater muscle activity in the more distal muscles and greater force in order to control the movement of the body over the stationary hands. As would be expected, the ability to perform transfers to and from a variety of surfaces (including bed, toilet, and the shower) is highly correlated with elbow extensor strength; however, the integrity of the wrist flexors is just as important.[73] Other muscles useful for more controlled transfers include wrist extensors and finger flexors. Thus, individuals with complete C7 or C8 SCI will be able to perform more difficult transfer skills than individuals with higher level injury who may not have wrist flexors and extensors or extrinsic hand muscles.

Grasp

Functional grasping patterns for individuals with cervical SCI may grossly be divided into four categories: inability to grasp, passive grasp, active grasp, and nonimpaired grasp.[4] The inability to grasp is characterized by the inability to hold objects through tenodesis or through active volitional control. Individuals without active wrist extension (such as individuals with motor-complete C5 SCI or higher) must rely on supination or pronation of the wrist to hold objects (Fig. 11-10). Passive grasp is defined as the ability to use tenodesis to grasp objects.[4] Individuals with active wrist extension (such as individuals with motor-complete C6 SCI or higher levels of motor-incomplete injury) may rely on passive grasp to grasp both small objects and larger light objects (Fig. 11-11). Both a power grip and key pinch grip are possible using tenodesis.[74] For a tenodesis grasp to be effective, the grasping power must exceed 2 newtons of force.[74] Baker et al.[75] measured the pinching force required to perform activities such as zipping a zipper, plugging in an electrical cord, stabbing food with a knife, and releasing a key from a lock, and found these activities require at least 2 newtons of key pinch grip force.[74,75] Individuals with active grasp have at least a muscle twitch in extrinsic or intrinsic muscles of the hand.[4] Individuals that fall into this category may have weakened grasp or difficulty with precision tasks (Fig. 11-12). Individuals with a lower level of injury have either nonimpaired grasp or only mildly impaired grasping function.[4] Individuals with this type of grasping function may have difficulty with tasks that require great speed or precision (Fig. 11-13).

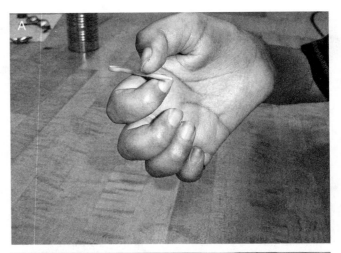

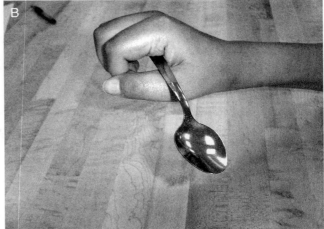

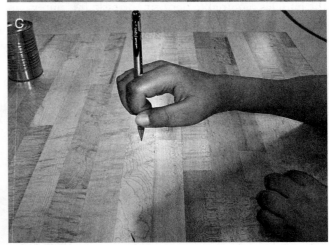

Figure 11-11. Grasping patterns of an individual with C6 motor-complete SCI. This individual does not have active extrinsic or intrinsic hand muscles and uses the mechanical properties of the shortened muscles to augment the grasp. (A) Strategy to replace pincer grasp, (B) strategy to replace key pincer grasp, and (C) strategy to replace tripod grasp.

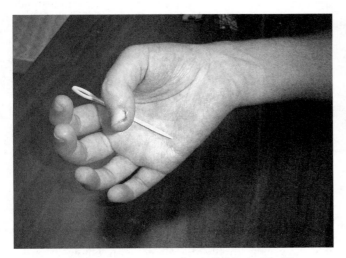

Figure 11-10. Grasping pattern of an individual with C5 motor-complete SCI. There is no wrist extension and therefore he cannot rely on tenodesis. The individual maintains the object in the hand by supinating the hand and releases using pronation. This strategy can be used to replace all grasping patterns.

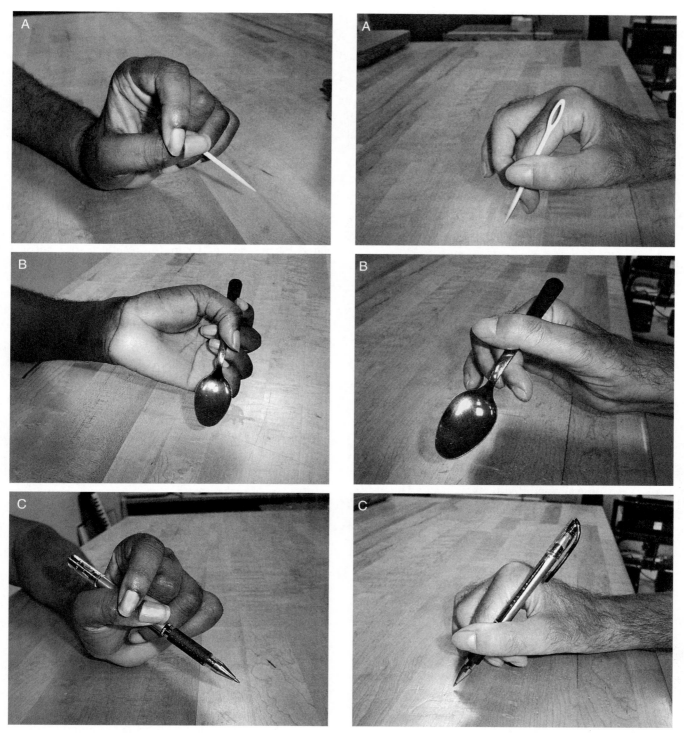

Figure 11-12. Grasping pattern of an individual with C7 motor-complete SCI. This individual has active thenar musculature and no active finger flexors or other small hand intrinsic muscles. (A) Strategy to replace pincer grasp, (B) strategy to replace key pincer grasp, and (C) strategy to replace tripod grasp.

Figure 11-13. Grasping pattern of an individual with C8 motor-incomplete SCI. This individual has active finger flexors, finger extensors, thenar muscles, dorsal interossei. (A) Strategy to replace pincer grasp, (B) strategy to replace key pincer grasp, and (C) strategy to replace tripod grasp.

Rehabilitation Interventions That Optimize Arm and Hand Function in Individuals With Cervical SCI

In the presence of abnormal cortical and spinal organization, the cortex is likely to be less than optimally effective in activating the spared descending pathways. Therefore, interventions that focus on the reversal of the maladaptive plastic reorganization may improve the effectiveness of the remaining corticospinal connections in individuals with SCI. In the subsequent section, the effect of nonsurgical intervention strategies and their impact on function, cortical neurophysiology and spinal neurophysiology will be discussed.

Interventions to Improve Function

In task-oriented training, the goal is to practice the particular task, not just the individual movements required to perform the task. There are several different strategies that may be implemented that achieve this goal, but this discussion is limited to massed practice training, including unimanual and bimanual training and functional electrical stimulation (FES).

Massed Practice Training

Massed practice is a form of task-oriented training that involves repetitive practice of discrete motor tasks. The most thoroughly investigated type of massed practice training is constraint-induced therapy in individuals with stroke.[76,77] Constraint-induced therapy involves intensive, repetitive practice of task-oriented activities using the more-affected upper extremity while the less-affected upper extremity is constrained.[76,77] However, evidence suggests that it is the intensity of the practice that accounts for the greatest improvement in hand and arm function.[78] While many constraint-induced therapy protocols require an intense training schedule—6 hours per day, 5 days per week, for 2 weeks[76,77]—less intense training has also been found to be effective.[78] Beekhuizen and Field-Fote[79,80] have investigated massed practice training in individuals with cervical SCI with a slightly less intensive training schedule: 2 hours per day, 5 days a week, for 3 weeks. To ensure a variety of training activities, each session was divided into five 20-minute sessions in which each session was dedicated to the performance of activities that focused on a different movement category. There were five movement categories: grip, grip with rotation, pinch, pinch with rotation, and gross motor movements.[79,80] Following massed practice training, individuals with tetraplegia demonstrated improvements in hand and arm function.[79–82]

Changes in Function Following Massed Practice Training

In individuals with stroke, massed practice training is associated with functional improvement as indicated by improvement in scores on functional tests.[76,77] Individuals with cervical SCI who were trained using massed practice training alone or in combination with somatosensory stimulation demonstrated improvements in sensory function, pinch grip force, and timed unimanual tasks.[79,80] Understanding the neurophysiological changes that are associated with skill acquisition in different subject groups may provide insight as to the mechanism in which individuals with SCI demonstrate functional recovery.

Changes in Cortical Neurophysiology Following Massed Practice Training

Plastic reorganization of the motor cortex is thought to be related to learning new, specialized fine motor movements.[83] Cortical motor reorganization may be investigated by measuring the motor response to a cortical stimulus (using TMS).[84,85] An increase in the size or amplitude of the motor response in response to the same stimulus intensity would suggest an increase in cortical excitability. Likewise, a decrease in the required stimulus intensity to elicit a minimal motor response would also suggest an increase in cortical excitability[84,85] (Fig. 11-14[81]). In nondisabled individuals, participation in a 4-week protocol of skill training has been shown to be associated with increased amplitude of maximum biceps MEP and decreased response threshold (level of stimulus required to elicit a minimum MEP).[86] This indicates that skill training is associated with increased corticospinal excitability, which may be important for improvements in performance.

A similar mechanism describes functional recovery in individuals with sensorimotor impairment. Several different investigations have provided evidence that the mechanism underlying the effectiveness of massed practice training in individuals with stroke is reversal of associated abnormalities in cortical organization.[76,77,87] Similar to the results observed in individuals with stroke, individuals with SCI who participated in massed practice training demonstrated cortical reorganization. Beekhuizen and Field-Fote[79,80] have shown that individuals with cervical SCI who were trained with either massed practice training or a combination approach using massed practice with somatosensory stimulation, demonstrated increased cortical excitability after the training.

A subsequent study investigated the cortical motor maps of an intrinsic hand muscle following either unimanual or bimanual massed practice training in individuals with cervical SCI.[81] Those individuals who were assigned to the unimanual group had greater increases in cortical map area and volume than either the control group or those in the bimanual group (Fig. 11-15).[81]

Changes in Spinal Neurophysiology Following Massed Practice Training

Spinal neurophysiology may be investigated by measuring responses and changes in spinal reflex pathways. The most commonly investigated spinal reflex is the Hoffman

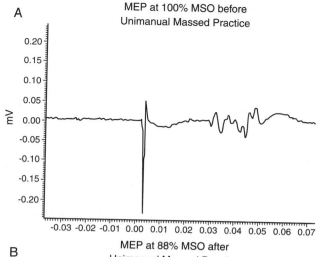

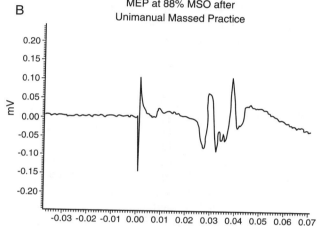

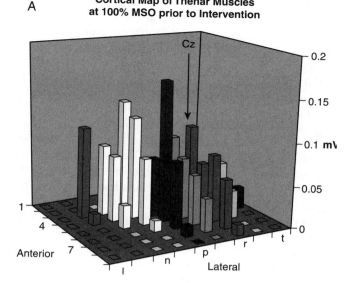

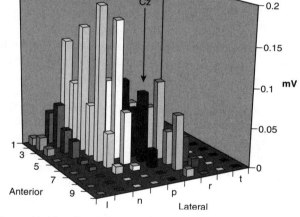

Figure 11-14. Motor evoked potential elicited from TMS before training and after training. Note the increase in size of the response following training.

Figure 11-15. Cortical motor maps in an individual with C4 incomplete SCI before and after unimanual massed practice training. Note the decrease in motor threshold required to map the MEPs, the increase in amplitude in the MEPs, and the shift of the potentials toward a more anterior location.

reflex (H-reflex), which is the electrical analog of the stretch reflex. In the well elderly, skilled hand training designed to improve pinch force steadiness and movement speed was associated with increased adductor pollicis H-reflex amplitudes,[88] meaning that the response of the reflex muscle is greater after training.

It is thought that individuals with SCI are not able to modulate the H-reflex excitability, and this loss of modulation is observed clinically as spasticity.[89,90] The impact of massed practice training or skill training on the excitability of spinal reflex pathways in the upper limb in individuals with cervical SCI is unknown. However, it has been shown that hyperreflexia in the upper limbs in these individuals can be modified through training.[91,92]

The excitability of the alpha motoneuron may also contribute to the ability to maximally activate a muscle. Individuals with cervical SCI have changes associated with the excitability of the alpha motoneuron. The F-wave amplitude is one way in which spinal motoneuron excitability may be measured. It is elicited by a supramaximal stimulation of the motor nerve and provides a measure of alpha motoneuron excitability. Following mass

practice training or a combination of massed practice training with somatosensory stimulation, there was a significant increase in F-wave amplitude.[93]

Bimanual Massed Practice Training

Previous studies of massed practice training have been primarily limited to unimanual task-oriented training. However, individuals with SCI most often have deficits in both upper limbs and therefore may benefit from bimanual training. In bilateral upper extremity tasks, the central nervous system must control a greater number of degrees of freedom, resulting in greater cortical activation.[94–96] There is both neurophysiological evidence and clinical evidence suggesting that bilateral movements may increase cortical excitability, thereby facilitating movement in nondisabled individuals,[97,98] and individuals with impaired movement.[99] The response of a muscle is greater when the contralateral homologous muscle is contracted.[97,98] Furthermore, there are more cortical motor areas active during bimanual tasks than unimanual tasks, even when the tasks are similar.[94] Finally, in individuals with sensorimotor impairment, the peak velocity is greater during a bilateral symmetrical ballistic movement than a unilateral movement.[100] If bimanual activities are associated with greater cortical drive, then bilateral massed practice training may be a strategy to improve functional arm and hand use in individuals with bilateral upper extremity dysfunction.

Using unimanual massed practice training as a model, a bimanual massed practice training model has been used in pilot studies.[81,82] This protocol uses a similar intensive training schedule of 5 days per week, 2 hours per day, for 3 weeks. Like the unimanual massed practice training, bimanual training divides each session into five movement categories: pinch, pinch with rotation, grip, grip with rotation, and finger isolation (Fig. 11-16).[81,82]

Changes in Function Following Bimanual Massed Practice Training

Preliminary data suggest that individuals participating in a combination intervention including both bimanual massed practice training and somatosensory stimulation improve in sensory function, strength, and timed unimanual and bimanual tasks.[81,82] Improvements in sensory function occurred within the zone of partial preservation, suggesting that through activation of spared pathways, improvements in sensory function can occur. Improvements in strength were seen both in muscles targeted by the submotor threshold stimulation as well as muscles that were not targeted by the stimulation. Finally, functional improvements were demonstrated both in terms of time to perform upper extremity tasks as well as the ability to perform functional tasks. In addition to these gains, there appears to be a trend in that those individuals who practice under a bimanual paradigm make greater gains on an outcome measure that measures bimanual hand function. Likewise, those individuals who practice unimanual tasks make greater improvements on tests that measure unimanual hand function.[81]

Changes in Cortical Neurophysiology Following Bimanual Massed Practice Training

Bimanual massed practice training is also associated with changes in cortical neurophysiology. Following this type of training, there is greater cortical excitability and the cortical map increases in size. Furthermore, the cortical map has been found to shift anteriorly following bilateral massed practice training, suggesting that with recovery of hand function, the associated cortical map moves progressively anterior.[82] Thus, individuals who were

relying on cortical spinal tract contributions from the sensory cortex may rely more heavily on cortical motor contributions.

Transcutaneous Functional Electrical Stimulation

Transcutaneous FES systems are electrical stimulating devices used to stimulate intact peripheral nerves or muscles during the performance of functional tasks. Factors influencing recovery of upper extremity function with use of FES are integrity of the peripheral nerve (or lower motoneuron) and volitional control of proximal limb muscles (FES systems are generally used for stimulating the distal extremity).[101] There are many transcutaneous devices that are used to improve grasp in individuals with SCI, including the Rebersk and Vodovnik FES unit, the Handmaster, the Bionic Glove, the Belgrade Grasping System, the ActiGrip System, and ETHZ ParaCare.[101–103] The primary differences between the systems are the type of grasp elicited (due to the stimulating electrode placement) and the switch that triggers the electrical stimulation.[101,103]

The system created by Rebersk and Vodovnik was one of the original systems used to improve hand function.[101,103,104] This device is activated through a variety of options for switches, including an EMG sensor, pressure sensor, or sliding resistor. The switch activates three stimulating channels that are set up to stimulate the finger flexors, finger extensors, and thumb flexors. With this system, key pinch as well as power grip and release functions can be triggered.[101,103,104]

The Bionic Glove is activated through a mechanical sensor that is triggered by actively extending the wrist, which elicits a power grasp by stimulating the finger flexors.[101,103,105] This system is only useful for individuals who have active wrist extension, and it essentially encourages the use of a tenodesis grasp.[101,103,105] Among individuals with tetraplegia, only 30% stated the device was useful for everyday use.[105] This may be due to its limitations, which include the placement of the stimulator (located on the forearm where it is subject to damage as the individual uses the forearm to push against objects) and the fragility of the mechanical, which must be replaced frequently.[101,103] The Bionic Glove is currently being remodeled to form a new system, the Tetron, which will address these limitations.[103]

Individuals with greater sensorimotor impairment may benefit from the Belgrade Grasping System. The Belgrade Grasping System is controlled using a push button that stimulates both finger flexors and triceps to induce both grasp and reaching functions.[101,103] The grasping function is divided into three stages: a preshaping phase, in which the individual adjusts the aperture of the hand in preparation for grasping; a relaxation phase, in which the hand is positioned over the object; and a grasping phase, in which the grasp takes place.[103] Reaching is achieved by measuring the velocity of shoulder movement and stimulating triceps

Finger Isolation	Grasp	Graps with Rotation	Pinch	Pinch with Rotation
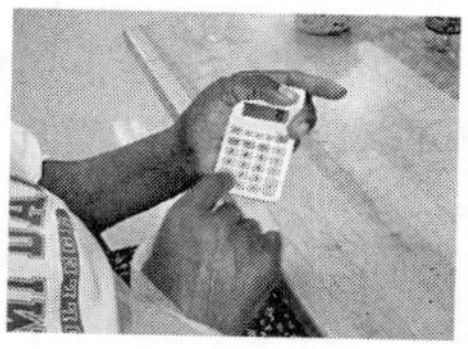	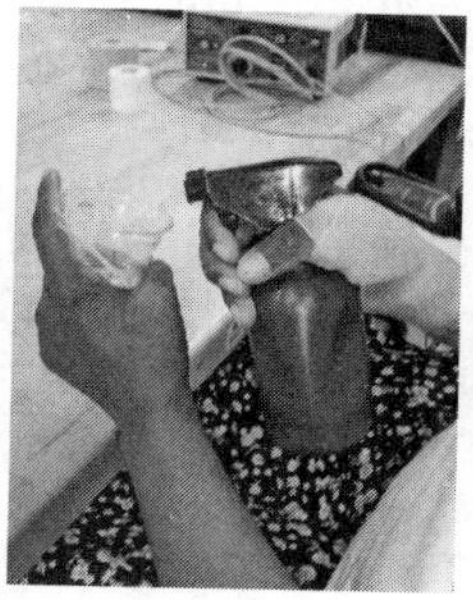	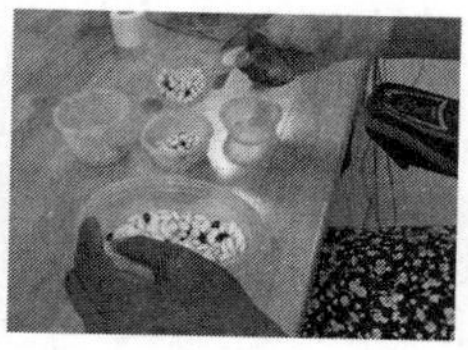	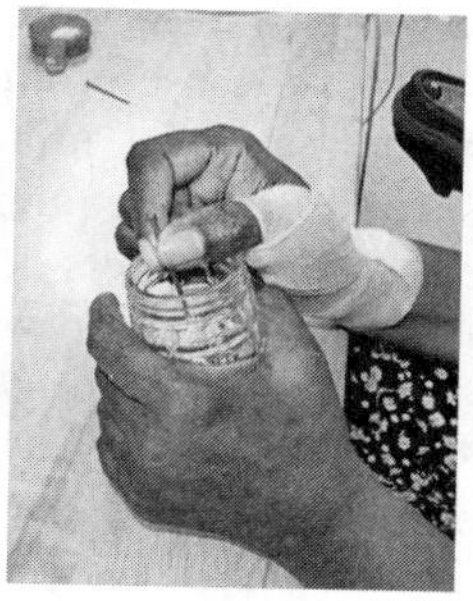	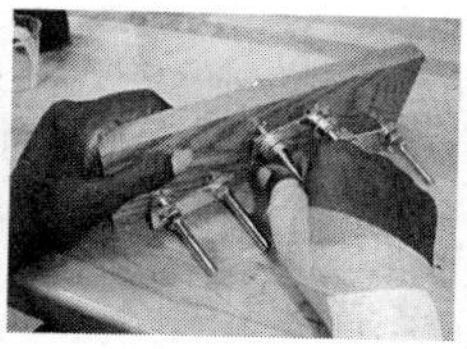
Keyboard: Typing on a keyboard with both hands, type a specified sequence of keys without activating multiple buttons.	**Extension Cords:** Plug two extension cords together and separate using both hands.	**Can Opener:** Squeeze the handle of a can opener together with one hand, while rotating the lever with the alternative hand.	**Picking Up Small Objects:** Hold container in one hand and pick up small objects such as nails and place in container.	**Tying Knots:** Using both hands, the different knots according to diagrams.
Phone: Stabilizing the phone with one hand, dial a list of phone numbers without depressing multiple buttons.	**Scissors:** Stabilize a piece of paper with one hand and cut out shapes with the other hand.	**Rubik's Cube:** Stabilize the Rubik's cube with one hand, while rotating the object with the other hand.	**Pipecleaner Shapes:** Using both hands, orient the pipecleaners to create preset shapes.	**Lace-up Cards:** Stabilizing the cards with one hand, thread the shoelace into the holes with the other hand.
Calculator: Stabilizing the calculator with one hand, depress the buttons of the calculator to calculate the solutions to set of math problems.	**Glue:** Using both hands, squeeze glue out of a large bottle, to create preset designs on paper.	**Scooping:** Stabilizing the container with one hand, scoop beans out of the container and into another container.	**Ziploc:** Using one hand to stabilize the Ziploc bag open and close the Ziploc with the other hand.	**String Beads:** Stabilizing the bead with one hand, thread string into bead with the other hand.
Punch Pad: Stabilizing a video game with one hand, depress the buttons to play the game with the other hand.	**Nesting Boxes:** Using both hands, separate nesting boxes, and place inside each other.	**Containers:** Stabilizing a container with one hand, unscrew the lid of the container with the other hand.	**Buttons:** Button and unbutton different-sized buttons on a strip.	**Twist Ties:** Stabilize the bag with one hand, and twist the twist tie around the bag with the other hand.
Clay: Poke holes into clay using each finger individually, and using both hands simultaneously.	**Building:** Using both hands, separate Legos and attach together.	**Measuring Cups:** Pour a predetermined amount of liquid into a measuring cup.	**Braiding Yarn:** Braid three pieces of yarn.	**Nuts and Bolts:** Stabilize the bolt with one hand and twist the nut on and off with the other hand.
Piano: Depress individual keys on the piano without activating multiple at one time.	**Clay:** Using both hands, shape clay into predetermined shapes.	**Flipping Cans:** Using two soda cans at one time, rotate both cans upside down simultaneously.	**Bubble Wrap:** Using both hands, pop bubbles in bubble wrap.	**Key and Padlock:** Using one hand to stabilize the lock, use key with other hand to open the lock.

Figure 11-16. List of training activities used for bimanual massed practice training.

to ensure the same rate of movement is achieved at the elbow.[103]

The ETHZ-ParaCare is used to stimulate palmar grasp and lateral grasping function.[103] The system has multiple options for switch activation: EMG, push button switch, or sliding resistor. The major limitation of the use of ETHZ-ParaCare is the time and assistance required to set up the system.[103]

Changes in Function Following Functional Electrical Stimulation

Many FES systems are used to improve hand grasp in individuals with SCI as a neural prosthesis; however, these systems may be associated with improved hand function even when the device is not in use, suggesting that it is useful as a training device.[102,106] This form of training has been shown to be effective in improving arm and hand function in individuals with cervical SCI[102,106] and stroke.[103,107] While stimulation parameters will vary depending on the device and tissue stimulated, Popovic et al.[101,103,106] advocate the use of biphasic pulse, with an intensity between 8 and 50 milliamps for a duration of 250 microseconds at a frequency of 20 to 70 Hertz.[101,103,106] Using these parameters and a training schedule of 45 minutes per session for 6 weeks, individuals practiced functional tasks, repeating the activity 35 to 50 times per session. Following this intervention, individuals demonstrated gains on the Functional Independence Measure and the Spinal Cord Independence Measure. The treatment effect, however, appears to depend on severity of injury, where individuals with less hand function demonstrate greater gains after use of FES than do individuals with more hand function.[106] It was hypothesized that individuals with more severe injuries may not be able to perform the tasks adequately in the absence of assistance (such as FES), and the performance of the task provides the central nervous system with greater sensorimotor feedback that is required for motor learning.[106]

Changes in Cortical Neurophysiology Following Functional Electrical Stimulation

Cortical neurophysiology associated with improvements in grasping function induced by FES have not been investigated; however, changes in cortical excitability following FES to the lower limb have been investigated. Kido et al.[108] investigated the changes in cortical excitability following 30 minutes of FES-assisted walking. The investigators found increased cortical motor excitability of the tibialis anterior after the intervention.[108] Thus, it is likely that training the upper limb through an intervention that uses FES will also result in increased cortical excitability.

Changes in Spinal Neurophysiology Following Functional Electrical Stimulation

Thompson et al.[109] investigated the impact of FES-assisted walking on spinal neurophysiology. The investigators found no change in H-reflex amplitude, reciprocal inhibition, and presynaptic inhibition. From these results, it was concluded that the changes in cortical excitability must be at the cortical level.[109] However, it may be that FES influences spinal reflex circuitry in individuals with hyperreflexia. Fung and Barbeau[110] found that FES has a modulating influence on the lower extremity for individuals with spastic gait, but not nondisabled individuals or individuals without spasticity. This may also be true for individuals with hypertonicity of the upper limb. While further investigations must be performed on the upper limb, it appears that changes in upper extremity function induced by FES are likely attributable to increased cortical excitability.

Interventions Aimed to Increase Strength

Performance of functional activities with the arm and hand are frequently limited by the inability to produce sufficient force to perform the task. Therefore, increasing muscle strength may be one way to increase arm and hand function, thereby increasing independence. A variety of interventions have been proposed to increase strength in individuals with SCI, including resistance training, neuromuscular electrical stimulation, biofeedback, and vibration.

Resistance Training

Upper extremity weakness is a common impairment among individuals with cervical SCI and thus resistance training is a common strategy for improving upper extremity motor function. In addition to deficits in force production, individuals with SCI exhibit great fluctuations in maximal force and the ability to grade force. Resistance training has been shown to decrease fluctuations in force at lower force levels.[111] Furthermore, both progressive resistance training programs (40% to 100% maximum voluntary contraction) and repetitive low-load training programs (10% maximum voluntary contraction) are accompanied by improved ability to perform rapid, coordinated movements to acquire a target. These changes are associated with differences in muscle coordination patterns, especially in muscles around the elbow.[112]

Resistance training of finger muscles has been shown to be associated with improved stability of coordination in performance of complex motor tasks. This improvement is accompanied by changes in recruitment pattern, suggesting that resistance training affects not only muscle physiology, but also neuroanatomical function.[113] Repetitive low-load training of finger muscles (10% maximum voluntary contraction), with emphasis on steadiness of contraction, has been shown to decrease fluctuations in movement acceleration in both concentric and eccentric contractions and decrease the variability of motor unit discharge rates. Subsequent training with higher loads (70% maximum voluntary contraction) did not result in further improvements in these parameters.[114] Based on evidence from nondisabled individuals and other clinical populations, resistance training has the potential for improving arm and hand strength in individuals with cervical SCI.

Changes in Function Following Resistance Training

There is little evidence for or against resistance training as an intervention in individuals with cervical SCI. The only published report concerns a strengthening program that focused on a single muscle group (either biceps or triceps), which compared resistance exercise to neuromuscular electrical stimulation (NMES). The investigators concluded that neither training regimen was effective in improving arm strength.[115] This finding is counter to other studies of

NMES-assisted exercise, which have shown improvements in upper extremity strength.[116] Furthermore, the notion that paretic muscles are amenable to training is evidenced by studies of training impaired respiratory muscles, which have been found to be successful in improving respiratory function in individuals with tetraplegia.[117,118]

Changes in Cortical Neurophysiology Following Resistance Training

Resistance training is associated with increased maximum voluntary contractions. In nondisabled individuals, resistance training is associated with a decrease in cortical motor excitability of the trained muscle.[86] As changes are not seen in cortical excitability, there must be changes in functional properties of the spinal cord or in the muscle.[119]

Changes in Spinal Neurophysiology Following Resistance Training

There is little information available regarding the effect of resistance training on spinal reflex properties of the upper limbs. In investigations in nondisabled individuals in the lower limb, resistance training has been shown to be associated with increased soleus H-reflex amplitude and no change in M-wave amplitude during a 90% maximum voluntary contraction.[120] This suggests that after resistance training, there may increases in the spinal reflex response during muscle contraction.

Biofeedback

Biofeedback therapy may be useful in rehabilitation to increase muscle activation for paretic muscles or decrease the motor response for spastic muscle.[121] Here we will discuss the use of biofeedback to increase voluntary motor output; however, further information regarding the use of biofeedback for decreasing spinal excitability will be discussed later in the chapter. It has been hypothesized that increasing attention to proprioceptive input, individuals with impaired sensorimotor function can learn to increase voluntary motor activation.

Changes in Function Following Biofeedback Training

Brucker et al.[122] investigated the effects of biofeedback training on triceps electromyography (EMG) in individuals with cervical SCI and found significantly greater EMG output following the intervention. However, when compared to other interventions, biofeedback training has been found to provide no additional benefit over traditional intervention. Kohlmeyer et al.[123] compared the effect of biofeedback training with task-oriented practice on the learning of tenodesis grasp in individuals with acute cervical SCI. Individuals were trained for 20 minutes per day, 5 days per week, for 6 weeks. Individuals in both groups demonstrated similar gains in manual muscle tests and performance of activities of daily living.[123] Thus, it is unclear if biofeedback is more beneficial than other therapies in increasing strength of paretic muscles.

Neuromuscular Electrical Stimulation

There are a variety of protocols that incorporate the use of NMES to elicit muscle contractions to strengthen weakened muscle. NMES may be applied to either a muscle or a nerve to increase motor output. Some protocols require some voluntary muscle activity, as in EMG-triggered NMES.[124] In this protocol, the individual must initiate the stimulation by creating a muscle contraction. Other protocols have the individual attempt to contract with the stimulation.[125] Finally, there are protocols designed to stimulate paralyzed musculature to reduce muscle atrophy.[126] This section will focus on the functional and neurophysiological changes associated with the application of NMES to weakened musculature.

Changes in Function Following Electrical Stimulation

Hatkopp et al.[125] investigated the effects of NMES on wrist extensor strength in individuals with tetraplegia. Individuals with C5 or C6 tetraplegia with some voluntary activity in their wrist extensors were trained 30 minutes per day, 5 days a week, for 12 weeks. The stimulation parameters were as follows: frequency was 30 Hertz, with a pulse duration of 250 microseconds at an intensity that elicited 100% of maximum load. Following the intervention, individuals trained with NMES demonstrated an 34% increase in force production. In addition, subjects reported improvements in grasp following the intervention.[125]

Changes in Cortical Neurophysiology Following Electrical Stimulation

In individuals with cervical SCI, the cortical changes associated with NMES have not been investigated; however, it has been shown that following NMES to the upper limb in individuals with stroke, there is increased activation in the sensory cortex. Kimberley et al.[124] investigated the effect of EMG-triggered NMES in individuals post-stroke. Individuals were trained 6 hours per day, for 10 days, over a period of 3 weeks. Following training, improvements in strength of finger and wrist extensors were found, as well as improvements in the performance of timed motor tasks. While improvements in function were found, there was no difference in activation of cortical motor areas; however, increased activation was seen in the sensory cortex as measured by fMRI. The authors suggest that in order to increase cortical motor activity, the training must incorporate problem solving into the intervention.[124]

Changes in Spinal Neurophysiology Following Electrical Stimulation

Neuromuscular electrical stimulation does not appear to alter spinal reflex activity when set at supramotor threshold levels. In nondisabled individuals, supramotor threshold electrical stimulation applied to either the tibialis anterior or the soleus does not affect the amplitude of response of spinal reflexes (H-reflex). However, when the stimulation is set to lower intensities, an increase in spinal reflexes is seen.[127] This is discussed in greater detail in subsequent sections.

Interventions Aimed to Increase Cortical Excitation

Individuals with cervical SCI have decreased cortical motor excitability related to both their sensory and motor impairment. Increasing cortical excitability is associated with the early signs of neural plasticity and learning.[128] Thus, interventions that focus on increasing cortical excitability may be essentially preparing the system for cortical reorganization and motor learning. Rehabilitation interventions that are associated with increasing cortical excitability include somatosensory stimulation, vibration, and motor imagery.

Somatosensory Stimulation

In individuals with stroke, one of the consequences of decreased movement is decreased movement-related afferent information to the sensory cortex. In individuals with SCI, the consequences of decreased movement are further complicated by varying degrees of central deafferentation due to the damage to ascending pathways that convey sensory information to the supraspinal centers. Consequently, in both populations, loss of afferent input to the sensory cortex may contribute to cortical changes that are detrimental to function. In published studies aimed at increasing cortical excitability, stimulation parameters used when applying somatosensory stimulation are trains of electrical stimulation delivered at a frequency of 1 Hertz, where one train consists of five pulses of 1 millisecond duration, at a frequency of 10 pulses per second, with the stimulus intensity just below that which evokes an observable muscle twitch.[129]

Changes in Function Following Somatosensory Stimulation

In individuals with impaired grasping function due to stroke, 2 hours of somatosensory stimulation applied to the median nerve induced increases in pinch grip strength.[129] In individuals with hand weakness due to SCI, 2 hours of somatosensory stimulation applied to the median nerve, 5 days per week, for 3 weeks, was found to increase pinch grip strength and somatosensory function, but not functional skills.[80] However, if the somatosensory stimulation is applied in conjunction with task-oriented training, such as massed practice training, the combination produces a powerful effect on function, greater than either intervention in isolation.[79,80]

Changes in Cortical Neurophysiology Following Somatosensory Stimulation

Somatosensory stimulation has been shown to increase cortical excitability in both nondisabled individuals[130] and individuals with sensorimotor impairment due to stroke[131] and SCI.[80] This type of stimulation is thought to preferentially activate the large sensory fibers associated with the Ia muscle afferents.[132] It may be that activity of muscle afferents plays a critical role in inducing cortical reorganization. The disruption of cutaneous and joint afferents alone does not result in a reduction in the corresponding cortical excitability;[133] whereas the disruption of muscle, joint, and cutaneous afferents has been found to decrease cortical excitability.[134] It may be that muscle afferents provide an important modulatory input that increases cortical excitability. Thus, prolonged stimulation that mimics muscle afferents may lead to increased cortical motor excitability, preparing the system for reorganization.

Changes in Spinal Neurophysiology Following Somatosensory Stimulation

Somatosensory stimulation alters spinal neurophysiology as well. In nondisabled individuals, 15 minutes of electrical stimulation set at low levels of intensity (sensory threshold) increases H-reflex amplitude.[127] This increase in spinal reflex excitability may be due to an increase in spinal motoneuron excitability. In individuals with cervical SCI, prolonged somatosensory stimulation applied to the median nerve increases spinal motoneuron excitability.[93]

Motor Imagery

Motor imagery is mental practice of a particular task in which the individual imagines he or she is performing the task. Individuals with cervical SCI report they experience a movement-related effort during motor imagery similar to that which they experience with executed movement.[135] Likewise, during motor imagery of the upper limb, individuals with tetraplegia have decreased cortical potentials of paralyzed muscles compared to either individuals with paraplegia or nondisabled individuals.[135] Imagining the performance of a motor task is thought to be controlled by the same neural substrate (motor cortex, supplementary motor cortex, and premotor cortex) as actually performing the same movements.[136] The use of motor imagery has long been used as a training strategy to improve performance for athletes and musicians, but has only recently been investigated as a tool for neurorehabilitation.[137]

Changes in Function Following Motor Imagery

Motor imagery has been shown to both increase strength and improve the performance of visual motor tasks. In nondisabled individuals, a 4-week motor imagery program increased strength of an intrinsic hand muscle similar to a resistance training program. The effect was specific to the targeted hand muscle and was not generalized to other muscles.[138] Motor imagery is also associated with improvements in performance of visual motor skills. In an investigation comparing physical training, mental imagery (imagining the task being performed by oneself), or control (visualizing the task being performed by another individual), nondisabled individuals who performed 45 minutes of either physical training or mental imagery improved in a visual motor task in speed and accuracy over individuals who performed the control activity of visualizing the task.[139]

Individuals with sensorimotor impairment may also benefit from motor imagery. Dijkerman et al.[140] compared the impact of physical practice with motor imagery in individuals with stroke. Individuals with stroke practiced either the motor activity of grasping small objects or participated in a daily routine of mental imagery of grasping small objects for 4 weeks. Subjects were all able to grasp a small object and lift it off of the table independently before the training. Both groups demonstrated improvements in their training tasks, but those in the physical training group demonstrated slightly greater gains. In addition, individuals in the physical training group were able to generalize their skills to tasks other than the training activities, whereas those in the mental imagery group were not.[140] Liu et al.[141] investigated the impact of either mental imagery or functional retraining in individuals with stroke who were independent in all activities of daily living. The training activities were different from that of Dijkerman et al.[140] in that individuals performed or imagined they were performing whole tasks, such as cleaning a room, preparing a meal, or taking transportation to a location. Liu et al.[141] found improvements in the ability to perform all the training tasks in both groups, with greater improvements in the imagery group. The investigators suggest that the improvements in the ability to perform the tasks are likely due to the improvements in motor planning, not sensorimotor function.[141] Thus, it appears that for individuals with sensorimotor impairment, tasks that require sequential steps and motor planning may improve more with motor imagery than do discrete tasks that require skill.

Changes in Cortical Neurophysiology Following Motor Imagery

In nondisabled individuals, imagining the performance of movements increases cortical excitability for those muscle representations targeted by the imagery.[142] Likewise, in individuals with stroke, motor imagery has been found to increase cortical excitability and increase the size of the cortical map of an intrinsic hand muscle during the imagery.[143]

Butler and Page[144] investigated the cortical changes following a training intervention in individuals poststroke. This case series compared mental practice, physical practice, and a combination of physical and mental practice over a 2 week time period. The individual who was assigned to mental practice alone demonstrated minimal gains in function and changes in cortical activity, whereas those assigned to the physical practice and the combined intervention made greater gains in both function and cortical activation.[144]

Changes in Spinal Neurophysiology Following Motor Imagery

While the excitability of the cortical motor system increases during motor imagery, there is no change in excitability of spinal motoneurons or spinal reflexes. The excitability of the spinal motoneurons (measured by the amplitude of the F-wave) is not significantly different during motor imagery, where the cortical excitability increased during the imagination of movement in nondisabled individuals.[145] Likewise, several investigators have found no change in H-reflex amplitude during motor imagery, where an increase in cortical excitability was found.[142,146]

Vibration

Vibration may be used to elicit a muscle contraction through the tonic vibratory response.[147] This response is mediated by vibration to the muscle or tendon that excites muscle spindle and Ia fiber.[147] Vibration may be used as an intervention strategy for individuals with muscle weakness to increase motor output and increase cortical motor excitability, but it may also be useful for individuals with severe spasticity to modulate spinal motor excitability.

Changes in Function Following Vibration

The impact of prolonged vibration as an intervention strategy to increase function has not been evaluated. In some individuals with cervical SCI, vibration increases motor output. Ribot-Ciscar et al.[148] found that, in individuals with cervical SCI and triceps weakness, vibration of the triceps brachii tendon resulted in increased elbow extension force output and triceps muscle activation; the response was greater in individuals who had stronger triceps muscles.[148] Thus, when paired with an intervention to increase function, vibration may be a strategy used to increase function in individuals with cervical SCI.

Changes in Cortical Neurophysiology Following Vibration

In nondisabled individuals, vibration to the wrist extensors increased cortical spinal excitability.[149,150] Smith and Brouwer[149] investigated 15 minutes of vibration applied at an amplitude of 0.5 mm, 100 Hertz, to extensor carpi radialis longus muscle. The investigators found that following 15 minutes of vibration to the muscle, the cortical excitability of the extensor carpi radialis longus muscle increased. The effect decreased 20 minutes after the vibration. Furthermore, the effect may be dependent on the frequency of vibration.[149] Steyvers et al.[150] found that lower frequency vibration (20 Hertz) and higher level frequency vibration (120 Hertz) had either no effect or less effect on corticospinal excitability, whereas moderate frequency vibration (75 Hertz) increased corticospinal excitability of flexor carpi radialis muscle.[150]

Changes in Spinal Neurophysiology Following Vibration

While prolonged muscle vibration appears to increase cortical excitability, this modality also appears to decrease spinal motoneuron excitability. Espiritu et al.[151] investigated the effect of vibration applied to the abductor policis brevis at a frequency of 50 Hertz for 10 minutes on the excitability of spinal motoneurons (by measuring F-waves) and spinal reflexes (by measuring H-reflexes). Vibration did not change the spinal motoneuron excitability, but was found to decrease the response of the H-reflex. The effect persisted for 5 minutes after the vibration.[151] Based on this evidence, vibration could be used not only to increase cortical excitability, but also to modulate the hyperexcitability of spinal reflexes in individuals with spasticity.

Interventions Aimed to Decrease Spinal Reflex Excitability

Many individuals with cervical SCI experience spasticity, muscle spasms, and hypertonicity that negatively impacts upper limb function.[39] In animal models of SCI, spinal reflexes are modifiable and amenable to training. In monkeys with cervical SCI, deep tendon reflexes and H-reflexes can be trained to either decrease or increase in amplitude.[152]

Biofeedback Combined With Operant Conditioning

Changes in Spinal Neurophysiology Following Biofeedback Training

Individuals with upper limb spasticity due to cervical SCI, were trained 3 days a week for 10 weeks. In each session, the subject's response to a stretch of the biceps brachii was elicited 250 times, and subjects received auditory feedback that indicated a successful or unsuccessful response. The response was considered successful if the amplitude was smaller than the average amplitude of the stretch reflex.[153] Following training, individuals had a reduction in the amplitude of the response of the biceps brachii to stretch.[153] Furthermore, the effect was maintained for up to 4 months after training.[92]

■ CASE STUDY 11-1　Individual With Asymmetric AIS A Tetraplegia

History

Dave is an 18-year-old man who received a gunshot injury to the neck 24 months ago and sustained a cervical SCI. He lives in a skilled nursing facility where he receives 24-hour nursing care. He uses a power chair for his community mobility and was right-handed prior to his injury. Dave relies on a caregiver to assist him with fine motor tasks such as writing, cutting food, and catheterization. He would like to decrease his reliance on his caregiver to allow him some independence with his friends on his community outings.

Motor Assessment

Dave transfers from his wheelchair to the treatment table with maximal assistance. The ASIA motor test is completed and his motor scores are as follows.

Key Muscle	Right	Left
Elbow flexors	5	5
Wrist extensors	2	5
Elbow extensors	2	5
Finger flexors	1	3
Finger abductors	0	2
Hip flexors	0	0
Knee extensors	0	0
Ankle dorsiflexors	0	0
Long toe extensors	0	0
Ankle plantarflexors	0	0

Based on this assessment, the therapist determines that Dave has a C5 motor level on the right and a C8 motor level on the left and that his injury would be classified as an AIS A injury.

Upon further manual muscle testing, the following results were obtained: right extensor digitorum = 1/5, left extensor digitorum = 5/5, right extensor indicis = 1/5, left extensor indicis = 4/5, right flexor carpi ulnaris = 1/5, left flexor carpi ulnaris = 4/5, right flexor carpi radialis = 1/5, left flexor carpi radialis = 4/5, right flexor digitorum superficialis = 2/5, left flexor digitorum superficialis = 2/5, right abductor pollicis brevis = 1/5, left abductor pollicis brevis = 2/5, right opponens pollicis = 1/5, left opponens pollicis = 2/5, right lumbricals = 0/5, left lumbricals = 1/5, right dorsal interossei = 0/5, and left dorsal interossei 1/5.

Sensory Assessment

The ASIA sensory test was completed, and his AIS sensory scores are as follows.

Dermatome	Light Touch Right	Light Touch Left	Pinprick Right	Pinprick Left
C2	2	2	2	2
C3	2	2	2	2
C4	2	2	2	2
C5	2	2	1	2
C6	2	2	2	2
C7	2	2	2	2

CASE STUDY 11-1   Individual With Asymmetric AIS A Tetraplegia—cont'd

Dermatome	Light Touch Right	Light Touch Left	Pinprick Right	Pinprick Left	Dermatome	Light Touch Right	Light Touch Left	Pinprick Right	Pinprick Left
C8	1	2	1	1	T11	0	0	0	0
T1	2	2	1	2	T12	0	0	0	0
T2	2	2	2	2	L1	0	0	0	0
T3	2	2	2	2	L2	0	0	0	0
T4	2	2	1	1	L3	0	0	0	0
T5	0	0	1	0	L4	0	0	0	0
T6	0	0	0	0	L5	0	0	0	0
T7	0	0	0	0	S1	0	0	0	0
T8	0	0	0	0	S2	0	0	0	0
T9	0	0	0	0	S3	0	0	0	0
T10	0	0	0	0	S4–5	0	0	0	0

Joint proprioception tests were completed with the following results regarding single joint directional awareness: shoulder = good, elbow = impaired, wrist = impaired, metacarpal phalangeal = impaired, and phalangeal = impaired.

The Ashworth Scale was completed on the muscles of the upper limb, with the following results: triceps = 0 (no increased tone); biceps = 0 (no increased tone); extrinsic finger extensors = 0 (no increased tone); and extrinsic finger flexors = 0 (no increased tone).

Range of motion of his upper and lower extremities were within normal limits. In sitting, Dave requires support of both upper extremities to maintain sitting balance.

To assess unimanual hand function, Dave completed the Jebsen Taylor hand function test with the following results.

To assess bimanual hand function, the Chedoke McMaster arm and hand inventory is used. This evaluation tool is scored similarly to the functional independence measure, where a score of 1 means "requires maximal assistance" and a score of 7 means "independent." The following results were obtained.

Task	Right Time	Left Time	Comments
Writing 1 sentence	unable	0:42.53	Right: Requires hand splint to hold pen. Left: Uses tripod grasp.
Turning 5 cards	0:28.29	0:10.37	Right: Slides cards over the edge of table and uses dorsum of hand to flip card over. Left: Grasps cards using key pinch and turns to flip.
Lifting 2 pennies, 2 caps, 2 paperclips	1:10.59	0:11.25	Right: Slides objects to edge of table and uses tenodesis to grasp and lift objects. Has difficulty with pennies, dropping frequently. Left: Slides objects to edge of table and uses tenodesis to lift objects.
Feeding 5 beans	1:22.93	0:12.75	Right: Uses tenodesis to grasp and hold spoon. Left: Grasps spoon with power grip.
Stacking 4 checkers	0:35.78	0:10.34	Right: Uses tenodesis to grasp and lift checkers. Left: Uses key pinch to grasp and lift checkers.
Lifting large empty cans	2:04.53	0:07.15	Right: Aperture between fingers and thumb is frequently not wide enough for can, and thus the light cans get pushed away from the hand. Left: Grasps cans using power grip.
Lifting large heavy cans	0:31.43	0:07.13	Right: Aperture is similar as before, but the weight of the can stabilizes object. Tenodesis is used to lift the can. Left: Grasps can using power grip.

Continued

CASE STUDY 11-1   Individual With Asymmetric AIS A Tetraplegia—cont'd

Task	Score	Comments
A. Open jar of coffee	5	Uses left hand to stabilize container and ulnar border of right hand to spin lid off container.
B. Call 911	4	Requires minimal assistance (of left hand) to grasp receiver, places in right hand, and dials with left using hyperextension of index finger.
C. Draw a line with ruler	4	Uses left hand to place ruler on paper. Stabilizes ruler with ulnar border of right hand and draws line with left hand.
D. Put toothpaste on toothbrush	3	Grasps toothbrush with left hand and places on the table. Grasps toothpaste with left hand and stabilizes with right arm against the trunk. With tube stabilized by right arm, uses left hand to remove cap. To squeeze toothpaste, both hands are used to press against each other (toothbrush remains on table).
E. Cut putty in 5 pieces	3	Uses left hand to place fork in putty and right hand to stabilize fork. Grasps knife with left hand and requires hand over hand to stabilize knife during cutting.
F. Pour a glass of water	4	Requires light touch assistance to place cup in right hand. Uses tenodesis to grasp handle of pitcher, lift, and pour.
G. Wring out washcloth	6	Grasps cloth with left hand and stabilizes with right hand (using tenodesis). Wrings cloth using left wrist extension. Takes excessive amount of time.
H. Clean both lenses on glasses	3	Grasps glasses with left hand and places in right hand. Grasps handkerchief with left hand and cleans lenses.
I. Zip up zipper	3	Requires assistance to start closure of zipper. Uses right hand to stabilize end of zipper and ulnar border of left hand to push zipper closed.
J. Do 5 buttons	1	Unable to fasten one button.

Dave's goals were to become more independent with tasks such as writing, cutting food, and catheterization. Writing is a unimanual task, and therefore unimanual massed practice training activities may best address this goal. Dave was previously right-hand dominant, so providing opportunity to practice unimanual skills with the right hand may be very beneficial. The cutting task may be best addressed through a bimanual program where each limb must perform specific aspects of the task. In this task, one extremity would perform the stabilizing function (using the fork), and the contralateral limb would perform the manipulative portion (using the knife). Both interventions could be combined with an intervention that increases cortical excitability (such as functional electrical stimulation, somatosensory stimulation, motor imagery, or vibration). Interventions that increase cortical motor representation would include massed practice training, bimanual training, and functional electrical stimulation.

CASE STUDY 11-2   Individual With AIS C Tetraplegia

History

Frank is a 42-year-old man who was hit by a subway train 4 months ago and suffered a cervical SCI. He currently lives with his sister in an apartment with an elevator. A caregiver comes to the house for 9 hours per day to assist in him in bathing, dressing, cooking, and transferring to and from the toilet. He currently uses a power wheelchair for mobility. Frank would like to decrease the number of hours the caregiver is needed. He feels that if he can transfer to and from his wheelchair to the toilet in his bathroom, it would vastly improve his independence during the day and decrease his reliance on others.

Motor Assessment

Frank transfers using a stand pivot transfer from his wheelchair to the treatment table with minimal assistance. The AIS motor test is completed, and his motor scores are as follows:

CASE STUDY 11-2   Individual With AIS C Tetraplegia—cont'd

Key Muscle	Right	Left
Elbow flexors	5	5
Wrist extensors	2	2
Elbow extensors	2	1
Finger flexors	1	0
Finger abductors	0	1
Hip flexors	3	2
Knee extensors	4	5
Ankle dorsiflexors	2	2
Long toe Extensors	2	2
Ankle plantarflexors	1	0

Based on this assessment, the therapist determines that Frank has C5 motor level bilaterally, and his injury would be classified as an AIS C injury.

Beyond using the AIS motor levels to classify the injury, the therapist tests additional muscles to obtain a fuller understanding of Frank's motor function. Additional muscles that may be useful for wheelchair transfers include pectoralis major, latissimus dorsi, deltoid, wrist flexors, and finger extensors. The proximal shoulder muscles may be useful by extending the shoulder and thereby assisting the triceps with the maintenance of elbow extension. The distal muscles are needed for grasping the surface and thereby stabilizing the hands.

Upon further manual muscle testing, the following results were obtained bilaterally:

pectoralis major = 4/5, deltoid = 5/5, brachioradialis = 5/5, serratus anterior = 3/5, supraspinatus = 5/5, subscapularis = 3/5, middle trapezius = 5/5, flexor carpi ulnaris = 2/5, flexor carpi radialis = 2/5, extensor digitorum = 1/5.

Based on these muscle scores, it is reasonable to expect that Frank will be able to achieve his goal of independent transfers. The muscles of the shoulder, wrist, and hand are weak, but intact. Given a rehabilitation intervention, he has the potential to improve these muscle scores and improve his transferring capabilities. In addition, he is in an acute stage of recovery that will further improve his chances of achieving his goal.

Sensory Assessment

The AIS sensory test was completed, and his sensory scores are as follows.

Dermatome	Light Touch Right	Light Touch Left	Pinprick Right	Pinprick Left
C2	2	2	2	2
C3	2	1	2	2
C4	2	1	1	2
C5	1	1	1	2
C6	1	1	0	1
C7	1	1	1	1
C8	1	1	0	0
T1	1	2	0	0
T2	2	1	1	0
T3	2	2	1	1
T4	1	1	1	1
T5	1	1	1	0
T6	1	1	1	0
T7	1	1	0	1
T8	0	1	0	1
T9	0	1	0	0
T10	1	1	0	0
T11	0	1	0	0
T12	1	1	0	0
L1	0	1	0	0
L2	0	1	0	1

Continued

CASE STUDY 11-2   Individual With AIS C Tetraplegia—cont'd

Dermatome	Light Touch Right	Light Touch Left	Pinprick Right	Pinprick Left
L3	I	I	0	0
L4	I	I	0	0
L5	I	I	0	0
SI	I	I	0	0
S2	I	I	0	I
S3	I	I	0	I
S4–5	I	I	0	I

Joint proprioception tests were completed with the following results regarding single joint directional awareness: shoulder = good, elbow = impaired, wrist = impaired, metacarpal phalangeal = impaired, and phalangeal = impaired.

These results suggest that dorsal column functions, which provide information such as proprioception, vibration, pressure, and discriminative touch, are impaired. This may impact the motor learning to some extent. While the sensory information is impaired, Frank is able to detect some information that will provide rudimentary position sense and aid in his performance of the task. The lateral pathways, which carry information regarding pain and temperature, are impaired to a greater extent than the dorsal columns, and this sensory function is absent in many locations in the lower extremity. This must be considered for protection of the lower extremity during transfers.

The Ashworth Scale was completed on the muscles of the upper limb with the following results: triceps = I (slight increased tone); biceps = 3 (considerable increased tone); extrinsic finger extensors = 0 (no increased tone); and extrinsic finger flexors = 3 (considerable increased tone). The abnormalities of tone in the flexors of the upper

extremity (indicated by greater resistance to passive stretch) may make it difficult for Frank to perform the reaching component of the transfer task as well as achieve the wrist extension required to grasp a surface. Transfers to a level surface will be easier to obtain, but higher level transfers may be more difficult.

Range of motion of his upper and lower extremities were within normal limits. In sitting, Frank does not require assistance or upper extremity support to maintain sitting balance for 2 minutes. He has difficulty reaching outside his base of support without the use of his upper extremities for balance. While Frank's trunk is weak, he has fair trunk strength, as demonstrated by his good static sitting balance; however, to complete the transfer task safely and independently, he should work on improving his dynamic sitting balance.

Based on this evaluation, the therapist designs a rehabilitation intervention that includes repetitive practice of transfers under various conditions. This task-oriented training is combined with interventions that enhance muscle activation in paretic muscles (resistance training, biofeedback, NMES, or motor imagery). If involuntary muscle activity limits functional performance, a trial of interventions to reduce involuntary activity may be beneficial (biofeedback or vibration).

Summary

Injury to the cervical spinal cord affects arm and hand function, which results in activity limitations and participation restrictions. Additional mechanisms may contribute to upper extremity dysfunction in individuals with cervical SCI by decreasing effectiveness of the remaining corticospinal tract connections. Furthermore, these changes are thought to occur rapidly after injury. Both the severity of injury and level of injury may be used as prognostic indicators for recovery of arm and hand function.

There are many different interventions used in the rehabilitation of hand and arm function in individuals with tetraplegia. The selection of the most appropriate intervention depends on the sensorimotor impairment, the activity limitation, and prognosis of the individual for recovery.

REVIEW QUESTIONS

1. What are the cortical changes that have been identified in individuals following cervical SCI and how are these changes likely to impact hand and arm function?

2. Compare and contrast the prognosis for recovery of arm and hand function in individuals with motor complete and motor-incomplete cervical SCI. How does the emphasis on teaching compensatory strategies early after injury impact individuals in each of these groups differently?

3. What two non-surgical interventions have been shown to be effective in improving hand function in individuals with chronic cervical SCI who have some voluntary thenar muscle control?

4. What are some examples of cortical and spinal mechanisms for recovery of function following non-surgical rehabilitation interventions for arm and hand function?

REFERENCES

1. Anderson KD. Targeting recovery: Priorities of the spinal cord-injured population. *J Neurotrauma.* 2004;21:1371–1383.

2. Snoek GJ, IJzerman MJ, Hermens HJ et al. Survey of the needs of patients with spinal cord injury: impact and priority for improvement in hand function in tetraplegics. *Spinal Cord.* 2004;42:526–532.

3. Darian-Smith I, Burman K, Darian-Smith C. Parallel pathways mediating manual dexterity in the macaque. *Exp Brain Res.* 1999;128:101–108.

4. Curt A, Dietz V. Traumatic cervical spinal cord injury: relation between somatosensory evoked potentials, neurological deficit, and hand function. *Arch Phys Med Rehabil.* 1996;77: 48–53.

5. Nudo RJ, Wise BM, SiFuentes F et al. Neural substrates for the effects of rehabilitative training on motor recovery after ischemic infarct. *Science.* 1996;272:1791–1794.

6. Nudo RJ. Role of cortical plasticity in motor recovery after stroke. *Neurol Rep.* 1998;22:61–67.

7. Bruehlmeier M, Dietz V, Leenders KL et al. How does the human brain deal with a spinal cord injury? *Eur J Neurosci.* 1998;10:3918–3922.

8. Calancie B, Alexeeva N, Broton JG et al. Distribution and latency of muscle responses to transcranial magnetic stimulation of motor cortex after spinal cord injury in humans. *J Neurotrauma.* 1999;16:49–67.

9. Cohen LG, Roth BJ, Wassermann EM et al. Magnetic stimulation of the human cerebral cortex, an indicator of reorganization in motor pathways in certain pathological conditions. *J Clin Neurophysiol.* 1991;8:56–65.

10. Curt A, Keck ME, Dietz V. Functional outcome following spinal cord injury: significance of motor-evoked potentials and ASIA scores. *Arch Phys Med Rehabil.* 1998;79:81–86.

11. Curt A, Alkadhi H, Crelier GR et al. Changes of non-affected upper limb cortical representation in paraplegic patients as assessed by fMRI. *Brain.* 2002;125: 2567–2578.

12. Curt A, Bruehlmeier M, Leenders KL et al. Differential effect of spinal cord injury and functional impairment on human brain activation. *J Neurotrauma.* 2002;19:43–51.

13. Green JB, Sora E, Bialy Y et al. Cortical sensorimotor reorganization after spinal cord injury: an electroencephalographic study. *Neurology.* 1998;50:1115–1121.

14. Green JB, Sora E, Bialy Y et al. Cortical motor reorganization after paraplegia: an EEG study. *Neurology.* 1999;53: 736–743.

15. Levy WJ, Amassian VE, Schmid UD et al. Mapping of motor cortex gyral sites non-invasively by transcranial magnetic stimulation in normal subjects and patients. *Electroencephalogr Clin Neurophysiol Suppl.* 1991;43:51–75.

16. Raineteau O, Schwab ME. Plasticity of motor systems after incomplete spinal cord injury. *Nat Rev Neurosci.* 2001;2: 263–273.

17. Topka H, Cohen LG, Cole RA et al. Reorganization of corticospinal pathways following spinal cord injury. *Neurology.* 1991;41:1276–1283.

18. Turner JA, Lee JS, Schandler SL et al. An fMRI investigation of hand representation in paraplegic humans. *Neurorehabil Neural Repair.* 2003;17:37–47.

19. Hoffman, L. R. and Field-Fote, E. C. Cortically evoked potentials from transcranial magnetic stimulation of muscles distal to the lesion are posteriorly shifted and of lower amplitude in individuals with cervical spinal cord injury. *J Neurol Phys Ther.* 2007;30:202–203.

20. Groos WP, Ewing LK, Carter CM et al. Organization of corticospinal neurons in the cat. *Brain Res.* 1978;143: 393–419.

21. Ralston DD, Ralston HJ, III. The terminations of corticospinal tract axons in the macaque monkey. *J Comp Neurol.* 1985;242:325–337.

22. Woolsey CN, Erickson TC, Gilson WE. Localization in somatic sensory and motor areas of human cerebral cortex as determined by direct recording of evoked potentials and electrical stimulation. *J Neurosurg.* 1979;51:476–506.

23. Davey NJ, Smith HC, Savic G et al. Comparison of input-output patterns in the corticospinal system of normal subjects and incomplete spinal cord injured patients. *Exp Brain Res.* 1999;127:382–390.

24. Brasil-Neto JP, Cohen LG, Pascual-Leone A et al. Rapid reversible modulation of human motor outputs after transient deafferentation of the forearm: a study with transcranial magnetic stimulation. *Neurology.* 1992;42:1302–1306.

25. Ziemann U, Corwell B, Cohen LG. Modulation of plasticity in human motor cortex after forearm ischemic nerve block. *J Neurosci.* 1998;18:1115–1123.

26. Zanette G, Manganotti P, Fiaschi A et al. Modulation of motor cortex excitability after upper limb immobilization. *Clin Neurophysiol.* 2004;115:1264–1275.

27. Thomas CK, Zijdewind I. Fatigue of muscles weakened by death of motoneurons. *Muscle Nerve.* 2006;33:21–41.

28. Liepert J, Classen J, Cohen LG et al. Task-dependent changes of intracortical inhibition. *Exp Brain Res.* 1998; 118:421–426.

29. Maynard FM, Jr., Bracken MB, Creasey G et al. International Standards for Neurological and Functional Classification of Spinal Cord Injury. American Spinal Injury Association. *Spinal Cord.* 1997;35:266–274.

30. Davey NJ, Romaiguere P, Maskill DW et al. Suppression of voluntary motor activity revealed using transcranial magnetic stimulation of the motor cortex in man. *J Physiol.* 1994;477(Pt 2):223–235.

31. Davey NJ, Smith HC, Wells E et al. Responses of thenar muscles to transcranial magnetic stimulation of the motor cortex in patients with incomplete spinal cord injury. *J Neurol Neurosurg Psychiatry.* 1998;65:80–87.

32. Smith HC, Savic G, Frankel HL et al. Corticospinal function studied over time following incomplete spinal cord injury. *Spinal Cord.* 2000;38:292–300.

33. Liepert J, Hamzei F, Weiller C. Motor cortex disinhibition of the unaffected hemisphere after acute stroke. *Muscle Nerve.* 2000;23:1761–1763.

34. Shimizu T, Hosaki A, Hino T et al. Motor cortical disinhibition in the unaffected hemisphere after unilateral cortical stroke. *Brain.* 2002;125:1896–1907.

35. Urasaki E, Genmoto T, Wada S et al. Dynamic changes in area 1 somatosensory cortex during transient sensory deprivation: a preliminary study. *J Clin Neurophysiol.* 2002;19: 219–231.

36. Jurkiewicz MT, Crawley AP, Verrier MC et al. Somatosensory cortical atrophy after spinal cord injury: a voxel-based morphometry study. *Neurology.* 2006;66:762–764.

37. Reisin HD, Colombo JA. Glial changes in primate cerebral cortex following long-term sensory deprivation. *Brain Res.* 2004;1000:179–182.

38. Jain N, Florence SL, Kaas JH. Reorganization of Somatosensory Cortex After Nerve and Spinal Cord Injury. *News Physiol Sci.* 1998;13:143–149.

39. Skold C, Levi R, Seiger A. Spasticity after traumatic spinal cord injury: nature, severity, and location. *Arch Phys Med Rehabil.* 1999;80:1548–1557.

40. Lance JW. The control of muscle tone, reflexes, and movement: Robert Wartenberg Lecture. *Neurology.* 1980;30: 1303–1313.

41. Nielsen J, Petersen N, Crone C et al. Stretch reflex regulation in health subjects and patients with spasticity. *Neuromodulation.* 2005;8:49–57.

42. Curt A, Keck ME, Dietz V. Clinical value of F-wave recordings in traumatic cervical spinal cord injury. *Electroencephalogr Clin Neurophysiol.* 1997;105:189–193.

43. Thomas CK, Broton JG, Calancie B. Motor unit forces and recruitment patterns after cervical spinal cord injury. *Muscle Nerve.* 1997;20:212–220.

44. Thomas CK, Nelson G, Than L et al. Motor unit activation order during electrically evoked contractions of paralyzed or partially paralyzed muscles. *Muscle Nerve.* 2002;25: 797–804.

45. Totosy de Zepetnek JE, Zung HV, Erdebil S et al. Innervation ratio is an important determinant of force in normal and reinnervated rat tibialis anterior muscles. *J Neurophysiol.* 1992;67:1385–1403.

46. Bodine SC, Roy RR, Eldred E et al. Maximal force as a function of anatomical features of motor units in the cat tibialis anterior. *J Neurophysiol.* 1987;57:1730–1745.

47. Marino RJ, Ditunno JF, Jr., Donovan WH et al. Neurologic recovery after traumatic spinal cord injury: data from the Model Spinal Cord Injury Systems. *Arch Phys Med Rehabil.* 1999;80:1391–1396.

48. Streletz LJ, Belevich JK, Jones SM et al. Transcranial magnetic stimulation: cortical motor maps in acute spinal cord injury. *Brain Topogr.* 1995;7:245–250.

49. Curt A, Dietz V. Electrophysiological recordings in patients with spinal cord injury: significance for predicting outcome. *Spinal Cord.* 1999;37:157–165.

50. Hiersemenzel LP, Curt A, Dietz V. From spinal shock to spasticity: neuronal adaptations to a spinal cord injury. *Neurology.* 2000;54:1574–1582.

51. Leis AA, Kronenberg MF, Stetkarova I et al. Spinal motoneuron excitability after acute spinal cord injury in humans. *Neurology.* 1996;47:231–237.

52. Kirshblum S, Millis S, McKinley W et al. Late neurologic recovery after traumatic spinal cord injury. *Arch Phys Med Rehabil.* 2004;85:1811–1817.

53. Kirshblum SC, O'Connor KC. Predicting neurologic recovery in traumatic cervical spinal cord injury. *Arch Phys Med Rehabil.* 1998;79:1456–1466.

54. Waters RL, Sie I, Adkins RH et al. Injury pattern effect on motor recovery after traumatic spinal cord injury. *Arch Phys Med Rehabil.* 1995;76:440–443.

55. Crozier KS, Graziani V, Ditunno JF, Jr. et al. Spinal cord injury: prognosis for ambulation based on sensory examination in patients who are initially motor complete. *Arch Phys Med Rehabil.* 1991;72:119–121.

56. Ditunno JF, Jr., Cohen ME, Hauck WW et al. Recovery of upper-extremity strength in complete and incomplete tetraplegia: a multicenter study. *Arch Phys Med Rehabil.* 2000;81:389–393.

57. Mange KC, Ditunno JF, Jr., Herbison GJ et al. Recovery of strength at the zone of injury in motor complete and motor incomplete cervical spinal cord injured patients. *Arch Phys Med Rehabil.* 1990;71:562–565.

58. Waters RL, Adkins RH, Yakura JS et al. Motor and sensory recovery following complete tetraplegia. *Arch Phys Med Rehabil.* 1993;74:242–247.

59. Ditunno JF, Jr., Burns AS, Marino RJ. Neurological and functional capacity outcome measures: essential to spinal cord injury clinical trials. *J Rehabil Res Dev.* 2005;42:35–41.

60. Hayes KC, Hsieh JT, Wolfe DL et al. Classifying incomplete spinal cord injury syndromes: algorithms based on the International Standards for Neurological and Functional Classification of Spinal Cord Injury Patients. *Arch Phys Med Rehabil.* 2000;81:644–652.

61. Pollard ME, Apple DF. Factors associated with improved neurologic outcomes in patients with incomplete tetraplegia. *Spine.* 2003;28:33–39.

62. Dvorak MF, Fisher CG, Hoekema J et al. Factors predicting motor recovery and functional outcome after traumatic central cord syndrome: a long-term follow-up. *Spine.* 2005;30:2303–2311.

63. Merriam WF, Taylor TK, Ruff SJ et al. A reappraisal of acute traumatic central cord syndrome. *J Bone Joint Surg Br.* 1986;68:708–713.

64. Roth EJ, Lawler MH, Yarkony GM. Traumatic central cord syndrome: clinical features and functional outcomes. *Arch Phys Med Rehabil.* 1990;71:18–23.

65. Ditunno JF, Jr., Stover SL, Freed MM et al. Motor recovery of the upper extremities in traumatic quadriplegia: a multicenter study. *Arch Phys Med Rehabil.* 1992;73:431–436.

66. Cameron T, Calancie B. Mechanical and fatigue properties of wrist flexor muscles during repetitive contractions after cervical spinal cord injury. *Arch Phys Med Rehabil.* 1995;76:929–933.

67. Krassioukov A, Wolfe DL, Hsieh JT et al. Quantitative sensory testing in patients with incomplete spinal cord injury. *Arch Phys Med Rehabil.* 1999;80:1258–1263.

68. Nicotra A, Ellaway PH. Thermal perception thresholds: Assessing the level of human spinal cord injury. *Spinal Cord.* 2006;44:617–624.

69. Hayes KC, Wolfe DL, Hsieh JT et al. Clinical and electrophysiologic correlates of quantitative sensory testing in patients with incomplete spinal cord injury. *Arch Phys Med Rehabil.* 2002;83:1612–1619.

70. Koshland GF, Galloway JC, Farley B. Novel muscle patterns for reaching after cervical spinal cord injury: a case for motor redundancy. *Exp Brain Res.* 2005;164:133–147.

71. van Drongelen S, van der Woude LH, Janssen TW et al. Glenohumeral contact forces and muscle forces evaluated in wheelchair-related activities of daily living in able-bodied subjects versus subjects with paraplegia and tetraplegia. *Arch Phys Med Rehabil.* 2005;86:1434–1440.

72. Mulroy SJ, Farrokhi S, Newsam CJ et al. Effects of spinal cord injury level on the activity of shoulder muscles during wheelchair propulsion: an electromyographic study. *Arch Phys Med Rehabil.* 2004;85:925–934.

73. Beninato M, O'Kane KS, Sullivan PE. Relationship between motor FIM and muscle strength in lower cervical-level spinal cord injuries. *Spinal Cord.* 2004;42:533–540.

74. Johanson ME, Murray WM. The unoperated hand: the role of passive forces in hand function after tetraplegia. *Hand Clin.* 2002;18:391–398.

75. Baker, B, Smaby, N, Johanson, ME. Identification of target key pinch forces for functional tasks. 2006. Proceedings of the 7th International Conference on Tetraplegia: Surgery and Rehabilitation. 2001.

76. Taub E. Constraint-induced movement therapy and massed practice. *Stroke*. 2000;31:986–988.

77. Wolf SL, Blanton S, Baer H et al. Repetitive task practice: a critical review of constraint-induced movement therapy in stroke. *Neurologist*. 2002;8:325–338.

78. Krakauer JW. Motor learning: its relevance to stroke recovery and neurorehabilitation. *Curr Opin Neurol*. 2006; 19:84–90.

79. Beekhuizen KS, Field-Fote EC. Massed practice versus massed practice with stimulation: effects on upper extremity function and cortical plasticity in individuals with incomplete cervical spinal cord injury. *Neurorehabil Neural Repair*. 2005;19:33–45.

80. Beekhuizen KS, Field-Fote EC. Sensory stimulation augments the effects of massed practice training in persons with tetraplegia. *Arch Phys Med Rehabil*. 2008;89:602–608.

81. Hoffman, L. R. and Field-Fote, E. C. Cortical reorganization in individuals with cervical spinal cord injury following two different hand training interventions. *Soc Neurosci Abstr*. 2006;228:29.

82. Hoffman LR, Field-Fote EC. Cortical reorganization following bimanual training and somatosensory stimulation in cervical spinal cord injury: a case report. *Phys Ther*. 2007;87:208–223.

83. Ioffe ME. Brain mechanisms for the formation of new movements during learning: the evolution of classical concepts. *Neurosci Behav Physiol*. 2004;34:5–18.

84. Rossini PM, Barker AT, Berardelli A et al. Non-invasive electrical and magnetic stimulation of the brain, spinal cord and roots: basic principles and procedures for routine clinical application. Report of an IFCN committee. *Electroencephalogr Clin Neurophysiol*. 1994;91:79–92.

85. Rossini PM, Pauri F. Neuromagnetic integrated methods tracking human brain mechanisms of sensorimotor areas 'plastic' reorganisation. *Brain Res Rev*. 2000;33:131–154.

86. Jensen JL, Marstrand PC, Nielsen JB. Motor skill training and strength training are associated with different plastic changes in the central nervous system. *J Appl Physiol*. 2005;99:1558–1568.

87. Liepert J, Bauder H, Wolfgang HR et al. Treatment-induced cortical reorganization after stroke in humans. *Stroke*. 2000;31:1210–1216.

88. Ranganathan VK, Siemionow V, Sahgal V et al. Skilled finger movement exercise improves hand function. *J Gerontol A Biol Sci Med Sci*. 2001;56:M518–M522.

89. Calancie B, Broton JG, Klose KJ et al. Evidence that alterations in presynaptic inhibition contribute to segmental hypo- and hyperexcitability after spinal cord injury in man. *Electroencephalogr Clin Neurophysiol*. 1993;89:177–186.

90. Schindler-Ivens SM, Shields RK. Soleus H-reflex recruitment is not altered in persons with chronic spinal cord injury. *Arch Phys Med Rehabil*. 2004;85:840–847.

91. Evatt ML, Wolf SL, Segal RL. Modification of human spinal stretch reflexes: preliminary studies. *Neurosci Lett*. 1989;105:350–355.

92. Wolf SL, Segal RL. Reducing human biceps brachii spinal stretch reflex magnitude. *J Neurophysiol*. 1996;75:1637–1646.

93. Beekhuizen, K. S. and Field-Fote, E. C. Massed practice and somatosensory stimulation improves hand/arm function in individuals with SCI. *Soc Neurosci Abstr*. 2004;231:8.

94. De Weerd P, Reinke K, Ryan L et al. Cortical mechanisms for acquisition and performance of bimanual motor sequences. *Neuroimage*. 2003;19:1405–1416.

95. Sadato N, Yonekura Y, Waki A et al. Role of the supplementary motor area and the right premotor cortex in the coordination of bimanual finger movements. *J Neurosci*. 1997;17:9667–9674.

96. Toyokura M, Muro I, Komiya T et al. Activation of pre-supplementary motor area (SMA) and SMA proper during unimanual and bimanual complex sequences: an analysis using functional magnetic resonance imaging. *J Neuroimaging*. 2002;12:172–178.

97. Hess CW, Mills KR, Murray NM. Responses in small hand muscles from magnetic stimulation of the human brain. *J Physiol*. 1987;388:397–419.

98. Stinear CM, Walker KS, Byblow WD. Symmetric facilitation between motor cortices during contraction of ipsilateral hand muscles. *Exp Brain Res*. 2001;139:101–105.

99. Renner CI, Woldag H, Atanasova R et al. Change of facilitation during voluntary bilateral hand activation after stroke. *J Neurol Sci*. 2005;239:25–30.

100. Rose DK, Winstein CJ. Bimanual training after stroke: are two hands better than one? *Top Stroke Rehabil*. 2004;11:20–30.

101. Popovic MR, Curt A, Keller T et al. Functional electrical stimulation for grasping and walking: indications and limitations. *Spinal Cord*. 2001;39:403–412.

102. Mangold S, Keller T, Curt A et al. Transcutaneous functional electrical stimulation for grasping in subjects with cervical spinal cord injury. *Spinal Cord*. 2005;43:1–13.

103. Popovic MR, Popovic DB, Keller T. Neuroprostheses for grasping. *Neurol Res*. 2002;24:443–452.

104. Rebersek S, Vodovnik L. Proportionally controlled functional electrical stimulation of hand. *Arch Phys Med Rehabil*. 1973;54:378–382.

105. Popovic D, Stojanovic A, Pjanovic A et al. Clinical evaluation of the bionic glove. *Arch Phys Med Rehabil*. 1999;80:299–304.

106. Popovic MR, Thrasher TA, Adams ME et al. Functional electrical therapy: retraining grasping in spinal cord injury. *Spinal Cord*. 2006;44:143–151.

107. Merletti R, Acimovic R, Grobelnik S et al. Electrophysiological orthosis for the upper extremity in hemiplegia: feasibility study. *Arch Phys Med Rehabil*. 1975;56:507–513.

108. Kido TA, Stein RB. Short-term effects of functional electrical stimulation on motor-evoked potentials in ankle flexor and extensor muscles. *Exp Brain Res*. 2004;159: 491–500.

109. Thompson AK, Doran B, Stein RB. Short-term effects of functional electrical stimulation on spinal excitatory and inhibitory reflexes in ankle extensor and flexor muscles. *Exp Brain Res*. 2006;170:216–226.

110. Fung J, Barbeau H. Effects of conditioning cutaneomuscular stimulation on the soleus H-reflex in normal and spastic paretic subjects during walking and standing. *J Neurophysiol*. 1994;72:2090–2104.

111. Keen DA, Yue GH, Enoka RM. Training-related enhancement in the control of motor output in elderly humans. *J Appl Physiol*. 1994;77:2648–2658.

112. Barry BK, Carson RG. Transfer of resistance training to enhance rapid coordinated force production by older adults. *Exp Brain Res*. 2004;159:225–238.

113. Carroll TJ, Barry B, Riek S et al. Resistance training enhances the stability of sensorimotor coordination. *Proc Biol Sci*. 2001;268:221–227.

114. Kornatz KW, Christou EA, Enoka RM. Practice reduces motor unit discharge variability in a hand muscle and improves manual dexterity in old adults. *J Appl Physiol*. 2005;98:2072–2080.

115. Seeger BR, Law D, Creswell JE et al. Functional electrical stimulation for upper limb strengthening in traumatic quadriplegia. *Arch Phys Med Rehabil*. 1989;70:663–667.

116. Peckham PH, Mortimer JT, Marsolais EB. Alteration in the force and fatigability of skeletal muscle in quadriplegic humans following exercise induced by chronic electrical stimulation. *Clin Orthop Relat Res*. 1976;326–333.

117. Hopman MT, van der Woude LH, Dallmeijer AJ et al. Respiratory muscle strength and endurance in individuals with tetraplegia. *Spinal Cord*. 1997;35:104–108.

118. Uijl SG, Houtman S, Folgering HT et al. Training of the respiratory muscles in individuals with tetraplegia. *Spinal Cord*. 1999;37:575–579.

119. Carroll TJ, Riek S, Carson RG. The sites of neural adaptation induced by resistance training in humans. *J Physiol*. 2002;544:641–652.

120. Aagaard P, Simonsen EB, Andersen JL et al. Neural adaptation to resistance training: changes in evoked V-wave and H-reflex responses. *J Appl Physiol*. 2002;92:2309–2318.

121. Glanz M, Klawansky S, Chalmers T. Biofeedback therapy in stroke rehabilitation: a review. *J R Soc Med*. 1997;90: 33–39.

122. Brucker BS, Bulaeva NV. Biofeedback effect on electromyography responses in patients with spinal cord injury. *Arch Phys Med Rehabil*. 1996;77:133–137.

123. Kohlmeyer KM, Hill JP, Yarkony GM et al. Electrical stimulation and biofeedback effect on recovery of tenodesis grasp: a controlled study. *Arch Phys Med Rehabil*. 1996;77:702–706.

124. Kimberley TJ, Lewis SM, Auerbach EJ et al. Electrical stimulation driving functional improvements and cortical changes in subjects with stroke. *Exp Brain Res*. 2004;154: 450–460.

125. Hartkopp A, Harridge SD, Mizuno M et al. Effect of training on contractile and metabolic properties of wrist extensors in spinal cord-injured individuals. *Muscle Nerve*. 2003;27:72–80.

126. Shields RK, Dudley-Javoroski S. Musculoskeletal plasticity after acute spinal cord injury: effects of long-term neuromuscular electrical stimulation training. *J Neurophysiol*. 2006;95:2380–2390.

127. Hardy SG, Spalding TB, Liu H et al. The effect of transcutaneous electrical stimulation on spinal motor neuron excitability in people without known neuromuscular diseases: the roles of stimulus intensity and location. *Phys Ther*. 2002;82:354–363.

128. Manto M, Oulad bT, Luft AR. Modulation of excitability as an early change leading to structural adaptation in the motor cortex. *J Neurosci Res*. 2006;83:177–180.

129. Conforto AB, Kaelin-Lang A, Cohen LG. Increase in hand muscle strength of stroke patients after somatosensory stimulation. *Ann Neurol*. 2002;51:122–125.

130. Ridding MC, Brouwer B, Miles TS et al. Changes in muscle responses to stimulation of the motor cortex induced by peripheral nerve stimulation in human subjects. *Exp Brain Res*. 2000;131:135–143.

131. Wu CW, Van Gelderen P, Hanakawa T et al. Enduring representational plasticity after somatosensory stimulation. *Neuroimage*. 2005;27:872–884.

132. Panizza M, Nilsson J, Roth BJ et al. Relevance of stimulus duration for activation of motor and sensory fibers: implications for the study of H-reflexes and magnetic stimulation. *Electroencephalogr Clin Neurophysiol*. 1992;85:22–29.

133. Duque J, Vandermeeren Y, Lejeune TM et al. Paradoxical effect of digital anaesthesia on force and corticospinal excitability. *Neuroreport*. 2005;16:259–262.

134. Rossi S, Pasqualetti P, Tecchio F et al. Modulation of corticospinal output to human hand muscles following deprivation of sensory feedback. *Neuroimage*. 1998;8: 163–175.

135. Lacourse MG, Cohen MJ, Lawrence KE et al. Cortical potentials during imagined movements in individuals with chronic spinal cord injuries. *Behav Brain Res*. 1999;104: 73–88.

136. Decety J. Do imagined and executed actions share the same neural substrate? *Brain Res Cogn Brain Res*. 1996;3: 87–93.

137. Lotze M, Halsband U. Motor imagery. *J Physiol (Paris)*. 2006;99:386–395.

138. Yue G, Cole KJ. Strength increases from the motor program: comparison of training with maximal voluntary and imagined muscle contractions. *J Neurophysiol*. 1992;67: 1114–1123.

139. Gentili R, Papaxanthis C, Pozzo T. Improvement and generalization of arm motor performance through motor imagery practice. *Neuroscience*. 2006;137:761–772.

140. Dijkerman HC, Letswaart M, Johnston M et al. Does motor imagery training improve hand function in chronic stroke patients? A pilot study. *Clin Rehabil*. 2004;18: 538–549.

141. Liu KP, Chan CC, Lee TM et al. Mental imagery for promoting relearning for people after stroke: a randomized controlled trial. *Arch Phys Med Rehabil*. 2004;85: 1403–1408.

142. Kasai T, Kawai S, Kawanishi M et al. Evidence for facilitation of motor evoked potentials (MEPs) induced by motor imagery. *Brain Res*. 1997;744:147–150.

143. Cicinelli P, Marconi B, Zaccagnini M et al. Imagery-induced cortical excitability changes in stroke: a transcranial magnetic stimulation study. *Cereb Cortex*. 2006;16: 247–253.

144. Butler AJ, Page SJ. Mental practice with motor imagery: evidence for motor recovery and cortical reorganization after stroke. *Arch Phys Med Rehabil*. 2006;87:S2–11.

145. Rossini PM, Rossi S, Pasqualetti P et al. Corticospinal excitability modulation to hand muscles during movement imagery. *Cereb Cortex*. 1999;9:161–167.

146. Hashimoto R, Rothwell JC. Dynamic changes in corticospinal excitability during motor imagery. *Exp Brain Res*. 1999;125:75–81.

147. Hagbarth KE, Eklund G. Tonic vibration reflexes (TVR) in spasticity. *Brain Res*. 1966;2:201–203.

148. Ribot-Ciscar E, Butler JE, Thomas CK. Facilitation of triceps brachii muscle contraction by tendon vibration after chronic cervical spinal cord injury. *J Appl Physiol*. 2003;94:2358–2367.

149. Smith L, Brouwer B. Effectiveness of muscle vibration in modulating corticospinal excitability. *J Rehabil Res Dev*. 2005;42:787–794.

150. Steyvers M, Levin O, Van Baelen M et al. Corticospinal excitability changes following prolonged muscle tendon vibration. *Neuroreport*. 2003;14:1901–1905.

151. Espiritu MG, Lin CS, Burke D. Motoneuron excitability and the F wave. *Muscle Nerve*. 2003;27:720–727.

152. Wolpaw JR, Seegal RF, O'Keefe JA. Adaptive plasticity in primate spinal stretch reflex: behavior of synergist and antagonist muscles. *J Neurophysiol*. 1983;50: 1312–1319.

153. Segal RL, Wolf SL. Operant conditioning of spinal stretch reflexes in patients with spinal cord injuries. *Exp Neurol*. 1994;130:202–213.

Lower Extremity Orthotic Prescription

12

Kelley L. Kubota, PT, MS, NCS

Valerie Eberly, PT, NCS

Sara J. Mulroy, PT, PhD

After reading this chapter, the reader will be able to:

- Describe the impact that level and completeness of spinal cord injury (SCI) has on walking potential
- Explain the influence of sensory and motor impairments on walking function after SCI
- List the critical events of the gait cycle and common gait deviations after SCI
- Describe how lower extremity orthoses can improve walking function and stabilize and assist with residual impairments after SCI
- List the advantages and disadvantages of each of the designs of lower extremity orthoses
- Discuss the decision-making process for selection of the most appropriate lower extremity orthosis for maximizing walking function based on the individual's level of injury, motor and sensory impairments, secondary deformities, and personal preferences

OBJECTIVES

OUTLINE

Introduction

The goal to walk is shared by most individuals following spinal cord injury (SCI). Walking is feasible at discharge from rehabilitation for approximately one-third[1] and is maintained at 1 year in less than one-third of the overall SCI population.[2,3] To achieve ambulation goals, assessing the appropriateness of walking, degree of impairment, and the advantages and disadvantages of the various lower extremity orthoses to maximize functional mobility is important. Clinicians are faced with making daily decisions and recommendations for orthotic prescription. The evidence supports use of orthoses such as ankle-foot orthoses (AFOs) and/or knee-ankle-foot orthoses (KAFOs) to improve walking ability after SCI.[4,5–8] Some clinicians, however, question the use of bracing to assist ambulation, believing that braces inhibit and limit muscle function. How does one determine when "to brace" or "not to brace"? Once a brace is deemed appropriate, how does one select the optimal settings for the brace? This chapter will address some of these questions as they relate to individuals with SCI. An algorithm to guide clinical decision making for AFO and KAFO prescription will be presented. Key determinants in appropriate orthosis selection for persons with motor incomplete SCI will be presented, as well. Case studies will be used to enhance concepts and demonstrate the principles introduced.

Potential for Ambulation

Complete Spinal Cord Injuries

Following SCI, the potential for walking function depends primarily on the level and completeness of injury.[9,10] Age, level of motivation, medical history, and body type also impact the feasibility of walking.[11] Persons diagnosed with complete motor and sensory tetraplegia (AIS A) as defined by the American Spinal Cord Injury Association (ASIA) Impairment Scale (AIS)[12] generally do not become functional ambulators.[13] For those diagnosed with complete motor and sensory paraplegia (AIS A), the potential for ambulation increases as level of injury descends caudally.[10,14]

Individuals with complete thoracic SCIs (T2–T12) have no volitional control of the lower extremities and limited trunk control, determined by the level of preserved innervation in the thoracic spine. At this level of SCI, individuals require external stabilization of the lower extremities and assistive devices for weight-bearing assistance by the upper extremities. They may have potential to ambulate with a reciprocating gait orthosis or bilateral KAFOs (lower thoracic injuries). Persons with complete thoracic level spinal injuries who are able to walk generally ambulate for exercise only.[11,15,16]

With SCIs at the lumbar level, trunk control is intact and partial motor and sensory function of the lower extremities is preserved, the extent increasing with descending level of injury.[17] A number of bracing combinations may be appropriate for an individual with a lumbar injury. The spinal cord generally ends at the L2 skeletal spine level, and persons with a cauda equina type injury (at or below L2) may have variable muscle and sensory involvement owing to the particular nerve roots affected. A person with a lumbar injury may require bilateral AFOs or KAFOs, an AFO/KAFO combination, or a single KAFO or AFO, depending on residual lower extremity muscle strength and proprioceptive involvement.

Immediately after SCI, a determination of neurological level and completeness of injury may be used to predict eventual potential for ambulation.[12,15] These early neurological status indicators are better predictors of long-term function for individuals with motor and sensory complete injuries owing to the greater likelihood of neurological recovery in the first year for those with motor or sensory incomplete injuries.[13,14,18] Waters and colleagues[18] tracked the recovery of ambulation in 61 individuals with complete tetraplegia (Frankel scale A) at 1 month and again at 1 year. All but 6 of the 61 individuals retained complete injury status at the 1-year post-injury follow-up. Of those individuals who had converted to incomplete injuries at 1 year, the average increase in upper extremity motor score was 9.7 points out of 50 possible. The average increase in the lower extremity motor score was 2.5 points. No persons were able to ambulate.

Individuals with initial motor and sensory complete paraplegia show infrequent conversion to incomplete injury. In a second study by Waters and colleagues[14] that recorded the recovery of 148 individuals who had complete paraplegia at 1 month post-injury, only 6 had converted to incomplete injury status at 1 year. None of the subjects with injury levels above T9 who retained a complete injury gained any lower extremity motor function or were ambulatory at follow-up. In the 71 individuals with injury levels below T9, the strength of hip flexor and knee extensor muscle groups recovered to manual muscle test grades of 3/5 or greater. Seven of these subjects with motor recovery and injury levels below T9 were community ambulators with reciprocal gait patterns, and 4 achieved a limited, swing-through gait with bilateral KAFOs, but used wheelchair propulsion as their primary means of ambulation.

The likelihood of neurological recovery is reduced after 1 year post-injury.[19] Ninety-four percent of 987 persons with traumatic SCI who had complete injuries at 1 year had complete injuries at 5 years post-injury, 3.5% improved to AIS B, and 2% improved to AIS C or D.

Incomplete Spinal Cord Injuries

The potential for ambulation in persons with motor incomplete SCIs is dependent on both the neurological level and severity of injury (AIS C or D). The degrees of motor and sensory impairment are the primary determinants of ability to walk. Persons with incomplete SCIs have a better prognosis for neurological recovery than do those with complete injuries, and this increases their potential for ambulation.[13,19–21] Preservation of pinprick sensation acutely after SCI is predictive of eventual recovery of walking function.[22–24] Crozier and colleagues[23] evaluated 27 individuals diagnosed with sensory incomplete SCIs (Frankel B) at 72 hours and assessed their ability to ambulate with reciprocal gait (with or without lower extremity orthoses and assistive devices) for more than 200 feet at discharge. Eighteen of these persons had preservation of light touch (but not pinprick) sensation and 9 individuals had intact light touch and partial or complete pain sensations assessed via pinprick below their level of injury. Eight of 9 individuals with some initial preservation of pinprick sensation were able to ambulate 200 feet or more at discharge, while only 2 of 18 individuals without any initial pinprick sensation were able to ambulate at his level. Similarly, Waters and colleagues[20] found that of 13 individuals with initial motor complete, sensory incomplete tetraplegia, motor recovery in the lower extremities occurred only in the 8 individuals with bilateral pinprick sensation.

Preserved neurological function is also indicated by somatosensory evoked potentials (SSEPs),[24,25] wherein the cortical activity evoked by sensory input is recorded. Both presence and strength of tibial nerve cortical SSEPs measured within 2 weeks of SCI were significantly associated with walking function at 2 years post-injury.[24] The SSEPs did not provide more accurate prediction of eventual ambulation, however, than the clinical measures of pinprick sensation and muscle grades.[24,25] Thus, presence of sacral pin sensation appears to be a simple, yet important, prognostic indicator for potential of walking recovery.

Impact of Sensory and Motor Impairments on Ambulation

Level of Injury, Paraplegia Versus Tetraplegia

In individuals with SCI, factors that may affect functional ambulation ability include level of injury, strength in both lower and upper extremities, proprioception, spasticity, and joint contractures. In persons with paraplegia, walking ability is less influenced by lower extremity strength than it is in those with tetraplegia.[13,26,27] Persons with tetraplegia must have stronger lower extremity strength to ambulate successfully, as upper extremity strength may be decreased, while those with paraplegia can rely more heavily on their strong upper extremities to substitute for deficits in leg strength.

Muscle Strength

Muscle strength after SCI is closely related to the neurological injury level both for individuals with motor complete and motor incomplete injuries, but within a given neurological level of injury, a range of muscle strength is possible.[15] The Ambulatory Motor Index (AMI) was defined in 1989 by Waters and colleagues.[28] The AMI is derived from the manual muscle test grades of both lower limbs (hip flexion, abduction, extension, knee flexion and extension) and can be used as an indicator of degree of paralysis. Waters and colleagues[28] documented that individuals with progressively increasing lower extremity paralysis exerted greater weight-bearing force on assistive devices and walked at slower speeds. The magnitude of upper extremity exertion as measured by the peak axial load (PAL) on the assistive device was proportional to the increase in physiological energy expenditure. The AMI was strongly correlated with rate of O_2 consumption, O_2 cost per meter, and cadence. AMI, in combination with the PAL, can help make a clinical prognosis for walking potential.

During the early 1990s, the ASIA motor-scoring system (the lower extremity motor score [LEMS] and upper extremity motor score [UEMS]) became accepted as the international standard for reporting muscle strength and degree of paralysis. The LEMS consists of the key muscles for neurological level classification of motor function: hip flexors (L2), knee extensors (L3), ankle dorsiflexors (L4), long toe extensors (L5), and ankle plantar flexors (S1).[17] There are only two muscle groups common to the AMI and the LEMS (hip flexors and knee extensors), but similar myotomes are represented. Waters and colleagues[29] found a strong linear relationship between LEMS and AMI and between LEMS and walking velocity (Fig. 12-1). Using the LEMS, they documented a curvilinear negative relationship between lower extremity muscle strength grades and the PAL during ambulation (Fig. 12-1). They also confirmed that as the LEMS decreased, O_2 rate and O_2 cost increased (Fig. 12-1). The LEMS is also strongly correlated ($r = 0.85$) with overall walking function, as reflected by the 20-point Walking Index for Spinal Cord Injury.[30] Thus, the ASIA LEMS, as well as the AMI, can be used to estimate ambulatory capability in persons with SCI.

The impact of strength in individual muscles on walking function after SCI has also been documented. Hussey and Stauffer[15] noted that for ambulation with a reciprocal gait in the home or community, good control of the pelvis, at least "fair" (3/5) manual muscle test grade of the hip flexor muscles, and at least "fair" (3/5) grade in the knee extensor muscles in one leg are important. A knee extensor grade of at least 3/5 in one leg also was identified as a critical determinant of reciprocal gait in two later studies.[21,31] Hip flexor muscle grade was the strongest predictor of gait speed and 6-minute walk distance in a study that evaluated the strength of all the major lower extremity muscle groups in 22 ambulatory subjects with incomplete SCI.[32] Pelvic control and hip flexion are critical for advancing the limb in swing,

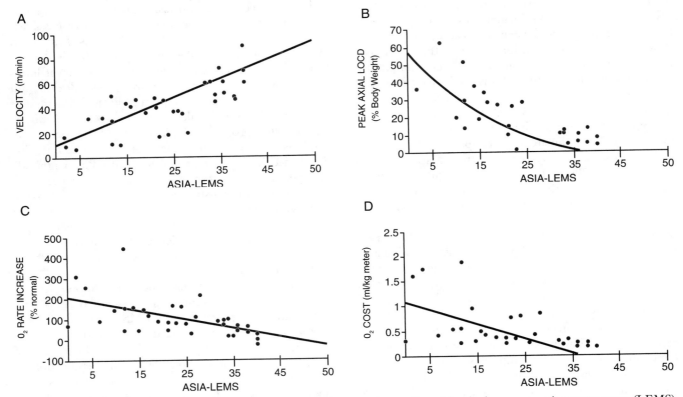

Figure 12-1. The relationships between lower extremity muscle strength as reflected by the lower extremity motor score (LEMS); (A, B) walking velocity and upper extremity weight bearing on assistive devices (peak axial load); (C, D) rate of oxygen consumption (percent increased above normal) and oxygen cost (rate of oxygen consumption normalized by walking velocity). Note that as lower extremity strength decreases, walking velocity decreases and the amount of weight on the upper extremities increases. Moreover, as lower extremity strength decreases, both the rate of energy consumption and the oxygen cost of waking increase. From Waters RL, Adkins R, Yakura J, Vigil D. Prediction of ambulatory performance based on motor scores derived from standards of the American Spinal Injury Association. *Arch Phys Med Rehabil.* 1994;75:756–760. Reprinted with permission from the *Archives of Physical Medicine and Rehabilitation.*

whereas lack of flexion at the ankle in swing can be corrected with an AFO.[33]

In neurologically intact individuals, the ankle plantar flexors and hip extensors provide the primary support for stance phase control in the sagittal plane and hip abductors in the frontal plane.[33,34] These muscle groups have sacral level innervation and, consequently, are typically the most impaired or absent after SCI. The impact of hip extensor and hip abductor weakness can be mitigated by weight bearing on an upper extremity assistive device. Knee extensor strength becomes more important to stance stability when the hip extensors and ankle plantar flexors are weak.[33,35] Hip extension weakness removes the normal posterior force on the femur, and plantar flexion weakness results in excessive anterior rotation of the tibia.[33,36] This combination requires excessive quadriceps activity (or an orthosis) to prevent collapse into knee flexion.[5,33,36] A reciprocal gait pattern is more energetically efficient than a swing-through pattern and can be achieved if one leg has an unlocked knee joint to permit flexion in swing. This requires muscle test grades of at least fair plus (3+/5) to good (4/5) for knee extensor strength.[15,21,37,38]

Ankle plantar flexor strength is influential for walking function in individuals with more intact levels of motor function since plantar flexion weakness can be augmented with an AFO. The key determinant separating those who could walk orthosis-free from those who ambulated with an AFO was standing ankle plantar flexor strength in a study of 97 individuals with incomplete SCI.[38] Thus, "good" (or 4/5 grade) in plantar flexor strength, as indicated by 10 standing single-limb heel raises, was required to walk without an AFO. Normal walking requires the plantar flexors to function at 70% of the maximum strength. A single heel rise uses 60% of the normal maximal strength of the plantar flexors, while the supine test for the plantar flexors generates at most 20% of the maximum torque-producing capability of the plantar flexors.[33,39] Consequently, the standing heel rise test is a more accurate reflection of functional plantar flexor strength than the supine test.

Proprioception/Sensation

Hussey and Stauffer[15] recognized proprioception as a key factor in ambulatory capability in a study of 164 individuals with ambulatory function. Only 1 of the 82 individuals in their community ambulatory group had absent proprioception at the hips and knees. They were unable to differentiate the effects of proprioception from that of muscle strength.[15] Proprioception at the hip joint was identified as the strongest determinant in separating nonambulatory individuals from those who could walk with a KAFO in a study of 97 individuals with incomplete SCI.[38] A stepwise discriminant analysis was utilized and all individual muscle strength and proprioception values were included as potential predictors. Those who were nonambulatory had impaired proprioception at the hip joint compared to the nearly normal proprioception in those who used a KAFO to walk. The nonambulatory group was also more likely to have complicating factors such as cardiovascular, orthopedic, decreased cognition, pain, or spasticity present. The combination of knee extensor manual muscle test grades and proprioception at the knee joint was the key determinant for those who could walk with an AFO versus those who required a KAFO to ambulate.

The influence of proprioception on walking function can be illustrated by contrasting the impact of severe quadriceps weakness in an individual with SCI to the effects in a person with post-polio sequelae or post-polio syndrome. Persons with post-polio sequelae have intact sensation, including proprioception. The ability to know where one's limbs are in space is critical to obtaining and maintaining a stable weight-bearing posture in stance and appropriate joint positions for efficient limb clearance in swing. With intact proprioception, individuals are often able to make useful substitutions despite a complete lack of muscle strength.[40] With severe quadriceps weakness, knee extensor strength is inadequate to support body weight in the normal knee flexion position of initial double limb support. With intact proprioception, the limb can be placed in a stable extended posture at initial contact, thus eliminating the demand on the quadriceps.[33] Individuals with SCIs who have deficits in strength combined with impairments in proprioception do not have the sense of when the joint is in a stable versus unstable posture, and they are unable to use these useful substitutions; therefore, a brace is necessary to allow successful walking.

Spasticity

Spasticity in lower extremity muscles may either limit or augment walking function.[15,41–43] The increased tension in muscles from mild to moderate spasticity is used by some individuals to substitute for absent or weak volitional control of lower extremity musculature. Extensor spasticity can be stabilizing, so the combination of spasticity in the quadriceps and ankle plantar flexors can be useful to assist with and to provide stability during single limb stance.[41] However, more severe spasticity impairs forward progression both in stance and swing. Common gait deviations such as equinovarus from spasticity in soleus or posterior tibialis muscles,[44–46] limited knee flexion in swing from spasticity of either the vasti or rectus femoris,[43,47–49] scissoring in swing from hip adductor spasticity, and limited knee extension in terminal swing from hamstring spasticity may result.[33] Generally, higher levels of spasticity in lower extremity muscles are associated with poor ambulatory function,[15,42,43] and antispasmodic drugs can improve walking in individuals with obstructive spasticity.[50–52]

Lower Extremity Joint Contractures

Adequate passive joint mobility is necessary to obtain a stable passive alignment during stance in order to effectively use lower extremity orthoses for walking. Using a mechanical modeling simulation, Kagaya and colleagues[53] confirmed the clinical impression of lower extremity postures for maximal passive stability during stance, which comprised 5 degrees of dorsiflexion at the ankle, 0 degrees flexion at the knee, and 15 degrees of extension at the hip. The model predicted significant increases in muscle demand for postures at or greater than 6 degrees of plantar flexion and 20 degrees of flexion at the knee or hip joints. In a subsequent mechanical modeling simulation, hip or knee flexion contractures of no greater than 15 degrees, or ankle plantar flexion contractures of less than 0 degrees, were required to maintain positive step length and forward movement of the center of gravity.[54] These theoretical models indicate that while moderate to severe contractures are destabilizing, mild contractures may be accommodated, and in fact, mild ankle plantar flexion tightness (0 to 5 degrees of dorsiflexion) can augment support for weak calf muscles in stance.[33,55,56] When using bilateral long leg orthoses (KAFOs), it is especially important to have an absence of contractures because the individual must rely on the position of the brace for stability. Full joint range of motion is key to allowing proper alignment of the segments.

Energy Cost

All of the previously discussed impairments can influence the energy cost of ambulation. Waters and Lunsford[57] evaluated the physiologic energy expenditure of the differing modes of mobility in a group of 151 individuals with paraplegia. They compared the energy demands of subjects who walked as their primary means of mobility to those who were primary wheelchair users and to nondisabled subjects. For those who used bilateral KAFOs to ambulate in a swing-through gait pattern, walking speed was slower when compared to those propelling a wheelchair as well as to those without disability. The average rate of oxygen consumption was 43% greater during walking with two long leg braces than for those who used a wheelchair for mobility and was 41% greater than in normal walking. Three subjects who used bilateral KAFOs were able to use a reciprocal gait pattern, but the rate of oxygen consumption was no better than in the swing-through gait. Individuals with at least one lower extremity with a free knee joint (using an AFO) preferred to walk using a reciprocal gait pattern. The reciprocal gait pattern with one AFO required a 27% lower rate of oxygen consumption and produced a 40% faster velocity than the swing-through gait with bilateral KAFOs.[57] There was no difference in speed, heart rate, or energy consumption between those who used the KAFO/AFO combination and those who used bilateral AFOs. Thus, the energy demands of repeatedly supporting body weight on the upper extremities in a swing-through gait pattern are high and require contribution from anaerobic metabolism.[28,58,59] For most individuals, this level of energy demand is not feasible for community mobility. Since knee extensor strength is the primary determinant of walking without a locked knee joint, this is also the critical factor in achieving community ambulation status.

The magnitude of the increased energy cost of walking after SCI is directly related to the extent of lower extremity weakness and the amount of weight borne on the upper extremities through an assistive device.[28,59] The weight of the orthosis also contributes to the increased energy demand.[60] Attempts to reduce the high rate of energy consumption during ambulation after SCI have met with limited success. Johnston and colleagues[61] demonstrated improved energy cost and walking speed with a year-long program of functional electrical stimulation (FES) during walking to strengthen selected lower extremity muscles, primarily at the hip, in three adolescents with incomplete SCI (AIS C). The program produced increased muscle strength, faster walking velocity (from 0.32 to 0.53 m/sec) and reduced energy cost (i.e., a reduction in the amount of oxygen consumed from 0.79 L/min to 0.44 L/min) during walking, both with and without the FES. Other trials of FES-assisted orthotic walking, however, did not improve the overall high energy cost of ambulation, even with reciprocating gait orthosis (RGO) systems that enabled the subjects to use a reciprocal gait pattern.[62,63] Thus, the combination of slow walking velocity and the high energy demands of walking limit the feasibility of community ambulation for most individuals after SCI.[59]

Gait Analysis

Critical Events During Normal Gait and Impact on Function

The gait cycle, which consists of two primary phases, stance and swing, can be further broken down into three functional tasks: weight acceptance, single limb support, and swing limb advancement.[33,64] During these functional tasks, there are task accomplishments that need to occur for gait to be smooth and efficient. During weight acceptance, the task accomplishments are forward progression, shock absorption, and stability. During single limb support, the task accomplishments are forward progression and stability, and during swing limb advancement, the task accomplishments are limb advancement and foot clearance. Critical events are key joint positions or motions, which allow the task accomplishments to be completed. When the critical events do not happen, the smoothness and efficiency of gait is affected. The critical event during initial contact is a neutral ankle, which allows for a heel-first contact and begins the progression of rockers (heel, ankle, and forefoot), contributing significantly to forward progression. During loading response, hip stability, controlled knee

Table 12-1
Waters/Lunsford Data for Gait Speed, Heart Rate, VO$_2$, Peak Axial Load for Primary Ambulators, Primary Wheelchair Users, and Nondisabled

	LEMS ≥30	LEMS ≤20	Able-bodied Controls
Gait speed	57.5 m/min	30.5 m/min	80 m/min
Heart rate	108 bpm	130 bpm	99.6 bpm
VO$_2$	14.6 ml/kg/min	15.23 ml/kg/min	12.1 ml/kg/min
Peak axial loadAL	PAL = 8.1% BW	PAL = 36.4% BW	
	1° Ambulators	1° W/C users	

Source: Waters and colleagues.[21]
Note: bpm = beats per minute; BW = body weight; W/C = wheelchair.

flexion, and ankle plantar flexion allow the task accomplishments of stability, shock absorption, and forward progression to occur.

Five degrees of dorsiflexion during mid-stance allows controlled tibial advancement and forward progression of body weight over the foot to continue. During terminal stance, 10 degrees of controlled dorsiflexion with a heel rise and a trailing limb (thigh extension behind the vertical) allow for continued forward progression. During pre-swing, passive knee flexion to 40 degrees and 15 degrees of plantar flexion contribute to prepositioning for foot clearance and limb advancement in swing. Fifteen degrees of hip flexion and continued knee flexion to 60 degrees allow limb advancement and foot clearance during initial swing. During mid-swing, hip flexion to 25 degrees and a neutral ankle position further contribute to limb advancement and foot clearance. During terminal swing, knee extension to at least 5 degrees flexion allows further limb advancement.

Common Gait Deviations in Individuals With SCI

The motor and sensory deficits of spinal injury result in characteristic gait deviations, depending on the combination of impairments. At initial contact, foot flat or forefoot contact may result from either inadequate knee extension (common with hamstring spasticity or tightness) or reduced ankle dorsiflexion in terminal swing (from calf spasticity, impaired ankle proprioception, plantar flexion tightness, or dorsiflexion weakness). Forward progression is impacted as the foot is not appropriately positioned for the heel rocker to occur. Another common deviation seen in the person with SCI is an extension thrust or a wobble of the knee position during stance secondary to proprioceptive deficits, spasticity, and/or weakness. There are two abnormal postures that typically occur during single limb stance. These common deviations are (1) increased flexion at the hip, knee, and ankle joints and (2) excessive plantar flexion with a relatively extended posture of the hip and knee joints. In both instances, a normal heel off is not achieved during terminal stance and pre-swing. This has a negative impact on forward progression. In the case of the flexed posture, stability would also be affected. The flexed posture would be typical of an individual with calf and hip extensor weakness and strong quadriceps. With strong quadriceps, the knee can maintain a flexed posture without collapse. The more extended posture at the knee combined with ankle plantar flexion is seen in an individual who has calf weakness combined with quadriceps weakness and needs to use joint positioning (rather than muscle control) for stability. Persons with proprioceptive deficits tend to position their ankle in plantar flexion during stance to maintain a position of stability. Excessive plantar flexion and knee extension in stance can also result from spasticity in the calf or quadriceps, or from an ankle plantar flexion contracture.[33] During swing, limited knee flexion secondary to quadriceps spasticity and excess plantar flexion due to weakness or spasticity can contribute to foot or toe drag.

An AFO (or KAFO) allows critical events to occur more readily and thus facilitates the task accomplishments. An individual with forefoot or foot flat initial contact may achieve heel-first initial contact with an AFO, thus allowing the heel, ankle, and forefoot rockers to progress more smoothly and for gait to occur in a more normalized fashion. An AFO with a dorsiflexion stop might promote heel off during terminal stance and pre-swing to allow the final forefoot rocker to occur. With dorsiflexion assistance in an AFO, foot clearance may no longer be a problem.

Orthoses

An RGO system may be used in an individual with a low cervical or thoracic complete injury[65] (see Fig. 12-2). The reciprocating gait orthosis is a specialized type of hip-knee-ankle-foot orthosis (HKAFO) that allows reciprocal motion to occur through the brace mechanism. There is a pelvic band with thoracic extensions to provide trunk stability and a cabling system to create hip

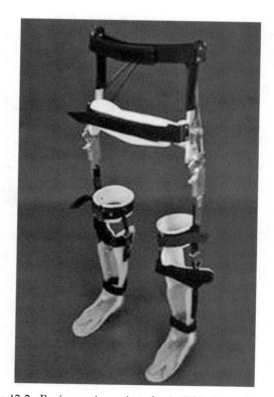

Figure 12-2. Reciprocating gait orthosis. This figure illustrates the different components of the RGO. There is a portion that is secured to the chest, along with a coupled cabling system that allows for, as the name implies, reciprocal versus step-to gait. As one limb swings forward into flexion, the other limb extends back via the cabled system.

motion. The cable allows a transfer of forces between the hips and allows reciprocal motion to occur.[66] This type of orthosis may be indicated in an individual with a weak trunk secondary to absence of abdominal musculature.

Persons with mid-level or lower complete thoracic injuries might be appropriate candidates for the Parastep system (Fig. 12-3).[8,67] The Parastep is a neuroprosthetic system that uses FES as a substitute for orthotic support during standing and stepping. It has been approved by the FDA for use in individuals with complete injuries, level T4 to T12.[68] To use the system, electrodes are placed over the quadriceps and select nerves. A cable box controls and delivers the electrical impulses, and the individual uses a walker for upper extremity support and to activate the electrical impulses with finger switches. There are hybrid systems that combine FES with an RGO-type system as well.[7] Bilateral KAFOs and a swing-through gait may be indicated for individuals who have complete lower thoracic or lumbar injuries, and have strong upper extremities and trunk muscles. Materials to consider for the KAFO are metal or plastic (*see* Fig. 12-4, 12-5).

An ankle component must be selected as part of a KAFO or for those individuals who require support only at the ankle and thus an AFO. AFOs can be either rigid

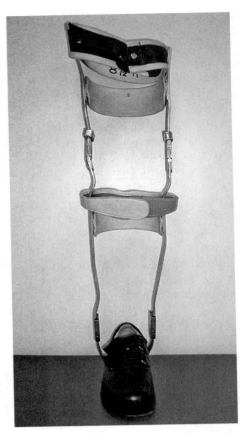

Figure 12-4. Metal KAFO. This KAFO consists of metal uprights, thigh cuff, calf band, a stirrup, and orthopedic shoe. The joint has drop locks at the knee. The thigh cuff and calf band are lined with leather for protection of the skin. The stirrup is attached to the shoe by a partial-length shank in the sole of the shoe. For those persons who walk with bilateral, locked KAFOs, a "spinal injury bottom" shoe can be used, which is heavily reinforced (and much heavier) to accommodate the repetitive forceful landing that occurs during this type of ambulation.

(solid) or articulated at the ankle joint. Articulating AFOs can be constructed of metal or plastic. While the choice of material is determined by several factors, the advantages of metal for the person with SCI are numerous. Many persons with SCI have impaired or absent sensation. A metal upright does not have any points of contact on the skin, so this type of brace would offer maximum protection for someone who is insensate. Metal uprights are attached to a shoe (or have a polypropylene [poly] foot plate that can be inserted into various shoes) and are appropriate for those who have swelling or edema issues, poor skin integrity, high body weight and/or are "heavy walkers" who load the limb forcefully, or problems with heat and sweating. These braces are heavier and tend to be more durable than plastic (Fig. 12-6, 12-7).

Some individuals with proprioceptive deficits report that they like the weight of the brace, as it gives them a sense of where their limb is in space. The heaviness of the brace may be a disadvantage in an individual with

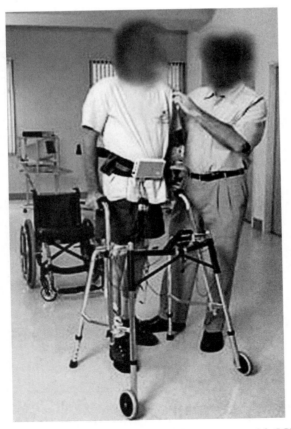

Figure 12-3. ParaStep. This system allows persons with SCI to achieve independent ambulation without the use of bracing. The Parastep system couples neuromuscular electrical stimulation with a walker that has finger-activated control switches.

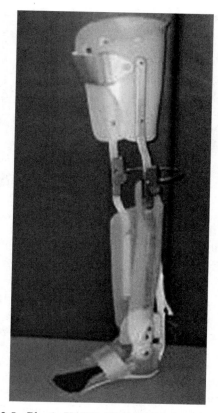

Figure 12-5. Plastic KAFO. This KAFO has plastic thigh and calf portions that have more points of contact on the skin than the previous metal KAFO. This knee joint has a bail lock mechanism. The ankle joints have Oklahoma joints, and the foot portion is lined with Drylex to protect the skin. There is also an additional strap over the dorsum of the foot to better secure the foot inside the orthosis and keep it firmly in the shoe.

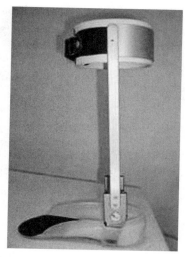

Figure 12-7. Metal AFO with poly footplate. This AFO is very similar to that in Figure 12-6 with the exception of a poly footplate, which allows placement of the AFO into different shoes. Modifications may be incorporated into the footplate such as a University of California Biomechanics Laboratory (UCBL) orthosis, which can control for excessive varus or valgus of the foot.

marginal strength, as he or she may have difficulty advancing the limb forward. These braces have a double adjustable ankle joint (DAAJ), so dorsiflexion motion can be controlled via the anterior channels and plantar flexion motion controlled via the posterior channels (Fig. 12-8).

Plastic or poly braces weigh less, are more cosmetic, and can be worn with a variety of shoes (Figs. 12-9, 12-10, 12-11). Poly braces can also be fabricated using a double adjustable ankle joint so that dorsiflexion

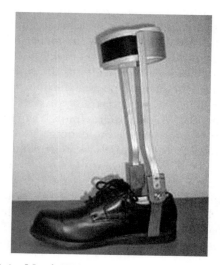

Figure 12-6. Metal AFO with shoe. This AFO has a double adjustable ankle joint, meaning there is ability to adjust both dorsiflexion and plantar flexion. There are stirrups, metal uprights, and a leather-lined calf band. The stirrup and uprights are attached via a partial-length shank placed in the sole of the shoe. The calf band portion may be secured with a pin-dot closure or Velcro, depending on patient preference. The heel may be beveled or cushioned to decrease the lever arm and forces during the loading response phase of gait.

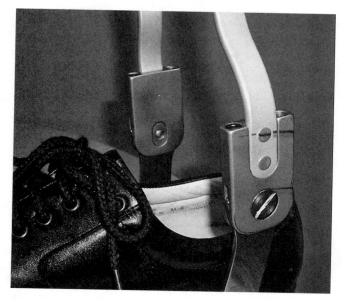

Figure 12-8. Close-up of the metal double adjustable ankle joint. This figure shows a close-up view of the joints used in the two previous figures. This joint allows for control of dorsiflexion and plantar flexion, including ability to include dorsiflexion assist. This joint is highly adjustable.

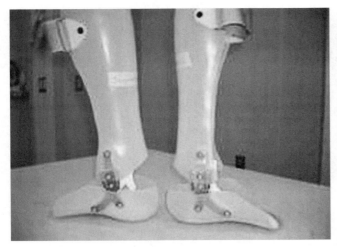

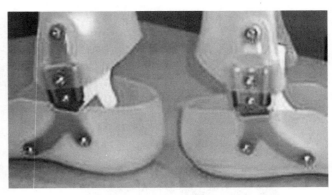

Figure 12-11. Close-up view of OttoBock joint that shows the anterior and posterior channels that allow for ability to control dorsiflexion (DF stop) and plantar flexion (PF stop). Springs may also be placed in the posterior channel to allow for dorsiflexion assist.

Figure 12-9. Polyarticulating AFO with OttoBock joint. The joint used in this type of AFO is also highly adjustable and allows the ability to control both dorsiflexion and plantar flexion. Dorsiflexion assist may also be included in this type of joint.

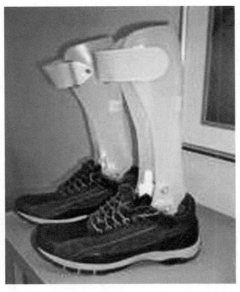

Figure 12-10. Polyarticulating AFO in shoe. This figure illustrates that these AFOs fit nicely into shoes. Note the design of the shoe, in that the heel is somewhat rounded (not square), and the toe box.

motion and plantar flexion motion can both be controlled. They may not be appropriate for the individual who is insensate or who has swelling or fluctuating levels of edema. To control excess medial or lateral movement of the foot, an in-shoe foot orthosis for the metal AFO or a build-up in the poly AFO is indicated. For individuals who have severe equinovarus posturing secondary to spasticity, the metal DAAJ AFO attached to a shoe holds the foot in the best position. Orthopedic ankle braces with straps and laces in combination with an AFO allow the option to bias the ankle into a more neutral position. A strap can also be placed on the anterior portion of an articulating poly AFO to try to hold

the ankle in a better position. A DAAJ AFO with a poly footplate is not recommended for persons with severe equinovarus secondary to spasticity as the foot tends to piston out of the brace.

A rigid or solid AFO can be fabricated and molded with plastic, or a metal and plastic AFO with double adjustable ankle joints can be locked to create a rigid AFO. The material of the in-shoe AFO impacts both the weight of the orthosis and the flexibility of the brace during walking. Carbon composite AFOs have the extra benefit of being very light. They are a nice cosmetic alternative to the double metal uprights attached to a shoe or poly foot plate.

A "semi-rigid" solid AFO constructed of a medium-thickness plastic or carbon composite restricts plantar flexion in swing and in the initial double limb support phase, and restricts dorsiflexion in single limb stance. Because the orthosis is solid, the ankle angle cannot be adjusted, making it difficult to allow the correct amount of resistance to plantar flexion in loading while providing adequate restraint of dorsiflexion in terminal stance, which requires more than twice the forces than those needed in loading.[69,70] Usually, if the orthosis is flexible enough to allow plantar flexion in loading, it will not be strong enough to control the tibia at the end of stance.[71] A more rigid orthosis can be constructed of thicker plastic that will provide sufficient resistance to dorsiflexion in stance, but would then not have flexibility to allow plantar flexion in loading response, increasing the external demand on the quadriceps.[36,72]

Rancho ROADMAP

The Rancho ROADMAP, the acronym for Recommendations for Orthotic Assessment, Decision Making, and Prescription, is an algorithm that reflects the culmination of many years of work conducted by a number of clinicians in the Physical Therapy Department of Rancho

Los Amigos National Rehabilitation Center (*see* Appendix 12-1). This tool uses information from the scientific literature, the experience of clinical experts, and individual client preferences to guide the decision-making process for orthotic prescription. However, the Rancho ROADMAP does not represent the only medically acceptable approach to treatment. Each clinician, along with the individual with SCI and other interdisciplinary team members, is responsible for determining the most appropriate, individualized approach to care.

Determining the appropriate orthosis for persons with a complete SCI is often more straightforward than it is for persons with an incomplete injury. Assessment of lower extremity strength, proprioception, sensation, spasticity, passive range of motion, and significant gait deviations is essential when determining bracing for individuals after SCI.

Muscle weakness can limit walking ability. Normal muscles work at approximately 25% of their maximum during ambulation.[73] Proprioceptive and sensory deficits, as discussed previously, make it difficult to know where the limb is in space and to substitute for weakness. Spasticity may assist with walking or, when severe, may interfere with walking. Individual preference is also an important issue to consider when recommending an orthosis and choosing the best option for the individual.

If a person has significant gait deviations, weakness, impaired proprioception, or ankle plantar flexion spasticity, a brace may be appropriate. First one must determine whether a KAFO or an AFO is most appropriate. If quadriceps manual muscle grade is greater than 3+/5, then an AFO should be considered[74] (*See* page 1 in Appendix 12-1). If knee extensor grade is less than 3+/5, then a long leg brace or KAFO is more appropriate. If the knee extensor -grade is less than 3+/5 bilaterally, bilateral KAFOs or an RGO is indicated. (*See* page 2 in Appendix 12-1.) Ambulation goals would likely be primarily for exercise or for household ambulation with these individuals. Due to the high energy cost of walking in two long leg braces and the corresponding high percentage of persons who do not continue walking after training, an ambulation trial based on criteria for successful ambulation may help to select individuals who are likely to be able to attain success with this challenging form of walking and continue ambulation in the future. Such criteria should include an assessment to ensure individuals have sufficient range of motion (no contractures in the lower extremities and a straight leg raise of 110 degrees). The hamstring range of 110 degrees is critical to be able to get off the ground with braces on. Other important criteria include adequate upper extremity strength as reflected by an individual's ability to perform 50 continuous full dips in the parallel bars. Adequate endurance is necessary due to the high energy cost of walking with bilateral locked KAFOs. Evidence of adequate endurance can be reflected through achieving a maximum VO_2 of greater than or equal to 20 ml/kg/min. Individuals should be independent with transfers, including wheelchair to floor. These are all important factors for ambulating successfully and safely in bilateral long leg braces.

An ambulation trial should include the following accomplishments: coming to stand with braces and upper extremity assistive devices independently, standing and walking in parallel bars with open hands independently, and walking with braces and assistive devices 20 continuous steps with supervision. Upon successful completion of the ambulation trial, braces can be ordered. The ambulation trial gives an individual an opportunity to experience standing and walking, and the effort required for these activities.

If knee extensor strength is less than 3+/5 in one limb and greater than 3+/5 in the other limb, a KAFO would be indicated only on the weak limb. A person with knee extensor strength grades of less than 3+/5 may not require a KAFO if hip extensor strength is at least 3+/5 and there is full range of knee extension and intact proprioception. In some instances, increased quadriceps tone or spasticity may effectively increase the strength of the quadriceps and augment the voluntary control of knee extension.

With knee extensor strength grades greater than 3+/5, an AFO should be considered. An AFO for this population has a number of options: rigid (or locked), plantar flexion stop, dorsiflexion assist, dorsiflexion stop, or a combination of the above. Joint movement should be provided whenever possible to decrease muscle demand, allow smoother transitions between phases, and to normalize gait. However, for individuals with impaired or absent proprioception, too much motion can be destabilizing. Persons with proprioceptive impairments tend to seek positions of stability, indicating a need to either limit motion or lock the brace. Another option for double adjustable ankle joint braces is to place pins inside of springs in both the anterior and posterior channels. The springs will slow the motion before the pins stop movement at the end of the desired joint position. This setup helps to prevent the abrupt change in motion that can sometimes happen with just a stop (pin). The gradual motion restraint at the ankle achieved through the spring and pin combination reduces the destabilizing effect an abrupt stop can create in individuals with proprioceptive deficits.

An AFO may be indicated if a person has decreased ankle strength, impaired or absent proprioception at the knee and/or ankle, or plantar flexor spasticity. If spasticity of the plantar flexors or a plantar flexion contracture is severe enough to affect placement of the foot during standing or gait, or proprioception at the ankle is absent, a rigid or locked AFO would be indicated. An orthosis with a locked ankle joint (or a solid, nonarticulating orthosis) causes the tibia to rotate forward at the same speed as the foot as it is lowered to the floor. The locked ankle joint creates a knee flexion thrust during loading response, resulting in an increased demand on the quadriceps.[36,75,76] An individual with quadriceps weakness may not be able to stabilize the knee with the excessive flexion torque created by a brace with a solid or locked ankle joint.

An articulating orthosis is indicated if spasticity or contracture do not interfere with foot placement and proprioception at the ankle is impaired to intact. A dorsiflexion stop is indicated if plantar flexion strength is less than or equal to 4/5 on a standing heel rise plantar flexor strength test (ability to perform 10 heel rises through full range of motion with the knee extended). Excessive dorsiflexion and knee flexion, or plantar flexion and knee extension during stance when walking, may also indicate the need for a dorsiflexion stop.

A dorsiflexion assist is indicated if dorsiflexion strength is 4/5 or less or if excess plantar flexion with a toe drag occurs during swing limb advancement. A leaf spring AFO (flexible polypropylene with trim lines posterior to the malleoli) may be appropriate if dorsiflexion assistance is all that is required.

If dorsiflexion and plantar flexion strengths are greater than or equal to 4/5, with little or no spasticity in the plantar flexors, an AFO would not be indicated unless endurance is a problem. An endurance problem is evident when increased gait deviations develop with prolonged walking. Marginal strength in the ankle plantar flexors may result in increased quadriceps activation to control tibial rotation in stance. Quadriceps fatigue may lead to limited knee flexion in loading and/or knee hyperextension or excess flexion in mid- and terminal-stance. Fatigue of the ankle dorsiflexors can produce a foot slap during loading response or a foot drag or exaggerated hip flexion in swing. In both instances, an AFO would be indicated for long-distance walking.

It is important to consider the preferences of the individual user in brace prescription. Discussions with the individual should explore the various options of design, settings, alternate treatment options, and the advantages and disadvantages of the orthotic recommendations. Individuals should be given the opportunity to compare different options, identify their preferences, discuss their expectations for use of the orthosis, and address any barriers they foresee in their use before ordering a brace.

Case Studies

The following case studies have been included to demonstrate application of the Rancho ROADMAP algorithm with clinical scenarios. Please refer to Appendix 12-1 as you work through the cases.

CASE STUDY 12-1   Individual With KAFO Unlocked

The first case study illustrates the impact of proprioception on walking ability. The unlocked KAFO can provide sensory input in individuals with impaired proprioception.

Tim is a 45-year-old man who had T10 incomplete paraplegia (AIS D) secondary to a T8–10 tumor resection and laminectomy. He was approximately 2 months post-injury. Muscle strength was decreased throughout both lower extremities with greater weakness on the right than on the left. Manual muscle test grades are presented below.

			Left	Right
MMT	Hip	Flexion	3+	2+
		Extension	2+	2+
		Abduction	3	2+
	Knee	Extension	5	4
	Ankle	Dorsiflexion	4	3−
		Plantar Flexion	3 (1 heel rise)	2− (0 heel rises)

Tim had no passive range limitations in either lower extremity. Proprioception was impaired at the hip, knee, ankle, and great toe, bilaterally. Spasticity was assessed in an upright standing position. His right ankle plantar flexors demonstrated reflex resistance (a catch) to rapid stretching at 25 degrees of plantar flexion, and bilateral knee extensors exhibited increased resistance at 25 degrees of flexion.

Tim's gait deviations included excessive weight bearing on his (front-wheeled walker) FWW and an exaggerated forward trunk lean. He also demonstrated an initial contact with a flat foot bilaterally, excessive plantar flexion during stance, and a knee extension thrust that was greater on the left side than on the right. All of these deviations impede forward progression. He was unable to achieve adequate extension of the hip in terminal stance, which decreased his step length. Knee flexion was reduced during pre-, initial-, and mid-swing, which creates a potential for a foot drag. His self-selected walking speed was 5.1 m/min, or 5.8% of normal speed.

To use the ROADMAP to assist with orthosis selection, start on page 1. Tim had gait deviations, lower extremity weakness, and impairments in proprioception at the knee and ankle joints as well as ankle plantar flexion spasticity. Beginning with assessment of the left lower extremity, Tim had 5/5 quadriceps strength, but proprioception was impaired. In this case the algorithm would guide the clinician to the section for long leg orthoses (see page 2 of Appendix 12-1). The first question, "Does the individual have <3+/5 quad strength?" can be answered "no," as his quadriceps strength was 5/5 on one side and 4/5 on the other. The next question is, "Does the individual have <3+/5 in reference side and ≥3+/5 quadriceps strength in the contralateral limb?" The

CASE STUDY 12-1   Individual With KAFO Unlocked—cont'd

answer, again, would be "no," but since proprioception was not intact at the left knee, the algorithm would recommend that an unlocked KAFO is indicated. The clinician would then need to make a decision whether an offset or free knee joint would be used. The offset knee joint, which places the knee axis of the orthosis anterior to the sagittal axis of the knee, can be used if the individual has knee hyperextension mobility. A free knee joint provides better medial/lateral control and can be used if the individual has adequate sagittal plane stability. A free knee joint would be most appropriate for Tim, as he did not have knee hyperextension mobility. The next decision is to select whether plastic or metal would be used.

Once the selection of the knee orthosis has been completed, the components of the ankle joint are selected using the AFO portion or the algorithm (see page 3 of Appendix 12-1). Tim had decreased strength at the ankle. With observational gait analysis, it was determined that Tim's spasticity and proprioception did not significantly affect his foot placement during gait, so the algorithm would recommend an ankle with an articulated joint. The clinician would next determine if a dorsiflexion stop is indicated. Tim had standing plantar flexor strength grades of 3/5 (one heel rise), and he demonstrated excessive plantar flexion during stance (Fig. 12-12). Based on these deficits a dorsiflexion stop would be indicated. Next, one would need to determine whether dorsiflexion assistance is needed. If dorsiflexor strength is less than 4/5, the individual would benefit from dorsiflexion assistance. For individuals whose dorsiflexor strength is 4/5, the dorsiflexion assistance may or may not be necessary. This level of strength may be adequate for short-distance ambulation, but insufficient for longer distances. A tendency to drag the foot with fatigue (either when walking longer distances or at the end of day) would indicate that dorsiflexion assistance might improve function. In Tim's case, it was determined to be helpful, so the orthosis would be selected, either from Group B or C (an unlocked KAFO with an articulated ankle joint having a dorsiflexion stop and dorsiflexion assistance). The same decision-making process would be conducted for the right lower extremity. Given Tim's deficits in the right leg, the algorithm would recommend the same type of brace (an unlocked KAFO with an articulated ankle with a dorsiflexion stop and dorsiflexion assistance).

When Tim walked with trial unlocked KAFOs, he demonstrated a more upright posture at the trunk with less weight bearing on his arms (Fig. 12-13). He had a heel-first initial contact, setting up his system of rockers to allow for improved forward progression. His knee extension thrust decreased bilaterally, and knee flexion during swing began to improve. Gait speed increased modestly to approximately 11.25 m/min or 12.8% of normal.

Finally, the last page of the algorithm describes Patient Involvement in Decision About Intervention (see page 4 of Appendix 12-1). A discussion with the individual with SCI regarding advantages and disadvantages of each brace including other treatment options is critical in selecting an orthosis that is acceptable and functional. Discussion of the individual's preferences and mobility needs should influence the decision of whether to order the orthosis as well as the particular design and settings. Tim preferred to use his own shoes, therefore KAFOs with poly foot plates were ordered. If he had chosen not to wear the orthosis or did not see value in the orthoses, the braces would not be ordered and consideration would be given to other treatment options.

In Tim's case, a question may be, why not AFOs? A trial with AFOs did not significantly improve his walking compared to that seen with shoes only, and Tim preferred the unlocked KAFO setup as he felt "better" and "more stable and secure" when walking.

Ordering orthoses should accommodate changes or recovery that might occur in the future. Continued reevaluation of strength in key muscle groups, proprioception, spasticity, other impairments, and gait should occur in the outpatient setting. KAFOs can be converted to AFOs fairly easily, and if ankle plantar flexion strength improves, it may be appropriate to discontinue use of an AFO. Tim had his KAFOs converted to AFOs approximately 6 months after he was discharged from the inpatient rehabilitation unit.

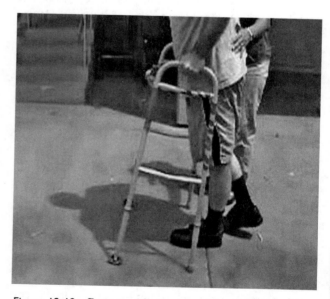

Figure 12-12. Person with proprioceptive deficits without unlocked KAFO. This picture demonstrates the patient's excess forward trunk lean combined with upper extremity weight bearing. The patient demonstrates excessive plantar flexion, which is impacting his forward progression.

Continued

CASE STUDY 12-1   Individual With KAFO Unlocked—cont'd

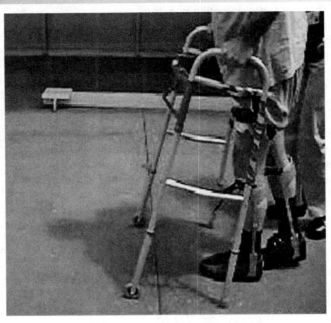

Figure 12-13. Person with proprioceptive deficits with unlocked KAFO. This picture illustrates an improved upright posture with less upper extremity weight bearing. The patient is now demonstrating tibial advancement and thus improved forward progression.

CASE STUDY 12-2   Individual With Locked KAFO and AFO

Marcelo is a 25-year-old man with T12 motor incomplete paraplegia (AIS D) secondary to a gunshot wound. He was evaluated at 6 weeks after his injury. He demonstrated reduced muscle strength bilaterally, with greater weakness in the left lower extremity than in the right. Manual muscle test grades are presented below.

			Left	Right
MMT	Hip	Flexion	2	3
		Extension	2	3
		Abduction	2	3
	Knee	Extension	2	4
	Ankle	Dorsiflexion	1	4
		Plantar Flexion (standing)	3 (1 heel rise)	2− (0 heel rises)

Marcelo had full passive mobility at the hip, knee, and ankle joints bilaterally and did not exhibit spasticity in any muscle groups. Proprioception was intact throughout the right lower extremity and left hip and ankle, but was impaired at the left knee and great toe. He walked with forward flexion of the trunk and demonstrated excessive weight bearing on his upper extremities. Deviations of the left leg included initial contact with the forefoot, excessive plantar flexion throughout stance, with no heel-off occurring in terminal stance, and a drag of the foot during initial and mid-swing. Deviations on the right included a flat foot initial contact, excessive knee flexion during loading response, excessive dorsiflexion throughout stance with no heel off, and limited knee flexion during swing.

Using the ROADMAP algorithm and beginning with the left lower extremity, Marcelo has gait deviations, muscle weakness, and impairments in proprioception. The next question, "Does the individual have <3+/5 quadriceps strength and or impaired/absent proprioception?" would be answered "yes," indicating the Long Leg Orthoses algorithm, page 2, should be used. Marcelo did not have less than 3+/5 quadriceps strength bilaterally, but he did have less than 3+/5 quadriceps strength in the tested side (in this case, the left) and greater than or equal to 3+/5 quadriceps strength in the contralateral limb (2/5 quadriceps strength in the test limb and 4/5 strength in the contralateral limb). With this combination of muscle strength values, a unilateral KAFO on the test side would be indicated. Since Marcelo did not have knee hyperextension mobility, a locked knee joint was also indicated. The options for the mechanism to lock the knee joint include drop locks or a bail lock (see Fig. 12-14, 12-15). The brace could be constructed of metal with leather for the thigh component or metal with plastic components at the thigh.

CASE STUDY 12-2   Individual With Locked KAFO and AFO—cont'd

Next, decisions regarding the orthotic ankle components would be made using page 3 of the algorithm. Again, Marcelo had decreased ankle strength. His foot placement during gait was not severely affected by his impairments, so an orthosis with an articulated ankle joint would be

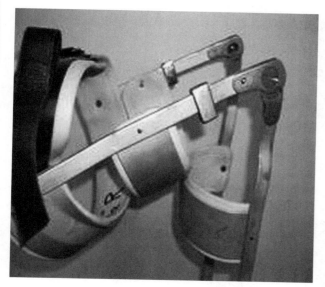

Figure 12-14. Drop lock KAFO. This image shows a close-up view of a knee joint on a KAFO with drop locks. The silver pieces can be moved distally to lock the knee joint when the knee is extended to maintain knee extension throughout gait. The drop locks can then be moved proximally to allow knee flexion for sitting.

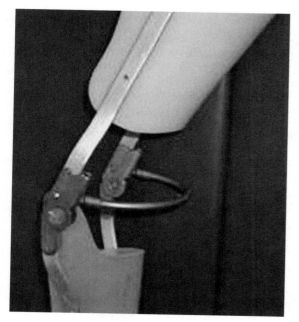

Figure 12-15. Bail lock KAFO. When the knee is fully extended, the mechanism locks and will then maintain knee extension throughout gait. To unlock the mechanism and to allow knee flexion for sitting, the client pulls up on the bail.

appropriate. The next step is to determine whether a dorsiflexion stop is indicated. Since Marcelo has plantar flexion strength of 2−/5 (standing grade), and he demonstrated excessive plantar flexion during stance, a dorsiflexion stop is indicated. The next decision is to determine whether dorsiflexion assistance is needed. Marcelo's dorsiflexion strength was 1/5, which is less than the threshold value of 4/5, and his foot dragged in swing, so dorsiflexion assistance would be indicated. The orthosis would be selected from "Group B with Group C, #2−4," either a plastic or metal AFO with a dorsiflexion stop and dorsiflexion assistance.

Start again on page 1 of the algorithm to select an orthosis for the right lower extremity. Marcelo had gait deviations and also right lower extremity weakness. He did not have less than 3+/5 quadriceps or proprioceptive deficits; therefore, the algorithm would not recommend a KAFO and would guide the clinician to the lower extremity algorithm for decisions regarding an AFO, page 3. Marcelo had decreased ankle strength, so an AFO would be indicated. His impairments did not affect his foot placement during gait, so an orthosis with an articulated joint is appropriate. Marcelo had 2−/5 standing plantar flexion strength, and he demonstrated excessive dorsiflexion during stance. Consequently, a dorsiflexion stop is needed. His dorsiflexion strength was 4/5, and he did not appear to drag his foot when walking longer distances, so dorsiflexion assistance is not needed. An orthosis from group B, an AFO with a dorsiflexion stop, would be selected. The brace should have free motion into plantar flexion. A spring to assist dorsiflexion can be added later (if deemed necessary) in an orthosis that has a double adjustable joint.

In summary, on the left, Marcelo had decreased strength and impaired proprioception; therefore, he required a locked KAFO for ambulation. On the right, an AFO was sufficient secondary to normal proprioception and better quadriceps strength. With the AFO/KAFO combination, gait speed was increased, and he demonstrated a more upright posture of his trunk. He was able to achieve initial contact with his heel, bilaterally. On the left, he no longer had excessive plantar flexion during stance or difficulty clearing his foot during swing. On the right, he no longer had excessive knee flexion during loading response or excessive dorsiflexion in stance. He now achieved heel off in single limb stance, and knee flexion was increased during swing (Fig 12-16).

The final step in selecting the orthoses is to discuss bracing options with the individual. Marcelo agreed to a trial with temporary bracing. Following the trial, he felt the braces were helpful to his walking, and he was confident he would wear them to assist his walking. An AFO/KAFO combination was ordered. He chose the metal bracing. Because the KAFO was locked during ambulation, creating a relative leg length discrepancy, a shoe lift was added to the AFO side to accommodate and allow clearance during swing of the KAFO side.

Continued

CASE STUDY 12-2   Individual With Locked KAFO and AFO—cont'd

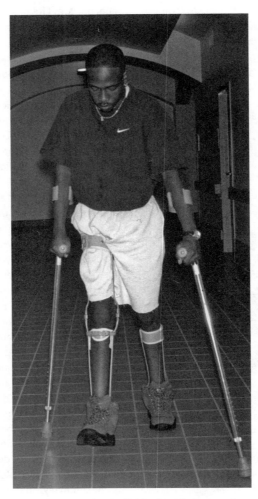

Figure 12-16. An individual with incomplete paraplegia ambulating with DAAJ AFO (with poly footplate), locked KAFO with DAAJ and poly foot plate, and bilateral forearm crutches. Note that the braces fit into the patient's preferred shoes. A lift has been added to the shoe with the AFO to allow for clearance of the KAFO limb during swing.

CASE STUDY 12-3   AFO Locked

The final case study illustrates how a locked AFO may be indicated in persons whose foot placement during ambulation is severely affected either by proprioceptive loss or spasticity. Gary is a 21-year-old man who had C1 motor incomplete tetraplegia (AIS D) secondary to multiple stab wounds. He was evaluated at 1 month following his injury. His lower extremity muscle strength was moderately reduced with greater weakness on the right side than on the left. His manual muscle test grades are presented below.

			Left	Right
MMT	Hip	Flexion	5	3+
		Extension	4	3
		Abduction	4	2
	Knee	Extension	5	4
	Ankle	Dorsiflexion	5	4
		Plantar Flexion (standing)	4 (10 heel rises)	2+ (partial heel rise)

CASE STUDY 12-3   AFO Locked—cont'd

Gary had full range-of-motion, and his proprioception was intact throughout bilaterally. Spasticity was assessed in an upright standing position (Fig. 12-17). His right ankle plantar flexors demonstrated reflex resistance to rapid stretching at 15 degrees of plantar flexion, and his right knee extensors exhibited increased resistance at 35 degrees of flexion.

During walking, he demonstrated excessive ankle plantar flexion on the right (Fig. 12-18), which resulted in an initial contact on lateral border of his foot. The excessive plantar flexion continued throughout stance, and heel off did not occur during terminal stance. Thus, all of his rockers for forward progression were disrupted (heel, ankle, forefoot rockers). His excessive plantar flexion continued in swing, and he occasionally demonstrated a foot drag during initial swing.

Gary did not need an orthosis on the left leg, but on the right he had significant gait deviations, lower extremity weakness, and ankle plantar flexor spasticity. Since his quadriceps strength was greater than 3+/5, he did not require bracing support at the knee. Use of the algorithm for selection of an ankle foot orthosis would begin on page 3. Gary had decreased ankle plantar flexor strength (2+/5) in addition to ankle plantar flexion spasticity. The spasticity did affect his foot placement during gait. The next question asks about a Berg Balance Score (more applicable in persons following stroke), the presence of severe spasticity or absent proprioception. Gary had severe spasticity, so the algorithm recommends an orthosis with a locked joint and an undercut or cushioned heel to reduce the knee flexion thrust. Specifically, the algorithm recommended an orthosis from Group A (rigid poly AFO or locked metal DAAJ AFO, either attached to shoe or with a poly footplate). A locked ankle joint promotes a quick succession of rockers from the heel to the ankle to the forefoot and also increases the demand on the quadriceps during loading response. An undercut, beveled, or cushioned heel can lessen the abruptness of the succession of rockers and thereby decrease the demand on the quadriceps. With a locked AFO, Gary attained a heel-first contact at initial contact and a heel off during terminal stance and pre-swing. Dragging of his foot no longer occurred, his step length was more symmetrical, and his gait speed was increased.

After discussing his needs, Gary stated that his ability to wear his own shoes was important. He did not have any issues with swelling, but he did have impaired pin-prick sensation. He therefore agreed to check his skin on a daily basis to prevent any potential skin breakdown. Gary stated that he felt "better" and "more stable" in the brace. He chose a polyarticulating AFO. The joint was locked in 5 degrees of dorsiflexion. Rather than order a solid poly AFO, we elected to order a polyarticulating brace and lock it. This option provides the potential to unlock the brace to introduce motion if the individual demonstrates recovery. Gary selected a shoe design with an undercut heel.

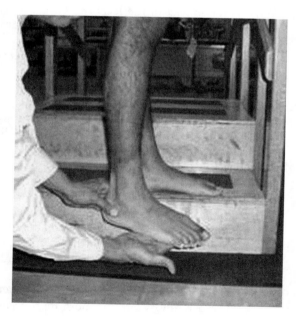

Figure 12-17. Testing spasticity of plantar flexors in upright position. This picture illustrates the upright testing position for the plantar flexors. A quick stretch into dorsiflexion is applied to determine where there might be resistance in the ankle plantar flexors. The joint angle (for example 15 degrees of plantar flexion) where the resistance occurs is recorded.

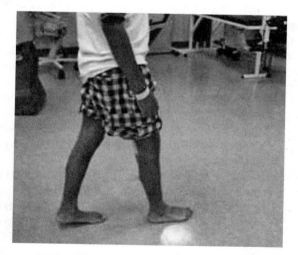

Figure 12-18. Person with incomplete spinal injury and without AFO. Note the flat foot initial contact of the right limb, which does not allow for the normal rocker system to occur (heel to ankle, to forefoot). This impacts forward progression.

Continued

CASE STUDY 12-3   AFO Locked—cont'd

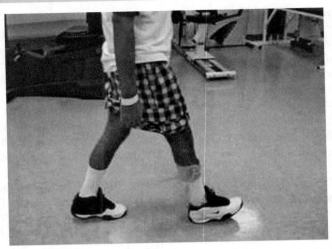

Figure 12-19. Person with incomplete spinal injury and with locked AFO. Note that the patient now gets heel-first contact during initial contact, setting up a better progression of his rocker systems. Forward progression is improved.

Summary

Walking is a primary goal for the majority of persons with SCI. Level and completeness of injury are important areas in determining an individual's potential for ambulation. Lower extremity orthoses are a commonly used and an effective intervention to improve the walking ability of persons with a SCI. It is helpful to have an awareness of clinical factors such as proprioception and spasticity, which may influence walking ability as well as how these factors may affect the type of brace most appropriate for an individual.

Our discussion has attempted to provide guidelines to assist with clinical decision making related to orthotic prescriptions for individuals with SCI. We have discussed critical events related to walking and how orthoses may facilitate the occurrence of these critical events more readily in individuals with neurologic impairment due to SCI. We have provided information on the orthoses available and advantages and disadvantages of the different options.

Individual preference is a key contributor to the final decision regarding the most appropriate bracing for an individual with SCI. When the clinician can provide expertise and evidence to support clinical recommendations and individual users are able express their preferences, a shared decision can be made that will be both beneficial and acceptable to the individual.

REVIEW QUESTIONS

1. What is the potential for ambulation in individuals with complete and incomplete spinal cord injuries?
2. What is the impact of the level of SCI and muscle strength of the trunk and lower extremities on walking function?
3. How does impairment or absence of proprioception impact walking function after SCI?
4. What are the positive and negative aspects of spasticity in lower extremity muscles on walking?
5. What are the optimal lower extremity joint positions for passive stability during single limb stance?
6. What magnitude of lower extremity joint contractures significantly increase the demands of walking and limit functional ambulation?
7. What are the critical events of the gait cycle and the most common gait deviations exhibited after SCI?
8. What are the lower extremity orthoses appropriate to assist walking after motor incomplete SCI and the advantages and disadvantages of each design?
9. What are the clinical factors that determine whether an AFO or a KAFO would be most appropriate to maximize walking function?
10. Compare the indications for rigid (solid) and articulated ankle joints in an AFO and discuss the impact of the presence or absence of mobility at the ankle during walking.

REFERENCES

1. Morganti B, Scivoletto G, Ditunno P et al. Walking index for spinal cord injury (WISCI): Criterion validation. *Spinal Cord.* 2005;43:27–33.
2. Subbarao JV. Walking after spinal cord injury. Goal or wish? *West J Med.* 1991;154:612–614.
3. Daverat P, Sibrac MC, Dartigues JF et al. Early prognostic factors for walking in spinal cord injuries. *Paraplegia.* 1988;26:255–261.
4. Sawicki GS, Domingo A, Ferris DP. The effects of powered ankle-foot orthoses on joint kinematics and muscle activation during walking in individuals with incomplete spinal cord injury. *J Neuroengineering Rehabil.* 2006;3:3.
5. Beekman C, Perry J, Boyd LA et al. The effects of a dorsiflexion-stopped ankle foot orthosis on walking in individuals with incomplete spinal cord injury. *Top Spinal Cord Inj Rehabil.* 2000;5:54–62.
6. Kim CM, Eng JJ, Whittaker MW. Effects of a simple functional electric system and/or hinged ankle-foot orthosis on walking in persons with incomplete spinal cord injury. *Arch Phys Med Rehabil.* 2004;85:1718–1723.
7. Sykes L, Campbell IG, Powell ES et al. Energy expenditure of walking for adult patients with spinal cord lesions using reciprocating gait orthosis and functional electrical stimulation. *Spinal Cord.* 1996;34:659–665.
8. Jacobs PL, Nash MS, Klose KJ et al. Evaluation of a training program for persons with SCI paraplegia using the Parastep 1 Ambulation System. Part 2. Effects on physiological responses to peak arm ergometry. *Arch Phys Med Rehabil.* 1997;78:794–797.
9. Dobkin B, Barbeau H, Deforge D et al. Spinal Cord Injury Locomotor Trial Group. The evolution of walking-related outcomes over the first 12 weeks of rehabilitation for incomplete traumatic spinal cord injury: The multicenter randomized spinal cord injury locomotor trial. *Neurorehabil Neural Repair.* 2007;21:25–35.
10. Vogel LC, Lubicky JP. Ambulation in children and adolescents with spinal cord injuries. *J Pediatr Orthop.* 1995;15:510–516.
11. Heinemann AW, Magiera-Planey R, Schiro-Geist C et al. Mobility for persons with spinal cord injury: An evaluation of two systems. *Arch Phys Med Rehabil.* 1987;68:90–93.
12. *International Standards for Neurological Classification of Spinal Cord Injury.* Chicago, IL: American Spinal Injury Association; 2002.
13. Wirz M, van Hedel HJ, Rupp R et al. Muscle force and gait performance: Relationships after spinal cord injury. *Arch Phys Med Rehabil.* 2006;87:1218–1222.
14. Waters RL, Yakura JS, Adkins RH et al. Recovery following complete paraplegia. *Arch Phys Med Rehabil.* 1992;73:784–789.
15. Hussey RW, Stauffer ES. Spinal cord injury: Requirements for ambulation. *Arch Phys Med Rehabil.* 1973;54:544–547.
16. Peterson MJ. Ambulation and orthotic management. In: Adkins HV, ed. *Spinal Cord Injury.* New York: Churchill Livingstone; 1985. pp. 199–218.
17. Maynard FM, Jr., Bracken MB, Creasey G et al. International standards for neurological and functional classification of spinal cord injury. *Spinal Cord.* 1997;35:266–274.
18. Waters RL, Adkins RH, Yakura JS et al. Motor and sensory recovery following complete tetraplegia. *Arch Phys Med Rehabil.* 1993;74:242–247.
19. Kirshblum S, Millis S, McKinley W et al. Late neurologic recovery after traumatic spinal cord injury. *Arch Phys Med Rehabil.* 2004;85:1811–1817.
20. Waters RL, Adkins RH, Yakura JS et al. Motor and sensory recovery following incomplete tetraplegia. *Arch Phys Med Rehabil.* 1994;75:306–311.
21. Waters RL, Adkins RH, Yakura JS et al. Motor and sensory recovery following incomplete paraplegia. *Arch Phys Med Rehabil.* 1994;75:67–72.
22. Oleson CV, Burns AS, Ditunno JF et al. Prognostic value of pinprick preservation in motor complete, sensory incomplete spinal cord injury. *Arch Phys Med Rehabil.* 2005;86:988–992.
23. Crozier K, Graziani V, Ditunno JF et al. Spinal CORD Injury: Prognosis for ambulation based on sensory examination in patients who are initially motor complete. *Arch Phys Med Rehabil.* 1991;72:119–121.
24. Jacobs SR, Yeaney NK, Herbison GJ et al. Future ambulation prognosis as predicted by somatosensory evoked potentials in motor complete and incomplete quadriplegia. *Arch Phys Med Rehabil.* 1995;76:635–641.
25. Curt A, Dietz V. Ambulatory capacity in spinal cord injury: Significance of somatosensory evoked potentials and ASIA protocol in predicting outcome. *Arch Phys Med Rehabil.* 1997;78:39–43.
26. Waters RL, Lunsford BR. Energy expenditure of normal and pathological gait: Application to orthotic prescription. In: Anonymous. *Atlas of Orthotics.* St. Louis: C.V. Mosby Co.; 1985; 151–9.
27. Kubota K, Furumasu J, Mulroy SJ. Muscle strength and proprioception in ambulatory and non-ambulatory incomplete spinal-injured patients. *Neurol Rep.* 1997;21:164. (Abstr.)
28. Waters RL, Yakura JS, Adkins R et al. Determinants of gait performance following spinal cord injury. *Arch Phys Med Rehabil.* 1989;70(12):811–818.
29. Waters RL, Adkins R, Yakura J et al. Prediction of ambulatory performance based on motor scores derived from standards of the American Spinal Injury Association. *Arch Phys Med Rehabil.* 1994;75:756–760.
30. Ditunno JF, Jr., Barbeau H, Dobkin BH et al. Spinal Cord Injury Locomotor Trial Group. Validity of the walking scale for spinal cord injury and other domains of function in a multicenter clinical trial. *Neurorehabil Neural Repair.* 2007;21(6):539–50.
31. Crozier K, Cheng LL, Graziani V et al. Spinal cord injury: Prognosis for ambulation based on quadriceps recovery. *Paraplegia.* 1992;30:762–767.
32. Kim CM, Eng JJ, Whittaker MW. Level walking and ambulatory capacity in persons with incomplete spinal cord injury: Relationship with muscle strength. *Spinal Cord.* 2004;42:156–162.
33. Perry J. *Gait Analysis, Normal and Pathological Function.* Thorofare, NJ: Charles B. Slack; 1992.
34. Sadeghi H, Sadeghi S, Prince F et al. Functional roles of ankle and hip sagittal muscle moments in able-bodied gait. *Clin Biomech.* 2001;16:688–695.
35. Yamaguchi GT, Hoy MG, Zajac FE. *Simulation of Knee Joint Mechanics in Two Dimensions. Proceedings of North*

American Congress on Biomechanics. Montreal, Quebec, 1986;2:95–6.

36. Lehmann JF, Condon SM, deLateur BJ et al. Ankle-foot orthoses: Effect on gait abnormalities in tibial nerve paralysis. *Arch Phys Med Rehabil.* 1985;66:212–218.

37. Kubota K, Furumasu J, Mulroy S. Criteria for orthosis type in ambulatory persons with spinal cord injury. *J Spinal Cord Med.* 1998;21:170. (Abstr.)

38. Kubota K, Furumasu J, Mulroy S. Criteria for orthosis selection in ambulatory persons with spinal cord injury. *Neurol Rep.* 1999;23:185. (Abstr.)

39. Mulroy SJ, Perry J, Gronley JK. A comparison of clinical tests for ankle plantar flexion strength. *Trans Orthop Res Soc.* 1991;16:667.

40. Perry J, Clark D. Biomechanical abnormalities of post-polio patients and the implications for orthotic management. *Neurorehabilitation.* 1997;8:119–138.

41. Dietz V, Wirz M, Jensen L. Locomotion in patients with spinal cord injuries. *Phys Ther.* 1997;77:508–516.

42. Dvorak MF, Fisher CG, Hoekema J et al. Factors predicting motor recovery and functional outcome after traumatic central cord syndrome: A long-term follow-up. *Spine.* 2005;30:2303–2311.

43. Krawetz P, Nance P. Gait analysis of spinal cord injured subjects: Effects of injury level and spasticity. *Arch Phys Med Rehabil.* 1996;77:635–638.

44. Fuller DA, Keenan MAE, Esquenazi A et al. The impact of instrumented gait analysis on surgical planning: treatment of spastic equinovarus deformity of the foot and ankle. *Foot Ankle Int.* 2002;22:738–743.

45. Edwards P, Hsu J. SPLATT combined with tendo achilles lengthening for spastic equinovarus in adults: Results and predictors of surgical outcome. *Foot & Ankle.* 1993;14:335–338.

46. Snyder M, Kumar SJ, Stecyk MD. Split tibialis posterior tendon transfer and tendo-Achilles lengthening for spastic equinovarus feet. *J Pediatr Orthop.* 1993;13:20–23.

47. Chantraine F, Detrembleur C, Lejune TM. Effect of the rectus femoris motor branch block on post-stroke stiff-legged gait. *Acta Neurol Belg.* 2005;105:171–177.

48. Kerrigan DC, Gronley JK, Perry J. Stiff-legged gait in spastic paralysis: a study of quadriceps and hamstring activity. *Am J Phys Med.* 1991;70(6):294–300.

49. Kerrigan DC, Karvosky ME, Riley PO. Spastic paretic stiff-legged gait: Joint kinetics. *Am J Phys Med Rehabil.* 2001;80:244–249.

50. Barbeau H, Norman KE. The effect of noradrenergic drugs on the recovery of walking after spinal cord injury. *Spinal Cord.* 2003;41:137–143.

51. Norman KE, Pepin A, Barbeau H. Effects of drugs on walking after spinal cord injury. *Spinal Cord.* 1998;36:699–715.

52. Fung J, Barbeau H. A dynamic EMG profile index to quantify muscular activation disorder in spastic paretic gait. *Electroencephalogr Clin Neurophysiol.* 1989;(73):233–244.

53. Kagaya H, Sharma M, Kobetic R et al. Ankle, knee, and hip moments during standing with and without joint contractures: simulation study for functional electrical stimulation. *Am J Phys Med Rehabil.* 1998;77:49–54.

54. Kagaya H, Ito S, Iwani T et al. A computer simulation of human walking in persons with joint contractures. *Tohoku J Exp Med.* 2003;200:31–37.

55. Siegler S, Moskowitz GD, Freedman W. Passive and active components of the internal moment developed about the ankle joint during human ambulation. *J Biomech.* 1984;17:647–652.

56. Broberg C, Grimby G. Measurement of torque during passive and active ankle movements in patient's with muscle hypertonia: A methodological study. *Scand J Rehabil Med.* 1983; Suppl 9:108–117.

57. Waters RL, Lunsford BR. Energy cost of paraplegic locomotion. *J Bone Joint Surg.* 1985;67A:1245–1250.

58. Lapointe R, Lajoie Y, Serresse O et al. Functional community ambulation requirements in incomplete spinal cord injured subjects. *Spinal Cord.* 2001;39:327–335.

59. Waters RL, Mulroy SJ. The energy expenditure of normal and pathological gait. *Gait & Posture.* 1999;9:207–231.

60. Barnett SL, Bagley AM, Skinner HB. Ankle weight effect on gait: Orthotic implications. *Orthop.* 1993;16:1127–1131.

61. Johnston TE, Finson RL, Smith BT et al. Functional electrical stimulation for augmented walking in adolescents with incomplete spinal cord injury. *J Spinal Cord Med.* 2003;26:390–400.

62. Spadone RMG, Bertocchi E, Mevio E et al. Energy consumption of locomotion with orthosis versus Parastep-assisted gait: A single case study. *Spinal Cord.* 2003;41:97–104.

63. Merati G, Sarchi P, Ferrarin M et al. Paraplegic adaptation to assisted-walking: Energy expenditure during wheelchair versus orthosis use. *Spinal Cord.* 2000;38:37–44.

64. The Pathokinesiology Service, the Physical Therapy Department. *Observational Gait Analysis Handbook.* 4th edition. 2001; Downey, CA: Los Amigos Research and Education Institute, Inc., Rancho Los Amigos National Rehabilitation Center.

65. Solomonow M, Reisin E, Aguilar E et al. Reciprocating gait orthosis powered with electrical muscle stimulation (RGO II). Part II. Medical evaluation of 70 paraplegic patients. *Orthop.* 1997;20:411–418.

66. Somers MF. Ambulation. In: Anonymous. *Spinal Cord Injury: Functional Rehabilitation.* Upper Saddle River, NJ: Prentice Hall; 2001. pp. 357–358.

67. Klose KJ, Jacobs PL, Broton JG et al. Evaluation of a training program for persons with SCI paraplegia using the Parastep 1 ambulation system. Part 1. Ambulation performance and anthropometric measures. *Arch Phys Med Rehabil.* 1997;78:789–793.

68. Umphred DA, Traumatic spinal cord injury. In: *Neurological Rehabilitation,* Vol. 3. Umphred DA, editor. St. Louis: C.V. Mosby Co.; 2001. pp. 522–524.

69. Chao EYS, Rim K. Application of optimization principles in determining the applied moments in human leg joints during gait. *J Biomech.* 1973;6:497–510.

70. Seireg A, Arvikar FJ. The prediction of muscular load sharing and joint forces in the lower extremities during walking. *J Biomech.* 1975;8:89–102.

71. Sumiya T, Suzuki Y, Kasahara T. Stiffness control in posterior-type plastic ankle-foot orthoses: Effect of ankle trimline. Part 2. Orthosis characteristics and orthosis/patient matching. *Prosthet Orthot Int.* 1996;20: 132–137.

72. Sutherland DH, Cooper L, Daniel D. The role of the ankle plantar flexors in normal walking. *J Bone Joint Surg.* 1980;62-A:354–363.

73. Perry J, Barnes G, Gronley J. The postpolio syndrome: An overuse phenomenon. *Clin Orthop Rel Res.* 1988;233: 145–162.

74. Waters RL, Miller L. A physiological rationale for orthotic prescription in paraplegia. *Clinical Prosthetics and Orthotics.* 1987;11:66–73.

75. Rao SS, Boyd LA, Mulroy SJ et al. Segment velocities in normal and trans-tibial amputees: Prosthetic design implications. *IEEE Trans Rehab Eng.* 1998;6:219–226.

76. Lehmann JF, Ko MJ, deLateur BJ. Knee moments: Origin in normal ambulation and their modification by double-stopped ankle-foot orthoses. *Arch Phys Med Rehabil.* 1982;63:345–351.

Appendix 12-1

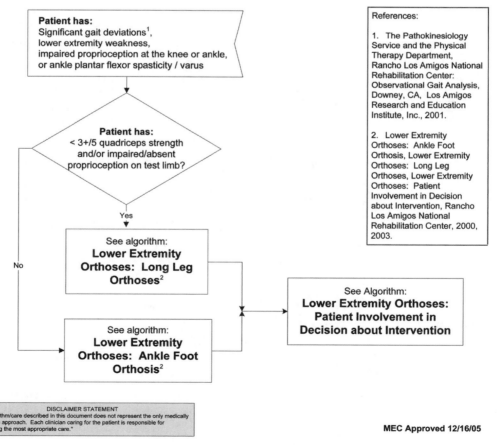

RANCHO LOS AMIGOS NATIONAL REHABILITATION CENTER
PHYSICAL THERAPY DEPARTMENT
RANCHO R.O.A.D.M.A.P.
   (**R**ecommendations for **O**rthotic **A**ssessment, **D**ecision-**M**aking, **A**nd **P**rescription)

Lower Extremity Orthoses: Overview

Page 1 of 4

Goal: Choose appropriate orthosis given patient's clinical picture and/or impairments.
Patient Population: Persons with neurological impairments who require orthoses to ambulate or to perform upright functional activities
In addition to the impairments indicated, before ordering orthoses, factors should be considered such as whether the patient has:
• Sufficient ROM in Lower Extremity joints to align segments
• The ability (including cognition) and desire to meet ambulation goals
• Adequate cardiovascular endurance and adequate Upper Extremity (UE) and Lower Extremity (LE) strength for the intended activity, i.e. ambulation
• Sufficient strength to advance the limb

Patient has:
Significant gait deviations[1],
lower extremity weakness,
impaired proprioception at the knee or ankle,
or ankle plantar flexor spasticity / varus

Patient has:
< 3+/5 quadriceps strength
and/or impaired/absent
proprioception on test limb?

No

Yes

See algorithm:
**Lower Extremity
Orthoses: Long Leg
Orthoses[2]**

See algorithm:
**Lower Extremity
Orthoses: Ankle Foot
Orthosis[2]**

See Algorithm:
**Lower Extremity Orthoses:
Patient Involvement in
Decision about Intervention**

References:

1. The Pathokinesiology Service and the Physical Therapy Department, Rancho Los Amigos National Rehabilitation Center: Observational Gait Analysis, Downey, CA, Los Amigos Research and Education Institute, Inc., 2001.

2. Lower Extremity Orthoses: Ankle Foot Orthosis, Lower Extremity Orthoses: Long Leg Orthoses, Lower Extremity Orthoses: Patient Involvement in Decision about Intervention, Rancho Los Amigos National Rehabilitation Center, 2000, 2003.

DISCLAIMER STATEMENT
"The algorithm/care described in this document does not represent the only medically acceptable approach. Each clinician caring for the patient is responsible for determining the most appropriate care."

MEC Approved 12/16/05

Appendix 12-2

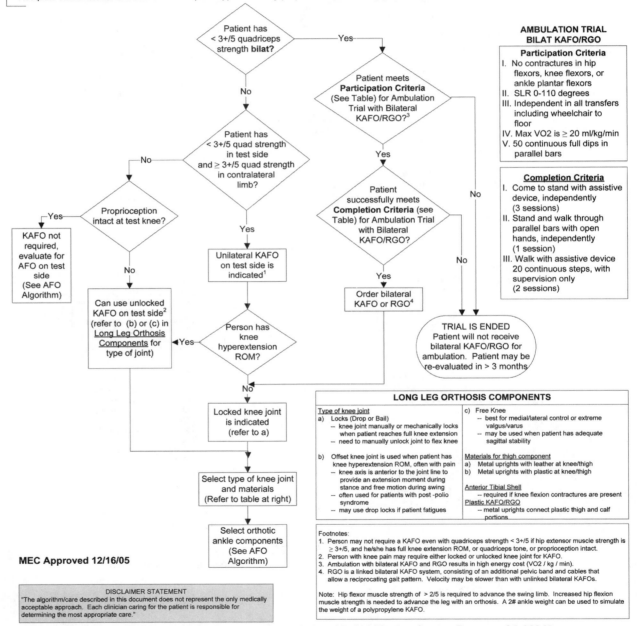

RANCHO LOS AMIGOS NATIONAL REHABILITATION CENTER
RANCHO R.O.A.D.M.A.P.   PHYSICAL THERAPY DEPARTMENT
(Recommendations for Orthotic Assessment, Decision-Making, And Prescription)
Lower Extremity Orthoses: Long-Leg Orthoses

Page 2 of 4

Goal: Choose appropriate orthosis given patient's clinical picture and/or impairments.
Patient Population: Persons with neurological impairments who require orthoses to ambulate or to perform upright functional activities
In addition to the impairments indicated, before ordering Knee Ankle Foot Orthoses (KAFO) or Reciprocating Gait Orthoses (RGO), other factors should be considered such as whether the patient has:
-- Sufficient ROM in Lower Extremity joints to align segments
-- The ability (including cognition) and desire to meet ambulation goals
-- Adequate cardiovascular endurance and adequate Upper Extremity (UE) and Lower Extremity (LE) strength for the intended activity, i.e. ambulation

Patient has < 3+/5 quadriceps strength **bilat**? — Yes →

Patient meets **Participation Criteria** (See Table) for Ambulation Trial with Bilateral KAFO/RGO?[3]

AMBULATION TRIAL
BILAT KAFO/RGO

Participation Criteria
I.   No contractures in hip flexors, knee flexors, or ankle plantar flexors
II. SLR 0-110 degrees
III. Independent in all transfers including wheelchair to floor
IV. Max VO2 is ≥ 20 ml/kg/min
V. 50 continuous full dips in parallel bars

Completion Criteria
I.   Come to stand with assistive device, independently (3 sessions)
II. Stand and walk through parallel bars with open hands, independently (1 session)
III. Walk with assistive device 20 continuous steps, with supervision only (2 sessions)

No →

Patient has < 3+/5 quad strength in test side and ≥ 3+/5 quad strength in contralateral limb?

Proprioception intact at test knee? — Yes →

KAFO not required, evaluate for AFO on test side (See AFO Algorithm)

Patient successfully meets **Completion Criteria** (see Table) for Ambulation Trial with Bilateral KAFO/RGO?

Yes →

Unilateral KAFO on test side is indicated[1]

Order bilateral KAFO or RGO[4]

TRIAL IS ENDED Patient will not receive bilateral KAFO/RGO for ambulation. Patient may be re-evaluated in > 3 months

Can use unlocked KAFO on test side[2] (refer to (b) or (c) in Long Leg Orthosis Components for type of joint) — Yes ←

Person has knee hyperextension ROM?

Locked knee joint is indicated (refer to a)

Select type of knee joint and materials (Refer to table at right)

Select orthotic ankle components (See AFO Algorithm)

MEC Approved 12/16/05

LONG LEG ORTHOSIS COMPONENTS

Type of knee joint
a) Locks (Drop or Bail)
   -- knee joint manually or mechanically locks when patient reaches full knee extension
   -- need to manually unlock joint to flex knee

b) Offset knee joint is used when patient has knee hyperextension ROM, often with pain
   -- knee axis is anterior to the joint line to provide an extension moment during stance and free motion during swing
   -- often used for patients with post -polio syndrome
   -- may use drop locks if patient fatigues

c) Free Knee
   -- best for medial/lateral control or extreme valgus/varus
   -- may be used when patient has adequate sagittal stability

Materials for thigh component
a) Metal uprights with leather at knee/thigh
b) Metal uprights with plastic at knee/thigh

Anterior Tibial Shell
   -- required if knee flexion contractures are present
Plastic KAFO/RGO
   -- metal uprights connect plastic thigh and calf portions

Footnotes:
1. Person may not require a KAFO even with quadriceps strength < 3+/5 if hip extensor muscle strength is ≥ 3+/5, and he/she has full knee extension ROM, or quadriceps tone, or proprioception intact.
2. Person with knee pain may require either locked or unlocked knee joint for KAFO.
3. Ambulation with bilateral KAFO and RGO results in high energy cost (VO2 / kg / min).
4. RGO is a linked bilateral KAFO system, consisting of an additional pelvic band and cables that allow a reciprocating gait pattern. Velocity may be slower than with unlinked bilateral KAFOs.

Note: Hip flexor muscle strength of > 2/5 is required to advance the swing limb. Increased hip flexion muscle strength is needed to advance the leg with an orthosis. A 2# ankle weight can be used to simulate the weight of a polypropylene KAFO.

© **Reviewed and modified 2005. Rancho Los Amigos National Rehabilitation Center, Downey, CA 90242**

Appendix 12-3

RANCHO LOS AMIGOS NATIONAL REHABILITATION CENTER
RANCHO R.O.A.D.M.A.P.   PHYSICAL THERAPY DEPARTMENT
(Recommendations for Orthotic Assessment, Decision-Making, And Prescription)
Lower Extremity Orthoses: Ankle Foot Orthoses (AFO)

Goal: Choose appropriate AFO given patient's clinical picture and/or impairments.

Patient Population: Persons with neurological impairments who require AFO to ambulate or to perform upright functional activities.   Page 3 of 4

In addition to the impairments indicated, other factors should be considered before ordering AFO:
1) Sufficient ROM in LE joints to align lower extremity segments
2) Patient's ability (including cognition) and desire to meet goals
3) Adequate cardiovascular endurance and adequate UE/LE strength for the intended activity, (e.g., ambulation)

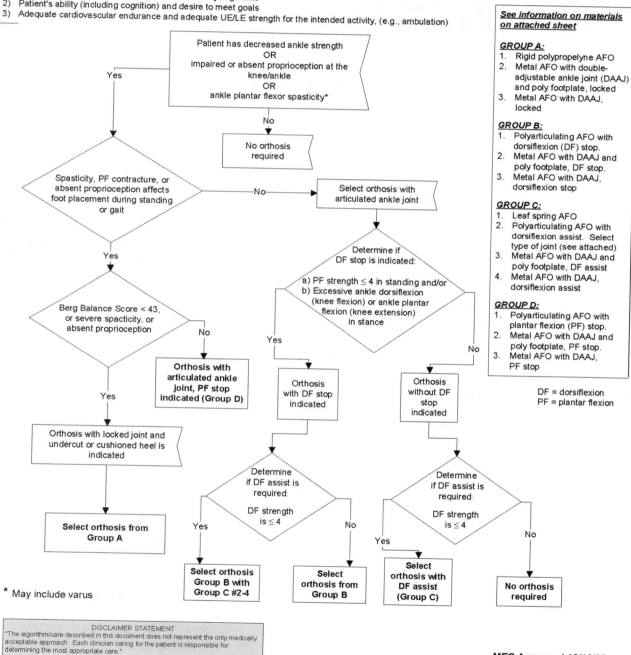

See information on materials on attached sheet

GROUP A:
1. Rigid polypropelyne AFO
2. Metal AFO with double-adjustable ankle joint (DAAJ) and poly footplate, locked
3. Metal AFO with DAAJ, locked.

GROUP B:
1. Polyarticulating AFO with dorsiflexion (DF) stop.
2. Metal AFO with DAAJ and poly footplate, DF stop.
3. Metal AFO with DAAJ, dorsiflexion stop

GROUP C:
1. Leaf spring AFO
2. Polyarticulating AFO with dorsiflexion assist. Select type of joint (see attached)
3. Metal AFO with DAAJ and poly footplate, DF assist
4. Metal AFO with DAAJ, dorsiflexion assist

GROUP D:
1. Polyarticulating AFO with plantar flexion (PF) stop.
2. Metal AFO with DAAJ and poly footplate, PF stop.
3. Metal AFO with DAAJ, PF stop

DF = dorsiflexion
PF = plantar flexion

* May include varus

MEC Approved 12/16/05

© **Reviewed and modified 2005. Rancho Los Amigos National Rehabilitation Center, Downey, CA 90242**

Appendix 12-4

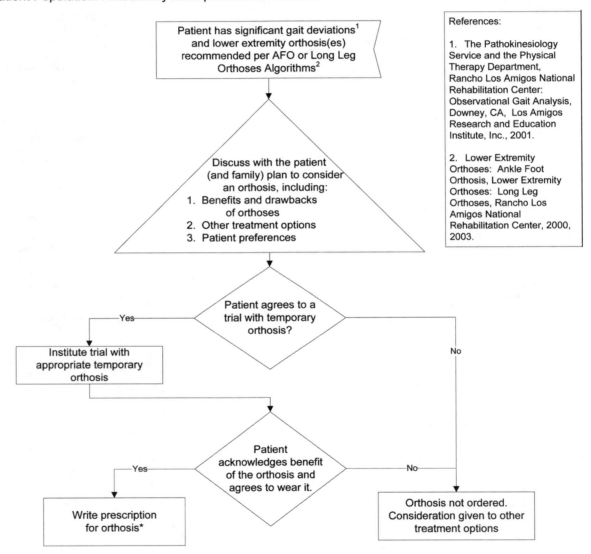

RANCHO LOS AMIGOS NATIONAL REHABILITATION CENTER
PHYSICAL THERAPY DEPARTMENT
RANCHO R.O.A.D.M.A.P.
    (**R**ecommendations for **O**rthotic **A**ssessment, **D**ecision-**M**aking, **A**nd **P**rescription)

Lower Extremity Orthoses: Patient Involvement in Decision About Intervention

Page 4 of 4

Goal: Include patient in the decision about use of a lower extremity orthosis
Patient Population: Ambulatory adult patients at RLANRC

Patient has significant gait deviations[1] and lower extremity orthosis(es) recommended per AFO or Long Leg Orthoses Algorithms[2]

Discuss with the patient (and family) plan to consider an orthosis, including:
1. Benefits and drawbacks of orthoses
2. Other treatment options
3. Patient preferences

Patient agrees to a trial with temporary orthosis?

Yes → Institute trial with appropriate temporary orthosis

No →

Patient acknowledges benefit of the orthosis and agrees to wear it.

Yes → Write prescription for orthosis*

No → Orthosis not ordered. Consideration given to other treatment options

References:

1. The Pathokinesiology Service and the Physical Therapy Department, Rancho Los Amigos National Rehabilitation Center: Observational Gait Analysis, Downey, CA, Los Amigos Research and Education Institute, Inc., 2001.

2. Lower Extremity Orthoses: Ankle Foot Orthosis, Lower Extremity Orthoses: Long Leg Orthoses, Rancho Los Amigos National Rehabilitation Center, 2000, 2003.

*Prescription is reviewed and initialed by clinical manager or designee.

MEC Approved 12/16/05

DISCLAIMER STATEMENT
"The algorithm/care described in this document does not represent the only medically acceptable approach. Each clinician caring for the patient is responsible for determining the most appropriate care."

© **Reviewed and modified 2005. Rancho Los Amigos National Rehabilitation Center, Downey, CA 90242**

Locomotor Training After Incomplete Spinal Cord Injury: Neural Mechanisms and Functional Outcomes

Edelle C. Field-Fote, PT, PhD

Andrea Behrman, PT, PhD

OBJECTIVES

After reading this chapter, the reader will be able to:

- Describe what is meant by the term *locomotor central pattern generator*
- Describe how a therapist might make optimal use of sensory information for promoting locomotor function
- Discuss placement of stimulating electrodes for use in eliciting a flexion withdrawal response
- List the advantages and disadvantages of each of the three forms of assisted stepping
- Describe currently available neuroprosthetic systems for assisted stepping
- Describe the mechanism by which epidural stimulation is thought to promote improved locomotor function

Introduction

The inability to walk is among the most apparent deficits that face an individual after spinal cord injury (SCI). For this reason, it is not surprising that "Will I be able to walk again?" is one of the first questions that an individual asks the physical therapist. Since the 1980s, developments in our understanding of the neural control of locomotion have brought renewed interest to the area of locomotor training after SCI. These developments represent an exciting new focus, as these are among the first rehabilitation techniques to grow out of work that began in the basic science laboratories. This work provides a physiological basis for training to restore and enhance walking recovery after SCI using the intrinsic mechanisms of the central nervous system (CNS), and it has challenged our assumptions concerning the potential for recovery. This focus is in contrast to conventional gait training, which is both currently and historically based on compensation for deficits of paralysis, weakness, balance, and coordination. Braces, assistive devices, and instruction in new strategies (e.g., loading upper extremities for weight bearing, knee extension via a brace) make up traditional rehabilitation practice to compensate for irremediable deficits and achieve bipedal mobility.[1] Severity and level of injury, the degree of voluntary motor control (e.g., manual muscle test scores), and sensory preservation are used to predict ambulatory potential.[2-6] Impairment-targeted training for strength and endurance in voluntarily activated muscles and requisite joint range of motion are also emphasized.[1,7]

Walking consists of three essential elements: (1) reciprocal stepping, (2) maintaining equilibrium during propulsion, and (3) adapting to the individual's own behavioral goals and environmental terrain and obstacles.[8,9] In this chapter, we will review the key basic science research that has contributed to our understanding of the control of locomotion. The application of this information to humans with SCI, recommendations related to optimizing training, and advantages and disadvantages of the various techniques for restoration of locomotor function will be discussed. Training to restore locomotor function using a body weight support (BWS) system and a treadmill, spinal cord stimulation, and locomotor prostheses will also be discussed. Furthermore, a model for the control of walking will be introduced to frame current developments and serve as a guide for assessing future strategies.

Spinal Cord Contributions to Control of Locomotor Function

The Role of Central Pattern Generators for Locomotor Output in Vertebrate Animals

Studies of cats that had undergone experimental spinal cord transection (*spinalization* or "spinal cats") have contributed greatly to the understanding of spinal cord control of locomotor function. In the early 1900s, Sherrington[10-12] demonstrated that complex rhythmic movements of the limbs could be produced in animals with complete transection of the spinal cord. While he erroneously attributed these movements to the "chaining" together of reflexes (i.e., stereotyped motor responses to afferent input), this work was among the first to demonstrate that the spinal cord is more than just a conduit for information traveling between the brain and the motor neurons. Later, Graham-Brown[11] demonstrated, by performing a dorsal rhizotomy in conjunction with the spinal transection, that the movements produced by spinal animals could not be merely reflexive. Dorsal rhizotomy prevents afferent input from entering the dorsal horn of the spinal cord, therefore reflex activation of the motor neurons is not possible. Despite this, the limbs of the spinalized animal produced rhythmic, albeit less-coordinated, motor patterns. This evidence demonstrated that the spinal cord is capable of producing complex rhythmic behaviors in the absence of phasic afferent input, even with complete isolation from descending supraspinal influences following spinal cord transection.

The neural output that elicits the appropriate pattern of muscle activation is inherent in the intraspinal connections of the spinal cord circuitry, giving rise to the term *central pattern generators* or CPGs. Graham-Brown is credited with conceiving the half-center model (Fig. 13-1) of the spinal cord CPG (although it was not until years later that the term *central pattern generators* came into use). In this model, each limb is controlled by a central (i.e., spinal) limb oscillator that is composed of two halves: one half drives the flexor motoneurons, and the other half drives the extensor motoneurons (hence the name, half-center). The two half-centers are coupled by inhibitory interneurons so that when one half is active, the other half is quiescent, thereby giving rise to alternating activity between them. This alternating drive produces the cyclic intralimb alternation between flexors and extensors that is observed with walking. The oscillator for one limb communicates with the oscillator of the opposite limb to control interlimb coordination. The oscillators receive tonic descending drive from supraspinal centers that is responsible for turning on the oscillator. Despite its limitations, this conceptualization offers a simple, straightforward first approximation of the control of rhythmic limb movement.

Further refinement of the role of the spinal cord in the generation of complex movements came with the influential work of Jankowska and colleagues,[14,15] who demonstrated the importance of monoaminergic agents such as DOPA to locomotor-related output. L-DOPA (levodopa, 3, 4-dihydroxy-L-phenylalanine, a precursor in the biosynthesis of dopamine in nerve cells) mimics the activity of the neurotransmitters from supraspinal centers that activate the spinal CPG during walking. After administration of DOPA in spinal cats, the usual response to activation of flexor reflex afferents (FRAs) is replaced by a longer latency flexion response ipsilaterally that is associated with a contralateral extensor response. These

works lent support to the half-center model of spinal cord organization as well as to the contribution of FRAs to the locomotor pattern-generating circuitry.

Grillner and Zangger[16] used DOPA to activate CPG circuitry in a curarized preparation, demonstrating conclusively that movement-related (proprioceptive) sensory input is not needed for the production of locomotor output. In this preparation, the neuromuscular junction is blocked such that no movement occurs (i.e., the preparation is "de-efferented"). In the absence of movement, there can be no phasic afferent feedback. Yet, direct recordings from motor nerves demonstrate that rhythmic locomotor output (termed *fictive locomotion*) is still produced by the spinal cord. Grillner[17] refined the concept of the locomotor CPG model with the development of the unit burst generator model (Fig. 13-2). Its modular design features a flexible arrangement of the components of the spinal CPG for locomotion in which control of each joint is coupled to that of the other joints in the limb in a flexible manner. This design allows for the variation in the intralimb coupling that is observed during movement. Furthermore, this arrangement is consistent

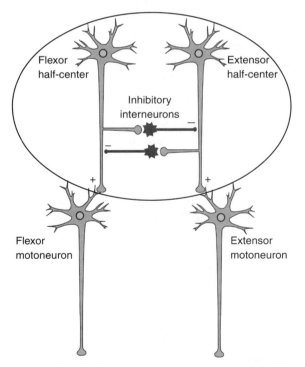

Figure 13-1. The half-center model of the locomotor CPG. In this model, each limb is controlled by a central oscillator composed of neurons that drive either the flexor motoneurons or the extensor motoneurons. Reciprocal inhibitory connections between the neurons produce alternation between the two halves of the central oscillator, thereby driving cyclic intralimb alternation between the limb flexor and extensor muscles.

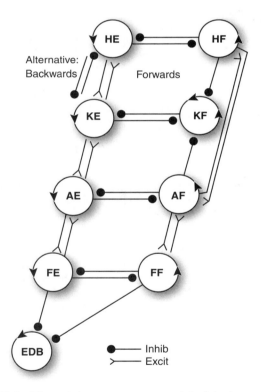

Figure 13-2. The unit burst generator model of the locomotor CPG. In this model, each limb is controlled by a central oscillator that controls each joint within a limb. The timing of activity between joints can be adjusted to produce different forms of a behavior, such as forward walking (wherein hip flexion and knee flexion occur at the start of swing phase) versus backward walking (wherein hip extension and knee flexion occur at the start of swing phase). From Grillner S. Biological pattern generation: The cellular and computational logic of networks in motion. *Neuron.* 2006;52:751–66. Reprinted with permission from Elsevier.

with the idea that every motor behavior need not have its own CPG. By merely altering the timing relationships between the various joints, diverse forms of movements may be produced.[18–20]

A further development of the CPG circuitry came with the work of Stein and colleagues[21] in the development of the bilateral shared core model (Fig. 13-3). Like the unit burst generator model, this model also suggests a modular organization of the CPG (based on evidence from the CPG for scratching), but has the advantage of illustrating how interlimb coordination may be achieved via coupling of the hip oscillators bilaterally. In this model, there is an inhibitory relationship between the circuitry controlling hip flexors and hip extensors that allow for the rhythmic alternation of flexion–extension within a limb. In addition, there is an inhibitory relationship between the circuitry controlling the hip flexors on one side and the hip flexors on the contralateral side, allowing for reciprocal alternation between limbs.

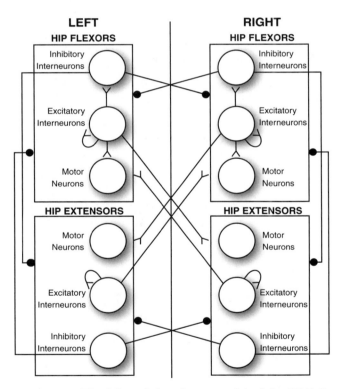

Figure 13-3. The bilateral shared core model of the CPG. In this model (developed to explain observations related to scratching behavior in spinal turtles), the control of a joint comprises a flexor and an extensor module. The modules controlling the hip on one side are coupled to those on the other side, allowing for coupling between limbs that is either alternating (e.g., as observed in walking) or synchronous (e.g., as observed in hopping). From Stein PS, Victor JC, Field EC, and Currie SN. Bilateral control of hindlimb scratching in the spinal turtle: Contralateral spinal circuitry contributes to the normal ipsilateral motor pattern of fictive rostral scratching. *J Neurosci.* 1995;15:4343–55. Reprinted with permission from the Society for Neuroscience.

Evidence for Spinal Locomotor CPG in Humans

Much of what is known about the organization of the locomotor CPG comes from studies of the cat model (for review *see* Duysens and Van de Crommert[22]). While the properties and organization of spinal cord circuitry in cats and humans are thought to be much alike,[23] it is also thought that the supraspinal centers exert greater influence on spinal circuitry in primates.[22] So, while the spinal cord CPG in many animal systems[17] (including primates[24]) is capable of producing locomotor output, evidence in humans has been less conclusive (or clear). This appears to be due partly to the difficulty in overcoming suppression of CPG circuitry in individuals with SCI. In spinal animals, for example, the CPG output becomes more vigorous when the animal is given a noxious stimulus (such as squeezing the tail).[25] A number of investigators[22,26,27] have offered reviews of the literature related to evidence for spinal locomotor CPG in humans. The following is a broad overview of this evidence.

Empirical support for the belief that humans have a CPG for locomotion at the spinal level comes from infants in the early postnatal period.[28] In this period of development, a stepping response is elicited if the infant is held suspended and the feet come in contact with a support surface. This response is attributed to spinal locomotor mechanisms, as the long tracts connecting the spinal and supraspinal centers are not fully myelinated at this stage of development.[29]

Calancie and colleagues[30] report the case of an individual with motor incomplete SCI who complained that his legs were waking him up at night by "walking" on their own. On radiological examination, it was discovered that the individual had severe degenerative disease of one hip. The investigators hypothesized that the bony degeneration was a source of noxious sensory input that was excitatory to a spinal locomotor CPG. Indeed, when the hip was anesthetized, the spontaneous "walking" activity stopped. Furthermore, while the individual complained that the walking activity occurred while he was sleeping, this was not the case. The activity was generated during the sleep–wake transition. This is a time when activity in the brainstem reticular centers is particularly high, and evidence from animal studies indicates that reticular activity is important in the activation of spinal CPGs.[31–34]

Studies by Bussel and colleagues[27,35,36] support the belief that cats and humans have similar organization of spinal cord circuitry related to locomotion. Their studies of flexion reflex activation in individuals with SCI have demonstrated that in a subset of these individuals, sensory input that activates the flexor reflex afferents produces rhythmic stepping movements of the lower extremities.[27,35,37] In a single case study,[35] they document rhythmic lower extremity movement in an individual with complete SCI who demonstrated myoclonus. While the movements involved bilateral, symmetric extensor contractions (rather than the alternating pattern associated with stepping), they were temporally regular and occurred in cyclic bursts. The pattern could be reset by activation of the flexor reflex afferents, as had previously been shown in spinal cats.[38]

Dimitrijevic and colleagues[39–41] have induced alternating stepping in individuals with SCI using tonic epidural stimulation. In individuals with chronic, complete SCI, the epidural stimulation produces rhythmically alternating flexion and extension phases in the bilateral lower extremities.[40] The application of this stimulation paradigm to training interventions will be discussed further in the related section below.

Behrman and colleagues[42] report a unique pattern of walking recovery in a 4-and-a-half-year-old boy following a severe, chronic cervical SCI. This child was nonambulatory, with an injury classified according to the American Spinal Cord Injury Association (AISA) impairment Scale (AIS) as AIS C, having a lower extremity motor score of 4/50, and 16 months post-SCI when he entered a locomotor training program. During the 23rd session, the boy demonstrated his first "step" immediately after a sensory-augmented step (i.e., manual stimulation of the tibialis anterior tendon). Eight sessions later, he voluntarily initiated his first seven steps over ground using a rolling walker, followed by a rapid rate of improvements, including the ability to start, stop, and step over ground. Several months after completion of training, he entered kindergarten as an ambulator, using a rolling walker. Interestingly, the boy was able to produce the rhythmic, alternating flexion and extension pattern associated with the swing and stance phases of walking, but his AIS lower extremity score remained unchanged after training; he was still unable to produce any voluntary, isolated movements in his legs. This finding provides indirect evidence of a human spinal pattern generator that may be activated via ascending afferent input associated with locomotor training and via descending supraspinal input in the absence of isolated movements control.

While the foregoing literature does not directly prove the existence of a spinal CPG in humans (direct proof is likely never to be available as studies in humans are limited to noninvasive techniques), it does supply strong support for this supposition. This belief is further supported by evidence that neural functions are preserved over the course of evolution as the nervous system develops phylogenetically, with the refinement of existing organization rather than the development of an entirely different organization.[43]

Sensory Input Contributes to the Refinement of Locomotor Output

While spinal CPGs are likely responsible for the generation of motor output related to the production of a rhythmical stepping pattern, sensory (or afferent) input is known to be important for the modulation and refinement of this output (for review of sensory contributions to locomotor

function *see* Van de Crommert and colleagues[44]). There is good evidence to suggest that sensory inputs are "gated" by the CPG so that the motor response to the sensory input is suited to the phase of the walking cycle in which the sensory input occurs. This gating results in a phase-dependent modulation of the influence of the sensory input. This gating mechanism has been demonstrated in lower vertebrate models of locomotor CPG circuitry,[45,46] and evidence for this gating has also been observed in studies of cats[47–50] and humans.[51–53] For example, sensory input that results in an inhibitory response when applied to the resting animal may produce an excitatory response when applied during locomotion.[54] Furthermore, in studies of spinalized animals, cutaneous stimulation to the dorsal surface of the foot during treadmill walking results in increased flexor muscle activity in the limb, while the same stimulus applied during stance phase results in increased extensor muscle activity.[50] This gating is thought to be important to ensure that inappropriate sensory input does not disrupt the rhythmicity of the motor pattern.

The fact that the influence of sensory input in CPG function is phase-dependent emphasizes its importance. Sensory input makes significant contributions to the quality and vigorousness of the motor output through the activation of reflexes and by influencing the excitability of spinal neural circuitry. In studies of locomotion in spinal animals, noxious sensory input is routinely used to facilitate a more vigorous walking pattern.[25] Locomotor output is known to be enhanced by sensory input such as that from load receptors and receptors that signal hip position.[52,55,56] Furthermore, experiments in the spinal cat have demonstrated that the pattern-generating circuitry adapts to partial loss of cutaneous sensory input from the foot, but some cutaneous input is needed for appropriate plantar foot placement and weight bearing.[52,57,58] Specific recommendations for optimizing appropriate sensory information during locomotor training will be discussed in a subsequent section.

Activity-Dependent Plasticity of Spinal Circuits

Wolpaw and colleagues[59–62] were among the first to demonstrate that spinal neural circuits are not immutable, but rather are modified in a training-dependent manner. Their investigations of the spinal stretch reflex (and its electrical analogue, the H-reflex) demonstrated that training-related changes are sustained for an extended time beyond the training period.[62,63] Using an operant conditioning paradigm, monkeys are able to increase or decrease the reflex response to a muscle stretch. They further demonstrated that these changes are retained at the level of the spinal cord,[61] as they persist after complete spinal transection. Similar effects have been found in individuals with SCI. Segal and Wolf[64,65] investigated the influence of an operant conditioning training paradigm on the stretch reflex amplitude of the biceps muscle in individuals with SCI who had spasticity of the elbow flexors. Subjects were trained to progressively decrease biceps electromyographic (EMG) activity during the application of an elbow extension torque that rapidly stretched the biceps. After training, subjects in the experimental group had significantly reduced biceps stretch reflexes, while those in the control (untrained) group showed no change.

Beyond training of simple reflexes, it is evident that even complex circuits such as the locomotor CPG respond to training. Edgerton and colleagues[66,67] have demonstrated in spinal cats that the stepping pattern becomes more vigorous with training. Furthermore, as was true with the stretch reflex modulation, the spinal cord circuitry appears to respond to training in a task-specific manner such that step-trained cats step, but do not stand well, and standing-trained cats stand, but do not step well.[68] Spinal cats can step on the treadmill with a pattern comparable to that of intact animals[69,70] and are able to coordinate complex patterns of movement such as stepping at different speeds with each leg[70] and coordinating stepping with paw shaking.[71,72] In the latter example, the animal lifts and shakes the swinging limb to remove piece of tape, but the paw shake occurs only during the swing phase. This indicates that the spinal circuitry responds to sensory input in a phase-appropriate manner. Similarly, the same afferent input (such as a tap to the dorsum of the foot) evokes different responses if the tapped limb is weight bearing (i.e., in stance phase) or non-weight bearing (i.e., in swing phase).[50] This phase-dependent modulation of responses to the sensory input result in increased extensor muscle activity if the tapped limb is in stance phase, but increased flexor muscle activity if the tapped limb is in swing phase.

The Role of Supraspinal Centers in Locomotor Function

Evidence of spinal cord control of complex innate behaviors such as walking, swimming, and scratching lends support to the idea that the spinal cord is much more than a passive conduit for descending motor commands and ascending sensory information. The findings that spinal circuits are capable of modulating motor output in a phase-dependent manner and that this circuitry is amenable to training opens the door to vast possibilities for improving locomotor function. The prevailing perspective about the role of the spinal cord in the generation of locomotor function is that the CPG circuitry manages the rhythm and timing of muscle activity. As such, it is not necessary for the supraspinal centers to be burdened with the task of activating the quadriceps muscles, turning off the hamstring muscles, etc. It is important to bear in mind, however, that supraspinal centers play an important role in activating the pattern generators in a manner that is consistent with a conscious goal (e.g., walk forward, walk fast, run to the ball, etc.)

and adapting the locomotor output to the environment based in visual and other sensory input (for review see Drew at al.[73]). Just as spinal circuits undergo activity-dependent plasticity with locomotor training, in individuals with motor incomplete SCI supraspinal centers are also modified by type of training.[74,75] This provides further evidence of the importance of these centers for locomotor function.

Applying Basic Neural and Engineering Science to Locomotor Rehabilitation

Contributions to rehabilitation of locomotor function have come not only from the neurosciences, but also from the engineering sciences as well. In most cases, the approach attempts to make use of the individual's own nervous system, either through activity-dependent plasticity or by directly activating the peripheral or central nervous system.

The following sections will discuss the three main approaches for rehabilitation of locomotor function in individuals with SCI: locomotor training, spinal cord stimulation, and neuroprostheses. Locomotor training, whether provided on a treadmill, overground, manual-assisted or robotic-assisted, attempts to use the evidence from both animal studies regarding the neural basis of locomotor function and human studies of locomotor training to improve the individual's ability to walk over ground. Spinal cord stimulation intervention involves the implantation of stimulating electrodes in the lumbar epidural space. The intent is to provide excitation to the spinal CPG to enhance the individual's ability to walk. Spinal cord stimulation is a newer approach that is not yet widely used. *Functional electrical stimulation (FES)* is the use of stimulation to provide neuroprosthetic support to the legs for walking function. Both superficial and implanted electrode systems have been used to improve walking function in individuals with SCI. These rehabilitation strategies add to the choices available to therapists as they evaluate the residual motor control available to persons after SCI and then decide among alternative therapies to optimize function and/or recovery. Next, a model for the control of walking will be introduced below to frame current developments and serve as a guide for assessing future strategies.

Locomotor Training for Individuals With Motor-Incomplete SCI

Barbeau[76] was the first to document the application of BWS (in which the lower extremities are partially unloaded by a harness and an overhead lift that supports a variable portion of the weight of the body) and a treadmill to individuals with motor incomplete SCI. Having studied locomotor function in the spinal cat model,[77,78] in addition to having clinical background as a physical therapist, Barbeau had a unique perspective. His seminal work has provided the foundation for others to further develop this approach. Since the early 1990s many other investigators have demonstrated that treadmill-based locomotor training results in improvements in walking function in individuals with chronic motor incomplete SCI.[79–87] This support provides an environment in which locomotor training can be initiated despite lower extremity paresis that prevents the individual from being able to support body weight when standing. Furthermore, this constrained, yet controlled, environment affords task-specific sensory experiences, control of speed and limb coordination, and the postural and weight-bearing conditions that are permissive for the nervous system to generate walking. The sensory-related input comprises the upright trunk posture; spatial-temporal coordination of the trunk, pelvic, and limb movements; interlimb and intralimb kinematics and coordination; and the resulting spatiotemporal gait pattern at designated speeds. The environment, with manual assistance from trainers, minimizes the compensatory gait strategies exhibited by persons with paresis that are often observed during overground walking with the use of braces and load bearing assistive devices.[88]

Influence of Chronicity and Injury Level on Locomotor Training Outcomes

In individuals with chronic (>1 year post-injury), motor incomplete SCI, in whom walking ability has been stable for some time, locomotor training in the treadmill-BWS system environment has been associated with several walking-related outcomes, including walking speed and distance[76,79–83,85,86,89–91] as well as other aspects of function, such as limb coordination,[82] strength,[81,82,86,87] muscle activation patterns,[90] and energy expenditure.[85] Subjectively, locomotor training in individuals with chronic, motor-incomplete SCI also improves sense of well-being.[91] However, among the investigations of locomotor training, a wide variety of training approaches and assisted-stepping protocols have been used. While it would seem intuitively obvious that individuals with acute SCI would benefit from this training as well, the inherent variability among individuals in the amount of spontaneous recovery makes it difficult to determine whether the early benefits of this form of training surpass those associated with standard rehabilitation practice.[92]

Injury level will also likely impact the outcomes associated with locomotor training. Individuals with injury to the cervical and thoracic levels of the spinal cord are likely to benefit from locomotor training that is aimed at promoting functional plasticity of the spinal cord circuits associated with walking. However, injury to the lower thoracic and lumbar levels is likely to be associated with lower motoneuron damage. This damage is associated with the denervation atrophy of the muscles innervated by the involved segments due to loss of all (or nearly all) of the spinal motoneurons innervating the muscle. In addition, and perhaps more importantly with regard to neural plasticity, there is the loss of the pathway through which sensory input reaches the spinal cord. The sensory input associated with training is likely to be as important for promoting neural plasticity as any other constituent of the spinal cord neural milieu.

Optimizing the Influence of Sensory Input

In light of the influence of sensory input on motor output, Behrman and Harkema[93] offer six recommendations regarding factors to consider in a locomotor training protocol, whether conducted in the treadmill-BWS system environment or the overground environment. While the veracity of these recommendations as they apply to locomotor training in people with SCI has not been systematically verified through comparative study, they do have a logical basis in the scientific literature. These recommendations are as follows: (1) train at the fastest tolerable speed (i.e., approximate normal walking speed); (2) allow as much load on the lower extremities as can be sustained; (3) maintain upright posture with extended trunk and neck; (4) approximate normal hip, knee, and ankle movements; (5) discourage upper extremity weight bearing while maximizing lower extremity weight bearing; and (6) synchronize terminal hip extension and unloading in one limb with loading of the contralateral limb. A brief review of the evidence for each of these recommendations is offered below.

Training Speed. While Visintin and Barbeau[94] offer observations about quality of gait and EMG with increased speed in those with SCI, quantitative assessment of the relationship between training speed and overground walking speed have, to date, been completed only in individuals with stroke.[95,96] Pohl and colleagues[95] have demonstrated a statistically significant effect of training speed in their study of individuals with stroke. Sullivan and colleagues[96] found trends toward greater improvement in those trained at faster speed, but differences were not statistically significant. Higher walking speeds have also been shown to be associated with higher levels of muscle activity in both animals and humans.[94,97] However, Oursler and Hidler[98] point out that increased muscle activity is not necessary beneficial, as much of this activity may be inappropriately timed, resulting in worsening of the EMG patterns in individuals with SCI.

Effects of Load. Increased lower extremity weight bearing is associated with more vigorous motor output, as evidenced by increased muscle EMG activity in both spinal animals and humans with SCI.[25,97] Therefore, theoretically, the lower extremities should be allowed to bear the maximum amount of body weight at which satisfactory quality of gait can be maintained. However, increased muscle activity is not necessary beneficial, as much of this activity may be inappropriately timed, resulting in agonist–antagonist muscle co-contraction EMG patterns in individuals with SCI.[98] Inadequate toe clearance during swing phase and excessive knee flexion during stance phase are examples of gait deviations that would indicate excessive load, and decreasing load by partially "unweighting" the lower extremities with BWS may result in a walking pattern that is more typical of normal gait.

Upright Posture With Trunk and Neck Extension. In decerebrate animals, neck extension is associated with a more vigorous walking pattern.[99] Furthermore, neck extension facilitates a generalized extension response in the limbs, perhaps due to vestibular influences (*compare* the asymmetrical tonic neck reflex). Adequate trunk extension also promotes increased hip extension, which has been shown to be a key sensory input for initiation of swing phase[100,101] (see below).

Joint Kinematics. The neural circuitry underlying locomotion is sensitive to movement-related (proprioceptive) sensory input from the moving limb.[102,103] In studies of locomotor output in the de-efferented cat model, passive flexion applied to the limb results in increased flexor motor output, while passive extension results in increased extensor motor output (i.e., entrainment). These movements were effective in making the motor output more vigorous only when they were applied during the appropriate phase of motor output (e.g., during a flexor burst passive extension, movement did not influence the motor output).

Upper Extremity Weight Bearing. The influence of handrails during treadmill training has been investigated primarily in individuals with asymmetrical paresis.[76,94] Barbeau and Blunt[76] report results from training three individuals with asymmetrical SCI. Their results indicate that the walking pattern becomes more symmetrical when upper extremities are not used for weight bearing. Visintin and Barbeau[94] studied the influence of using handrails in individuals with spastic paresis due to SCI. In those who had asymmetrical involvement, allowing the upper extremities to swing freely was associated with improved gait symmetry. In a small number of subjects with symmetrical involvement, there was inappropriately prolonged activation of muscle activity during stance phase when handrails were not used. They note that there are clear differences in response to use of parallel bars in those with gait asymmetry and those with symmetrical gait. Conrad and colleagues[104,105] encourage the use of parallel bars in order to improve stability and achieve a more normal gait pattern. The use of handrails during training in individuals with SCI therefore requires further investigation before a definitive, evidence-based recommendation can be made. The role of arm swing relative to retraining, not only in stepping, but as the co-requisite balance for walking, is also warranted. Whether arm swing adds to the sensory experience of walking and can facilitate lower extremity stepping requires investigation, though preliminary evidence is supportive of this potential training effect.[106,107]

Hip Position and Load at Terminal Stance. In studies of walking in spinalized cats, there is clear evidence that the transition from stance phase to swing phase is critically dependent upon hip position and load.[100,101] At terminal stance, full hip extension and low load create the most favorable conditions for initiation of the ensuing step. The application of these recommendations to humans is supported by studies of stepping in infants who are in the pre-walking period.[52,108]

Locomotor Training on the Treadmill

For many individuals, locomotor training on a treadmill (typically with BWS) is performed with assistance to promote achievement of the appropriate stepping pattern and upright posture. The following sections discuss the various forms of assistance that are currently used in the locomotor training of individuals with SCI.

Manual-Assisted Stepping

The manual assistance of a human trainer is the most commonly employed approach for providing assistance for stepping (Fig. 13-4). There are a number of reports of manual assistance for locomotor training in individuals with SCI;[79–87] however, no comparative studies have been performed to assess whether one approach is superior to others. The common element in all reports of manual training is that trainers assist the individual in moving the legs through the stepping pattern. In one conceptualization of this approach, a trainer assists at the trunk and pelvis to help the individual with SCI achieve an upright posture of the trunk and to aid the pelvis in the rotation consistent with limb advancement, loading, and hip extension.[93]

In all forms of assisted training, but particularly with manual-assisted stepping, the sensory input associated with stepping deserves particular consideration. In this regard, placement of the hands during the provision of assistance is considered important. To provide the phase-appropriate sensory cues, therapists are encouraged to place their hands on the extensor surface of the limb only during the extensor phase of the movement and then on the flexor surface of the limb during the flexor phase. Therapists position themselves facing the opposite direction relative to the individual being trained in order to promote extension and flexion movements (*see* Fig. 13-4). In addition to leg trainers, manual assistance may be provided to promote an upright posture and pelvic rotation consistent with the transfer of weight from one limb to the other, coordinated with the stepping pattern; in this case, the trunk/pelvic trainer stands directly behind the individual being trained, often using handholds on the harness to coordinate the pelvis rotation and stepping.

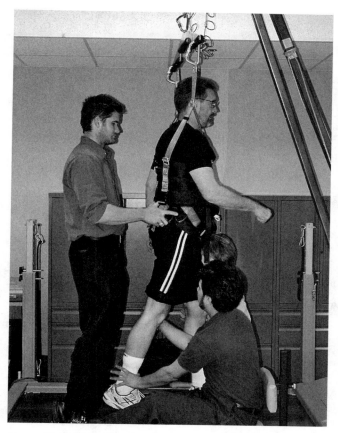

Figure 13-4. Manual-assisted stepping. The therapist provides assistance for stepping during swing phase, while BWS decreases the effort required of paretic muscles during stance phase.

Advantages/Disadvantages. One of the primary advantages of the manual-assisted approach is that the trainer is able to adapt the amount of assistance provided to the needs of the individual on a cycle-by-cycle basis. This allows the individual to perform the components of walking that he or she is able to execute independently and receive assistance for those components that are more difficult. Furthermore, the feedback provided through the manual contact allows the individual being trained to receive additional cues for determining appropriate timing of progression. The main disadvantage of this form of training is that it is strenuous work on the part of the trainer, especially when the individual being trained has a high degree of spasticity. For these reasons, the assistance is likely to be inconsistent when the trainer becomes fatigued, thereby making the training inconsistent. Body mechanics during training, rotation of training positions, and responding to fatigue become critical elements of manual-assisted locomotor training. The training environment for manual trainers is particularly important in order to promote upright posture with ergonomic seating and back support, adjustable seating to afford easy access to the limbs while maintaining an upright trunk without rotation, and foot stabilization support.

Manufactured BWS systems may or may not include a seating system for manual trainers. Without support, trainers are at a disadvantage and may be more susceptible to injury during the repetitive task of training.

Case examples demonstrating application of the training variables recommended by Behrman and Harkema[93,109] within a locomotor training protocol using manual-assistance for persons post-SCI have been published previously. According to these recommendations, the progression entails two training environments, treadmill and overground, with the guidelines for training applied to both environments. Attention is paid to (1) the type and timing of sensory information that the individual is given by the trainer within the training environment and (2) the experience of upright posture and good stepping pattern (e.g., spatial–temporal pattern that is kinematically consistent with walking). Accommodations are made with BWS, treadmill speed, and manual assistance to achieve this pattern. An early training goal is for the person to achieve an upright posture and to achieve 20 minutes of total stepping time, thus a training effect. Progression advances by decreasing the BWS and manual assistance in order for the person to gain endurance and independent control of his or her limb(s) and trunk. Late in training, and with increased independence, varying the treadmill speed, walking at slow speeds, and negotiating inclines are addressed on the treadmill and during overground training. Following daily step training on the treadmill, an assessment is made of walking skills acquired on the treadmill and exhibited during overground walking. See the section on overground training for details.

Stimulation-Assisted Stepping

Individuals with SCI retain intact spinal reflex circuitry. The connections among the sensory receptors, the spinal reflex arc, and the motor output are intact. Furthermore, because of the loss of descending control, these reflexes are typically hyperactive (hence, the presence of hyperreflexia). One of these spinal reflex circuits, the flexion withdrawal reflex, is thought to be a component of the pattern-generating circuitry associated with locomotion.[14,15,27,35,38]

Field-Fote[81,82] was the first to document the use of flexor reflex activation in conjunction with BWS treadmill training for individuals with SCI, although it had previously been used in individuals with stroke.[110] She demonstrated that subjects trained with this combined approach improved walking speed, walking distance, lower extremity strength, and inter-limb coordination. The application of this technique involves placing a pair of stimulating electrodes on each limb (if bilateral assistance is required) over sites that elicit a vigorous flexion withdrawal response. There are multiple sites from which this response can be elicited, and these are described in Table 13-1. Optimal electrode placements (Fig. 13-5a and 13-5b) vary considerably between individuals and may

Table 13-1

Electrode Placement and Stimulus Parameters for Stimulation-assisted Stepping

Cathode Position	Anode Position	Pulse Width	Train Duration	Voltage or Current	Comments
1–2 cm distal to fibular head	1–2 cm proximal to popliteal fossa, lateral to midline	0.3–1 msec pulse duration	250–500 msec	As determined by response and patient tolerance	Vigorous response that is typically well tolerated
As above	Medial tibial plateau	As above	As above	As above	Often a less vigorous response relative to site above, but easier to elicit in some individuals
As above	5–8 cm distal to cathode	As above	As above	As above	Least likely to elicit hip and knee flexion, but produces vigorous dorsiflexion
Medial aspect of plantar arch	Medial dorsal surface of foot	As above	As above	As above	Vigorous response, but may be poorly tolerated due to compression inside shoes

differ for each leg for an individual (*note* in Fig. 13-5b that the optimal site for the anode is more distal and lateral than on the left leg). For this reason, it may be necessary to evaluate the response at multiple sites in order to ascertain which of these evokes the best response in the individual.

Advantages/Disadvantages. The advantage to using this form of assistance is that it makes use of a spinal reflex that may be a component of the pattern-generating circuitry for walking.[14,15,27,35,38] As such, the repetitive activation of this circuit may be associated with improvements in the circuit's efficacy. By this means, the individual's own nervous system may become more effective in producing the neural output necessary for walking. There is evidence to suggest that this form of stimulation may influence the spinal neural circuitry such that reflexes, which are commonly hyperactive in individuals with SCI, and reflex modulation become more normal.[111–113] The disadvantage to this technique is that, as it is currently applied, it is an open-loop system (no feedback from the current step to modulate output in the ensuing step) that provides the same level of assistance from step to step regardless of the requirements of the individual. While the reflex may become less effective over the course of a

session due to habituation, this problem is easy to address by simply making small adjustments to the stimulus parameters.

Robot-Assisted Stepping

In the early part of the millennium, Colombo and colleagues[114,115] developed a motorized gait orthosis that operates in conjunction with a treadmill to provide mechanical assistance to stepping (Fig. 13-6). When used by individuals with SCI[115] and nondisabled individuals,[116] physiologic gait patterns and locomotor-related EMG have been comparable to that obtained with human assistance.[115] Hidler and Wall[117] demonstrate that, at least in nondisabled subjects, the activation patterns may differ from those typically associated with walking.

Studies by Hornby and colleagues[84] suggest that use of the device is associated with improvements in locomotor function. Robotic-assisted stepping was followed by manual-assisted locomotor training, thus sequencing training based on the type of assistance and ability, using first robotic training, then manual-assisted training to progress elements of balance and adaptability. This sequence may be a successful strategy in some individuals with SCI. However, the greatest improvements may be in

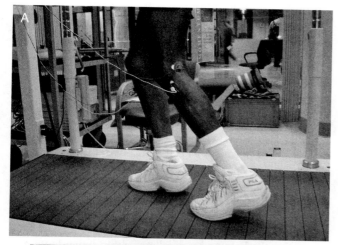

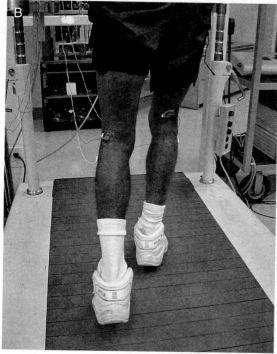

Figure 13-5. Stimulation-assisted stepping. Electrical stimulation is used to provide assistance for stepping during swing phase, while BWS decreases the effort required of paretic muscles during stance phase. The optimal electrode placement may vary, depending on the individual (*see* Table 13-1). When a flexion withdrawal reflex is desired to assist stepping, placing the cathode below the fibular head (A) and the anode on the distal hamstrings (B) is often effective.

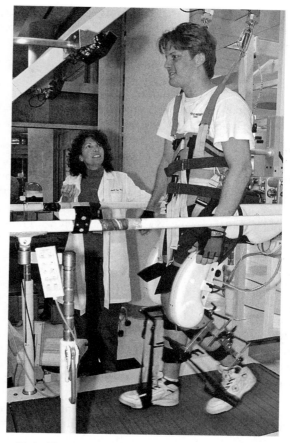

Figure 13-6. Training with the Lokomat robotic gait orthosis. The Lokomat provides mechanical assistance for stepping in a kinematically correct pattern. The device is coupled to the treadmill so that walking speed can be adjusted. BWS decreases the effort required of paretic muscles during stance phase.

individuals who have the potential for some locomotor function, but who have some lower extremity motor function but who are not yet able to walk over ground. Transfer to overground walking will be important, whether applying manual-assisted or robotic-assisted locomotor training.

Advantages/Disadvantages. The primary advantage to using this device is that it provides a highly consistent stepping pattern throughout the walking session. As such, the sensory information related to muscle length, load, and joint position are all highly consistent as well. Whereas consistency of input appears important, some degree of variability may be a critical element in the retraining of limb control or be important at a later stage of training. The major disadvantage to the use of this device is that it currently has a maximum speed of 3.2 km/h (2.0 mph), which is lower than the range of normal comfortable walking speed. The manufacturer will customize the treadmill and robotic exoskeleton motors to allow a speed up to 4.5 km/h (2.8 mph), but this is not a usual option. As such, it may not be appropriate for training individuals who are already able to walk at normal walking speeds. Furthermore, since the device requires no active assistance on the part of the user, it is conceivable that it does not optimally engage the nervous system in the act of walking. Accommodations to changes in limb movement independence are more difficult in the robotic environment as the exoskeleton remains in place regardless of the degree of independence achieved by the user. Additionally, the development of the requisite equilibrium control for walking may be limited within the robotic training environment. The back support may be removed and BWS decreased to progress postural control; however, the absence of pelvic and trunk rotation may limit the development of such control.

Locomotor Training Overground

A Contemporary Approach to Overground Locomotor Training

The treadmill environment (whether manual, robotic, or electrical stimulation assisted) provides a controlled environment in which to relearn and develop the capacity to step. The treadmill affords (1) a consistent speed that is often faster than that which can be achieved over ground and (2) a means to assist repetitively with posture and stepping. When the individual with SCI steps off the treadmill, these elements quickly change. The sensory experience of walking must be driven from within the task of walking itself, without the speed and the repetitive, rhythmic sensory contact of the soles of the feet afforded by the treadmill. If overground training is done in the absence of BWS, then gravity has its full effect and the comfort and security from the overhead safety is absent. Providing manual cues while moving over ground becomes difficult to coordinate; robotic devices have not yet extended to overground use.

The approach consistent with conventional physical therapy when training overground walking and a more contemporary approach whereby locomotor training is provided over ground differ considerably. A detailed comparison and contrast of these two approaches is available,[118] as is a case report demonstrating the training progression.[109] Some researchers refer to overground training as part of the locomotor training program;[85-87] however, only a few have delineated a process of extending the training guidelines from treadmill to overground training, thus altering the process of overground training.[92,93,118] Differences between the treadmill and the overground walking environments would suggest there may be a need for training in both environments.

A determination of the abilities the individual needs to acquire for overground locomotion consists of comparing the performance on the treadmill to the performance of the same skills over ground. For instance, can the individual stand upright and maintain extension upon loading and weight transfer? Does "hip hiking" return in the overground environment, or are the proper kinematics sustained? This assessment identifies skills for continued refinement in the treadmill/BWS environment. Instructions are provided for walking over ground as well. When overground training is performed in the absence of BWS, assistance with balance, posture, and support is provided by handhold assistance or the use of horizontal poles. With such support, trainers focus on advancing upright postural control within the task of walking and promoting a faster speed than that which could be achieved without support and assistance. Verbal

instructions are provided for altering kinematics and posture. Independence in walking function achieved on the treadmill is evaluated over ground for carryover. Training over ground may advance the patient's confidence in his or her skills and capacity and allow the patient to understand the relationship between posture/kinematics and walking successfully.

The final aspect of this contemporary approach requires that the therapist work with the individual to extend the use of his or her locomotor skills to the home and community. At this point, the use of assistive devices or a brace may be introduced. Instructions in using the assistive device incorporate each aspect of the training guidelines, thus encouraging upright posture and minimal weight bearing on the arms. The specifics of such carryover are dictated by the degree of independence and skill level of the individual. Extending the training program to the home may consist of attempts to stand upright in a walker without load bearing on the arms. Alternatively, it may be walking within the home with two forearm crutches, rather than a walker, while focusing on upright posture, hip extension, and minimizing use of the crutches for support.

Building on the overground training program, the subsequent locomotor training session on the treadmill takes advantage of the knowledge gained from the previous overground training session, with goals for the training targeting the gait deviations observed as well as other skills necessary to progress independence in overground walking. Thus, the cycle of training in the BWS treadmill and overground environment continues. The BWS/treadmill environment is the primary environment for increased walking capacity, whereas the overground environment is necessary for transfer of skill, building the confidence and context to training for transfer of walking skills, and maximizing walking abilities in the home and community.

BWS and Assistance for Stepping in Overground Training

As with locomotor training on the treadmill, in the overground environment, there are available options for both partially unloading the limbs and for providing assistance for stepping. There are currently several devices on the market, such as the LiteGait (Fig. 13-7) and the Biodex Unweighting System (Fig. 13-8), which are designed to provide a mobile system of BWS for use in overground locomotor training. In most cases, these devices offer the option to position the BWS system over the treadmill for use in treadmill locomotor training, assuming the treadmill does not have an elevated base. The advantages to using BWS systems for overground locomotor training is that, as with treadmill locomotor training, they provide a safe environment by decreasing the risk for falls and allow for walking with decreased load on paretic lower extremities. However, the inherent disadvantage is that the individual may not develop the appropriate postural

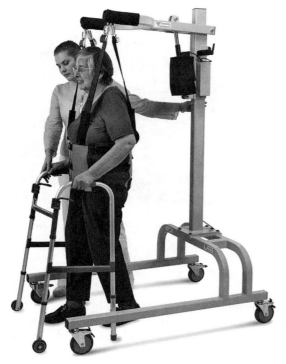

Figure 13-7. Overground training with BWS. The LiteGait 300MX allows overground walking while providing assistance for balance and partial support of body weight. The device may be positioned over a treadmill to allow body weight-supported locomotor training on a treadmill. (Photo courtesy of Mobility Research, used with permission.)

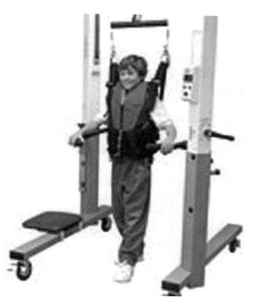

Figure 13-8. Overground training with body weight support. The Biodex Unweighting System allows overground walking while providing assistance for balance and partial support of body weight. The device may be positioned over a treadmill to allow body weight-supported locomotor training on a treadmill; however, note that the position of the upright supports may make it difficult to provide assistance for stepping. (Photo courtesy of Biodex Medical Systems, used with permission.)

control strategies needed for independent overground walking. As such, these systems may be most appropriate for use early in the locomotor training program.

Surface electrical stimulation has been used for decades to provide assistance for dorsiflexion[119] during walking. This application is most effective for individuals who have relatively good control over the other components of walking and who simply require some assistance for toe clearance during the swing phase of walking. As indicated earlier, the literature suggests that this form of stimulation may modify spinal neural circuitry, resulting in more normal reflex modulation.[111–113] There are currently several devices on the market specifically made for use as a dorsiflexion-assist device. The WalkAide II[120,121] provides assistance by stimulation of the common peroneal nerve (Fig. 13-9). The stimulation can be triggered at the onset of the swing phase by any of three means: a footswitch inserted into the shoe, a manual trigger button, or a tilt sensor. The use of the tilt sensor is individualized to the user's walking pattern by means of a computer program that "teaches" the stimulator to recognize the shank angle at which the stimulation should be triggered. Two other available devices that make use of a foot switch to trigger stimulation for dorsiflex assistance include the Ness L300 (Fig. 13-10) and the Odstock Dropped-Foot Stimulator (ODFS)[122] (Fig. 13-11). The assistance provided by a foot drop stimulator for overground walking has been found to be comparable to that provided by an ankle-foot orthosis (AFO)[122] and to be associated with decreased metabolic cost of walking.[123] The stimulators may be preferred by users for reasons of cosmesis.

As just illustrated, there are many options available for improving walking function in individuals with motor incomplete SCI. To date, however, there have been few

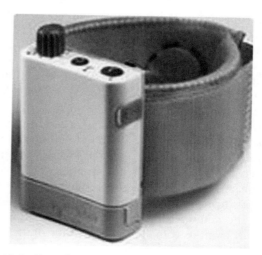

Figure 13-9. Foot drop stimulators activate the common peroneal nerve through surface electrodes to provide assistance for dorsiflexion during the swing phase of walking. There are a number of commercially stimulators available, including the WalkAide system (Photo courtesy of Innovative Neurotronics, Inc., Austin, Texas.)

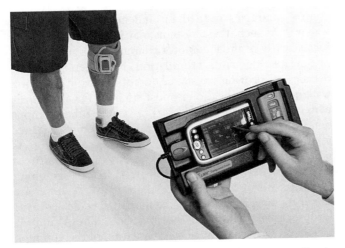

Figure 13-10. The Ness L300. (Bioness. permission pending.)

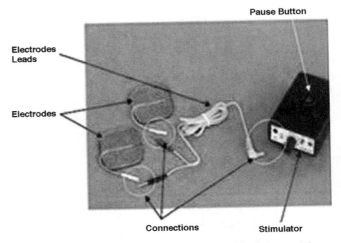

Figure 13-11. The Odstock Drop-Foot Stimulator (Photo courtesy of Odstock Medical, Ltd. Salisbury, Wiltshire, UK. Permission pending.)

studies to directly compare outcomes associated with different training approaches. Dobkin and colleagues[92] compared locomotor training on the treadmill to conventional training over ground in individuals with SCI who were within 8 weeks of injury. For individuals who were motor-incomplete at the time of entry into the study, no differences were found between the two training groups in terms of walking speed; however, both groups achieved a mean walking speed of 1.0 m/sec. For individuals who were motor complete at the time of entry into the study, no differences were found between the two training groups in terms of scores on a standardized test of functional ability.

Whether one modality or treatment approach for locomotor training is better than another for persons with chronic motor-incomplete SCI remains to be answered. The current study by Field-Fote and colleagues[124] is comparing four forms of locomotor training, consisting of (1) treadmill training with manual assistance, (2) treadmill training with FES, (3) overground training with FES, and (4) treadmill training with robotic assistance. Walking-related outcome measures assessed include overground walking speed, training speed, step length, and step symmetry. Preliminary data indicate a trend toward greater increases in walking speed in the group trained over ground with FES and the group trained on the treadmill with FES, but the overall differences between groups were small. Step symmetry was increased to a greater extent in the groups trained on the treadmill with manual assistance or with robotic assistance. While the definitive findings and interpretations from this study await its completion, at the time of the preliminary report this study contained a larger number of subjects than most other locomotor training studies, with a study sample that was relatively homogeneous (consisting only of individuals with chronic SCI), and with stratified randomization based upon degree of impairment. In addition, it is one of only a few studies to compare different training approaches in a randomized trial.

Understanding the limits and benefits of each environment and training strategy relative to the movement dysfunction of the individual, as well as its inherent advantages and disadvantages, will aid in developing better clinical decision-making and optimize walking recovery. As demonstrated by Hornby et al.,[84] the choice of training environments may even change during the process of recovery and be dictated not only by ability, but also possibly by the nature of the limiting factor for achieving ambulation. Thus, the "therapeutic toolbox" for walking recovery may hold several alternative activity-based tools that will require appropriate selection and sequencing during the course of an individual's recovery.

Promoting Locomotor Function in Individuals With Motor-Complete SCI

While the focus of locomotor training has been on those with some volitional control of the lower extremities, there have been several investigations of training for those with motor complete SCI. Dietz and colleagues[79,80] were the first to assess the effects of locomotor training on a treadmill in individuals with severe SCI associated with motor complete lesion (i.e., no motor function below the level of injury). In some of these individuals, treadmill-based training is associated with improved stepping ability while on the treadmill, but there was no transfer of this stepping to overground walking conditions. While others have come to similar conclusions,[80,93] Harkema and colleagues[97,125] have shown that even individuals with motor complete SCI exhibit locomotor-appropriate muscle responses while walking on the treadmill and, furthermore, that these responses adapt according to the amount of weight (load) on the limbs.[97] While these studies suggest that individuals with chronic motor complete SCI are able to generate locomotor-appropriate muscle activity while walking on the treadmill, these individuals have not been shown to be able to walk over ground despite training.

Despite the absence of change in walking-related outcome measures, individuals with motor complete SCI do benefit from this training as there are many benefits to walking that go beyond the restoration of locomotor function. For example, Nash and colleagues[126] have demonstrated that there is a metabolic cost associated with treadmill walking in an individual with motor-complete SCI. This would suggest that there may be cardiorespiratory benefits to walking. Furthermore, walking is likely to be associated with improved bone health and, perhaps, improved pulmonary function,[126,127] bowel motility, and tissue health.[128]

While treadmill-based locomotor training may not be the intervention of choice for improving walking function in individuals with motor complete SCI, there is a long history of the use of bracing and FES for individuals with motor complete SCI. While issues related to bracing and orthotics are not within the scope of this chapter, a brief mention of available surface and implanted electrical stimulation systems that have been used by those with motor complete SCI is given here and below.

The Parastep system[129] is an FDA-approved FES system for individuals with complete thoracic-level SCI. The high level of stimulation provided by this device is uncomfortable for individuals with spared sensory function, therefore the use of the device is limited to those with complete SCI. In the present state of knowledge, the lack of volitional control of the lower extremities in those with complete SCI precludes locomotor training with respect to the goal of restoration of walking function. While the device does allow these individuals to walk for exercise,[130] the high physiologic cost[131] limits its applicability for functional locomotion.

The Future of Assisted Locomotion for Individuals With SCI

Implanted FES Systems

Implanted FES systems represent a possible means of promoting locomotor function in individuals with SCI. These systems are used as neuroprostheses, providing multichannel stimulation to activate the peripheral nervous system in a functionally appropriate manner during walking. While these systems are typically regarded as devices to compensate for decreased or lost volitional control, there is evidence in individuals with stroke that the use of these devices is associated with a training effect such that improved walking and voluntary muscle function persists after the stimulator is turned off or removed.[132,133] One of the major limitations of this approach to locomotion is the high metabolic cost.[131] Recent developments with implantable systems appear to remedy some of these problems, but electrical stimulation for walking as a primary means of locomotion is currently used by only a small proportion of individuals with SCI. Multichannel FES for individuals with complete SCI received much attention in the popular media in the 1980s

based on the work of Petrofsky.[134,135] In this use, a complex computer-based algorithm activated multiple muscles at the appropriate time in the gait cycle. Since that time, there have been significant developments in systems that stimulate multiple muscles. Badj and Kralj[136,137] have been involved in the development of both surface and implanted systems of electrical stimulation for restoration of walking function in individuals with SCI. They report that difficulty associated with using the systems and the competing needs of adjusting to SCI are among the factors limiting continued use of these systems[136] and make recommendations for patient selection and training prior to use of stimulators as neuroprostheses.[138]

While percutaneous muscle stimulation (using electrodes that penetrate the skin to reach the target muscle)[139] were used at one time, these were met with complications such as infection and electrode breakage. Currently available systems[140,141] employ implanted electrodes that are inserted through a common incision approximately at the level of the umbilicus. The stimulus parameters are determined by an implanted multichannel microprocessor that is controlled with an external transmitter. In addition to applications in individuals with SCI, these systems are also used in individuals with stroke and other upper motor neuron disorders. According to one report,[141] users report a moderate to high degree of satisfaction with the capabilities of the system.

Spinal Cord Stimulation

In animal models of SCI, spinal cord stimulation is accomplished via indwelling electrodes implanted into the gray matter of the spinal cord, either into the intermediate zone (the region where the chief components of the locomotor CPG are thought to be located) or into the ventral horn (the region where the motoneurons are located). Studies of intraspinal stimulation in cats[142,143] have shown that the electrodes are stable over long periods of time. The stimulation is well tolerated by the animals and can produce complex multijoint movements such as those associated with standing and walking.

Intraspinal stimulation has not been documented in humans, but studies of epidural stimulation are in early phases.[40,41,144,145] In this application, stimulating electrodes are inserted into the dorsal epidural space over the lumbar enlargement. At this time, published reports are limited to a case report of a single subject.[144,145] In this report, the subject was able to walk farther following the implantation of the device and reported increased ease of walking when the stimulator was active. Positive results were associated with the use of specific stimulus parameters. These parameters were intensity above sensory threshold, but below motor threshold; pulse duration of 0.8 msec; and stimulus frequency of 20 to 60 hertz. The report indicates that the subject was able to walk farther within a specified time period with the stimulator in place. However, the gain in walking speed (distance/time) was similar to what has been reported with locomotor training alone in individuals with comparables type of injury.[146]

CASE STUDY 13-1   Locomotor Training for an Individual With Motor-Incomplete SCI

The following case study demonstrates the evaluation process and the locomotor training guidelines and progression for the treadmill and overground environments.

History and evaluation

Jeremy is a 22-year-old man injured in a motor vehicle accident 20 months earlier, sustaining a T4 SCI with an upper extremity ASIA motor score of 50/50 and lower extremity motor score of 44/50. Sensory testing indicated impaired pinprick perception below T5, with the right side pinprick score of 39/56 and left side pinprick score of 36/56, as well as impaired light touch, with a score on the right of 35/56 and on the left of 28/56. Quick passive stretch of the plantar flexors resulted in clonus, hyperactive quadriceps deep tendon reflexes were elicited, and a positive Babinski reflex was present bilaterally.

Jeremy was a full-time community ambulator and used a straight cane for balance. He walked with a forward flexed trunk and wide base of support. At 0.56 m/sec, his self-selected overground walking speed was approximately one-half that typical for a nondisabled individual (Fig. 13-12). He could increase his walking speed to 0.92 m/sec by increasing his step length to 0.62 m and 0.61 m, left and right, and decreased double limb support time to 0.21 sec.

Jeremy was evaluated initially while walking on the treadmill with BWS at 0%, but with an overhead support that would provide safety from falling. He could not walk independently on the treadmill, even at 0.2 m/sec, without using a parallel bar or arm support. On the treadmill, Jeremy's steps were short and staggering, and he quickly fell forward, holding onto the BWS apparatus frame to catch himself. He compensated for lack of dynamic equilibrium with prolonged double limb support (0.34 sec) and short step lengths (0.48 m, 0.47 m, left and right, respectively). Subsequently during the evaluation on the treadmill, the BWS was increased to 30%, treadmill speed to 0.83 m/sec and assistance was provided by three trainers. One trainer advanced the right lower extremity during the swing phase of walking. A second trainer assisted with achieving pelvic rotation for hip extension, loading during terminal stance, and an adequate push-off for forward propulsion. A third trainer stood in front of Jeremy, with her hands in front of his shoulders to remind him to maintain an upright posture (Fig. 13-13). A trainer was not necessary on the left lower extremity as Jeremy was able to maintain the spatial-temporal pattern of walking independently in this leg. With partial BWS, increased speed, and the three trainers assisting, Jeremy produced a symmetrical stepping pattern and upright trunk posture. Having established this motor response during the evaluation, training would be initiated with these parameters.

Goal

The primary locomotor training goals of this individual were to walk faster and with better balance and endurance. From the therapist's perspective, this meant achieving a normal walking speed and the corequisite dynamic equilibrium that would afford elimination of a cane on even terrain. Furthermore, the goal of increasing his adaptability to different environments was added. This included the ability to negotiate obstacles, start and stop suddenly, and adapt to gait speed changes without upper extremity support by using the cane.

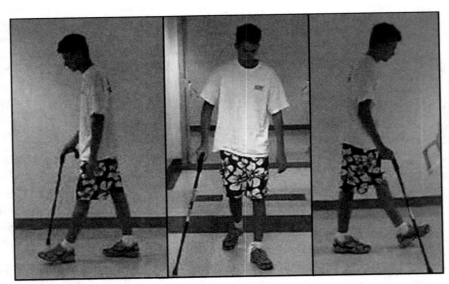

Figure 13-12. Case study pretraining overground walking. Note short step length, lack of knee flexion on weight acceptance in early stance, and wide base of support despite use of the cane.

CASE STUDY 13-1   Locomotor Training for an Individual With Motor-Incomplete SCI—cont'd

Training

Jeremy participated in daily training on the treadmill, with a target goal of 30 minutes of stepping time, followed by 15 min of overground walking and instruction. The overground training component encouraged transfer of skills acquired on the treadmill to the overground environment. He participated in a total of 45 training sessions. Training was initiated using the parameters established during the treadmill-based evaluation that promoted a kinematically-appropriate stepping and posture. Training speed with assisted stepping was quickly increased and maintained near 1.2 m/sec.

By session 5, the trainer providing assistance for upright posture was no longer required. At this time, the 30-min session duration was achieved and sustained for the duration of the 45 sessions, though the length of each individual bout increased across training sessions. At session 12, the trainer for the right leg was eliminated. BWS was decreased incrementally, with 20% BWS achieved by session 16 and 10% BWS achieved by session 25. The pelvis and trunk trainer was not required from session 24 onward; therefore, only a single trainer was needed from this time onward. By session 27, adaptability training was initiated and included starting and stopping the treadmill abruptly, walking at varying speeds from slow to fast as the speeds were changed slowly or rapidly, and stepping over obstacles. Independent stepping trials during each session often required slowing the speed, but independent stepping at 1.2 m/sec was achieved by session 35, with 10% BWS. This trainer did not need to touch the subject, but now provided verbal cueing and challenges for adaptability training to the treadmill and overground environment.

Outcome

Jeremy completed training on the treadmill, having achieved the ability to walk 30 min continuously at 1.2 m/sec with 5% BWS. Following completion of training, Jeremy walked over ground without a cane, demonstrating good balance and lower extremity kinematics (Fig. 13-14). His self-selected walking speed was 0.96 m/sec, and his fast walking speed was 1.2 m/sec. Double limb support time decreased from 0.34 to 0.18 sec for self-selected speed and from 0.21 sec to 0.14 sec for fast speed. Concomitantly, step lengths increased from 0.48 m to 0.60 m and from 0.62 m to 0.68 m for self-selected and fast speeds. One month later, his self-selected walking speed had increased to 1.2 m/sec and fast speed to 1.5 m/sec, indicating continued improvement in community ambulation, even after the treadmill-based training had ceased.

This case study demonstrates a locomotor recovery program targeting stepping, dynamic equilibrium, and adaptability while training in both the treadmill and overground environments for an individual with a motor-incomplete SCI. Though this person had a relatively mild injury reflected in his AIS motor/sensory scores, the impact on his self-selected walking speed was certainly disabling for this 22-year-old man. His pretraining walking speed (0.56 m/sec) was 50% slower than an age-matched noninjured adult (1.2 m/sec). To achieve a normal walking speed through training was a significant clinical and meaningful achievement. Post-training, he was also able to walk without a cane and sustain forward propulsion with an upright posture at normal speeds for a 30-min duration, as well as change speeds and sustain his balance. In addition, he could now adapt to self-directed changes in speed and step length, as well as negotiate obstacles without dependence on a cane.

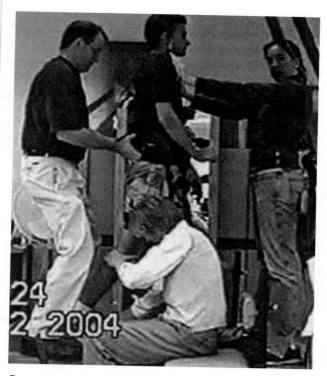

Figure 13-13. Trainer positions during locomotor training is the subject of the case report. Trainers assist with limb advancement, pelvic rotation, and maintenance of upright posture.

Continued

CASE STUDY 13-1   Locomotor Training for an Individual With Motor-Incomplete SCI—cont'd

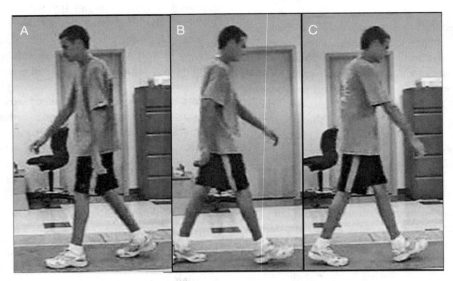

Figure 13-14. Case study post-training overground walking. Note improved step length and knee flexion on weight acceptance in early stance; subject is able to walk without use of a cane. Self-selected (A) and fast walking speeds (B, C) are illustrated.

Summary

In animal models of SCI, much is known about the properties and organization of the CPG associated with locomotion. While the evidence for spinal CPG for locomotion in humans is indirect, its existence clearly has support in the scientific literature. Despite the complex patterns of movement that can be produced autonomously by spinal CPGs, they do not function in isolation and are strongly influenced by sensory input.

From simpler circuits, such as the monosynaptic stretch reflex, to more complex networks, like the locomotor pattern generator, spinal cord circuits respond to training in a task-specific way. Locomotor training for individuals with SCI ostensibly requires engaging either the central or peripheral nervous system or both. Locomotor training using the permissive BWS-treadmill environment makes use of current knowledge about the neural control of locomotion and activity-dependent plasticity to improve walking function in individuals with SCI. Assistance for stepping may be accomplished by several means: providing manual assistance, electrically activating a flexor reflex response, or by a motorized robotic device. There is currently much interest in the possible applications of spinal cord stimulation in individuals with SCI. While this work is still in its early stages, it has the potential to make a meaningful contribution to improving walking function by increasing the effectiveness of the spinal circuitry underlying locomotion.

While this discussion has targeted the scientific evidence for means and mechanisms to restore and recover stepping for walking after SCI, walking is not limited to achieving a rhythmical stepping pattern. Functional walking requires the ability to produce reciprocal stepping, maintain balance and posture, and adapt to the environment. Advances in rehabilitation strategies to promote walking function and quality of life after SCI will also need to address achievement of the corequisite task of equilibrium while walking and train for adaptability within the locomotor task.

REVIEW QUESTIONS

1. What are locomotor CPGs, and what are their fundamental features within the nervous system?
2. What is the evidence for a locomotor CPG in humans?
3. What types of sensory information contribute to the control of locomotion?
4. How may sensory cues be used to promote activation of stepping responses in persons with SCI aiming to recover walking ability?
5. Compare and contrast overground versus treadmill-based locomotor training, and describe four ways that assistance for stepping may be provided.
6. What are the recommendations for training parameters for locomotor training?

7. What is the procedure for electrode placement for use in eliciting a flexion withdrawal response?

8. What are the forms of therapy or devices that currently provide upright mobility to persons with motor-complete SCI (including neuroprosthetic systems), what are their future directions, and how do these systems work to achieve walking?

9. What is the mechanism by which epidural stimulation is thought to promote improved locomotor function?

REFERENCES

1. Atrice MB, Morrison S, McDowell S et al. Traumatic spinal cord injury. In: Umphred DA, editor. *Neurological Rehabilitation*. 5th edition St. Louis: Mosby; 2005. pp. 605–657.

2. Burns SP, Golding DG, Rolle WA, Jr. et al. Recovery of ambulation in motor-incomplete tetraplegia. *Arch Phys Med Rehabil*. 1997;78(11):1169–1172.

3. Crozier KS, Cheng LL, Graziani V et al. Spinal cord injury: Prognosis for ambulation based on quadriceps recovery. *Paraplegia*. 1992;30(11):762–767.

4. Burns AS, Ditunno JF. Establishing prognosis and maximizing functional outcomes after spinal cord injury: A review of current and future directions in rehabilitation management. *Spine*. 2001;26:S137–S145.

5. Waters RL, Adkins R, Yakura J et al. Prediction of ambulatory performance based on motor scores derived from standards of the American Spinal Injury Association. *Arch Phys Med Rehabil*. 1994;75(7):756–760.

6. Waters RL, Adkins RH, Yakura JS et al. Motor and sensory recovery following incomplete tetraplegia. *Arch Phys Med Rehabil*. 1994;75(3):306–311.

7. Somers M. *Spinal Cord Injury: Functional Rehabilitation*. London: Prentice-Hall; 2001.

8. Barbeau H. Locomotor training in neurorehabilitation: Emerging rehabilitation concepts. *Neurorehabil Neural Repair*. 2003;17:3–11.

9. Forssberg H. Spinal locomotor functions and descending control. In: Sjolund B, Bjorklund RA, editors. *Brainstem Control of Spinal Mechanisms*. Amsterdam: Elsevier Science Publications; 1982. pp. 253–71.

10. Sherrington, C. S. Reflexes excitable in the cat from the pinna, vibrissae, and jaws. *J Physiol*. 1917;51:401–431.

11. Sherrington CS. Notes on the scratch reflex of the cat. *J Physiol*. 1910;3:213–220.

12. Sherrington CS. Observations on the scratch reflex in the spinal dog. *J Physiol*. 1906;34:1–50.

13. Graham-Brown TG. The intrinsic factors in the act of progression in the mammal. *Proc Roy Soc Lond*. 1911;84:308–319.

14. Jankowska E, Jukes MG, Lund S et al. The effect of DOPA on the spinal cord. 5. Reciprocal organization of pathways transmitting excitatory action to alpha motoneurones of flexors and extensors. *Acta Physiol Scand*. 1967;70(3):369–388.

15. Jankowska E, Jukes MG, Lund S et al. The effect of DOPA on the spinal cord. 6. Half-centre organization of interneurones transmitting effects from the flexor reflex afferents. *Acta Physiol Scand*. 1967;70(3):389–402.

16. Grillner S, Zangger P. On the central generation of locomotion in the low spinal cat. *Exp Brain Res*. 1979;34:241–261.

17. Grillner S. Control of locomotion in bipeds, tetrapods and fish. In: Brookhart JM, Mountcastle VB, Brooks VB et al editors. *Handbook of Physiology—The Nervous System. Motor Control*. Bethesda. MD: American Physiological Society; 1981. pp. 1179–1236.

18. Field EC, Stein PS. Spinal cord coordination of hindlimb movements in the turtle: Interlimb temporal relationships during bilateral scratching and swimming. *J Neurophysiol*. 1997;78:1404–1413.

19. Field EC, Stein PS. Spinal cord coordination of hindlimb movements in the turtle: intralimb temporal relationships during scratching and swimming. *J Neurophysiol*. 1997;78:1394–1403.

20. Perreault MC, Enriquez-Denton M, Hultborn H. Proprioceptive control of extensor activity during fictive scratching and weight support compared to fictive locomotion. *J Neurosci*. 1999;19:10966–10976.

21. Stein PS, Victor JC, Field EC et al. Bilateral control of hindlimb scratching in the spinal turtle: Contralateral spinal circuitry contributes to the normal ipsilateral motor pattern of fictive rostral scratching. *J Neurosci*. 1995;15:4343–4355.

22. Duysens J, Van de Crommert HW. Neural control of locomotion; The central pattern generator from cats to humans. *Gait Posture*. 1998;7(2):131–141.

23. Jankowska E, Hammar I. Spinal interneurones; How can studies in animals contribute to the understanding of spinal interneuronal systems in man? *Brain Res Brain Res Rev*. 2002;40:19–28.

24. Fedirchuk B, Nielsen J, Petersen N et al. Pharmacologically evoked fictive motor patterns in the acutely spinalized marmoset monkey (Callithrix jacchus). *Exp Brain Res*. 1998;122:351–361.

25. Edgerton VR, Roy RR, Hodgson JA et al. Potential of adult mammalian lumbosacral spinal cord to execute and acquire improved locomotion in the absence of supraspinal input. *J Neurotrauma*. 1992;9 Suppl 1:S119–S128.

26. Dietz V. Spinal cord pattern generators for locomotion. *Clin Neurophysiol*. 2003;114:1379–1389.

27. Bussel B. Evidence for a spinal stepping generator in man. Electrophysiological study. *Acta Neurobiol Exp*. 1996;56(1):465–468.

28. Yang JF, Lam T, Pang MY et al. Infant stepping: A window to the behaviour of the human pattern generator for walking. *Can J Physiol Pharm*. 2004;82:662–674.

29. Paus T, Collins DL, Evans AC et al. Maturation of white matter in the human brain: A review of magnetic resonance studies. *Brain Res Bull*. 2001;54:255–266.

30. Calancie B, Needham-Shropshire B, Jacobs P et al. Involuntary stepping after chronic spinal cord injury. Evidence for a central rhythm generator for locomotion in man. *Brain*. 1994;117(Pt 5):1143–1159.

31. Basso DM, Beattie MS, Bresnahan JC. Descending systems contributing to locomotor recovery after mild or moderate spinal cord injury in rats: Experimental evidence and a review of literature. *Restor Neurol Neurosci*. 2002;20:189–218.

32. Whelan PJ. Control of locomotion in the decerebrate cat. *Prog Neurobiol*. 1996;49:481–515.

33. Drew T, Rossignol S. Phase-dependent responses evoked in limb muscles by stimulation of medullary reticular formation during locomotion in thalamic cats. *J Neurophysiol.* 1984;52:653–675.

34. Shik ML, Orlovsky GN. Neurophysiology of locomotor automatism. *Physiol Rev.* 1976;56(3):465.

35. Bussel B. Late flexion reflex in paraplegic patients. Evidence for a spinal stepping generator. *Brain Res Bull.* 1989;22(1):53–56.

36. Roby-Brami A. Effects of flexor reflex afferent stimulation on the soleus H reflex in patients with a complete spinal cord lesion: Evidence for presynaptic inhibition of Ia transmission. *Exp Brain Res.* 1990;81(3):593–601.

37. Bussel B, Roby-Brami A, Azouvi P et al. Myoclonus in a patient with spinal cord transection. Possible involvement of the spinal stepping generator. *Brain.* 1988;111 (Pt 5):1235–1245.

38. Schomburg ED, Petersen N, Barajon I et al. Flexor reflex afferents reset the step cycle during fictive locomotion in the cat. *Exp Brain Res.* 1998;122:339–350.

39. Minassian K, Jilge B, Rattay F et al. Stepping-like movements in humans with complete spinal cord injury induced by epidural stimulation of the lumbar cord: Electromyographic study of compound muscle action potentials. *Spinal Cord.* 2004;42:401–416.

40. Dimitrijevic MR. Evidence for a spinal central pattern generator in humans. *Ann N Y Acad Sci.* 1998;860:360–376.

41. Jilge B, Minassian K, Rattay F et al. Initiating extension of the lower limbs in subjects with complete spinal cord injury by epidural lumbar cord stimulation. *Exp Brain Res.* 2004;154:308–326.

42. Behrman AL, Nair PM, Bowden MG et al. Locomotor training restores walking in a nonambulatory child with chronic, severe, incomplete cervical spinal cord injury. *Phys Ther.* 2008;88:580–590.

43. Slotine JJ, Lohmiller W. Modularity, evolution, and the binding problem: A view from stability theory. *Neural Networks.* 2001;14:137–145.

44. Van de Crommert HW, Mulder T, Duysens J. Neural control of locomotion: Sensory control of the central pattern generator and its relation to treadmill training. *Gait Posture.* 1998;7:251–263.

45. Sillar KT. Spinal pattern generation and sensory gating mechanisms. *Curr Opin Neurobiol.* 1991;1:583–589.

46. Li WC, Soffe SR, Roberts A. Spinal inhibitory neurons that modulate cutaneous sensory pathways during locomotion in a simple vertebrate. *J Neurosci.* 2002;22: 10924–10934.

47. Andersson O, Grillner S. Peripheral control of the cat's step cycle. I. Phase dependent effects of ramp-movements of the hip during "fictive locomotion". *Acta Physiol Scand.* 1981;113:89–101.

48. Forssberg H. Stumbling corrective reaction: A phase-dependent compensatory reaction during locomotion. *J Neurophysiol.* 1979;42(4):936–953.

49. Pearson KG. Modification of transmission in reflex pathways during locomotion. *Curr Opin Neurobiol.* 1995;5: 786–791.

50. Forssberg H, Grillner S, Rossignol S. Phase dependent reflex reversal during walking in chronic spinal cats. *Brain Res.* 1975;85(1):103–107.

51. Duysens J, Tax AA, Nawijn S et al. Gating of sensation and evoked potentials following foot stimulation during human gait. *Exp Brain Res.* 1995;105:423–431.

52. Pang M, Yang J. Sensory gating for the initiation of the swing phase in different directions of human infant stepping. *J Neurosci.* 2002;22(13):5734–5740.

53. Dietz V. Gating of reflexes in ankle muscles during human stance and gait. *Prog Brain Res.* 1993;97:181–188.

54. Pearson KG, Collins DF. Reversal of the influence of group Ib afferents from plantaris on activity in medial gastrocnemius muscle during locomotor activity. *J Neurophysiol.* 1993;70(3):1009–1017.

55. Dietz V, Muller R, Colombo G. Locomotor activity in spinal man: Significance of afferent input from joint and load receptors. *Brain.* 2002;125:2626–2634.

56. Pang M, Yang JF. The initiation of the swing phase in human infant stepping: Importance of hip position and leg loading. *J Physiol.* 2000;528(2):389–404.

57. Bouyer LJ, Rossignol S. Contribution of cutaneous inputs from the hindpaw to the control of locomotion: 2. Spinal cats. *J Neurophysiol.* 2003;Aug 27.

58. Marco YCP, Jaynie P. Interlimb co-ordination in human infant steeping. *J Physiol.* 2001;533.2:617–625.

59. Wolpaw JR, Kieffer VA, Seegal RF et al. Adaptive plasticity in the spinal stretch reflex. *Brain Res.* 1983;267(1):196–200.

60. Wolpaw JR, O'Keefe JA. Adaptive plasticity in the primate spinal stretch reflex: Evidence for a two-phase process. *J Neurosci.* 1984;4:2718–2724.

61. Wolpaw JR, Lee CL. Memory traces in primate spinal cord produced by operant conditioning of H-reflex. *J Neurophysiol.* 1989;61(3):563–572.

62. Wolpaw JR. Operant conditioning of primate spinal reflexes: The H-reflex. *Neurophysiology.* 1987;57(2):443–459.

63. Wolpaw JR, O'Keefe JA, Noonan PA et al. Adaptive plasticity in primate spinal stretch reflex: Persistence. *J Neurophysiol.* 1986;55(2):272–279.

64. Segal RL, Wolf SL. Operant conditioning of spinal stretch reflexes in patients with spinal cord injuries. *Exp Neurol.* 1994;130(2):202–213.

65. Wolf S, Segal RL. Conditioning of the spinal stretch reflex: Implications for rehabilitation. *Physical Therapy.* 1990; 70(10):652–660.

66. Lovely RG, Gregor RJ, Roy RR et al. Effects of training on the recovery of full-weight-bearing stepping in the adult spinal cat. *Exp Neurol.* 1986;92(2):421–435.

67. de Leon RD, Hodgson JA, Roy RR et al. Full weight-bearing hindlimb standing following stand training in the adult spinal cat. *J Neurophysiol.* 1998;80(1):83–91.

68. Edgerton VR, de Leon RD, Tillakaratne N et al. Use-dependent plasticity in spinal stepping and standing. *Adv Neurol.* 1997;72:233–247.

69. Forssberg H. The locomotion of the low spinal cat. I. Coordination within a hindlimb. *Acta Physiol Scand.* 1980;108(3):269–281.

70. Forssberg H. The locomotion of the low spinal cat. II. Interlimb coordination. *Acta Physiol Scand.* 1980;108(3):283–295.

71. Carter MC, Smith JL. Simultaneous control of two rhythmical behaviors. II. Hindlimb walking with paw-shake response in spinal cat. *J Neurophysiol.* 1986;56:184–195.

72. Carter MC, Smith JL. Simultaneous control of two rhythmical behaviors. I. Locomotion with paw-shake response in normal cat. *J Neurophysiol.* 1986;56:171–183.

73. Drew T, Prentice S, Schepens B. Cortical and brainstem control of locomotion. *Prog Brain Res.* 2004;143:251–261.

74. Dobkin BH. Spinal and supraspinal plasticity after incomplete spinal cord injury: Correlations between functional magnetic resonance imaging and engaged locomotor networks. *Prog Brain Res.* 2000;128:99–111.

75. Winchester P, McColl R, Querry R et al. Changes in supraspinal activation patterns following robotic locomotor therapy in motor-incomplete spinal cord injury. *Neurorehabil Neural Re.* 2005;19:313–324.

76. Barbeau H, Blunt R. A novel interactive locomotor approach using body weight support to retrain gait in spastic paretic subjects. In: Wernig A, editor. *Plasticity of Motoneuronal Connections.* Amsterdam: Elsevier Science Publishers; 1991. pp. 461–74.

77. Barbeau H, Rossignol S. Recovery of locomotion after chronic spinalization in the adult cat. *Brain Res.* 1987;412: 84–95.

78. Barbeau H, Rossignol S. The effects of serotonergic drugs on the locomotor pattern and on cutaneous reflexes of the adult chronic spinal cat. *Brain Res.* 1990;514:55–67.

79. Dietz V, Colombo G., Jensen JL. Locomotor activity in spinal man. *Lancet.* 1994;344(8932):1260–1263.

80. Dietz V. Locomotor capacity of spinal cord in paraplegic patients. *Ann Neurol.* 1995;37(5):574–582.

81. Field-Fote E, Tepavac D. Combined use of body weight support, functional electric stimulation, and treadmill training to improve walking ability in individuals with chronic incomplete spinal cord injury. *Arch Phys Med Rehabil.* 2001;82(6):818–824.

82. Field-Fote EC, Tepavac D. Improved intralimb coordination in people with incomplete spinal cord injury following training with body weight support and electrical stimulation. *Phys Ther.* 2002;82:707–715.

83. Gardner MB, Holden MK, Leikauskas JM et al. Partial body weight support with treadmill locomotion to improve gait after incomplete spinal cord injury: A single-subject experimental design. *Phys Ther.* 1998;78(4):361–374.

84. Hornby TG, Zemon DH, Campbell D. Robotic-assisted, body-weight-supported treadmill training in individuals following motor incomplete spinal cord injury. *Phys Ther.* 2005;85(1):52–66.

85. Protas EJ, Holmes SA, Qureshy H et al. Supported treadmill ambulation training after spinal cord injury: A pilot study. *Arch Phys Med Rehabil.* 2001;82(6):825–831.

86. Wernig A, Muller S. Laufband locomotion with body weight support improved walking in persons with severe spinal cord injuries. *Paraplegia.* 1992;30(4):229–238.

87. Wernig A, Nanassy A, Cagol E. Laufband therapy based on "rules" of spinal locomotion' is effective in spinal cord injured persons. *Eur J Neurosci.* 1995;7(4):823–829.

88. Visintin M, Barbeau H. The effects of body weight support on the locomotor pattern of spastic paretic patients. *Can J Neurol Sci.* 1989;16(3):315–325.

89. Barbeau H, Ladouceur M, Mirbagheri MM et al. The effect of locomotor training combined with functional electrical stimulation in chronic spinal cord injured subjects: Walking and reflex studies. *Brain Res Rev.* 2002;40(1–3):274–291.

90. Barbeau H, Danakas M, Arsenault B. The effects of locomotor training in spinal cord injured subjects: A preliminary study. *Restor Neurol.* 1993;5:81–84.

91. Hicks AL, Adams MM, Martin GK et al. Long-term body-weight-supported treadmill training and subsequent follow-up in persons with chronic SCI: Effects on functional walking ability and measures of subjective well-being. *Spinal Cord.* 2005;43:291–298.

92. Dobkin B, Apple D, Barbeau H et al. Weight-supported treadmill vs over-ground training for walking after acute incomplete SCI. *Neurology.* 2006;66:484–493.

93. Behrman AL, Harkema SJ. Locomotor training after human spinal cord injury: A series of case studies. *Phys Ther.* 2000;80(7):688–700.

94. Visintin M, Barbeau H. The effects of parallel bars, body weight support, and speed on the modulation of the locomotor pattern of spastic paretic gait. A preliminary communication. *Paraplegia.* 1994;32(8):540–553.

95. Pohl M, Mehrholz J, Ritschel C et al. Speed-dependent treadmill training in ambulatory hemiparetic stroke patients: A randomized controlled trial. *Stroke.* 2002;33:553–558.

96. Sullivan KJ, Knowlton BJ, Dobkin BH. Step training with body weight support: Effect of treadmill speed and practice paradigms on poststroke locomotor recovery. *Arch Phys Med Rehabil.* 2002;83(5):683–691.

97. Harkema SJ, Hurley SL, Patel UK et al. Human lumbosacral spinal cord interprets loading during stepping. *J Neurophysiol.* 1997;77(2):797–811.

98. Oursler M, Hidler J. Effects of walking speed and body-weight support on walking ability in individuals with spinal cord injury. *Proceedings of the Annual Meeting of the American Physical Therapy Association.*, 2003.

99. Wetzel MC, Stuart DG. Ensemble characteristics of cat locomotion and its neural control. *Prog Neurobiol.* 1976;7: 1–98.

100. Duysens J. Inhibition of flexor burst generation by loading ankle extensor muscles in walking cats. *Brain Res.* 1980;187(2):321–332.

101. Grillner S, Rossignol S. On the initiation of the swing phase of locomotion in chronic spinal cats. *Brain Res.* 1978;146(2):269–277.

102. Andersson O, Grillner S. Peripheral control of the cat's step cycle. II. Entrainment of the central pattern generators for locomotion by sinusoidal hip movements during "fictive locomotion." *Acta Physiol Scand.* 1983;118:229–239.

103. Andersson O, Grillner S, Lindquist M et al. Peripheral control of the spinal pattern generators for locomotion in cat. *Brain Res.* 1978;150(3):625–630.

104. Conrad B, Benecke R, Carnehl J et al. Pathophysiologic aspects of human locomotion. In: Desmedt JE, editor. *Motor Control Mechanisms in Health and Disease.* New York: Raven Publishing; 1983. pp. 717–26.

105. Conrad B, Benecke R, Meinck HM. Gait disturbances in paraspastic patients. In: Delwaide PJ, Young RR, editors. *Clinical Neurophysiology in Spasticity. Vol. 1 Restorative Neurology.* Amsterdam: Elsevier Science Publishers; 1985. pp.155–174.

106. Ferris DP, Huang HJ, Kao PC. Moving the arms to activate the legs. *Exerc Sport Sci Rev.* 2006;34:113–120.

107. Kawashima N, Nozaki D, Abe MO et al. Effects of upper limb motions on locomotive motor outputs in persons with spinal cord injuries. *Soc Neurosci Abstr.* 2005;865.

108. Pang MY, Yang JF. Interlimb co-ordination in human infant stepping. *J Physiol.* 2001;533:617–625.

109. Behrman AL, Lawless-Dixon AR, Davis SB et al. Locomotor training progression and outcomes after incomplete spinal cord injury. *Phys Ther.* 2005;85: 1356–1371.

110. Hesse S, Malezic M, Schaffrin A et al. Restoration of gait by combined treadmill training and multichannel electrical stimulation in non-ambulatory hemiparetic patients. *Scand J Rehabil Med.* 1995;27:199–204.

111. Carnstam B, Larsson LE, Prevac TS. Improvement of gait following functional electrical stimulation. I. Investigations on changes in voluntary strength and proprioceptive reflexes. *Scand J Rehabil Med.* 1977;9(1):7–13.

112. Crone C, Nielsen J, Petersen N et al. Disynaptic reciprocal inhibition of ankle extensors in spastic patients. *Brain.* 1994;117(Pt 5):1161–1168.

113. Fung J, Barbeau H. Effects of conditioning cutaneomuscular stimulation on the soleus H-reflex in normal and spastic paretic subjects during walking and standing. *J Neurophysiol.* 1994;72:2090–2104.

114. Colombo G, Joerg M, Schreier R et al. Treadmill training of paraplegic patients using a robotic orthosis. *J Rehabil Res Dev.* 2000;37:693–700.

115. Colombo G, Wirz M, Dietz V. Driven gait orthosis for improvement of locomotor training in paraplegic patients. *Spinal Cord.* 2001;39:252–255.

116. Dietz V, Colombo G, Muller R. Single joint perturbation during gait: Neuronal control of movement trajectory. *Exp Brain Res.* 2004;158:308–316.

117. Hidler J, Wall A. Alterations in muscle activation patterns during robotic-assisted walking. *Clinical Biomech.* 2005;20:184–193.

118. Behrman AL, Bowden MG, Nair PM. Neuroplasticity after spinal cord injury and training: An emerging paradigm shift in rehabilitation and walking recovery. *Phys Ther.* 2006;86:1406–1425.

119. Stillings D. Electrical stimulation for drop foot, 1772. *Med Instrum.* 1975;9:276–277.

120. Kido TA, Stein RB. Short-term effects of functional electrical stimulation on motor-evoked potentials in ankle flexor and extensor muscles. *Exp Brain Res.* 2004;159:491–500.

121. Dai R, Stein RB, Andrews BJ et al. Application of tilt sensors in functional electrical stimulation. *IEEE Trans Rehabil Eng.* 1996;4:63–72.

122. Sheffler LR, Hennessey MT, Naples GG et al. Peroneal nerve stimulation versus an ankle foot orthosis for correction of footdrop in stroke: Impact on functional ambulation. *Neurorehabil Neural Repair.* 2006;20:355–360.

123. Burridge JH, Taylor PN, Hagan SA et al. The effects of common peroneal stimulation on the effort and speed of walking: A randomized controlled trial with chronic hemiplegic patients. *Clin Rehabil.* 1997;11:201–210.

124. Field-Fote EC, Lindley SD, Sherman AL. Locomotor training approaches for individuals with spinal cord injury: A preliminary report of walking-related outcomes. *J Neurol Phys Ther.* 2005;29:127–137.

125. Dobkin BH, Harkema S, Requejo P et al. Modulation of locomotor-like EMG activity in subjects with complete and incomplete spinal cord injury. *J Neurol Rehabil.* 1995;9:183–190.

126. Nash MS, Jacobs PL, Johnson BM et al. Metabolic and cardiac responses to robotic-assisted locomotion in motor-complete tetraplegia: A case report. *J Spinal Cord Med.* 2004;27:78–82.

127. Cohen MI, Beckley CD, Perez MX et al. Effect of locomotor training on respiratory function in individuals with incomplete cervical or thoracic spinal cord injury. *Cardiopulmonary Phys Ther.* 2005;31.

128. Bogie KM, Triolo RJ. Effects of regular use of neuromuscular electrical stimulation on tissue health. *J Rehabil Res Dev.* 2003;40:469–475.

129. Chaplin E. Functional neuromuscular stimulation for mobility in people with spinal cord injuries. The Parastep I System. *J Spinal Cord Med.* 1996;19:99–105.

130. Klose KJ, Jacobs PL, Broton JG et al. Evaluation of a training program for persons with SCI paraplegia using the Parastep 1 ambulation system. Part 1. Ambulation performance and anthropometric measures. *Arch Phys Med Rehabil.* 1997;78:789–793.

131. Winchester P. Physiologic costs of reciprocal gait in FES assisted walking. *Paraplegia.* 1994;32(10):680–686.

132. Daly JJ, Ruff RL. Electrically induced recovery of gait components for older patients with chronic stroke. *Am J Phys Med Rehab.* 2000;79(4):349–360.

133. Daly JJ, Ruff RL, Haycook K et al. Feasibility of gait training for acute stroke patients using FNS with implanted electrodes. *J Neurol Sci.* 2000;179:103–107.

134. Petrofsky JS. Functional electrical stimulation and the rehabilitation of the spinal cord-injured patient. *Adv Clin Rehabil.* 1987;1:115–136.

135. Petrofsky JS, Phillips CA. The use of functional electrical stimulation for rehabilitation of spinal cord injured patients. *Cent Nerv Syst Trauma.* 1984;1:57–74.

136. Kralj A, Bajd T, Turk R. Enhancement of gait restoration in spinal injured patients by functional electrical stimulation. *Clin Orthop Relat Res.* 1988;233:34–43.

137. Kralj A, Bajd T. *Functional Electrical Stimulation: Standing and Walking after Spinal Cord Injury.* Boca Raton, FL: CRC Press; 1989.

138. Kralj A, Bajd T, Turk R. Electrical stimulation providing functional use of paraplegic patient muscles. *Med Prog Technol.* 1980;7:3–9.

139. Marsolais EB, Kobetic R. Functional electrical stimulation for walking in paraplegia. *J Bone Joint Surg-Am.* 1987;69:728–733.

140. Creasey GH, Ho CH, Triolo RJ et al. Clinical applications of electrical stimulation after spinal cord injury. *J Spinal Cord Med.* 2004;27:365–375.

141. Agarwal GC, Gottlieb GL. Effect of vibration of the ankle stretch reflex in man. *Electroencephalogr Clin Neurophysiol.* 1980;49(1–2):81–92.

142. Mushahwar VK, Aoyagi Y, Stein RB et al. Movements generated by intraspinal microstimulation in the intermediate gray matter of the anesthetized, decerebrate, and spinal cat. *Can J Physiol Pharmacol.* 2004;82:702–714.

143. Prochazka A, Mushahwar V, Yakovenko S. Activation and coordination of spinal motoneuron pools after spinal cord injury. *Prog Brain Res.* 2002;137:109–124.

144. Carhart MR, He J, Herman R et al. Epidural spinal-cord stimulation facilitates recovery of functional walking following incomplete spinal-cord injury. *IEEE Trans Neural Syst Rehabil Eng.* 2004;12:32–42.

145. Herman R. Spinal cord stimulation facilitates functional walking in a chronic, incomplete spinal cord injured. *Spinal Cord.* 2002;40(2):65–68.

146. Field-Fote E. Spinal cord stimulation facilitates functional walking in a chronic, incomplete spinal cord injured subject. *Spinal Cord.* 2002;40:428.

Management of Respiratory Dysfunction

14

Jane L. Wetzel, PT, PhD

After reading this chapter, the reader will be able to:

OBJECTIVES

- Determine critical areas to prioritize in the physical therapy plan of care for individuals with spinal cord injury (SCI) based on respiratory function examination data
- Select interventions to address specific areas of respiratory dysfunction in individuals with spinal injuries
- Recognize signs and symptoms of respiratory muscle fatigue and inadequate ventilation in individuals with SCIs and suggest modifications to the physical therapy plan of care
- List important principles required for successful physical therapy treatment of the individual with SCI who requires mechanical ventilator support
- Discuss essential information with the health-care team, family, and individual with SCI in order to achieve optimal recovery of respiratory function
- Determine components of a comprehensive respiratory care program for lifetime management of respiratory dysfunction in individuals with spinal injuries

OUTLINE

Introduction

Respiratory dysfunction is one of the most devastating effects occurring after an injury to the spinal cord. Respiratory insufficiency is the primary cause of death in individuals sustaining high cervical spinal cord injuries (SCIs).[1] Paralysis of the respiratory muscles and poor ventilatory mechanics lead to atelectasis and decreased expiratory flow.[2] There is a decreased ability to mobilize secretions, allowing bacteria to accumulate and setting the stage for pneumonia. Among all respiratory causes of mortality in individuals with SCI, pneumonia is the most common.[1,3,4] However, recent reports indicate that individuals with chronic SCI have an increased prevalence of pathological vascular conditions due to inactivity while living with a disability.[5,6] Diseases of the cardiovascular system contribute to recurrent pulmonary emboli, pulmonary hypertension, and ischemic heart disease in those with long-standing tetraplegia.[5,7] Although the risk for mortality from respiratory disorders is greatest among individuals with tetraplegia, and especially older individuals, most individuals with paraplegia will also have decreased ventilatory capacity and limited airway clearance compared to their nondisabled counterparts.[3] Jackson and Groomes[3] reported more than 65% of those with paraplegia (T1 and below) had respiratory complications (pleural effusion, atelectasis, and pneumohemothorax) compared to 60% for those with injuries at C5–C8 (atelectasis, pneumonia, and ventilatory failure); however, the risks were highest in those with injuries at C1–C4, in whom 84% had respiratory complications.[3]

The role of the therapist includes implementing strategies for prevention of atelectasis and pneumonia as well as methods for optimizing the recovery of weakened muscles responsible for ventilation. In some cases, the effects of functional training may be limited by low ventilatory reserve and poor gas exchange. Therefore, the therapist must be aware of the individual's ventilatory limitation in order to modify treatment, select equipment that will enhance ventilation, and achieve quality cost-effective care. It is also important for the therapist to recognize the impact of chronic diseases of the cardiovascular and respiratory system in those living with SCI so

that long-term lifestyle modification strategies and education are offered to reduce the risk for mortality. The respiratory problems of the individual with a SCI will vary across the continuum of care, and the goals of therapeutic plan will need to be modified according to the stage of the injury (acute, rehabilitation, or chronic).

This chapter assumes that the reader has a thorough understanding of normal ventilation and respiration, a firm grasp of methods used to evaluate respiratory function, and a working understanding of how these methods would be applied to individuals with spinal cord injury. An on-line guide to these aspects of respiratory function and care, entitled *Respiratory Evaluation of Individuals with SCI*, is given on the FA Davis website (http://www.davisplus.fadavis.com). As a review, a glossary of common respiratory terms is provided in Appendix A. For ease of reading, only frequently recurring abbreviations will be used in this chapter.

Respiratory System Functions

The respiratory system has two components: (1) the gas exchanging organ (the lungs) and (2) the ventilatory pump (the contraction of respiratory muscles acting to deform a compliant chest wall to change the intrathoracic and intra-abdominal pressures).[8,9] As the respiratory muscles act on the chest wall, the resulting pressure changes cause air to move between the atmosphere and the lungs.[9] The muscles of ventilation are designed to work in a coordinated manner to expand the chest wall during inspiration and relax the chest wall during quiet expiration.

Normally, the muscles of respiration act on a mobile skeleton to create changes in pressure in the thorax, resulting in air movement into and out of the lungs. Air moving between the atmosphere and the lungs is referred to as *ventilation*, and gas exchange between the alveoli and pulmonary circulation is referred to as *respiration*. An individual must ventilate in order to respire. Most individuals with SCI will have ventilatory dysfunction due to muscle paralysis, while only those individuals with atelectasis, pneumonia, or lung tissue disorders will have respiratory dysfunction. Often, a problem with ventilation will lead to limitations in gas exchange and thereby respiratory impairment. When the chest expands, the intrathoracic pressure decreases and air moves into the lungs. Poor ventilatory pump mechanics and immobility are the underlying problems leading to atelectasis and pneumonia in the individual with SCI.[10] Understanding the mechanics of ventilation is critical to identifying the cause of respiratory problems and selecting effective therapeutic interventions in individuals who have sustained a SCI.

Impact of Spinal Injury Level on Mechanics of Breathing

Most breathing problems in individuals with SCI are the result of weakness or paralysis disrupting breathing mechanics. The clinical manifestations arising from muscle impairment will vary according to level and completeness of the injury.[23] Individuals with higher levels of injury having motor complete lesions have greater impairment than those with lower levels of injury or those with motor incomplete lesions.[13,23] Additionally, the ventilatory capacity will be influenced by age, pre-morbid conditions (lung disease or heart failure), and musculoskeletal injuries that may be unrelated to the SCI yet impact the ability to breathe.[50] Nevertheless, an understanding of the impact of level of injury on respiratory muscle function, lung volume, and breathing kinematics is important to lay the foundation for clinical decision making for individuals with SCI (*see* Table 14-1).

Respiratory function in individuals with SCI may be classified according to the amount of residual respiratory muscle function and ventilatory reserve available.[23,24] In these individuals, the ventilatory reserve is considered to be the volume by which the vital capacity (VC) exceeds tidal volume (TV). The more active residual respiratory muscle available, the larger the ventilatory reserve to support activity. Individuals with high cervical, motor complete injuries (C1–C4) will have little to no ventilatory reserve and consequently have the greatest risk for respiratory insufficiency or failure. These individuals may require at least part-time mechanical ventilator support.[51] Those with motor complete injuries between C1–C2 will have the least residual muscle function and require full-time ventilatory support. These individuals have no active diaphragm, abdominal, or intercostal muscles, but may have partial innervation of a few accessory muscles (sternocleidomastoid, upper trapezius, capital/cervical extensors). If the individual is briefly disconnected from the ventilator, the sternocleidomastoid muscles will actively lift the sternum if the head is stabilized. In this condition, VC = TV and falls well below 500 mL (comparatively, VC normally reaches approximately 5000 mL in nondisabled young men). These individuals have inadequate voluntary ventilation to support resting metabolism and no ability to cough.

Table 14-1
Level of Spinal Injury and Respiratory Functions[13,17,18,54,55,58,126,132,133]

Level of Injury	Muscles of Respiration	% Predicted FVC	MIP or NIF cm H₂O	MEP cm H₂O	Breathing Pattern	Chest Wall Expansion
C1–C2	Sternocleidomastoid (SCM) Upper trapezius, Capital extensors Cervical extensors	<10%	<−25 cm	<20 cm	SCM prominent with sternal rise if head is fixed.	Elevates sternum with minimal anterior-posterior expansion.
C3–C4	Scalenes, Levator scapulae, Upper trapezius Partial diaphragm	10%–40%	−20 to −35 cm	20–60 cm	SCM, scalenes lift sternum and first two ribs. Active diaphragm results in rib retraction (Litten's sign).	Sternum elevates, expands inferiorly and superiorly with minimal A-P expansion. Slightly negative (−1/4 inch)
C5	Diaphragm Pectoralis major Serratus anterior Rhomboids	35%–55%	−25 to −60 cm	30–70 cm	Diaphragmatic Belly rise with inspiration. Uses neck breathing and arm support when fatigued.	Negative (−1/4 to −1/2) Mostly expansion superiorly. Paradoxical breathing

Continued

Table 14-1

Level of Spinal Injury and Respiratory Functions—cont'd

Level of Injury	Muscles of Respiration	% Predicted FVC	MIP or NIF cm H$_2$O	MEP cm H$_2$O	Breathing Pattern	Chest Wall Expansion
C6–C8	Diaphragm Pectoralis major/minor Serratus anterior (upper and lower) Latissimus dorsi	40%–70%	−40 to −120 cm	30–80 cm	As above.	As with C5
T1–T4	Diaphragm & most accessory muscles Intercostals (few) Erector spinae	45%–75%	−50 to −120 cm	30–95 cm	Diaphragmatic Moderate belly rise Intercostal action promotes expansion.	Decreased anterior and lateral chest expansion (1/4–1-1/2 inches)
T5–T10	Diaphragm Intercostals Abdominal through segmental level	60%–95 %	>−75 cm*	50–160 cm	Diaphragmatic and chest wall movement. Minimal belly rise due to intact abdominal	Chest wall expansion is still slightly decreased. (1–2-1/2 inches)
T11 and below	All of the above	>80%	>−90 cm*	>120 cm	Equal diaphragm and chest wall motion	Chest wall expansion may be diminished slightly due to bowel impaction or decreased pelvic floor tone (2-1/2–3-1/2 inches)

*Extrapolated, no published reports. % Predicted FVC = forced vital capacity as %-age of normal predicted (varies with time of onset of injury; becomes stable 6–18 months post-injury). NIF = negative inspiratory force. MIP = maximal inspiratory pressure. MEP = maximal expiratory pressure (values vary with body position as vital capacity in sitting is less than in supine by 15–25 ml for cervical and high thoracic injuries, while vital capacity in sitting is greater than in supine by 10 ml for other thoracic injuries).

An individual with a motor complete cervical SCI at C3–C4 will have more accessory muscle activity (scalenes, levator scapulae, middle and lower trapezius) and will use a partially innervated diaphragm to generate an inspiratory effort. This individual may tolerate part-time removal from the ventilator but will fatigue easily. The VC may be greater than TV at rest for brief periods until the muscles of respiration fatigue. The breathing pattern includes neck breathing and some diaphragm activity. However, when the diaphragm contracts in the absence of abdominal and intercostal muscles, there may be slight negative chest wall expansion. Inward displacement or retraction of the intercostal muscles will confirm the presences of weak diaphragmatic contraction (Litten's sign).[52] Energy requirements for neck breathing may exceed the amount of oxygen supplied by the individual's inefficient effort, such that neck breathing opposes the goal of increasing oxygen supply to the body. Therefore, this type of breathing has been referred to as *paradoxical breathing*, since more energy is consumed by the respiratory muscles than is delivered to the individual (*see* Fig. 14-1a).[53]

As respiratory muscle fatigue occurs, neck breathing and respiratory rate (RR) increases, and head bobbing may be exhibited. The individual may appear lethargic, with the onset of hypercapnia (increased partial pressure of carbon dioxide [PaCO$_2$]). These are signs the individual needs to be returned to mechanical ventilation.

Individuals who use a ventilator will initially have an endotracheal tube connected to tubing that is connected to a mechanical ventilator. The endotracheal tube is temporary and is approximately 6 inches long, running from the mouth, past the glottis and vocal cords, and into the trachea. Most individuals who have a cervical or high

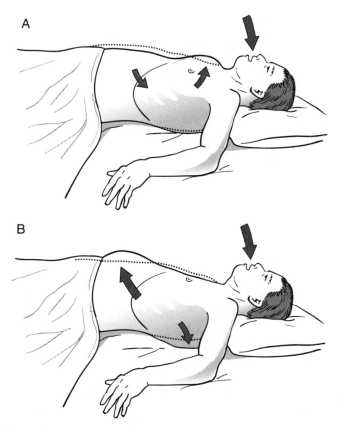

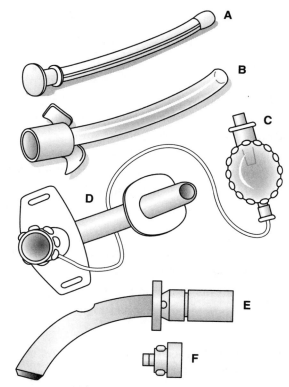

Figure 14-1. Paradoxical breathing patterns. (A) The individual with C2–C4 injury will display neck accessory breathing. (B) The individual with C5–C8 injury will display diaphragmatic breathing. (Redrawn with permission from: Massery M. The patient with neuromuscular or musculoskeletal dysfunction. In: *Principles and Practice of Cardiopulmonary Physical Therapy*, 4th edition Elsiever Mosby, 1996; Chapter 37.)

Figure 14-2. Tracheostomy tube and component parts. (A) Obturator (used to pass the tracheal tube into the trachea); (B) inner cannula; (C) pilot balloon (lies external to the patient to determine cuff inflation); (D) outer cannula with cuff in the inflated state; (E) fenestrated tracheostomy tube (allows airflow to vocal cords above); (F) decannulation cap or button (usually red in color).

thoracic injury will require intubation with an endotracheal tube until they are medically stable, at which time the tube will be removed (called *extubation*). Individuals requiring prolonged ventilator support will receive a tracheostomy (also called *tracheotomy*). A tracheostomy is a surgical incision in the trachea below the glottis and vocal cords through which a shorter tube is placed. A tracheostomy tube and component parts are shown in Figure 14-2. The characteristics of the different component parts are described in Table 14-2. If the individual is receiving part-time ventilation, then the tracheostomy may be "capped off" (usually with a red decannulation cap) when disconnected from the mechanical ventilator.

The individual with a motor complete cervical lesion between the levels of C5 and C8 will have a much improved ventilatory capacity relative to higher level injuries, as there is innervation of the functional scapular stabilizers, the pectoralis major and minor, and serratus anterior muscles that assist with ventilation. VC exceeds TV, and inspiratory volume is adequate for deep breathing, freeing most individuals from need for mechanical

ventilation. Although the diaphragm may be fully innervated, diaphragmatic contraction is not optimal due to the lack of abdominal muscle tone and lack of intercostal muscle activation. VC, maximal inspiratory pressure (MIP), and maximal expiratory pressure (MEP) are well below normal values,[18,54,55] especially in the acute stage.[56–58]

In the sitting position, VC is further diminished compared to supine position because the dome of the diaphragm is flattened as the abdominal contents fall forward and pull down on the central tendon (into which the muscles of the diaphragm insert). This positioning therefore disturbs the length–tension relationship of the diaphragm and limits its excursion, resulting in an inefficient pattern of ventilation. As the diaphragm contracts, it pulls the lower ribs inward without opposition from the abdominal or intercostal muscles. A decrease in transverse chest wall motion occurs with inspiration. Because the chest wall dimension decreases, this motion works against the desired chest wall expansion during inspiration and increases the oxygen cost of breathing for individuals with tetraplegia.[59,60] This breathing pattern is another form of paradoxical breathing (see Fig. 14-1b).[53] In the sitting position, both the breathing pattern and VC can be improved for those with motor complete

Table 14-2
Types of Tracheotomy Tubes and Components

Cuffed Tube

Used initially after formation of the tracheostomy

Cuff is inflated, providing protection of the airway from excess secretions

In individuals on mechanical ventilation, ensures that air reaches the lungs and does not escape through the larynx

Cuff pressure dynamically adjusted at the points of contact with the trachea during the breathing cycle, thereby minimizing trauma to the trachea

Used when there is a risk of secretions entering the airway as inflated cuff reduces the risk of aspiration

May be fenestrated or nonfenestrated

Decannulation caps not used with an inflated cuff as the individual would be unable to breathe

Uncuffed Tube

Used when the patient does not need precisely controled ventilation parametrs

Used when no risk of patient aspirating

Used on patients with head and neck tumours

May be fenestrated and nonfenestrated

Fenestrated Tube

Has a hole in the back wall of the tube allowing air to pass through the oral/nasal pharynx as well as the tracheal stoma when breathing

Assists in return to normal breathing as can breathe through the fenestrations of the tube as well as around it

May be used with cuffed or uncuffed tubes

An uncuffed fenestrated tube used in ventilator discontinuation training

Inner Cannula

Reduces risk of tracheostomy tube becoming blocked by secretions

Increases ease of secretion removal

Reduces frequency of need for change of full tracheostomy tube

Speaking Valve

A one-way valve that closes upon exhalation, redirecting exhaled gas into the upper airway, thereby allowing for vocalization

Different types of speaking valves available, each with different characteristics

Speaking valves not used with tubes having an inflated cuff as the individual would be unable to breathe

---

cervical and high thoracic injuries through the use of an abdominal binder to contain the abdominal contents (Fig. 14-3; abdominal binders will be discussed in detail below.)[24,61-64] Absence of abdominal muscle contraction also contributes to weak cough function that may be inadequate for airway clearance. Therefore, the risk for respiratory complications remains high even though most individuals with SCI between C5 and C8 are eventually able to breathe without mechanical ventilation.[55]

Individuals with a high thoracic injury (T1–T4) will have some intercostal muscle function to provide modest stability of the chest wall during inspiration. Some individuals with injury at this level may still have negative chest wall expansion, but most will achieve some outward expansion during inspiration. Overall, the literature suggests that there is little difference in tests of pulmonary function

and respiratory muscle pressures for those with high paraplegia compared to cervical-level injuries.[18,54,55] However, the increase in amount of residual respiratory muscle function may provide protection against respiratory muscle fatigue by decreasing the inspiratory time (T_i) within the total breath cycle (T_{TOT}).[65] The RR may be lower than the rate observed in those with cervical injuries, but it is still elevated compared to nondisabled individuals.

The force-length and force-velocity principles of skeletal muscle also apply to the muscles of respiration.[9] Respiratory muscles can become weaker if the muscle fiber length–tension dynamics are altered. This occurs when the dome of the diaphragm is lost because there is no opposing abdominal muscle tone. The abdominal contents pull down on the central tendon of the diaphragm, thereby flattening this muscle when the individual is seated upright. This occurs in individuals with

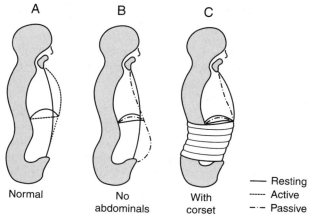

Figure 14-3. Influence of abdominal binder breathing dynamics. (A) Breathing pattern in an nondisabled individual. (B) Breathing pattern in an individual without diaphragm or abdominal muscle control. (C) Impact of the binder on the breathing pattern. (Redrawn with permission from: Alverez SE, Peterson M, Lundsford BR. Respiratory treatment of the adult patient with spinal cord injury. *Phys. Ther.* 1981;61(12): 1742.)

motor complete cervical or high thoracic SCI. Cough function remains markedly reduced with high thoracic injury, as there is limited inspiratory volume due to abnormal muscle length–tension relationships from poor breathing mechanics and absent abdominal muscle function for forced expiration.

Unlike other skeletal muscles, the respiratory muscles do not rest and are subjected to both elastic and resistive loads. The respiratory muscles will fatigue if the load demand is greater than the ability to supply repetitive force generation.[66] The fatigue may be one of two types: either neuromuscular transmission fatigue or skeletal muscle fatigue.[67] Skeletal muscle fatigue can occur when the rate of energy consumed by the muscle is greater than the rate of energy supplied to the muscle. When respiratory muscles carry a greater load (e.g., when they must work against a stiff chest wall or against secretions that restrict airflow), or if weaker muscles are acting excessively to substitute for the diaphragm, signs of fatigue may appear.

In individuals with cervical and high thoracic SCI, respiratory muscle fatigue may result in respiratory insufficiency. Since the respiratory muscles are life sustaining, fatigue may lead to the development of hypercapnia, respiratory insufficiency, and failure. (Fig. 14-4).[68] Respiratory muscle fatigue is a common occurrence in individuals with tetraplegia.[67,69] Signs of fatigue may not be noticeable upon initial examination; therefore the therapist reexamines each individual after he or she has been seated upright and functioning for awhile. One of the earliest signs of fatigue is an increase in RR and a change in breathing pattern.[67] It is especially important to monitor individuals who have recently been extubated or who have the tracheostomy site capped off.

Most individuals who have a thoracic injury below T5 will not require ventilatory support for survival in the acute stage. These individuals will usually not have had a tracheostomy. However, the expiratory function is not normal, and the cough may not be forceful. Chest wall expansion

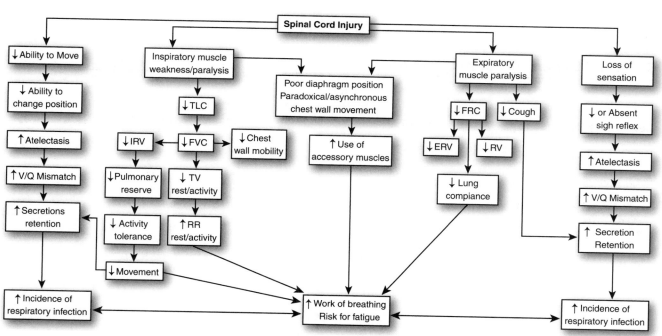

Figure 14-4. Factors contributing to respiratory insufficiency in patients with high thoracic and cervical SCIs. A person with a SCI will have multiple issues contributing to respiratory dysfunction. V/Q = Ventilation/perfusion; TLC = total lung capacity; FVC = forced vital capacity; IRV = inspiratory reserve volume; TV = tidal volume; RR = respiratory rate; FRC = functional residual capacity; ERV = expiratory reserve volume; RV = residual volume; ↑ = increase; ↓ = decrease. Reproduced in modified form with permission from: Peat M, editor. *Current Physical Therapy.* Philadelphia: BC Decker; 1988. p. 34.

measures may be diminished by weak pelvic floor muscles as well as by abdominal muscle weakness. Additionally, bowel impaction occurring in the acute stage can contribute to improper descent of the diaphragm and lower the VC.

Classification of Respiratory Dysfunction

Individuals with SCI have muscle paralysis that impairs lung volume and capacity for breathing; they may be at risk for acquiring respiratory complications and will need a program that includes interventions to prevent them. The problem is primarily one of poor ventilation, which can result in secondary respiratory complications, producing hypercapnia and hypoxemia (decreased partial pressure of oxygen [PaO_2], the gas pressure of oxygen in the arterial blood). Hypercapnia is a sign that the individual is underventilated (musculoskeletal pump failure), whereas hypoxemia usually indicates a problem with lung tissue and gas exchange. The therapist uses the clinical presentation to assist in classifying the individual for physical therapy diagnoses and selection of interventions using the *Guide to Therapist Practice*.[70] Individuals with a SCI who have impaired ventilation and respiration may classified as having either *impaired ventilation and respiration associated with ventilatory pump dysfunction or failure* (practice pattern 6E) or *impaired ventilation and respiration associated with respiratory failure* (practice pattern 6F).[20,51]

Using the guide's classification system, if muscle paralysis is the core reason for the breathing problem, then the individual with SCI would be classified as having impaired ventilation and respiration associated with ventilatory pump dysfunction or failure.[20] Ventilatory pump failure is distinct from ventilatory pump dysfunction; ventilatory pump dysfunction occurs when the respiratory muscle function is abnormal, resulting in limitations to exercise training and higher functioning, while ventilatory pump failure restricts routine activities of daily living.[20,51,71] In such cases, TV breathing is sustainable without ventilator support, but TV may not be adequate during activity. The VC in an individual with ventilatory pump dysfunction or failure is usually more than 10 to 15 mL/kg of ideal body weight ($\geq$500 to 1000 mL). Individuals with SCI can comfortably sustain function when they have a VC of at least 1500 mL, or 30% of the normative value. Individuals who are free from ventilator support may be using inefficient paradoxical breathing patterns or have difficulty sustaining activities of daily living due to limited ventilatory reserve. These individuals require respiratory muscle reeducation and training as a significant part of their rehabilitation program.

Conversely, individuals will be classified as having impaired ventilation and respiration associated with respiratory failure if the examination reveals an elevated RR (>35 breaths per minute), a low VC (<10 to 15 mL/kg of ideal body weight), and/or low MIP (<–25 cm H_2O), or any other signs and symptoms suggestive of respiratory muscle fatigue and failure. Individuals falling into this classification will require close monitoring by the health-care team (physicians, nurses, and respiratory therapists) and assistance from a mechanical ventilator. The signs and symptoms associated with respiratory muscle fatigue that may determine the need for mechanical ventilation are summarized Table 14-3.[10]

Table 14-3
Signs and Symptoms of Respiratory Muscle Fatigue[51,101,102]

Respiratory Parameters	Signs	
	Normal	Mechanical Ventilation with O₂ Necessary
$PaCO_2$ (mm Hg)	35–45	>50
PaO_2 (mm Hg)	75–100	<50
Respiratory rate (breaths per minute)	12–20	>35
VC (ml/kg IBW)	60–75	<10–15
MIP (cm H₂O)	–75 to –100	0 to –25
PaO_2/FiO_2 ratio	$\geq$380	<250

Symptoms

Increased use of accessory muscles
Dyssynchronous breathing
Respiratory alternans (shifting between muscle groups for breathing)

> ### Table 14-3
> ## Signs and Symptoms of Respiratory Muscle Fatigue[51,101,102] —cont'd
>
> Paradoxical breathing (new onset)
> Increased RR
> Shallow breathing; decreased TV
> Head bobbing
> Gray appearance
> Lethargy
> Decrease memory or cognitive functioning
> Inability to use upper extremities effectively for function
> Frequent requests for repositioning
>
> $PaCO_2$ = partial pressure of arterial blood carbon dioxide tension; PO_2 = Partial pressure of arterial oxygen tension; VC = vital capacity; ml/kg/IBW = volume in milliliters per kilogram of body weight for the individual's ideal body weight; MIP = maximum inspiratory pressure; FiO_2 = fraction of oxygen in the inspired air

This classification also applies when atelectasis, pneumonia, or other respiratory complications (e.g., trauma, pneumothorax, effusions, or other airway clearance dysfunction) overwhelm a weakened ventilatory system, producing high RR (>35 breaths/minute) and elevated $PaCO_2$ (>50 mm Hg), with dyssynchronous or paradoxical breathing and dyspnea at rest.[51] In such cases, at least partial ventilator support is necessary to manage respiratory failure. When airways are compromised or there is extensive atelectasis, the result may be a ventilation–perfusion mismatch, as well as low PaO_2 and low oxyhemoglobin saturation (SaO_2, a measure of the proportion of hemoglobin-carrying sites that are occupied by oxygen) in arterial blood. Supplemental oxygen may be required in these cases. Often, ventilator support is sufficient to correct the blood gas levels and reverse temporary hypercapnia and hypoxemia; this support may be delivered noninvasively, using a mask rather than a tracheostomy.

During the acute and subacute stages of recovery, it is the goal of the health-care team to advance the respiratory function of the individual classified as having respiratory failure to the classification of ventilatory pump dysfunction.[70] The therapist must be cognizant of the fact that individuals may revert from one classification to another and be prepared to estimate a longer period of rehabilitation for those with marginal respiratory status. Individuals who have recurrent respiratory illnesses, elevated temperatures, inconsistent breathing strategies, signs of respiratory muscle fatigue with elevated RRs, poor arterial blood gas (SaO_2 or end tidal carbon dioxide [$ETCO_2$]), and abnormal lab values (white blood cells or hematocrit) will require more time to recover.

Physical Therapy Diagnosis and Prognosis

The purpose of establishing a physical therapy diagnosis is to use the information obtained from the examination to determine which problems may be improved through physical therapy and to identify issues that need to be managed in order to achieve the best outcome during the rehabilitation period. Possible problems that may be identified in the examination session include the following:

- Decreased vital capacity
- Impaired or absent cough function
- Respiratory complications (present or increased risk)
- Decreased chest wall expansion
- Intolerance to upright sitting position
- Increased work of breathing and risk of respiratory muscle fatigue, including
  - Increased RR
  - Inefficient breathing pattern
  - Chest wall stiffness and poor breathing mechanics
- Limited respiratory muscle endurance and reserve for activity

When determining the prognosis for the individual with SCI, the time required for rehabilitation of the respiratory system will vary with the level of injury and the severity of the injury (i.e., degree of completeness or incompleteness).[14,18] While there is ample evidence documenting the relationship between severity of respiratory dysfunction and the level of injury (high cervical through midthoracic), the therapist must consider the examination findings for each individual when projecting the required rehabilitation time and potential for recovery. Individuals with less ventilatory reserve will be those with decreased VC, paradoxical breathing patterns, negative or limited chest wall mobility, poor airway clearance, dyspnea, and elevated RRs at rest or during usual activities of daily living. These individuals will require greater emphasis on recovery of respiratory function within the therapeutic plan of care as well as education for development of a lifelong strategy for management of their respiratory function.

The therapist will also need to consider other confounding factors such as co-morbidities (obesity, multisystem injuries), smoking history, and age-related factors that may prolong the time to recovery. When developing the plan of care, the therapist considers whether the individual will be chronically living with respiratory impairments and marginal airway protection or whether he or she will recover enough ventilatory reserve to support community level functioning. This is determined by asking questions such as: Does the individual have potential to recover a lot of residual muscle? Can the individual return to activities that require a high volume of air exchange (i.e., high minute ventilation) (walking and functioning upright)? Adequate ventilatory reserve will need to be developed to support higher activity levels. Incorporating exercise training and conditioning into the therapeutic plan can accomplish this goal.

The recommended plan of care will also vary depending on the individual's stage of recovery and the point in the continuum of health-care delivery at which the referral for physical therapy is initiated. Some therapists will examine individuals with SCI the day after injury in the acute care setting, and other therapists may be performing an evaluation in the home or in an outpatient clinic months after the initial injury. The acuity of the injury and the prior medical and rehabilitation management offered to the individual will influence the plan of care. The stage of recovery will also dictate which tests and measures the therapist will select to determine the status of the respiratory system and monitor the efficacy of the therapeutic plan.

To improve respiratory function for individuals with SCI, the plan of care is generally directed toward

- optimizing ventilation and gas exchange,
- clearing secretions,
- preventing respiratory infections,
- mobilizing the chest wall,
- providing optimal musculoskeletal alignment and posture,
- preventing respiratory muscle fatigue, and
- improving respiratory muscle performance.

The priorities in treatment will shift as different impairments pose limitations for the individual. Limiting factors are best determined by integrating the examination findings from physical therapy with those of other disciplines. In many cases, other health-care professionals may provide information from their assessments that will influence the overall plan for respiratory management. The stage of recovery may be acute, subacute/ rehabilitative, or chronic, and the respiratory management plan will change as the individual moves through each stage.

It is critical to address respiratory dysfunction at the onset of a SCI; therefore, most of the interventions are offered in the acute stage and are continued through the subacute or early rehabilitation stage of recovery. Further enhancement of respiratory function is continued during the rehabilitation stage, where more aggressive techniques are employed. Once the respiratory status has stabilized and the rehabilitation goals are met, the discharge plan will include family and caregiver training for lifetime management of respiratory function.

The Acute Stage

When the therapist receives a request to evaluate an individual in the acute stage after a SCI, it is important to identify the role of physical therapy within the context of the entire scope of care and all the medical management priorities. The role of physical therapy will vary depending on the individual's medical status. Initially in acute care, the individual may be in one of three stages with respect to respiratory function and medical stability.

1. Survival stage
2. Optimization of ventilation and gas exchange stage
3. Functional training stage

The first stage is the survival stage. During this stage, the health-care team is focused on keeping the individual alive. The individual is likely to have extensive invasive support. Here, the role of the physical therapist is that of prevention. The therapist provides range-of-motion exercise for contracture prevention, muscle protection strategies to avoid overstretch, body positioning for prevention of pressure sores, and positioning as treatment for any atelectasis and/or pneumonia. Enhancement of ventilation and perfusion occurs through passive positioning, postural drainage, and gentle external manipulation (percussion and vibration if there are no spinal- or trauma-related precautions). Some individuals will be on paralytic agents and ventilation support to decrease metabolic demands associated with breathing. Exercise requiring active contraction of peripheral muscle is unwanted during this period as the potential increase in energy requirements may result in anaerobic metabolism that damages the cells.

Once it has been determined that survival is likely, the focus turns toward the second stage: optimizing gas exchange. The therapist can now offer active airway-clearance training (coughing techniques), breathing exercises (progressing from facilitation of active efforts, to active exercise, and then to resistive breathing retraining), more aggressive body positioning, and mobilization to the upright position in the wheelchair. When and if the individual has achieved optimal ventilation and gas exchange at rest, the individual may be considered ready for the functional training; breathing strategies for optimizing ventilation during upright functioning are offered at this time.

During the third stage, functional training treatments are designed to challenge the neuromuscular system in an effort to restore function. Ventilation needs are increased, and the therapist incorporates physiological monitoring of the cardiovascular and pulmonary system responses to determine safe progression of activity. Training activities designed to improve strength in residual muscle increase the metabolic demand for oxygen and requirements for ventilation, thus increasing the work of breathing. The respiratory muscles need to be supp-orted during functional training, and any ventilator support should not be discontinued during this time. To optimize the treatment session, the therapist should plan to keep any individual with marginal respiratory function on the ventilator during functional training. Therefore, respiratory muscle rehabilitation initially occurs at a time dif-ferent from that of functional train-ing. Programs designed to increase respiratory muscle performance need to occur during a time when the individual can attend fully to the action of breathing. This is important initially during the acute stage so that all muscles are appropriately stressed but also given an opportunity to rest. In this next section, each thera-peutic intervention will be described, including qualify-ing the evidence and correctly identifying which individuals may benefit from the use of each therapeutic strategy.

Therapeutic Interventions

Regardless of the intervention, the principles of treat-ment for the individual with respiratory dysfunction are constant. Three areas must be addressed in proper sequence.[23] The three areas are

- bronchial hygiene,
- chest mobility, and
- respiratory muscle performance.

The airways must be clear and free from secretions prior to offering any breathing retraining activities or before beginning ventilator discontinuation.[167] Similarly, the chest wall must be mobile and relatively easy to deform if the respiratory muscles are to func-tion optimally. For this reason, chest mobilization interventions will follow treatment of bronchial hygiene and precede efforts to improve respiratory muscle performance.

Many interventions address more than one of the three areas and may offer different benefits or outcomes depending on the individual's potential for recovery and presenting respiratory issues. Improving bronchial hygiene and chest mobility may decrease the ventilatory load, while techniques focused on increasing respiratory muscle performance improve the ventilatory capacity. The correct selection and use of therapeutic interven-tions will restore the balance between load and capacity, provide for a good ventilatory reserve, and prevent respi-ratory muscle failure. Other interventions, such as body positioning, are directed toward improving gas transfer across the alveoli to the pulmonary capillary rather than ventilatory functions. Complete details citing the quality of the evidence supporting each intervention are beyond the scope of this chapter. There are several extensive evidence-based reports on respiratory management for individuals with SCI.[142,156,168]

Prescriptive Body Positioning

When the therapist receives a referral for rehabilitation for an individual with SCI, the initial thoughts may be of strength and functional assessments. While much of the examination will include assessments of strength, range of motion, and sensation, these tests cannot be performed effectively if the individual cannot breathe. Rehabilitation sessions can be maximized when the therapist optimally manages respiratory status; recog-nizing the importance of selecting a body position that will optimize ventilation as the first step for any physi-cal therapy session. Most individuals with SCI will breathe better in supine than upright or seated posi-tions,[18] therefore it is important to keep the individual in supine position initially.

Functional assessments typically begin with assess-ment of range of motion, strength testing, and bed mobility as the therapist works within the medical pre-cautions related to spine stabilization and restrictions associated with surgical postoperative protocols. These very actions are also important to assist recovery of the respiratory system. Even if the individual is dependent in bed mobility, gentle turning and repositioning in bed may offer excellent therapeutic benefits to the individual who has significant respiratory dysfunction.[169,170] Turning in bed will "stir up" the respiratory system, encourage coughing, and move secretions from dependent regions of the lungs.[171] Turning and prescriptive positioning are recommended for those who are supported with a venti-lator as well as those who are free from ventilator sup-port.[172] These actions are designed to improve gas exchange, clear secretions, and prevent infection.

The therapist uses heart rate (HR), RR, and SaO_2 as outcome measures to identify optimal positions. This approach is referred to as *response-dependent treatment*,[172] wherein the therapist interprets the measures of physio-logic status (HR, RR, SaO_2, or electrocardiogram [EKG]), along with any medical information (chest x-rays, ventilation–perfusion studies, arterial blood gasses, pulmonary function tests) to determine the effec-tiveness of each change in position. The optimal position and tolerance to treatment can be documented and pre-scribed for the individual. The therapist allows at least 2 minutes for recovery after a change in position before interpreting and documenting new baseline measures.[167] The therapist also observes the breathing pattern to determine if the proper muscles are being recruited for specific position (e.g., greater use of diaphragm and chest muscles, and less use of neck and accessory muscles of breathing if sensory testing and muscle exam indicate the presence of diaphragm function). Later, when the indi-vidual is medically cleared for extreme changes in intrathoracic pressure and vigorous coughing, the ideal body position can be further evaluated by testing the VC or MIP/MEP in various positions. This usually occurs in the rehabilitation stage.

Mechanical ventilation preferentially ventilates and distends the uppermost or least-dependent airways, neglecting expansion of more dependent regions.[9,173] This places the dependent airways at risk for atelectasis and respiratory complications. In order to address this problem, the individual can be placed in a modified head-down position so that the effects of gravity are used to increase opening pressure in the lower regions. The shallow Trendelenberg position (15 degrees) has been shown to improve recruitment of the lower airways in those with cervical SCI who require ventilator assistance for respiration.[167] Cameron et al[174] first reported VC was increased with head-down positioning in individuals with tetraplegia. Initially, the individual with motor complete tetraplegia, striving to breathe independently from the ventilator, will benefit from a supine position. Conversely, the individual with a midthoracic or lumbar injury will breathe more efficiently in the upright position.[18] In individuals with more caudal levels of injury, more residual muscle is available, so breathing mechanics are normalized and ventilation is facilitated by elevation of the head or sitting upright.

Although research has demonstrated that prone positioning offers advantages over supine positioning in those with acute lung injury and respiratory failure,[51,175] there are no studies specifically addressing these benefits in individuals with SCI. Prone positioning may be difficult for individuals who have spine precautions.[175] However, rotational beds are effective in managing spine precautions while turning the individual and will reduce the incidence of respiratory complications.[176,177] Once the individual is wearing a halo vest that stabilizes the spine, prone positioning is possible.[51] The health-care team must be well coordinated and understand the complications and adjuncts that must be managed during turning and positioning.[175] The prone position may limit diaphragmatic excursion in some individuals, whereas it may improve diaphragmatic excursion in others. Theoretically, the abdominal contents are contained when the individual is in the prone position, and therefore there should be improvement in diaphragm excursion in those with higher injuries. This is because when the abdominal contents are contained in the prone position, the resting position of the diaphragm moves up in the thoracic cavity. Careful monitoring of the RR, $ETCO_2$, and SaO_2 assist in determining whether this position is efficacious. Lying prone may also assist in preventing flexion contractures of the hips and knees, as well as provide an alternative position for pressure relief.

Tracheal Suctioning and Postural Drainage

Early in the acute stage, positioning will assist in opening the alveoli in the uppermost regions. Passive drainage of airways will occur, facilitating the transport of secretions toward major airways (main-stem bronchi and trachea). Many individuals with higher spinal cord lesions will have hyperresponsive airways and increased mucous production.[142,156] SCI results in a loss of effective cough function for most individuals. Yet, the medical status of the individual may be too acute (having spine precautions or chest trauma and medical management with paralytic agents) to permit training in manual cough techniques (discussed below). Initially, individuals with cervical injuries are intubated with an endotracheal tube, which is subsequently converted to a tracheostomy within 3 weeks if ventilator support becomes prolonged.[142] If this is the case, the individual then receives a tracheostomy with an inflated cuff and is placed on a form of positive pressure ventilation (wherein air is pushed into the lungs). The cuff provides accurate ventilation management and prevents aspiration of fluid into the lungs. Prevention of fluid aspiration is important, as the prevalence of swallowing dysfunction and potential aspiration is reported in about 22.5% of individuals with cervical SCI[178] after discharge from the acute care setting. The therapist plans for suctioning of the individual's tracheostomy prior to mobilization, body positioning, or application of interventions for respiratory muscle conditioning.

Infection is a major concern for those with a tracheostomy. The condition of the tracheostomy is described as being either acute or chronic. Acute tracheostomies have not been colonized (bacteria are not yet established, no antibodies developed), and the risk for infection is high (for about 8 weeks). Sterile suctioning procedures must be used. Later, after the tracheostomy has healed, risk of infection declines, and a clean technique may be used during suctioning. Suctioning is performed by nursing staff in many acute care settings. However, therapists and, eventually, caregivers may be trained to suction the individual, especially when there is a chronic tracheostomy. In many acute care settings, a multidisciplinary suction catheter may be used for suctioning. This type of catheter is not disposed of after each use, but lies in line at a 90-degree angle with the ventilator tubing to allow immediate secretion removal (see Fig. 14-5). The suction line is attached to wall suction. Suction pressures are usually set at approximately 120 mm Hg in most adults. If the individual is being treated on the rehabilitation floor or at home, a portable suction unit may be used.

Precautions must be considered whenever suctioning is applied to an individual with a tracheostomy. Tracheal suctioning can produce transient hypoxia that may lower oxygen in the arterial blood, precipitating cardiac arrhythmias. Additionally, stimulation of the vagus nerve may occur, producing a bradycardic rhythm. Manual hyperinflation of the lungs, using an insufflation device or bag (discussed in detail below), can add inspiratory volume to prevent decreased SaO_2, as well as provide adequate airflow through collateral airways.[179] Removal of secretions is optimized when air moves behind secretions prior to expulsion. This technique is often applied prior to suctioning airways, as suctioning will likely

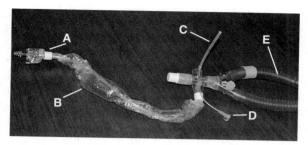

Figure 14-5. Multidisciplinary suction catheter. (A) Control valve for applying suction manually; (B) plastic sleeve to facilitate operation when advancing the catheter; (C) catheter tip advanced forward halfway would enter the trache;a (D) the port to instill flushing solution or saline; (E) tubing connecting ventilator to the individual.

stimulate a coughing reflex. After hyperinflation and preoxygenation is provided, suctioning is used as part of a postural drainage and airway clearance program to clear secretions. If the individual has been medically cleared for high intrathoracic pressures, then a manual cough (discussed below) may be applied.

Postural drainage positions with manual external manipulation techniques (such as percussion and vibration) may assist the individual in removing secretions if these positions and techniques are tolerated. Proper hydration and humidification of the airways is critical for keeping the secretions thin and mobile. Humidification may be managed by external nebulizer treatments or through a device set up within the ventilator tubing. Any respiratory therapy treatments should be performed prior to implementing the postural drainage program.

Prior to positioning, the therapist confirms radiographic reports of infiltrates and identifies areas to treat using auscultation. The postural drainage positions are modified depending on the individual's physiologic responses and medical precautions. For example, to adhere to spine precautions, the individual may be turned using log roll techniques. It is important to adhere to spine precautions and note the presence of rib fractures and other injuries to the thoracic cage when modifying procedures. Manual techniques will need to be gentle, yet applied with appropriate force. For individuals who have been fitted with a halo vest, a portion of the halo vest may be pulled back to expose the region of the chest requiring manual clearance techniques (gentle percussion or vibration).[51]

If the individual needs the abdomen to be unencumbered to maintain an optimal breathing strategy, then the prone position may not be tolerated. These individuals may be placed in a position that is three-quarters prone. The side-lying position may need to be modified to allow easy movement of the diaphragm. If the upper lung lobes are involved and upright positioning is indicated, then an abdominal binder may be necessary to maintain inspiratory volumes in those with tetraplegia. Upon completion of an airway clearance program, the color, quality, and

quantity of the secretions, as well as the region or lobe treated, are documented. Auscultation is performed after completion of the treatment. The therapist documents the presence of normal or clear breath sounds in the chart because bronchoscopy will be necessary in some individuals if airways do not clear with chest physical therapy.[51]

Early Management of Ventilator Support and Discontinuation (Weaning) Strategies

The physical therapist views the individual requiring ventilator support as someone who can greatly benefit from all the usual physical therapy treatments. Although the method by which the individual receives oxygen to support working muscles and metabolism has changed, the individual with SCI who needs ventilation support will still have the same rehabilitation goals as an individual with the similar level of injury who may not be supported by mechanical ventilation. These individuals should not be designated as "too sick" for physical therapy or seen as people whose needs can only be addressed by respiratory therapy. The therapist will want to consult with the members of the health-care team who are providing respiratory therapy, nursing, and medical care concerning management considerations (changes in ventilator settings, suctioning, timing of medications and assistance for mobilization activities, etc.) and request their assistance throughout the rehabilitation program. Early mobilization may be the key to success in freeing the individual from the ventilator. Because mobilization and exercise are the most efficacious treatments that can be offered to improve oxygen transport, it will be critical to get the individual upright and tolerant of the sitting position.[171] Additionally, for individuals who initially require mechanical ventilation, survival rate is greatly enhanced (84%) for those who are able to be discontinued from mechanical ventilation compared to survival rates (33%) for those who remain ventilator dependent.[180]

The health-care team will determine the ventilator discontinuation protocol, and it will be important for the therapist to understand whether the individual is succeeding with the protocol and what time of day ventilator discontinuation trials are scheduled. The therapist can then arrive at the right time and receive adequate support from the interdisciplinary team so the treatment session will be optimal. Individuals with spinal injury at C5 and below have intact diaphragm function and will probably achieve independent breathing. Those with C3–C4 have variable diaphragm function and may differ in their ability to discontinue ventilatory support. Individuals with a motor complete C1–C2 level of injury are not likely to be successful with ventilator discontinuation trials.[142] The mode of ventilator support (see Table 14-4) varies depending on the amount of spontaneous breathing the individual can perform and the presence of respiratory complications.

Individuals with high cervical injuries (C1–C2) with no diaphragm function will require complete ventilator support and will use control mode ventilation. Sometimes, respiratory muscle training programs are offered to such individuals with the goal of developing the ability to prolong the endurance time off the ventilator in case of accidental ventilator disconnection.[167] This out-come may also be achieved through the use of EMG biofeedback using electrode sensors on the neck accessory muscles, which are easily accessible for training.[181] Glossopharyngeal breathing may also offer the ability to spend some time off the ventilator (discussed below).[165] Ultimately, the individual with a high level of motor complete tetraplegia will need to remain on the ventilator full time and will achieve only brief periods of ventilator discontinuation during the acute and subacute rehabilitation periods. Later, some of these individuals may consider phrenic nerve or diaphragmatic electrical or magnetic stimulation (discussed below).[182]

For the individual with a C3–C4 level of injury, the approach to ventilator discontinuation requires constant monitoring for signs of fatigue, balancing periods of ventilator discontinuation with periods of rest. Peterson et al[183] described ventilator weaning methods in 52 subjects having C3 or C4 level injuries; 67.6% of subjects were successfully weaned with progressive ventilator-free breathing (i.e., T-piece) methods versus 34.6% who were weaned using intermittent mandatory ventilation methods.[2,183] Therefore, ventilator discontinuation trials preferentially use ventilator-free breathing sessions followed by periods of rest on mechanical ventilation using the high volume assist control mode. This strategy is recommended in the *Clinical Practice Guidelines* developed by the Consortium for Spinal Cord Medicine and is therefore the most common approach to ventilator discontinuation for individuals with high SCI.[2] Synchronized intermittent mandatory ventilation with pressure support ventilation, another common approach to ventilator discontinuation, provides a gradual lowering of the amount of ventilation support. This strategy does not offer as much rest for the respiratory muscles. Regardless of the mode used, therapists can recommend methods for supporting the head and trunk and positioning

Table 14-4
Ventilator Support Modes

	Parameters	Purpose	Clinical Considerations
Full Ventilatory Support Pressure-controlled ventilation	Preset: • Pressure limits • RR • Inspiratory time or inspiration-expiration (I/E) ratio Volume varies	Provides constant airway pressure, controlling for excessive damaging pressures.	May offer too little volume if lung compliance decreases. No guaranteed V_E Patient can initiate some breaths. Ventilator will deliver minimum number of breaths and does most of the work of breathing.
Full Ventilatory Support Volume-controlled ventilation or control mode ventilation	Preset: • TV • RR • Minute ventilation (V_E)	Provides a reliable V_E. All breaths are delivered by the ventilator.	Ventilator does all of the work of breathing. Respiratory muscles may rest; improved alveolar ventilation. Airway pressure increases during inspiration. Risk of barotrauma is increased.
Partial Support Assist control	Preset: • Number of breaths/min • Sensitivity: Amount of negative pressure required to trigger a breath • TV	The ventilator will support every breath, yet the patient may participate in initiating an increase in the number of breaths. The ventilator supports the patient-initiated breaths.	Allows the patient who is recovering some respiratory function to recruit muscles. May prevent atrophy. Some patients can work on diaphragmatic breathing.

Table 14-4
Ventilator Support Modes—cont'd

	Parameters	Purpose	Clinical Considerations
Partial Support Synchronized intermittent mandatory ventilation (SIMV)	Pre-set: • V_E: respiratory rate and TV will be delivered to meet minimum V_E • Sensitivity levels	Patient can initiate breaths that will be unassisted. The ventilator will synchronize some assisted breaths with the patient efforts.	Avoids breath-stacking and improves patient comfort over only intermittent mandatory ventilation. Allows increased patient participation. SIMV may contribute to respiratory muscle fatigue. Usually used in conjunction with PSV. Some patients can work on diaphragmatic breathing.
Partial Support Pressure support ventilation (PSV)	Pre-set: • Inspiratory pressure • Flow rate limits	Allows increased TV and lower respiratory rate. Assists spontaneous breathing more comfortably	Provides assistance to inspiratory muscles and decreases the work of breathing. Some patients can work on deep breathing and segmental breathing
Noninvasive Ventilation (NIV) or Noninvasive Positive Pressure Ventilation (NIPPV or NPPV) Continuous positive airway pressure (CPAP) also called "mouth positive"	Pre-set: • Pressure level: usually 5–10 cm H_2O	Delivers air during both inspiration and expiration as patient breathes spontaneously. Supports work of breathing and stabilizes airways.	May reduce risk of infection since patient does not have to have a tracheostomy. May use CPAP to resolve symptoms related to sleep apnea or assist with glossopharyngeal breathing training and assisted cough. Can be delivered via mask, mouthpiece or nasally.
Noninvasive Ventilation (NIV) or Noninvasive Positive Pressure Ventilation (NIPPV or NPPV) Bi-level positive airway pressure (Bi-PAP)	Preset: • Pressure levels: Separate settings for Inspiration (10–20 cm H_2O) Expiration (5–10 cm H_2O	Can add more support to inspiration during patient's spontaneous efforts than CPAP. Decreases work of breathing.	May reduce risk of infection since patient does not have to have a tracheostomy. May use Bi-PAP to resolve symptoms related to sleep apnea. Can be delivered via mask, mouthpiece, or nasally.

the arms, pelvis, and lower extremities, thereby increasing the chance for successful weaning.

When beginning ventilator discontinuation training in the individual with a C3–C4 injury, a supine position with elevation of the head and upper torso to about 15 degrees is recommended to keep the abdominal contents from encroaching on the diaphragm and to improve diaphragmatic function for early strengthening. Eventually, it will be necessary for the individual to tolerate ventilator discontinuation while in the sitting position. Therefore, the angle of the bed may be gradually progressed toward 60 degrees. As the individual with an injury at this level assumes a more erect posture, an abdominal binder is applied to assist diaphragm mechanics during the early stages of mobilization.[63] An intermittent abdominal compression system consisting of a bladder placed externally over the abdomen and inflated via noninvasive mechanical support, called a pneumobelt or exsufflation belt (Lifecare Inc., Lafayette, CO), may be applied for those with C3–C5 lesions to provide active assistance to the diaphragm while seated (Fig. 14-6).[23,24,184] The pneumobelt allows the diaphragm to be repositioned further up in the thoracic cavity, improving the length–tension relationship of a weakened diaphragm and using gravitational effects for inspiration.[185] The pneumobelt has been shown to increase TV breathing by 300 to 1200 mL.[184]

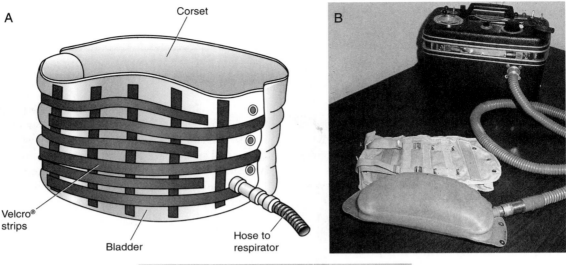

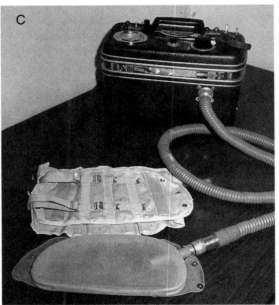

Figure 14-6. (A) A pneumobelt may be used to assist the diaphragm back to an optimal resting position. (B) The bladder inflates during exhalation pushing the diaphragm up in the thoracic cavity, and (C) deflates during inspiration. This device is helpful for individuals with impaired or partially innervated diaphragm (C3–C5).

Ventilatory muscle training, applying resistance to respiratory muscles, has been successfully used to improve respiratory muscle performance and assist in ventilator discontinuation, even in the acute care stage.[129,167,186] Gutierrez et al[167] developed a treatment protocol for improving respiratory muscle strength and endurance for ventilator-dependent individuals undergoing ventilator discontinuation trials. Individuals with C1–C2 injuries were not successful with long-term weaning, whereas those with injuries at levels C4 and below were able to wean within 2 months of training, using an inspiratory muscle trainer attached through the endotracheal or ventilator tubing. Individuals in this trial viewed the bedside monitor for visual biofeedback of SaO_2 and $ETCO_2$ to assist them in maintaining adequate RR and TV during the training period. Similarly, the

therapist can use these measures during mobilization sessions and during early stages when the goal is directed toward building sitting tolerance. Bedside monitoring is also useful for evaluation of the efficacy of an abdominal binder and various sitting postures and to monitor fatigue during breathing retraining sessions. When providing ventilatory muscle training to individuals in the acute stage, it is imperative that the therapist document VC; inspiratory muscle strength (either via negative inspiratory force [NIF] or via MIP); SaO_2; HR; training time; and resistance level applied. The TV, RR, and ventilator setting should also be recorded. Offering resistive breathing exercises to individuals who are at risk for ventilatory failure is controversial and may be contraindicated. Resistive breathing is known to produce an "immune challenge" to the body, increasing oxidative stress that can stimulate the production of cytokines in the diaphragm.[187,188] A decrease in TV or change in RR (increase in rate initially and, if fatigue occurs later, then a decrease in rate) for those who are able to breath spontaneously, with or without ventilator support, may indicate the resistive breathing exercises are excessive.

The respiratory muscle training protocol recommended by Gutierrez et al[167] also includes a pretraining optimization procedure. Prior to positioning and training the respiratory muscles, each individual was placed in a shallow Trendelenberg position (15 degrees) for 15 to 20 minutes to increase transpulmonary pressure at the base of the lungs. Suctioning was performed in this position and was effective in preparing the airways for a respiratory muscle training program. Each individual also received aerosolizing bronchodilators to reverse atelectasis and hyperinflation to the lungs to increase the chest wall mobility. This research confirms the importance of proper sequencing of interventions (bronchial hygiene, chest mobilization, followed by respiratory muscle training) for improving ventilation in those individuals with SCI.

When working to develop respiratory muscle function in the individual who is supported by mechanical ventilation, reviewing the mode of mechanical ventilation gives clues to the therapist as to the degree of participation and the ability of the individual to actively participate in breathing retraining tasks. An individual who is breathing on assist control mode has at least some active inspiratory effort, while the individual who is using control mode ventilation is relying entirely on the ventilator. The individual who is on synchronized intermittent mandatory ventilation and/or pressure support ventilation can participate in deep breathing activities because they are able to breathe spontaneously. Often, breathing retraining activities can begin while the individual is still on some form of mechanical ventilation. Individuals who are on synchronized intermittent mandatory ventilation or assist control mode can attempt diaphragmatic breathing, and those on pressure support ventilation may participate in segmental breathing. Those who are able to use noninvasive positive pressure ventilation also have the ability to breathe spontaneously. Noninvasive positive pressure ventilation allows air to be delivered without using a tracheostomy, minimizing the risk of infection.[189] In some centers, individuals with acute SCI are now being placed directly on this form of ventilation support after extubation of the endotracheal tube.[179] Continuous positive airway pressure (CPAP) is a form of noninvasive positive pressure ventilation that delivers airflow via the tracheostomy, by mouth via a mouthpiece (also referred to as *mouth positive*), or by mask to the nose and mouth. The pressure (5 to 10 cm H_2O) is constant throughout inspiration and expiration; this form of positive pressure ventilation is often used for glossopharyngeal breathing training.[165] Bi-level positive airway pressure (Bi-PAP) is another form of noninvasive positive

pressure ventilation that offers two levels of pressure, one higher level of pressure (10 to 20 cm H_2O) during inspiration and one lower level of pressure (5 to 10 cm H_2O) during expiration.

When the individual begins functional training, the therapist keeps in mind the total plan of care, especially when training upper extremity function for the individual with motor complete tetraplegia or when walking with individuals who have a motor incomplete injury but who may still be receiving mechanical ventilation. If pressure levels delivered by the ventilator are being decreased as part of the ventilator discontinuation strategy, then it would be inappropriate to offer a challenging activity during the therapy session. Challenging activities are reserved for times when the respiratory muscles are resting in assist control mode or control mode ventilation. Discussing the physical therapy plan with all members of the health-care team will provide optimal scheduling of all components of the individual's program.

Optimizing Ventilation for Function: Seating and Positioning Upright

Abdominal Support for Upright Postures

When the abdominal muscles are weak and the contents of the viscera are not supported, the diaphragm sits in a descended position when the individual is sitting or in the upright posture. This results in poor diaphragm mechanics. Linn et al[14] reported a significant decrease in VC when individuals with a tetraplegia assume an upright position compared to supine position. There are multiple reports that VC drops between 8% and 28% of the predicted value when individuals with cervical injuries move from supine to sitting position.[11,17,18,86,190] Chen et al[11] proposed that the weight of the abdominal contents put the diaphragm in a lower position, decreasing the excursion during inspiration. There is good evidence that abdominal binders effectively reposition the diaphragm, thereby providing a more effective resting position in the thorax. This support results in increased inspiratory capacity, VC, and decreased functional residual capacity (the volume of air remaining in the lungs at the end of an ordinary TV expiration) when the individual with tetraplegia or high thoracic injury assumes the upright posture.[24,62–64,191] Dyspnea levels are known to decrease as VC and inspiratory capacity improve in individuals with SCI when they are wearing an abdominal binder.[62]

Individuals with injury at the level of T6 or above may benefit from abdominal support provided by either an elastic abdominal binder with Velcro closures or a corset with adjustable straps. The corset is made of cloth, has a felt lining, and has several closure buckles that allow custom fittings. When an individual begins using abdominal support, the therapist evaluates the fit of the abdominal binder or corset in both supine and routine sitting postures. The upper portion of the binder should rest over the last two floating ribs, and the lower portion should cover the iliac crest over the anterior superior iliac spines. The upper portion should be loose enough to allow thoracic expansion. One hand should slip easily between the abdominal binder and the abdomen.[23] Conversely, if more than one hand can be placed between the binder and the abdomen, it may be too loose to be effective. Some abdominal binders may offer too much stretch to adequately contain the abdominal contents and cannot reposition the diaphragm effectively. The abdominal binder is evaluated for wear, and replacement binders are provided so that the binder can be washed; the elastic component of any binder eventually wears out. The skin will need to be examined and pressure areas relieved, if present. The individual should not wear any abdominal support device that has metal stays or components that put pressure or shear force on the skin.

The use of abdominal binders is evaluated using the response-dependent model described previously. The binder should be applied while the individual is supine in bed and breathing comfortably. The head of the bed should be gradually inclined and breathing observed. Clinical decisions regarding use or discontinuation of an abdominal binder may be confirmed by noting the RR and breathing pattern, and by measuring chest wall expansion and pulmonary functions. Research has demonstrated improved inspiratory capacity in individuals with tetraplegia wearing an abdominal binder when sitting at an angle of 37 degrees or higher.[63] There are also reports of reduced dyspnea, increased VC, diaphragm activation (as indicated by transdiaphragmatic pressure), increased rib cage dimensions, and lower functional residual capacity and residual volume (the volume of air remaining in the lungs after a maximal expiration) when abdominal binding is used in those with SCI.[17,62,63] Abdominal support may also be important when a halo vest is required. There is evidence that application of the halo vest decreases predicted VC in both the supine (6% to 8%) and sitting (2.5%) positions.[86] However, there are no reports evaluating the benefits of abdominal binders during halo vest use.

Some individuals with motor-incomplete lesions may rely on intercostal muscle breathing for thoracic expansion. These individuals will find abdominal binders restrictive and will demonstrate elevated RR and/or decreased VC if the abdominal binder is not helpful. Additionally, an individual may develop spasticity in the abdominal and intercostal muscles that is adequate for supporting diaphragm mechanics and supporting the rib cage.[76,156] In these cases, it may be possible to discontinue the abdominal binder if pulmonary functions and respiratory muscle strength tests (assessed in sitting) indicate adequate ventilatory support for coughing and activities of daily living. There are no long-term studies documenting the effects of prolonged abdominal binder use.[142] However, the long-term incidence of respiratory complications in individuals with motor complete tetraplegia and motor complete high thoracic injuries

suggests that wearing a abdominal binder may be important conservative management. Likewise, when a thoracolumbar orthosis is removed in the individual with a high thoracic injury, the therapist reevaluates respiratory function and considers whether an abdominal binder is necessary. Proper use of tests and measures documenting respiratory function in appropriate positions assist in evaluating the need for abdominal support for each case individually. No two individuals will present with exactly the same physical attributes or residual motor control.

In addition to supporting mechanics of breathing, the abdominal binder also offers improved cardiovascular support for cardiac output; therefore, vital signs (HR and blood pressure (BP)) should be assessed prior to discontinuing use of the abdominal binder.[23] Use of the binder may initially be necessary during bathing. This is especially true if the individual uses a bath bench or shower chair and is seated upright for bathing. Care must be taken in these situations, as changes in body temperature may shift the blood to the periphery. This, along with the decreased diaphragmatic excursion resulting from removal of the abdominal binder, can result in decreased venous return and fainting.

Wheelchair Positioning

Sitting position in the wheelchair has different effects in individuals with SCI, depending on the level of injury, posture, and the amount of residual respiratory muscle function. An individual with a high cervical injury (C1–C4) who uses a mechanical ventilator may depend on neck accessory muscle function, either to trigger a breath from the ventilator or to permit independent breathing. Adequate head support assists with accessory muscles action. Slight backward recline (15 degrees from upright, or sitting with the hips at 75 degrees) in the wheelchair will assist in stabilizing the occiput, so the sternocleidomastoid muscles may work in reverse, lifting the sternum. If the individual with injury at this level requires neck accessory muscle action in order to operate electric wheelchair activation systems, then a full control mode of ventilation support may be necessary. In these cases, the therapist works with the respiratory therapist to provide the optimal setup. When noninvasive ventilation is in use, a pneumobelt may be effective during sitting, freeing the neck accessory muscles for function (e.g., mouthstick activities).

The therapist takes note of the habitual sitting posture used by the individual and evaluates the impact on ventilation. Amodie-Storey et al[192] evaluated habitual sitting postures in individuals with cervical SCI and demonstrated higher VC and maximal voluntary ventilation measures with habitual forward head posture compared to the more aligned postures. Therefore, changing the posture toward one of less kyphosis may decrease ventilatory reserve in some individuals with SCI. However, an individual may need a good postural base to build new ventilation strategies for long-term ventilatory gains.[20,88] Bodin et al[193] also evaluated respiratory function with positioning and reported variable responses in four individuals with chronic cervical injuries. After positioning with correction for excessive kyphosis and pelvic obliquity, only one subject reported subjective improvement in breathing, and there were no objective improvements in VC. Therefore, restoring normal posture through therapeutic stretching and muscle elongation must be considered carefully in those with marginal respiratory status. Overstretch of already weakened accessory muscles may cause posturing that may lead to inability to use a valuable compensatory strategy. Conversely, tight chest muscles will lead to increases in the work of breathing. The effects of any postural program should be evaluated by consistent monitoring of chest wall expansion measures, VC, MIP and MEP, and maximal voluntary ventilation. In this way, the therapist can use the actual outcome measures to assist in making the best clinical decision for each individual.

The goals of respiratory intervention in the acute stage of SCI are highly dependent upon the individual's level and severity of injury. With optimal care and education in the acute stage, individuals will be able to provide as much self-management of respiratory care as their function will afford. Individuals will also know how to direct others in those activities that they are not able to accomplish themselves. The role of each component of respiratory care in improving respiratory function is summarized in Table 14-5.

Rehabilitation Stage

Once the individual is medically stable, the rehabilitation stage begins. In this stage, more aggressive strategies are used to improve respiratory function. A major effort is directed toward complete discontinuation of mechanical ventilation and complete removal of the tracheostomy tube (decannulation), if possible. Individuals who are no longer receiving mechanical ventilation will benefit from further enhancement of respiratory muscles and will need strategies to prevent respiratory complications. Once mechanical ventilation is discontinued, the chest wall does not receive the stretch applied by the ventilator. Paradoxical breathing may appear. Some individuals with

Table 14-5
Primary Role of Interventions

Intervention	↓ Ventilatory Load	↑ Ventilatory Capacity	↑ Gas Exchange
Mechanical ventilation	√		√++
Prescriptive body positioning	√	√	√+
Tracheal suction	√		√
Postural drainage	√		√
Abdominal binder		√++	√
Pneumobelt		√+	√
Chest wall stretching	√+		√−
Wheelchair positioning		√	√−
Airway clearance	√+		√
Glossopharyngeal breathing	√	√	√
Functional electrical stimulation	√	√	√
Coordinated breathing	√	√	√
Facilitated breathing		√++	√
Ventilatory muscle training		√ +++	√
Conditioning		√+	

Key: √−: Offers minimal support to enhance the component
√ : Offers moderate support to enhance the component
√+: Offers maximum support to enhance the component

a tracheostomy will progress from cuffed to uncuffed or to fenestrated tracheostomies, or they may be evaluated for a speaking valve or qualify for decannulation. These changes increase the dead space ventilation and the work of breathing. It will be important to begin teaching effective coughing, initiate chest mobilization techniques, and continue respiratory muscle conditioning while encouraging development of efficient breathing strategies.

Airway Clearance

Higher level injuries to the spinal cord result in a loss of sympathetic nervous system innervation and a parasympathetic dominance in the lungs that leads to bronchoconstriction and increased mucous secretion.[142,156,194] These factors, combined with the loss of abdominal muscle contraction for forced expiration, result in poor airway clearance in most individuals with SCI.[195] The cough function will be impaired even in those with paraplegia. All individuals with paraplegia are encouraged to perform deep breathing and perform self-assisted coughing regularly to prevent infection.

Individuals with high paraplegia and tetraplegia will also have a significant loss of inspiratory volume, which will increase the risk of respiratory complications. Voluntary activation of any muscles involved in coughing will be an important component of the respiratory rehabilitation program. There are several reports confirming that an improvement in MIP in those with cervical injuries is important for achieving effective expiratory flow rates during coughing.[46,196] Also of interest is the fact that some accessory muscles typically known for inspiratory function may also work to improve forced expiration.[197] Fujiwara et al[197] reported peak expiratory flow rate (the fastest speed of airflow generated during maximal expiration, which is used to detect airway restriction due decreased speed of expiratory muscle contraction) and MEP were correlated with pectoralis major and latissimus dorsi muscle activity in individuals with motor complete tetraplegia. Estenne et al[198] have demonstrated that strengthening the pectoralis muscles improves cough function in individuals with tetraplegia. This may be true for strengthening of other accessory muscles as well and should be considered when developing the respiratory rehabilitation program. The therapist analyzes all intact residual muscles, their actions, and reverse muscle actions to determine their potential to participate in the production of an effective cough.

Coughing

Airway clearance is normally achieved by producing a strong cough (release of 2.3 ± 0.5 L with flow rates of 6 to 20 L/sec; 300 to 700 L/min).[153–156,199] Individuals who have vital capacities lower than 1500 mL will not generate adequate peak cough flows voluntarily.[200] The therapist observes the individual's cough effectiveness during four phases:[39,161,162]

1. The first phase involves observing for good inspiration and noting the individual's ability to use trunk extension or *breath-stacking* (also called *air-stacking*) to augment the inspiratory volume.[106,161] Breath-stacking occurs when the individual takes a second, third, or fourth inspiratory breath on top of the first breath without releasing air.
2. The second phase requires glottis closure and holding for about 2 seconds.
3. The third phase is the force-generating phase, wherein the individual generates force behind the closed glottis.
4. Finally, during the fourth phase, the glottis must open and release air smoothly.[161]

The individual is instructed to cough two to six times forcefully within one breath using trunk flexion or intact abdominal muscle. Alternately, the individual may manually compress the abdomen just above the umbilicus as a self-assistance strategy if abdominal muscles are weak. The therapist observes the timing and coordination of any compensatory motion or self-assisted strategies. The quality of the cough is classified as *functional*, *weak-functional*, or *nonfunctional*.[23,24] The cough is functional if the individual can clear all secretions using several powerful expulsions within one breath without using any cough-assist techniques. The cough is weak-functional if there is partial clearing of secretions or clearing of the throat during one breath attempt. Here, a cough assist would be necessary to mobilize mucus and clear the airways during an infection. The cough is classified as nonfunctional if the effort is not forceful enough to produce any expiratory airflow.[23,24] (*See* the online resource *Respiratory Evaluation of Individuals with SCI* on the DavisPlus website (http://www.davisplus.fadavis.com) for more information related to cough evaluation).

When designing a program to improve cough function, the therapist determines which of the four phases of coughing are impaired and develops a therapeutic plan to address the specific problem. Training activities related to improving cough function may include strategies to increase inspiratory volume, to increase glottis control, and/or to improve expiratory force generation and release.[20] Almost all individuals with a SCI will have a diminished expiratory component to their cough, and those with high paraplegia and tetraplegia will have abnormal inspiratory and expiratory components. Therefore, strategies to improve expiratory force generation and airflow are critical for most individuals at any level of injury. Glottal control problems often appear following extubation or in those with very high lesions, where there may be bulbar muscle involvement. Thus, individuals with higher cervical injuries need more work on strategies to improve inspiration and glottal control. Weak or absent cough function is usually managed by teaching one of several cough-assist techniques as summarized in Table 14-6. Cough-assist techniques may be performed by caregivers, or the individual may learn one of several self-assist manual cough strategies.[161,199]

Table 14-6
Cough-Assist Strategies

Methods	Description	Clinical Considerations
Abdominal thrust	Applied over the abdomen. Heel of one or both hands (interlocking) of caregiver or therapist is applied in a downward and inward motion. Quick thrust action is applied with air expulsion (phase 4)	Contraindicated with the presence of vena cava filters, unstable spine, lower abdominal injuries, or gastrointestinal tubes.
Costophrenic assist[161,198]	Performed in supine, sitting, or side-lying position. Hands are placed over the costophrenic angles of the rib cage. Quick stretch applied at the end of exhalation (phase 4, expiratory assist, and phase 1, facilitation). Used with breath-stacking and hold (phase 1, 2, and 3).	Provides facilitation for inspiratory phase of coughing. Can be applied as a series of repetitive quick stretches. Helpful for lower airway clearance, but not upper airways unless combined with individual effort/assist. Good for acute stage when individuals need modified assist.
Anterior chest compression[161,198]	One arm across upper and lower chest or may be applied with two hands across upper chest (tussive squeeze). Upper arm rests across pectoral region while lower arm rests over midabdominal region midway between umbilicus and xiphoid. Force applied downward and back or up and back with air expulsion.	More effective than abdominal thrust for those with weak upper chest muscles. Provides greater force to upper airways. Can offer some facilitation to inspiration. May not be appropriate for those with cavus deformity of chest.
Counter-rotation assist[161]	Performed with the individual in side-lying position. The therapist places one hand on shoulder and one on pelvis and prepares to diagonally move the pelvis, rotating it forward and up while moving the shoulder so the scapular rotates down and back. The individual attempts to expel air. The motions are reversed and the individual inspires.	Can facilitate inspiration and expiration. Will also offer chest mobilization prior to recruitment of inspiratory effort. Person must not have any orthopedic precautions to rib cage, pelvis, shoulder, or spine. May be more difficult to coordinate and perform effectively.
Inspiratory assist/ glossopharyngeal breathing[24,154,164,199,202]	When inspiratory volume is low, the individual uses the tongue to pump air from the mouth and pharynx into the lungs. Each stroke is held behind a functional glottis (phase 1 and 2). A manual assist is applied during the expulsion phase to move air rapidly up and out.	Useful for the person with tetraplegia who has poor inspiratory volume. The person must have good glottis control and therefore needs a "speaking valve" or tracheostomy button or be fully decannulated and well healed.
Inspiratory assist/ insufflation[46,154,155,158,199]	Air is delivered to the lungs as the individual attempts inspiration. This can be offered manually with a resuscitation bag via tracheostomy or mask or mechanically by volume-cycled ventilator (called *insufflation*). Pressure delivered mechanically during inspiration is around 40–70 cc H_2O.	Individual takes deep breaths, and additional air is added. The person must have a functional glottis

Continued

Table 14-6
Cough-Assist Strategies—cont'd

Methods	Description	Clinical Considerations
Mechanical insufflator-exsufflator (MI-E)[154] **(also called the cough-a-lator)**[154,198,204]	Positive pressure delivered during inspiration is followed by negative pressure "suction" during expiration to draw secretions out. Both cycles are mechanically delivered via tracheostomy or mask over mouth and nose.	Used when glottis/laryngeal control is weak or absent. Used when there are contraindications to vigorous manual compression of the epigastric region or chest wall (invasive tubes, fractures). Useful when lungs are overwhelmed with mucus and decrease in SaO_2 is significant.
Functional electrical stimulation[201,202,212]	Electrodes are placed on the abdominal muscles. No device currently available on U.S. market. Previously, devices have been developed that allow stimulation to abdominal muscle contraction to be triggered by person with SCI or caregiver.	Requires proper electrode placement and good tolerance. May allow independence from caregiver assistance for coughing. Observe skin under electrodes. May affect BP.
Combinations[46,54,158,201]	Both inspiratory and expiratory components of cough are augmented to increase total peak cough flow rate.	Evaluation of each individual and caregiver team is warranted to assist in determining optimal cough. Outcome measures to consider include peak cough flow rate measures, individual comfort, caregiver preference, and effectiveness, as well as overall ability to clear airways.
Self-Assist Methods **Upper extremity/torso abdominal thrust assist**	The individual places interlocking hands across epigastric region and applies force inward and upward toward the head. This is timed with the expulsion or air (phase 4). Head and trunk flexion may be used to assist with air expulsion. In sitting or side-lying position, head and trunk extension may assist with inspiratory phase (phase 1).	May be performed in most positions. Typically, performed in supine or sitting in wheelchair. Individual needs to be sure wheelchair is stable if using head and trunk accessory motions. Person with SCI must be cleared for high intrathoracic pressure changes.
Self-Assist Methods **Long-sitting**[161]	Individual sitting with legs fully extended on mat table or in bed. Upper extremities may be positioned in supportive propping posture. Individual can use head, neck, and trunk extension during inspiratory phase (phase 1) and head, neck, and trunk flexion during expulsion (phase 3, 4). If arms are functional, they may be used over epigastric region to assist expulsion.	Useful for those with higher levels of injury who do not have hand function and need to generate some inspiratory lung volume and expiratory flow. Those with arm function may use butterfly posture with hands clasped behind head during inspiration to open anterior chest wall and close elbows together during expiration to enhance movement of out of upper airways.

Manual-Assisted Cough Techniques

Manual-assisted coughing involves the application of several firm, quick thrusts, using various positions for hand and arm placements over the abdomen or chest during expiration.[161,202] The most common form of manual-assisted coughing (also called the "quad" cough) is a method wherein the heel of the hand(s) is applied over the abdominal region as the individual attempts to cough (Fig. 14-7a). The thrusting motion is applied in a manner similar to the Heimlich maneuver. The hand placement must be at least 2 inches below the xiphoid process and just above the umbilicus. The therapist instructs the individual to inhale deeply (phase 1) prior to closing the glottis (phase 2) and then holding briefly (pressure-building phase 3). The individual then releases the glottis (phase 4) at the same time the therapist applies manual assistance.[161] The force is applied in a direction that moves inward and up at an angle toward the head. This must be a quick action that is well timed with the individual's cough effort. Cough function has been known to increase as much as 33% with this technique.[156,201]

Complications can occur when using the abdominal thrust if proper precautions are not taken. Pressure on the xiphoid process should be avoided. Individuals should be medically cleared for high intra-abdominal and intrathoracic pressures. It is also important to consider the presence of any vena cava filters or epigastric tubes that may contraindicate the use of this technique.[161,198] Manual-assisted coughing is initially applied while the individual is supine. If the individual is seated in a wheelchair, the chair must be stable. The therapist or caregiver may want to assume a position behind the chair and reach around or over the individual if using the abdominal thrust technique. This may be an effective approach for improving body mechanics while maintaining wheelchair stability. Alternative techniques to consider when the abdominal compression is contraindicated may include the costophrenic assist (Fig. 14-7b), anterior chest compression (also applied as a tussive squeeze), and counter-rotation assist.[23,24,161,198,199]

Self-Assisted Coughing

Most individuals with paraplegia will have a weak cough that can be assisted by interlocking the hands and pushing over the epigastric region in an inward and upward direction toward the head. The individual is encouraged to inhale deeply and may perform several breath-stacking maneuvers using a strong glottis to hold the air with each breath. Then, after the lung volume is fully enhanced, the individual pushes on the epigastric region while releasing the air. The head and trunk may flex forward if the individual is lying on his or her side or supine or may fall forward if sitting to assist in the expulsion of air during the cough.[161] Individuals having strong biceps and some wrist extension (C5–C6) can position the arms and hands appropriately and learn an effective epigastric push for self-assisted coughing (Fig. 14-8).

Head and trunk motions become more important for self-assisted coughing in individuals with higher levels of injuries. In sitting, the individual can also

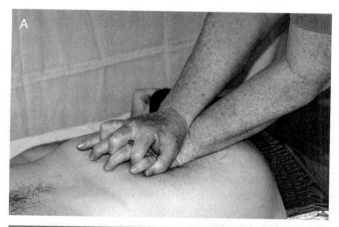

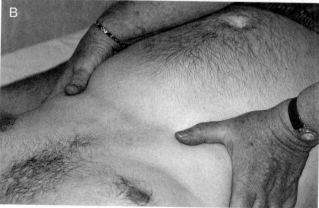

Figure 14-7. Manual-assisted coughing techniques. (A) Abdominal thrust technique. (B) Costophrenic assist technique.

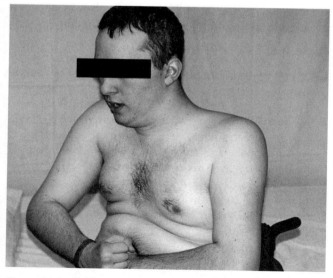

Figure 14-8. Self-assisted manual coughing. Manual coughing may be performed by individuals with adequate upper extremity function to apply a coordinated force during the cough effort.

increase inspiratory volume by extending the trunk during breath-stacking and flexing the trunk while moving the head forward during expulsion.[202] Some individuals will need to use glossopharyngeal breathing if they cannot generate sufficient volume during several inspiratory holds with breath-stacking.[20] The individual in a wheelchair may need to back the chair up against a wall, keeping the caster wheels forward to ensure stability, when using accessory trunk motions for coughing. Most individuals learn to perform the self-assisted cough in several positions. Alternative positions that may be considered for self-assisted cough include being prone on the elbows, long sitting, and being in the quadruped position and rocking on the hands and knees.

Strategies to Augment Cough Function: Inspiratory Volume and Glottis Control

Individuals who have a tracheostomy will not be able to generate the same effective force as those who do not have a tracheostomy.[164] There are two reasons for this. First, they will lack the inspiratory volume, and second, they will not have the ability to close the glottis and generate force behind a functional glottis. Once the individual has a tracheostomy that allows speech, he or she can participate in building inspiratory volume by taking a deep breath and then stacking several breaths one after the other, using the glottis to hold a larger and larger inspiratory volume. The therapist may need to teach the individual how to improve glottis control. Training of glottis control may be as simple as asking the individual to say "ah, ah, ah" in repetitive fashion.[85,203] Often, a feather is held at the mouth to show air movement. After the individual performs several breath-stacking efforts, he or she can release the air and see a large perturbation of the feather, demonstrating correct release of a larger volume of air. If breath-stacking is still difficult after several sessions, the therapist can begin glossopharyngeal breathing training to improve inspiratory volume.[164]

Glossopharyngenal Breathing

Glossopharyngeal breathing is preferable to neck accessory muscle breathing for building inspiratory volume in individuals with high SCIs.[164] The technique is often called "frog" breathing and involves using the tongue to pump air into the lungs. It was originally developed to assist individuals with polio who were dependent on the "iron lung" to leave this large enclosed mechanical ventilation system. To teach this technique, the therapist must demonstrate the action of gulping air and using the tongue to move the air into the lungs, then have the individual imitate the action. Each gulp of air delivers 60 to 200 mL of air to the inspiratory volume.[204] The individual repeats the gulps sequentially so that six to nine gulps are stacked together. Montero et al[205] demonstrated that training in glossopharyngeal breathing improved peak expiratory flow rate (39% to 92% predicted), maximal voluntary ventilation, and VC (35% to 65% predicted) in 14 subjects with cervical SCIs. Two excellent training resources are available for therapists wanting to learn the steps required to teach this technique (see Dail et al and Los Amigos Research and Education Institute Inc.)[203,206]

Huff Coughing

Complete decannulation of the tracheostomy can occur when the individual has the ability to breathe through the upper airway (using a tracheostomy that is fenestrated or has a speaking valve) for a prolonged period of time without signs of fatigue (see Table 14-3). The individual must also be able to clear the airways using an effective cough strategy and have adequate swallowing function to avoid aspiration. Communicating with the speech therapist and coordinating the care with the entire health-care team is critical for appropriately managing this stage of the respiratory rehabilitation program. The therapist assists by determining the most effective cough strategy and reporting any signs of fatigue or positions that cause respiratory distress to the health-care team. Vigorous coughing should be avoided while the tracheostomy site is still healing. During this period, the individual is encouraged to build inspiratory volume and use forced expiratory technique or "huff" coughing (discussed below).[207] When the tracheostomy site is difficult to heal, negative pressure mechanical ventilation systems applied to the body (chest cuirass) or rocking beds (a bed that tilts the individual upright and then back to horizontal, so that the resulting shift in abdominal contents causes inspiration) may be considered.[202]

Insufflation

If an individual has difficulty learning glossopharyngeal breathing, the therapist can use other methods to assist inspiration. As long as the individual has a functional glottis and laryngeal control, the inspiratory volume can be assisted by insufflation. *Insufflation* occurs when air is forced into the lungs rather than using muscle activation to expand the thorax. Insufflation occurs through breath-stacking, glossopharyngeal breathing, manual resuscitation bagging, or by using a volume-cycled positive pressure portable ventilator.[23,24,202,204] Closure of the glottis holds the insufflated volume of air. The maximum insufflation capacity is measured to designate strength of glottis closure.[155]

Insufflation using a manual resuscitation bag is a common approach to assisting inspiratory volume. In an individual who does not have a tracheostomy, the bag is attached to a mask that is fitted over the individual's nose and mouth. In an individual who has a tracheostomy, the bag is attached to the tracheostomy through an adapter. The individual with a tracheostomy may have a one-way valve as part of their tracheostomy to allow air to flow out through the mouth, or it may be possible to inflate the lungs using a bag with a one-way valve, leaving the bag in place during cough attempts (Fig. 14-9).

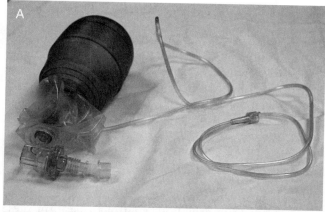

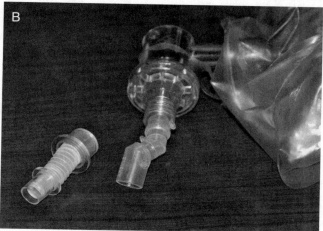

Figure 14-9. Manual resuscitation bag with swivel adapters. (A) A manual resuscitation bag may be connected to the tracheostomy with an adapter. Squeezing the bag during inspiration adds volume. (B) Swivel adapters may be used to avoid stress to the tracheostomy site if the individual is ambulatory or needs ventilation with a bag during mobility sessions.

When using the manual resuscitation bag, the therapist notes the individual's size, considers the person's tidal volume, and squeezes the bag so that the correct volume is released to the individual. After the individual attempts inspiration, additional air is delivered by squeezing the manual resuscitation bag. The individual holds the air with the glottis. Diaphragm activation can also be encouraged by providing manual/tactile cues, squeezing downward and inward at the end of expiration. The therapist then verbally encourages sniffing and breath-stacking during inspiration. Several small breaths may be "stacked," followed by manual insufflation with a resuscitation bag. Two people may be required to provide both appropriate timing with the bag and tactile cues.

When insufflation is used prior to assisted coughing, the individual holds the extra air with the glottis until the therapist or caregiver signals the individual to release the air while a manual assist to expiration is offered over the epigastric region, lateral costal region, or upper chest. As the expiratory assist is applied, the individual releases the glottis. Kang et al[46] evaluated 40 individuals with cervical SCI and compared four cough conditions: (1) unassisted coughing, (2) assisted cough after volume insufflation using a bag, (3) assisted abdominal thrust coughing, and (4) combined volume insufflation followed by abdominal thrust expiratory assist. Mean peak cough flow rates were greatest during combined cough-assist efforts (362 ± 82 L/min) compared to independently applying only an abdominal thrust assist (324 ± 77 L/min) or only assisted volume insufflation with a resuscitation bag (277 L/min). This research supports the importance of treating both inspiratory and expiratory components of coughing.

Accessory Devices to Assist Cough

Mechanical Insufflation

A volume-cycled ventilator offers the same benefit as the manual resuscitation bag. Pressurized air (40 to 70 cc H_2O) is delivered during inspiration only, and the air is held behind a strong glottis.[199] Again, the manual thrust is used to assist expiration as the glottis is released. Most assisted-cough techniques bring the levels of peak flow beyond the minimal 160 L/min required for effective mobilization of secretions.[154,199] Kirby et al[158] demonstrated that individuals with a C5–C6 injuries could optimally improve their cough function to near normal levels (78% improvement from unassisted cough levels) when using the combination of positive pressure insufflation, an abdominal binder, and manual abdominal thrust assist.

Mechanical Insufflation/Exsufflation

When the glottis is weak or there is significant bulbar dysfunction (individual is unable to hold air at 40 to 70 cc H_2O), then the CoughAssist mechanical insufflator-exsufflator (commonly referred to as the "cough-a-lator"; Philip Respironics; Amsterdam, The Netherlands) should be considered.[20,199] A deep insufflation or positive air pressure is delivered during inspiration, followed by a forceful exsufflation, thereby creating a negative pressure in the lungs on expiration. A pause occurs between insufflation and exsufflation. The levels of each pressure and the pause time is set according to comfort. Chatwin et al[208] recently demonstrated that coughing with the assistance of a mechanical insufflator-exsufflator device increased the peak cough flow rate from 169 L/min to 235 L/min in individuals having a weak cough due to neuromuscular conditions resulting in bulbar dysfunction. Clinical trials in individuals with neuromuscular weakness have demonstrated that the use of mechanical insufflation/exsufflation assists in the normalization of SaO_2 and improvements in VC and peak expiratory flow rate as mucus clears.[204,209] Complications occurring from mechanical insufflation/exsufflation use are rare, but may include dry mouth, nose bleeds, and chest discomfort.[20]

In individuals with intact bulbar function and strong glottis control, the use of mechanical insufflation/exsufflation should not be necessary, even when there is complete paralysis of both inspiratory and expiratory muscles.[199] Bach[154] reported mean peak expiratory flow rates in 21 ventilator-assisted individuals having neuromuscular weakness. Four conditions were evaluated: unassisted coughing; breath-stacking (glossopharyngeal breathing or alternative); manual-assisted coughing (abdominal thrust or anterior compression); and mechanical insufflation/exsufflation. Although the mechanical insufflation/exsufflation resulted in the greatest mean peak expiratory flow rate (7.47 ± 1.02 L/sec), the mean peak expiratory flow rate was also adequately enhanced above the critical 2.7 L/sec with breath-stacking (3.37 ± 1.07 L/sec) and assisted coughing (4.27 ± L/sec) techniques. Mean peak expiratory flow rate for unassisted coughing was inadequate (1.81 ± 1.03 L/sec). This research suggests that with the assistance of a properly trained caregiver, most individuals can learn to generate adequate cough function. Each individual and caregiver team should have their coughing strategies evaluated for effectiveness. The actual peak cough flow rate may be measured to confirm appropriate force for airway clearance. It is also important to determine that the caregiver is able to properly use mechanical devices to assist cough.

Functional Electrical Stimulation for Cough

Functional electrical stimulation (FES) to the abdominal muscles can improve cough function as well as enhance TV for individuals with tetraplegia.[158,200,201,210–212] In this technique, four to eight electrodes are placed on the abdominal wall over abdominal muscle motor points.[200,212] Electrodes may be placed in a corset to assist in securing the proper location.[213] Research has demonstrated an increase in MEP from 27.3 ± 6.4 to 60 ± 22.8 cm H_2O[200] and improvement of peak expiratory flow rate from 275 L/min to 425 L/min[212] when abdominal muscle stimulation was used. Optimal surface electrode placement has been confirmed as being associated with abdomino-intercostal nerves T9–T12 for producing contractions related to improved ventilation.[214] FES-assisted cough requires some practice to develop appropriate timing after the electrodes are activated. Additionally, some individuals may not be able to tolerate the stimulation. However, the benefit offered by FES-assisted cough is that there is potential for the individual to be independent.

Secretion Mobilization Techniques

While a variety of coughing options exist for clearing the upper airways, the cough or cough assist will only move secretions from the seventh generation of bronchioles and above. Therefore, the therapist incorporates approaches that mobilize secretions below this level. During the rehabilitation stage, individuals are medically stable and are able to tolerate a variety of positions for postural drainage, as well as receive percussion and vibration.[215] The contemporary approach to secretion mobilization uses active breathing to move the inspiratory volume to regions that may be closed off by mucus.[216] Airway-clearance strategies are designed to assist air movement into the regions that are obstructed by providing flow through collateral airways. The techniques emphasize slow, controlled breathing with adequate pause time between inspiration and expiration. Expiratory flow during initial stages occurs at a low rate to prevent airway irritation and bronchospasm, which might restrict the upward flow of mucus. Some of the techniques provide vibration during expiration to assist in loosening of mucus. A list of the most common techniques for mobilization of secretions is provided in Table 14-7.

While many individuals with SCI may not be able to generate adequate expiratory control to perform these techniques effectively,[20] it is especially important for those with low thoracic and lumbar paraplegia who have premorbid lung problems to be trained and encouraged in their use. Likewise, those with motor incomplete injuries will vary in their expiratory control ability, and some may benefit from these techniques. Individuals having motor complete tetraplegia may require mucolytics, bronchodilators, postural drainage with percussion and vibration, humidification treatments and hydration. This may be especially true once they are removed from the ventilator.[2] Secretion mobilization strategies may be combined with most traditional chest physical therapy positions and protocols. The effectiveness of each technique is evaluated on an individual basis. A recent report by Bodin et al[217] documented significantly increased functional residual capacity and alveolar ventilation during positive expiratory pressure (10 cm H_2O) exercise in individuals with motor complete C5–C8 injuries. This study demonstrated that changes occur at the alveolar level when positive expiratory pressure maneuvers are implemented in those with cervical injuries. Outcomes demonstrating success with airway clearance include volume of sputum collected over a 24-hour period, comparison of pre- and posttreatment chest x-ray and lung sounds, SaO_2, and changes in any of the signs of respiratory fatigue (see Table 14-3). Again, the individual should be well rested after the airway clearance treatment before the therapist assesses these outcome measures.

Chest Mobilization

Individuals become physically more active during the rehabilitation stage. Many individuals in this stage are able to breathe free from the ventilator and spend much of the time sitting upright, challenging the respiratory system. Musculoskeletal limitations to rib cage expansion may arise from muscular atrophy, spasticity, pain, impaired breathing mechanics, poor posture, scar tissue, soft tissue tightness, and contractures. Compliance in the lung tissues may also be diminished due to atelectasis.[204,218] Individuals cannot change an inefficient breathing strategy to a more appropriate ventilatory pattern if the chest wall is stiff.[116] Chest wall stiffness increases the

Table 14-7
Secretion Mobilization Approaches[216]

Secretion Mobilization Technique	Description
Forced expiratory technique, also called "Huff" coughing. • Low volume • High volume	The individual inhales deeply and the releases air through an open glottis. The air is released slowly for low-volume and quickly for high-volume huffing. Low-volume huffing occurs from deep inspiration to tidal volume and mobilizes secretions in peripheral airways. High-volume huffing is quick and forceful and mobilizes secretions in upper airways.
Active cycle breathing	The individual is instructed in a sequence of breathing designed to alternate rest phase diaphragmatic breathing with deep lateral costal breathing and diaphragmatic breathing. Deep breathing is facilitated to encourage inspiration to different levels or volumes prior to using a low-volume huff. After several low-volume huffs are performed (mobilizing secretions from peripheral airways) from a position of deep inspiration, then a larger, more forceful high-volume huff is used for expulsion of mucus.
Positive expiratory pressure (PEP) therapy	The individual inhales deeply and then exhales slowly into a mask or mouthpiece. Valves releasing the expired air are under pressure. Usually low pressure is 10–20 cm H_2O.
Flutter valve PEP	The individual inhales deeply and then exhales slowly into a pipelike device housing a metal ball. As exhaled air moves forward, the ball moves and sends vibration down the airways to assist in loosening of mucus.
Acapella PEP	The individual inhales deeply and then exhales slowly into a small football-shaped device. As expired air enters the device, a magnetic system opens and closes, creating vibrations in the pulmonary airways to assist in loosening of mucus.
High-frequency chest wall oscillator	A vest worn externally can deliver vibrations and predetermined frequency.

ventilatory load requirements to already weakened respiratory muscles.[219] Respiratory muscle weakness and abnormal breathing mechanics increase the likelihood of respiratory muscle fatigue. Therefore, the therapist incorporates chest mobility into the respiratory care program for individuals with respiratory dysfunction. Strategies for improving chest wall motion include deep breathing, breath-stacking, glossopharyngeal breathing, coordinated breathing, air-shift maneuvers, segmental breathing, positional stretching, manual chest stretching, rib mobilization, and insufflation (manual bagging or mechanical insufflation).

Deep Breathing, Breath-Stacking, and Glossopharyngeal Breathing

Periodic deep breathing to encourage active range of motion of the chest wall is a key component of instruction in self-management of respiratory care for the individual with SCI. Routine TV breathing occurring with activity will not expand the chest fully. Each individual should achieve at least 2 inches (5 cm) of chest wall expansion with deep breathing.[23,108] Together, deep breathing and coughing will help prevent respiratory complications. Many individuals with SCI will not achieve adequate chest wall expansion with deep breathing. However, if the individual can perform breath-stacking or glossopharyngeal breathing, he or she can increase chest wall motion beyond the dimensions achieved with TV breathing.[220] Nygren-Bonnier et al[220] recently demonstrated significant improvements in chest wall expansion in 20 subjects with chronic tetraplegia after 8 weeks of training in glossopharyngeal breathing (10 repetitions, four times per week).

Coordinated Breathing

Individuals with SCI learn to coordinate their breathing during functional activities and with movements that expand and open up different regions of the chest. If the individual has functional upper extremities, then he or she can be positioned in a short-sitting position and the arms placed with hands clasped behind the head in a butterfly position.[116,221] The individual leans forward to exhale or cough while bringing the elbows together and collapsing the anterior chest, then inhale while returning to upright sitting, moving the elbows apart and opening the anterior chest.[116] The individual can also rotate to one side or lean laterally to one side to increase the arc of motion and overall mobility in the chest wall. The therapist analyzes most therapeutic activities performed by the individual and encourages an appropriate, coordinated breathing strategy. Trunk flexion is paired with exhalation and extension with inhalation.[116] The added movements promote mobility in the chest wall and increase the volume of air moved into the lungs with deep breathing. Later, the individual can incorporate these breathing strategies into the activities of daily living routine, breathing in when reaching up to put an arm through the shirt sleeve or when reaching for a cup on a shelf, and then breathing out when reaching down.

Some individuals will not have full upper extremity function and will need the assistance of the therapist to use the coordinated breathing approach. In some cases, the individual may have shoulder motion but lack full voluntary control of the elbow and wrist. The therapist must support the distal portions of the extremities and work within functional patterns to assist the individual, yet allow him or her to perform as much of the activity as possible.[116] Timing inspiration with the motion of reaching the arm up or forward into shoulder flexion can translate to increased thoracic motion. Many cough-assist techniques will naturally incorporate chest mobility into the breathing pattern. Counter-rotation and costophrenic cough-assist techniques work on axial rotation and lateral rib mobility. These techniques also provide facilitation/cuing to muscles of respiration, encouraging increased inspiratory volume, which further improves the expansion of the rib cage.

Air-Shift Maneuver and Segmental Breathing

The greatest changes in pressures are localized under the regions where the respiratory muscles act, therefore manual techniques used with segmental breathing may elicit pressure changes or may cue muscle activation and influence air distribution.[9,222,224] Although many individuals with a SCI do not have sensation over the upper thorax and rib cage, segmental breathing may be effective for expanding selected segments of the lungs and chest wall.[221] The therapist can offer manual cues through pressure sensation or vibratory sensations that may be detected by some individuals. A mirror may also be added to allow the individual to observe manual techniques during segmental breathing. Manual cues are provided over the region of the chest wall that is not expanding well. The individual is instructed to "take in a deep breath under my hand" as the therapist presses in, and the therapist releases as the individual attempts inspiration. The therapist can place the individual's hand under the therapist's own hand, over the affected area, and repeat the command. Through multiple cues and alternative sensory inputs, some individuals may learn to move air into poorly expanding areas. However, evidence supporting this technique is limited.[221]

Any individual with paradoxical breathing (see Fig. 14-1) or a poorly expanding chest wall during inspiration should learn to perform an air-shift maneuver. When an individual has a dominant diaphragmatic breathing pattern that results in collapse of the anterior chest wall (as occurs in those with C4–T4 motor complete injuries), the volume of air moving into the lungs does not act to expand the chest wall but instead moves in a caudal direction. The air-shift maneuver is a technique that allows the individual to move the air upward toward the middle and upper lobes of the chest and creates expansion of these regions. This technique may increase the chest wall motion at the xiphoid level from one-half inch (1.25 cm) to 2 inches (5 cm) and provide a method for self range-of-motion exercise.[23,24] Individuals should be instructed to perform this maneuver daily.

When teaching an individual how to perform an air-shift maneuver, the individual should lie in the supine position. The therapist places one hand on the upper part of the chest wall and the second hand over the epigastric area. The individual takes a deep breath in and is asked to hold that breath. While holding the breath, the belly rises, and the therapist asks the individual to move the air upward (giving a tactile cue over the upper chest) as the breath hold is maintained. The therapist may say, "relax your belly," or "suck in," to encourage the individual to draw the air upward toward the anterior and upper chest. The technique requires strong closure of the glottis, which must remain closed throughout the maneuver. The individual exhales between attempts and should rest frequently throughout the training session to avoid consequences associated with breath holding and hyperventilation.[23,24]

Positional Stretching

Positional stretching of the chest wall is a passive process that allows a gradual lengthening of muscles and soft tissue structures around the rib cage, shoulders, and spine. The therapist must determine what areas of the chest wall are tight. Typically, for many individuals with cervical or high thoracic injuries, the anterior chest wall is collapsed due to poor breathing mechanics. To open the anterior chest wall, the individual is positioned in supine position and a towel roll placed longitudinally under the thoracic spine.[116] If the individual has been sitting and collapsing into a slumped posture with excessive kyphosis, then a towel roll is placed transversely across the spine, at the level of the axilla, to assist in realignment of the thoracic vertebrae. Skin must be monitored periodically when using towel rolls and static positioning. Likewise, the impact of each position must be monitored for signs of respiratory muscle fatigue.

Many individuals with motor incomplete injuries or those with asymmetrical motor complete lesions have muscle imbalances creating torsion (lateral bending with rotation) to the thoracic cage. The individual may be placed in sidelying over a pillow, with the more restricted side of the chest wall positioned upward. In this position, the individual can add deep breathing and shoulder flexion and abduction overhead to elongate the shortened aspects of the trunk. The therapist can add manual techniques to assist in lengthening the chest wall (discussed below). Individuals are encouraged to inspire fully and use a series of breath-stacking maneuvers as passive stretching continues. Some individuals may add active motions to further increase the range of motion. Passive-positioning principles should be carried over to apply when the individual is sitting in the wheelchair to encourage the proper breathing pattern.

Manual Chest Stretching and Rib Mobilization

For an individual who is in the early rehabilitation process, general chest-mobilizing techniques are often adequate for mobilizing a tight chest wall. At this stage, the therapist actively assists the individual through motions that elongate the rib cage and expand the anterior chest wall. The therapist can passively stretch the thorax by using a wringing motion, with the hands moving in opposite directions. With the individual positioned in supine or side-lying position, the therapist places one hand on the posterior wall of the thorax and the other on the anterolateral surface. The therapist places pressure through the heels of the hands or through the ulnar surfaces as the hands are brought together, applying a counter-rotation motion to move the rib segments. As pressure is applied, the individual with SCI exhales to assist expiration. The therapist's upper hand (on the posterior surface of the thorax, closest to the head and shoulders) may stabilize, as the lower hand (located on the anterolateral surface of the thorax, closest to the pelvis) assists the ribs to move in the downward and inward direction during expiration.[23,24] A variety of hand placements may be effective in mobilizing the chest. The

important aspect is to realize that individuals with paralysis are just as vulnerable to loss of range in the thoracic cage as they are to forming contractures in the extremities.

The individual with a SCI can also have the thoracic cage and vertebra mobilized while seated in the short-sitting position. The individual's feet must be firmly in contact with the floor, and the pelvis must be level. The therapist sits at one side or directly behind the individual and works on aligning the spine. This action begins by moving the individual's posteriorly tilted pelvis forward toward neutral. Once the pelvis is aligned at neutral, the therapist applies manual pressure inward and upward to move each section of the spine into a more neutral alignment. The front of the chest is stabilized by the therapist's nondominant arm, which is placed across the upper torso while pressure is applied to the posterior aspect of each spinal segment. The dominant hand applies a graded force moving slowly up the back from the pelvis up to the mid- and upper-thoracic regions. These actions help lengthen the soft tissues, making it easier for the muscles of respiration to work.

If a contracture or specific area of muscle tightness develops, more specific and specialized techniques may be indicated, such as rib and vertebral mobilization methods. When applying more specific mobilizations, the therapist modifies the techniques for individuals with impaired sensation; in such cases, mobilization strategies are applied gradually and with caution.

Insufflation Techniques

Chest wall stretching can also be performed by using insufflation techniques, since insufflation increases the volume of air accepted into the lungs (discussed above). Insufflation programs encourage individuals to use their own strategies to inhale as much air as possible before adding more volume to the lungs with a resuscitation bag or mechanical positive pressure ventilation. The individual uses a strong glottis to hold the air in place, thereby stretching the chest wall. The stronger the glottis, the larger the volume of air placed in the lungs. Progress is documented by reporting the maximal volume held by the glottis, which is referred to as the *maximal insufflation capacity*. The maximal insufflation capacity is measured by releasing the air held by the glottis into a spirometer.[155,204] Chest wall expansion can also be measured with a tape measure to document the impact of these techniques on expansion of the chest.

When a portable positive pressure device is used for insufflation, approximately 5 to 40 cm H_2O pressurized air may be delivered.[23,209,224] This technique is also referred to as intermittent positive pressure breathing. High pressures (beyond 20 cm H_2O) may be contraindicated in individuals with premorbid lung conditions or when there are injuries to the thoracic cage. This technique may be implemented in a variety of ways and offered by several disciplines. In some cases, respiratory therapy may offer intermittent positive pressure breathing and instill medications into the airways as the chest is expanded. Respiratory muscle weakness is an indication for positive pressure insufflation; however, it is costly to administer chest mobilization in this manner if alternative techniques are effective.[225] Reasons for implementing an intermittent positive pressure breathing program include treatment of atelectasis, normalization of blood gases, improving cough function, and chest mobility.[225]

If the goal of intermittent positive pressure breathing is to expand the chest wall and maintain lung compliance, then the therapist evaluates the breathing pattern with and without the insufflation volume. If the individual takes in air from a positive pressure device, then the air may enter the lungs without expanding the chest wall (the air moves caudally). The individual may need to wear an abdominal binder to restrict the abdominal wall and force the air to expand the chest. The therapist may also place one hand over the abdomen if a binder is not available. The individual is given the instruction to "let the air flow into the lungs like releasing pressure from a balloon." The applied pressure level is initially low (5 to 10 cm H_2O) and increases in increments of 5 to 20 cm H_2O as the individual adapts to the airflow, until a maximum of 40 cm H_2O is reached.[23,24,224] There are two reports in the literature documenting significant increases in VC after several sessions of insufflation were offered to individuals with cervical spinal cord lesions.[209,226] Reports on the immediate effects of one intermittent positive pressure breathing treatment suggest only small, nonsignificant increases in VC (43 mL),[227] with no change in total respiratory system compliance.[228] This technique can be taught to caregivers; it is valuable for those individuals who have not yet learned how to perform an air-shift maneuver or for individuals who have difficulty learning glossopharyngeal breathing, breath-stacking, or other self range-of-motion strategies to maintain chest mobility. Regardless of the technique used, chest wall mobilization is important for preventing restrictions and maintaining efficient use of respiratory muscle function.[218] Mobilization of the chest wall should be performed daily and should be part of the home program.

Strategies to Enhance Respiratory Muscle Performance

Respiratory muscle performance encompasses a variety of dimensions. Initially, the goal is for the individual to develop adequate respiratory function to allow comfortable breathing without a ventilator. To do this, the individual must not only have sufficient respiratory muscle strength, but also have sufficient muscle endurance. Accordingly, the muscles of ventilation must develop a resistance to fatigue. The individual must also perceive a level of comfort and report no dyspnea at rest. Removal from ventilator support or positioning in stressful postures

may provoke anxiety responses. Such responses may increase the work of breathing. Therefore, relaxation techniques may also play a role in assisting these individuals. Breathing control and eccentric muscle contraction is required for speech in the individual who has become at least partially independent from ventilation support. A comprehensive respiratory muscle conditioning program will also include eccentric exercise.

The ability to develop adequate reserve for activity is important, especially for individuals who are ambulatory or those who use a manual wheelchair for community mobility. These individuals may be comfortable at rest, but fatigue easily during functional tasks or with positioning in upright postures. Respiratory muscle strength and endurance must be adequate to support activity needs over an entire day; the individual may have a goal of returning to work or participation in recreational sports. Exercise training programs will be necessary in order to fully condition the respiratory muscles. In the following section, facilitation/cuing of muscle activation, respiratory muscle strength and endurance training, and respiratory muscle conditioning through exercise training will be discussed.

Individuals who participate in respiratory muscle conditioning programs must be monitored closely for signs of fatigue (*see* Table 14-3). The initial breathing pattern is noted, baseline physiological measures are recorded (HR, RR, BP, and SaO_2), and the rating of perceived exertion and dyspnea are documented. Criteria for terminating the respiratory muscle training activity include the following:

- RR increased to >30 breaths per minute during rest phase
- SaO_2 decreased 5% from baseline
- SaO_2 <90%
- Unwanted accessory muscle use present or increased
- Paradoxical breathing when not previously present
- Perceived exertion rating of >6/10 (on a 0 to 10 scale) or >14/20 (on a 6 to 20 scale)
- Elevation in $ETCO_2$
- Disproportionate rise in HR associated with hypoxemia
- Complaints of headache

Although HR rarely increases excessively with respiratory muscle training, it may indicate the degree of physiologic stress being introduced by the exercise, or HR may be elevated in association with hypoxemia.

Facilitation of Respiratory Muscle Actions

Individuals who have low MIP, low VC, and/or a strength score of 3/5 or less in muscles of ventilation may benefit from muscle facilitation to both accessory muscles and the diaphragm. The therapist considers the individual's breathing pattern and his or her potential for recovery when deciding which muscles to facilitate and the methods to use in the breathing retraining program. For example, an individual who has an injury at C3–C4 will have some diaphragm activity. Unfortunately, the diaphragm may not be adequate to sustain breathing, therefore compensatory accessory muscle activity will be necessary if the individual is to develop adequate ventilatory capacity for independent breathing. Alternatively, the individual with a C5 level of injury will likely have full innervation to the diaphragm. Accessory muscle use in this case may initially hinder recruitment of a weakened diaphragm. The therapist may choose to discourage the activation of the scalenes, upper trapezius, and sternocleidomastoid muscles for this individual. Conversely, if an overactive diaphragm is contributing to paradoxical breathing and distortion of the chest wall, then inhibition of the diaphragm may be considered,[20] especially if paradoxical motion occurs after an abdominal is applied. The therapist must recognize the overall impact of strengthening specific muscles and consider their influence on the mechanics of breathing and balance of chest wall motion.

Once the individual's breathing pattern and potential for recovery has been determined, the individual is positioned so that the appropriate muscles are facilitated.[229] If diaphragm activation is desired, then positioning the individual in a supine position with a 15- to 20-degree incline of the head and slight knee flexion will maintain the pelvis in a posterior tilt, shifting the abdominal contents away from the diaphragm.[23,116] Positioning of the pelvis in a posterior tilt is recommended for encouraging diaphragm activation.[116] The therapist can encourage diaphragmatic breathing by reaching under the anterior costal margins at the level of ribs 6 to 8 and providing manual cues. The therapist follows the actions of inspiration and expiration with the hand and provides a gentle squeeze at the end of inspiration along with the instruction, "breathe into my hand," or "sniff."[116,221] Sniffing is encouraged if the individual has trouble recruiting the diaphragm.[221] Often a mirror or biofeedback methods may be combined with verbal and manual cues to encourage diaphragm activation.[180] The neck accessory muscles can be inhibited by placing the head in capital flexion while the upper chest muscles can be inhibited by shoulder internal rotation and adduction.[116] If the individual needs to develop strength in the accessory muscles, then the individual may need positioning of the head and neck in neutral and the shoulders in external rotation and abduction.[22,116] Monitoring the individual's breathing pattern, RR, and physiologic measures (HR, SaO_2, etc.) will be important to confirm the optimal position. Later, the individual can gradually be progressed to more challenging positions (e.g., sitting upright >60 degrees in bed) and combining the positional stress with breathing maneuvers (e.g., deep breathing or resistive breathing).

Any program designed to improve muscle function begins with facilitation and progresses toward adding active-assisted techniques to elicited muscle contractions. Once the muscle is activated, the therapist uses the muscle action to develop a pattern of movement with the individual participating; because upper extremity and trunk movements influence ventilation, this is especially true for the muscles of ventilation in individuals with SCI who have little voluntary movement in the upper extremities.[20] Therapeutic movement patterns that incorporate the arms and trunk during functional training may also be used to facilitate breathing. There are muscle spindles and proprioceptive control mechanisms in the intercostal muscles and surrounding scapulothoracic muscles; however, there is no evidence of such motor control systems in the diaphragm.[12,230] Therefore, facilitation/cuing strategies applying proprioceptive techniques are directed toward the recruiting intercostal, scapulothroacic, and neck muscles rather than the diaphragm. Any individual who has marginal diaphragm function can use a pneumobelt for active assistive exercise (discussed above[23,94]). The pneumobelt bladder fills under pressure from a machine that has predetermined pressure limits. Therefore, early in the training, the pressure inside the bladder is high so that there will be firm compression of the abdominal contents to allow the diaphragm to be passively moved to a high place in the thoracic cavity. The bladder inflation pressure applied is gradually decreased as diaphragm function improves. Eventually, only an abdominal binder may be necessary.

Facilitation/cuing techniques can also be applied during the coordinated breathing activities mentioned earlier. For example, a quick stretch to the pectoral muscles prior to reaching up and across during rolling from supine to side-lying position can facilitate and/or cue inspiration as the trunk extends.[20] A firm manual contact encouraging isometric stabilization of the thorax can offer stability during breath holding for repositioning in the wheelchair. Another facilitation/cuing strategy uses a series of quick stretches applied on the lateral costal boarders of the thorax as the individual attempts breath-stacking. The individual is usually in a supine position initially when learning the technique, but the technique may also be used while in the sitting position. The manual cues are applied down and inward quickly at the end of expiration and the end of each stacking attempt. The therapist instructs the individual by saying, "breathe in, breath in, breath in," as the quick stretch is applied to the intercostals and various other muscles acting on the chest wall. Hand position is modified to provide cues at the region of the thorax with the most potential for muscle activation. Pectoralis muscle facilitation/cuing has been recommended to assist with both inspiratory and expiratory function.[51,116,196,197] Later, the manual cues can offer resistance to inspiration as the individual's ventilatory muscle control improves.[221] Alternatively, a belt or towel can be wrapped around the thorax and the level of ribs 8 to 12 and held firmly in place as the individual inspires. This action will resist inspiration during breath-stacking attempts if the individual is seated or an abdominal binder is in place to restrain any caudal movement of the diaphragm.

Expiration may use concentric contractions, eccentric contractions, or relaxation of inspiratory muscle.[20,116]

Teaching the individual with SCI vocalization patterns or singing is a method for training the diaphragm for eccentric breathing control. One way to develop this control is to ask the individual to take a deep breath and count aloud or sing a song. The higher the number or more syllables in the song that can be vocalized during a single expiration, the greater the eccentric control (normal is 8 to 10 syllables per breath).[20] The individual can also be asked to hold one syllable, such as "ohooo," for as long as possible, and the therapist records the time for the period of phonation in seconds (normal is 15 seconds).[47] This eccentric control is useful not only for phonation, but may also assist in using inspiratory volume for air-shifts and for effective performance of contemporary secretion mobilization strategies. Again, the therapist can observe the influence of body positioning or the application of an abdominal binder on eccentric control by asking the individual to count or hold a vowel sound and then comparing the differences in performance.

Respiratory Muscle Training: Strength and Endurance

Once the muscles of ventilation are 3+/5 in strength, with a VC of greater than 10 mL/kg of ideal body weight (500 to 1000 mL) or MIP greater (more negative) than –30 cm H_2O, then a progressive resistive exercise training program can be implemented. Progressive resistive exercise training may begin with something as simple as deep breathing with or without an incentive spirometer. This training may also prevent atelectasis in some individuals. Ward et al[231] found deep breathing that incorporated a 3-second breath hold (i.e., sustained maximal inspiration) was more effective in preventing postoperative atelectasis than was having each individual perform multiple deep breaths. Therefore, breathing with an inspiratory hold or pause at the end of a deep breath may be important.

Incentive spirometers can be used to encourage deeper sustained breaths. Although a recent systematic review reported incentive spirometry to be ineffective in preventing postoperative pulmonary complications after abdominal or cardiothoracic surgery,[232] these findings may have little relevance to the potential benefits for reducing pulmonary complications in individuals who have weakness of the respiratory muscles. Cheshire and Flack[233] reported improved mean differences in VC (>2000 mL) for individuals with both acute and chronic tetraplegia after ventilatory muscle training when using an approach that combined biofeedback and incentive spirometry. Bodin et al[217] compared breathing at rest to deep breathing maneuvers in 20 individuals with C5–C8 motor complete spinal injuries and found deep breathing resulted in significantly greater TV, alveolar ventilation, peak inspiratory volume, and reduced the RR. Incentive spirometry or any deep breathing action that provokes expansion of the lungs in individuals with SCI will be important for developing respiratory muscle strength and endurance and may enhance cough function.[23,116]

The therapist provides guidance in proper positioning and instructs the individual in the correct breathing patterns to use during any deep breathing exercises. Adding an abdominal binder during deep breathing exercise will be important in those with tetraplegia or high paraplegia who perform exercises in an upright position.[234]

Once the individual can complete 15 minutes of deep breathing with the proper breathing pattern, more challenging resistive exercises can begin. The most common methods used to offer resistance to breathing include manual resistance, diaphragmatic training with weights, breathing into devices that resist airflow generated by the individual (e.g., respiratory muscle trainers, fluid-filled bottles), or breathing against positive mechanical airflow.[226] Manual resistance is often a natural progression in strength training programs. Ventilatory muscles can be strengthened using hand placements similar to those described for facilitation/cuing, with the difference being that pressure is applied against the inspiratory effort rather than applying a facilatory cue at the end of expiration. For example, when the hands are placed over the lateral costal boarders of the thorax, the therapist actually resists inspiration instead of applying a quick stretch to the intercostal muscles at the end of expiration as described earlier. Likewise, when individuals are working on extremity patterns as part of coordinated breathing during therapeutic activities or while performing functional tasks, manual resistance can be added to challenge movement when the individual is ready. Manual resistance can also be applied directly to the epigastric region to resist the diaphragmatic descent during inspiration. Manual resistance techniques have the advantage of being individualized and allow the therapist to modify the amount of resistance according to tolerance. This is especially helpful if the individual experiences pain or fatigues easily.

Resistive training with diaphragmatic weights is initially performed with the individual lying in the supine position. Weight may be applied by placing a sandbag or cuff weight directly onto the abdomen. A wooden weight pan with a dowel in the middle may be used to hold disc weights. Initially, a very light weight (3 to 5 lbs) or the weight pan itself may be used. The individual is instructed to "breathe in deeply while keeping your upper chest quiet." The breath is held for several seconds. Ten maximal breaths are performed in three to four sets.[23,24,135] Resting breaths can be performed between the maximal efforts. The therapist observes the amount of epigastric rise during inspiration with deep breathing prior to applying any weight. The epigastric region should continue to rise to the same level after any weight is applied, indicating full unrestricted excursion of the diaphragm. More weight can be applied as long as the breathing pattern is maintained.

The therapist also determines the appropriate amount of weight by measuring inspiratory capacity and adding weights to a maximal level that does not alter the baseline inspiratory capacity.[135] The exercise should not provoke a decrease in SaO_2 or excessive neck or accessory muscle breathing[24]; these may be signs of respiratory muscle fatigue indicating that the weight applied is excessive. Usually, the individual can tolerate 15 minutes of weighted breathing.[23,221] To progress the strengthening program, the weight is gradually increased until measures of respiratory muscle strength (VC and MIP) plateau.[23,135] The number of repetitions and the time for weighted breathing can be decreased when more weight is applied. As long as the individual is able to generate good diaphragmatic action with a complete epigastric rise, then the repetitions and time are gradually increased again with the new weight.

Ventilatory muscle training uses resistive breathing by offering resistance to either inspiration (inspiratory muscle training) or expiration (expiratory muscle training) or both. For individuals with SCI, ventilatory muscle training usually focuses on increasing inspiratory muscle work initially. This is because many individuals with SCI do not have active abdominal muscles, so expiration is passive or is too weak for resistive training. Individuals with some expiratory function (moderate cough force or 3+/5 abdominal muscle strength) can also work on expiratory muscle strengthening using resistive breathing devices. Individuals having motor incomplete cervical, midthoracic, or lumbar injuries will participate in ventilatory muscle training, whereas most individuals with motor complete cervical or high thoracic lesions will primarily focus on inspiratory muscle training. Pressure, flow, or volume loads are used separately or in combinations to train the muscles of ventilation. Using a training stimulus that combines maximal flow and pressure is recommended for individuals with neuromuscular weakness to prevent respiratory muscle fatigue.[134]

Several handheld devices are commercially available to improve strength and endurance of the respiratory muscles.[20,142] The devices available may be linear (Threshold Trainer, available from Philips Respironics; Amsterdam, The Netherlands) or nonlinear (P-Flex Resistive Trainer; Philips Respironics; Amsterdam, The Netherlands) and can offer resistance to flow and/or determine a pressure threshold. Linear devices have a spring-loaded valve to set a negative pressure threshold load and maintain a consistent load regardless of breathing pattern. The amount of negative pressure can be increased by winding the spring more tightly. Nonlinear devices such as P-Flex, DHD Medical Products IMT (DHD Medical Products, Canastoga, NY), The Breather (PN Medical; Orlando, FL) often have a variable load because they offer resistance to flow through a small hole. The amount of resistance is increased when the diameter of the hole is decreased. A disadvantage of the nonlinear device is that the individual can simply change the breathing pattern and breathe more slowly to decrease the challenge to the muscles of ventilation (nontargeted training). A target RR or target flow rate must be set for the individual when using nonlinear devices to ensure consistent resistive challenge (targeted training).

When a target is set, the individual can see the pressure level generated (by oscilloscope or viewing a needle gauge attached to manometer). Both linear and nonlinear devices may be used with supplemental oxygen if the SaO_2 declines; however, this is not usually necessary when training individuals with SCI. Resistive breathing may be contraindicated for use in individuals who are at risk for intracranial hemorrhage or seizures (e.g., those with head trauma), are hypertensive with cardiac instability, or for anyone for whom it is not safe to perform a Valsalva maneuver.

Respiratory muscles do not rest; for this reason, endurance training may be more important than strength training. While respiratory muscle strength training involves using high, near-maximal inspiratory or expiratory maneuvers, which include some isometric holding, respiratory muscle endurance training involves repetitive submaximal contractions using a desired breathing pattern.[26] For individuals with SCI, an initial endurance training load is usually 20% to 40% of MIP or 5% to 10% of MEP.[20] The resistance is increased based on the individual's rating of perceived exertion during the training period.[127] The individual should work toward 15 to 20 minutes of loaded breathing. The breathing sessions initially begin with short 3- to 5-minute bouts, with rest periods,[26] and require the individual to breathe deeply with the diaphragm. Gradually, the length of time for loaded breathing is increased and the rest period decreased until 20 continuous minutes are achieved without a change in breathing pattern. Typically, the training sessions are offered two to three times per day, 5 to 7 days per week, for 6 to 8 weeks.[20,26,167] Guidelines for progressing ventilatory muscle resistance during training are given in Table 14-8.

It is important to demonstrate the benefit of the ventilatory muscle training program by examining dyspnea levels during stressful activities of daily living (especially activities involving arm work). Progress may also be demonstrated by measuring repetitive MIP and/or MEP, measuring maximal voluntary ventilation, using maximal sustainable volume technique, or by performing a progressive incremental threshold loading (determining threshold loading maximum) test. Simply measuring VC or MIP one time or taking the best of three measures will only reflect improvement in respiratory muscle strength; it will not demonstrate change or improvement in respiratory muscle endurance or demonstrate the impact of any improvement on performance of activities of daily living. Although ventilatory muscle training protocols have been described for people with spinal injuries,[20] optimal prescription parameters have yet to be confirmed due to the wide discrepancy in ventilatory muscle training techniques and limitations in research design.[142,167,235]

Preliminary reports on ventilatory muscle training and abdominal weight training suggest that these approaches have potential for improved respiratory function in individuals with SCI. Loveridge et al[236] reported improved MIP and sustained inspiratory pressure in both control

Table 14-8

Guidelines for Progressing Ventilatory Muscle Training Loads While Using Resistive Threshold Loading Device in Individuals with Neuromuscular Weakness[267]

Initial IMT Training Session

Beginning IMT level is to be set at 30% of MIP

If symptomatic: decrease resistance by 2 cm H_2O until no symptoms persist

If RPE >15: decrease resistance by 2 cm H_2O until within 13–15 range

SaO_2 will be monitored and kept above 90% during training.

Weekly IMT Progression

MIP <50 cm H_2O		MIP >50 cm H_2O	
RPE <13	+2	RPE <13	+4
RPE 13–15	+1	RPE 13–15	+2
RPE <15	+0	RPE <15	+0

↑ Resistance by 2 cm H_2O if RPE <13

↓ Resistance by 2 cm H_2O if RPE ≥15

Once MIP > 50 cm H_2O, the increments of progression are 4 cm H_2O (see left side)

IMT= inspiratory muscle training; RPE = rating of perceived exertion

and inspiratory muscle training groups (no target, 85% sustained inspiratory pressure training for 15 minutes, two times daily, for 8 weeks) with no post-training differences. Derrickson et al[135] compared training with abdominal weight to inspiratory muscle training (using no target). In 11 individuals with cervical injuries, significant improvements in VC, maximal voluntary ventilation, peak expiratory flow rate, and MIP were observed after 7 weeks of training for both techniques, with no significant difference between the techniques. Lane[237] reported statistically significant increases in VC for 16 individuals with tetraplegia who received abdominal weight training (three times a week for 6 weeks) compared to 15 individuals who had routine therapy. Liaw et al[238] reported greater changes in VC compared to control when using inspiratory muscle training (targeted, 15 to 20 minutes, twice a day, for 6 weeks). Thus, it appears that offering some respiratory muscle training stimulus provides an improvement over baseline, but no one technique is superior to the others. When subjects with chronic injuries (≥1 year after injury) are offered inspiratory muscle training (no target, twice daily), improvements in MIP and VC achieved with 8 weeks of training are not retained 4 months later if training is not continued.[133] This research indicates that individuals with SCI are also susceptible to de-training of the respiratory muscles.[133,134]

Most of the respiratory muscles respond to principles of exercise training, acquiring physiological adaptations similar to other skeletal muscles.[239] However, the diaphragm is composed primarily of fatigue-resistant (type I) muscle fibers[9] and requires a different training regimen (e.g., endurance training) compared to abdominal muscles or intercostal muscles, which have a more equal composition of type I and type II muscle fibers.[239] Muscle fiber action is also dependent upon nervous system signaling. The respiratory motor control system may also have latent pathways that emerge after a SCI and assist in greater respiratory muscle fiber activation and recovery of ventilatory capacity.[240] Additionally, there appears to be some evidence that ventilatory muscle training effects can transfer to functional outcomes.[239] Functional outcomes achieved through expiratory muscle training include enhanced cough due to increased speed of vocal cord closure, with increased driving force behind a closed glottis providing faster flow rates for airway clearance.[239] Improved glottis control also assists in speech production. Speech improves after expiratory muscle training by strengthening the muscles responsible for generating positive pressure and prolonged pressure release. Additionally, swallowing function improves due to improved subglottal pressure control and increased airway protective actions resulting from increased strength in the muscles involved in swallowing. Wang et al[140] reported that inspiratory muscle training improved MIP and maximal voluntary ventilation, but also resulted in decreased CO_2 retention and increased SaO_2 during sleep. Perhaps ventilatory muscle training should be included in the home program for some individuals as part of their lifetime management of their respiratory dysfunction. It may be that those who maintain good respiratory muscle strength and endurance will be more successful in preventing the occurrence of respiratory complications in the long term.

Respiratory Muscle Conditioning: Exercise Training

For healthy individuals, activity challenges and aerobic exercise increase the metabolic demands for oxygen resulting in an increased ventilatory response. The RR and TV increase to support higher minute ventilation. Respiratory muscle demands are increased during activity and exercise. Individuals with SCI often return to very active lives despite requiring a wheelchair for mobility. Most individuals do not recover normal pulmonary function, yet they may want to return to full-time work and social roles. Aerobic exercise training can be helpful in conditioning the respiratory muscles to support the ventilation necessary for an active lifestyle. Cardiovascular health can be improved through increased activity and aerobic conditioning.[142] There are a variety of therapeutic approaches used to condition the muscles of respiration. Common approaches include arm ergometry, wheelchair ergometry, or endurance propulsion as aerobic training modes.[80,241,242] These approaches may be used alone or combined with other breathing control techniques.[80] Exercise training has been shown to improve pulmonary function in individuals with tetraplegia[243] as well as those with paraplegia.[80]

The prescription for aerobic exercise training must include high-intensity activity (i.e., 80% HR maximum) maintained for 20 to 30 minutes at least three times a week for 6 weeks if the goal is to improve pulmonary function, peak minute ventilation, TV, and overall ventilatory reserve in those with SCI.[142] Studies of healthy individuals and those with chronic obstructive pulmonary disease and multiple sclerosis suggest that MIP and peak minute ventilation values change in association with arm activity.[244-246] During arm activity, the accessory muscles are involved in moving and stabilizing the arms and cannot participate effectively in ventilation.[246,247] This shifts the ventilatory demand to the diaphragm, especially when the arms are unsupported.[245] Uijl et al[78] found that training the respiratory muscles with a targeted ventilatory muscle training protocol twice a day for 15 minutes improved arm cycle aerobic exercise performance (peak oxygen consumption [VO_2] increased from 870 mL to 980 mL; arm ergometry protocol) in nine individuals with C3–C7 tetraplegia. Thus respiratory muscle function and arm function are related; therefore, interventions involving either arm ergometry or ventilatory muscle training may influence performance of the other. Individuals who wish to participate in wheelchair sports programs may include combinations of ventilatory muscle training and arm work (wheelchair ergometry or

propulsion) to further challenge the respiratory muscles. When implementing any aerobic exercise program, the therapist must provide complete physiological monitoring and be cognizant of the risks of exercise training (i.e., thermal dysregulation, hypotension, autonomic dysreflexia, and musculoskeletal injury) for an individual with SCI.[248] Details pertaining to the appropriate aerobic exercise prescription for muscle conditioning and aerobic training for individuals with SCI are reported elsewhere (see chapter 16).[248]

Discharge Planning

Education is the primary role of the therapist who is preparing an individual with SCI for discharge. During this time, the therapist reexamines the respiratory function of the individual and determines which therapeutic activities are important for the home program. The therapist determines whether each measure of respiratory function has reached a plateau or whether there is room for continued improvement. Individuals who are continuing to improve in their MIP, MEP, and VC should be offered the opportunity for follow-up during their outpatient or home health visits. Gains in respiratory function may be lost if the individual or the family do not continue with a lifetime program. The individual, family, and/or caregiver will need to learn good bronchial hygiene, strategies for maintaining chest mobility, and effective positioning, as well as continue with breathing exercises.[23] Training of the individual, family, and caregiver can begin as soon as they are ready to learn. Early training allows time for practice throughout the rehabilitation period.

Prevention of pulmonary complications is the most important goal of any home program for respiratory care in individuals with SCI. Deep breathing and applying air shifts and/or glossopharyngeal breathing techniques are performed daily to maintain chest wall expansion and good inspiratory volume. The family should be instructed in general chest-stretching procedures as part of the overall range-of-motion program. The individual and family should demonstrate a good manual cough assist that is adequate to remove secretions effectively. Coughing is encouraged even if the airways are not productive or if the individual is to be discharged home on ventilator support. The family and caregiver need to learn any postural drainage and airway clearance strategies that have been effective for the individual. For the individual who is continuing with partial or full-time ventilator support, the appropriate family member or caregiver will need to learn how to suction the airways. However, it should be noted that the training of various levels of health-care providers in suctioning techniques differs according to state practice acts.[249] Once the appropriate caregiver has been identified, those who are responsible for suctioning will need to practice and be able to use proper technique before the individual is discharged. The therapist provides education in recognizing the signs of infection and excessive respiratory muscle fatigue, as well as in the importance of aggressively seeking medical assistance at the first sign of respiratory compromise. Demonstrating breathing exercises and requesting that the individual demonstrate in return is one method for continuing to keep the respiratory system strong and resistant to illness. Additionally, providing an oximeter at home assists in detecting early signs of pneumonia.[106] Criteria for determining medical stability and readiness for discharge is further described in the "Statement on Home Care for Patients with Respiratory Disorders," approved by the American Thoracic Society.[250]

Individuals who are ventilator assisted may go home if there is adequate family or caregiver support. A minimum of three caregivers will need to be trained in management of respiratory program.[249] Caregivers need to have good coping skills. The family will need to be trained in emergency management in the event of a power failure or improper functioning of the ventilator.[23] Portable ventilators have an internal battery that can operate for a limited time. The internal battery will remain fully charged if the ventilator is properly plugged into the wall whenever the individual returns from any outing. The individual's home will need to be equipped with a minimum of 100 amp electrical service and have three-pronged industrial-grade outlets.[249] A backup generator should be available, as should the phone number of a local home health team with expertise in servicing individuals on ventilator support. Additionally, letters of special consideration should be sent to the power company, telephone company, and fire departments, alerting them to the possibility of an emergency call for a ventilator-dependent individual.[249]

Today's interdisciplinary environment requires a team effort to coordinate all the necessary training for discharge. The family and caregivers will need to meet with a number of members of the team. The therapist may not be the primary educator when training family or caregivers of individuals who are leaving with ventilator support. However, it is important for the family or caregivers to understand that the training for respiratory care is occurring and that the program as a whole is critically important for increasing life expectancy and reducing the incidence of respiratory complications. The therapist may be more involved in training family and caregivers in techniques for transferring the individual from the bed to wheelchair and wheelchair to car or van. The therapist determines that the caregivers know how to manage the ventilation support during transfers, that the wheelchair is set up with a portable ventilator, and that the family understands how to maintain and charge both the wheelchair and ventilator batteries. In addition, the therapist will ascertain that the family understands the importance of proper positioning in the wheelchair, proper fitting and use of the abdominal binder, and other aspects of the respiratory management. Encouraging the use of airway-clearance techniques as part of a routine home program should be included, along with chest mobility and breathing exercises. Prior to discharge, all ventilator-assisted individuals should have a complete 24-hour caregiver stay that includes an overnight home visit and evaluation by a qualified health-care provider.[249] The evaluation should review the home environment, emergency system, and all caregiver respiratory management skills.

For therapists working in home health who may visit the individual after discharge, it will be important to assess the capacity of the caregivers to attend to the needs of the individual with SCI. The therapist ensures that the caregiver has the needed skills to participate in manual coughing, chest stretching, positioning of the individual in the wheelchair, and proper setup for breathing exercises and that the caregiver can safely manage the ventilation equipment during changes in positions. Practice is one of the most important components of education for emergencies;[251] the therapist provides the caregiver with an opportunity to practice handling an emergency, providing artificial ventilation to the individual via tracheostomy using a manual resuscitation bag. Caregivers who have practiced emergency management skills are more likely to respond correctly in a true emergency. It will be important to know the level of experience the caregiver holds and his or her comfort level in performing all "hands-on" skills. Essential caregiver respiratory care management skills are summarized in Table 14-9.

Table 14-9
Essential Caregiver Respiratory Care Management Skills
Managing Ventilation Equipment
Suctions and applies good technique prior to mobility
Provides effective manual cough or cough-assist technique
Manages ventilation equipment appropriately during
repositioning in bed
transfers to wheelchair

Table 14-9

Essential Caregiver Respiratory Care Management Skills—cont'd

Providing Artificial Ventilation

Able to perform mouth-to-mouth/tracheostomy/mask ventilation with protective shield

Correctly uses a manual resuscitation bag to
    tracheostomy
    mouth (via mask) if closed tracheostomy

Has practiced on a manikin

Responding to Emergencies

CPR training is current

Has an emergency management plan

Knows how long the back-up battery will last

Knows how to maintain the battery, recharge, etc.

Knows the correct method to activate EMS

Encourages/supports Home Respiratory Care Program

Bronchial hygiene

Chest mobility

Respiratory muscle conditioning

The Chronic Stage

Respiratory concerns continue long after the individual with SCI is discharged from the rehabilitation stay. Respiratory symptoms (e.g., wheezing, dyspnea with activities of daily living, phlegm, and cough) are known to contribute to lower health-related quality of life scores in individuals with chronic SCI.[252] Individuals with SCI who have been breathing on their own for years may unexpectedly develop ventilatory failure.[2,156] Health-care professionals should be aware of sudden changes in the respiratory demands of individuals with SCI. If the individual gains weight, starts smoking, develops a fever, or has a cold or asthma, then the load on the respiratory muscles is increased. Any decline in neurologic function that may occur from cervical instability, the development of a syrinx, or the accumulation of excessive scar tissue around the cord could have an impact on the muscles of respiration. In those with SCI, the incidence of neurological decline after a period of stability has been reported to be as high as 10% in individuals with tetraplegia.[253]

Changes in the medication regimen can also affect respiratory function. For example, if spasticity medication is reduced, then the tone in the intercostal muscles will likely be decreased and paradoxical breathing may appear.[9,55] Any individuals who become sedentary or decide not to continue participating in the respiratory care program may be at risk for pulmonary complications, especially as they begin to age.[254] Signs and symptoms associated with late ventilatory failure include changes in mental alertness, daytime drowsiness, elevated RR, unexplained dyspnea, and increased stressful ventilation

concerns with changes in position.[156] Individual who have these symptoms should be immediately referred to their physician for a thorough examination.

Individuals with motor complete tetraplegia between C1 and C3 will most likely remain ventilator dependent. Once the individual with high cervical SCI survives beyond the first year of ventilator dependency, there is a cumulative survival rate of 61.4% over the next 14 years.[255] Forty-nine percent of deaths occurring in ventilator-dependent individuals are due to respiratory conditions.[255] Individuals who remain ventilator dependent are generally satisfied with their quality of life.[256] Today, there are assisted ventilatory care centers to support individuals who are living with invasive ventilator support. These centers have been successful in increasing the amount of ventilator-free time by specifically attending to evaluation of the ventilatory reserve, monitoring gas exchange, and providing nutritional support.[257] Some individuals requiring ventilator assistance can eventually be decannulated and discharged to the community, and others progress from cuffed to uncuffed tracheostomies. Delayed diaphragm recovery and freedom from the ventilator occurs in 21% of individuals having motor complete C1–C4 injuries. This has resulted in the recommendation that phrenic nerve testing be performed every 3 months for the first year after discharge with ventilator support.[258]

Individuals with low VCs who are unable to breathe without the ventilator will have either invasive or noninvasive support. If the individual using invasive support continues with a tracheostomy, then the parameters of ventilation support may change. This change may include increasing the volume of air delivered by the ventilator while the individual learns to permit airflow to escape to the oral cavity for speech.[48,259] This increase in volume accelerates the flow through the fenestrated tubing and permits the use of speaking valves for communication. Unfortunately, it may also result in hypocapnia and cause the individual to become lightheaded. Yet, communication is a priority for those who are living at home on ventilator support.

For some, ventilation may be managed by noninvasive support that may include either negative- or positive pressure support.[106] Negative pressure devices are less common and include total body chambers (iron lung), chest cuirass (plastic shell over the anterior chest), or chest wrap (plastic bag around the body).[156] Negative pressure ventilators create an outward pull on the abdomen and/or thoracic cage during the negative pressure cycle so that inspiration occurs. Positive pressure devices (CPAP or BiPAP) are more common with air delivery occurring via a mask or mouthpiece. The advantage of using noninvasive support is that the individual no longer has a tracheostomy, and this reduces the risk of infection. The disadvantage of noninvasive support is that there may be leaks around the interfacing and less-precise ventilation management. Headaches may occur with some forms of positive pressure ventilation. Tzeng et al[106] documented a successful home protocol using noninvasive support and manual-assisted cough, which resulted in reduced hospital days and numbers of pulmonary complications in 14 individuals with neuromuscular disease.

Some individuals who require full-time ventilator support may feel confined as they depend on family members or caregivers to properly maintain the equipment, position the tubing correctly, suction the airways, and attend to alarm systems. Phrenic nerve or diaphragm pacing may be offered to appropriate individuals to improve speech control, increase comfort, and allow a more portable system for ventilation.[181] Phrenic nerve pacing involves stimulation of the phrenic nerve to elicit contraction of the diaphragm. Electrophysiologic assessment of phrenic nerve function may also be useful to assist in determining the prognosis for weaning from ventilator support.[260] Candidates for phrenic nerve pacing must have no current aspiration problems, a strong immune system for fighting infection, unimpaired cognitive processing, good lung function, a compliant chest wall, and an intact phrenic nerve.

Several methods of stimulation may be considered for phrenic nerve pacing. Electrodes may be placed directly on the phrenic nerve surgically via a thoracotomy.[181,261] Electrodes may be positioned intramuscularly within both hemidiaphragms or in combination with the intercostal muscles.[262,263] Placement of intramuscular electrodes may be done laparoscopically, which offers less risk and shorter hospital stays than does a thoracotomy.[262] The number of electrodes may vary, with greater numbers of electrodes providing greater improvements in volume achieved under stimulation.

Therapists will be involved in the postsurgical examination and treatment of individuals who may be readmitted for a phrenic nerve or diaphragm-pacing procedure after months or years of living with ventilator support. Mobility precautions that apply to any individual who has had a surgery will apply to these individuals as well. Therapists may be asked to attend training sessions to learn about the stimulators. The pacing system does not usually allow removal of the tracheostomy tube due to the high likelihood for development of obstructive sleep apnea.[73] Reconditioning of the diaphragm must occur in the early postsurgical period. The pacing system is turned on for gradually increasing periods of time. Charting of the individual's response to stimulation is critical during this period. Initially, prior to the reconditioning period, the inspiratory volume may be 400 to 1000 mL post-surgery. This may increase to 1100 to 1300 mL after conditioning has occurred.[262] Approximately, 15 to 25 weeks may be needed for the period of reconditioning. On average, the individual will achieve 20 or more hours per day off the ventilator after the reconditioning period. The duration of the training period may be shorter when stimulation is provided by four electrodes rather than two electrodes.[73]

Although respiratory concerns are predominant in the individual who has a high cervical injury, the therapist recognizes that individuals with high thoracic injuries (T1–T6) also have a high incidence of respiratory complications and elevated risk for mortality.[264] Individuals living with a chronic SCI, who are ambulatory or functioning in the community in a wheelchair, complain of dyspnea during dressing when the arms are unsupported.[147] Therapists treating individuals with SCI in the home environment can assist these individuals by emphasizing the importance of continuing with a respiratory care program and teaching energy conservation and breathing control as the individual works on activities of daily living such as dressing. Generally, across the population of individuals with SCI, fatigue is a greater symptomatic concern than dyspnea and is most responsible for limiting the return to full community-level participation.[265]

Most individuals with SCI have respiratory concerns that continue after discharge. It will be important for the therapist to emphasize the respiratory management plan as part of the home program and to stress the importance of adapting a routine that includes continuation of preventative exercises. Family members and caregiver skills must be practiced and must be performed competently to avoid respiratory complications in those with motor complete cervical lesions, especially if the individual with SCI requires ventilatory assistance. The individual with SCI, the family, and the caregivers should be able to recognize the signs and symptoms of ventilatory failure and know when and how to contact the health-care team. Although a few ventilator-dependent individuals may qualify for phrenic nerve or diaphragm pacing, a tracheostomy may still be necessary to prevent sleep apnea.[73] Many individuals with high SCI develop sleep apnea and require nighttime ventilation support. Any onset of new symptoms (headaches, lethargy, fever, etc.) could result from sleep apnea or indicate late ventilatory failure and should be reported to the health-care team.[156] Implementing a good respiratory management program and following the guidelines for prevention will result in fewer respiratory complications, decrease the number of readmissions to the hospital, and improve the quality of life for the individual with SCI.[2,106]

CASE STUDY 14-1   Respiratory Training for an Individual Requiring Mechanical Ventilation

José is a 35-year-old agricultural worker who was traveling in the trunk of a car while crossing the border when the car was involved in a rear-end collision. He was triaged at the scene and transported to the emergency room at a Level 1 trauma center. Upon arrival in the emergency room, he was intubated and placed on control mode ventilation. Spine x-rays revealed he had sustained anterior compression fractures of C3–C4 vertebrae. There were several rib fractures and small abrasions. José had no family in the United States, spoke only Spanish, and was unemployed. He had cigarettes in his jacket. A summary of the acute care stay medical events and examinations are summarized in Table 14-10. A physical therapy consultation was requested and an examination began on day 2. The therapist reviewed the medical chart and noted that José was receiving mechanical ventilation, had a chest tube, feeding tube, urinary catheter, arterial line, and pulmonary artery line, and he was stabilized with cervical traction. History of vital signs and the time of pain medications were noted. Review of laboratory values indicated significant blood loss, but no risk of bleeding. Internal injuries had been repaired.

A physical therapy examination was initiated within 24 hours of admission to the intensive care unit (ICU). During the early acute care stage, the therapist recognized that the priority for medical management would be to ensure individual survival and optimize ventilation and oxygenation. Therefore, the initial examination session involved documenting the baseline measures available from the hemodynamic monitor and the ventilator (see Table 14-11).

The therapist proceeded with the examination while respecting the line and tube precautions. The therapist noted the individual's body position, auscultated lobes of the lungs, evaluated passive range of motion and tone, observed grimacing to pain, and examined the skin. Any changes in the physiologic measures from baseline were noted. The therapist communicated with José throughout the session. The therapist used hand signals and had command of a few key words in Spanish. The goals of the respiratory care program at this early time were to support metabolism, prevent lung infection, and optimize ventilation. The physical therapy goals were to prevent contractures and prevent pressure sores while monitoring and reporting

Table 14-10   Case History 35-Year-Old Male With C4 Tetraplegia

History and Medical Status: Acute Care	Hospital Day	Medical Management	Implication for Physical Therapy
• Admitted to emergency department; IV access, 100% O$_2$ via face mask, no significant external bleeding. HR = 120 bpm RR = 36 br/min BP = 100/60 mm/Hg • Spine and rib fracture • Pneumothorax • Emergent laparotomy to stop bleeding/repair internal injuries • Orthopedic consult • Neurology consult • Pulmonary consult • Transferred to ICU	Day 1	• Spine and head x-ray revealed C3–C4 vertebral fractures. No head injury. • Spine stabilization with traction. • Fracture ribs 8–10 left side • Chest x-ray small lungs on left • Chest tube on left • Intubated and placed on CMV	• Respiratory muscle involvement likely. • Chest wall injuries increase pain if innervated, look for signs and symptoms of pneumo/hemothorax. • Check positioning orders and evaluate in 15-degree supine position. • Communication limited • Infection control: gloves, hand washing

Continued

CASE STUDY 14-1 Respiratory Training for an Individual Requiring Mechanical Ventilation—cont'd

History and Medical Status: Acute Care	Hospital Day	Medical Management	Implication for Physical Therapy

• ICU nursing evaluation
• Medications: Heparin
• Halo vest applied
	Day 2	• Arterial line on left radial artery
		• Subclavian access for pulmonary artery monitoring
		• EKG: 12 lead
		• Pulse oximetry
		• Continuing with CMV
		• $ETCO_2$ monitor
		• IV lines
		• Feeding tubes
		• Pleurvac
		• Intermittent pneumatic compression devices to lower extremities
			• Invasive monitoring can assist PT during evaluation.
			• PT notes all baseline measures for:
			  • HR/EKG
			  • BP/MAP
			  • respiratory rate (set by mechanical ventilation)
			  • SaO_2
			  • $ETCO_2$
			• MV settings indicate individual is not participating at this time.
			• PT is familiar with MV and EKG alarm settings
			• Communication occurs with nursing; provides system to communicate with José

• Tracheostomy performed: Cuffed
• Arterial blood gases
  • PaO_2 = 90 mm Hg
  • $PaCO_2$ = 40 mm Hg
  • pH = 7.42
  • SpO_2 = 95%
	Day 3	• Continues with CMV mode
		  FiO_2 = 40%
		  RR = 18 br/min
		  Pressure = 30 mm Hg
			• Increased risk of infection
			• Positioning program
			• PROM program
			• PT examination continues

MV mode changed to SIMV
SIMV = 14 breaths/min
PSV = 15 cm H_2O
PEEP = 6 cm H_2O
	Day 4–6	• Continue with all of the above.
		• Use $ETCO_2$, SaO_2, EKG and MAP to evaluate tolerance to new mode.
		• Oxygen FiO_2 = 40%
			• Begin diaphragm breathing.
			• Develop rapport with José.
			• Initiate sitting program in bed.
			• Use bedside hemodynamic monitor and "response dependent" analysis to position change.
			• Orthostatic BP noted
			  Supine 30 degrees
			  = 112/85 mm Hg
			  Sitting 90 degrees
			  = 80/65 mm Hg

Remove chest tube	Day 7	Chest x-ray	• Modify mobility program: no excessive challenge immediately after chest tube removed. Sitting balance program deferred • Observe for signs of distress; ↑ neck breathing • Measure for wheelchair

CASE STUDY 14-1 Respiratory Training for an Individual Requiring Mechanical Ventilation—cont'd

History and Medical Status: Acute Care	Hospital Day	Medical Management	Implication for Physical Therapy
Orders for out of bed (OOB)	Day 8	• a.m. chest x-ray clear • Labs = no ↑ in white blood cells • Fio$_2$ = 40%	• Diaphragm breathing, PROM in a.m. • Mobility, transfer to wheelchair in p.m.
MV discontinuation trials Medical clearance for manual cough training	Day 9–12	Fio$_2$ = 35% via tracheostomy mask for several hours.	• Do not provide diaphragmatic breathing during discontinuation • Teach manual cough
Fever = 102°	Day 11	• Chest x-ray-Lower right lobe infiltrates • Labs = ↑ in WBC • HR = 96 bpm • Sao$_2$, = 92% • Increase Fio$_2$, = 45%	• Weakness to respiratory muscles; reduce training load. • Auscultation, sputum analysis, HR elevations expected, Sao$_2$, • Implement postural drainage and airway clearance program
Fever resolves	Day 14		• Consider increasing exercise training resistance • Reassess VC, NIF • Reinstitute positioning program, balance training and mobility program.
Progressed to tracheostomy mask full time during the day. Discharge to rehab floor	Day 15	• Sleep study notes: desaturation and periods of apnea at night • Evaluate for speaking value • CPAP ordered for nighttime	• VMT program for endurance • Individual and caregiver learn manual coughing • Teach GPB and air-shifts when trach closed off. • Implement chest stretching as MV is discontinued.

Table 14-11   Physical Therapy Evaluation in ICU

Examination Component	Early ICU	Late ICU
Chart review	Review of vital signs José not communicating Alert & oriented ↓ Tolerance to positioning Meds/labs/timing of each Chest x-ray	Coordination of care Note sitting tolerance MV discontinuation trials – strategy. Medications Sputum cultures Cigarettes = ↑ wean time and ↑ infection risk

MV Settings
• Mode
• TV or V$_E$
• RR
• PEEP
Oxygen needs
	Control Mode
	18 br/min
	10 PEEP
	40% Fio$_2$
		SIMV = 10
		5 PEEP
		Can tolerate time off ventilator support
		   RR off vent = 28 br/min
		   Neck breathing

Continued

CASE STUDY 14-1   Respiratory Training for an Individual Requiring Mechanical Ventilation—cont'd

Examination Component	Early ICU	Late ICU
HR/EKG	80 b/min; Normal sinus rhythm	70 b/min on vent 86 b/min during wean
BP/MAP arterial line	ABP = 110/80 mm Hg ; MAP = 95 mm Hg	116/78 mm Hg (manual)
SaO$_2$	95%	97%; ↓ 94% with weaning
Breath sounds	Decreased on right and in basal regions	Off ventilator = Diminished bilaterally
Sputum color	Clear	Yellow
Pain/facial grimacing	Yes; with passive range of motion to right side extremities	5/10 pain with PROM on right shoulder.
Breathing pattern	No spontaneous breathing	Off vent breathing: Neck = 3; Diaph = 1
Cough/airway clearance	Intubated → Tracheostomy with cuff Stimulated by suction catheter	Manual assist = Abdominal thrust with tracheal suction. Weak self assist
Positional changes	Improved vitals/oxygenation with left side down	Poor tolerance to upright; Off ventilator VCsupine = 450 ml NIF supine = −20 cm H$_2$O RR supine = 26 br/min
Muscle exam	No tone noted/spinal shock Intact neck accessory observed spontaneously	Sternocleido, trapezius, scalenes = intact (halo limits testing) Deltoid = 3/5 bilat Biceps = 2/5 left 1/5 right
Integumentary	Observable areas intact	Intact; no pressure areas after sitting for 5 hours.

interventions that improve oxygenation. Once José was placed in the halo vest, the therapist worked with the team, assisting in implementing a positioning program. Turning José required that the therapist attend to line and tube management as well as spine precautions (accomplished by directly handling the individual and not pulling on the halo vest).

A prescriptive body-positioning program was established. This intervention assists in improving oxygenation. José could breathe effectively in the supine position with slight head elevation (15 degrees) to prevent aspiration. Positioning José on his side required management of the chest tube and pleurovac. When premedicated for pain, José was able to tolerate rib pressure and shoulder pain, thus he could be placed in a modified position on the right side to assist in reducing amount of negative intrapleural pressure.

If the therapist noted significant decrease in SaO$_2$ or excessive elevation in RR or HR when José was lying on the right, the therapist changed his position. Later, after discussing options with the health-care team, José was placed in modified side-lying position on the left to optimize ventilation–perfusion matching and open collapsed airways on the right for brief therapeutic periods (30 minutes). The chest tube was sutured in place and did not move during position changes. The physiologic responses were evaluated after 2 minutes in the new position and documented in the medical chart. Chest percussion and vibration were not appropriate and were not indicated because there are no infiltrates during the early period in ICU. The therapist communicated with the team, modified therapeutic sessions according to medical management plan, and then initiated a positioning

CASE STUDY 14-1   Respiratory Training for an Individual Requiring Mechanical Ventilation—cont'd

program. The therapist worked with José in a variety of positions and used a supine position for diaphragm reeducation. Aggressive coughing was avoided for 8 to 10 days, until the chest x-ray and auscultation exam revealed complete right lung re-expansion, without air in the pleural space.

On subsequent visits to the ICU, the therapist continued with the examination according to José's tolerance. Therapeutic sessions were short and lasted between 15 and 20 minutes. The therapist performed a neurologic exam, a muscle exam, and continued with a passive range-of-motion and positioning program. The sensory test indicated intact sharp dull sensation on the C4 dermatomes, impaired sensation over C5, and no sensation at C6 and below. The therapist observed any changes in the ventilator settings and discussed the responses to changes in body position with the team. SaO_2 gradually improved. The therapist noted the ventilatory settings for RR, TV, and positive end-expiratory pressure levels (PEEP), and auscultated before and after each therapeutic session. When the ventilator settings were changed on day 4 to synchronized intermittent mandatory ventilation with PEEP, the therapist started a deep breathing program in addition to the positioning program. José was taught to activate the diaphragm and to assist in mobilization of secretions with huff coughing as the therapist applied a gentle tussive squeeze over the upper chest. Sputum color was recorded. Coordination of care was arranged so that medications for pain and bronchodilation could be offered well in advance of any therapy session. Tube feedings were discontinued at least 30 minutes before therapy sessions, and suctioning was provided before any breathing retraining sessions. Airway clearance and breathing exercises were scheduled during a time when the ventilator discontinuation program was not occurring.

After José had adjusted to the ventilator and the routine in the ICU, the therapist checked with the nursing and respiratory therapy staff and learned that José had been weaning by gradual decrease in PEEP and the number of Synchronized intermittent mandatory ventilation ventilator-supported breaths. The team discussed preparing José for wheelchair sitting and transfers. José was gradually placed in a more upright position during ventilator discontinuation trials. An abdominal binder was applied to assist with breathing mechanics and BP during upright periods. Pneumatic air splints, used to prevent thromboemboli, were periodically removed, and elastic hose were placed on the lower extremities to support the vascular system when sitting and mobile. The therapist progressed José on days 4 to 6 by implementing a short-sitting balance program at bedside. All physiologic responses were documented as the therapist observed the hemodynamic monitor for values. Clinical decision making occurred according to response-dependent analysis.

On occasion, José became lightheaded with sitting and was returned to supine in bed when the therapist noted a drop in BP. José remained on ventilation support for all mobility sessions.

By the second week, José was able to tolerate some time off the ventilator, so the therapist planned to reexamine his respiratory function. The therapist had developed good rapport with José by communicating throughout all therapy sessions. Nursing reported he was now able to accomplish 5 minutes of ventilator-free breathing in supine position (15 degrees). José had developed trust in the therapist and gave permission to be removed briefly from the ventilator. The therapist observed and documented RR, breathing pattern, took VC and NIF measures, and auscultated the lungs during ventilator-free breathing. The therapist reassured José by reattaching the ventilator periodically and thoroughly explaining each action taken. Initially, there was a high RR (26 breaths/minute), low VC (450 cc), and negative inspiratory pressures (-20 cm H_2O). The therapist arranged the bedside to have mirrors placed overhead to assist in providing feedback as José learned ventilator-independent diaphragmatic breathing. A portable biofeedback unit was brought to the bedside, and surface electrodes were applied to the sternocleidomastoid muscles. José was encouraged to keep the neck muscles quiet while activating the diaphragm during inspiration. After José had rested, the therapist returned to arrange for mobility training.

On day 8, the team planned for wheelchair-to-bed transfers. Initially, mechanical ventilation was applied in synchronized intermittent mandatory ventilation (nonweaning protocol) as José was transferred from bed to upright and then transferred to a wheelchair. Because José had a high cervical injury, the therapist selected a wheelchair with a high back and headrest extension. The angle of the chair was tilted far back (about 45 degrees), and the leg rests were elevated during the first session in the wheelchair. During the first session, only an arterial line, urinary catheter, and ventilator tubing were in place. Since most hemodynamic monitoring lines were removed, the therapist manually measured BP, HR, and SaO_2 with changes in position or mobility challenges. The RR, TV, and minute ventilation could be observed on the ventilator. The manual BP measures could be compared to the hemodynamic monitor values for accuracy. José progressed to 3 hours of sitting tolerance at 80 degrees upright in wheelchair over the next 2 days.

Respiratory muscle training continued during the morning therapy session, and mobility training occurred in the afternoon. By day 10, José was able to tolerate 2 hours of ventilator-free breathing. He received O_2 via a tracheostomy mask during free breathing. Biofeedback training continued with José in a more upright position and an abdominal binder in place. Deep sustained breathing was

Continued

CASE STUDY 14-1   Respiratory Training for an Individual Requiring Mechanical Ventilation—cont'd

encouraged. José was able to perform two sets of 10 deep breaths with proper diaphragmatic control.

Unfortunately, on day 11, secretions increased, and José developed pneumonia with right lower lobe infiltrates and a fever. The therapist auscultated and heard sonorous rhonchi over the right lower and posterior lobes. Sputum was yellow. The positioning program was directed toward airway clearance. José was able to tolerate being positioned head down on the left side in a three-quarters prone position. José remained on the ventilator during airway clearance sessions. The therapist encouraged deep inspirations prior to assisting coughing attempts. The therapist received medical clearance to implement gentle vibration and percussion and to perform manual cough assist with abdominal thrust. The therapist initially used one hand over the abdomen and braced the right side (over rib fractures) using a blanket splint and firm pressure with other hand. Suctioning occurred frequently during all sessions. José could not tolerate diaphragmatic reeducation during this period and resorted to neck breathing with higher RR during weaning trials. Mobility sessions continued with José supported by the ventilator while sitting upright in the wheelchair.

Three days later the pneumonia resolved. José's respiratory management included mucolytics, bronchodilators, proper humidification, and ample intravenous fluids to maintain hydration. He was no longer febrile and was therefore evaluated for a speaking tracheostomy. Eventually, José began tolerating brief periods of having the tracheostomy capped off. By the end of the third week, José could tolerate a full manual-assist cough with pressure over the umbilicus. He had some further return of strength in his biceps (scoring 3/5), and was impaired to light touch in sporadic areas throughout the body. José was taught how to perform a self-assisted cough by using his biceps. The therapist continued to work on diaphragmatic breathing, emphasizing sniffing, facilitation techniques, and breath-stacking with glottis control. Resistive training began with an incentive spirometer while José's tracheostomy was capped. Next, when the inspiratory capacity was approximately 900 mL, José was progressed to using diaphragm weights. The training was done with José in a supine position. The therapist observed José's breathing pattern as the weight pan was applied during the first session. A full epigastric rise was observed, and José was encouraged to inhale deeply and hold the breath at full inspiration. José was instructed to slowly release the breath during exhalation to develop eccentric control. The diaphragm weights were progressed in 5-pound increments as long as the epigastric rise was full and the inspiratory capacity under the new weight did not drop significantly below baseline (900 mL).[135] Specific segmental breathing, directed at the right lower lobe, posterior division, was performed while using a mirror so that José could observe his efforts during deep inspiration. Daily deep-breathing techniques were emphasized. Teaching of air-shift maneuvers were added in preparation for full discontinuation of the mechanical ventilator.

Mobility sessions and periods of positioning upright in the wheelchair occurred without ventilator support. José was transferred to the rehabilitation floor and received only nighttime ventilation. Upon arrival at the rehabilitation floor, a reexamination of respiratory function was performed. Results are given in Table 14-12.

The therapeutic plan continued with diaphragmatic breathing, and José progressed to 30 pounds of weighted breathing without any neck breathing. The therapist monitored the breathing pattern and recorded HR, RR, and SaO_2 before and after resistive training. José now had a speaking valve and had expiration through the oral cavity. Since he had airflow over the vocal cords and glottis, he could speak, and he began working on glottal control through vocalization exercises. The therapist discussed appropriate eccentric control activities with the speech and respiratory therapists.

Table 14-12   Rehabilitation Stage Physical Therapy Examination Initial and Discharge

Examination Component	Intial Rehab	Discharge
Respiratory rate:	Supine: 18 br/min	Sitting with binder: 16 br/min
	Sitting: 24 br/min	Sitting no binder: 20 br/min
Breathing pattern:	Supine: 2 neck; 2 diaphragm	Supine: 1 neck; 3 diaphragm
	Sitting: 3 neck; 1 diaphragm	Sitting with binder: 0 neck
Chest expansion: All measures taken with VC breathing	Supine: UCWE (axillary = +0.75 cm MCWE (xiphoid) = −1.10 cm LCWE (lower ribs) = +1.35 cm	Sitting with binder: UCWE = +1.25 cm MCWE = −0.50 cm LCWE = +2.50 cm

Key: CWE = chest wall expansion, U = upper, M = middle, L = lower

CASE STUDY 14-1   Respiratory Training for an Individual Requiring Mechanical Ventilation—cont'd

Examination Component	Intial Rehab	Discharge
Chest expansion (cont'd)	Sitting: UCWE = NT MCWE = NT LCWE = +0.50 cm	Sitting no binder UCWE = +0.75 MCWE = −0.60 LCWE = +1.75 cm Xiphoid level (MCWE) Supine = +0.50 cm Supine with airshift = +4 cm Supine with GPB = +6 cm
Cough function Type assist: Abdominal thrust	Sitting with halo and binder Weak functional without assist With caregiver assist functional PCFR = 1.7 L/s without assist = 2.5 L/s with assist	Sitting with binder: Weak PCFR = 2.7 L/s Assisted PCFR = 4.2 L/s Sitting no binder: Weak PCFR = 2.4 L/s
Sputum color	Clear	Clear
Auscultation	Diminished bilateral basal regions	Diminished bilateral basal regions
Eccentric control/phonation	Sitting with halo and binder 4 syllables/br; 5 sec vowel sound	Sitting with binder = 7 syllables/br 8 sec vowel Sitting no binder = 5 syllables/br 6 sec vowel
Vital capacity (ml)	Supine: 750 mL Sitting with halo and binder: 700 ml	Sitting with binder : 2800 mL Sitting no binder: 2500 mL GPB : 3200 mL
MIP cm H_2O Measured at RV	Sitting with halo and binder: −35 cm H_2O	Sitting with binder : −45 cm H_2O Sitting no binder: −35 cm H_2O
MEP cm H_2O Measured at TLC	Sitting with halo and binder: 10 cm H_2O	Sitting with binder: 40 cm H_2O Sitting no binder: 30 cm H_2O

UCWE = Upper chest wall expansion; MCWE = midchest wall expansion; LCWE = lower chest wall expansion; VC = vital capacity; GPB = glossopharyngeal breathing; PCFR = peak cough flow rate; MIP = maximal inspiratory pressure, MEP = maximal expiratory pressure.

A more specific respiratory muscle training program was subsequently implemented so that muscles other than the diaphragm could be strengthened. The therapist used 30% of maximal inspiratory pressure and began implementing a threshold loaded respiratory muscle exercise program two times per day, for 10 minutes. Initially, the tracheostomy was fitted with an adapter to allow interfacing with the inspiratory muscle training device so resistive breathing would be imposed at the level of the tracheostomy. Later, José was able to accept resistance with the tracheostomy closed. The training program was adjusted to increase the length of time to 15 to 30 minutes to incorporate endurance training into the program. Progression was determined by observing the breathing pattern, monitoring HR, and rating the perceived exertion, SaO_2, and postexercise RR.

Functional mobility exercises began to focus on learning to roll, coming to sitting position, and developing balance in short- and long-sitting. During therapeutic sessions, the therapist worked on strengthening all the shoulder musculature, especially the pectoralis major. Coordinated breathing strategies were emphasized using facilitation of weaker accessory muscles and resistance to stronger muscles. During upper extremity shoulder flexion for rolling from supine to side-lying position, José was taught to reach his right arm across his body and over his head, well above his left shoulder. He was taught to inhale with this motion and

Continued

CASE STUDY 14-1   Respiratory Training for an Individual Requiring Mechanical Ventilation—cont'd

to use his eyes to follow his arm motions as he breathed. When returning to supine from side-lying position, he was taught to look down and exhale when placing his arms at his side. The therapist observed José for signs of fatigue by examining the respiratory function at the end of mobility sessions. Occasionally, the therapist used the manual resuscitation bag on the back of the wheelchair and provided a few deep breaths through the tracheostomy site. This was done to increase the level of alertness, to improve SaO_2 and to assist in cough function at the end of a long period off ventilator support.

The therapist also evaluated José's sitting posture in the wheelchair to be sure he was well aligned, with a neutral pelvis, to permit good diaphragmatic breathing. Although José was stronger and able to tolerate inspiratory muscle training with a resistance at −30 cm H_2O by the end of his rehabilitation stay, he continued to be at risk for respiratory complications. The therapist used respiratory examination measures to demonstrate the improvement in the respiratory care program and the benefits of using an abdominal binder. This helped to justify the purchase of a respiratory muscle trainer and an extra abdominal binder to wear during cleaning. The therapist wrote notes to document important seating principles related to respiratory function. José was discharged to an extended care facility that had expertise in management of respiratory disorders.

José will continue to be at risk for respiratory complications his entire life. Training in airway clearance was provided but was not as effective as routine deep breathing, breath-stacking, and caregiver-assisted coughing. Caregiver training specific to respiratory function would need to include the following:

- Education in the signs of fatigue and pneumonia and what to do, including when to call the physician
- Manual cough assist (suctioning if tracheostomy still present)
- Airway-clearance strategies that are effective (vibration, percussion, postural drainage, deep inspiration with pause followed by costophrenic and abdominal thrust cough-assist strategies)
- Glossopharyngeal breathing and breath-stacking prior to cough
- Air-shift maneuvers and general chest stretching
- Wheelchair positioning for optimal ventilation
- Inspiratory muscle training program
- Use of coordinated breathing during dressing, bed mobility, wheelchair transfers, and repositioning
- Setup of CPAP machine at night
- Use of manual resuscitation bag (via mask or via tracheostomy)
- Being alert for signs of depression and understanding how to interpret them:

José should be scheduled for routine follow-up once a month during the first year for proper coordination of care and to continue to have his respiratory care program adjusted and progressed.

Summary

After SCI, most individuals have some degree of respiratory dysfunction. Expiratory function is impaired in almost all individuals, even those with low thoracic paraplegia. This loss affects cough function and the ability to clear the airways. Further loss of respiratory function is related to the completeness of injury and the level at which it occurs. Individuals with high paraplegia (T6 and above) lose inspiratory function and will have an increased risk of respiratory complications and mortality. The individual with a high motor complete cervical injury has the greatest loss of respiratory function and will likely require ventilator assistance. Therapists can provide information about the respiratory status by performing a thorough examination of the muscles of ventilation, the chest wall motion, and breathing kinematics. A comprehensive respiratory care program that is coordinated among all disciplines is critical to survival of the individual with SCI. Progression of the treatment program should continue based on the physiologic responses and measures of respiratory performance. The respiratory care program should be progressed until outcome measures plateau. Emphasis on continuation of therapeutic strategies after discharge will increase the life expectancy and reduce hospitalizations for most individuals with SCI. Education in self-management, as well as caregiver education and practice, are essential. The individual should then continue with a maintenance and prevention program for respiratory function similar to the therapeutic home program offered for contracture prevention, skin protection, and the general program for mobility and good healthy living.

REVIEW QUESTIONS

1. How do the mechanics of breathing differ for the various levels of injury? Compare those with high tetraplegia (C1–C4) to those with low tetraplegia (C5–C8), to those with high paraplegia (T1–T6), and those with thoracic injuries at T7 and below?

2. What are the signs of respiratory muscle fatigue in individuals with SCI?

3. What medical tests are commonly performed in individuals with SCI that indicate the degree of respiratory muscle impairment? Which tests indicate the degree of lung tissue impairment?

4. Describe phases of a normal cough. What interventions could be offered to improve cough function?

5. How do an abdominal binder and a pneumobelt each assist the individual with SCI? Who could benefit from these devices?

6. How can body position influence respiratory function?

7. How should you develop a ventilatory muscle training program?

8. What is the difference between an individual who is receiving control mode ventilation and one who is receiving continuous positive airway pressure ventilation support?

9. How would you work on increasing chest wall expansion in an individual with a C5 motor complete tetraplegia?

REFERENCES

1. Hartkopp A, Bronnum-Hansen H, Seidenschnur A et al. Survival and cause of death after traumatic spinal cord injury. A long-term epidemiological survey from Denmark. *Spinal Cord.* 1997;35(2):76–85.

2. Consortium for Spinal Cord Medicine. Respiratory management following spinal cord injury: A clinical practice guideline for health-care professionals. *J Spinal Cord Med.* 2005;28(3):259–293.

3. Jackson AB, Groomes TE. Incidence of respiratory complications following spinal cord injury. *Arch Phys Med Rehabil.* 1994;75(3):270–275.

4. DeVivo M, Kartus P, Stover S et al. Cause of death for patients with spinal cord injuries. *Arch Intern Med.* 1989;149(8):1761–1766.

5. Garshick E, Kelley A, Cohen SA et al. A prospective assessment of mortality in chronic spinal cord injury. *Spinal Cord.* 2005;43(7):408–416.

6. Zeilig G, Dolev M, Weingarden H et al. Long-term morbidity and mortality after spinal cord injury: 50 years of follow-up. *Spinal Cord.* 2000;38(19):563–566.

7. Frisbie JH, Sharma GV, Brahma P et al. Recurrent pulmonary embolism and pulmonary hypertension in chronic tetraplegia. *Spinal Cord.* 2005;43(10):625–630.

8. Widmaier EP Raff H, Strang KT. *Vander's Human Physiology. The Mechanisms of Body Function.* 10th edition. New York: McGraw Hill; 2006.

9. Derenne J, Macklem PT, Roussos CH. The respiratory muscles: Mechanics, control, and pathophysiology. Part I. *Am Rev Respir Dis.* 1978;118:119–133.

10. Peat M. *Current Physical Therapy.* Philadelphia: BC Decker; 1988.

11. Chen CF, Lien IN, Wu MC. Respiratory function in patients with spinal cord injuries: Effects of posture. *Paraplegia.* 1990;28(2):81–86.

12. De Troyer A, Heilporn A. Respiratory mechanics in quadriplegia. The respiratory function of the intercostal muscles. *Am Rev Respir Dis.* 1980;122:591–600.

13. Anke A, Aksnes AK, Stanghelle JK et al. Lung volumes in tetraplegic patients according to cervical spinal cord injury level. *Scand J Rehabil Med.* 1993;25(2):73–77.

14. Linn WS, Adkins RH, Gong H, Jr et al. Pulmonary function in chronic spinal cord injury: A cross-sectional survey of 222 southern California adult outpatients. *Arch Phys Med Rehabil.* 2000;81(6):757–763.

15. Vilke GM, Chan TC, Neuman T et al. Spirometry in normal subjects in sitting, prone, and supine positions. *Respir Care.* 2000;45(4):407–410.

16. Craig AB. Effects of position on expiratory reserve volume of the lungs. *J Appl Physiol.* 1960;15:59–61.

17. Estenne M, DeTroyer A. Mechanism of the postural dependence of vital capacity in tetraplegic subjects. *Am Rev Respir Dis.* 1987;135:367–371.

18. Baydur A, Adkins RH, Milic-Emili J. Lung mechanics in individuals with spinal cord injury: Effects of injury level and posture. *J Appl Physiol.* Feb 2001;90(2): 405–411.

19. Cherniack R, Cherniack L. *Respiration in Health and Disease.* 3rd edition. Philadelphia: W.B. Saunders; 1983.

20. Massery M. Physical therapy associated with ventilatory pump dysfunction and failure. In: DeTurk W, Cahalin, LP, editors. *Cardiovascular and Pulmonary Physical Therapy: An Evidence-Based Approach.* New York: McGraw Hill; 2004. pp. 593–646.

21. Verschakelen JA, Deschepper K, Demedts M. Relationship between axial motion and volume displacement of the diaphragm during VC maneuvers. *J Appl Physiol.* 1992; 72(4):1536–1540.

22. Massery MP, Dreyer HE, Bjornson AS et al. Chest wall excursion and tidal volume change during passive positioning in cervical spinal cord injury. *Cardiopulmonary Phys Ther J.* 1997;8(4):27. (Abstr.)

23. Wetzel JL, Lunsford BR, Peterson MJ et al. Respiratory rehabilitation of the patient with a spinal cord injury. In: Irwin S, Techlin JS, editors. *Cardiopulmonary Physical Therapy.* 3rd edition. St. Louis: Mosby; 1995. pp. 579–603.

24. Alvarez SE, Peterson M, Lunsford BR. Respiratory treatment of the adult patient with spinal cord injury. *Phys Ther.* 1981;61(12):1737–1745.

25. Harty HR, Corfield DR, Schwartzstein RM et al. External thoracic restriction, respiratory sensation, and ventilation during exercise in men. *J Appl Physiol.* 1999;86(4): 1142–1150.

26. Reid D, Dechman G. Considerations when testing and training the respiratory muscles. *Phys Ther.* 1995;75: 971–982.

27. Flaminiano LE, Celli BR. Respiratory muscle testing. *Clin Chest Med.* 2001;22(4):661–677.

28. DeTroyer A, Estenne M. Coordination between rib cage muscles and diaphragm during quiet breathing in humans. *J Appl Physiol.* 1984;57:899–906.

29. Dean E. Cardiopulmonary anatomy. In: Frownfelter D, Dean E, editors. *Cardiovascular and Pulmonary Physical Therapy: Evidence and Practice.* 4th edition. St. Louis: Mosby Elsevier; 2006. pp. 53–72.

30. Carter RE. Medical management of pulmonary complications of spinal cord injury. *Adv Neurol.* 1979;22:261–269.

31. Morris JF, Koski A, Johnson LC. Spirometric standards for healthy nonsmoking adults. *Am Rev Respir Dis.* 1971;103: 57–67.

32. Bergofsky EH. Mechanism for respiratory insufficiency after cervical cord injury; A source of alveolar hypoventilation. *Ann Intern Med.* 1964;61:435–447.

33. Loring SH, DeTroyer A. Actions of the respiratory muscles. In: Roussos CH, Macklem PT, editors. *The Thorax.* New York: Marcel Dekker Inc.; 1985. pp. 327–349.

34. Grimby G, Goldman, M, Mead, J. Respiratory muscle action inferred from rib cage and abdominal V-P partitioning. *J Appl Physiol.* 1976;41:739.

35. Goldman G, Mead J. Mechanical interaction between the diaphragm and the rib cage. *J Appl Physiol.* 1973;35:197.

36. Goldman M, Grimby, G, Mead, J. Mechanical work of breathing derived from rib cage and abdominal V-P partitioning. *J Appl Physiol.* 1976;41:752.

37. Roussos C, Macklem PT. The respiratory muscles. *N Engl J Med.* 1982;307:786–797.

38. Black LF, Hyatt RE. Maximal respiratory pressures: Normal values and relationship to age and sex. *Am Rev Respir Dis.* 1969;99:696 –702.

39. ATS/ETS. ATS/ETS Statement on Respiratory Muscle Testing. *Am J Resp Crit Care Med.* 2002;166(4):518–624.

40. Taylor A. Contribution of intercostal muscles to the effort of respiration in man. *Am J Physiol.* 1960;151:390.

41. Campbell EJM. The role of scalene and sternocleidomastoid in breathing in normal subjects. *J Anat.* 1955;89: 378–386.

42. Hislop HJ, Montgomery J, Connelly B et al. *Daniels and Worthingham's Muscle Testing.* 6th edition. Philadelphia: W.B. Saunders Company; 1995.

43. Aliverti A, Cala SJ, Duranti R et al. Human respiratory muscle actions and control during exercise. *J Appl Physiol.* 1997;83:1256–1269.

44. Braun SR, Giovannoni R, O'Connor JR. Improving cough in patients with spinal cord injury. *Am J Physl Med.* 1984; 63:1–10.

45. Wang AY, Jaeger RJ, Yarkony GM et al. Cough in spinal cord injured patients: The relationship between motor level and peak expiratory flow. *Spinal Cord.* 1997;35(5): 299–302.

46. Kang SW, Shin JC, Park CI et al. Relationship between inspiratory muscle strength and cough capacity in cervical spinal cord injured patients. *Spinal Cord.* 2006;44(4): 242–248.

47. Deem JF, Nukker L. *Manual of Voice Therapy.* 2nd edition. Austin, Tex: Pro-Ed; 2000.

48. Hoit JD, Banzett RB, Brown R et al. Speech breathing in individuals with cervical spinal cord injury. *J Speech Hear Res.* 1990;33(4):798–807.

49. Apfelbaum RI, Kriskovich MD, Haller JR. On the incidence, cause, and prevention of recurrent laryngeal nerve palsies during anterior cervical spine surgery. *Spine.* 2000;25(22):2906–2912.

50. Gausch P, Linder S, Williams T et al. A functional classification of respiratory compromise in spinal cord injury. *SCI Nurs.* 1991;8(1):4–10.

51. Ciesla N. Physical therapy associated with respiratory failure. In: DeTurk WE, Cahalin LP, editors. *Cardiovascular and Pulmonary Physical Therapy: An Evidence-Based Approach.* New York: McGraw Hill; 2004 pp. 541–592.

52. Dail CW. Muscle breathing patterns. *Med Arts and Sci.* 1956;10(Second Quarter):64.

53. Massery M. The patient with neuromuscular or musculoskeletal dysfunction. In: Frownfelter D, Dean E, editors. *Principles and Practice of Cardiopulmonary Physical Therapy.* 3rd edition. St. Louis: MosbyYear Book; 1996 pp. 679–702.

54. Tully K, Koke K, Garshick E et al. Maximal expiratory pressures in spinal cord injury using two mouthpieces. *Chest.* 1997;112(1):113–116.

55. Roth EJ, Lu A, Primack S et al. Ventilatory function in cervical and high thoracic spinal cord injury. Relationship to level of injury and tone. *Am J Phys Med Rehabil.* 1997;76(4): 262–267.

56. Ball PA. Critical care of spinal cord injury. *Spine.* 15 2001; 26;24 Suppl:S27–30.

57. Ledsome JR, Sharp JM. Pulmonary function in acute cervical cord injury. *Am Rev Respir Dis.* 1981;124(1):41–44.

58. McMichan JC, Michel L, Westbrook PR. Pulmonary dysfunction following traumatic quadriplegia. Recognition, prevention, and treatment. *JAMA.* 1980;243(6):528–531.

59. Manning H, McCool FD, Scarf SM et al. Oxygen cost of resistive-loaded breathing in quadriplegia. *J Appl Physiol.* 1992;73(3):825–831.

60. Silver JR. The oxygen cost of breathing in tetraplegic patients. *Paraplegia.*1963;17:204–214.

61. Maloney FP. Pulmonary function in quadriplegia: Effects of a corset. *Arch Phys Med Rehabil.* 1979;60:261–265.

62. Hart N, Laffont I, de la Sota AP et al. Respiratory effects of combined truncal and abdominal support in patients with spinal cord injury. *Arch Phys Med Rehabil.* 2005; 86(7):1447–1451.

63. McCool FD, Pichurko B, Slutsky A et al. Changes in lung volume and rib cage configuration with abdominal binding in quadriplegia. *J Appl Physiol.* 1986;60(4): 1198–1202.

64. Goldman JM, Rose LS, Williams SJ et al. Effect of abdominal binders on breathing in tetraplegic patients. *Thorax.* 1986;41(12):940–945.

65. Bellemare F, Grassino A. Effect of pressure and timing of contraction on human diaphragm fatigue. *J Appl Physiol.* 1982;53(5):1190–1195.

66. Vassilakopoulos T, Zakynthinos S, Roussos CH. Respiratory muscles and weaning failure. *Eur Respir J.* 1996;9:2383–2400.

67. Derenne J, Macklem PT, Roussos CH. The respiratory muscles: Mechanics, control, and pathophysiology. Part III. *Am Rev Respir Dis.* 1978;118:581–601.

68. Begin P Grassino A. Inspiratory muscle dysfunction and chronic hypercapnia. *Am Rev Respir Dis.* 1991;143: 905–912.

69. Gross D, Grassino A, Scott G et al. Respiratory muscle fatigue in quadriplegic patients. *Clin Res.* 1977;25:713A.

70. American Physical Therapy Association. *Guide to Therapist Practice.* 2nd edition. Alexandria, VA: American Physical Therapy Association; 2003.

71. Cahalin LP. Pulmonary evaluation. In: DeTurk WE, Cahalin LP, editors. *Cardiovascular and Pulmonary Physical Therapy. An Evidence-Based Approach.* New York: McGraw Hill; 2004. pp. 221–269.

72. American Thoracic Society. Standardization of spirometry, 1994 update. *Am J Resp Crit Care Med.* 1995;152: 1107–1136.

73. Brown R, DiMarco AF, Hoit JD et al. Respiratory dysfunction and management in spinal cord injury. *Respir Care.* 2006;51(8):853–867.

74. DeLorey DS, Wyrick BL, Babb TG. Mild-to-moderate obesity: Implications for respiratory mechanics at rest and

during exercise in young men. *Int J Obes*. 2005;29(9): 1039–1047.

75. Varon J, Marik P. Management of the obese critically ill patient. *Crit Care Clin*. 2001;17(1):187–200.

76. Menter RR, Bach J, Brown DJ et al. A review of the respiratory management of a patient with high level tetraplegia. *Spinal Cord*. 1997;35:805–808.

77. Burns SP, Kapur V, Yin KS et al. Factors associated with sleep apnea in men with spinal cord injury: A population-based case-control study. *Spinal Cord*. 2001;39(1):15–22.

78. Uijl SG, Houtman S, Folgering HT et al. Training of the respiratory muscles in individuals with tetraplegia. *Spinal Cord*. 1999;37(8):575–579.

79. Cerny FJ, Ucer C. Arm work interferes with normal ventilation. *Appl Ergonomics*. 2004;35(5):411–415.

80. Sutbeyaz ST, Koseoglu BF, Gokkaya NK. The combined effects of controlled breathing techniques and ventilatory and upper extremity muscle exercise on cardiopulmonary responses in patients with spinal cord injury. *Int J Rehabil Res*. 2005;28(3):273–276.

81. Ciesla ND, Murdock KR. Lines, tubes, catheters, and physiologic monitoring in the ICU. *Cardiopulmonary Phys Ther J*. 2000;11(1):16–25.

82. Hergenroeder AL. Implementation of a competency-based assessment of interpretation of laboratory values. *Acute Care Perspect*. 2006;15(1):7–15.

83. Poponick JM, Jacobs I, Supinski G et al. Effect of upper respiratory tract infection in patients with neuromuscular disease. *Am J Respir Crit Care Med*. 1997;156(2 Pt 1): 659–664.

84. Knott P. Imaging of the chest. In: Frownfelter D, Dean E, editors. *Cardiovascular and Pulmonary Physical Therapy. Evidence and Practice*. 4th edition. St. Louis: Mosby Elsevier; 2006. pp. 163–168.

85. Zablotny C. Evaluation and management of swallowing dysfunction. In: Montgomery J, editor. *Clinics in Physical Therapy. Physical Therapy for Traumatic Brain Injury*. New York: Churchill Livingstone; 1995. pp. 99–115.

86. Maeda CJ, Baydur A, Waters RL et al. The effect of the halo vest and body position on pulmonary function in quadriplegia. *J Spinal Disord*. 1990;3(1):47–51.

87. Noble-Jamieson CM, Heckmatt JZ, Dubowitz V et al. Effects of posture and spinal bracing on respiratory function in neuromuscular disease. *Arch Dis Child*. 1986;61(2):178–181.

88. Massery M. Multisystem consequences of impaired breathing mechanics and/or postural control. In: Dean E, Frownfelter D, editors. *Cardiovascular and Pulmonary Physical Therapy: Evidence and Practice*. 4th edition. St. Louis: Mosby Elsevier; 2006. pp. 695–717.

89. Dean E, Frownfelter D. Individuals with chronic secondary cardiopulmonary dysfunction. In: Dean E, Frownfelter D, editors. *Cardiovascular and Pulmonary Physical Therapy. Evidence and Practice*. 4th edition. St. Louis: Mosby Elsevier; 2006. pp. 569–593.

90. Gardner BP, Watt JW, Krishnan KR. The artificial ventilation of acute spinal cord damaged patients: A retrospective study of forty-four patients. Paraplegia. 1986;24(4): 208–220.

91. Como JJ, Sutton ER, McCunn M et al. Characterizing the need for mechanical ventilation following cervical spinal cord injury with neurologic deficit. *J Trauma*. 2005;59(4): 912–916.

92. Harrop JS, Sharan AD, Scheid EH, Jr. et al. Tracheostomy placement in patients with complete cervical spinal cord injuries: American Spinal Injury Association Grade A. *J Neurosurg*. 2004;100 Suppl 1:20–23.

93. Fagon J, Chastre J, Hance AJ et al. Nosocomial pneumonia in ventilated patients: A cohort study evaluating attributable mortality and hospital stay. *Am J Med*. 1993;94: 281–288.

94. Bach JR. Alternative methods of ventilatory support for the patient with ventilatory failure due to spinal cord injury. *J Am Paraplegia Soc*. 1991;14(4):158–174.

95. Bach JR, Alba AS. Noninvasive options for ventilatory support of the traumatic high level quadriplegic patient. *Chest*. 1990;98(3):613–619.

96. Burns SP, Rad MY, Bryant S et al. Long-term sleep apnea in persons with spinal cord injury. *Am J Phys Med Rehabil*. 2005;84(8):620–626.

97. McEvoy RD, Mykytyn I, Sajkov D et al. Sleep apnea in patients with quadriplegia. *Thorax*. 1995;50(6):613–619.

98. Tobin MJ, Mador MJ, Guenther SM et al. Variability of resting respiratory drive and timing in healthy subjects. *J Appl Physiol*. 1988;65(1):309–317.

99. Eason JM. Cardiopulmonary assessment. *Cardiopulmonary Phys Ther J*. 1999;10(4):135–142.

100. Schmitz TJ. Vital signs. In: O'Sullivan SB, Schmitz TJ, editors. *Physical Rehabilitation: Assessment and Treatment*. 4th edition. Philadelphia: F.A. Davis; 2001. pp. 77–100.

101. Gerold K. Therapists' guide to the principles of mechanical ventilation. *Cardiopulmonary Phys Ther J*. 1992;3: 8–13.

102. MacIntyre NR, Cook DJ, Guyatt GH, editors. Evidence-based guidelines for weaning and discontinuing ventilatory support: A collective task force facilitated by the American College of Chest Physicians; the American Association for Respiratory Care; and the American College of Critical Care Medicine. *Chest*. 2001;120(6): 375S–395S.

103. Yang KL, Tobin MJ. A prospective study of indexes predicting the outcome of trials of weaning from mechanical ventilation. *N Engl J Med*. 1991;324:1445–1450.

104. Clanton TL, Diaz PT. Clinical assessment of the respiratory muscles. *Phys Ther*. 1995;75:983–995.

105. Shapiro BA. Evaluation of blood gas monitors: Performance criteria, clinical impact, and cost/benefit. *Crit Care Med*. 1994;22(4):546–548.

106. Tzeng AC, Bach JR. Prevention of pulmonary morbidity for patients with neuromuscular disease. *Chest*. 2000; 118(5):1390–1397.

107. Threethambal P, Vareshree AL, Shivani M et al. Thoracolumbar corsets alter breathing pattern in normal individuals. Int *J Rehabil Res* 2005;28(1):81–85.

108. Oatis CA. Structure and function of the bones and joints of the thoracic spine. In: Oatis CA, editor. *Kinesiology. The Mechanics and Pathomechanics of Human Movement*. Philadelphia: Lippincott, Williams & Wilkins; 2004. pp. 488–514.

109. Harris J, Johansen J, Pedersen S et al. Site of measurement and subject position affect chest excursion measurements. *Cardiopulmonary Phys Ther J*. 1997;8(4):12–17.

110. LaPier TK, Cook A, Droege K et al. Intertester and intratester reliability of chest excursion measurements in subjects without impairment. *Cardiopulmonary Phys Ther J*. 2000;11(3):95–98.

111. Moll JM, Wright V. An objective clinical study of chest wall expansion. *Ann Rheum Dis.* 1972;31:1–8.

112. Carlson B. Normal chest wall expansion. *Phys Ther.* 1973;53:10–14.

113. Burgos-Vargas R, Castelazo-Duarte G, Orozco JA et al. Chest wall expansion in healthy adolescents and patients with the seronegative enthesopathy and arthropathy syndrome or juvenile ankylosing spondylitis. *J Rheumatol.* 1993;20:1957–1960.

114. Feldman D, Ouellette M, Villamez A et al. The relationship of ventilatory muscle strength to chest wall excursion in normal subjects and persons with cervical spinal cord injury. *Cardiopulmonary Phys Ther J.* 1998;9(4):20.(Abstr.)

115. Mellin G, Harjula R. Lung function in relation to thoracic spine mobility and kyphosis. *Scand J Rehabil Med.* 1987; 19:89–92.

116. Frownfelter D, Massery M. Facilitating ventilation patterns and breathing strategies. In: Frownfelter D, Dean E, editors. *Cardiovascular and Pulmonary Physical Therapy. Evidence and Practice.* 4th edition. New York: Mosby Elsevier; 2006. pp. 377–403.

117. Frownfelter D, Massery M. Body mechanics–The art of positioning and moving patients. In: Frownfelter D, Dean E, editors. *Cardiovascular and Pulmonary Physical Therapy. Evidence and Practice.* 4th edition. St. Louis: Mosby Elsevier; 2006. pp. 749–758.

118. Crosbie W, Myles S. An investigation into the effect of postural modification on some aspects of normal pulmonary function. *Physiotherapy.* 1985;7:311–314.

119. Rahn H, Otis AB, Chadwick LE et al. The pressure-volume diagram of the thorax and lung. *Am J Physiol.* 1946;146:161.

120. Troosters T, Gosselink R, Decramer M. Respiratory muscle assessment. *Eur Respir Mon.* 2005;31:51–71.

121. Hamnegard CH, Wraggs S, Kyroussis D et al. Portable measurement of maximum mouth pressures. *Eur Respir J.* 1994;7:398–401.

122. Roth EJ, Nussbaum SB, Berkowitz M et al. Pulmonary function testing in spinal cord injury: Correlation with vital capacity. *Paraplegia.* 1995;33(8):454–457.

123. Gardner RM, Hankinson JL, West BJ. Evaluation commercially available spirometers. *Am Rev Respir Dis.* 1980;121(1):73–82.

124. Nelson SB, Gardner RM, Crapo RO et al. Performance evaluation of contemporary spirometers. *Chest.* 1990; 97(2):288–297.

125. Rebuck DA, Hanania NA, D'Urzo AD et al. The accuracy of a handheld portable spirometer. *Chest.* 1996; 109(1):152–157.

126. Kelley A, Garshick E, Gross ER et al. Spirometry testing standards in spinal cord injury. *Chest.* 2003;123(3): 725–730.

127. Cruzado D, Jones MJ, Segebart S et al. Resistive inspiratory muscle training improves inspiratory muscle strength in subjects with cervical spinal cord injury. *Neurol Rep.* 2002;26(1):3–7.

128. Black LF, Hyatt RE. Maximal static respiratory pressures in generalised neuromuscular disease. *Am Rev Respir Dis.* 1971;103:641–650.

129. Gross D, Ladd HW, Riley EJ et al. The effect of training on strength and endurance of the diaphragm in quadriplegia. *Am J Phys Med.* 1980;68(1):27–35.

130. Enright PL, Kronmal RA, Manolio TA et al. Respiratory muscle strength in the elderly. Correlates and reference values. Cardiovascular health study research group. *Am J Resp Crit Care Med.* 1994;149:430–438.

131. Fishman A, Elias J, Fishman J. *Fishman's Pulmonary Diseases and Disorders.* 3rd edition. New York: McGraw Hill; 1998.

132. Gounden P. Static respiratory pressures in patients with post-traumatic tetraplegia. *Spinal Cord.* 1997;35(1): 43–47.

133. Rutchik A, Weissman AR, Almenoff PL et al. Resistive inspiratory muscle training in subjects with chronic cervical spinal cord injury. *Arch Phys Med Rehabil.* 1998;79(3):293–297.

134. McCool FD, Tzelepis GE. Inspiratory muscle training in the patient with neuromuscular disease. *Phys Ther.* 1995;75:1006–1114.

135. Derrickson J, Ciesla ND, Simpson N et al. A comparison of two breathing exercise programs for patients with quadriplegia. *Phys Ther.* 1992;72:763–769.

136. Lin KH, Wu HD, Chang CW et al. Ventilatory and mouth occlusion pressure responses to hypercapnia in chronic tetraplegia. *Arch Phys Med Rehabil.* 1998; 79(7):795–799.

137. Mueller G, Perret C, Spengler CM. Optimal intensity for respiratory muscle endurance training in patients with spinal cord injury. *J. Rehabil Med.* 2006;38(6): 381–386.

138. Gosselink R. Controlled breathing and dyspnea in patients with chronic obstructive pulmonary disease (COPD). *J Rehab Res Dev.* 2003;40(5):S25–34.

139. Aldrich TK, Arora NS, Rochester DF. The influence of airway obstruction and respiratory muscle strength on maximal voluntary ventilation in lung disease. *Am Rev Respir Dis.* 1982;126:195–199.

140. Wang TG, Wang YH, Tang FT et al. Resistive inspiratory muscle training in sleep-disordered breathing of traumatic tetraplegia. *Arch Phys Med Rehabil.* 2002; 83(4):491–496.

141. Almenoff PL, Spungen AM, Lesser M et al. Pulmonary function survey in spinal cord injury: Influences of smoking and level and completeness of injury. *Lung.* 1995;173(5):297–306.

142. Sheel AW, Reid WD, Townson AF et al. Respiratory management following spinal cord injury. In: Eng JJ, Teasell RW, Miller WC et al., editors. *Spinal Cord Injury Rehabilitation Evidence.* Vancouver: International Collaboration on Repair Discoveries (ICORD); 2006. pp. 8.1–8.30.

143. McKenzie DK, Gandevia SC. Influence of muscle length on human inspiratory and limb muscle endurance. *Respir Physiol.* 1987;67:171–182.

144. Nickerson BG, Keens TG. Measuring ventilatory muscle endurance in humans as sustainable inspiratory pressure. *J Appl Physiol.* 1982;52(3):768–772.

145. Spungen AM, Grimm DR, Lesser M et al. Self-reported prevalence of pulmonary symptoms in subjects with spinal cord injury. *Spinal Cord.* 1997;35(10):652–657.

146. Ayas NT, Garshick E, Lieberman SL et al. Breathlessness in spinal cord injury depends on injury level. *J Spinal Cord Med.* 1999;22(2):97–101.

147. Grandas NF, Jain NB, Denckla JB et al. Dyspnea during daily activities in chronic spinal cord injury. *Arch Phys Med Rehabil.* 2005;86(8):1631–1635.

148. Wien MF, Garshick E, Tun CG et al. Breathlessness and exercise in spinal cord injury. *J Spinal Cord Med.* 1999;22(4):297–302.

149. Rabinstein AA, Wijdicks EF. Warning signs of imminent respiratory failure in neurological patients. *Semin Neurol.* 2003;23(1):97–104.

150. Frownfelter D, Ryan J. Dyspnea: Measurement and evaluation. *Cardiopulmonary Phys Ther J.* 2000;11(1):7–15.

151. Koga T, Watanabe K, Sano M et al. Breathing intolerance index. *Am J Phys Med Rehabil.* 2006;85(1):24–30.

152. Manning HL, Brown R, Scharf SM et al. Ventilatory and P0.1 response to hypercapnia in quadriplegia. *Resp Physiol.* 1992;89:97–112.

153. Leith DE. Cough. In: Brain JD, Proctor D, Reid L, editors. *Lung Biology in Health and Disease: Respiratory Defense Mechanisms.* Vol 2. New York: Marcel Dekker; 1977. pp. 545–592.

154. Bach JR. Mechanical insufflation-exsufflation: Comparison of peak expiratory flows with manually assisted and unassisted coughing techniques. *Chest.* 1993; 104:1553–1562.

155. Kang SW, Bach JR. Maximum insufflation capacity. *Chest.* 2000;118:61–65.

156. Agency of Healthcare Research and Quality. Treatment of Pulmonary Disease Following Cervical Spinal Cord Injury. Summary. Evidence Report/Technology Assessment, Number 27. AHRQ Publication No. 01–E013. June 2001. Available at: http://www.ahrq.gov/clinic/epcsum/spinalsum.htm

157. Bach JR, Saporito L. Criteria for extubation and tracheostomy tube removal for patients with ventilatory failure: A different approach to weaning. *Chest.* 1996;110:1566–1571.

158. Kirby NA, Barnerias MJ, Siebens AA. An evaluation of assisted cough in quadriparetic patients. *Arch Phys Med Rehabil.* 1966;46:705–710.

159. Lin KH, Lai YL, Wu HD et al. Cough threshold in people with spinal cord injury. *Phys Ther.* 1999;79(11):1026–1031.

160. Dicpinigaitis PV, Grimm DR, Lesser M. Cough reflex sensitivity in subjects with cervical spinal cord injury. *Am J Respir Crit Care Med.* 1999;159(5 Pt 1):1660–1662.

161. Frownfelter D, Massery M. Facilitating airway clearance with coughing techniques. In: Frownfelter D, Dean E, editors. *Cardiovascular and Pulmonary Physical Therapy. Evidence and Practice.* 4th edition. St. Louis: Mosby Elsevier; 2006. pp. 363–376.

162. Bouros D, Siafakas N, Green M. Cough: Physiology and pathophysiological considerations. In: Roussos CH, editor. *The Thorax.* New York: Marcel Dekker; 1995. pp. 1335–1354.

163. Wilkins RL, Hodgkin JE, Lopez B. *Lung Sounds.* St. Louis: Mosby; 1988.

164. Warren VC. Glossopharyngeal and neck accessory muscle breathing in a young adult with C2 complete tetraplegia resulting in ventilator dependency. *Phys. Ther.* 2002; 82(6):590–600.

165. Hoit JD, Banzett RB, Brown R. Binding the abdomen can improve speech in men with phrenic nerve pacers. *Am J Speech Lang-Pathol.* 2002;11(1):71–76.

166. Gutierrez CJ, Harrow J, Haines F. Using an evidence-based protocol to guide rehabilitation and weaning of ventilator-dependent cervical spinal cord injury patients. *J Rehabil Res Dev.* 2003;40(5 Suppl 2):99–110.

167. Brooks D, O'Brien K, Geddes EL et al. Is inspiratory muscle training effective for individuals with cervical spinal cord injury? A qualitative systematic review. *Clin Rehabil.* 2005;19(3):237–246.

168. Dean E. Effect of body position on pulmonary function. *Phys. Ther.* 1985;65(5):613–618.

169. Pape H, Remmers D, Weinberg A et al. Is early kinetic positioning beneficial for pulmonary function in multiple trauma patients? *Injury.* 1998;29(3):219–225.

170. Dean E. Body positioning. In: Frownfelter D, Dean E, editors. *Cardiovascular and Pulmonary Physical Therapy: Evidence and Practice.* 4th edition. St. Louis: Mosby Elsevier; 2006. pp. 307–324.

171. Perme C, Dean E. An evidence-based approach to weaning ICU patients from mechanical ventilation. Paper presented at: World Confederation of Physical Therapy; June 2–6, 2007; Vancouver, Canada.

172. Froese AB, Bryan AC. Effects of anesthesia and paralysis on diaphragmatic mechanics in man. *Anesthesiology.* 1974;41:242.

173. Cameron G, Scott J, Jousse AT et al. Diaphragm respiration in the quadriplegic patient and the effect of position on his vital capacity. *Ann Surg.* 1955;141:451–456.

174. Messerole E, Peine P, Wittkopp S et al. The pragmatics of prone positioning. *Am J Respir Crit Care Med.* 2002; 165:1359–1363.

175. Lemons VR, Wagner FC, Jr. Respiratory complications after cervical spinal cord injury. *Spine.* 1994;19(20):2315–2320.

176. Borkowski C. A comparison of pulmonary complications in spinal cord-injured patients treated with two modes of spinal immobilization. *J Neurosci Nurs.* 1989;21(2):79–85.

177. Kirshblum S, Johnston MV, Brown J et al. Predictors of dysphagia after spinal cord injury. *Arch Phys Med Rehabil.* 1999;80(9):1101–1105.

178. Bach JR, Hunt D, Horton JA, III. Traumatic tetraplegia: Noninvasive respiratory management in the acute setting. *Am J Phys Med Rehabil.* 2002;81(10):792–797.

179. Wicks AB, Menter RR. Long-term outlook in quadriplegic patients with initial ventilator dependency. *Chest.* 1986;90(3):406–410.

180. Morrison SA. Biofeedback to facilitate unassisted ventilation in individuals with high-level quadriplegia. A case report. *Phys Ther.* 1988;68(9):1378–1380.

181. DiMarco AF. Restoration of respiratory muscle function following spinal cord injury. Review of electrical and magnetic stimulation techniques. *Respir Physiol Neurobiol.* 28 2005;147(2–3):273–287.

182. Peterson WP, Charlifue W, Gerhart A et al. Two methods of weaning persons with quadriplegia from mechanical ventilators. *Paraplegia.* 1994;32:98–103.

183. Bach JR, Alba AS. Total ventilatory support by the intermittent abdominal pressure ventilator. *Chest.* 1991;99:630–636.

184. Miller HJ, Thomas E, Wilmot CB. Pneumobelt use among high quadiplegic population. *Arch Phys Med Rehabil.* 1988;69(5):369–372.

185. Hornstein S, Ledsome J. Ventilatory muscle training in acute quadriplegia. *Physiotherapy.* 1986;28:145–149.

186. Vassilakopoulos T, Zakynthinos S, Roussos C. The immune response to resistive breathing: Implications for respiratory failure. *Clin Intensive Care.* 2004;15(4): 131–144.

187. Reid WD, Belcastro AN. Time course of diaphragm injury and calpain activity during resistive loading. *Am J Respir Crit Care Med.* 2000;162(5):1801–1806.

188. Bach JR, Rajaraman R, Ballanger F et al. Neuromuscular ventilatory insufficiency: Effect of home mechanical ventilator use v oxygen therapy on pneumonia and hospitalization rates. *Am J Phys Med Rehabil.* 1998;77(1):8–19.

189. Fugl-Meyer AR. Effects of respiratory muscle paralysis in tetraplegic and paraplegic patients. *Scand J Rehabil Med.* 1971;3(4):141–150.

190. Scott MD, Frost F, Supinski G et al. The effect of body position and abdominal binders in chronic tetraplegia subjects more than 15 years post injury. *J Am Paraplegia Soc.* 1993;16(2):117.

191. Amodie-Storey C, Nash MS, Roussell PM et al. Head position and its effect on pulmonary function in tetraplegic patients. *Spinal Cord.* 1996;34(10):602–607.

192. Bolin I, Bodin P, Kreuter M. Sitting position - posture and performance in C5 - C6 tetraplegia. *Spinal Cord.* 2000;38(7):425–434.

193. Dicpinigaitis PV, Spungen AM, Bauman WA et al. Bronchial hyperresponsiveness after cervical spinal cord injury. *Chest.* 1994;105(4):1073–1076.

194. Estenne M, Pinet C, De Troyer A. Abdominal muscle strength in patients with tetraplegia. *Am J Respir Crit Care Med.* 2000;161(3 Pt 1):707–712.

195. Ehrlich M, Manns PJ, Poulin C. Respiratory training for a person with C3-C4 tetraplegia. *Aust J Physiother.* 1999;45(4):301–307.

196. Fujiwara T, Hara Y, Chino N. Expiratory function in complete tetraplegics: Study of spirometry, maximal expiratory pressure, and muscle activity of pectoralis major and latissimus dorsi muscles. *Am J Phys Med Rehabil.* 1999;78(5):464–469.

197. Estenne M, Knoop C, Vanvaerenbergh J et. al. The effect of pectoralis muscle training in tetraplegic subjects. *Am Rev Respir Dis.* 1989;139:1218–1222.

198. Bach JR. Update and perspective on noninvasive respiratory muscle aids. Part 2: The Expiratory Aids. *Chest.* 1994;105:1538–1544.

199. Bach JR. Mechanical insufflation/exsufflation: Has it come of age? A commentary. *Eur Respir J.* 2003;21: 385–386.

200. Linder SH. Functional electrical stimulation to enhance cough in quadriplegia. *Chest.* 1993;103(1):166–169.

201. Jaeger RJ, Turba RM, Yarkony GM et al. Cough in spinal cord injured patients: Comparison of three methods to produce cough. *Arch Phys Med Rehabil.* 1993;74(12): 1358–1361.

202. Bach JR. Update and perspectives on noninvasive respiratory muscle aids. Part 1: The inspiratory aids. *Chest.* 1994;105:1230–1240.

203. Dail C, Rodgers M, Guess V et al. *Glossopharyngeal Breathing Manual.* Downey, CA.: Rancho Los Amigos Hospital Inc.; 1979.

204. Kang SW. Pulmonary rehabilitation in patients with neuromuscular disease. *Yonsei Med J.* 2006;47(3): 307–314.

205. Montero JC, Feldman DJ, Montero D. Effects of glossopharyngeal breathing on respiratory function after cervical cord transection. *Arch Phys Med Rehabil.* 1967;48(12):650–653.

206. Los Amigos Research and Education Institute Inc. *Glossopharyngeal Breathing for Patients with High Quadriplegia.* Downey, CA: Los Amigos Research and Education Institute Inc.; 1989.

207. Ishii M. Benefit of forced expiratory technique for weak cough in a patient with bulbar onset amyotrophic lateral sclerosis. *J Phys Ther Sci.* 2004;16:137–141.

208. Chatwin M, Ross E, Hart N et al. Cough augmentation with mechanical insufflation/exsufflation in patients with neuromuscular weakness. *Eur Respir J.* 2003;21: 502–508.

209. Pillastini P, Bordini S, Bazzocchi G et al. Study of the effectiveness of bronchial clearance in subjects with upper spinal cord injuries: Examination of a rehabilitation programme involving mechanical insufflation and exsufflation. *Spinal Cord.* 2006;44:614–616.

210. Stanic U, Kandare F, Jaeger R et al. Functional electrical stimulation of abdominal muscles to augment tidal volume in spinal cord injury. *IEEE Trans Rehabil Eng.* 2000; 8(1):30–34.

211. DiMarco AF, Kowalski KE, Geertman RT et al. Spinal cord stimulation: A new method to produce an effective cough in spinal cord injured patients. *Am J Respir Crit Care Med.* 2006;173(12):1386–9.

212. Taylor PN, Tromans AM, Harris KR et al. Electrical stimulation of abdominal muscles for control of blood pressure and augmentation of cough in a C3/4 level tetraplegic. *Spinal Cord.* 2002;40:34–36.

213. Lin VW, Singh H, Chitkara RK et al. Functional magnetic stimulation for restoring cough in patients with tetraplegia. *Arch Phys Med Rehabil.* 1998;79(5):517–522.

214. Bell S, Shaw-Dunn J, Gollee H et al. Improving respiration in patients with tetraplegia by functional electrical stimulation: An anatomical perspective. *Clin Anat.* 2007;20:1–5.

215. Braverman JM. EP guide to every body, part 5. Respiratory compromise: A barrier to recovery after spinal cord. *Exceptional Parent.* 2001;118:120–124.

216. Pryor JA. Physiotherapy for airway clearance in adults. *Eur Respir J.* 1999;14:1418–1424.

217. Bodin P, Kreuter M, Bake B et al. Breathing pattens during breathing exercises in persons with tetraplegia. *Spinal Cord.* 2003;41:290–295.

218. Estenne M, Gevenois PA, Kinnear W eet al. Lung volume restriction in patients with chronic respiratory muscle weakness: The role of microatelectasis. *Thorax.* 1993;48:698–701.

219. Estenne M, Heilporn A, Delhez L et al. Chest wall stiffness in patients with chronic respiratory muscle weakness. *Am Rev Respir Dis.* 1983;128:1002–1007.

220. Ngyren-Bonnier M, Wahman K, Lindholm P et al. *Long-term effects of glossopharyngeal insufflation in persons with cervical spinal cord injury.* 15th International WCPT Congress. Vancouver, Canada: The World Confederation for Physical Therapy; 2007.

221. Kisner C, Colby LA. Management of pulmonary conditions. In: Kisner C, Colby LA, editors. *Therapeutic Exercise: Foundation and Techniques.* 4th edition. Philadelphia: F.A. Davis; 2002.

222. Roussos CS, Fixley M, Genest J et al. Voluntary factors influencing the distribution of inspired gas. *Am Rev Respir Dis.* 1977;116:457.

223. D'Angelo E, Sant' Ambrogio G, Agostoni E. Effect of diaphragm activity or paralysis on distribution of pleural pressure. *J Appl Physiol.* 1977;37:311.

224. Dohna-Schwake C, Ragette R, Teschler H et al. IPPB-assisted coughing in neuromuscular disorders. *Pediatr Pulm.* 2006;41:551–557.

225. Sorenson HM, Shelledy DC. AARC clinical practice guideline. Intermittent positive pressure breathing—2003 revision & update. *Respir Care.* 2003;48(5):540–546.

226. Huldtgren AC, Fugl-Meyer AR, Jonasson E et al. Ventilatory dysfunction and respiratory rehabilitation in post-traumatic quadriplegia. *Eur J Respir Dis.* 1980;61(6):347–356.

227. Stiller K, Simionato R, Rice K et al. The effect of intermittent positive pressure breathing on lung volumes in acute quadriparesis. *Paraplegia.* 1992;30(2):121–126.

228. McCool FD, Natewsju RF, Shayne DS et al. Intermittent positive pressure breathing in patients with respiratory muscle weakness. Alterations in total respiratory system compliance. *Chest.* 1986;90(4):546–552.

229. Massery MP. What's positioning got to do with it? *Neurology Report.* 1994;18(3):11–14.

230. Derenne J, Macklem PT, Roussos CH. The respiratory muscles: Mechanics, control, and pathophysiology. Part II. *Am Rev Respir Dis.* 1978;118:373–390.

231. Ward RJ, Damzoger F, Bonica JJ et al. An evaluation of postoperative respiratory maneuvers. *Surg Gynecol Obstet.* 1966;123:51–54.

232. Overend TJ, Anderson CM, Lucy SD et al. The effect of incentive spirometry on postoperative pulmonary complications. A systematic review. *Chest.* 2001;120:971–978.

233. Cheshire DJ, Flack WJ. The use of operant conditioning techniques in the respiratory rehabilitation of the tetraplegic. *Paraplegia.* 1978;16(2):162–174.

234. Bodin P, Olsen MF, Bake B et al. Effects of abdominal binding on breathing patterns during breathing exercises in persons with tetraplegia. *Spinal Cord.* 2005;43:117–122.

235. Van Houtte S, Vanlandewijck Y, Gosselink R. Respiratory muscle training in persons with spinal cord injury: A systematic review. *Respir Med.* 2006;100:1886–1895.

236. Loveridge B, Badour M, Dubo H. Ventilatory muscle endurance training in quadriplegia: Effects on breathing pattern. *Paraplegia.* 1989;27(5):329–339.

237. Lane IS. Inspiratory muscle weight training and its effect on the vital capacity of patients with quadriplegia. *Cardiopulmonary Quarterly.* 1982;5(10):13.

238. Liaw MY, Lin MC, Cheng PT et al. Resistive inspiratory muscle training: Its effectiveness in patients with acute complete cervical cord injury. *Arch Phys Med Rehabil.* 2000;81(6):752–756.

239. Sapienza CM, Wheeler K. Respiratory muscle strength training: Functional outcomes versus plasticity. *Semin Speech Lang.* 2006;27(4).

240. Goshgarian HG. The crossed phrenic phenomenon: A model for plasticity in the respiratory pathways following spinal cord injury. *J Appl Physiol.* 2003;94(2):795–810.

241. Silva AC, Neder JA, Chiurciu MV et al. Effect of aerobic training on ventilatory muscle endurance of spinal cord injured men. *Spinal Cord.* 1998;36(4):240–245.

242. Le Foll-de Moro D, Tordi N, Lonsdorfer E et al. Ventilation efficiency and pulmonary function after a wheelchair interval-training program in subjects with recent spinal cord injury. *Arch Phys Med Rehabil.* 2005;86(8):1582–1586.

243. Crane L, Klerk K, Ruhl A et al. The effect of exercise training on pulmonary function in persons with quadriplegia. *Paraplegia.* 1994;32(7):435–441.

244. Foglio K, Cini E, Facchetti D et al. Respiratory muscle function and exercise capacity in multiple sclerosis. *Eur Respir J.* 1994;7(23–28).

245. Takahashi T, Jenkins SC, Strauss GR et al. A new unsupported upper limb exercise test for patients with chronic obstructive pulmonary disease. *J Cardiopulmonary Rehabil.* 2003;23(430–437).

246. Cerny FJ, Ucer C. Arm work interferes with normal ventilation. *Appl Ergonomics.* 2004;35(5):411–415.

247. Celli BR. The clinical use of upper extremity exercise. *Clin Chest Med.* 1994;15(2):339–349.

248. Jacobs PL, Nash MS. Exercise recommendations for individuals with spinal cord injury. *Sports Med.* 2004;34(11):727–751.

249. Pancotto C. Preparing for discharge and transitioning care: Family/patient education and home modification. Paper presented at: Rehabilitation and Long-Term Ventilation: An Interdisciplinary Approach; 2006; Chicago, Illinois.

250. ATS. Statement on home care for patients with respiratory disorders. *Am J Respir Crit Care Med.* 2005;171:1443–1464.

251. American Heart Association Guidelines for Cardiopulmonary Resuscitation and Emergency Cardiovascular Care. Part 8: Interdisciplinary Topics. *Circulation.* 2005;112(24):III 100–III 108.

252. Jain NB, Sullivan M, Kazis LE et al. Factors associated with health-related quality of life after chronic spinal cord injury. *Am J Phys Med Rehabil.* 2007;86(5):387–396.

253. Harrop JS, Sharan AD, Vaccaro AR et al. The cause of neurologic deterioration after acute cervical spinal cord injury. *Spine.* 2001;26(4):340–346.

254. Janssens JP, Pache JC, Nicod LP. Physiological changes in respiratory function associated with ageing. *Eur Respir J.* 1999;13(1):197–205.

255. DeVivo MJ, Ivie CS, 3rd. Life expectancy of ventilator-dependent persons with spinal cord injuries. *Chest.* 1995;108(1):226–232.

256. Bach JR, Saporito LR. Life satisfaction and well-being measures in ventilator assisted individuals with traumatic tetraplegia. *Arch Phys Med Rehabil.* 1994;75(6):626–632.

257. Wijkstra PJ, Avendano MA, Goldstein RS. Inpatient chronic assisted ventilatory care: A 15-year experience. *Chest.* 2003;124(3):850–856.

258. Oo T, Watt JW, Soni BM et al. Delayed diaphragm recovery in 12 patients after high cervical spinal cord injury. A retrospective review of the diaphragm status of 107 patients ventilated after acute spinal cord injury. *Spinal Cord.* 1999;37(2):117–122.

259. Hoit JD, Banzett RB, Lohmeier HL et al. Clinical ventilator adjustments that improve speech. *Chest.* 2003;124(4):1512–1521.

260. Strakowski JA, Pease WS, Johnson EW. Phrenic nerve stimulation in the evaluation of ventilator-dependent individuals with C4- and C5-level spinal cord injury. *Am J Phys Med Rehabil.* 2007;86(2):153–157.

261. Vanderlinden SW, Epstein SW, Hyland RH. Management of chronic ventilatory insufficiency with electrical diaphragm pacing. *Can J Neurol Sci.* 1988;15:63–67.

262. DiMarco AF, Onders RP, Ignagni A et al. Phrenic nerve pacing via intramuscular diaphragm electrodes in tetraplegic subjects. *Chest.* 2005;127(2):671–678.

263. DiMarco AF, Takaoka Y, Kowalski KE. Combined intercostal and diaphragm pacing to provide artificial ventilation in patients with tetraplegia. *Arch Phys Med Rehabil.* 2005;86(6):1200–1207.

264. Cotton BA, Pryor JP, Chinwalla I et al. Respiratory complications and mortality risk associated with thoracic spine injury. *J Trauma.* 2005;59(6):1400–1407; discussion 1407–1409.

265. Jensen MP, Kuehn CM, Amtmann D et al. Symptom burden in persons with spinal cord injury. *Arch Phys Med Rehabil.* 2007;88:638–645.

266. Strakowski JA, Pease WS, Johnson EW. Phrenic nerve stimulation in the evaluation of ventilator-dependent individuals with C4- and C5-level spinal cord injury. *Am J Phys Med Rehabil.* 2007;86(2):153–157.

267. Fry DK, Pfalzer LA, Chokshi AR, Wagner MT, Jackson ES. Randomized control trial of effects of a 10-week inspiratory muscle training program on measures of pulmonary function in persons with multiple sclerosis. *J Neurol Phys Ther.* 2007;31(4):162–172.

Appendix A

Respiratory Function Terminology

Word	Abbreviation	Definition/
Vital capacity	VC	The maximum volume of air that can be expelled after a maximum inspiration, i.e., from total lung capacity (TLC) to residual volume (RV).
Total lung capacity	TLC	The total amount of air in the lungs after a maximal inspiration. TLC = RV + ERV + TV + IRV.
Inspiratory capacity	IC	The maximal volume of air that can be inhaled (sum of TV and IRV).
Functional residual capacity	FRC	The volume of air remaining in the lungs at the end of an ordinary TV expiration. FRC = ERV + RV
Tidal volume	TV	The volume of air inhaled or exhaled during breathing (at rest or durig exercise).
Inspiratory reserve volume	IRV	The maximum volume of air that can be inhaled to total lung capacity over and above tidal volume inspiration.
Expiratory reserve volume	ERV	The maximum volume of air that can be exhaled from the end expiratory level or from functional residual capacity to residual volume.
Residual volume	RV	The volume of air remaining in the lungs after a maximal expiration.
Ventilatory muscle training	VMT	Resistive training for the respiratory muscles; includes both inspiratory and expiratory muscle work.
Inspiratory muscle training	IMT	Resistive training for the muscles responsible for inspiration.
Expiratory muscle training	EMT	Resistive training for the muscles responsible for expiration.
Threshold loading maximum	TL_{max}	The highest resistive load that can be sustained for at least 2 minutes during progressive incremental resistive loading test. Used to define the endurance capacity of the respiratory muscles.
Maximal voluntary ventilation	MVV	The volume of air breathed when a person breathes as deeply and as quickly as possible for a given time (15 seconds). Usually extrapolated to what could be breathed over 1 minute.
Sustained (maximal) inspiratory pressure	SIP or SMIP	The highest pressure a subject can generate in each breath for 10 minutes without a decline in force or onset of adverse effects.
Maximal sustainable ventilation	MSV	The level of isocapnic hyperpnea that the individual can maintain for 12 minutes. During a period of volitional hyperpnea, various amounts of carbon dioxide are added to the inspired air to maintain isocapnia (in arterial blood) as measured by monitoring of ET_{CO_2}.

Forced expiratory volume in the first second	FEV1	The volume of air released during the first second of a VC maneuver. This indicates the speed of air movement out of the lungs. Used to detect resistance to lung flow or poor expiratory flow.
Peak expiratory flow rate	PEFR	The fastest speed of airflow in liters per second or liters per minute generated during a maximal VC maneuver. This measure is used to detect any airway restriction or loss of rapid expiratory flow due to decreased speed of expiratory muscle contraction.
Peak cough flow rate	PCFR	A measure of speed of airflow in liters per second or liters per minute generated during rapid forced expiration such as occurs with coughing. Normal PCFR = 6–20 L/sec or 300–700 L/min.
Partial pressure of arterial carbon dioxide	$Paco_2$	The gas pressure of carbon dioxide found in arterial blood. Normal $Paco_2$ = 35–45 mm Hg
End tidal carbon dioxide	$ETco_2$	Provided the patient has a stable cardiac status, stable body temperature, absence of lung disease, and a normal capnographic trace, end tidal carbon dioxide ($ETco_2$) approximates the partial pressure of CO_2 in arterial blood ($Paco_2$) The measure is taken noninvasively (without needles)
Partial pressure of arterial oxygen	Pao_2	The gas pressure of oxygen found in arterial blood. Normal Pao_2 = 80–100 mm Hg
O_2 saturation of Hgb	Sao_2	The percentage of hemoglobin carrying sites that are occupied by oxygen. Fully saturated = 100%.
Diffusion capacity	DL_{co}	The ability of the lungs to transfer gas (carbon monoxide) across the alveoli to the pulmonary circulation. Used to detect lung tissue thickening or disease.
Negative inspiratory pressure/force	NIP or NIF	A measure of inspiratory muscle strength. The subject inhales against a device that occludes airflow. A negative pressure in generated and recorded in cubic centimeters or centimeters of H_2O.
Maximal inspiratory pressure	MIP	A measure of maximal pressure created by inspiratory muscle force. The subject inhales maximally from a predetermined lung volume (usually RV). A negative pressure is generated and recorded in cubic centimeters or centimeters of H_2O.
Peak inspiratory pressure	PIP or PI max	Same as MIP above. Different terms used to denote peak or maximal inspiratory pressure generated during a maximal inspiratory maneuver against occluded airflow. A negative pressure is generated and recorded in cubic centimeters or centimeters of H_2O.
Maximal expiratory pressure	MEP	A measure of maximal pressure created by expiratory muscle force. The subject exhales maximally from a predetermined lung volume (usually TLC). A positive pressure is generated and recorded in cubic centimeters or centimeters of H_2O.
Peak expiratory pressure	PEP or PE_{max}	Same as MEP above. They are different terms used to denote peak or maximal expiratory pressure generated during a maximal expiratory maneuver against occluded airflow. A positive pressure is generated and recorded in cubic centimeters or centimeters of H_2O.
Minute ventilation	V_E	The volume of air moved in 1 minute. Typically used to determine the ability of the person to move air in and out of the lungs during exercise. V_E = TV × RR
Inspiratory duty cycle; inspiratory time/ total time for one breath	Ti/T_{TOT}	Method for detecting the increase in inspiratory muscle activation during the respiratory cycle. Increase in Ti suggests the muscles of inspiration are working harder and have the potential to fatigue.
Transdiaphragmatic pressure	Pdi	Difference between pressure generated at the esophageal level (pleural pressure) and pressure generated at the gastric level (abdominal pressure). The difference in pressure suggests the ability of the diaphragm to contract and generate force.
Pressure at the level of the esophagus (Sometimes called Ppl for pleural pressure)	Pes (Ppl)	A pressure reading taken in the esophagus to detect pressure during various phases of the respiratory cycle and used to infer pleural pressure.

Pressure at the level of the gastric region (Sometimes called Pab for intra-abdominal pressure)	Pgs (Pab)	A pressure reading taken in the stomach or gastric region to detect pressure during various phases of the respiratory cycle and used to infer intra-abdominal pressure.
Mouth occlusion pressure	$P_{0.1}$	Measure used to indicate central respiratory motor drive. Airway pressure developed at the mouth that occurs 0.1 seconds after the onset of inspiration. The airway is occluded at the mouth. The time parameter suggests that this measure occurs before volitional contraction of respiratory muscles and reflects nervous system activation.
Rapid shallow breathing index	RR/TV	Method used to determine volitional breathing ability. Breaths per minute divided by tidal volume in liters (breaths/min/L). Normal = 50

Bowel and Bladder Function and Management

15

Catherine Warms, PhD, RN, CRRN
Diana D. Cardenas, MD, MHA

After reading this chapter, the reader will be able to:

OBJECTIVES

- Review the neurophysiologic basis of bladder and bowel dysfunction in spinal cord injury (SCI)
- Describe upper motor neuron and lower motor neuron lesions and delineate the effects of these lesions on bowel and bladder function
- Discuss current management options for neurogenic bladder and bowel
- Name factors to consider when developing an individualized management plan for neurogenic bowel and bladder
- Apply knowledge of potential complications of neurogenic bladder and bowel to educate individuals and families about long-term management
- Describe areas of controversy related to neurogenic bowel and bladder dysfunction

OUTLINE

Neural Basis for Bowel and Bladder Dysfunction

Normal Bowel and Bladder Function and Innervation

Voluntary control of the bladder and bowel requires intact neural pathways from the S2 through S4 spinal segments through the pelvic nerves and from the sacral cord to and from the pontine level of the brain. Both organs are innervated through complex sympathetic and parasympathetic systems that operate at various levels of the spinal cord and are coordinated by centers in the brainstem.

Bladder Innervation and Control

The most important peripheral pathways affecting bladder function are the parasympathetic nerve supply to the detrusor through the pelvic nerve, the sympathetic nerve supply to the bladder neck through the hypogastric nerve, and the somatic innervation of the external urethral sphincter through the pudendal nerve. The sympathetic nerve supply is by the hypogastric postganglionic outflow from T12 to L2. The afferent and efferent neurons supplying the external sphincter via the pudendal nerve arise at the S3–S4 level. In neurologically normal individuals, the volume of the bladder and the normal voiding reflex is routed via the afferent Aδ fibers. In individuals with SCI, vanilloid receptor stimulation excites C-afferent fibers that may mediate the bladder dysfunction due to inflammatory reactions. In individuals with SCI above the sacral levels, these capsaicin-sensitive vanilloid receptors and C-afferents have a major role in the pathogenesis of bladder hyperactivity.[1,2]

The reflex center for the bladder lies in the pons, along with the other autonomic centers. Sensory information from the bladder wall travels through the pelvic nerve to the S2–S4 spinal segments and from there ascends to the pontine mesencephalic reticular formation. A reflex with afferent axons originating from the bladder and synapsing on the pudendal nerve nucleus at S2, S3, and S4 (Onuf's nucleus) allows inhibition of pelvic floor activity during normal voiding (micturition). Another important reflex is the local segmental innervation of the external sphincter with afferents from the urethra, sphincter, and pelvic floor and efferents in the pudendal nerve. Higher (voluntary) control over the pelvic floor is achieved through afferents that ascend to the sensory cortex. Descending fibers from the motor cortex synapse with the pudendal motor nucleus and control external urethral sphincter activity. The simple act of voiding is thus a complex and coordinated activity involving the central as well as the peripheral nervous system pathways.

Bladder continence is maintained by coordination of two functions at the sacral level of the cord (the *sacral micturition center*). First, alpha-adrenergic receptors contract the bladder neck and internal sphincter to close the bladder outlet. Second, beta-adrenergic receptors relax the detrusor muscle, which allows the bladder to fill without contraction. Voluntary voiding is a complex action that is a result of coordination between the pontine and sacral micturition centers and sympathetic control via preganglionic neurons at the T10–L2 spinal cord segments. With an intact nervous system, the pontine micturition center signals the need to void and stimulates sympathetic, parasympathetic, and somatic pathways. Detrusor muscle contraction is mediated mainly by parasympathetic control via preganglionic axons in the pelvic nerve with cell bodies in the S2–4S spinal segments.[3] The internal bladder sphincter, which is smooth muscle, relaxes in response to parasympathetic stimulation, and the external bladder sphincter, which is striated muscle, relaxes in response to somatic impulses via the pudendal nerve. Thus, an intact pathway between the pontine and sacral micturition centers allows for coordinated and voluntary voiding.[4]

Clinically, the *upper urinary tract* is a term used to describe the kidneys and the ureters. The *lower urinary tract* is a term used to describe the following anatomic structures: (1) the fundus of the bladder, (2) the trigone and neck of the bladder, (3) the pelvic diaphragm, and (4) the urethra. The effect of SCI is more profound on the lower urinary tract. The detrusor muscle of the fundus is a collection of interconnected muscle bundles that allow a smooth contraction. Parasympathetic receptors are scattered throughout the bladder, with a greater concentration in the fundus. The parasympathetic nerve input to the bladder arises from the sacral spinal cord segments S2–S4. The smooth muscle of the bladder neck also contains parasympathetic end organs, but these are of minimal clinical significance (*see* Fig. 15-1).

Bowel Innervation and Control

In a manner similar to that of the bladder, the neural control of the gastrointestinal system involves complex interactions between autonomic and somatic nervous systems operating in a coordinated manner. Myenteric reflexes operate independently within the colon walls and do not require central nervous system (CNS) innervation for ongoing function. These intrinsic reflexes maintain local segmental peristalsis whereas more global colonic movement relies on spinal cord-mediated reflexes. The colon is extrinsically innervated through multiple pathways. Parasympathetic fibers from the vagus nerve in the brainstem and pelvic nerve at the S2–S4 levels of the cord influence the entire gut and the colon, respectively. Sympathetic innervation is provided to the colon via the mesenteric nerves at the T5–T12 and the hypogastric nerve at the T12–L3 spinal levels. Finally, somatic innervation to the external anal sphincter is supplied by the sacral nerve and the somatic pudendal nerve (S2–S4)[5] (*see* Fig. 15-2).

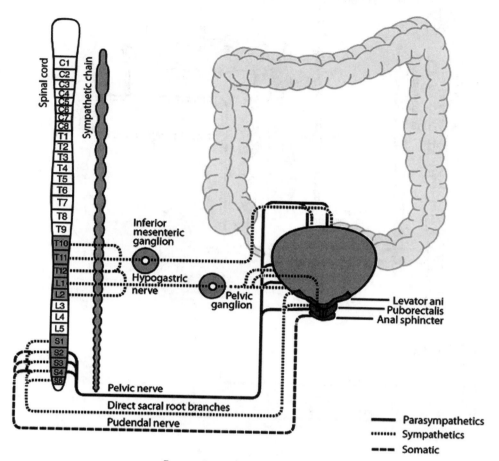

Figure 15-1. Bladder innervation.

Similar to the bladder, two sphincters operate in coordination to maintain bowel continence. The internal anal sphincter (IAS; consisting of smooth muscle) maintains a baseline state of contraction intrinsically, and the external anal sphincter (EAS; consisting of striated muscle) is under voluntary control.[6] Normal defecation, like micturition, involves coordination of involuntary reflexes and voluntary mechanisms. As stool moves into the rectum and begins to distend the rectal wall, the wall distention stimulates the intrinsic reflex that causes giant peristaltic waves in the colon. The rectoanal inhibitory reflex causes contraction of the EAS and relaxation of the IAS as the rectum fills, triggering voluntary inhibition of defecation until appropriate. Once voluntary relaxation of the EAS is initiated, the parasympathetic defecation reflex intensifies the peristaltic waves and further relaxes the IAS, and voluntary contraction of the levator ani muscles, external abdominals, and diaphragm aid in propelling the stool out.[5,7]

SCI Effects on Bladder and Bowel

SCI level and completeness determine the type of dysfunction in bladder and bowel. An injury above the sacral segments of the spinal cord produces an upper motor neuron (UMN) or *reflexic* bladder and bowel. An injury at the sacral segments (or cauda equina) produces a lower motor neuron (LMN) or *areflexic* bowel and bladder. Incomplete injury at any level may modify the typical patterns of dysfunction, often conferring greater voluntary control over urination or defecation or allowing reflex activity in LMN injuries.

UMN injury effects on the bladder typically include hyperreflexia of the detrusor muscle, resulting in

- contraction, with small volumes of urine;
- excessive pressures when it contracts;
- increased tone or spasticity of the sphincter; and
- dyssynergia (lack of coordination between the detrusor and sphincters that is often, but not always, present).[3,7]

LMN injuries are likely to result in a flaccid bladder with low sphincter tone. The three main types of voiding dysfunction seen in people with SCI are: (1) failure to store urine due to either detrusor hyperactivity or a flaccid bladder outlet, (2) failure to empty due to either a flaccid detrusor or a hyperactive sphincter, and (3) detrusor–sphincter dyssynergia (DSD) due to a lack of coordination between bladder muscle contraction and

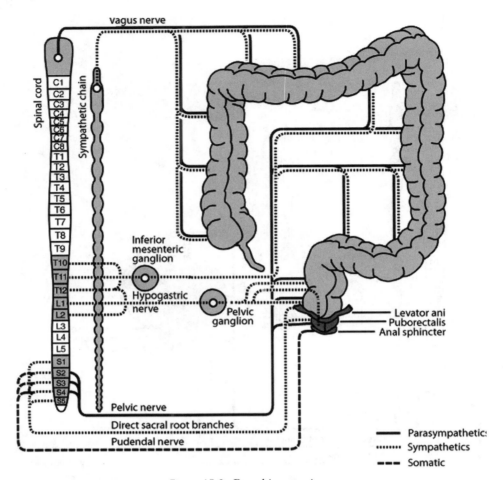

Figure 15-2. Bowel innervation.

sphincter relaxation, causing high voiding pressures and incomplete emptying.[4]

UMN injury effects on the bowel sphincters result in an overall increase in tone similar to the effects on the bladder sphincters. UMN produces a bowel in which baseline colonic activity is higher than normal but peristalsis is poorly coordinated (hyperactive segmental activity but underactive propulsive activity). The overall result is slow transit of stool through the entire gut, predisposing the individual to constipation.[8] LMN injury disrupts parasympathetic control over defecation and causes decreased tone in the IAS and loss of EAS control, predisposing the individual to fecal incontinence. The absence of spinal cord-mediated reflex peristalsis means that stool propulsion is produced only by the myenteric plexus, and as a result, there is sluggish movement and dry stools.[8]

Neurogenic Bladder

Acute Phase Management and Evaluation

Typically, immediately after a SCI, an indwelling catheter is inserted. It is useful for handling large urine output commonly found in the early days after SCI. The caliber of the catheter should be less than that of the urethra, but large enough to allow a free flow of urine. In the adult, a caliber of 14 to 16 French is common. In the male, the catheter should be strapped over the abdomen to prevent erosion of the urethra at the penoscrotal junction. An indwelling catheter should be changed every 3 to 4 weeks. Any individual with an indwelling catheter soon develops bacteria in the urine, a condition called *bacteriuria*. Treatment with antibiotics is not generally recommended for asymptomatic bacteriuria.[9]

An indwelling catheter is usually maintained until the individual's medical state is stable and fluid intake can be regulated to achieve a urine output of 1500 to 2000 mL/day. At that time, intermittent catheterization (IC) may be started. IC refers to the method of in-and-out urethral catheterization performed at regular intervals throughout a 24-hour period. However, some individuals will continue to have large urine outputs despite fluid restrictions for many weeks, and some will have large urine outputs during the night due to retention of interstitial fluid in the lower limbs while in the upright position, delaying the start of IC. The individual should learn self-catheterization when able to do so. A sterile technique is generally used in the hospital by nursing staff, based more on tradition than on evidence.[10] Three randomized, controlled trials have not shown any significant increase in the incidence of symptomatic bacteriuria using clean versus sterile technique.[11–13] A clean technique is often used in the hospital when the individual is able to do self-IC and before being discharged home. Maximum allowable bladder volume is 500 mL to 600 mL. An ultrasound to determine bladder volume assists in creating the appropriate IC schedule.[14] Starting with IC every 4 hours will allow the individual to participate in therapies during rehabilitation while avoiding overdistension of the bladder. For the individual who does not have sufficient hand function to perform self-IC, who does not have the cognitive ability to learn the technique, or who decides not to do so, an indwelling catheter may be continued beyond the acute phase. The potential problems associated with chronic indwelling catheters include an increased risk for epididymitis, fistula formation, calculi, and carcinoma.[9]

A neurological examination will assist in determining if the bladder can be expected to develop reflex activity; however, the period of spinal shock is variable and longer in the case of the bladder than in the motor system. Thus, the individual may start to demonstrate spasticity in the lower extremities but not yet have any reflex bladder activity. Episodes of overdistension may also slow the return of reflex activity of the bladder. The urinary system is usually evaluated in the acute phase to be certain that there are no undiagnosed medical problems such as a congenital anomaly, renal calculi, etc. present. This evaluation includes renal imaging (a radiograph of kidneys, ureters, and bladder [KUB], ultrasound, or computed tomography [CT]) and assessment of renal function (serum creatinine and creatinine clearance).

Urodynamic evaluation is recommended after the bladder is out of spinal shock or by 6 months post-injury, unless otherwise indicated, to evaluate treatment changes.[15] After the early period, follow-up urodynamic evaluation has been recommended on a yearly basis for the first 5 to 10 years and every other year thereafter if the individual is doing well;[15] however, the evidence for the frequency of repeat testing is based primarily on expert opinion. The benefit of determining the pressure within the bladder produced by contractions should not be discounted because high pressures in the bladder associated with outlet obstruction, such as in DSD, may lead to upper urinary tract damage. Without urodynamic evaluation, one cannot reliably determine the cause of urinary incontinence nor the presence or absence of DSD. Urodynamic evaluation is also helpful in determining the effect of anticholinergics, drugs commonly used to reduce bladder pressure and reduce urinary incontinence, and is needed to determine the value of certain surgeries to the lower tract.

Influence of the Level of Injury

The functional level achievable by the individual also influences the selection of bladder management technique.

Typically, more hand function is required to apply a condom catheter in the case of male individuals than to perform intermittent catheterization; thus, some men with complete C6 tetraplegia are able to perform self-catheterization using a tenodesis splint, but may need assistance with clothing. More recently, a simple assistive device, the HouseHold (available from Flexlife Medical, Kingwood, TX) enabled a group of men with C5–C7 tetraplegia, who had been unable to perform clean IC independently, to become independent in IC.[16] Typically, a male with C6 tetraplegia is not able to apply a condom catheter. Women with C6 or higher levels of tetraplegia will likely require continued assistance with IC and may choose to use an indwelling urethral catheter. Women with C7 or lower may become independent in IC, although devices such as a labia spreader or a splint may be required for those with impaired hand function. Spasticity in the hip adductors may also make IC more difficult.

Individuals with lesions at the level of C7 and below who are able to do self-catheterization can continue this in the long term. If the detrusor reflex cannot be suppressed with medications, the individual should consider bladder augmentation, which remains the standard method today for achieving a low-pressure reservoir if medications fail.[17] Augmentation involves surgically opening the bladder and sewing in a detubularized segment of bowel to produce a reservoir of 600 mL capacity. Intravesical therapy with Botox or with instillations of anticholinergics may also be an option. Intravesical capsaicin and resiniferatoxin, which block transmission through C-afferent fibers for several months, have been used experimentally to treat hyperactivity when it does not respond to the usual pharmacological agents (Table 15-1).[1,2]

In men with SCI who are unable or unwilling to do self-catheterization, and for those who refuse augmentation, external urethral sphincterotomy followed by use of an external catheter is probably the best alternative. Urodynamic evaluation is necessary to determine if external urethral sphincterotomy is appropriate. Ablation of the sphincter is usually done by incision anteriorly to avoid damage to the cavernous artery and nerve. In some individuals, a bladder neck ablation is also necessary to relieve outflow resistance. An implantable stainless steel stent is another alternative to a sphincterotomy.[18] Stents avoid the risk of damage that may lead to impotency, a rare complication of sphincterotomy. Other options include intermittent catheterization by an attendant, although this has a greater risk of febrile urinary tract infections (UTIs) and is not recommended.[19] Wearing an external collector alone may be considered, but only 15% of men with SCI have a suitable, truly "balanced" bladder with coordination of the detrusor and sphincter to achieve voiding at low pressure. Some men with tetraplegia end up with an indwelling catheter because of sphincterotomy failure, inadequate detrusor contractions, or skin breakdown on the penile shaft.

Table 15-1

Medications Commonly Used in the Management of the Neurogenic Bladder

Class	Type	Agent/Trade Name	Mechanism of Action	Cautions
Anticholinergic/antispasmodic	Oral	Oxybutynin (Ditropan) (also available transdermally) Propantheline bromide (Pro-Banthine) Dicyclomine (Bentylol, Bentyl) Flavoxate HCL (Urispas) Hyoscyamine sulfate (Cystospaz, Levsin) Emepronium (Cetiprin) Darifenacin (Enablex) Trospium (Sanctura)	Smooth muscle relaxants, suppresses bladder contractions, increases bladder capacity.	Common side effects: dry mouth, constipation, tachycardia, blurred vision.
	Intravesicular	Oxybutynin		Inconvenient due to need to crush tablets and instill via catheter.
Calcium channel blockers	Oral	Tolterodine (Detrol) (also available transdermally) Verapamil hydrochloride (Isoptin)		Verapamil may decrease blood pressure.
Neurotoxins	Intravesicular	Capsaicin Resiniferatoxin		Treatments last 3–6 months. Requires instillation by urologist and local anesthesia due to local discomfort.
Adrenergic blocking agents	Oral	Phenoxybenzamine HCl (Dibenzyline) Prazosin HCL (Minipress) Terbutaline (Bricanyl) Terazosin (Hytrin)	Decrease bladder outlet pressure, decrease external sphincter spasticity	May decrease blood pressure. Other side effects: fatigue, tachycardia, inhibited ejaculation.
Striated muscle relaxants	Oral	Dantrolene (Dantrium) Baclofen (Lioresal) (may also be delivered intrathecally)		Often taken for muscle spasticity, may have significant bladder effects.
Toxin	Injection	Botulinum A toxin (Botox)		Requires cystoscopic injection by a urologist, treatments last 2–10 months.

Long-term Management Options

The choice of bladder management depends on a variety of factors, including type of bladder, functional level of the individual, individual preference, and physician bias. Data from the Model SCI Systems in the United States suggest that the most common method of management at the time of discharge from initial rehabilitation is IC,[20] the single technique most responsible for decreased morbidity and mortality after SCI since WWII. The exact proportion of individuals that continue on IC long term is unknown, but data suggest that the use of IC significantly decreases with time and the use of condom catheters in males increases.[21] The goal is for the individual with a SCI to be catheter-free and to empty with low post-void residuals without excess bladder pressure elevations. (*see* Fig. 15-3 for examples of bladder management supplies).

Techniques that are employed in addition to IC, indwelling catheters, and (in males) condom catheters, include suprapubic tapping and Valsalva and Credé maneuvers. Suprapubic tapping works only for individuals with UMN bladders and no dyssynergia. Tapping involves lightly tapping with the fingertips directly over the bladder in a rhythmic manner. This technique triggers a bladder contraction, emptying the bladder as long as the sphincter opens normally. Individuals with areflexia and some denervation of the pelvic floor are able to void by doing a Valsalva maneuver, or straining. This is most effective in women because even the partially paralyzed pelvic floor descends with straining, and the bladder neck opens. Over time, however, the pelvic floor descent increases as the paralyzed muscles atrophy and stretch, and the individual complains of worsening stress incontinence. In men, complete flaccidity of the pelvic floor may allow emptying by straining. The Credé maneuver, which is often performed by an attendant, mechanically pushes urine out by manual pressure over the bladder in individuals with tetraplegia. The abdominal wall and suprapubic area must be relaxed to allow the Credé maneuver to be effective; it is no longer recommended because there is a theoretical risk of producing ureteral reflux by the long-term use of this method.

Other Options

Electrical stimulation has been used to stimulate the anterior roots at the sacral level to produce bladder emptying at acceptable intravesical pressures.[22] Usually, bilateral S2–S4 dorsal rhizotomies are performed to prevent spontaneous hyperactive contractions and antidromic reflex contractions. Such rhizotomies, however, abolish reflex erections. Bowel evacuation is improved in many individuals with the use of such stimulation. For a detailed discussion of this approach see chapter 5.

Complications

In addition to possible DSD, autonomic dysreflexia, and UTIs, individuals may develop bladder stones, which are treated with cystoscopy and lithotripsy. Small stones can

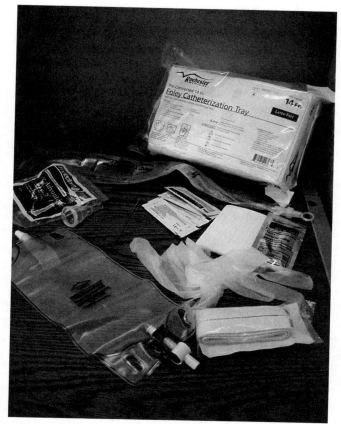

Figure 15-3. Bladder management supplies. Typical disposable medical supplies required for management of the neurogenic bladder.

be dissolved by daily bladder irrigations with hemiacidrin solution. Another complication is renal stone formation, which occurs in approximately 8% of individuals with SCI, many secondary to infection. Treatment generally includes lowering the pressure with IC and anticholinergics, or if this fails, surgery to repair the reflux or otherwise reduce the pressure.

Periodic Monitoring and Evaluation

A regular long-term urinary tract surveillance program is recommended for individuals with SCI.[15] Prevention of UTIs is also important to prevent silent damage to the kidneys. There is evidence that individual education,[23] good personal hygiene,[24] and, potentially, certain types of catheters can reduce the incidence of UTIs in individuals with SCI. Bladder overdistention, vesicoureteral reflux, high-pressure voiding, large post-void residual urine volumes, stones in the urinary system, and outlet obstruction are important risk factors that increase the risk of UTIs.[9]

Neurogenic Bowel

Acute Phase Management and Evaluation

Immediately after SCI, there is a sudden and usually complete lack of neural regulation of the gut. The complex coordinated system of transport, secretion, and blood flow is disrupted. Intrinsic gut function is preserved, but both voluntary and reflex activity may be absent or significantly impaired. The result is ileus (prolonged time for digestion and for gastrointestinal transit), constipation (slow colonic transit time), and passive leakage of stool.[6] During this acute phase, manual evacuation of stool will be required for people with all levels of injury. Reflex defecation usually returns as the period of spinal shock begins to resolve, approximately 4 to 8 weeks after injury, except for those with LMN injuries at the sacral level of the spinal cord or conus medularis injuries.[6]

Once spinal shock begins to resolve, sacral reflexes return. A careful neurological exam should be done to assess anal tone and presence or absence of the sacral reflexes (i.e., the anocutaneous, bulbocavernosus, and internal anal sphincter reflexes; see Table 15-2). Some centers may use anorectal manometry to identify sphincter dyssynergia. Such testing can help to plan the best method of future management.[25] For example, those whose sphincter relaxes reflexively when the rectum fills can use digital stimulation to initiate reflexive defecation. Those with a compliant (relaxed) rectum and low sphincter tone will require ongoing manual evacuation. And finally, individuals with dyssynergia may need to use caution with digital stimulation to avoid sphincter spasm and autonomic dysreflexia.

The entire gastrointestinal system is prone to complications during the acute period of spinal shock. These complications include paralytic ileus, gastric dilatation, peptic ulcer disease, pancreatitis, and superior mesenteric artery syndrome.[8] These complications result from unopposed parasympathetic activity from the vagus nerve and transient loss of sympathetic innervation, as well as from prolonged bed rest and metabolic imbalances precipitated by the abrupt physiological changes related to SCI.

Long-term Management Goals, Principles, and Options

Surveys of people with SCI indicate that bowel dysfunction is rated as one of the most distressing aspects of living with SCI. A well-managed bowel is thus extremely important for both health and social reasons. Goals for bowel management include both safety and acceptability of bowel care routines. Safety goals include continence for maintaining healthy and intact skin, prevention of damage to colorectal structures, and prevention of autonomic dysreflexia. Goals for an acceptable bowel care routine include achieving continence in order to avoid embarrassment, bowel care that is reasonable in duration and sustainable over time, and bowel care that is carried out in privacy, allowing maintenance of dignity.

There is no single bowel care routine or bowel management plan that will fit every person with SCI. Basic principles for management of both UMN-type and

Table 15-2
Sacral Reflexes

Reflex	Description
Bulbocavernosus reflex	External anal sphincter contraction in response to squeezing the glans penis or tugging on the Foley catheter.
Anocutaneous reflex ("anal wink")	Reflex contraction of the external anal sphincter upon stroking the skin around the anus.
Internal anal sphincter reflex	Relaxation of the internal anal sphincter on insertion of a gloved, lubricated finger.

LMN-type neurogenic bowel need to be aligned with characteristics of the injury, functional abilities, lifestyle, and preferences to derive a plan tailored to the individual. Teaching the individual with SCI and the individual's caregivers that various factors can affect the success of bowel care routines and that changes and adjustments may be required is important. Teaching bowel management principles rather than a specific program provides the individual with tools needed to more successfully self-manage neurogenic bowel over the years. Important factors include timing, position, equipment, stimulation or evacuation techniques, and use of medications.

Timing

Bowel movement patterns prior to injury offer the best information for establishing the optimal time of day and frequency for bowel care. Regularity of timing and routine is the key to continence.[26] Individuals with well-established bowel regularity prior to injury may find that mimicking the pre-morbid pattern will help to achieve continence sooner. Anyone with preexisting bowel disorders will have these same disorders, and they may complicate a post-injury program.[5] Personal routines and caregiver schedules must also be considered in the selection of a time of day for bowel care.

A frequent complaint of people with SCI is the prolonged time required for completion of bowel care. A survey of people with SCI found wide variability in the amount of time spent on bowel care each week.[27] In this sample, the mean time spent was 10.3 hours/week, with extremes of "all day" and less than 30 minutes every other day. A reasonable goal is less than 1 hour per bowel care episode.[28] People with UMN injuries often do best on an every other day schedule, whereas people with

LMN injuries require daily or even two times per day bowel care.

Although there is some controversy over whether the gastrocolic reflex is completely functional in people with SCI,[5,8] it is recommended that timing bowel care about 30 minutes after a meal or warm beverage may help increase the speed and completeness of evacuation. The gastrocolic reflex is a mass contraction in the sigmoid and descending colon segments that is generated after meals. There are also giant peristaltic waves that occur often in the morning,[8] suggesting the possibility that a morning routine might be more efficient than one performed at another time of day. Nevertheless, the time of day and frequency selected need to be optimal for the individual's lifestyle. Consistency of timing and routine is more important than the time of day chosen.

Positioning and Equipment

Acutely after injury, and until the individual's spine is stable and he or she is ready to sit up, bowel care will be done in bed. If possible, the left side-lying position will facilitate defecation because the descending colon will be gravity-dependent, allowing the benefits of gravity to assist stool transit. It is well known that prolonged bed rest interferes with bowel motility, so as soon as it is safe and feasible to perform bowel care in the seated position, the individual should be encouraged to do so. The seated position is known to reduce the anorectal angle, allowing both gravity and better alignment to facilitate defecation.[5] People with UMN injuries should avoid Valsalva maneuvers because they can trigger reflex sphincter spasm. The seated position allows forward and sideways bending that can be used to increase intra-abdominal pressure by generating muscle spasms in the abdominal wall.[29]

Appropriate equipment for bowel care includes a padded shower or commode chair or padded raised toilet seat. The best selection for a given individual depends on his or her functional abilities (independent versus dependent transfers), trunk stability (usually determined by level and completeness of injury), need for assistance from others, and the environment where bowel care will take place. People with lower injury levels who can transfer and do their bowel care independently will often be able to use a raised toilet seat. People with tetraplegia will need a wheeled chair with removable armrests and footrests that can be placed over the toilet or used with a plastic receptacle for stool. After bowel care is completed, this type of chair can be wheeled into a roll-in shower for ease of care. Padded seats are required for all to prevent skin damage and pressure ulcers. The necessity for individually prescribed and adjusted commode chairs needs to be stressed. A recent survey of people with SCI regarding their equipment suggests that there may be significant risks from using shower or commode chairs that are not appropriate. The survey found that 25% of those surveyed reported development of pressure ulcers from a commode seat and 35% reported having fallen from the chair (23% of whom required hospitalization as a direct result of the fall).[30]

In addition to toileting equipment, specific disposable medical supplies are required for bowel care. These include water-soluble lubricant, nonsterile examination gloves, and for those who do bowel care in bed, disposable underpads. Many people are allergic to latex, so it is recommended that nonlatex gloves be used. People with tetraplegia and some larger people with short arms may need a device called a digital stimulator to extend their reach in order to accomplish digital stimulation. These devices are commercially available and can be modified by an occupational therapist to accommodate varying levels of hand function. (*See* Figs. 15-4 and 15-5 for examples of bowel care equipment and supplies.)

Bowel Care Routines

LMN injuries cause loss of rectal tone resulting in a flaccid accommodating rectum that fills with stool. Along with this, there is decreased tone of the anal sphincter muscle. There is no reflex activity to initiate bowel movements and nothing to prevent incontinence if the stool is too soft or the rectum is allowed to fill for too long. These characteristics make it necessary to empty the bowel frequently, keep the stool fairly firm, and use the technique of manual evacuation for stool removal.[28] Manual evacuation consists of inserting a gloved, lubricated finger into the rectum, hooking into any stool that is present, and gently pulling it out. The procedure can be repeated until the rectum is empty. The Valsalva maneuver and transabdominal massage of the colon in a clockwise manner may be helpful for advancing the stool.[5] Although massage is commonly suggested for LMN bowel, there have been no studies of its efficacy. It is recommended that the bowel care routine for a LMN bowel be done at least daily, and many people will choose

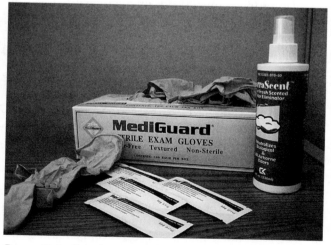

Figure 15-4. Bowel care supplies. Supplies required for management of the neurogenic bowel.

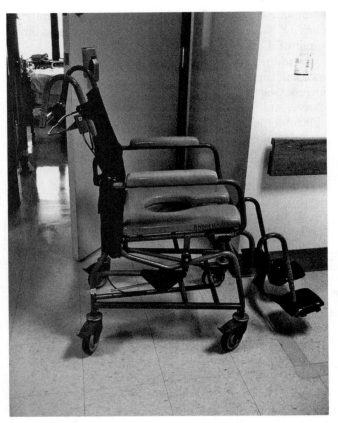

Figure 15-5. Padded shower commode chair. Typical padded commode chair for bowel care. Padding is essential for skin protection.

to do a digital rectal check several times per day in conjunction with bladder emptying or hygiene activities.

UMN bowels rely on reflex relaxation of the internal and external anal sphincters to trigger bowel emptying. Stimulation of this reflex, known as the *rectocolic reflex*, may trigger both giant rectal contractions and the rectoanal inhibitory reflex at the same time.[31] Two methods of stimulating this reflex are commonly used, chemical stimulation (by a suppository or mini-enema placed in the rectum) and digital stimulation.

Bowel care is frequently initiated to occur at a planned time by insertion of a suppository or by a mini-enema. The choice of which to use is often determined by standard practice in a given hospital, but standard practice should be used only as a place to begin since individuals will respond differently to the various stimulants and delivery vehicles. Rectal stimulants are one of the few aspects of SCI bowel care that have been studied. Two studies of docusate mini-enemas compared to bisacodyl suppositories have shown that they decrease the overall time spent in evacuation.[32,33] An open-label trial of four bowel stimulants (bisacodyl suppositories, glycerin suppositories, mineral oil enemas, and docusate mini-enemas) in seven people with UMN SCI compared colonic transit time, bowel evacuation time, and questionnaire responses about various associated symptoms after a

1-week trial of each stimulant.[34] Both docusate and mineral oil enemas decreased total and left-sided colonic transit time, but docusate was superior in terms of decreasing bowel evacuation time and symptom reduction. Based on this evidence, docusate mini-enemas are recommended. It is helpful to know the characteristics of the various suppository options in order to guide individuals with SCI in their selection. Bisacodyl suppositories are typically delivered in a vegetable oil base, which may dissolve slowly, prolonging overall bowel care time. Bisacodyl is also available in a polyethylene glycol base (Magic Bullet). There is some evidence that this base may produce more rapid onset of stool evacuation and reduced bowel care time.[33,35,36] Glycerin suppositories provide a less-potent chemical stimulus but may work well in individuals with mucosal irritation or delayed results from bisacodyl. Another type of suppository (Ceo-Two) produces CO_2 gas when it is inserted, causing distention of the rectum and an increase in colon peristalsis when activated. Some people may prefer these, but they may not produce predictable results due to leakage of the gas through the anal sphincter.[5]

Digital stimulation is usually required to further stimulate the rectocolic reflex and complete bowel evacuation. Digital stimulation consists of gentle insertion of a lubricated gloved finger or a digital stimulator adapted for the individual with decreased hand function. The finger is inserted in the direction of the sacrum, with gentle but sustained pressure in a circular, rotating motion, past the spastic EAS and pelvic muscles.[5,37] The rotating motion will initiate the rectoanal inhibitory reflex, relax the IAS, and stimulate the rectocolic reflex, promoting pelvic nerve-mediated peristalsis. As the IAS relaxes, flatus passes and stool comes down. This procedure is repeated about every 10 minutes until no further stool is palpated and the IAS tone is palpably increased, a sign that defecation is complete.[5] It is important to avoid both Valsalva maneuvers and rapid or excessive stretching of the anal sphincter because these may provide sphincter spasms and dyssynergia.[8]

A list of the knowledge and skills required by the individual and/or caregiver is provided in Table 15-3. A very sensitive issue to resolve is who will be performing bowel care if the individual with SCI is unable to do so. Having a significant other or family member perform this intimate routine can be emotionally difficult and may significantly affect family relationships.[5] Teaching and paying for outside caregivers can also be challenging. Frank discussion during the acute hospitalization and rehabilitation period is necessary.

Regulation of Stool Transit Time and Consistency: Food, Fiber, Fluid, and Medications

The time required for stool to pass through the colon depends on stool bulk and consistency in addition to the underlying colonic peristalsis. Softer, bulkier stools

Table 15-3

Individual and Family Education Requirements for Neurogenic Bowel Management

Planning	Knowledge	Skills
1. What interventions will be used? 2. When will bowel care be done? 3. Who will be performing bowel care interventions? 4. Where will bowel care take place? 5. What equipment, supplies, and adaptations are needed? 6. How to obtain supplies and equipment as needed?	1. Basic anatomy and physiology of the gastrointestinal system, elimination, and the effect of SCI. 2. The role of food, fiber, and fluid in bowel management. 3. Mode of action, dosage, and common side effects of rectal and oral medications to be used. 4. Recognition and treatment of potential problems, including autonomic dysreflexia, constipation, and hemorrhoids. 5. Safe disposal of waste. 6. How to get help and support.	1. Monitoring and evaluating bowel program results. 2. Safe and effective performance or capable direction of recommended techniques. 3. Basic problem solving and management of AD (if appropriate). 4. How to protect and preserve skin integrity during bowel management. 5. Transfer skills (or safe direction of others). 6. Safe and effective use of equipment and medical supplies.

Adapted from: Ash D. Sustaining safe and acceptable bowel care in spinal cord injured individuals. *Nurs Stand.* 2005;20(8):55–64. Used by permission.

promote more rapid colon transit time. To a certain extent, food and fluid intake can be modified to regulate stool consistency in people with SCI. A fluid intake of at least 2 liters per day is helpful to soften stool. Specific fluids, especially prune juice and apricot nectar, promote stool transit due to mild chemical irritation. In most people, fiber hastens stool transit by increasing stool bulk, which, in turn, distends the colon, promoting propulsive activity. The effect of fiber on colonic transit time in people with SCI is a matter of controversy. One study demonstrated no improvement in transit time from fiber supplementation.[38] Nevertheless, a high-fiber diet and/or fiber supplementation are often recommended for people with SCI because fiber improves stool consistency by absorbing fluid and adding bulk.[5,25] Certain foods are known to slow stool transit (bananas, high-fat foods, dairy products, especially cheese) and thus may be helpful for treating diarrhea or regulating stools that are too loose.

In addition to the rectal stimulants discussed earlier, there are three major classes of medications for regulating the neurogenic bowel (Table 15-4). These are bulk-forming agents, stool softeners, and laxatives. Bulk-forming agents include natural and manufactured fiber supplements. Examples are bran, psyllium, methylcellulose, and calcium polycarbophil. They are available as granules to be dissolved in liquid or sometimes in a pill form to be taken with a full glass of liquid. An adequate fluid intake is essential for these agents to work successfully. Side effects, including bloating and flatulence, may

develop, but they often resolve over time or by switching from one type of fiber to another. Stool softeners work by decreasing the surface tension of the stool, allowing fluid to be combined with stool, producing a softer stool. They do not directly affect bowel motility, but softer stools move more easily through the colon. Stool softeners are most useful for prevention of constipation or when straining should be avoided. People with LMN bowels will need to use them carefully to avoid stool that is too soft in order to be able to maintain continence.

Use of laxatives by people with SCI is common, but indiscriminate use can be problematic due to adverse effects. Laxatives produce their effects by increasing intestinal motility. There are three classes of laxatives: (1) osmotic laxatives, (2) saline laxatives, and (3) stimulant laxatives. Osmotic laxatives are indigestible carbohydrates that work by osmotically drawing fluid into the colon. Examples are lactulose and polyethylene glycol. They usually work quickly, and doses are easily adjusted to regulate stool consistency, making them a good choice for a person with SCI.[29] Saline laxatives include milk of magnesia, magnesium citrate, and sodium phosphate/biophosphate. They work in the small intestine, drawing fluid into the lumen and inducing mixing actions and stimulation of colonic motility.[5] Saline laxatives are good choices for occasional constipation that does not resolve with use of an osmotic laxative. Stimulants work directly on the myenteric plexus to chemically stimulate peristalsis. Stimulant laxatives include bisacodyl, senna, cascara, aloe, rhubarb, and phenolphthalein. In people with SCI,

Table 15-4
Medications Commonly Used in Management of the Neurogenic Bowel

Class	Type	Agent/Trade name	Mechanism of Action	Cautions
Rectal stimulants	Mini-enemas	Docusate (Enemeez)	Chemical stimulation of rectocolic reflex	
	Suppositories	Bisacodyl (Dulcolax, Magic Bullet) CO_2 (Ceo-Two) Glycerin	Chemical stimulation of rectocolic reflex	Slow dissolution may prolong bowel care.
Stool softeners	Oral capsules	Docusate sodium/calcium (DOSS) (Colace, Surfak)	Decrease surface tension of stool, allowing greater water content thus causing softer stool.	Careful use in LMN bowels required to prevent incontinence.
Bulking agents	Natural fiber supplements Manufactured fiber supplements	Bran Psyllium (Metamucil, Citrucel, Per Diem) Calcium polycarbophil (Fibercon)	Improves stool consistency and adds bulk.	May cause bloating and gas. Requires adequate fluid intake.
Laxatives	Osmotic	Lactulose (Constulose) Polyethylene glycol (MiraLax)	Draws water into the colon via osmosis.	Can deplete electrolytes if overused.
	Saline	Milk of magnesia (MOM, Phillips) Magnesium citrate (Citroma, Citrate of Magnesia)	Draws fluid into small intestine and induces mixing action and stimulation of colonic motility.	Cramping, diarrhea. Magnesium citrate can be used as bowel prep.
	Stimulant	Bisacodyl (Dulcolax) Phenolphthalein (Ex-Lax) Senna (Senokot) Cascara	Chemical stimulation of colonic motility.	Cramping, diarrhea. Chronic use may cause sluggish bowel and megacolon. Reserve for times when other agents do not work.
	Herbal agents	Aloe Rhubarb Burdock root Dandelion Dong quai Flaxseed	Various, mainly chemical stimulation of motility.	No research evidence supporting use in SCI.
Prokinetic agents	Oral tablets	Metoclopramide (Reglan)	Increases rate of gastric emptying and small intestine transit. No effect on colon.	May cause drowsiness.

chronic use of stimulant laxatives may cause the colon to become unresponsive and more sluggish over time. Senna is particularly implicated in this harmful effect and has also been shown to lead to megacolon and colonic mucosal staining (melanosis coli).[39]

Complications

The three most common problems related to SCI neurogenic bowel management are constipation, incontinence, and prolonged time required for bowel care. In addition, there are several conditions associated with neurogenic bowel for which people with SCI are known to be at risk, including hemorrhoids, diverticuli, and chronic abdominal pain. Management of constipation, fecal incontinence, and prolonged bowel care in people with SCI requires obtaining a thorough history of the problem, evaluation of any indications of serious medical problems, and methodical problem solving, changing only one element at a time and allowing at least a week to evaluate the impact of changes before making other changes.[29]

Symptoms of constipation include hard, dry stools that are small in size and occur less frequently than usual. Causes of constipation are usually multifaceted and include sluggish colonic propulsion and dysmotility related to the neurological injury, medications (especially opioids and anticholinergics) that slow colonic motility, low fiber intake, poor fluid intake, and inactivity. Recent surveys of people with SCI found 46% of people reported constipation and 58% reported two or fewer bowel movements in a week.[40,41] Preventing constipation should be a goal of every bowel management plan. Severe constipation can lead to impaction or cause autonomic dysreflexia. Treatment of constipation depends on the duration and severity of symptoms. Hard stools should trigger an increase in the dose of stool softener or fiber and fluids. If stool becomes so hard that it is difficult to pass or there has been no stool output for 24 hours after a planned bowel evacuation, a laxative is indicated, usually beginning with an osmotic laxative and progressing to a saline laxative and, finally, a stimulant laxative, if constipation persists. It is best to carefully titrate laxative dose in order to avoid diarrhea and fecal incontinence, common outcomes of laxative use. Occasionally, constipation alternating with diarrhea may be an indication of a partial bowel obstruction, with liquid stool flowing around an impaction.[5] Abdominal plain films will aid in diagnosis of this condition.

Incontinence of stool can be an indication of a number of different problems, including a management plan that does not match the person's injury level/completeness or lifestyle, a program that is not correctly carried out or is skipped, overuse of laxatives, poor titration of stool softeners, dietary indiscretions, food intolerances, or foodborne illness, as well as any health condition that can cause diarrhea. One very large survey of people

with SCI found that more unplanned bowel evacuations were associated with use of oral laxatives and fewer unplanned evacuations were associated with manual removal of stool.[42] Another survey study suggested an association with higher levels of anxiety,[41] though it may be that anxiety is due to the fecal incontinence rather than causing it. Similarly, prolonged bowel care times are multicausal and are known to be associated with use of oral laxatives, chronic constipation, incorrectly managed bowel care (especially overly vigorous and too frequent digital stimulation in people with UMN lesions), and rectal sphincter dyssynergia.

Autonomic dysreflexia (AD) associated with bowel care is a significant concern for anyone with an injury level at T6 or above. Guidelines for management of AD are published and should be followed.[43] In some people, AD may occur subacutely (without the usual symptoms of headache, increase in blood pressure, etc.) during bowel care and cause unusual symptoms such as fatigue or dizziness that contribute to a general feeling of "unwellness" on bowel care days.[44] Avoiding constipation and overly vigorous digital stimulation are important ways to prevent AD. Also, using local anesthetic agents such as lidocaine gel instead of a plain lubricant may help to prevent AD.

Medical complications of neurogenic bowel are common. For example, up to 75% of individuals with SCI have reported hemorrhoids,[8] and 33% in another survey reported regular abdominal pain.[40] Hemorrhoids can be managed conservatively by treating constipation and using a hemorrhoidal cream or ointment, unless they bleed profusely or contribute to AD. Banding, an outpatient surgical procedure, can be done to remove them.[5] Abdominal pain warrants evaluation to determine if there is an acute medical problem requiring immediate intervention, a chronic medical problem requiring ongoing management (diverticuli, irritable bowel syndrome), or if the pain is chronic, SCI-related pain that might be best addressed with pain management medications and treatments.

Surgical and Other Alternatives

Most people with SCI will be able to manage their bowel without surgery or technology. However, there are some cases where diverting the stool to a surgically created stoma in the abdominal wall (colostomy) is helpful or necessary. The two most common reasons for colostomy in people with SCI are treatment of sacral or perineal pressure ulcers and to decrease the amount of time required for bowel care. Recent interview studies of people with SCI who had colostomy surgery found very positive effects on quality of life.[27,45] These studies reported significantly shorter times for bowel care, greater independence, high levels of satisfaction, and a large percentage of people who stated they would have liked to have had the surgery sooner.

As with any surgical procedure, there are risks of complications associated with colostomy. One survey of individuals with SCI who had a colostomy reported complications in 44% of 32 individuals interviewed.[27] Complications reported include bowel obstruction, peristomal hernias, stomal stenosis, and leakage of mucus from the rectum. A common cause of leakage of mucus and blood from the rectum is diversion colitis, a condition requiring further surgery or medical management with short-chain free fatty acid enemas or steroid enemas.[27]

An alternative to colostomy surgery is a surgical diversion procedure called the *antegrade continence enema (ACE)* procedure. The surgeon creates a catheterizable channel by attaching the appendix to the right lower abdominal wall. Once the stoma has healed, bowel care is done by inserting a catheter into the stoma, instilling fluid, waiting 15 minutes, then beginning digital rectal stimulation and continuing it every 10 minutes until the rectum is empty.[46] These periodic rectal washouts are accomplished because the fluid is instilled before (antegrade to) the stool, pushing the stool out as it travels. Case reports document less toileting time and fewer episodes of incontinence after this procedure.[46,49] But complications, including stomal stenosis and less efficiency of the irrigations over time, are frequently reported.[46,48]

Electrical stimulation of defecation is possible, but so far has only been done in conjunction with implantation of a sacral anterior nerve root stimulator for bladder emptying.[49,50] This procedure requires a very motivated individual with good hand function and a complete UMN SCI above the sacral level. A posterior sacral rhizotomy is done along with surgical implantation of electrodes on the sacral nerves. A receiver–stimulator is implanted under the abdominal skin and is controlled by radio transmission. The stimulator triggers bladder emptying, and once stimulation stops, the EAS relaxes quickly while the rectum relaxes slowly, causing defecation. To date, 17 cases have been reported.[49,50] Most individuals who underwent the procedure had much shorter bowel care time without increased frequency of fecal incontinence.

A final technological option reported in the literature is the pulsed irrigation evacuation (PIE). This is a machine designed to deliver pulsed tap water to the rectum through a catheter that is held in place by a retention cuff.[51] The pulsed enema loosens the stool and suspends it in water, and it is removed through a drain conduit that runs through the center of the catheter. There are no reports of its long-term efficacy, risks, or individual satisfaction, so no recommendation can currently be made.

Periodic Monitoring and Evaluation

As part of each annual or bi-annual SCI evaluation, questions addressing current bowel function should be included. It is important to note the frequency, method(s), and outcomes of bowel care. Outcomes queried should address the length of time required for bowel care as well as stool amount and frequency and consistency of stool. Medications taken for bowel management, as well as those that have a potential effect on bowel motility, should be reviewed, and the individual's understanding of medication effects and use should be tested. Questions designed to detect common potential problems are also necessary, including those regarding diarrhea, constipation, hemorrhoids, anal or rectal bleeding, stool incontinence, and abdominal pain. Equipment availability and condition may also be assessed, and prescriptions for new or replacement equipment provided as appropriate.

The most recent and largest study of colon cancer risk in people with SCI found no significantly different degree of risk or higher incidence of colon cancer in this group,[52] although an earlier, smaller study did find a greater incidence of colon cancer.[53] The clinical practice guideline developed by the U.S. Consortium for Spinal Cord Medicine in 1998[28] emphasizes the need for routine colorectal cancer screening as per general population guidelines. The current general population guidelines for those who are age 50 or older with average risk (i.e., no first-degree relatives with colon cancer) emphasize yearly stool hemoccult testing, with flexible sigmoidoscopy every 5 years and/or colonoscopy every 10 years.[54] It is very important to ensure that individuals with SCI obtain routine screening because symptoms of colorectal cancer may not be apparent due to sensory changes or they may be attributed to neurogenic bowel. Significant delay in obtaining treatment is associated with increased likelihood of poor outcomes.

▌CASE STUDY 15-1   Neurogenic Bladder

Rick is a 21-year-old man with T6 paraplegia, ASIA A (complete motor and sensory), since an automobile accident 9 months earlier. He was discharged from initial rehabilitation using clean IC every 6 hours during the day. During the past week, he began to notice increasing urinary incontinence each afternoon and is distressed by this. He seeks help from his health-care provider who obtains an otherwise negative history and negative laboratory evidence for a UTI. His urine volumes range from 400 to 500 mL and average a total daily output of 1700 mL. Urodynamic evaluation is requested and indicates that Rick has a hyperactive detrusor with no evidence for DSD. How would you manage Rick's bladder?

Management for Rick

Rick was asked to add another catheterization during the afternoon. After 2 weeks, he was having fewer episodes of

CASE STUDY 15-1   Neurogenic Bladder—cont'd

incontinence but still was wetting his pants and was unhappy. Tolterodine once a day was then begun and the dose increased to the maximum recommended, but Rick still had occasional urinary incontinence, not only in the afternoon, but also at night. He stopped doing the additional catheterization since it no longer seemed to help. Tolterodine was discontinued, and a second smooth muscle relaxant, oxybutynin, was begun, and after gradual dose adjustments, Rick no longer was incontinent.

Discussion

Since Rick did not have signs or symptoms of a UTI, he did not need to be treated with antibiotics. He did have urodynamic evidence of detrusor hyperactivity and moderately high urine volumes despite the incontinence. The first change to consider is adding an additional catheterization around the time of day that Rick is usually incontinent. This might reduce the incidence of incontinence and is worth trying. If, despite adding another catheterization, Rick continues to have incontinence,

then a trial of an anticholinergic would be the next step. Rick also began having incontinence at other times, which is not unusual since his bladder was in the process of developing detrusor activity and he is still in the early stages of SCI. The first smooth muscle relaxant did not prevent incontinence, and a second drug was tried. This is not atypical, but it is important to keep in mind that smooth muscle relaxants also slow down bowel motility. Simply increasing the dose of a smooth muscle relaxant to prevent incontinence may lead to a dangerous bowel emergency, that is, bowel obstruction. Such medications also have side effects that individuals may not tolerate, and these medications may be contraindicated in certain circumstances. Finally, since Rick already had a modest urine output (1700 mL per 24 hours), reducing his fluid intake would be contraindicated. Review of the *timing* of his fluid intake should be part of his assessment, but with urodynamic data of detrusor hyperactivity, the most direct management approach would be to reduce the activity in the bladder with medication.

CASE 15-2   Neurogenic Bowel

Jeremy is a 20-year-old male with C6 AIS B tetraplegia due to a skiing accident. Initially, post-injury he was in the ICU for 2 weeks on a ventilator and had a brief period of paralytic ileus that resolved in 2 days after placement of a nasogastric tube. Bowel care during the acute period was done daily by manual evacuation of stool by the nurses, usually in the early morning hours when he was sleeping. He was transferred directly to the rehabilitation unit after his ICU stay, where daily manual evacuation was continued, but the timing was changed to occur after breakfast now that Jeremy was eating regular meals.

Prior to his injury, Jeremy would typically have a bowel movement daily, usually in the early evening after dinner. As a college student, his usual diet consisted of two meals per day (lunch and dinner) and snacks, with a heavy predominance of fast food, sandwiches, pasta and noodles, with few fruits or vegetables. He had no pre-morbid history of gastrointestinal problems and had never thought much about his bowels prior to his injury. Education about neurogenic bowel was started immediately by the rehabilitation staff, with the daily manual evacuation being used as an optimal "teachable moment" to discuss bowel management.

At 5 weeks post-injury, JC's anal tone returned and a neurological examination showed that he had anocutaneous and bulbocavernosus reflexes. Bowel management was changed to a daily bisacodyl suppository followed by digital stimulation every 10–15 minutes until defecation was complete. JC was now able to sit on a commode chair for bowel care and became more active in his own care. The following were goals for his long-term bowel management plan: (1) switch to an every-other-day program, (2) change to an after dinner program since this fit best with his lifestyle,

(3) learn to do bowel care independently, and (4) have trained caregivers to assist as needed with bowel care after discharge. When the daily evening routine was successfully established, a trial of every-other-day bowel care was started. For the initial 3 days, JC experienced small stool incontinences on the day he did not have bowel care, but by the fourth day the routine was established without further incontinence. JC began learning to use a suppository inserter and digital stimulator while in the rehabilitation unit. He chose to have his mother and a hired attendant trained to do his bowel care. He was discharged on a daily dose of Metamucil fiber and a single dose of 250 mg of stool softener (DOSS) daily.

At his 1-month follow-up after rehabilitation, JC complained of bowel care requiring 2 hours to complete and stools that were becoming hard. He had returned to his usual diet and discontinued the Metamucil fiber because he disliked the texture, but continued to take the stool softener. His attendant was inserting the suppository but JC was able to perform digital stimulation safely and independently with his digital stimulator. Three changes to the program were made: (1) changing to DOSS mini-enemas to initiate bowel care, (2) discussion and education about dietary fiber and a decision to switch to a less gritty fiber supplement, and (3) increasing use of the stool softener to twice daily. These changes decreased his bowel care time to 45 to 60 minutes, softened his stool, and he continued this plan for years without difficulty. JC should return for yearly evaluations including an assessment of his bowel program and gastrointestinal function. Regular monitoring will help guarantee early detection and/or prevention of complications as well as allow his health care providers to teach him about anticipated changes with aging.

Summary

Both the bladder and bowel are innervated through complex sympathetic and parasympathetic systems that operate at various levels of the spinal cord and are coordinated by centers in the brainstem. SCI may disrupt the coordinated activities at these various levels that allow normal urination and defecation. SCI level and completeness determine the type of dysfunction in bladder and bowel. An injury above the sacral segments of the spinal cord produces a UMN or reflexic bladder and bowel. An injury at the sacral segments (or cauda equina) produces a LMN or areflexic bowel and bladder. Incomplete injury at any level may modify the typical patterns of dysfunction.

The choice of bladder management depends on a variety of factors, including type of bladder, functional level of the individual with SCI, the individual's preference, and physician bias. The goal is for the individual with a SCI to be catheter-free and to empty the bladder with low postvoid residuals without excess bladder pressure elevations. Intermittent catheterization is the most common management technique. Additional methods that are employed include indwelling catheters, suprapubic tapping, Valsalva and Credé maneuver, and (in males) condom catheters (often after a sphincterotomy) that help to decrease outflow resistance and prevent elevation of bladder pressures. Prevention of UTIs and other urological complications, including autonomic dysreflexia, urinary stones, and reflux, are important in order to prevent long-term renal damage. A regular long-term urinary tract surveillance program is recommended for individuals with SCI.

Because bowel dysfunction is rated as one of the most distressing aspects of living with SCI, a well-managed bowel is important for both health and social reasons. Goals for bowel management include both safety and acceptability of bowel care routines. Basic principles for management of UMN-type and LMN-type neurogenic bowel need to be aligned with the characteristics of the individual and that person's functional abilities, lifestyle, and preferences. Teaching bowel management principles rather than a specific program provides the individual with tools needed to more successfully self-manage the neurogenic bowel over the years. Important factors include timing, position, equipment, stimulation or evacuation techniques, and use of medications. The three most common problems related to SCI neurogenic bowel management are constipation, incontinence, and prolonged time required for bowel care. Management of these problems requires obtaining a thorough history of the problem, evaluation of any indications of serious medical problems, and methodical problem solving, changing only one element at a time and allowing at least a week to evaluate the impact of the change before making other changes. Most people with SCI will be able to manage their bowel without surgery or technology; however, surgical options, including colostomy, may provide improved quality of life for some individuals.

REVIEW QUESTIONS

1. Where are the micturition control centers located?
2. Describe innervation of the two bladder sphincters and the two bowel sphincters. How do these sphincters work to maintain continence?
3. How do involuntary reflexes and voluntary mechanisms work in a coordinated manner during defecation?
4. Define upper and lower motor neuron lesions as relates to bowel and bladder function in individuals with SCI and describe the effect of each on bowel and bladder function.
5. What methods of bladder and bowel management are usually used during the first days after SCI and why?
6. List the tests that will help determine the most appropriate long-term bladder management plan.
7. What factors must be considered in selecting the best bladder management plan for a given individual with SCI?
8. Explain why periodic monitoring and evaluation are important for people with neurogenic bladder. What are the most common complications of neurogenic bladder?
9. Why do you think that bowel dysfunction is rated one of the "most distressing" aspects of living with SCI?
10. Name at least two bowel management principles for each of the following: timing, position, equipment, stimulation or evacuation techniques and medications.
11. What is meant by teaching "principles" rather than a "specific program" in neurogenic bowel management?
12. Identify the three most common complications related to SCI bowel management and suggest interventions to address each of these.
13. Discuss pros and cons of surgical procedures for bowel management including colostomy, ACE procedure, and electrical stimulation of defecation.

REFERENCES

1. Kim JH, Rivas DA, Shenot PJ et al. Intravesical resiniferatroxin for refractory detrusor hyperreflexia: A multicenter, blinded, randomized, placebo-controlled trial. *J Spinal Cord Med.* 2003;26(4):358–363.
2. Giannantoni A, Di Stasi SM, Stephen RL et al. Intravesical resiniferatroxin versus botulinum-A toxin injections for neurogenic detrusor overactivity: A prospective randomized study. *J Urol.* 2004;172(1):240–243.
3. Potter PJ. Disordered control of the urinary bladder after human spinal cord injury: What are the problems? *Prog Brain Res.* 2006;152:51–57.
4. Benevento BT, Sipski ML. Neurogenic bladder, neurogenic bowel, and sexual dysfunction in people with spinal cord injury. *Phys Ther.* 2002;82:601–612.
5. Stiens SA, Bergman SB, Goetz LL. Neurogenic bowel dysfunction after spinal cord injury: Clinical evaluation and rehabilitative management. *Arch Phys Med Rehabil.* 1997;78:S86–S102.

6. Brading AF, Ramalingam T. Mechanisms controlling normal defecation and the potential effects of spinal cord injury. *Prog Brain Res.* 2006;152:345–358.

7. Nout YS, Leedy GM, Beattie MS et al. Alterations in eliminative and sexual reflexes after spinal cord injury: Defecatory function and development of spasticity in pelvic floor musculature. *Prog Brain Res.* 2006;152:359–372.

8. Chung EAL, Emmanuel AV. Gastrointestinal symptoms related to autonomic dysfunction following spinal cord injury. *Prog Brain Res.* 2006;152:317–333.

9. Cardenas DD, Hooton TM. Urinary tract infection in persons with spinal cord injury. *Arch Phys Med Rehabil.* 1995;75(3):272–280.

10. Lemke JR, Kasprowicz K, Worral PS. Intermittent catheterization for individuals with a neurogenic bladder: Sterile versus clean: Using evidence-based practice at the staff nurse level. *J Nurs Care Qual.* 2005;20(4):302–306.

11. Prieto-Fingerhut T, Banovac K, Lynne CM. A study comparing sterile and nonsterile urethral catheterization in individuals with spinal cord injury. *Rehabil Nurs.* 1997;22(6):299–302.

12. Duffy LM, Cleary J, Ahern S et al. Clean intermittent catheterization; safe, cost-effective bladder management for male residents of VA nursing homes. *J Am Geriatr Soc.* 1995;43(8):865–870.

13. King RB, Carlson CE, Mervine J et al. Clean and sterile intermittent catheterization methods in hospitalized individuals with spinal cord injury. *Arch Phys Med Rehabil.* 1992;73:798–802.

14. Cardenas DD, Kelly E, Krieger JN et al. Residual urine volumes in individuals with spinal cord injury. Measurement with a portable ultrasound instrument. *Arch Phys Med Rehabil.* 1988;69(7):514–526.

15. Linsenmeyer TA, Culkin D. APS recommendations for the urological evaluation of individuals with spinal cord injury. *J Spinal Cord Med.* 1999;22(2):139–142.

16. Adler US, Kirshblum SC. A new assistive device for intermittent self-catheterization in men with tetraplegia. *J Spinal Cord Med.* 2003;26(2):155–158.

17. Cardenas DD, Mayo MI. Management of bladder dysfunction. In: Braddom RL, editor. *Textbook of Physical Medicine and Rehabilitation.* 3rd edition. Philadelphia: W.B. Saunders; (2007).

18. McInerney DD, Vanner TF, Harris SF et al. Permanent urethral stent for detrusor sphincter dyssynergia. *Br J Urol.* 1991;67(3):291–294.

19. Cardenas DD, Mayo ME. Bacteriuria with fever after spinal cord injury. *Arch Phys Med Rehabil.* 1987;68:291–293.

20. Stover SL, Fine PR, editors. *Spinal Cord Injury: The Facts and Figures.* Birmingham, AL: University of Alabama; 1986.

21. Cardenas DD, Farrell-Roberts L, Sipski M et al. Management of gastrointestinal, genitourinary and sexual function. In: *Spinal Cord Injury. Clinical Outcomes from the Model Systems.* Gaithersburg, MD: Aspen; 1995. pp. 12–144.

22. Brindley GS, Rushton DN. Long-term follow-up of individuals with sacral anterior root stimulator implants. *Paraplegia.* 1990;28(8):469–475.

23. Cardenas DD, Hoffman JM, Kelly E et al. Impact of a urinary tract infection educational program in persons with spinal cord injury. *J Spinal Cord Med.* 2004;27:47–54.

24. Waites KB, Canupp KC, DeVivo MJ. Epidemiology and risk factors for urinary tract infection following spinal cord injury. *Arch Phys Med Rehabil.* 1993;74(7):691–695.

25. Lynch AC, Antony A, Dobbs BR et al. Bowel dysfunction following spinal cord injury. *Spinal Cord.* 2001;39:193–203.

26. Multidisciplinary Association of Spinal Cord Injury Professionals. *MASCIP Guidelines for Bowel Management after Spinal Cord Injury. Part 4: Rehabilitation and Discharge Guidelines.* Available at: www.mascip.co.ukpdfs/Part4-Bowel Management.pdf. Accessed: June 14, 2006.

27. Branagan G, Tromans A, Finnis D. Effect of stoma formation on bowel care and quality of life in individuals with spinal cord injury. *Spinal Cord.* 2003;41:680–683.

28. U.S. Consortium for Spinal Cord Medicine. Neurogenic Bowel Management in Adults with Spinal Cord Injury. 1998; Washington DC, Paralyzed Veterans of America.

29. Ash D. Sustaining safe and acceptable bowel care in spinal cord injured individuals. *Nurs Stand.* 2005;20(8):55–64.

30. Nelson A, Malassigne P, Cors MW et al. Promoting safe use of equipment for neurogenic bowel management. *SCI Nurs.* 2000;17(3):119–124.

31. Krogh K, Olsen N, Christensen P et al. Colorectal transport during defecation in individuals with lesions of the sacral spinal cord. *Neurogastroenterol Motil.* 2003;15:25–31.

32. Dunn KL, Galka ML. A comparison of the effectiveness of Therevac SB and bisacodyl suppositories in SCI individuals' bowel programs. *Rehabil Nurs.* 1994;19:334–338.

33. House JG, Stiens SA. Pharmacologically initiated defecation of persons with spinal cord injury: Effectiveness of three agents. *Arch Phys Med Rehabil.* 1997;78:1062–1065.

34. Amir I, Sharma R, Bauman WA et al. Bowel care for individuals with spinal cord injury: comparison of four approaches. *J Spinal Cord Med.* 1998;21:21–24.

35. Stiens SA, Luttrel W, Binard J. Reduction in bowel program time with polyethylene glycol-based bisacodyl suppositories: An open label study. *J Spinal Cord Med.* 1995;18:299.

36. Stiens SA. Reduction in bowel program duration with polyethylene glycol-based bisacodyl suppositories. *Arch Phys Med Rehabil.* 1995;76:674–677.

37. Lynch AC, Frizelle FA. Colorectal motility and defecation after spinal cord injury in humans. *Prog Brain Res.* 2006;152:335–343.

38. Cameron KJ, Nyulasi IB, Collier GR et al. Assessment of the effecty of increased dietary fiber intake on bowel function in individuals with spinal cord injury. *Spinal Cord.* 1996;34:277–283.

39. Harari D, Minaker KL. Megacolon in individuals with chronic spinal cord injury. *Spinal Cord.* 2000;38:331–339.

40. Delooze D, VanLaere M, De Muynck et al. Constipation and other chronic gastrointestinal problems in spinal cord injury individuals. *Spinal Cord.* 1998;36:63–66.

41. Ng C, Prot G, Rutkowski S et al. Gastrointestinal symptoms in spinal cord injury: Relationships with level of injury and psychologic factors. *Dis Colon Rectum.* 2005;48(8):1562–1568.

42. Haas U, Geng V, Evers GCM et al. Bowel management in individuals with spinal cord injury–A multicentre study of the German speaking society of paraplegia (DMGP). *Spinal Cord.* 2005;43:724–730.

43. Consortium for Spinal Cord Medicine. *Acute Management of Autonomic Dysreflexia: Adults with Spinal Cord Injuries Presenting to Health-Care Facilities [clinical practice guideline].* 1997; Washington, DC, Paralyzed Veterans of America.

44. Yoshimura O, Maejima H, Saski H et al. Bowel dysfunction and disturbance of physical condition after evacuation in individuals with chronic cervical spinal cord injuries. *J Phys Ther Sci.* 2001;13(2):145–148.

45. Safadi BY, Rosito O, Nino-Murcia M et al. Which stoma works better for colonic dysmotility in the spinal cord injured individual? *Am J Surg.* 2003;186:437–442.

46. Teichman JMH, Zabihi N, Kraus SR et al. Long-term results for Malone antegrade continence enema for adults with neurogenic bowel disease. *Urology.* 61:502–506.

47. Yang C, Stiens SA. Antegrade continence enema for the treatment of neurogenic constipation and fecal incontinence after spinal cord injury. *Arch Phys Med Rehabil.* 2000;81:683–685.

48. McAndrews HF, Malone PS. Continent catheterizable conduits: Which stoma, which conduit and which reservoir? *BJU Int.* 2002;89:86–89.

49. Creasey GH, Grill JH, Korsten M et al. An implantable neuroprosthesis for restoring bladder and bowel control to individuals with spinal cord injuries: A multicenter trial. *Arch Phys Med Rehabil.* 2001;82:1512–1519.

50. Creasey GH, Dahlberg JE. Economic consequences of an implanted neuroprosthesis for bladder and bowel management. *Arch Phys Med Rehabil.* 2001;82:1520–1525.

51. Puet TA, Phen L, Hurst DL. Pulsed irrigation enhanced evacuation: New method for treating fecal impaction. *Arch Phys Med Rehabil.* 1991;72:935–936.

52. Stratton MD, McKirgan LW, Wade TP et al. Colorectal cancer in individuals with previous spinal cord injury. *Dis Colon Rectum.* 1996;39:865–968.

53. Frisbie JH, Chopra S, Foo D et al. Colorectal carcinoma and myelopathy. *J Am Paraplegia Soc.* 1984;7:33–36.

54. Ko C, Hyman NH. Practice parameter for the detection of colorectal neoplasms: An interim report *Dis Colon Rectum.* 2006;49:299.

Cardiovascular Health and Exercise Prescription

16

Mark S. Nash, PhD, FACSM

After reading this chapter, the reader will be able to:

OBJECTIVES

- Identify the major causes for accelerated cardiovascular disease in persons with spinal cord injuries (SCIs)
- Discuss co-morbid states and conditions that worsen the cardiovascular disease prognosis for persons with SCI
- Discuss causes and consequences of physical deconditioning after SCI
- Identify the prevalent lipid profile that predisposes persons with SCI to premature cardiovascular disease
- Identify components of the exercise prescription for persons with SCI and guidelines used to prescribe safe, effective exercise programs
- Contrast benefits of endurance and resistance training programs for persons with SCI
- Identify unique limitations and risks for exercise after SCI and the precautions that can be adopted to minimize them

OUTLINE

Cardiovascular Disease After Spinal Cord Injury

More than two decades have passed since cardiovascular diseases emerged as a major health concern for persons with SCI.[1-3] In the years that immediately followed World War II, genitourinary complications accounted for 43% of deaths after SCI, although mortality from these causes was reduced to 10% of cases in the 1980s and 1990s.[2,4] Cardiovascular diseases (CVDs) currently represent the most frequent cause of death among persons surviving more than 30 years after injury (46% of deaths) and among persons more than 60 years of age (35% of deaths).[5] Of special concern is the accelerated rate at which CVD appears in those with SCI.[4,6,7] Asymptomatic CVD after SCI appears at an earlier age[8] and may have symptoms that are masked by interruption of sensory pain fibers that normally convey warnings of cardiac ischemia and imminent cardiac damage.[9,10] The latter makes delays in emergent treatment needed to prevent impending myocardial damage and cardiac dysfunction a strong possibility, especially for those with higher levels of SCI and greater loss of sensory function.[11]

Several major risk factors commonly reported in persons with SCI have been linked with their accelerated course of CVD; these include an atherogenic dyslipidemia,[12] hyperinsulinemia,[13-15] and visceral obesity.[16,17] An atherogenic lipid profile has been widely reported in persons with chronic SCI.[15-23] The most consistent finding of this dyslipidemia is a depressed blood plasma concentration of the high-density lipoprotein cholesterol (HDL-C),[6,17,24,25] whose functions include protection against development of vascular disease.[26] More than 40% of young persons with SCI have HDL-C levels that failed to meet authoritative targets. This risk is commonly accompanied by other health hazards, including visceral obesity,[16,17] elevated body mass indices,[16] physical inactivity,[27,28] reduced lean body mass,[5,29-31] diabetes,[6,32] insulin resistance with obesity and dyslipidemia (metabolic syndrome X),[33] and advancing age,[34,35] all of which are recognized as independent risks for accelerated disease progression and early cardiovascular morbidity.[36-38]

Insulin resistance occurring in a high percentage of persons with SCI was first reported in 1980[32] and has since been confirmed by other investigations.[14,39] As many as half the persons with SCI live in a state of carbohydrate intolerance or insulin resistance.[9,13,32] A reason for prevalent insulin resistance in persons with SCI has not been firmly identified, although physical inactivity,[39] obesity,[14,16,17] and sympathetic dysfunction[15] have all been suggested as causes. An association may also exist between abnormal lipid profiles and insulin resistance, as persons without disability having low HDL-C are also especially prone to insulin resistance.[40-42]

The Metabolic Syndrome

The frequent clustering of CVD risks poses a serious health hazard for persons with SCI. While criteria for

---

diagnosis of a *metabolic syndrome* (formerly *metabolic X*) differ among authorities, 64 of 201 million U.S. individuals aged 20 years and older have CVD risk clustering that significantly increases their risk both for future CVD and diabetes. When assessed by standards of the National Cholesterol Education Project, Adult Treatment Panel (III), a recent report found that the combination of abdominal obesity, elevated fasting triglycerides, low levels of fasting HDL-C, hypertension, and fasting hyperglycemia was observed in more than one of three young, healthy persons with paraplegia (*see* Box 16-1). No evidence suggests that higher levels of SCI or time since injury will improve this scenario, and thus, aggressive primary prevention in the SCI population must match lifestyle and medical efforts already initiated among persons without disability to offset this risk.

Alterations in Cardiovascular Structure and Function After SCI

Circulatory Dysregulation After SCI

Different patterns of circulatory dysregulation are common among persons with SCI,[43] as injuries occurring above the T1 spinal level disrupt sympathetic nervous system functions and result in resting hypotension.[44] Low mean arterial pressures challenge the ability of persons with cervical SCI to regulate systemic blood pressure during orthostatic challenge and physical activity[45-47] and diminish cardiac ventricular chamber sizes and functions.[48] In those with tetraplegia, a chronic reduction of cardiac preload and myocardial volume, coupled with chronic hypotension, cause the left ventricle to atrophy, which further limits their ability to mount a cardiac output response needed for effective blood pressure regulation.[48,49] By contrast, long-term survivors of paraplegia have normal (or slightly elevated) blood pressure, left ventricular mass, and resting cardiac output, although the cardiac output has elements of elevated resting heart rate (HR) and depressed resting stroke volume.[50,51] This lowered stroke volume is attributed to decreased venous return from the immobile lower extremities accompanying loss or diminished efficiency of venous pumps or to venous insufficiency of the paralyzed limbs.[52,53]

Peripheral Vascular Structure and Function in Persons With Paraplegia and Tetraplegia

Blood volume and velocity of lower extremity arterial circulation are significantly lowered after SCI, with volume flow of about half to two-thirds that reported in healthy individuals without paralysis.[54,55] This so-called circulatory hypokinesis[56,57] results from loss of autonomic control of blood flow as well as diminished regulation of local blood flow by vascular endothelium.[54] The lowering of volume and velocity contribute to increased thrombosis, which is most often reported in those with acute and subacute SCI.[58] A contributing factor to thrombosis risk also appears to be a markedly hypofibrinolytic response to venous occlusion of the paralyzed lower extremities, a poor response explained by low blood flow conditions[54,59] or interruption of adrenergic pathways that normally regulate fibrinolysis in those without neurological dysfunction.[60]

Physical Deconditioning After SCI

Diminished levels of fitness probably account for a large part of accelerated disease after SCI. A sedentary lifestyle either imposed on, or adopted by, persons with SCI has ranked them at the lowest end of the human fitness continuum.[61] In cases of high cervical SCI, muscle paralysis is extensive enough to make voluntary exercise impossible or ineffective. In other cases, persons with SCI simply adopt a sedentary lifestyle or fail to secure personnel and equipment needed to assist them with exercise. Notwithstanding an identified cause for exercise abstention, one in four healthy young persons with SCI fails to satisfy a level of fitness needed to perform many essential activities of daily living.[62] While those with sparing of upper extremity sensorimotor functions have far greater capacities for activity and more extensive exercise options, they are hardly more fit than persons with tetraplegia.[61,63]

It is widely reported that young persons with SCI sustain diseases and disorders often associated with accelerated aging.[2,34] Characteristic conditions of this accelerated state occurring early after SCI include atherogenic dyslipidemia and vascular disease,[2,59,64,65] arterial circulatory insufficiency,[57,59,66] diabetes and related endocrine disorders,[6,14,15,32,67] bone and joint diseases,[68] immune dysfunction,[69,70] and pain of musculoskeletal and neuropathic origins.[71–75]

Exercise Prescription After SCI

An exercise prescription is a detailed plan of fitness-related activities designed to achieve specific health goals. In most cases, this goal specifically targets improved fitness, which can be measured using benchmarks of heightened peak oxygen consumption or peak power output. Well-designed exercise programs normally incorporate the four components of exercise programming into a synergistic plan that specifies an exercise mode, intensity, duration, and frequency. Because a thoughtful, well-considered exercise prescription serves as an effective countermeasure to both physical deconditioning and CVD progression in persons without SCI, it is reasonable to assume that a well-considered and executed exercise prescription will achieve the similar goals for persons with SCI. The following section addresses the design of exercise prescriptions for arm exercise to achieve improved fitness, with specific reference to exercise as a countermeasure to development or progression of CVD in persons with SCI.

Various studies that have reported successful exercise conditioning of persons with SCI have been detailed in monographs addressing a wide range of complexities for exercise design. A simplified view of the exercise prescription for persons with SCI suggests that the undertaking of *any* physical activity is preferable to a sedentary lifestyle. The perception that high levels of fitness are required for cardiovascular protection is a common misconception in exercise programming, as most persons derive cardioprotection and related benefits from low and moderate levels of fitness. High levels of fitness actually afford little additional benefit and impose the risks of overuse and injury. Moreover, persons who are living a sedentary lifestyle generally obtain levels of fitness relatively easily, which suggests that *any* physical activity performed above levels needed for daily subsistence and performance of activities of daily living would be beneficial.

Exercise Mode

The selection of an accessible and engaging exercise mode is the bedrock of well-designed exercise programming, as activities that are mundane build barriers to both adoption and continuation of exercise as a lifestyle choice. In many cases involving SCI, either total or subtotal paralysis of the lower extremities limits regular use of ambulation, treadmills, or other exercise modes that require weight-bearing contractions of the lower extremities. Body weight support is an option is these cases, but it requires specialized equipment to carry out. Because lower extremity exercise activities often require expensive equipment and/or several assistive personnel, upper extremity modes of exercise such as arm ergometry, swimming, wheelchair locomotion, or resistance activities represent more reasonable and available exercise options. Key in the selection of an exercise mode is the ability of the activity to hold the interest of the user on a regular basis, as long-term compliance with exercise programs is notoriously poor and is obviously influenced by the pleasure derived from exercise activities. Availability of resources and reasonable cost both factor into an equation that ultimately determines whether or not persons with SCI will be compliant with long-term exercise.

Exercise Frequency and Duration

Universal guidelines for selection of optimal exercise frequency and duration are incompletely developed for persons with SCI. Authorities such as the American College of Sports Medicine recommend that persons perform 30 to 60 minutes of physical activity on most days of the week, although these guidelines are typically developed for persons without disability. In addition, these guidelines do not consider that the upper extremities undergoing training will also be used for functional activities such as wheelchair propulsion, and that damage from overuse or injury might profoundly diminish personal independence. In almost all instances, exercising two to three times weekly for 30 minutes each session is sufficient to significantly increase maximal oxygen uptake and, in some cases, improve the lipid profile. More frequent exercise may be needed to attain fitness, and once attained, moderate exercise is probably sufficient to maintain it. Those exercising for competition will probably need more frequent and longer exercise sessions, although the risk of overuse or injury increases with prolonged exercise activity. Preservation of upper extremity function should be considered within the exercise plan so that chronic fatigue and injury do not interrupt the consistency of activity and independent lifestyle.

Exercise Intensity

In most cases, an exercise intensity of 50% to 80% of peak oxygen uptake is sufficient to significantly improve fitness and to reduce CVD risks. In significantly deconditioned persons, this percentage may be as low as 40% of peak capacity at the beginning of training and increased with the acquisition of higher levels of fitness. For ease of application, the exercise intensity is generally specified as target HR ranges to be maintained during physical activity. However, work performed by the upper extremities generally elicits higher HR response than lower extremity work. Persons with SCI injuries above the levels of sympathetic nervous system outflow at the T1 level may have altered HR responses to exercise. Therefore, HR may not be an accurate reflection of exercise intensity.

The measurement of energy expenditure and assessment of exercise intensity pose novel challenges for persons with SCI. Oxygen consumption measurements during movement have been used to evaluate energy cost per unit of distance traveled; however, these measurements require collection of expired air and metabolic analysis performed by equipment not available in the home or most clinical settings. An option is to use HR, time, and distance measures to compute a physiological cost index (PCI) or to use the perceived exertion (RPE) method of Borg, the latter based upon somatic ratings of effort.[76] Both methods have shortcomings when used to assess human performance after SCI. The PCI was developed by MacGregor (1979)[77] as a surrogate for energy expenditure when assessing locomotor efficiency. While the method has been used for gait assessment in healthy adults, adults ambulating with prostheses, individuals with stroke, and children with cerebral palsy, it assumes a linear relationship between HR and exertion not always observed in persons with cervical or high thoracic SCI. While several small studies have used the PCI as a study outcome, it has not been validated for use in persons with SCI. Similarly, the Borg range model postulates a relationship between somatic sensations and HR response, but assumes a body habitus both uncompromised by loss of sensation and cardiovascular dysregulation. There is limited evidence to suggest that it is valid and reliable for use by persons with SCI, and a recent study has challenged its use as an index of work intensity in persons with both paraplegia and tetraplegia.

An underused yet simple method of intensity determination is the so-called talk test[76]. This method is advocated by the Centers for Disease Control and Prevention and can be readily adopted for persons with disability. When using the method, it is understood that a person who is active at a *light* intensity level should be able to sing while doing the activity. One who is active at a *moderate* intensity level should be able to carry on a conversation comfortably while engaging in the activity. If a person becomes winded or too out-of-breath to carry on a conversation, the activity can be considered *vigorous*. Another method of intensity determination include use of the Karvonen method, which bases exercise intensity on a percentage of the HR reserve (HRR; $HR_{max} - HR_{rest}$), rather than estimation of an age-adjusted maximal HR. The latter method will often have compromised validity for many persons with SCI, as it fails to consider effects of adrenergic dysfunction on peak HR during activity. In such cases, HR will generally not exceed 120 beats per minute for those with injuries above T1. It also fails to consider the resting HR as an important determinant in establishing HR targets.

Unique Features of the Exercise Response That Influence Exercise Prescription

Injury to the spinal cord dissociates homoeostatic mechanisms whose integrated functions regulate physiological responses needed to sustain exercise. To varying degrees, it further disrupts essential signal integration among motor, sensory, and autonomic targets and thus profoundly influences acute adjustments to activity and peak exercise capacity. Thus, physiological responses to exercise in persons with SCI differ from those of persons without injury.[78–80] Exercise limitations are also associated with the level of SCI and are explained by various factors:

1. Progressively higher levels of injury cause greater loss of mass in those muscles that serve as prime movers and stabilizers of the trunk. Therefore, in individuals with higher levels of injury, the arms must simultaneously generate propulsive forces and steady the trunk during exercise.

2. Progressively higher levels of injury are associated with greater degrees of adrenergic dysfunction and, at key spinal levels, totally dissociate adrenal, cardiac, and sympathetic nervous system regulation from central command. Because the adrenergic and noradrenergic systems normally adjust key metabolic functions during physical activity, their diminished regulatory input alters the cardiovascular and metabolic efficiencies achieved by individuals whose exercise is regulated by an intact neuraxis.

Evidence strongly supports a direct relationship among level of injury, peak workload, and peak oxygen uptake (VO_{2peak}) attained during arm crank testing. Peak work under exercise conditions is delimited by suboptimal circulatory adjustments,[57,76,79,81–82] as individuals with injuries below the level of sympathetic outflow at T6 have significantly lower resting stroke volumes and higher resting heart rates than persons without disability.[82,84,85] The significant elevation of resting and exercise HR is thus thought to compensate for a lower cardiac stroke volume imposed by pooling of blood in the lower extremity venous circuits, diminished venous return, and cardiac end-diastolic volumes, or frank circulatory insufficiency.[57,86] Compensatory upregulation of the intact adrenergic system after SCI may also invoke excessive HR responses observed during exercise, which have been observed in individuals with paraplegia having middle thoracic (T5) cord injuries.[87] These HR responses exceed resting and exercise levels of those with high-level paraplegia and healthy persons without SCI.[84,88] Hypersensitivity of the supralesional spinal cord is believed to regulate this atypical adrenergic state and dynamic, which contrasts the downregulation of adrenergic functions observed in persons with high thoracic and cervical cord lesions.[88] The exaggerated HR response to endurance exercise in persons with paraplegia[87] may limit their ability to achieve high work intensities, as these persons consume higher levels of oxygen to perform at the same work intensity as persons without SCI.[56,84,89] As the sympathetic nervous system regulates hemodynamic and metabolic changes during activity, the elevated oxygen consumption and HR response to endurance exercise in individuals with injuries below T5 may be due to adrenergic overactivity accompanying their paraplegia.[87,88]

Exercise Conditioning Programs

Despite experiencing physical and homeostatic limitations, many persons with SCI can still undertake and benefit from exercise reconditioning. Those who retain upper extremity function have the opportunity to participate in a wide variety of exercise activities and sports[90,91] and ambulate with the assistance of orthoses and with surface or implanted electrical neuroprostheses (Fig. 16-1).[92–95] Individuals with upper motor neuron lesions have pedaled ergometers using surface electrical stimulation of selected lower extremity muscle groups delivered under computer control.[96,97] Furthermore, many body organs and tissues respond to exercise despite dissociation of their control from central command, and because many survivors of SCI experience complete sensory loss or significantly diminished nociceptive responses, electrically stimulated muscle contractions can often be used without pain.

Arm Endurance Training

In most cases, SCI leaves the lower limbs either entirely paralyzed or with insufficient strength, endurance, or

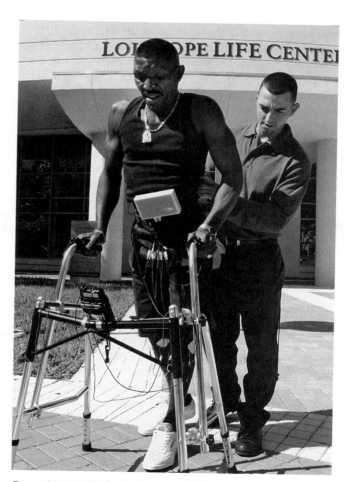

Figure 16-1. An individual with paraplegia using an ambulation neuroprosthesis with surface electrical stimulation (Parastep system) triggered via buttons on the walker.

motor control to support safe and effective physical training. It is for this reason that most exercise training after SCI employs the upper extremity exercise modes of arm crank ergometry, wheelchair ergometry, and swimming. All of these training modes improve physical conditioning in those with SCI by an average of 15% to 25%,[89,98–103] with a magnitude of fitness improvement usually inversely proportional to level of spinal lesion. While persons with low levels of tetraplegia can train on an arm ergometer, special measures must be taken to affix the hands to the equipment. Also, their gains in peak oxygen uptake fail to approach those of counterparts with paraplegia.[104] Thus, level of injury is a key to predicting benefits obtained from endurance training.[105,106]

Resistance Training After SCI

Prevalent upper extremity weakness and pain after SCI justifies a need for increased strength of the shoulders, upper back, chest, and arms. Surprisingly, however, far less is known about resistance than endurance training for persons with SCI. In a study of Scandinavian men (most having incomplete low thoracic lesions), a weight training program emphasizing triceps strengthening needed for crutch walking yielded modest but significant increases in peak exercise capacity accompanied by increased strength of the triceps brachii.[107] Others[108] have examined effects of arm cycle ergometry in subjects assigned to 70% or 40% of their peak work capacity. Strength gains were limited to subjects assigned to high-intensity training and occurred only in the shoulder extensor and elbow flexor muscles. Otherwise, no changes in shoulder abductor or adductor muscle strengths were reported, and none of the muscles that move or stabilize the scapulothoracic articulation or chest were stronger after training. These results suggest that arm crank cycle exercise is a poor choice for use as a training mode for upper extremity strengthening because it fails to target the muscles most involved in performance of daily activities. Similar limitations in strengthening were reported after conditioning of five persons with paraplegia and five with tetraplegia who trained three times weekly for 9 weeks using a hydraulic fitness machine. Exercises performed were chest press, rowing, shoulder press, and latissimus pull.[109] Significant increases in upper extremity work and power output were observed, although direct measurement of strength in muscle groups undergoing training was not performed. A recent study observed reduced shoulder pain following a series of shoulder resistance exercises using elastic bands.[110]

Circuit Resistance Training

As both endurance and resistance exercises benefit those without SCI, the effects of circuit resistance training (CRT)[111] on various attributes of fitness, dyslipidemia, and shoulder pain have been studied in young and middle-aged subjects with paraplegia. The exercise program incorporated periods of low-intensity fast-paced movements interposed within activities performed at a series of resistance training stations (see Fig. 16-2). The CRT exercise program adapted for individuals with paraplegia consisted of three circuits of six resistance stations encompassing three pairs of agonist/antagonist movements (e.g., overhead press and pull) and three 2-minute periods of free-wheeling arm cranking performed between resistance maneuvers. No true rest periods were allowed during the performance of CRT, with active recovery limited to the time necessary for the individual to propel the wheelchair to the next exercise station. Three weekly sessions were completed, with each session lasting approximately 45 minutes. Participants undergoing 16 weeks of mixed resistance and endurance exercise increased their upper extremity oxygen consumption by 29%, with accompanying upper extremity strength gains of 13% to 40%, depending on the site tested.[112] Subjects undergoing CRT also lowered their total and low-density lipoprotein cholesterol while increasing their HDL-C by nearly 10%.[12] Subjects over the age of 40 years undergoing the same treatment for 12 weeks experienced significant gains in endurance, strength, and anaerobic power, even though training did not specifically target the latter (M.S. Nash, unpublished data). Shoulder pain reported in these subjects before training was significantly reduced and was eliminated in 4 of 10 individuals. This circuit has been replicated using elastic bands[113] so that access to expensive weight-lifting equipment would not impose a limitation to participation in training. Evidence thus supports health and fitness advantages of CRT over either endurance or resistance exercises alone for persons with paraplegia.

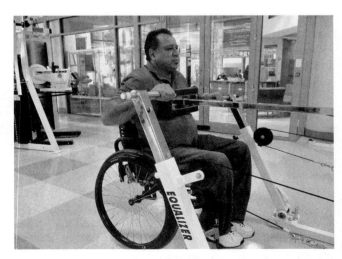

Figure 16-2. Resistance exercise performed by a person with paraplegia. The horizontal row strengthens muscles that stabilize the shoulder girdle. The bolster positioned on the chest stabilizes the body during lifting.

Limitations and Risks of Exercise After SCI

Special precautions are typically recommended when persons with SCI undertake exercise programs for physical conditioning. While usual risks of exercise injury and overuse apply, the consequences of imprudent exercise may be far more serious, potentially irreversible, and will likely compromise daily activities to a far greater extent than similar injuries arising in persons without SCI. A summary of these potential hazards is shown in Table 16-1.

Table 16-1

Risks of Exercise When Undertaken by Persons With SCI: Possible Causes and Possible Prevention

Risk	Probable Cause	Possible Prevention
Fracture	More than 50% of sublesional bone is lost within the first 6 months after injury. Sublesional bone remains permanently rarefied and susceptible to fracture, even with trivial injury.	No systematic evaluation for fracture susceptibility has been developed. Care should be exercised in wheelchair seating. Attention should be paid to severe chronic muscle spasm or those with exacerbation of tone from urinary tract infection or other causes.
Musculoskeletal overuse/injury	Musculoskeletal overuse may be undetectable in areas where sensation of pain is diminished. For the upper extremities, bearing excessive weight for prolonged periods (such as during locomotion)	The lower extremities should be monitored for cardinal signs of injury. Heightened spasticity may cue injury, even in the absence of swelling, pain warmth, or erythema. Adequate range of motion of the upper extremities, strength, and balance must be achieved and maintained. Individuals using the upper extremities for sports must be skilled in the mechanics of ballistic wheelchair locomotion. Use a wheelchair and appropriate cushion that will minimize injury.
Thermal dysregulation	Loss of vasomotor and sudomotor responses below the level of injury. Altered blood flow redistribution during exercise. Absence of sweating reflex below level of injury.	Exercise in intemperate environment should be avoided. Attention should be given to hydration, clothing, and signs and symptoms of heat stress.
Autonomic dysreflexia	Loss of central autonomic control results in reflex adrenergic responses to noxious stimuli.	Bowel routine and bladder emptying should be performed on schedule. External catheters should be inspected for outflow obstruction. Exercise should be avoided when autonomic episodes are increasing. Boosting of exercise responses using intentional urinary outflow obstruction must be discouraged.
Skin burn	Use of poorly hydrated or gelled conducting electrodes. Use of galvanic current for long duration or intense stimulation increases risk of burn.	Replace electrodes regularly and inspect for bubbles or drying at the edges.

Continued

Table 16-1

Risks of Exercise When Undertaken by Persons With SCI: Possible Causes and Possible Prevention—cont'd

Risk	Probable Cause	Possible Prevention
Pressor decompensation during and after exercise	Loss of sympathetic reflex responses to exercise or post-exercise pooling of blood in the lower extremities.	Careful prevention of orthostatic decompensation through conservative exercise progression and hydration. Active cool down after exercise to support venous return. Anticipation of the need to recline subjects to prevent syncope.

Adrenergic Dysregulation After SCI

Limitations in physical function after SCI are typically explained by profound sensorimotor deficits accompanying cord damage, although tracts of the sympathetic nervous system also descend in the spinal cord within the intermediolateral columns and exit with motor nerves in the thoracolumbar segments. This makes these nerve tracts equally susceptible to damage and the targets they control highly vulnerable to dysregulation after injury. As sympathetic autonomic tracts exit the cord at T1–L2 spinal levels, individuals with complete cervical level injuries often lose all central command over sympathetic nervous system functions, while loss of autonomic outflow to the adrenals and their sympathomedullary cell targets is also observed in persons with paraplegia above the T6 spinal level.

Autonomic dysfunction that results from injury above the thoracolumbar levels of sympathetic nerve outflow is associated with cardiac and circulatory dysfunction,[48,49] clotting disorders,[58] altered insulin metabolism,[15] resting and exercise immunodysfunction,[12,114] orthostatic incompetence,[115] osteoporosis and joint deterioration,[116] and thermal dysregulation at rest and during exercise.[117,118] A blunted HR response to exercise in persons with tetraplegia is well documented and usually yields peak HR in the mid-120 beats per minute range—similar in magnitude to persons without SCI who exercise under conditions of pharmacological beta-adrenergic blockade.[49] Absence of exercise, or limited catecholamine responses to it,[88] explains attenuated HR responses as well as the widely variable pressor, fuel, peripheral circulatory, thermal, and work capacity responses after SCI. When compared with individuals exercising after sustaining paraplegia, the combination of diminished muscle mass and adrenergic dysfunction experienced by individuals with tetraplegia roughly halves their peak exercise capacity.[65,100] For those with paraplegia from T2 to T5 (or T6), sparing of sympathetic efferents to the heart with resulting noradrenergic-mediated cardiac acceleration will be observed. A more typical exercise response is observed in persons having

injuries below the T6 level,[119] as central inhibitory control of the adrenal glands (innervated from T6 to T9) is maintained below these levels.[87]

Perhaps the most worrisome of adverse responses to exercise involves potentially life-threatening episodes of autonomic dysreflexia (hyperreflexia) in persons having injuries above the T6 spinal level.[120] The neurological basis for these episodes involves loss of supralesional sympathetic inhibition after injury, which normally suppresses the unrestricted autonomic reflex in persons having an intact neuraxis. The most common stimuli evoking autonomic dysreflexia are bladder and bowel distention before they are emptied. Other stimuli include venous thromboembolism, bone fracture, sudden temperature change, febrile episodes, and exercise. The disposition to autonomic dysreflexia during exercise is especially heightened when electrical current is used to generate muscle movement, or when exercising while febrile, or during bladder emptying. Episodes of autonomic dysreflexia are characterized by hypertension and bradycardia, supralesional erythema, piloerection, and headache.[121] In some cases, hypertension can rise to the point where crisis headache results and cerebral hemorrhage and death ensue. Recognition of these episodes, withdrawal of the offending stimulus, and the possible administration of a fast-acting peripheral vasodilator may be critical in preventing serious medical complications. It is known that wheelchair racers have intentionally induced dysreflexia as an ergogenic aid by restricting urine outflow through a Foley catheter.[122] Such so-called boosting of performance represents a dangerous and potentially life-threatening practice.

Fracture Precautions for Persons With SCI

Post-injury osteopenia is a common concern after SCI and may result in bone fracture following nominal skeletal stress or trauma.[70,123–126] The magnitude of the clinical problem posed by osteopenia and fracture is best revealed by the many attempts to increase sublesional bone mineral density (BMD) using physical activity,[127–130] weight bearing,[131,132] physical agents,[133,134] and drugs.[135,136] Despite best attempts to slow bone loss and reduce fracture after SCI, none of these methods has been shown sufficiently effective to justify widespread use in clinical practice.

Considerable sublesional bone demineralization is expected in the first year after SCI,[124,137–139] after which bone density levels continue to slowly decay. Bone loss is likely the result of physical, endocrine, and nervous system changes accompanying injury.[64] Contributing factors may include depression of serum growth hormone and insulin-like growth factor 1 accompanying SCI,[140] as well as low levels of serum testosterone[140] and a suppressed parathyroid hormone (PTH)–vitamin D axis, resulting in lowered PTH, 1,25-dihydroxyvitamin D, and nephrogenous cyclic adenosine monophosphate levels.[141–143] Nutritional deficiencies of vitamin D, deprivation of sunlight, or vitamin D loss from medication effects on accelerated hepatic vitamin D metabolism may contribute to widespread osteopenia after SCI.[144]

Notwithstanding the known causes for osteopenia, early urinary excretion of calcium and hydroxyproline and progressive rarefying of sublesional bone on radiographs are clearly evident after SCI.[145–147] During the initial period after SCI, markers of bone formation remain in the reference range, although at 10 to 16 weeks post-injury, resorption is elevated to 10 times the typical level.[148] During these times, decreased osteoblastic activity is associated with a rapid increase in bone resorption.[149,150] While bone of most persons with SCI remains innervated,[151] the differentiation of bone marrow osteoprogenitor cells becomes impaired.[152] Thus, about one-third to one-half of BMD is lost by 1 year after injury, with primary losses occurring in the supracondylar femur and proximal tibia.[70,107,123,124,137] During this time, bone becomes underhydroxylated and hypocalcific,[149,150,153] with permanently heightened susceptibility to fracture, even with trivial or imperceptible trauma.[154–156] Joints suffer similar deterioration and heightened injury susceptibility brought on by cartilage atrophy and joint space deformities.

Musculoskeletal Injury

Persons with SCI risk bone fracture and joint dislocation of the lower extremities and serious injury to the upper extremities. Bone fracture and joint dislocation may be caused by asynergistic movement of spastic limbs against co-contractive forces imposed by electrical stimulation of paralyzed muscles or by inertia developed by devices used for exercise.[157] These risks explain why exercise involving electrically stimulated muscle activity is contraindicated for individuals having severe spasticity when at rest or uncontrolled spastic responses when electrical current is used.

Precautions to prevent overuse injuries of the arms and shoulders are essential for those participating in upper extremity exercise.[110,158,159] As the shoulder joints are mechanically ill-suited to perform locomotor activities,

but must do so in individuals using a manual wheelchair for transportation, these injuries may ultimately compromise performance of essential daily activities, including wheelchair propulsion, weight relief, and depression transfers.[160,161]

Thermal Dysregulation

Loss of sublesional vasomotor and sudomotor control after SCI poses a special challenge to temperature regulation during exercise and often results in hyperthermia.[80,117,162–164] Hyperthermia is more pronounced in persons with higher level injuries[165,166] and when exercising in a hot, humid environment.[163,167] Thus, attention should be paid to clothing, hydration, and limiting the duration and intensity of activities performed in intemperate environments.

Pain as a Common Problem After SCI

Both nociceptive and neuropathic pain are highly prevalent after SCI. Upper limb pain is the most common symptom of physical dysfunction reported by those with SCI,[73,168,169] and the shoulder the most common site for pain.[170,171] It is also the location for commonly experienced rotator cuff dysfunction, tears, and impingement.[72,158] A large segment of the paralyzed population lives with pain in the shoulders, arms, and wrists, with complaints reported in 35%[172] to 73%[169] of persons with chronic paraplegia. These figures cause special concern because onset of pain occurs earlier than observed in persons without disability and because pain from muscle and joint overuse worsens with passing time and advancing age.[168] Upper limb pain must be prevented if function is to be enhanced by exercise and incipient disability avoided.

While a single cause for shoulder pain has not been identified, many studies attribute pain to deterioration and injury resulting from insufficient shoulder strength, range, and muscle endurance.[110,158,171,173–175] Pain that accompanies wheelchair locomotion and other wheelchair activities interferes with functional performance, including upper extremity weight bearing for transfers, high-resistance muscular activity in extremes of limb range, wheelchair propulsion up inclines, and frequent overhead activity.[171,176,177] Wheelchair propulsion and transfers requiring shoulder girdle depression cause the most pain and increase the intensity of existing pain more than other daily activities.[103] As many as half of persons with SCI experience significant shoulder pain intensified by wheelchair propulsion and body transfers,[176] which represent activities critical to activity and health maintenance. The severity of upper limb pain increases during common transfer activities and increases as time following injury lengthens,[168] although exercises focusing on the posterior shoulder and upper back appear to lessen the pain.[110]

Persons with paraplegia must depend on their upper extremities for transportation, body transfers, and other activities. Thus, the consequences and necessary treatments for shoulder pain and injury ultimately dictate the degree of their independence. While some report that surgical repair of the shoulder results in full recovery of musculoskeletal function and remedy of pain,[178] others report not.[170] Regardless, upper extremity surgery would require special post-operative and rehabilitative convalescent strategies and deny personal independence in performing many essential daily functions. These factors make injury prevention an essential part in planning for exercise by those with SCI.

CASE STUDY 16-1   Circuit Resistance Training for Treating CVD Risks Clustering as Metabolic Syndrome

Daniel is a 51-year-old, nonsmoking man, who was in excellent health until 1983, when he was involved in a motor vehicle accident and sustained T5 motor complete (AIS A) paraplegia. His pre-morbid history was unremarkable. After injury, he underwent a posterior decompressive laminectomy with bone fusion and then a 5-month in-patient rehabilitation program. He was then discharged home. His post-injury course has been complicated by significant weight gain from a pre-injury weight of 140 pounds to a current 192 pounds and by a diagnosis of type 2 diabetes. Waist circumference is 44 inches, and body mass index is 29.6. Resting blood pressure is 144/92. To control his diabetes, Daniel takes 500 mg of Metformin nightly. A fasting blood sample was obtained and analyzed as follows:

Fasting blood glucose: 165 mg/dL
Total cholesterol (TC): 190 mg/dL
Triglycerides: 150 mg/dL
Low-density lipoprotein cholesterol (LDL-C): 130 mg/dL
HDL-C: 32 mg/dL
TC/HDL-C ratio: 5.9
Risk assessment (death or myocardial infarction): 14%

Case Analysis

The fasting blood glucose above 110 mg/dL confirms the diagnosis of diabetes by all authoritative guidelines. Lipid levels reflect the common profile of isolated low HDL. While the TC below 200 mg/dL is in the low risk range, the interplay of TC and HDL-C has a computed value above the high risk criterion of 4.5. The risk assessment tool uses recent data from the PROCAM Study to estimate a 10-year risk for "hard" coronary heart disease outcomes (myocardial infarction and coronary death). Unlike the Framingham Risk calculator, the PROCAM is appropriate for use by persons with diabetes. Age-appropriate and gender-specific risk for Daniel should be in the 4% to 6% range. Presence of truncal obesity, hypertension, borderline elevated triglycerides, and depressed HDL-C provides more than the three risk factors needed to confirm a diagnosis of metabolic syndrome.

Key Concerns

1. Daniel states that he is not feeling well and knows that he is badly out of shape.
2. He states that he is concerned about the increasing difficulty in the performance of his daily activities. He acknowledges that his body mass and physical deconditioning are contributing to these problems.
3. He states that he is concerned that his worsening cardiovascular health will contribute to early heart disease and that either his disease or the cost of medication will become a future burden upon his daughter.

Treatment Plan

Daniel underwent a 16-week program of resistance and endurance activities conducted three times weekly. Resistance settings were set to 50% of one-repetition maximum (1-RM) measured at the start of training and were escalated to 55% and 60% of 1-RM by the fourth week of each month. At this point, the strength was retested and the new 1-RM value used to anchor resistance settings for the next month. Daniel noted improvements in upper body strength and an easing in the difficulty of daily activities. These activities were no longer an impediment to wheelchair locomotion while propelling his wheelchair up inclines and pulling himself up into his van. In the eighth week of conditioning, Daniel complained of post-exercise lightheadedness and was referred to his physician for examination. Fasting blood glucose showed a reduction from preconditioning levels to 145 mg/dL, which caused his physician to halve his Metformin dosage to remedy post-exercise hypoglycemia. Body mass was unchanged by the eighth training week, although changes in body appearance emphasized an increase in lean mass and a reduction in body fat. An additional 8 weeks of training resulted in loss of 16 pounds in body mass and reoccurrence of the post-exercise hypoglycemia. At this point, his fasting blood glucose was 122 mg/dL and the Metformin was discontinued. Daniel reported that daily activities were easy and he could now pull himself in and out of his swimming pool without assistance from his daughter. This permitted him greater latitude in recreation with his children and the use of swimming as an endurance activity for fat loss without fear of being trapped in his swimming pool without assistance. A home program of resistance conditioning was continued twice weekly using elastic bands and a peg board Daniel mounted to a bedroom door. After 16 weeks, his waist circumference was 39 inches. A fasting blood sample was repeated and analyzed as follows:

Fasting blood glucose: 112 mg/dL
TC: 170 mg/dL
Triglycerides: 136 mg/dL
LDL-C: 120 mg/dL
HDL-C: 46 mg/dL
TC/HDL-C ratio: 3.7
Risk assessment (death or myocardial infarction): 6%

CASE STUDY 16-1   Circuit Resistance Training for Treating CVD Risks Clustering as Metabolic Syndrome—cont'd

Summary

This training program emphasizes some key benefits with people with SCI. While endurance activity alone has been shown to improve levels of cardiovascular fitness, these activities are limited in their ability to significantly improve strength and anaerobic power. While body weight is generally not lost early in the training program, the shift in body composition toward increased lean mass and decreased fat mass may offset each other so that the total weight is not changed. Continued training generally results in a reduction in body fat, which is a desirable training outcome and will further ease the performance of key daily activities such as transfers and weight shifts. Loss of body fat may also decrease strain on the upper limbs, thus reducing discomfort in the shoulder joint and girdle. Attention should be paid to post-exercise hypoglycemia within 4 to 8 weeks of training. Exercise conditioning improves insulin sensitivity

rather rapidly and can result in post-exercise hypoglycemia. For individuals who monitor their blood glucose with a glucometer, the adequacy of pre-exercise blood sugar and the observation of low post-exercise blood sugar can be a cue for referral to a physician and reduction of glucose-lowering medications. In this instance, the reduction was sufficient to warrant termination of pharmacological treatment with a glucose-lowering agent. All lipids and lipoproteins are now in reference range, and there has been a significant reduction in CVD risk of death and myocardial infarction. Reduction of waist girth, fasting triglycerides, and systolic blood pressure, coupled with elevation of HDL-C above 40 mg/dL, reduced the risk of metabolic syndrome. A home program of recreational swimming and twice-weekly resistance exercise was sufficient to maintain the conditioning benefits 1 year after the start of the conditioning program.

Summary

Many persons with SCI already benefit from a lifestyle that incorporates habitual physical activity. Despite special needs, equipment, qualifications, and risks, evidence collected across the spectrum of available training modes supports the ability of exercise to reduce multisystem disease in persons with SCI. Evidence further suggests that habitual exercise reduces fatigue, pain, weakness, musculoskeletal decline, and incipient neurological deficits that accompany aging with disability. Because these deficits challenge the ability of those with SCI to perform essential daily activities first mastered after injury, their prevention likely fosters fullest health and life satisfaction when aging with a disability. Thus, health-care professionals should encourage persons with SCI to adopt or continue their use of therapeutic or recreational exercise as a health-enhancing strategy after SCI. Risks of injury associated with imprudent exercise must be managed to ensure that physical activity and daily activities can be sustained without interruption. If carefully prescribed, exercise has the demonstrated ability to enhance the activity, life satisfaction, and health of those with disability from SCI.

REVIEW QUESTIONS

1. What are the major causes underlying accelerated CVD in persons with SCI?
2. What are the co-morbid states and conditions that worsen the CVD risk prognosis for persons with SCI?
3. What is the lipid profile that predisposes persons with SCI to premature CVD?
4. What are the key components of exercise prescription for individuals with SCI, and what are the guidelines used to prescribe safe, effective exercise programs?
5. Compare and contrast benefits of endurance and resistance training programs for persons with SCI.
6. What are the unique limitations and risks for exercise after SCI, and what precautions can be adopted to remedy them?

REFERENCES

1. DeVivo MJ, Black KJ, Stover SL. Causes of death during the first 12 years after spinal cord injury. *Arch Phys Med Rehabil.* 1993;74:248–254.
2. Gerhart KA, Bergstrom E, Charlifue SW et al. Long-term spinal cord injury: Functional changes over time. *Arch Phys Med Rehabil.* 1993;74:1030–1034.
3. Le CT. Survival from spinal cord injury. *J Chron Dis.* 1982;35:487–492.
4. Whiteneck GG, Charlifue SW, Frankel HL et al. Mortality, morbidity, and psychosocial outcomes of persons spinal cord injured more than 20 years ago. *Paraplegia.* 1992;30:617–630.
5. Bauman WA, Kahn NN, Grimm DR et al. Risk factors for atherogenesis and cardiovascular autonomic function in persons with spinal cord injury. *Spinal Cord.* 1999;37:601–616.
6. Bauman WA, Spungen AM, Adkins RH et al. Metabolic and endocrine changes in persons aging with spinal cord injury. *Assist Technol.* 1999;11:88–96.
7. Bauman WA, Spungen AM, Raza M et al. Coronary artery disease: Metabolic risk factors and latent disease in individuals with paraplegia. *Mt Sinai J Med.* 1992;59:163–168.
8. Bauman WA, Raza M, Spungen AM et al. Cardiac stress testing with thallium-201 imaging reveals silent ischemia in

individuals with paraplegia. *Arch Phys Med Rehabil.* 1994;75:946–950.

9. Bauman WA, Raza M, Spungen AM et al. Cardiac stress testing with thallium-201 imaging reveals silent ischemia in individuals with paraplegia. *Arch Phys Med Rehabil.* 1994;75:946–950.

10. Bauman WA, Spungen AM, Flanagan S et al. Blunted growth hormone response to intravenous arginine in subjects with a spinal cord injury. *Horm Metab Res.* 1994;26:152–156.

11. Groah SL, Menter RR. Long-term cardiac ischemia leading to coronary artery bypass grafting in a tetraplegic patient. *Arch Phys Med Rehabil.* 1998;79:1129–1132.

12. Nash MS, Jacobs PL, Mendez AJ et al. Circuit resistance training improves the atherogenic lipid profiles of persons with chronic paraplegia. *J Spinal Cord Med.* 2001;24:2–9.

13. Bauman WA, Spungen AM. Disorders of carbohydrate and lipid metabolism in veterans with paraplegia or quadriplegia: A model of premature aging. *Metabolism.* 1994;43:749–756.

14. Karlsson AK. Insulin resistance and sympathetic function in high spinal cord injury. *Spinal Cord.* 1999;37:494–500.

15. Karlsson AK, Attvall S, Jansson PA et al. Influence of the sympathetic nervous system on insulin sensitivity and adipose tissue metabolism: A study in spinal cord-injured subjects. *Metabolism.* 1995;44:52–58.

16. Maki KC, Briones ER, Langbein WE et al. Associations between serum lipids and indicators of adiposity in men with spinal cord injury. *Paraplegia.* 1995;33:102–109.

17. Zlotolow SP, Levy E, Bauman WA. The serum lipoprotein profile in veterans with paraplegia: The relationship to nutritional factors and body mass index. *J Am Paraplegia Soc.* 1992;15:158–162.

18. Alberti KG, Zimmet PZ. Definition, diagnosis and classification of diabetes mellitus and its complications. Part 1. Diagnosis and classification of diabetes mellitus provisional report of a WHO consultation. *Diabetic Med.* 1998;15: 539–553.

19. Bauman WA, Adkins RH, Spungen AM et al. Is immobilization associated with an abnormal lipoprotein profile? Observations from a diverse cohort. *Spinal Cord.* 1999;37: 485–493.

20. Report of the Second Task Force on Blood Pressure Control in Children—1987. Task Force on Blood Pressure Control in Children. National Heart, Lung, and Blood Institute, Bethesda, Maryland. *Pediatrics.* 1987;79:1–25.

21. Chobanian AV, Bakris GL, Black HR et al. Seventh report of the Joint National Committee on Prevention, Detection, Evaluation, and Treatment of High Blood Pressure. *Hypertension.* 2003;42:1206–1252.

22. Goran MI, Gower BA. Longitudinal study on pubertal insulin resistance. *Diabetes.* 2001;50:2444–2450.

23. Hickman TB, Briefel RR, Carroll MD et al. Distributions and trends of serum lipid levels among United States children and adolescents ages 4–19 years: Data from the Third National Health and Nutrition Examination Survey. *Prev Med.* 1998;27:879–890.

24. Washburn RA, Figoni SF. High density lipoprotein cholesterol in individuals with spinal cord injury: The potential role of physical activity. *Spinal Cord.* 1999;37:685–695.

25. Zhong YG, Levy E, Bauman WA. The relationships among serum uric acid, plasma insulin, and serum lipoprotein levels in subjects with spinal cord injury. *Horm Metab Res.* 1995;27:283–286.

26. Grundy SM. Atherogenic dyslipidemia: Lipoprotein abnormalities and implications for therapy. *Am J Cardiol.* 1995;75:45B–52B.

27. Noreau L, Shephard RJ. Spinal cord injury, exercise and quality of life. *Sports Med.* 1995;20:226–250.

28. Washburn RA, Figoni SF. Physical activity and chronic cardiovascular disease prevention in spinal cord injury: A comprehensive literature review. *Top Spinal Cord Injury Rehabil.* 1998;3:16–32.

29. Jones LM, Goulding A, Gerrard DF. DEXA: A practical and accurate tool to demonstrate total and regional bone loss, lean tissue loss, and fat mass gain in paraplegia. *Spinal Cord.* 1998;36:637–640.

30. Spungen AM, Bauman WA, Wang J, Pierson RN Jr. Measurement of body fat in individuals with tetraplegia: A comparison of eight clinical methods. *Paraplegia.* 1995;33: 402–408.

31. Cerneca F, Crocetti G, Gombacci A et al. Variations in hemostatic parameters after near-maximum exercise and specific tests in athletes. *J Sports Med Phys Fitness.* 1999;39:31–36.

32. Duckworth WC, Solomon SS, Jallepalli P et al. Glucose intolerance due to insulin resistance in patients with spinal cord injuries. *Diabetes.* 1980;29:906–910.

33. Kuhne S, Hammon HM, Bruckmaier RM et al. Growth performance, metabolic and endocrine traits, and absorptive capacity in neonatal calves fed either colostrum or milk replacer at two levels. *J Anim Sci.* 2000;78: 609–620.

34. Ohry A, Shemesh Y, Rozin R. Are chronic spinal cord injured patients (SCIP) prone to premature aging? *Med Hypotheses.* 1983;11:467–469.

35. Ragnarsson KT. The Cardiovascular System. In: Whiteneck G, editor. *Aging with Spinal Cord Injury.* New York: Demos Medical Publishing; 1993:73–92.

36. Third Report of the National Cholesterol Education Program (NCEP) Expert Panel on Detection, Evaluation, and Treatment of High Blood Cholesterol in Adults (Adult Treatment Panel III) final report. *Circulation.* 2002;106: 3143–3421.

37. Grundy SM, Pasternak R, Greenland P et al. Assessment of cardiovascular risk by use of multiple-risk-factor assessment equations: A statement for healthcare professionals from the American Heart Association and the American College of Cardiology. *Circulation.* 1999;100: 1481–1492.

38. Rocker L, Gunay S, Gunga HC et al. Activation of blood platelets in response to maximal isometric exercise of the dominant arm. *Int J Sports Med.* 2000;21:191–194.

39. Burstein R, Zeilig G, Royburt M et al. Insulin resistance in paraplegics—Effect of one bout of acute exercise. *Int J Sports Med.* 1996;17:272–276.

40. Cominacini L, Zocca I, Garbin U et al. High-density lipoprotein composition in obesity: Interrelationships with plasma insulin levels and body weight. *Int J Obesity.* 1988;12:343–352.

41. Hashimoto R, Adachi H, Tsuruta M et al. Association of hyperinsulinemia and serum free fatty acids with serum high density lipoprotein-cholesterol. *J Atheroscler Thromb.* 1995;2:53–59.

42. Jeppesen J, Facchini FS, Reaven GM. Individuals with high total cholesterol/HDL cholesterol ratios are insulin resistant. *J Intern Med.* 1998;243:293–298.

43. Nash MS. Exercise reconditioning of the heart and peripheral circulation after spinal cord injury. *Top Spinal Cord Inj Rehabil.* 1997;3:1–15.

44. King ML, Lichtman SW, Pellicone JT, et al. Exertional hypotension in spinal cord injury. *Chest.* 1994;106:1166–1171.

45. Figoni SF. Cardiovascular and haemodynamic responses to tilting and to standing in tetraplegic patients: A review. *Paraplegia.* 1984;22:99–109.

46. Figoni SF. Perspectives on cardiovascular fitness and SCI. *J Am Paraplegia Soc.* 1990;13:63–71.

47. Lopes P, Figoni SF, Perkash I. Upper limb exercise effect on tilt tolerance during orthostatic training of patients with spinal cord injury. *Arch Phys Med Rehabil.* 1984;65:251–253.

48. Kessler KM, Pina I, Green B et al. Cardiovascular findings in quadriplegic and paraplegic patients and in normal subjects. *Am J Cardiol.* 1986;58:525–530.

49. Nash MS, Bilsker MS, Kearney HM et al. Effects of electrically-stimulated exercise and passive motion on echocardiographically-derived wall motion and cardiodynamic function in tetraplegic persons. *Paraplegia.* 1995;33:80–89.

50. Davis GM. Exercise capacity of individuals with paraplegia. *Med Sci Sports Exerc.* 1993;25:423–432.

51. Nash MS, Bilsker S, Marcillo AE et al. Reversal of adaptive left ventricular atrophy following electrically-stimulated exercise training in human tetraplegics. *Paraplegia.* 1991;29:590–599.

52. Hopman MT. Circulatory responses during arm exercise in individuals with paraplegia. *Int J Sports Med.* 1994;15:126–131.

53. Hopman MT, van Asten WN, Oeseburg B. Changes in blood flow in the common femoral artery related to inactivity and muscle atrophy in individuals with long-standing paraplegia. *Adv Exp Med Biol.* 1996;388:379–383.

54. Nash MS, Montalvo BM, Applegate B. Lower extremity blood flow and responses to occlusion ischemia differ in exercise-trained and sedentary tetraplegic persons. *Arch Phys Med Rehabil.* 1996;77:1260–1265.

55. Taylor PN, Ewins DJ, Fox B et al. Limb blood flow, cardiac output, and quadriceps muscle bulk following spinal cord injury and the effect of training for the Odstock functional electrical stimulation standing system. *Paraplegia.* 1993;31:303–310.

56. Davis GM, Shephard RJ. Cardiorespiratory fitness in highly active versus inactive paraplegics. *Med Sci Sports Exerc.* 1988;20:463–468.

57. Hjeltnes N. Oxygen uptake and cardiac output in graded arm exercise in paraplegics with low level spinal lesions. *Scand J Rehabil Med.* 1977;9:107–113.

58. Green D, Hull RD, Mammen EF et al. Deep vein thrombosis in spinal cord injury. Summary and recommendations. *Chest.* 1992;102:633S–635S.

59. Jacobs PL, Mahoney ET, Robbins A et al. Hypokinetic circulation in persons with paraplegia. *Med Sci Sports Exerc.* 2002;34:1401–1407.

60. Winther K, Gleerup G, Snorrason K et al. Platelet function and fibrinolytic activity in cervical spinal cord injured patients. *Thromb Res.* 1992;65:469–474.

61. Dearwater SR, LaPorte RE, Robertson RJ et al. Activity in the spinal cord-injured patient: An epidemiologic analysis of metabolic parameters. *Med Sci Sports Exerc.* 1986;18:541–544.

62. Noreau L, Shephard RJ, Simard C et al. Relationship of impairment and functional ability to habitual activity and fitness following spinal cord injury. *Int J Rehabil Res.* 1993;16:265–275.

63. Bostom AG, Toner MM, McArdle WD et al. Lipid and lipoprotein profiles relate to peak aerobic power in spinal cord injured men. *Med Sci Sports Exerc.* 1991;23:409–414.

64. Bauman WA, Spungen AM. Metabolic changes in persons after spinal cord injury. *Phys Med Rehabil Clin N Am.* 2000;11:109–140.

65. Phillips WT, Kiratli BJ, Sarkarati M et al. Effect of spinal cord injury on the heart and cardiovascular fitness. *Curr Prob Cardiol.* 1998;23:641–716.

66. Hopman MT, Monroe M, Dueck C et al. Blood redistribution and circulatory responses to submaximal arm exercise in persons with spinal cord injury. *Scand J Rehabil Med.* 1998;30:167–174.

67. Hawkey CM, Britton BJ, Wood WG et al. Changes in blood catecholamine levels and blood coagulation and fibrinolytic activity in response to graded exercise in man. *Br J Haematol.* 1975;29:377–384.

68. Rodriguez GP, Claus-Walker J, Kent MC et al. Collagen metabolite excretion as a predictor of bone- and skin-related complications in spinal cord injury. *Arch Phys Med Rehabil.* 1989;70:442–444.

69. Nash MS. Known and plausible modulators of depressed immune functions following spinal cord injuries. *J Spinal Cord Med.* 2000;23:111–120.

70. Segatore M. The skeleton after spinal cord injury. Part 2: Management of sublesional osteoporosis. *SCI Nurs.* 1995;12:115–120.

71. Galanis DJ, McGarvey ST, Sobal J et al. Relations of body fat and fat distribution to the serum lipid, apolipoprotein, and insulin concentrations of Samoan men and women. *Int J Obes Relat Metab Disord.* 1995;19:731–738.

72. Lal S. Premature degenerative shoulder changes in spinal cord injury patients. *Spinal Cord.* 1998;36:186–189.

73. Sie IH, Waters RL, Adkins RH et al. Upper extremity pain in the postrehabilitation spinal cord injured patient. *Arch Phys Med Rehabil.* 1992;73:44–48.

74. Widerstrom-Noga EG, Felipe-Cuervo E, Yezierski RP. Relationships among clinical characteristics of chronic pain after spinal cord injury. *Arch Phys Med Rehabil.* 2001;82:1191–1197.

75. Widerstrom-Noga EG, Turk DC. Types and effectiveness of treatments used by people with chronic pain associated with spinal cord injuries: Influence of pain and psychosocial characteristics. *Spinal Cord.* 2003;41:600–609.

76. Lewis JE, Nash MS, Hamm LF, Martins SC, Groah SL. The relationship between perceived exertion and physiological indicators during graded arm exercise in persons with spinal cord injuries. *Arch Phys Med Rehabil* 2007;88:1205–1211.

77. MacGregor J. The objective measurement of physical performance with long term ambulatory physiological surveillance equipment. In: Stott FD, Raftey EB and Goulding L, editors. *Proceedings of the Third International Symposium on Ambulatory Monitoring.*1979. pp. 29–39.

78. Hopman MT, Oeseburg B, Binkhorst RA. Cardiovascular responses in persons with paraplegia to prolonged arm

exercise and thermal stress. *Med Sci Sports Exerc.* 1993;25:577–583.

79. Hopman MT, Pistorius M, Kamerbeek IC et al. Cardiac output in paraplegic subjects at high exercise intensities. *Eur J Appl Physiol.* 1993;66:531–535.

80. Sawka MN, Latzka WA, Pandolf KB. Temperature regulation during upper body exercise: Able-bodied and spinal cord injured. *Med Sci Sports Exerc.* 1989;21:S132–S140.

81. Hjeltnes N. Cardiorespiratory capacity in tetra- and paraplegia shortly after injury. *Scand J Rehabil Med.* 1986;18:65–70.

82. Hooker SP, Greenwood JD, Hatae DT et al. Oxygen uptake and heart rate relationship in persons with spinal cord injury. *Med Sci Sports Exerc.* 1993;25:1115–1119.

83. Hopman MT, Kamerbeek IC, Pistorius M et al. The effect of an anti-G suit on the maximal performance of individuals with paraplegia. *Int J Sports Med.* 1993;14:357–361.

84. Hopman MT, Oeseburg B, Binkhorst RA. Cardiovascular responses in paraplegic subjects during arm exercise. *Eur J Appl Physiol.* 1992;65:73–78.

85. Van Loan MD, McCluer S, Loftin JM et al. Comparison of physiological responses to maximal arm exercise among able-bodied, paraplegics, and quadriplegics. *Paraplegia.* 1987;25:397–405.

86. Houtman S, Thielen JJ, Binkhorst RA et al. Effect of a pulsating anti-gravity suit on peak exercise performance in individual with spinal cord injuries. *Eur J Appl Physiol Occup Physiol.* 1999;79:202–204.

87. Bloomfield SA, Jackson RD, Mysiw WJ. Catecholamine response to exercise and training in individuals with spinal cord injury. *Med Sci Sports Exerc.* 1994;26:1213–1219.

88. Schmid A, Huonker M, Barturen JM et al. Catecholamines, heart rate, and oxygen uptake during exercise in persons with spinal cord injury. *J Appl Physiol.* 1998;85:635–641.

89. Hoffman MD. Cardiorespiratory fitness and training in quadriplegics and paraplegics. *Sports Med.* 1986;3:312–330.

90. Curtis KA, McClanahan S, Hall KM et al. Health, vocational, and functional status in spinal cord injured athletes and nonathletes. *Arch Phys Med Rehabil.* 1986;67:862–865.

91. Nash MS, Horton JA. Recreational and therapeutic exercise after SCI. In: Kirshbaum S, Campagnolo DI, DeLisa JS, editors. *Spinal Cord Injury Medicine.* Philadelphia: Lippincott, Williams, and Wilkins; 2002: pp. 331–337.

92. Davis R, Houdayer T, Andrews B et al. Paraplegia: Prolonged closed-loop standing with implanted nucleus FES-22 stimulator and Andrews' foot-ankle orthosis. *Stereotact Funct Neurosurg.* 1997;69:281–287.

93. Jacobs PL, Nash MS, Klose KJ et al. Evaluation of a training program for persons with SCI paraplegia using the Parastep 1 ambulation system: Part 2. Effects on physiological responses to peak arm ergometry. *Arch Phys Med Rehabil.* 1997;78:794–798.

94. Triolo RJ, Bieri C, Uhlir J et al. Implanted functional neuromuscular stimulation systems for individuals with cervical spinal cord injuries: Clinical case reports. *Arch Phys Med Rehabil.* 1996;77:1119–1128.

95. Klose KJ, Jacobs PL, Broton JG et al. Evaluation of a training program for persons with SCI paraplegia using the Parastep 1 ambulation system: Part 1. Ambulation performance and anthropometric measures. *Arch Phys Med Rehabil.* 1997;78:789–793.

96. Glaser RM. Functional neuromuscular stimulation. Exercise conditioning of spinal cord injured patients. *Int J Sports Med.* 1994;15:142–148.

97. Ragnarsson KT. Physiologic effects of functional electrical stimulation-induced exercises in spinal cord-injured individuals. *Clin Orthop.* 1988;53–63.

98. Cowell LL, Squires WG, Raven PB. Benefits of aerobic exercise for the paraplegic: A brief review. *Med Sci Sports Exerc.* 1986;18:501–508.

99. Davis GM, Kofsky PR, Kelsey JC et al. Cardiorespiratory fitness and muscular strength of wheelchair users. *Can Med Assoc J.* 1981;125:1317–1323.

100. Franklin BA. Exercise testing, training and arm ergometry. *Sports Med.* 1985;2:100–119.

101. Sairyo K, Katoh S, Sakai T et al. Characteristics of velocity-controlled knee movement in patients with cervical compression myelopathy: What is the optimal rehabilitation exercise for spastic gait? *Spine.* 2001;26:E535–E538.

102. Hooker SP, Wells CL. Effects of low- and moderate-intensity training in spinal cord-injured persons. *Med Sci Sports Exerc.* 1989;21:18–22.

103. Taylor AW, McDonell E, Brassard L. The effects of an arm ergometer training programme on wheelchair subjects. *Paraplegia.* 1986;24:105–114.

104. Yim SY, Cho KJ, Park CI et al. Effect of wheelchair ergometer training on spinal cord-injured paraplegics. *Yonsei Med J.* 1993;34:278–286.

105. DiCarlo SE. Effect of arm ergometry training on wheelchair propulsion endurance of individuals with quadriplegia. *Phys Ther.* 1988;68:40–44.

106. Drory Y, Ohry A, Brooks ME et al. Arm crank ergometry in chronic spinal cord injured patients. *Arch Phys Med Rehabil.* 1990;71:389–392.

107. Nilsson S, Staff PH, Pruett ED. Physical work capacity and the effect of training on subjects with long-standing paraplegia. *Scand J Rehabil Med.* 1975;7:51–56.

108. Davis GM, Shephard RJ. Strength training for wheelchair users. *Br J Sports Med.* 1990;24:25–30.

109. Cooney MM, Walker JB. Hydraulic resistance exercise benefits cardiovascular fitness of spinal cord injured. *Med Sci Sports Exerc.* 1986;18:522–525.

110. Curtis KA, Tyner TM, Zachary L et al. Effect of a standard exercise protocol on shoulder pain in long-term wheelchair users. *Spinal Cord.* 1999;37:421–429.

111. Gettman LR, Ayres JJ, Pollock ML et al. The effect of circuit weight training on strength, cardiorespiratory function, and body composition of adult men. *Med Sci Sports.* 1978;10:171–176.

112. Jacobs PL, Nash MS, Rusinowski JW. Circuit training provides cardiorespiratory and strength benefits in persons with paraplegia. *Med Sci Sports Exerc.* 2001;33: 711–717.

113. Nash MS, Jacobs PL, Woods JM et al. A comparison of 2 circuit exercise training techniques for eliciting matched metabolic responses in persons with paraplegia. *Arch Phys Med Rehabil.* 2002;83:201–209.

114. Campagnolo DI, Bartlett JA, Keller SE. Influence of neurological level on immune function following spinal cord injury: A review. *J Spinal Cord Med.* 2000;23:1 21–128.

115. King ML, Freeman DM, Pellicone JT et al. Exertional hypotension in thoracic spinal cord injury: Case report. *Paraplegia.* 1992;30:261–266.

116. Minaire P. Immobilization osteoporosis: A review. *Clin Rheumatol.* 1989;8 Suppl 2:95–103.

117. Gass GC, Camp EM, Nadel ER et al. Rectal and rectal vs. esophageal temperatures in paraplegic men during prolonged exercise. *J Appl Physiol.* 1988;64:2265–2271.

118. Hopman MT, Oeseburg B, Binkhorst RA. The effect of an anti-G suit on cardiovascular responses to exercise in persons with paraplegia. *Med Sci Sports Exerc.* 1992;24:984–990.

119. Gass GC, Camp EM. The maximum physiological responses during incremental wheelchair and arm cranking exercise in male paraplegics. *Med Sci Sports Exerc.* 1984;16:355–359.

120. Ashley EA, Laskin JJ, Olenik LM et al. Evidence of autonomic dysreflexia during functional electrical stimulation in individuals with spinal cord injuries. *Paraplegia.* 1993;31:593–605.

121. Donaldson N, Perkins TA, Fitzwater R et al. FES cycling may promote recovery of leg function after incomplete spinal cord injury. *Spinal Cord.* 2000;38:680–682.

122. Davis SE, Mulcahey MJ, Smith BT et al. Outcome of functional electrical stimulation in the rehabilitation of a child with C-5 tetraplegia. *J Spinal Cord Med.* 1999;22:107–113.

123. Garland DE, Adkins RH, Stewart CA et al. Regional osteoporosis in women who have a complete spinal cord injury. *J Bone Joint Surg-Am.* 2001;83-A:1195–1200.

124. Garland DE, Stewart CA, Adkins RH et al. Osteoporosis after spinal cord injury. *J Orthop Res.* 1992;10:371–378.

125. Hunt AH, Civitelli R, Halstead L. Evaluation of bone resorption: A common problem during impaired mobility. *SCI Nurs.* 1995;12:90–94.

126. Kiratli BJ, Smith AE, Nauenberg T et al. Bone mineral and geometric changes through the femur with immobilization due to spinal cord injury. *J Rehabil Res Dev.* 2000;37:225–233.

127. Bloomfield SA, Mysiw WJ, Jackson RD. Bone mass and endocrine adaptations to training in spinal cord injured individuals. *Bone.* 1996;19:61–68.

128. Hangartner TN, Rodgers MM, Glaser RM et al. Tibial bone density loss in spinal cord injured patients: Effects of FES exercise. *J Rehabil Res Dev.* 1994;31:50–61.

129. Mohr T, Podenphant J, Biering-Sorensen F et al. Increased bone mineral density after prolonged electrically induced cycle training of paralyzed limbs in spinal cord injured man. *Calcif Tissue Int.* 1997;61:22–25.

130. Leeds EM, Klose KJ, Ganz W et al. Bone mineral density after bicycle ergometry training. *Arch Phys Med Rehabil.* 1990;71:207–209.

131. Kaplan PE, Roden W, Gilbert E et al. Reduction of hypercalciuria in tetraplegia after weight-bearing and strengthening exercises. *Paraplegia.* 1981;19:289–293.

132. Scremin AM, Kurta L, Gentili A et al. Increasing muscle mass in spinal cord injured persons with a functional electrical stimulation exercise program. *Arch Phys Med Rehabil.* 1999;80:1531–1536.

133. Sloan KE, Bremner LA, Byrne J et al. Musculoskeletal effects of an electrical stimulation induced cycling programme in the spinal injured. *Paraplegia.* 1994;32:407–415.

134. Belanger M, Stein RB, Wheeler GD et al. Electrical stimulation: Can it increase muscle strength and reverse osteopenia in spinal cord injured individuals? *Arch Phys Med Rehabil.* 2000;81:1090–1098.

135. Chappard D, Minaire P, Privat C et al. Effects of tiludronate on bone loss in paraplegic patients. *J Bone Miner Res.* 1995;10:112–118.

136. Sniger W, Garshick E. Alendronate increases bone density in chronic spinal cord injury: A case report. *Arch Phys Med Rehabil.* 2002;83:139–140.

137. Dauty M, Perrouin VB, Maugars Y et al. Supralesional and sublesional bone mineral density in spinal cord-injured patients. *Bone.* 2000;27:305–309.

138. de Bruin ED, Frey-Rindova P, Herzog RE et al. Changes of tibia bone properties after spinal cord injury: Effects of early intervention. *Arch Phys Med Rehabil.* 1999;80:214–220.

139. Demirel G, Yilmaz H, Paker N et al. Osteoporosis after spinal cord injury. *Spinal Cord.* 1998;36:822–825.

140. Tsitouras PD, Zhong YG, Spungen AM et al. Serum testosterone and growth hormone/insulin-like growth factor-I in adults with spinal cord injury. *Horm Metab Res.* 1995;27:287–292.

141. Campagnolo DI, Bartlett JA, Chatterton R Jr et al. Adrenal and pituitary hormone patterns after spinal cord injury. *Am J Phys Med Rehabil.* 1999;78:361–366.

142. Mechanick JI, Pomerantz F, Flanagan S et al. Parathyroid hormone suppression in spinal cord injury patients is associated with the degree of neurologic impairment and not the level of injury. *Arch Phys Med Rehabil.* 1997;78:692–696.

143. el-Sayed MS, Davies B. A physical conditioning program does not alter fibrinogen concentration in young healthy subjects. *Med Sci Sports Exerc.* 1995;27:485–489.

144. Bauman WA. Endocrinology and metabolism after spinal cord injury. Kirshblum S, Campagnolo DI, DeLisa JA, editors. In: *Spinal Cord Medicine.* Philadelphia: Lippincott Williams and Wilkins; 2002. pp. 164–180.

145. Claus-Walker J, Halstead LS. Metabolic and endocrine changes in spinal cord injury: II (Section 2). Partial decentralization of the autonomic nervous system. *Arch Phys Med Rehabil.* 1982;63:576–580.

146. Garland DE, Adkins RH, Matsuno NN et al. The effect of pulsed electromagnetic fields on osteoporosis at the knee in individuals with spinal cord injury. *J Spinal Cord Med.* 1999;22:239–245.

147. Lazo MG, Shirazi P, Sam M et al. Osteoporosis and risk of fracture in men with spinal cord injury. *Spinal Cord.* 2001;39:208–214.

148. Roberts D, Lee W, Cuneo RC et al. Longitudinal study of bone turnover after acute spinal cord injury. *J Clin Endocrinol Metab.* 1998;83:415–422.

149. Uebelhart D, Demiaux-Domenech B, Roth M et al. Bone metabolism in spinal cord injured individuals and in others who have prolonged immobilisation. A review. *Paraplegia.* 1995;33:669–673.

150. Uebelhart D, Hartmann D, Vuagnat H et al. Early modifications of biochemical markers of bone metabolism in spinal cord injury patients. A preliminary study. *Scand J Rehabil Med.* 1994;26:197–202.

151. Iversen PO, Nicolaysen A, Hjeltnes N et al. Preserved granulocyte formation and function, as well as bone marrow innervation, in subjects with complete spinal cord injury. *Br J Haematol.* 2004;126:870–877.

152. Iversen PO, Hjeltnes N, Holm B et al. Depressed immunity and impaired proliferation of hematopoietic progenitor cells in patients with complete spinal cord injury. *Blood.* 2000;96:2081–2083.

153. Chantraine A, Nusgens B, Lapiere CM. Bone remodeling during the development of osteoporosis in paraplegia. *Calcif Tissue Int.* 1986;38:323–327.

154. Vestergaard P, Krogh K, Rejnmark L et al. Fracture rates and risk factors for fractures in patients with spinal cord injury. *Spinal Cord.* 1998;36:790–796.

155. Naftchi NE, Viau AT, Sell GH et al. Mineral metabolism in spinal cord injury. *Arch Phys Med Rehabil.* 1980;61:139–142.

156. Ragnarsson KT, Sell GH. Lower extremity fractures after spinal cord injury: A retrospective study. *Arch Phys Med Rehabil.* 1981;62:418–423.

157. Jacobs PL, Nash MS, Klose KJ et al. Evaluation of a training program for persons with SCI paraplegia using the Parastep 1 ambulation system: Part 2. Effects on physiological responses to peak arm ergometry. *Arch Phys Med Rehabil.* 1997;78:794–798.

158. Burnham RS, May L, Nelson E et al. Shoulder pain in wheelchair athletes. The role of muscle imbalance. *Am J Sports Med.* 1993;21:238–242.

159. Olenik LM, Laskin JJ, Burnham R et al. Efficacy of rowing, backward wheeling, and isolated scapular retractor exercise as remedial strength activities for wheelchair users: Application of electromyography. *Paraplegia.* 1995;33:148–152.

160. Ballinger DA, Rintala DH, Hart KA. The relation of shoulder pain and range-of-motion problems to functional limitations, disability, and perceived health of men with spinal cord injury: A multifaceted longitudinal study. *Arch Phys Med Rehabil.* 2000;81:1575–1581.

161. Bayley JC, Cochran TP, Sledge CB. The weight-bearing shoulder. The impingement syndrome in paraplegics. *J Bone Joint Surg-Am.* 1987;69:676–678.

162. Gerner HJ, Engel P, Gass GC et al. The effects of sauna on tetraplegic and paraplegic subjects. *Paraplegia.* 1992;30:410–419.

163. Ishii K, Yamasaki M, Muraki S et al. Effects of upper limb exercise on thermoregulatory responses in patients with spinal cord injury. *Appl Human Sci.* 1995;14:149–154.

164. Takada A, Takada Y, Urano T. The physiological aspects of fibrinolysis. *Thromb Res.* 1994;76:1–31.

165. Muraki S, Yamasaki M, Ishii K et al. Relationship between core temperature and skin blood flux in lower limbs during prolonged arm exercise in persons with spinal cord injury. *Eur J Appl Physiol.* 1996;72:330–334.

166. Muraki S, Yamasaki M, Ishii K et al. Effect of arm cranking exercise on skin blood flow of lower limb in people with injuries to the spinal cord. *Eur J Appl Physiol Occup Physiol.* 1995;71:28–32.

167. Price MJ, Campbell IG. Thermoregulatory responses of spinal cord injured and able-bodied athletes to prolonged upper body exercise and recovery. *Spinal Cord.* 1999;37:772–779.

168. Gellman H, Sie I, Waters RL. Late complications of the weight-bearing upper extremity in the paraplegic patient. *Clin Orthop.* 1988;132–135.

169. Subbarao JV, Klopfstein J, Turpin R. Prevalence and impact of wrist and shoulder pain in patients with spinal cord injury. *J Spinal Cord Med.* 1995;18:9–13.

170. Goldstein B, Young J, Escobedo EM. Rotator cuff repairs in individuals with paraplegia. *Am J Phys Med Rehabil.* 1997;76:316–322.

171. Pentland WE, Twomey LT. Upper limb function in persons with long term paraplegia and implications for independence: Part I. *Paraplegia.* 1994;32:211–218.

172. Silfverskiold J, Waters RL. Shoulder pain and functional disability in spinal cord injury patients. *Clin Orthop.* 1991;141–145.

173. Donovan WH, Brown DJ, Ditunno JF Jr et al. Neurological issues. *Spinal Cord.* 1997;35:275–281.

174. Winther K, Gleerup G, Snorrason K et al. Platelet function and fibrinolytic activity in cervical spinal cord injured patients. *Thromb Res.* 1992;65:469–474.

175. Curtis KA, Tyner TM, Zachary L et al. Effect of a standard exercise protocol on shoulder pain in long-term wheelchair users. *Spinal Cord.* 1999;37:421–429.

176. Nichols PJ, Norman PA, Ennis JR. Wheelchair user's shoulder? Shoulder pain in patients with spinal cord lesions. *Scand J Rehabil Med.* 1979;11:29–32.

177. Pentland WE, Twomey LT. The weight-bearing upper extremity in women with long term paraplegia. *Paraplegia.* 1991;29:521–530.

178. Robinson MD, Hussey RW, Ha CY. Surgical decompression of impingement in the weightbearing shoulder. *Arch Phys Med Rehabil.* 1993;74:324–327.

Pain After Spinal Cord Injury: Etiology and Management

17

Eva Widerström-Noga, DDS, PhD

OBJECTIVES

After reading this chapter, the reader will be able to:

- Understand the clinical characteristics and classifications of the various chronic pain types associated with spinal cord injury (SCI)
- Understand ideas concerning the underlying pathophysiological mechanisms of chronic pain associated with SCI
- Understand the role of common psychosocial factors involved in the experience of chronic pain associated with SCI
- Understand the various components of a comprehensive assessment of chronic pain associated with SCI
- Understand the role of recent clinical trials in providing guidelines for clinical management of chronic pain associated with SCI

Introduction

Prevalence of Pain

In the aftermath of a spinal cord injury (SCI), chronic pain is unfortunately a common and often severe and persistent consequence.[1-7] Moreover, pain commonly interferes with both routine daily activities and physical functioning, including sleep,[8-11] making chronic pain one of the major contributors to reduced quality of life after SCI.[12-14] In addition to a background of spontaneous chronic pain, persons with SCI also frequently experience pain exacerbation induced by a variety of common emotional as well as physical stimuli, such as negative mood, fatigue, prolonged sitting, cold weather, muscle spasms, constipation, etc.[15]

Persons who suffer from pain associated with SCI rarely report complete remission of their pain. In a study by Störmer et al,[16] only 5.8% of those who suffered from chronic pain or other distressing sensory abnormalities following SCI completely recovered spontaneously or due to a treatment. Similarly, several recent studies have confirmed the refractory nature of SCI.[17–19] Thus, pain continues to be a significant problem for large numbers of individuals living with a SCI despite the availability of treatments that have proven effective in other chronic pain populations.

Pain Classification

The chronic pain conditions that develop following a SCI are heterogeneous,[20–23] and most persons experience more than one type of pain simultaneously.[4,6,24] This heterogeneity complicates both the diagnosis and the subsequent treatment of pain and has therefore prompted the development of special pain classifications, or *taxonomies*, for SCI-related pain. The development of a standard mechanism-based taxonomy for SCI-related pain is an important step toward the development of treatment strategies that are tailored to specific mechanisms of pain.[23,25,26] A standardized taxonomy would facilitate comparisons among research studies and communication among professionals involved in the care of patients with SCI. Moreover, a consistent classification system for SCI-related pain would also improve the interpretation and translation of basic research findings by facilitating the development of clinically relevant animal models of

pain. However, a taxonomy based exclusively on pathophysiological mechanisms is not realistic until the relationship between specific mechanisms of pain and clinical signs and symptoms is better understood.

Several attempts have been made to categorize the chronic pain conditions associated with SCI into specific classification systems.[27–30] Although these taxonomies have many similarities with respect to the broad categories, such as the division into nociceptive and neuropathic pain, the specific terminologies differ. The first level of the taxonomy suggested by the International Association for the Study of Pain task force on SCI pain[29] divides pain into nociceptive and neuropathic types (Fig. 17-1).

While nociceptive pain in a region of sensory preservation may be described as dull, aching, and cramping, neuropathic pain in a region of sensory dysfunction may be described as sharp, shooting, electric, or burning. Neuropathic pain is usually associated both with sensory deficits and abnormal sensory phenomena, such as allodynia or hyperalgesia.[7,31] *Allodynia* is pain that is evoked by a normally innocuous (nonpainful) stimulus, such as touch, cooling, or warmth (*see* Table 17-1). *Hyperalgesia* is pain that is abnormally intense and evoked by a mild to moderately intense nociceptive stimulus. Both hyperalgesia and allodynia can be evoked by thermal or mechanical stimuli. The classification into specific pain types is based on a combination of pain characteristics (e.g., pain locations and pain descriptors) and other injury characteristics (e.g., level of injury). Identification of level of

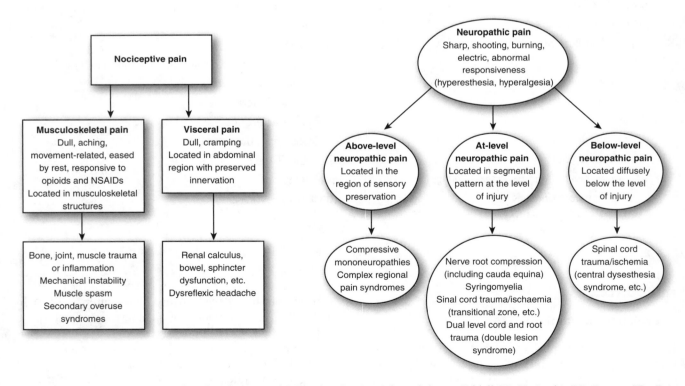

Figure 17-1. The IASP system for classification of SCI-related pain. Adapted from: Siddall PJ, Yezierski, RP, Loeser JD. Pain following spinal cord injury: Clinical features, prevalence, and taxonomy. *IASP Newsletter*. 2000;3:3–7.

Table 17-1

Pain Terminology

Pain Terms	Definition*
Pain	An unpleasant sensory and emotional experience associated with actual or potential tissue damage, or described in terms of such damage.
Allodynia	Pain due to a stimulus that does not normally provoke pain. The term *allodynia* was originally introduced to differentiate it from hyperalgesia and hyperesthesia, the conditions seen in patients with lesions of the nervous system where touch, light pressure, or moderate cold or warmth evoke pain when applied to apparently normal skin.
Central pain	Pain initiated or caused by a primary lesion or dysfunction in the central nervous system.
Dysesthesia	An unpleasant abnormal sensation, whether spontaneous or evoked. Special cases of dysesthesia include hyperalgesia and allodynia.
Hyperalgesia	An increased response to a stimulus which is normally painful. *Hyperalgesia* reflects increased pain on suprathreshold stimulation.
Hyperesthesia	Increased sensitivity to stimulation, excluding the special senses. *Hyperesthesia* may refer to various modes of cutaneous sensibility, including touch and thermal sensation without pain, as well as to pain. The word is used to indicate both diminished threshold to any stimulus and an increased response to stimuli that are normally recognized.
Hypoalgesia	Diminished pain in response to a normally painful stimulus.
Hypoesthesia	Decreased sensitivity to stimulation, excluding the special senses.
Neuropathic pain	Pain initiated or caused by a primary lesion or dysfunction in the nervous system.
Nociceptor	A receptor preferentially sensitive to a noxious stimulus or to a stimulus that would become noxious if prolonged.
Paresthesia	An abnormal sensation, whether spontaneous or evoked. *Paresthesia* should be used to describe an abnormal sensation that is not unpleasant and *dysesthesia* should be used preferentially for an abnormal sensation that is considered to be unpleasant.
Peripheral neuropathic pain	Pain initiated or caused by a primary lesion or dysfunction in the peripheral nervous system.

*Pain terminology from: Merskey H, Bogduk N, editors. *Classification of Chronic Pain*, 2nd edition. , Seattle, WA: IASP Press; 1994. pp. 209–214.

injury in the classification is important since it is specific to SCI and thus improves both the diagnosis and the evaluation of SCI-related pain. The second level of the International Association for the Study of Pain taxonomy includes a further categorization of nociceptive pain into musculoskeletal and visceral pain types. This level in the classification scheme also divides neuropathic pain into pain that is located above, at, or below the neurological level of SCI. It is important to recognize that as the knowledge base concerning mechanisms responsible for the origin and maintenance of the chronic pain conditions associated with SCI evolves, the classification systems for SCI-related pain will need to be revised accordingly.

Pain Types

Nociceptive Pain

Nociceptive pain is caused by normal activation of the nociceptive system by a noxious stimulus. Thus, a noxious stimulus activates a nociceptor, and the signal is transmitted in primary afferent fibers (Aδ- and C-fibers). This incoming nociceptive information is subsequently processed in the dorsal horn of the spinal cord and in ascending neural pathways, including brain structures such as the thalamus and cortex. It is important to recognize that nociception is not equivalent to pain. Nociception is merely the sensory process that includes the activation of a nociceptor and transmission of this signal in the nervous system. Although nociception may contribute to the experience of pain, pain may arise in the absence of nociception, as in the case of neuropathic pain (*see* below). Pain is defined by the International Association for the Study of Pain as an unpleasant sensory and emotional experience associated with actual or potential tissue damage, or described in terms of such damage.

Nociceptive pain in persons with SCI is primarily caused by damage or inflammation that may involve bones, ligaments, or muscles. Nociceptive pain is also caused by visceral stimuli, such as urinary tract infections or bowel impaction, and may be transmitted via the autonomic nervous system.[32] As a contrast, genital pain may be caused by damage to the cauda equine[29] and thus be neuropathic in origin. In persons with SCI, nociceptive pain is usually located in a region with preserved sensation above or near the level of injury. However, in persons with incomplete injuries, nociceptive pain may also occur below the level injury, providing that the nociceptive pathways are spared. One commonly occurring nociceptive pain type after SCI is chronic musculoskeletal pain that is caused by overuse or "abnormal" use of the arm and shoulder.[33]

Neuropathic Pain

Neuropathic pains result from injury or disease of the peripheral or central nervous system. Neuropathic pain is initiated or caused by a primary lesion or dysfunction in the nervous system and is located in areas with sensory abnormalities *above*, *at*, or *below* the level of injury. This type of pain may be generated by hyperactive neurons involved in pain transmission at the spinal level[34–37] or in the thalamus,[38] or by decreased endogenous pain inhibitory function.[39]

Neuropathic pain associated with SCI can be divided into three categories: above, at, or below the level of injury. Above-level neuropathic pain is located above the level of injury and includes pain types that may not necessarily be exclusive to SCIs. Examples of such pains are complex regional pain syndromes and pain caused by peripheral nerve compression. At-level neuropathic pain is located within two segments above or below the level of injury and is often associated with allodynia or hyperalgesia. This pain may also be called *segmental*, *transitional zone*, *border zone*, *end zone*, or *girdle zone* pain. The neuropathic at-level pain may be due to damage of either nerve roots or of the spinal cord itself; however, the exact cause may be difficult to determine.[33] Below-level neuropathic pain may be defined as *central pain*, *dysesthetic*, or *deafferentation* pain. Below-level neuropathic pain is located three or more dermatomes below the level of injury and is often associated with allodynia or hyperalgesia.

Mechanisms of Pain

The refractory nature of neuropathic pain associated with SCI highlights the need for a greater understanding of both the pathophysiological and the psychosocial mechanisms underlying the generation and maintenance of SCI-related pain Although basic research has made many important discoveries concerning pathophysiological phenomena associated with SCI, it is unclear how these mechanisms translate into clinical signs and symptoms in the individual with chronic pain.

Pathophysiology

Recent clinical research suggests that hyperexitability caused by loss of inhibitory neurons above the level of spinal injury in combination with spinothalamic tract lesions may result in the development of neuropathic pain in persons with SCI.[40,41] Two primary mechanisms are hypothesized to trigger this hyperexcitability: *central disinhibition* (resulting from the loss of function of spinal cord inhibitory interneurons) and *central sensitization* (increased responses of spinothalamic neurons to mechanical or thermal stimulation). Both these mechanisms are capable of causing neuronal hyperactivity of spinal as well as supraspinal neurons.[42,43] These ideas are consistent with basic research studies that have shown that pain behaviors in animals were associated with lesions in areas where cell bodies are located, that is, the gray matter of the spinal cord in combination with hyperexcitable and hyperactive neurons in the dorsal horn of the spinal cord.[35,44] Furthermore, lesions in the anterolateral white matter (location of the spinothalamic tract) resulted in allodynia and hyperalgesia only when combined with gray matter damage.[45] For a recent review concerning pathophysiology of neuropathic pain associated with SCI, *see* Yezierski.[46] In the patient with chronic neuropathic pain, common clinical signs of decreased spinothalamic function are higher thresholds for cool or warm sensation, or heat pain,[31,40,41] whereas allodynia, hyperalgesia, or wind-up pain in painful skin areas in denervated regions may be signs of hyperexcitability.[26,41] Thus, the existing body of research suggests that neuronal hyperexcitability, clinically manifested as hypersensitivity to various stimuli (such as mechanical and cold) at the lesion level, is an important mechanism underlying neuropathic pain at or below the level of injury.

Finnerup and Jensen[43] recently grouped the pathophysiological mechanisms of neuropathic pain associated with SCI into several different categories (i.e., anatomic, neurochemical and excitotoxic, and inflammatory changes). These are briefly summarized below.

Anatomic Changes

The damage or loss of nervous tissue as a result of a traumatic injury such as a SCI can potentially cause reorganization of neurons located at multiple levels in the central nervous system. Several lines of research show that significant changes take place after a SCI and that some of these changes are linked to the development of neuropathic pain. Specifically, deafferentation and sprouting of spinal afferents containing calcitonin gene-related peptides and substance P are possible causes of increased excitability of central neurons.[47,48] Similarly, results from a study by Crown et al[49] indicate that activation of intracellular signaling cascades (the main ways of communication between the plasma membrane and intracellular targets) traditionally associated with long-term potentiation (lasting enhancement of synaptic transmission) are also associated with the transition of acute to chronic pain and with the development of chronic neuropathic pain following SCI.

When an injury is incomplete, some spinal cord tracts are more damaged than others. This imbalance between pathways is hypothesized to be another possible generator of neuropathic pain. For example, if descending pain inhibitory pathways are more injured than pathways transmitting nociceptive information, the resulting imbalance may amplify nociceptive activity. Plastic changes induced by a SCI are also possible in higher centers. For example, Hubsher and Johnson[50] suggested that neurons in specific regions of the thalamus undergo significant changes in responsiveness following severe chronic SCI. They concluded that the observed plasticity and hypersensitivity are likely to be part of a central reorganization producing a multitude of sensory disturbances after SCI. Further evidence for changes in central structures has also been provided by Pattany et al.[51] In this study, metabolite concentrations were assessed in the right and left thalami in people with SCI and chronic pain using magnetic resonance spectroscopy (see discussion below). The conclusions from this study were that the relationship between metabolic activity in the thalamus and perceived pain intensity suggested anatomic, functional, and biochemical changes in the thalamus associated with the presence of chronic neuropathic pain.

Neurochemical and Excitotoxic Changes

Several neurochemical and neurotoxic changes are hypothesized to be contributors to the development of neuropathic pain. For example, the excitatory amino acid glutamate is suggested to exert excitotoxic actions (transsynaptic injury due to release of excitatory amines) on both spinal and descending inhibitory control systems involving γ-aminobutyric acid.[52] The resulting decreased inhibitory control is thought to be the cause of hyperexcitability of spinal neurons. A number of other neurochemical changes have been implicated as generators of neuropathic pain associated with SCI. For example, upregulated expression of sodium channel Nav1.3 has

been observed within second-order spinal cord dorsal horn neurons (ascending neurons that originate in the spinal cord) and third-order thalamic neurons (ascending neurons that originate in the thalamus) along the pain pathway after SCI.[53] This upregulation appears to contribute to neuronal hyperresponsiveness and pain-related behaviors. The authors of this study suggested that the abnormal expression of sodium channels makes both spinal and thalamic neurons hyperexcitable so that they act as amplifiers as well as generators of pain.

Inflammatory Changes

Both inflammatory and immune activations are also suggested to be important for the generation of chronic neuropathic pain following a SCI.[54] In a recent study by Nesic et al,[55] the authors suggested that chronic neuropathic pain develops partly due to dysfunctional and chronically "overactivated" spinal astrocytes. Similarly, glial cells in the dorsal root ganglion and spinal dorsal horn synthesize and release small secreted proteins, or so-called cytokines, which may mediate inflammation. Tumor necrosis factor-alpha, an inflammatory cytokine with both growth-stimulating properties and growth-inhibitory processes, appears to be related to development of neuropathic below-level pain and associated mechanical allodynia.[56] This is also supported by other basic research, suggesting that Wallerian degeneration (degeneration of the axon distal to a site of injury) following a peripheral axon injury contributes to the development of neuropathic pain by stimulating the production of cytokines and nerve growth factors.[57] Tumor necrosis factor-alpha, in particular, appears to play a significant role in the development of peripheral neuropathic pain and hyperexcitability of sensory neurons leading to allodynia and hyperalgesia.[58]

Psychosocial Contributors

The biopsychosocial view on pain incorporates a dynamic interaction between physical, psychological, and social factors that evolve over time. This perspective includes not only the pathophysiological mechanisms underlying the cause of pain, but also the psychological and psychosocial factors of importance for maintaining and exacerbating chronic pain conditions. Since all people with pain may differ on important variables that influence coping and adaptation, this model provides a theoretical foundation that can be helpful for the development of tailored therapeutic options in the psychological realm.

Although the different types of pain following SCI are caused by multiple pathophysiological mechanisms,[28,29] the maintenance and aggravation of the chronic pain condition depends on a variety of factors, some of them unrelated to the pathophysiology of pain. This is true for both heterogeneous pain populations[59] and for those with SCI.[60–62] Similar to observations in other pain populations, the severity of SCI-related pain tends to be associated with affective distress such as depressed mood.[63] Indeed, psychological factors such as anxiety, sadness, and perceptions of excessive fatigue are commonly acknowledged by people experiencing SCI-related pain.[60,64,65] These factors have also been shown to significantly affect coping and adjustment to SCI in general.[66–68] Thus, the refractory nature of the painful conditions following SCI suggests that personal characteristics related to adaptation and coping skills are crucial for improving quality of life.[69]

People living with a SCI obviously have many aspects of their life altered by their injury. An important determinant for quality of life following SCI is successful independent living.[70] This may include the perception of having control over one's life, having a satisfying social function, such as being employed, being minimally dependent on others for daily life activities, etc. Consequently, people with SCI who are also suffering from chronic pain are more likely to have a diminished quality of life[12,71] since chronic pain may further compromise their independence by interfering with daily activities, including social activities and work.[8–10] In addition, greater life satisfaction following SCI has been shown to display positive relationships with factors such as level of education, income, employment, and social/recreational activities, whereas the presence of medical complications are often related to decreased satisfaction with life.[72,73]

Another factor important for coping and living with SCI is social support. However, *low* levels of perceived support have been reported by persons with SCI and chronic pain.[63] This study indicated that the pattern of perceived responses and support from significant others may be different in the SCI chronic pain population compared to able-bodied heterogeneous chronic pain populations, but similar to populations with a known organic underlying disease, such as post-polio syndrome and cancer. McColl et al[74] found that the relationship between social support and coping with SCI changed over time. For example, early after SCI, there was a positive association between social support and positive coping, whereas follow-up data (collected 12 months after discharge) indicated a reversed relationship (i.e., a high level of social support was negatively associated with coping capability). The authors suggested that this pattern may be specific to the SCI population wherein high levels of support might deter the individual from developing independent coping strategies in the chronic stages.

Although similarities among various chronic pain populations clearly exist, it is apparent that the multiple medical consequences (e.g., paralysis; decreased bowel, bladder, and sexual function; spasticity, etc.) that are associated with SCI may influence the adaptation patterns to chronic pain in this population. Two different patterns of coping and adaptation to chronic pain following SCI were identified in a study by Widerström-Noga et al.[63] A cluster analysis and a discriminant analysis divided persons with SCI and chronic pain into one of two different adaptational patterns based on their responses on the

Multidimensional Pain Inventory.[75] The clusters, or subgroups, consisted of (1) *dysfunctional*, that is, those who have high levels of pain, affective distress, and perceived interference and low levels of perceived control and activity, and (2) *adaptive copers*, that is, those who have lower levels of pain, affective distress, and life interference and higher sense of control and activity. The dysfunctional cluster in individuals with SCI was almost identical to the dysfunctional group described in heterogeneous chronic pain patients,[59] both with respect to the subscale scores and the proportion of participants classified as dysfunctional. In contrast, the adaptive coper cluster of the SCI chronic pain population constituted a much larger percentage of the total sample compared to other populations with chronic pain.[59,76,77] For example, 29.5% belonged to this subgroup in a study including heterogeneous chronic pain[59] compared to 57.5% in persons with SCI.[63] Interestingly, the interference caused by pain was lower following SCI compared to both chronic headache and heterogeneous chronic pain in able-bodied populations. One possible explanation is that persons with SCI often have significant impairments caused by their injury and therefore must deal with frequent medical complications that interrupt their lives. For these people, chronic pain is superimposed on these other restrictions and may not be viewed as interfering as much with their lives compared to able-bodied persons who have chronic pain. A stepwise discriminant analysis was performed to define the combination of factors that best discriminated between the adaptive coper and dysfunctional subgroups. Variables representing sociodemographic factors, injury characteristics, and pain characteristics were included in the analysis. The combination of variables that best predicted the dysfunctional cluster was (1) presence of allodynia or hyperalgesia; (2) presence of "burning" pain; (3) tetraplegia; (4) male gender; and (5) not working or studying. The inclusion of neurological abnormalities such as allodynia and hyperalgesia combined with burning quality of pain in this analysis suggests that persons who have neuropathic pain are more likely to have a dysfunctional (DYS) psychometric profile.

The effects of gender observed in the study by Widerström-Noga and colleagues[63] parallel the findings reported by Spertus et al,[78] revealing that a history of trauma was associated with particularly poor adjustment to chronic pain in men. The authors suggested that men and women differ in the way they adjust to chronic pain following trauma. Similarly, men with chronic pain and SCI reported more frequent pain interference with daily activity, including sleep.[10] The role of gender in coping and adaptation to chronic pain is obviously one that is in need of additional investigation. Moreover, having a higher level of injury (i.e., cervical versus lower level) was associated with the dysfunctional cluster. Indeed, life satisfaction has been reported to be lower in persons with higher levels of injury and lower levels of functional independence and greater handicap.[79]

Assessment of Pain

Despite the high prevalence of chronic pain within the SCI population, the low incidence of SCI makes it difficult to obtain sufficient numbers of participants for definitive clinical trials. Few large, randomized, controlled clinical pain trials have been conducted in the SCI population. In order to expedite the development of beneficial treatments, it is important to evaluate the outcomes of treatments in a comprehensive and consistent manner. The use of comparable sets of outcome measures would increase efficiency and greatly facilitate the translation, interpretation, and application of results to improve management of SCI-related pain.

The Initiative on Methods, Measurement, and Pain Assessment in Clinical Trials is a consortium of governmental representatives, academic investigators, consumer advocates, and representative of the pharmaceutical industry with the mission to develop consensus recommendations for improving the design, execution, and interpretation of clinical pain trials in general. In a recent publication,[80] this group suggested that in addition to pain, specific measures of the core health-related quality of life domains should be considered in all clinical trials of the efficacy and effectiveness of chronic pain interventions. This recommendation was based on studies suggesting that three primary domains, namely, *pain severity*, *physical functioning*, and *emotional functioning*, were required to capture the multidimensionality of the pain experience.[81,82] Although these recommendations did not specifically include chronic pain populations with SCI, the general domains also seem appropriate for use in this population.[83]

Health-related quality of life is based on preferences and values specific to each individual and concerns multiple dimensions of life, including well-being and enjoyment of life. Specifically, health-related quality of life refers to those domains that are specifically related to health and that can be potentially influenced by the health-care system.[84,85] In people with physical impairments, the inclusion of additional health-related quality of life domains (e.g., changed roles due to physical problems and general health) may be important for evaluating outcome. Thus, an increased understanding of the interaction between these various domains is important for the understanding and subsequent management of the complex pain syndromes associated with SCI.

Pain

Verbal Report

Because of the heterogeneity of pain associated with SCI and multiple putative mechanisms involved, it is essential to conduct a thorough pain history. Pain is subjective, and peoples' perceptions of their pain are critical for a comprehensive pain evaluation.[85] Therefore, both the evaluation and treatment strategy for people with chronic pain and SCI should rely on an assessment procedure reflecting psychosocial factors and behavioral factors, as well as pathophysiological mechanisms.[83] The assessment of pain following SCI is complicated by the fact that SCI results in a number of medical consequences.[5,20] For example, common medical consequences, such as constipation and muscle spasms, are frequently reported to increase the severity of pain.[62]

A number of assessment instruments have been developed for chronic pain patients in general.[87] However, these may not be appropriate for those with SCI because of the limitations caused by consequences of injury other than pain. Therefore, it is inappropriate to assume that measures developed for use with other chronic pain populations can be generalized without adaptation to people with SCI. Several important factors need to be considered in the evaluation of SCI-related pain. For example, the nature of the pain needs to be defined because different types of pain may respond differently to treatment.[25,26,88] Thus, attempts should be made to determine whether the pain is nociceptive or neuropathic. A classification of pain can be made based on a comprehensive pain history in combination with a neurological examination defining the extent of neurological deficit. The evaluator should obtain information regarding the location and quality of pain, temporal pattern, pain intensity, aggravating and pain-relieving factors, effects of medication and treatments, changes in location and intensity, etc. In addition to changes in intensity, changes in temporal pattern may also provide valuable information concerning the pain-relieving efficacy of a particular therapy. Because of the complexity associated with the chronic pain conditions after a SCI, collection of pain history information is best obtained by interview. Efforts should be made to develop a good rapport between the interviewer and the individual with SCI, since some persons may find it difficult to describe their pain experience (Fig. 17-2).

In clinical trials, rating scales designed to assess pain severity[89] are commonly used as primary outcome measures. These scales may be numerical (0 to 10), categorical (e.g., mild, moderate, severe), or visual analog (a 100-mm line with anchors of no pain and worst possible pain). The instructions to patients may be designed to ask about their "usual pain," "pain at its worst," "pain at its least," or pain over some time period (e.g., over the past week). Rating scales are sometimes combined with both location of pain and adjectives describing qualities of pain in instruments such as in the McGill Pain Questionnaire.[90] When the use of concomitant pain treatments is permitted during the course of a clinical treatment or a trial, these should be assessed and considered as outcome measures.[91] Effects of a pain therapy may be continuously evaluated in a pain diary, which may be written or electronic.[92] The diary may record the intensity, location, and description of pain at regular intervals. It may also include ratings of alleviating and aggravating factors, use of medication, mood state, and activities.[93] Recording

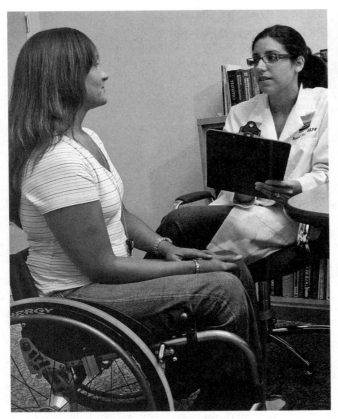

Figure 17-2. The pain history information should be obtained in a personal and relaxed manner.

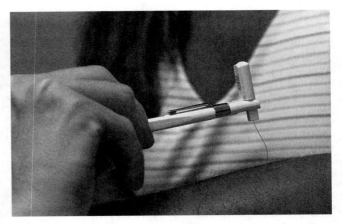

Figure 17-3. The von Frey filament used for determining the sensory threshold for light touch.

levels of pain and related factors with a short delay, as is possible when using diaries, reduces the risk of recall bias.[94]

Quantification of Neurological Dysfunction

In addition to the evaluation of chronic spontaneous pain, a comprehensive pain evaluation may include the assessment of evoked pain and abnormal sensations, since sensory dysfunction is an integral part of the neuropathic pain condition associated with SCI and can provide insights into the mechanisms of a pain condition.[31,40] A comprehensive assessment of pain may include quantitative sensory testing that can detect sensory dysfunction, such as hypo- or hyperesthesia (revealed by measurement of thresholds), or qualitative abnormalities, such as allodynia, dysesthesia, or paresthesia.[95]

In neuropathic pain conditions, the neurological dysfunction may be manifested as abnormal sensory, motor, and autonomic functions.[96] Assessment of sensory thresholds may include detection of light touch by using a graded set of von Frey monofilaments (Fig. 17-3).

Used frequently in clinical settings, von Frey filaments are used to diagnose sensory pathologies associated with various neurological disorders. As the tip of the filament is pressed against the skin at a right angle, the force of the application increases only to the level at which the filament bends. Thus, a specific size of filament produces a

reproducible force and can be used for research purposes. Hypoalgesia and hyperalgesia to vibration and thermal stimuli (e.g., thresholds to cool sensation, warm sensation, and cold and heat pain) can be assessed with a thermal and vibratory sensory analyzer. Testing sites are usually located in painful areas, but usually include nonpainful areas or areas with normal sensory function for comparison (Fig. 17-4).

Several investigators have provided information concerning potential pain-generating mechanisms and suggested that these responses may serve as a diagnostic basis for prescribing pain treatment.[31,41,97] Interestingly, self-reports of various types of sensory dysfunctions have been found to correspond well with standard quantitative sensory assessments.[98] Results from a study in 120 persons with SCI and chronic pain suggest that pain aggravation due to various factors, situations, and behaviors is common in people who experience neuropathic pain.[62] In this study, the extent of self-reported evoked pain was significantly associated with specific pain characteristics indicative of neuropathic pain as well as greater psychosocial impact. Assessment of the neurological dysfunction associated with chronic pain is an important diagnostic tool. However, it is not clear to what extent quantitative sensory assessments will be useful as outcome measures in clinical trials. Additional research is required to establish the reliability of these methods in assessing and quantifying specific types of neurological dysfunction. In addition, the relationship between neurological dysfunction and severity of spontaneous pain also needs to be clearly established.

Imaging of the Brain

The availability of noninvasive brain imaging has resulted in more opportunities to examine the brain processes that are critical to the understanding of the neuronal mechanisms involved in human chronic pain conditions. The subjective experience of pain (i.e., the intensity and affective nature) is a result of a complex interaction

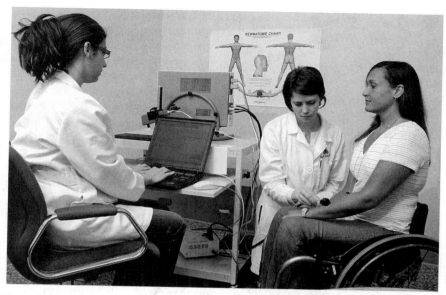

Figure 17-4. The assessment of the sensory threshold of warm sensation using a computerized sensory analyzer.

between the incoming nociceptive information and the modulation of this information at multiple levels along the neuroaxis, that is, in the spinal cord and in higher brain structures such as the thalamus and cortex. While both spinal and medullary mechanisms of pain and pain modulation have been researched extensively since the ground-breaking work by Melzack and Wall,[99] Basbaum and Fields,[100] and Le Bars and colleagues,[101] the supraspinal processing of pain has been much less studied. Recent results from neuroimaging studies strongly support the idea that pain perception is dependent on a network consisting of cortical (primary and secondary somatosensory cortices), limbic (anterior cingulate and insular cortices), associative (prefrontal cortex), and subcortical structures (thalamus).[102] Thus, dysfunction in these networks may be the cause of both the generation and the maintenance of chronic pain and associated conditions.[103] Unfortunately, the extent to which these basic mechanisms translate into clinical signs and symptoms in people with chronic neuropathic pain associated with SCI is not conclusively known.

While the strong affective-motivational character of pain is assumed to be reflected in activation of regions within the anterior cingulate and insular cortices,[104–106] both experimental and clinical studies show multiple interactions between the sensory and affective dimensions of pain in a central network of brain structures.[107] Since sensory stimulation triggers inhibitory activity in the thalamus,[108,109] and inhibitory neurons compose a significant proportion of the thalamic neurons in primates,[110,111] it is reasonable to assume that the thalamus is not only important for the processing, but also for the modulation of nociceptive signals.[102,112] These inhibitory neurons also appear to be highly susceptible to pathological changes following SCI,[113] and decreased function or loss of inhibitory neurons may therefore contribute to the development of neuropathic pain conditions after injury.

Magnetic resonance spectroscopy (MRS) is a noninvasive method to assess metabolic activity in the brain. MRS measures chemicals within the body and brain without removing tissue or blood samples and without using any tracers. MRS is based on the fact that different chemicals vibrate at different frequencies when stimulated by a magnet. MRS uses the signal from hydrogen protons to determine the concentration of brain metabolites such as N-acetyl aspartate, choline, and creatine. Clinically, MRS is mostly used in the evaluation of central nervous system disorders. Both the anatomical structure investigated and metabolic concentrations can be visualized as an image or spectrum (Fig. 17-5).

The advantage of MRS for potential utility in research and clinical trials is the stability of the signals analyzed.[102] Thus, when changes are detected, they are presumed to reflect long-term plasticity. A metabolite of interest is N-acetyl aspartate, which is a free amino acid thought to be localized in neurons and neuronal processes in the mature brain. N-acetyl aspartate is commonly thought of as a neuronal marker; however, it is also assumed to reflect temporary neuronal dysfunction since recovery of N-acetyl aspartate levels have been observed.[114] Decreased level of these metabolites have also been demonstrated in various cerebral pathologies (e.g., brain tumors,[115] epilepsy,[116,117] and neurological disorders such as Alzheimer's and Parkinson's diseases and amyotrophic lateral sclerosis.[118–120] Another metabolite detected by MRS scans is myo-inositol, which is thought to be a glial marker possibly indicating gliosis. Myo-inositol acts as an organic osmolyte, which is a small organic neutral solute that reacts minimally with the contents of a cell while

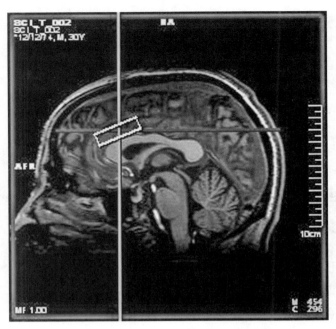

Figure 17-5. Positioning of the 2-dimensional chemical shift imaging slice over the region of the left and right thalamus. The central 8 × 8 voxels highlighted in the white square are processed, and one of the sub-voxels within the region of the thalamus is indicated by the square.

protecting it from drying out. Myo-inositol has a major role in the volume and osmoregulation of astrocytes.[114,121]

A recent MRS study in people with low back pain and depression showed overlapping chemical changes in various brain areas supportive of the relationships between the sensory and affective aspects of pain.[122] In another study using MRS, Phillips and colleagues[123] suggested that negative affect increased pain-related activity in the limbic region, including the anterior cingulate cortex. Furthermore, evidence from single-neuron recordings, electrical stimulation, electroencephalogram, positron emission tomography, functional magnetic resonance imaging, and lesion studies indicate that the anterior cingulate cortex has an important role in emotional self-control as well as in focused problem solving, error recognition, and adaptive responses to challenging conditions.[124] These functions have been suggested to be intimately correlated,[124] and activity in the limbic structures are, therefore, likely to be important for an individual's ability to cope with pain. Because chronic pain associated with SCI is both heterogeneous and often refractory to available treatments, personal characteristics related to adaptation and coping are critical determinants for quality of life.

Studies involving imaging of the brain and central neuropathic pain are few. However, a recent case study using magnetic resonance and diffusion tensor imaging in a patient with central post-stroke pain showed a reduction in thalamocortical fibers and an increase in pain-specific responses in the anterior cingulate cortex.[125] The authors suggested that a combination of reduced nociceptive

thalamocortical function and increased activation of the anterior cingulate cortex was associated with central post-stroke pain. This idea concurs with a study in which MRS was used to assess metabolic activity in persons with SCI who had chronic pain.[51] In this study, metabolite concentrations were assessed in the right and left thalami using single-voxel stimulated echo acquisition mode 1.5 tesla MRS. In participants with neuropathic pain, the concentration of N-acetyl aspartate was significantly and negatively associated with the intensity of pain. In contrast, myo-inositol was positively correlated with pain intensity. The low levels of N-acetyl aspartate in persons with neuropathic pain were hypothesized to be related to a decreased function of inhibitory neurons in the thalamic region, whereas higher concentrations of myo-inositol were hypothesized to reflect gliosis. Gliosis is a proliferation of astrocytes in damaged areas of the central nervous system. Astrocytes are relatively large glial cells and are the connective tissue cells of the central nervous system. These cells have various functions, including accumulating in areas where nerve cells have degenerated or have been damaged. The idea that gliosis would be present in the thalamus of those with SCI and chronic neuropathic pain is based on the hypothesis that neuropathic pain causes neurodegenerative changes. Thus, data demonstrating increased myo-inositol levels may indicate thalamic nerve cell degeneration. The results from this study suggest that anatomic, functional, and biochemical changes in the thalamus may be associated with the presence of chronic neuropathic pain in individuals with SCI.

Physical Functioning

In many chronic pain conditions, physical activity is accompanied by increased pain. However, the way people respond to pain varies between individuals. For example, while some people may limit their physical functioning because of pain, other people will tolerate an increased pain level in order to maintain a certain level of function. Although a general measure of physical functioning applicable to all heterogeneous pain populations would allow for better comparisons among chronic pain populations, it is usually the case that physical functioning after a SCI is more influenced by the neurological impairment than by chronic pain per se. Physical functioning in the SCI population may, therefore, not be accurately assessed by a generic measure, and disease-specific measures may be more likely to reveal a clinically important improvement or decline in function.

Pain Interference

The term *pain interference* refers to the extent to which pain hinders or interferes with common activities in a person's daily life. Many of the consequences of SCI impose limitations on a person's ability to perform and participate in daily activities. Furthermore, studies in people with SCI demonstrate that chronic pain significantly decreases quality of life.[2,13] Therefore, pain-related interference with daily activities may be particularly important to evaluate in individuals with SCI. For example, interference caused by pain during daily activities can result in decreased independence, ultimately leading to affective distress[59] and reduced motivation for participation in activities essential for reaching optimal levels of functional independence following SCI.[126,127] In fact, high levels of pain interference assessed by the SCI version of the Multidimensional Pain Inventory,[128] and not actual severity of pain, was one of the predictors of decreased quality of life in a recent study in 161 persons with SCI and chronic pain.[129] Therefore, pain interference measures may provide more useful and relevant alternatives or compliments to instruments that assess general physical function. The extent to which chronic pain (as distinct from other consequences of SCI) hinders or interferes with activities of daily life may provide more specific information in populations afflicted with physical impairment.[128]

Some SCI-specific measures of pain interference have been psychometrically tested for validity and reliability. For example, the Multidimensional Pain Inventory[75] was recently adapted to the SCI chronic pain population[128] and psychometrically evaluated. The Life Interference and the Pain Interference with Activity subscales of the Multidimensional Pain Inventory were found to be both valid and reliable.[129] Similarly, the Pain Interference subscale of the Brief Pain Inventory[130] was also found to be valid and reliable for use with SCI chronic pain populations.[131]

Emotional Functioning

Emotional distress, such as depressed mood, anxiety, and anger, is intimately linked to the experience of chronic pain. Similarly, individuals experiencing SCI-related pain report higher levels of psychological distress and excessive fatigue.[64,65] While the ability to cope with and adjust to the injury is negatively associated with pain in those with SCI,[67,68] no consistent causal relationship has been demonstrated. The presence of emotional distress in people with chronic pain and SCI presents a challenge when assessing symptoms such as fatigue, reduced activity level, decreased libido, appetite change, sleep disturbance, weight change, and memory and concentration deficits. Although improvements or deterioration in such symptoms may be due to changes in either pain or emotional distress, another possibility is that these changes are also dependent on changes in other aspects of the injury. Despite the difficulty in interpreting changes in emotional functioning, this domain is central to a person's assessment of his/her well-being and satisfaction with life.

Using a factor analysis, Widerström-Noga and Turk[62] detected five different sets of factors that were associated with exacerbation of chronic pain. In particular, two of these factors (i.e., *negative mood* and *prolonged afferent activity*) were commonly and significantly associated with both specific pain characteristics and psychosocial issues. The factor that accounted for the largest proportion of the variation, that is, negative mood, included anxiety, sadness, anger, and feelings of fatigue as reasons for increased pain. This factor was significantly associated with both specific characteristics, such as widespread pain and multiple pain descriptors, and the Life Interference, Affective Distress, and Decrease in Activities Due to Pain subscales of the Multidimensional Pain Inventory (SCI version).[127] In people classified as *dysfunctional* (e.g., those who had high levels of pain severity, emotional distress, and interference with activities, and low levels of life control and general activity), the number of aggravating factors was significantly higher than in people classified as *adaptive copers* (e.g., those with lower levels of pain severity, affective distress, and high levels of life control and activity). Thus, the dysfunctional profile is not only associated with more severe spontaneous pain after SCI[63] and poorer treatment outcome,[132] but it is also associated with more evoked pain. The extent to which pain itself contributes to affective distress in the complex pain conditions associated with SCI is not clear. Because affective distress is important for the overall experience of pain, additional research in this area is warranted.

Clinical Trials for Management of Pain in Individuals With SCI

The refractory nature of the chronic pain conditions associated with SCI increases the risk for a significantly diminished quality of life that adds to the burdens imposed by the other consequences of SCI. Although many pharmacological and nonpharmacological treatments have been used to relieve pain following SCI, treatment is often inadequate.[132,133] One explanation for the failure of adequate pain control is that, although knowledge about the mechanisms involved in causing, exacerbating, and sustaining pain is accumulating,[23,46,134] there remain many gaps in the understanding of how these mechanisms translate into specific clinical signs and symptoms.

The most widely used pharmacological treatment strategies in neuropathic pain include the tricyclic antidepressants and anticonvulsants.[135] The analgesic effects of these two agents are based on fundamentally different mechanisms of action. The inhibition of monoamine uptake in the central nervous system by tricyclic antidepressants is thought to mediate their pain-relieving effects.[135,136] In contrast, the analgesic effects of anticonvulsants are thought to depend on their ability to suppress aberrant electrical activity throughout the nervous system.[137] Anticonvulsants have been shown to be effective in several types of neuropathic pain conditions, such as carbamazepine in trigeminal neuralgia[138] and gabapentin in diabetic peripheral neuropathy[139] and post-herpetic neuralgia.[140] In addition, retrospective studies[141,142] also suggest that gabapentin may provide some relief for neuropathic pain following SCI. Two randomized, controlled trials in persons with SCI suggest beneficial results for anticonvulsants for subgroups of neuropathic pain in the SCI population.[143,144] A recent Australian multicenter trial in SCI concluded that pregabalin was effective in relieving central neuropathic pain and improving sleep, anxiety, and overall patient status.[145] The analgesic properties of another class of pharmacological agents, sodium channel blockers (i.e., lidocaine), have also been examined in patients with SCI. One clinical trial demonstrated that lidocaine delivered into the subarachnoid space significantly relieved SCI-related pain.[146] In a sample with either stroke- or SCI-related pain,[147] intravenous lidocaine decreased spontaneous pain and mechanical allodynia and hyperalgesia, but had no significant effect on thermal allodynia and hyperalgesia.

Clinical trials involving tricyclic antidepressants suggest that approximately 60% to 70% of people with heterogeneous neuropathic pain report at least moderate reductions in pain with these agents.[136] A problem with older tricyclic antidepressants, such as imipramine and amitriptyline, however, is the presence of significant side effects that may hinder effective dosing.[148] The effects of tricyclic antidepressants are thought to be mediated by enhancing endogenous modulatory systems that involve neurotransmitters such as serotonin and norepinephrine.[149] Although a number of clinical trials using tricyclic antidepressants have shown significant relief of neuropathic pain for several different neuropathic pain conditions (e.g., post-herpetic neuralgia, diabetic neuropathy[150–152]), only one large, randomized controlled trial has been conducted in SCI. This study[153] found no significant pain-relieving effect of amitriptyline compared to active placebo. The dosing was limited by side effects and may have been too low to produce optimal analgesia.[154] For a recent review of clinical pharmacological pain trials in SCI, *see* Finnerup and Jensen.[43]

There is a great need for conclusive and large-scale, randomized, controlled trials investigating pain-relieving treatments for chronic pain associated with SCI. Unfortunately, there is limited availability of participants, which emphasize the importance of standardized pain classification and evaluation in order to facilitate multicenter trials. Because the current literature pertaining to SCI and chronic pain is limited, a rational approach is to test interventions that have proven efficacious in other neuropathic pain populations in individuals with SCI.[135] In addition to pharmacological trials, the results from a recent study using transcranial stimulation for the management of neuropathic pain associated with SCI suggested that this type of therapy may be effective in some patients.[155]

More than 40% of a sample of 120 people with SCI who had chronic pain reported that they did not use any treatments to relieve their pain.[132] Regrettably, people who used treatments to control their pain perceived their pain to be significantly more severe than those who did not use treatments despite ongoing treatment. The most commonly used pain medications in the chronic stages of SCI were opioids, nonsteroidal anti-inflammatory drugs, and acetaminophen, closely followed by anticonvulsants, antispasticity medication, and sedatives (Table 17-2).

Although opioids are considered to be far less effective for the relief of neuropathic pain than for nociceptive pain,[154,156] their frequent use and the perceived usefulness of this drug[132] reported by some patients deserve further investigation (Table 17-3).

The idea that opioids may relieve neuropathic pain associated with SCI is supported by Yamamoto et al[157] and Jensen and Sindrup,[158] who suggested that specific subgroups of neuropathic pains may respond well to opioids. Another possibility is that opioids are effective in relieving the less-resistant pain types such as nociceptive musculoskeletal pain. Unfortunately, the specific pain types were not evaluated separately in the study by

Table 17-2
Reported Frequency Treatment Use for SCI-Related Chronic Pain

Nonpharmacological	%	Pharmacological Intervention	%
Massage	26.7	Opioids	22.5
Heat therapy	16.7	Nonsteroidal anti-inflammatory drugs	20.0
Other physiotherapy	15.0	Acetaminophen	18.3
Ice therapy	13.3	Anticonvulsants	17.5
Meditation	10.0	Antispasticity medication	16.7
		Sedatives	15.0
		Antidepressants	12.5

Adapted from: Widerström-Noga EG, Turk DC. Types and effectiveness of treatments used by people with chronic pain associated with spinal cord injuries: Influence of pain and psychosocial characteristics. *Spinal Cord.* 2003;41:600–609.

Table 17-3
Reported Effectiveness of Some Commonly Used Treatments

Interventions	Worse	No Effect	Slightly Better	Considerably Better	Pain-free
Physical therapy		7.5 %	42.5%	47.5%	2.5%
Psychological		23.1 %	61.5%	15.4%	
Opioids		18.5%	48.1%	22.2%	11.1%
Anticonvulsants		33.3%	42.9%	19.0%	4.8%
Antidepressants	6.6%	66.7 %	13.3%	13.3%	
Nonsteroidal anti-inflammatory drugs		29.2%	50.0%	20.8%	
Antispasticity medication		45.0%	40.0%	15.0%	
Sedatives	5.6%	16.7%	55.6%	22.2%	
Acetylsalicylic acid		54.6%	36.4%	9.1%	
Acetaminophen		36.4%	45.4%	18.2%	

Adapted from: Widerström-Noga EG, Turk DC. Types and effectiveness of treatments used by people with chronic pain associated with spinal cord injuries: Influence of pain and psychosocial characteristics. *Spinal Cord.* 2003;41:600–609.

Widerström-Noga and Turk.[132] Similar to findings by Warms et al,[133] massage and various physiotherapeutic interventions were among the most commonly used nonpharmacological pain treatments.[132] Various forms of physiotherapeutic interventions were reported to provide considerable to complete pain relief in 50% of people using these therapies, although the effects may only have been temporary. Thus, these types of interventions may potentially be useful as adjunct treatments in combination with pharmacotherapy for some people with SCI and chronic pain, even long after their injury.

The use of prescription medication has been shown to be associated with a number of pain characteristics as well as with specific psychosocial and behavioral responses to pain. In one study,[132] the use of prescription medication was not only associated with more intense pain, but also with a significantly greater number of painful areas and a significantly greater number of descriptive adjectives. In addition, pain that could either be evoked or aggravated by non-noxious stimuli was common among those who used prescription medication. Although these results suggest that the use of prescription medication is associated with having neuropathic pain, the results also show that the presence of multiple types of pain is associated with the use of prescription medication. Both spontaneous and evoked pain in the frontal aspects of the torso and genital area were found to be strongly related to the use of prescription medicine, suggesting that pain in this area is particularly bothersome. In summary, these findings suggest that people with SCI who experience intense neuropathic pains have a difficult time coping with them despite the use of prescription medicine and other types of treatments. Because different types of pain were not assessed separately in this study, it was not possible to determine whether people were using "appropriate" treatments, such as anticonvulsants for neuropathic pain.[159]

The chronic pain conditions associated with SCI are both complex and resistant to available treatments. People with SCI experience pain of various origins that are usually inadequately relieved by prescribed or self-initiated treatments, even many years after injury. Similar treatments and medications appear to be used for various types of pain; whereas high pain severity and impact on functioning are more likely to be related to the use of prescription medication. Important areas for future research include the development of standardized evaluation protocols with valid and reliable methods specific to the SCI population. Future research should also evaluate the efficacy of pharmacological treatments used in combination with nonpharmacologic treatments (e.g., physical therapy, cognitive behavioral therapy). Another important area of research and clinical work involves the development of multidisciplinary pain management programs[160] that are both tailored to type of pain (since the mechanisms underlying different pains are likely to differ) and to psychosocial factors. Despite the fact that evidence for clinical efficacy for most treatments is limited in this population, the development of standardized evidence-based clinical management strategies for pain following SCI is critical for progress in this area. Indeed, a clinical algorithm for the treatment of the various pain types associated with SCI was recently proposed by Siddall and Middleton.[161]

Summary

Chronic pain is a significant problem associated with SCI. An interdisciplinary perspective of pain associated with SCI that incorporates epidemiology, taxonomy, pathophysiological and psychosocial mechanisms of pain, pain evaluation, and clinical pain trials represents an optimal approach to this problem. Published research studies relevant for the understanding of these complex pain conditions give clinicians a framework upon which to base their treatments. It is hoped that this information will encourage the reader to appreciate the difficulties associated with chronic pain that the person with SCI encounters on a daily basis. Furthermore, it is hoped that the material presented here will trigger interest in the study of this important clinical problem that has the potential to significantly influence the quality of life in a person with SCI.

REVIEW QUESTIONS

1. What makes chronic pain a significant contributor to a decreased quality of life after a SCI?
2. What are the types of pain experienced after SCI, and how do they differ?
3. What is the difference between nociception and pain?
4. What are the known main pathophysiological mechanisms responsible for the development of neuropathic pain after a SCI?
5. What psychosocial factors are relevant for the maintenance and aggravation of chronic pain associated with SCI?
6. What assessment domains are important for capturing the multidimensional nature of pain?
7. What factors may evoke or aggravate pain associated with SCI?
8. How can imaging of the brain contribute to an increased understanding of pain?
9. What are the most common classes of pharmacological agents that have proven to be efficacious in various neuropathic pain conditions?

REFERENCES

1. Demirel G, Yllmaz H, Gencosmanoglu B et al. Pain following spinal cord injury. *Spinal Cord*. 1998;36:25–28.
2. Rintala DH, Loubser PG, Castro J et al. Chronic pain in a community-based sample of men with spinal cord injury: Prevalence, severity, and relationships with impairment, disability, handicap, and subjective well-being. *Arch Phys Med Rehabil*. 1998;79:604–614.
3. Siddall PJ, Taylor DA, McClelland JM, et al. Pain report and the relationship of pain to physical factors in the first 6 months following injury. *Pain*. 1999;81:187–197.
4. Turner JA, Cardenas DD. Chronic pain problems in individuals with spinal cord injuries. *Semin Clin Neuropsychiatry*. 1999;4:186–194.
5. Widerström-Noga EG, Felipe-Cuervo E, Broton JG et al. Perceived difficulty in dealing with consequences of spinal cord injury. *Arch Phys Med Rehabil*. 1999;80:580–586.
6. Turner JA, Cardenas DD, Warms CA et al. Chronic pain associated with spinal cord injuries: A community survey. *Arch Phys Med Rehabil*. 2001;82:501–509.
7. Finnerup NB, Johannesen IL, Sindrup SH et al. Pain and dysesthesia in patients with spinal cord injury: A postal survey. *Spinal Cord*. 2001;39:256–262.
8. Dalyan M, Cardenas DD, Gerard B. Upper extremity pain after spinal cord injury. *Spinal Cord*. 1999;37:191–195.
9. Ravenscroft A, Ahmed YS, Burnside IG. Chronic pain after SCI. A patient survey. *Spinal Cord*. 2000;38:611–614.
10. Widerström-Noga EG, Felipe-Cuervo E, Yezierski RP. Chronic pain following spinal cord injury: Interference with sleep and activities. *Arch Phys Med Rehabil*. 2001;82:1571–1577.
11. Norrbrink BC, Hultling C, Lundeberg T. Quality of sleep in individuals with spinal cord injury: A comparison between patients with and without pain. *Spinal Cord*. 2005;43:85–95.
12. Stensman R. Adjustment to traumatic spinal cord injury. A longitudinal study of self-reported quality of life. *Paraplegia*. 1994;32:416–422.
13. Westgren N, Levi R. Quality of life and traumatic spinal cord injury. *Arch Phys Med Rehabil*. 1998;79:1433–1439.
14. Kennedy P, Lude P, Taylor N. Quality of life, social participation, appraisals, and coping post spinal cord injury: A review of four community samples. *Spinal Cord*. 2006;44:95–105.
15. Widerström-Noga EG. Chronic pain and nonpainful sensations after spinal cord injury: Is there a relation? *Clin J Pain*. 2003;19:39–47.
16. Stormer S, Gerner HJ, Gruninger W et al. Chronic pain/dysesthesiae in spinal cord injury patients: Results of a multicentre study. *Spinal Cord*. 1997;35:446–455.
17. Rintala DH, Hart KA, Priebe MM. Predicting consistency of pain over a 10-year period in persons with spinal cord injury. *J Rehabil Res Dev*. 2004;41:75–88.
18. Cruz-Almeida Y, Martinez-Arizala A, Widerström-Noga EG. Chronicity of pain associated with spinal cord injury: A longitudinal analysis. *J Rehabil Res Dev*. 2005;42:585–594.
19. Jensen MP, Hoffman AJ, Cardenas DD. Chronic pain in individuals with spinal cord injury: A survey and longitudinal study. *Spinal Cord*. 2005;43:704–712.
20. Levi R, Hulting C, Nash M et al. The Stockholm spinal cord injury study 1. Medical problems in a regional SCI population. *Paraplegia*. 1995;33:308–315.
21. Bowsher D. Central pain: Clinical and physiological characteristics. *J Neurol Neurosurg Psychiatry*. 1996;61:62–69.
22. Siddall PJ, Cousins MJ. Spinal pain mechanisms. *Spine*. 1997;22:98–104.
23. Siddall PJ, Loeser JD. Pain following spinal cord injury. *Spinal Cord*. 2001;39:63–73.

24. Widerström-Noga EG, Felipe-Cuervo E, Yezierski RP. Relationships among clinical characteristics of chronic pain following spinal cord injury. *Arch Phys Med Rehabil.* 2001;82:1191–1197.

25. Ragnarsson KT. Management of pain in persons with spinal cord injury. *J Spinal Cord Med.* 1997;20:186–199.

26. Eide PK. Pathophysiological mechanisms of central neuropathic pain after spinal cord injury. *Spinal Cord.* 1998; 36:601–612.

27. Donovan WH, Dimitrijevic MR, Dahm L et al. Neurophysiological approaches to chronic pain following spinal cord injury. *Paraplegia.* 1982;20:135–146.

28. Bryce TN, Ragnarsson KT. Pain after spinal cord injury. *Phys Med Rehabil Clin N Am.* 2000;11:157–168.

29. Siddall PJ, Yezierski, RP, Loeser JD. Pain following spinal cord injury: Clinical features, prevalence, and taxonomy. *IASP Newsletter.* 2000;3:3–7.

30. Cardenas DD, Turner JA, Warms CA et al. Classification of chronic pain associated with spinal cord injuries. *Arch Phys Med Rehabil.* 2002;83:1708–1714.

31. Eide PK, Jorum E, Stenehjelm AE. Somatosensory findings in patients with spinal cord injury and central dyesthesia pain. *J Neurol Neurosurg Psychiatry.* 1996;60:411–415.

32. Komisaruk BR, Gerdes CA, Whipple B. "Complete" spinal cord injury does not block perceptual responses to genital self-stimulation in women. *Arch Neurol.* 1997;54:1513–1520.

33. Siddall PJ, McClelland JM, Rutkowski SB et al. A longitudinal study of the prevalence and characteristics of pain in the first 5 years following spinal cord injury. *Pain.* 2003; 103:249–257.

34. Loeser JD, Ward AA, White LE. Chronic deafferentation of human spinal cord neurons. *J Neurosurg.* 1968;29:48–50.

35. Yezierski RP, Park SH. The mechanosensitivity of spinal sensory neurons following intraspinal injection of quisqualic. *Neuroscience Lett.* 1993;157:115–119.

36. Edgar RE, Best LG, Quail PA et al. Computer assisted DREZ microcoagulation: Post traumatic spinal deafferentation pain. *J Spinal Disord.* 1993;6:48–56.

37. Wiesenfeld-Hallin Z, Hao J-X, Aldskogius H et al. Allodynia-like symptoms in rats after spinal cord ischemia: An animal model of central pain. In: Boivie J, Hansson P, Lindblom U, editors. *Touch, Temperature and Pain in Health and Disease: Mechanisms and Assessments. Progress in Pain Research and Management.* Seattle, WA: IASP Press; 1994. pp. 355–372.

38. Lenz FA, Kwan HC, Martin R et al. Characteristics of somatotopic organization and spontaneous neuronal activity in the region of the thalamic principal sensory nucleus in patients with spinal cord transection. *J Neurophysiol.* 1994;72:1570–1587.

39. Pertovaara A, Kontinen VK, Kalso, EA. Chronic spinal nerve ligation induces changes in response characteristics of nociceptive spinal dorsal horn neurons and in their descending regulation originating in the periaqueductal grey in the rat. *Exp Neurol.* 1997;147:428–436.

40. Defrin R, Ohry A, Blumen N et al. Characterization of chronic pain and somatosensory function in spinal cord injury subjects. *Pain.* 2001;89:253–263.

41. Finnerup NB, Johannesen IL, Fuglsang-Frederiksen A et al. Sensory function in spinal cord injury patients with and without central pain. *Brain.* 2003;126:57–70.

42. Boivie J, Leijon G, Johansson I. Central post-stroke pain— A study of the mechanisms through analyses of the sensory abnormalities. *Pain.* 1989;37:173–185.

43. Finnerup NB, Jensen TS. Spinal cord injury pain— Mechanisms and treatment. *Eur J Neurol.* 2004;11:73–82.

44. Hao JX, Kupers RC, Xu XJ. Response characteristics of spinal cord dorsal horn neurons in chronic allodynic rats after spinal cord injury. *J Neurophysiol.* 2004;92:1391–1399.

45. Vierck CJ Jr, Light AR. Effects of combined hemotoxic and anterolateral spinal lesions on nociceptive sensitivity. *Pain.* 1999;83:447–547.

46. Yezierski RP. Spinal cord injury: A model of central neuropathic pain. *Neurosignals.* 2005;14:182–193.

47. Christensen MD, Hulsebosch CE. Spinal cord injury and anti-NGF treatment results in changes in CGRP density and distribution in the dorsal horn in the rat. *Exp Neurol.* 1997;147:463–475.

48. Gwak YS, Nam TS, Paik KS et al. Attenuation of mechanical hyperalgesia following spinal cord injury by administration of antibodies to nerve growth factor in the rat. *Neurosci Lett.* 2003;336:117–120.

49. Crown ED, Ye Z, Johnson KM et al. Increases in the activated forms of ERK 1/2, p38 MAPK, and CREB are correlated with the expression of at-level mechanical allodynia following spinal cord injury. *Exp Neurol.* 2006;199: 397–407.

50. Hubscher CH, Johnson RD. Chronic spinal cord injury induced changes in the responses of thalamic neurons. *Exp Neurol.* 2006;197:177–188.

51. Pattany PM, Yezierski RP, Widerström-Noga EG et al. Proton magnetic resonance spectroscopy of the thalamus in patients with chronic neuropathic pain after spinal cord injury. *Am J Neuroradiol.* 2002;23:901–905.

52. Wiesenfeld-Hallin Z, Aldskogius H, Grant G et al. Central inhibitory dysfunctions: Mechanisms and clinical implications. *Behav Brain Sci.* 1997;20:420–425.

53. Hains BC, Waxman SG. Activated microglia contribute to the maintenance of chronic pain after spinal cord injury. *J Neurosci.* 2006;26:4308–4317.

54. DeLeo JA, Yezierski RP. The role of neuroinflammation and neuroimmune activation in persistent pain. *Pain.* 2001;90:1–6.

55. Nesic O, Lee J, Johnson KM et al. Transcriptional profiling of spinal cord injury-induced central neuropathic pain. *J Neurochem.* 2005;95:998–1014.

56. Peng XM, Zhou ZG, Glorioso JC et al. Tumor necrosis factor-alpha contributes to below-level neuropathic pain after spinal cord injury. *Ann Neurol.* 2006;59:843–851.

57. George A, Buehl A, Sommer C. Wallerian degeneration after crush injury of rat sciatic nerve increases endo- and epineurial tumor necrosis factor-alpha protein. *Neurosci Lett.* 2004;372:215–219.

58. Wieseler-Frank J, Maier SF, Watkins LR. Glial activation and pathological pain. *Neurochem Int.* 2004;45:389–395.

59. Turk DC, Rudy TE. Toward an empirically derived taxonomy of chronic pain patients: Integration of psychological assessment data. *J Consult Clin Psychol.* 1988; 56:233–238.

60. Summers JD, Rapoff MA, Varghese G et al. Psychosocial factors in chronic spinal cord injury pain. *Pain.* 1991;47:183–189.

61. Richards JS. Chronic pain and spinal cord injury: Review and comment. *Clin J Pain*. 1992;8:119–122.

62. Widerström-Noga EG, Turk DC. Exacerbation of chronic pain following spinal cord injury. *J Neurotrauma*. 2004;21:1384–1395.

63. Widerström-Noga EG, Duncan R, Turk DC. Psychosocial profiles of people with pain associated with spinal cord injury: Identification and comparison with other chronic pain syndromes. *Clin J Pain*. 2004;20:261–271.

64. Jacob KS, Zachariah K, Bhattacharji S. Depression in individuals with spinal cord injury: Methodological issues. *Paraplegia*. 1995;33:377–380.

65. Kennedy P, Frankel H, Gardner B et al. Factors associated with acute and chronic pain following traumatic spinal cord injuries. *Spinal Cord*. 1997;35:814–817.

66. Scivoletto G, Petrelli A, Di Lucente L et al. Psychological investigation of spinal cord injury patients. *Spinal Cord*. 1997;35:516–520.

67. King C, Kennedy P. Coping effectiveness training for people with spinal cord injury: Preliminary results of a controlled trial. *Br J Clin Psychol*. 1999;38:5–14.

68. Kemp BJ, Krause JS. Depression and life satisfaction among people ageing with post-polio and spinal cord injury. *Disabil Rehabil*. 1999;21:241–249.

69. Haythornthwaite JA, Benrud-Larson LM. Psychological aspects of neuropathic pain. *Clin J Pain*. 2000;16: S101–105.

70. Harker WF, Dawson DR, Boschen KA et al. A comparison of independent living outcomes following traumatic brain injury and spinal cord injury. *Int J Rehabil Res*. 2002;25: 93–102.

71. Ville I, Ravaud JF. Subjective well-being and severe motor impairments: The Tetrafigap survey on the long-term outcome of tetraplegic spinal cord injured persons. *Soc Sci Med*. 2001;52:369–384.

72. Vogel LC, Klaas SJ, Lubicky JP et al. Long-term outcomes and life satisfaction for adults who had pediatric spinal cord injuries. *Arch Phys Med Rehabil*. 1998;79:1496–1503.

73. Anderson CJ, Vogel LC. Employment outcomes of adults who sustained spinal cord injuries as children or adolescents. *Arch Phys Med Rehabil*. 2002;83:791–801.

74. McColl MA, Stirling P, Walker J et al. Expectations of independence and life satisfaction among aging spinal cord injured adults. *Disabil Rehabil*. 1999;21:231–240.

75. Kerns RD, Turk DC, Rudy TE. The West Haven-Yale Multidimensional Pain Inventory (WHYMPI). *Pain*. 1985; 23:345–356.

76. Jamison RN, Rudy TE, Penzien DB et al. Cognitive-behavioral classifications of chronic pain: Replication and extension of empirically derived patient profiles. *Pain*. 1994;57:277–292.

77. Bergström G, Bodin L, Jensen IB et al. Long-term, non-specific spinal pain: Reliable and valid subgroups of patients. *Behav Res Ther*. 2001;39:75–87.

78. Spertus IL, Burns J, Glenn B et al. Gender differences in associations between trauma history and adjustment among chronic pain patients. *Pain*. 1999;82:97–102.

79. Dijkers MP. Correlates of life satisfaction among persons with spinal cord injury. *Arch Phys Med Rehabil*. 1999; 80:867–876.

80. Turk DC, Dworkin RH, Allen RR et al. Core outcome domains for chronic pain clinical trials: IMMPACT recommendations. *Pain*. 2003;106:337–345.

81. De Gagné TA, Mikail SF, D'Eon JL. Confirmatory factor analysis of a 4-factor model of chronic pain evaluation. *Pain*. 1995;60:195–202.

82. Holroyd KA, Malinoski P, Davis MK et al. The three dimensions of headache impact: Pain, disability and affective distress. *Pain*. 1999;83:571–578.

83. Widerström-Noga, Turk DC. Outcome measures in chronic pain trials involving people with spinal cord injury. *SCI Psychosocial Process*. 2004;17:258–267.

84. Varni JW, Seid M, Kurtin PS. Pediatric health-related quality of life measurement technology: A guide for healthcare decision makers. *JCOM*. 1999;6:33–40.

85. Seid M, Varni JW, Jacobs J. Pediatric health-related quality-of-life measurement technology: Intersections between science, managed care, and clinical care. *J Clin Psychol Med Settings*. 2000;7:17–27.

86. Wincent A, Liden Y, Arner S. Pain questionnaires in the analysis of long lasting (chronic) pain conditions. *Eur J Pain*. 2003;7:311–321.

87. Turk DC, Melzack R, editors. *Handbook of Pain Assessment*. New York: Guilford Press; 2001.

88. Siddall PJ, Middleton JW. A proposed algorithm for the management of pain following spinal cord injury. *Spinal Cord*. 2006;44:67–77.

89. Jensen MP, Karoly P, Braver S. The measurement of clinical pain intensity: A comparison of six methods. *Pain*. 1986;27:117–126.

90. Melzack R. The short-form McGill Pain Questionnaire. *Pain*. 1987;30:191–197.

91. Kieburtz K, Simpson D, Yiannoutsos C et al. A randomized trial of amitriptyline and mexiletine for painful neuropathy in HIV infection. AIDS Clinical Trial Group 242 Protocol Team. *Neurology*. 1988;51:1682–1688.

92. Jamison RN, Fanciullo GJ, Baird JC. Computerized dynamic assessment of pain: Comparison of chronic pain patients and healthy controls. *Pain Med*. 2004;5: 168–177.

93. Feldman SI, Downey G, Schaffer-Neitz R. Pain, negative mood, and perceived support in chronic pain patients: A daily diary study of people with reflex sympathetic dystrophy syndrome. *J Consult Clin Psychol*. 1999;67:776–785.

94. Smith WB, Safer MA. Effects of present pain level on recall of chronic pain and medication use. *Pain*. 1993;55: 355–361.

95. Lindblom U. Analysis of abnormal touch, pain, and temperature sensation in patients. In: Boivie J, Hansson P, Lindblom U, editors. *Touch, Temperature, and Pain in Health and Disease: Mechanisms and Assessments. Progress in Pain Research and Management*. Seattle, WA: IASP Press; 1994. pp. 63–84.

96. Cruccu G, Anand P, Attal N et al. EFNS guidelines on neuropathic pain assessment. *Eur J Neurol*. 2004;l: 153–162.

97. Jörum E, Warncke T, Stubhaug A. Cold allodynia and hyperalgesia in neuropathic pain: The effect of N-methyl-D-aspartate (NMDA) receptor antagonist ketamine—a double-blind, cross-over comparison with alfentanil and placebo. *Pain*. 2003;101:229–235.

98. Bouhassira D, Attal N, Fermanian J et al. Development and validation of the Neuropathic Pain Symptom Inventory. *Pain*. 2004;108:248–257.

99. Melzack R, Wall PD. Pain mechanisms: A new theory. *Science*. 1965;150:971–979.

100. Basbaum AI, Fields HL. Endogenous pain control mechanisms: Review and hypothesis. *Ann Neurol.* 1987;4: 451–462.

101. Le Bars D, Dickenson AH, Besson JM. Diffuse noxious inhibitory controls (DNIC). Effects on dorsal horn convergent neurons in the rat. *Pain.* 1979;6:283–304.

102. Apkarian AV, Bushnell CM, Treede RD et al. Human brain mechanisms of pain perception and regulation in health and disease. *Eur J Pain.* 2005;9:463–484.

103. Dubner R. The neurobiology of persistent pain and its clinical implications. *Suppl Clin Neurophysiol.* 2004;57:3–7.

104. Rainville P, Duncan GH, Price DD et al. Pain affect encoded in human anterior cingulate but not somatosensory cortex. *Science.* 1997;277:968–971.

105. Tolle TR, Kaufmann T, Siessmeier T et al. Region-specific encoding of sensory and affective components of pain in the human brain: A positron emission tomography correlation analysis. *Ann Neurol.* 1999;45:40–47.

106. Fulbright RK, Troche CJ, Skudlarski P et al. Functional MR imaging of regional brain activation associated with the affective experience of pain. *Am J Roentgenol.* 2001;77:1205–1210.

107. Price DD. Psychological and neural mechanisms of the affective dimension of pain. *Science.* 2000;288:1769–1772.

108. Salt TE. Gamma-aminobutyric acid and afferent inhibition in the cat and rat ventrobasal thalamus. *Neuroscience.* 1989;28:17–26.

109. Roberts WA, Eaton SA, Salt TE. Widely distributed GABA-mediated afferent inhibition processes within the ventrobasal thalamus of rat and their possible relevance to pathological pain states and somatotopic plasticity. *Exp Brain Res.* 1992;89:363–372.

110. Ohara PT, Chazal G, Ralston HJ III. Ultrastructural analysis of GABA immunoreactive elements in the monkey thalamic ventrobasal complex. *J Comp Neurol.* 1989;283:541–558.

111. Williamson AM, Ohara PT, Ralston DD et al. An analysis of gamma-aminobutyric acidergic synaptic contacts in the thalamic reticular nucleus of the monkey. *J Comp Neurol.* 1994;349:182–192.

112. Bowsher D. Representation of somatosensory modalities in pathways ascending from the spinal anterolateral funiculus to the thalamus demonstrated by lesions in man. *Eur Neurol.* 2005;54:14–22.

113. Ralston HJ III, Ohara PT, Meng XW et al. Transneuronal changes of the inhibitory circuitry in the macaque somatosensory thalamus following lesions of the dorsal column nuclei. *J Comp Neurol.* 1996;371:325–335.

114. Govindaraju V, Young K, Maudsley AA. Proton NMR chemical shifts and coupling constants for brain metabolites. *NMR Biomed.* 2000;13:129–153.

115. Jeun SS, Kim MC, Kim BS et al. Assessment of malignancy in gliomas by 3T 1H MR spectroscopy. *Clin Imaging.* 2005;29:10–15.

116. Savic I, Osterman Y, Helms G. MRS shows syndrome differentiated metabolite changes in human-generalized epilepsies. *Neuroimage.* 2004;21:163–172.

117. Mueller SG, Laxer KD, Barakos JA et al. Metabolic characteristics of cortical malformations causing epilepsy. *J Neurol.* 2005;252:1082–1092.

118. Bowen BC, Block RE, Sanchez-Ramos J et al. Proton MR spectroscopy of the brain in 14 patients with Parkinson disease. *Am J Neuroradiol.* 1995;6:61–68.

119. Castillo M, Kwock L, Mukherji SK. Clinical applications of proton MR spectroscopy. *Am J Neuroradiol.* 1996;17:1–15.

120. Rule RR, Suhy J, Schuff N et al. Reduced NAA in motor and non-motor brain regions in amyotrophic lateral sclerosis: A cross-sectional and longitudinal study. *Amyotroph Lateral Scler Other Motor Neuron Disord.* 2004;5:141–149.

121. Isaacks RE, Bender AS, Kim CY et al. Effect of osmolality and myo-inositol deprivation on the transport properties of myo-inositol in primary astrocyte cultures. *Neurochem Res.* 1997;22:1461–1469.

122. Grachev ID, Ramachandran TS, Thomas PS et al. Association between dorsolateral prefrontal N-acetyl aspartate and depression in chronic back pain: An in vivo proton magnetic resonance spectroscopy study. *J Neural Transm.* 2003;110:287–312.

123. Phillips ML, Gregory LJ, Cullen S et al. The effect of negative emotional context on neural and behavioural responses to oesophageal stimulation. *Brain.* 2003;126:669–684.

124. Allman JM, Hakeem A, Erwin JM et al. The anterior cingulate cortex. The evolution of an interface between emotion and cognition. *Ann N Y Acad Sci.* 2001;935:107–117.

125. Seghier ML, Lazeyras F, Vuilleumier P et al. Functional magnetic resonance imaging and diffusion tensor imaging in a case of central poststroke pain. *J Pain.* 2005;6: 208–212.

126. Kishi Y, Robinson RG, Forrester AW. Prospective longitudinal study of depression following spinal cord injury. *J Neuropsychiatry and Clin Neurosci.* 1994;6:237–244.

127. Fuhrer MJ. The subjective well-being of people with spinal cord injury: Relationships to impairment, disability, and handicap. *Top Spinal Cord Inj Rehabil.* 1996;1:56–71.

128. Widerström-Noga EG, Duncan R, Felipe-Cuervo E et al. Assessment of the impact of pain and impairments associated with spinal cord injuries. *Arch Phys Med Rehabil.* 2002;83:395–404

129. Widerström-Noga EG, Cruz-Almeida Y, Martinez-Arizala A et al. Internal consistency, stability, and validity of the spinal cord injury version of the multidimensional pain inventory. *Arch Phys Med Rehabil.* 2006;87:516–523.

130. Cleeland CS, Ryan KM. Pain assessment: Global use of the brief pain inventory. *Ann Acad Med Singapore.* 1994;23:129–138.

131. Raichle KA, Osborne TL, Jensen MP et al. The reliability and validity of pain interference measures in persons with spinal cord injury. *J Pain.* 2006;7:179–186.

132. Widerström-Noga EG, Turk DC. Types and effectiveness of treatments used by people with chronic pain associated with spinal cord injuries: Influence of pain and psychosocial characteristics. *Spinal Cord.* 2003;41:600–609.

133. Warms CA, Turner JA, Marshall HM et al. Treatments for chronic pain associated with spinal cord injuries: Many are tried, few are helpful. *Clin J Pain.* 2002;18:154–163.

134. Vierck CJ Jr, Siddall P, Yezierski RP. Pain following spinal cord injury: Animal models and mechanistic studies. *Pain.* 2000;89:1–5.

135. Sindrup SH, Jensen TS. Efficacy of pharmacological treatments of neuropathic pain: An update and effect related to mechanism of drug action. *Pain.* 1999;83: 389–400.

136. Sindrup SH. Antidepressants as analgesics. In: Yaksh TL, Lynch C, Zapot WM et al., editors. *Anesthesia:Biological Foundations.* Philadelphia: Lippincott-Raven; 1997. pp. 987–997.

137. Dickenson AH, Matthews EA, Suzuki R. Neurobiology of neuropathic pain: Mode of action of anticonvulsants. *Eur J Pain*. 2002;6 Suppl A:51–60.

138. Campbell F, Graham J, Zilkha K. Clinical trial of carbamazepine in trigeminal neuralgia. *J Neurol Neurosurg Psychiatry*. 1966;29:265–267.

139. Backonja M, Beydoun A, Edwards K et al. Gabapentin for the symptomatic treatment of painful neuropathy in patients with diabetes mellitus: A randomized controlled trial. *JAMA*. 1998;280:1831–1836.

140. Rowbotham M, Harden N, Stacey B et al. Gabapentin for the treatment of postherpetic neuralgia: A randomized controlled trial. *JAMA*. 1998;280:1837–1842.

141. To TP, Lim TC, Hill ST et al. Gabapentin for neuropathic pain following spinal cord injury. *Spinal Cord*. 2002;40:282–285.

142. Putzke JD, Richards JS, Kezar L et al. Long-term use of gabapentin for treatment of pain after traumatic spinal cord injury. *Clin J Pain*. 2002;18:116–121.

143. Tai Q, Kirshblum S, Chen B et al. Gabapentin in the treatment of neuropathic pain after spinal cord injury: A prospective, randomized, double-blind, crossover trial. *J Spinal Cord Med*. 2002;25:100–105.

144. Finnerup NB, Sindrup SH, Bach FW et al. Lamotrigine in spinal cord injury pain: A randomized controlled trial. *Pain*. 2002;96:375–383.

145. Siddall PJ, Cousins MJ, Otte A et al. Pregabalin in central neuropathic pain associated with spinal cord injury: A placebo-controlled trial. *Neurology*. 2006;67:1792–800

146. Loubser PG, Donovan WH. Diagnostic spinal anaesthesia in chronic spinal cord injury pain. *Paraplegia*. 1991;29:25–36.

147. Attal N, Gaude V, Brasseur L et al. Intravenous lidocaine in central pain: A double-blind, placebo-controlled, psychophysical study. *Neurology*. 2000;54:564–574.

148. Ansari A. The efficacy of newer antidepressants in the treatment of chronic pain: A review of current literature. *Harv Rev Psychiatry*. 2000;7:257–277.

149. Millan MJ. The induction of pain: An integrative review. *Prog Neurobiol*. 1999;57:1–164.

150. Magni G. The use of antidepressants in the treatment of chronic pain: A review of the current evidence. *Drugs*. 1991;42:730–748.

151. Onghena P, Van Houdenhove B. Antidepressant-induced analgesia in chronic non-malignant pain: A meta-analysis of 39 placebo-controlled studies. *Pain*. 1992;49:205–219.

152. Max MB, Culnane M, Schafer SC et al. Amitriptyline relieves diabetic neuropathy pain in patients with normal or depressed mood. *Neurology*. 1987;37:589–596.

153. Cardenas DD, Warms CA, Turner JA et al. Efficacy of amitriptyline for relief of pain in spinal cord injury: Results of a randomized controlled trial. *Pain*. 2002;96:365–373.

154. McQuay HJ. Neuropathic pain: Evidence matters. *Eur J Pain*. 2002;6 Suppl A:11–18.

155. Fregni F, Boggio PS, Lima MC et al. A sham-controlled, phase II trial of transcranial direct current stimulation for the treatment of central pain in traumatic spinal cord injury. *Pain*. 2006;122:197–209.

156. Arner S, Meyerson BA. Lack of analgesic effect of opioids on neuropathic and idiopathic forms of pain. *Pain*. 1988;33:11–23.

157. Yamamoto T, Katayama Y, Hirayama T et al. Pharmacological classification of central post-stroke pain: Comparison with the results of chronic motor cortex stimulation therapy. *Pain*. 1997;72:5–12.

158. Jensen TS, Sindrup SH. Opioids: A way to control central pain? *Neurology*. 2002;58:517–518.

159. Jensen TS. Anticonvulsants in neuropathic pain: Rationale and clinical evidence. *Eur J Pain*. 2002;6 Suppl A:61–68.

160. Norrbrink Budh C, Kowalski J, Lundeberg T. A comprehensive pain management programme comprising educational, cognitive, and behavioural interventions for neuropathic pain following spinal cord injury. *J Rehabil Med*. 2006;38:172–180.

161. Siddall PJ, Middleton JW. A proposed algorithm for the management of pain following spinal cord injury. *Spinal Cord*. 2006;44:67–77.

Spasticity After Human Spinal Cord Injury

18

Christine K. Thomas, PhD
Edelle C. Field-Fote, PT, PhD

After reading this chapter, the reader will be able to:

OBJECTIVES

- Differentiate among spasticity, tone, hyperreflexia, and rigidity
- Describe spasticity and its associated signs
- Discuss ways that spasticity may be beneficial and ways that spasticity can be problematic
- Explain clinical tests that are used to quantify spasticity
- Discuss some of the physical treatments that have been shown to reduce spasticity
- Compare and contrast the medications that are commonly used to treat spasticity

Introduction

Tone, Hyperreflexia, and Spasticity

Damage to the central nervous system frequently results in pathophysiology of the motor control system. One consequence of this pathophysiology is an alteration in the regulation of muscle tone, such that tone is increased (i.e., *hypertonia*) or decreased (i.e., *hypotonia*). *Muscle tone* is the resting tension in a muscle that is evidenced by its resistance to the elongation associated with imposed movement at a joint. Tone reflects both the balance of excitatory and inhibitory influences on the spinal motoneuron innervating the muscle and the intrinsic elastic properties of the muscle itself. When the neuropathology involves damage to the upper motor neurons or their descending pathways, there is a loss of modulation of spinal reflexes such that these reflexes become more responsive to afferent (sensory) input. This increased responsiveness of spinal reflex activity is termed *hyperreflexia* and contributes to involuntary muscle contractions (spasms) in response to afferent input.

One form of hyperreflexia, *spasticity*, has historically been associated with increased responsiveness of the monosynaptic stretch reflex. The monosynaptic stretch reflex (also called the *deep tendon reflex*, the *Ia reflex*, and the *phasic stretch reflex*) is one of many spinal reflexes, but by virtue of being monosynaptic (i.e., having only a single synapse between the afferent and efferent limb of the reflex arc), it gives rise to motor responses to afferent input (in this case the afferent input being muscle stretch) that are among the fastest responses in the nervous system. The classical definition of spasticity as being "a velocity-dependent increase in resistance to passive stretch,"[1] reflects the supposed relationship between the monosynaptic stretch reflex and spasticity.

Characterizing Spasticity

Despite the historical attribution of spasticity to impaired regulation of the monosynaptic stretch reflex, it is well recognized that the signs associated with spasticity may occur in response to forms of afferent input other than muscle stretch (e.g., cutaneous input such as touch of the skin or prick from a sharp object and mechanical input such as pulling of the hair on the limb). Thus, in the clinic, involuntary contractions and other associated signs (i.e., clonus, clasped-knife phenomenon, flexor reflexes, extensor spasms, irradiation of spasms, unusual co-contractions during movements) have also been labeled as spasticity, thereby extending the classical definition.[2-6] This group of signs in combination with muscle weakness due to impaired voluntary control in those with motor incomplete injury is termed *spastic paresis*, or in cases wherein there is an absence of voluntary muscle control in individuals with motor complete injury, *spastic paralysis*. For reasons that are not entirely clear, spasticity seems to be more problematic for individuals with motor incomplete injury compared to those with motor complete injury.[7] This may be because the residual descending supraspinal inputs are no longer appropriate for the spinal circuits that have reorganized after SCI.

In spasticity, the muscles on one side of the joint demonstrate increased responsiveness to afferent input. Unless the length and range of motion of the spastic muscle is maintained with a consistent program of stretching, this prolonged static posturing of the limb results in shortening of the soft tissue (both muscles and tendons), making it resistant to stretch and resulting in muscle contractures. Spastic muscles and their tendons are known to undergo intrinsic, structural changes that make them more resistant to stretch.[8-11] This may explain why spastic muscles seem to develop more tension when stretched compared to muscles that are not spastic.[12]

Spasticity is not evident in the early stages after spinal cord injury (SCI). In fact, within the first weeks after trauma, the nervous system may be relatively unresponsive to afferent input; this period has been referred to as *spinal shock*. However, even in individuals with acute SCI, there is typically not a complete absence of reflexes.[13] This transient period of relative areflexia is a physiologic response to trauma and may involve areas that were not directly affected by the injury. The period of spinal shock typically resolves within 2 to 6 weeks after trauma and, in those who do not have purely lower motor neuron damage, is usually followed by the development of spastic paresis or spastic paralysis.

Spasticity is also observed in cases where the upper motor neurons have been damaged, such as in stroke and cerebral palsy; in cases where the conduction in the descending pathways from these upper motor neurons is impaired, such as occurs in multiple sclerosis; and in cases where there has been injury to the brainstem. However, there are differences between spasticity of spinal origin and that of cerebral origin.[6,14] Rigidity is another disorder of movement associated with hypertonia that is sometimes confused with spasticity. However, rigidity is not associated with SCI. Differences between spasticity and rigidity can be observed in their respective responses to externally imposed movement (i.e., stretch) as well as other characteristic signs as summarized in Table 18-1 (*see* Sanger et al[15] for review).

Some individuals with SCI learn to use their spasticity to perform functional tasks such as transferring from a chair to a bed by initiating or "triggering" their spasms at the appropriate time. However, other individuals find that spasticity interferes with their mobility and ability to perform activities of daily living; for individuals who must rely on a caregiver for assistance, spasticity may make care more difficult. From a clinical perspective it is important to know how these symptoms of spasticity can be evaluated reliably, when they are problematic, and how they can be managed. In this chapter, we will summarize the incidence of problematic spasticity after human SCI

Table 18-1

Characteristics of Spasticity Versus Rigidity

	Spasticity	Rigidity
Associated with SCI	Yes, and other upper motor neuron disorders	No, associated with disorders of the basal ganglia
Onset of resistance to stretch	Resistance initiated at a threshold speed of imposed movement and/or joint angle	Resistance encountered at all speeds of imposed movement regardless of joint angle
Influence of rate of stretch	Resistance to externally imposed movement (stretch) increases as a function of the speed of the stretch.	Resistance is not dependent on speed, and resistance is present even at low speeds.
Influence of direction of stretch	Greater in one particular direction of imposed movement (i.e., toward flexion versus toward extension)	Resistance encountered regardless of direction of imposed movement
Tendency for posturing of limbs	If present, arises from the increased muscle activity on one side of a joint	Tonic posturing of the limbs due to increased muscle activity on both sides of the joint
Typical posturing	The upper extremities tend to adopt a posture of flexion; the lower extremities usually adopt a posture of extension.	The trunk and the upper and lower extremities tend to adopt a flexed posture.
Neural origin	Reflects a loss of spinal reflex modulation that results in hyperreflexia	Reflects increase in tonic excitation from the extrapyramidal systems (primarily the basal ganglia)
Babinski sign	Positive	Negative

and describe how certain aspects of spasticity can be measured in the clinic. We will review the relative importance of changes in spinal inhibition, neuron excitability, and neuromuscular properties to spasticity, drawing on the most pertinent research performed on either animals or humans. Then we will examine the treatments currently used to ameliorate spasticity, a process that requires us to explore the scientific rationale behind these interventions and to critically evaluate whether these treatments are effective.

For additional insight on spasticity, including how it is defined and assessed, physical and pharmacological interventions for spasticity management, and evidence for the factors involved in spasticity, there are other informative reviews.[16–24]

Incidence of Spasticity in Humans With SCI

Most individuals with SCI (60% to 80%) report signs of spasticity at 1 year post-injury. For 30% to 40% of these individuals, particularly those with cervical SCI, the symptoms are problematic (see Table 18-2). Variation in the incidence of spasticity is to be expected for a number

of reasons. First, spasticity is defined in different ways, both in the clinic and by the injured individual. Second, each of the symptoms of spasticity is assessed using tests that measure different parameters. Third, the severity and distribution of spasticity can vary for different joints or muscles, may change during the day, and may vary over the long term. Fourth, responses may depend on the stimulus used to initiate the response (e.g., the speed at which a joint is moved) and the position of the limb.[8] Finally, whether individuals with SCI judge spasticity as problematic also depends on whether they use symptoms of spasticity to help them perform tasks such as turning in bed or whether these changes in their limbs and muscle behavior interfere with everyday activities.[3,7,16]

Multiple Factors Contribute to Spasticity

Neural Contributions

After a SCI, various descending pathways may be damaged (corticospinal, vestibulospinal, reticulospinal, rubrospinal), and different pathways may be damaged to

Table 18-2
Incidence of Spasticity After Human Spinal Cord Injury

Subject Sample, %	Incidence, %	Problematic Spasticity, %	Injury Duration, yrs	Number of Subjects	Reference
C, AIS A: 17	93	36	0–18+	55	Sköld et al[5]
C, AIS B–D: 28	78	43		90	
T, AIS A: 24	72	23		78	
T, AIS B–D: 16	73	25		51	
L–S, AIS A: 2	0	0		5	
L–S, AIS B–D: 13	26	5		43	
Complete: 52	88	50	1–44	25	Little et al[7]
Incomplete: 48	78	82		23	
All	82	91		48	
C: 48–53		34	1	357	Johnson et al[166]
T1–T6: 11–12		31	3	269	
T7–T12: 19-24		28	5	170	
L–S: 15–16					
C1–C8: 48	89	52	118 ± 7	46	Maynard et al[167]
T1–7:11	82	45	days	11	
T8–12: 21	45	20		20	
L1–S5: 20	26	10		19	
All:				96	
Comp. tetraplegia		50	>1	117	Noreau et al[168]
Comp. paraplegia		39		183	
Incomp. tetraplegia		40		94	
Incomp. paraplegia		29		88	
All		40		482	
All levels		12	± 4	270	Westgren and Levi[169]

C = cervical; T = thoracic; L = lumbar; S = sacral; Comp = complete; Incomp = incomplete

different extents. Descending signals may be eliminated, reduced, or changed, all of which will alter the type and/or strength of inputs that reach the spinal cord. Any disruption of descending input not only results in decreased voluntary drive to the motoneurons (and therefore paresis and varying amounts of paralysis[25]), but also leads to changes in the discharge rates of motoneurons.[26] Modulation of spinal reflex activity is also altered, not so much because of the decreased input to the motoneurons themselves, but as a result of the change in input to the interneurons that regulate motoneuron

activity. Likewise, disruption or damage to afferent and intraspinal pathways will influence the balance of spinal excitation and inhibition (e.g., changes in presynaptic inhibition of Ia terminals, group II afferents, autogenic inhibition from Golgi tendon organs via Ib afferents, recurrent inhibition via motor axon collaterals and Renshaw cells, reciprocal inhibition from Ia afferents from antagonistic muscles, and propriospinal fibers). With time, the strength of intact synaptic inputs may change, new inputs may arise from collateral (dendritic) sprouting, the sensitivity of receptors in the neuronal membranes may increase, the excitability of the various spinal neurons may be enhanced (i.e., alpha motoneurons, interneurons, propriospinal neurons, gamma motoneurons), and there may be alterations in the intrinsic properties of muscle fibers, sensory receptors (e.g., muscle spindles), connective tissue, and joints. All of these factors have the potential to influence the transmission in spinal pathways, the excitability of reflexes, and muscle tone and spasms. We now consider these possibilities in more detail, starting with afferent inputs to the spinal cord.

Weeks after SCI, increases in muscle tone are likely. In addition, trivial inputs (e.g., pushing a wheelchair over a bumpy pavement) can evoke reflex contractions in paralyzed muscles. Despite this, there is little evidence for excessive afferent activity (impulses in Ia afferent or cutaneous fibers) at rest in the nerves of individuals who experience spasticity.[27–30] However, few recordings have been made. Overall, the data suggest that prolonged inputs are not necessary to evoke hyperexcitable reflex responses after SCI, that the sensitivity of peripheral sensors has not changed, and that the spasms probably reflect an exaggerated central response to incoming signals, from whatever source.

Changes in neuron excitability may enhance reflexes, but these changes are difficult to examine in humans, even for motoneurons. One way to measure motoneuron excitability is to evaluate the amplitude and the persistence of F-waves (the antidromic impulse induced by a single stimulus to a peripheral nerve can re-excite the motoneuron to elicit a second, smaller orthodromic electromyographic [EMG] potential, termed an *F-wave*.) [31] F-wave magnitude and persistence are reduced immediately after SCI, but usually recover with time.[4,32,33] However, F-wave data vary widely across subjects and for different motor units,[34,35] making it likely that the excitability of only some motoneurons has increased.

In animals, it is possible to examine changes in the intrinsic properties of neurons. The voltage-dependent, persistent inward sodium and calcium currents that amplify and prolong the response of motoneurons to synaptic excitation are depressed following SCI, but later recover.[36] These currents may themselves change. They may also be facilitated by long excitatory postsynaptic potentials[37] and the lack of inhibition needed to terminate them.[22,38,39] Although not yet documented, similar changes may also occur in interneurons, gamma motoneurons, and propriospinal neurons. One indication of the operation of these persistent currents in humans with SCI may be the prolonged motor unit activity observed in paralyzed muscles[40,41] after vibration or electrical stimulation,[42–44] during spasms,[25,45] and during voluntary contractions of muscles weakened by injury.[46] Individuals with SCI have difficulty terminating this activity, so the source of the spontaneity may be the motoneuron itself. This would be consistent with the changes in resting membrane potential of

lumbar motoneurons and the changes in the level at which spikes are triggered in rats after weeks of spinal transection.[47] However, only some neurons may be influenced, as other reports indicate decreases in motoneuron excitability after months of cord transection in cats.[48,49]

Disturbances in excitatory and inhibitory inputs, known to occur after chronic human SCI, must contribute to the enhancement of reflexes, muscle tone, and spasms. At rest, there are reports of reductions in presynaptic inhibition of primary afferent terminals after SCI,[50] decreases in postactivation depression of the Ia afferent–motoneuron synapse,[51–54] reductions in corticospinal inhibition onto propriospinal neurons and associated interneurons, interruption of the usual gating of monoaminergic inputs from the brainstem to group II afferents,[55] decreases in inhibition from activation of Ib afferents from Golgi tendon organs,[56,57] and reductions in reciprocal Ia inhibition,[58,59] although the latter seems less pronounced when recovery is improved and spasticity is reduced.[60,61] Reciprocal Ia inhibition can even increase, depending on muscle, injury completeness, or conditioning test interval.[62,63]

These measurements made are at rest and are important in that they allow examination of how reflexes respond to relatively well-defined inputs. However, reflex modulation is also task dependent (e.g., at rest impulses from Ib afferents of ankle extensors are inhibitory, but reverse their effects to become excitatory when a cat locomotes[64]). Thus, reflexes also need to be examined in a behavioral context, although these recordings are more difficult to obtain and to interpret. Many movements involve excitation of agonist and antagonistic muscles. For movements to be smooth, the changes in the gain and the amplitude of reflexes during contractions have to be balanced across muscles. For example, the soleus H-reflex usually increases during the stance phase of walking and decreases during swing,[65] as descending inputs modulate interneurons that enhance presynaptic inhibition of Ia terminals on motoneurons antagonist to contracting muscle. After SCI, this modulation of the soleus H-reflex is absent or reduced,[66] suggesting that poor modulation of presynaptic inhibition of Ia terminals is one factor that must underlie the functional impairment. Similarly, reciprocal Ia inhibition of the soleus H-reflex from dorsiflexors typically occurs at the onset of dorsiflexion in nondisabled individuals.[67] Abnormal reciprocal inhibition may reduce or delay relaxation of antagonistic muscles and disrupt voluntary contractions.[68,69] Furthermore, Ib afferent activity from Golgi tendon organs produced by the contraction of agonist muscles can facilitate co-contraction of antagonists, which may disrupt voluntary movement.[63] In individuals with spasticity, all of these factors contribute to changes in the typical task-dependent modulation of reflex excitability observed in nondisabled individuals.[53,59,66] Thus, the extent to which spasticity impairs movement depends on the excitability of the reflexes in all of the involved muscles, as this will potentially alter the timing and extent of activation of agonist and antagonist muscles. Muscle activity left unchecked may also result in reflex irradiation because of the widespread heteronymous Ia connections between muscles.

Muscle, Connective Tissue, and Joint Contributions

Changes in muscle properties after human SCI (weakness, slowness, fatigability, altered activity [reviewed by Thomas and Zijdewind[41]]), connective tissues,[70] and joints may also constrain movements, change muscle tone, and increase resistance of the muscle to passive stretch. There is evidence to indicate that changes in the intrinsic properties of the muscle contribute to the increased stiffness observed in spasticity.[8-11] The extended periods of limb immobility that are typical in individuals with spasticity[71] likely lead to the many of the same connective tissue changes that are observed in studies of limb immobilization[72,73] and may result in the development of contractures.[74] Reliable distinction between the changes in passive tissue properties and changes that relate to neural processes is difficult to assess in the clinic. Their contribution to spasticity usually requires other biomechanical and EMG analyses.

The Clinical Measurement of Spasticity

Reliable assessments of the various presentations of spasticity are important, both to evaluate possible treatment options and to judge whether any treatment is effective. In the clinic, muscle tone is usually graded subjectively in response to movement at one velocity. Reliability depends on the consistent implementation of the assessment and consistent judgment of the examiner. Because of this, inter-rater reliability of the tests varies considerably. Clinical tests of spasticity include the Ashworth scale or Modified Ashworth Scalethe Tardieu Scale or Modified Tardieu Scale, the pendulum test, the Spinal Cord Assessment Tool for Spastic reflexes (SCATS), and the Penn Spasm Frequency Scale or Snow Spasm Frequency Scale. We describe each of these assessments, with some comments on the advantages and disadvantages of each measure. The evaluation criteria and the scoring systems vary across the tests; therefore, the test results are not necessarily comparable. In addition, we describe the Hoffman reflex (H-reflex), which is considered the electrical equivalent of the stretch reflex. While not a clinical measure, this electrophysiological test is frequently used in rehabilitation-related research and is reported in relation to the maximal evoked response of the same muscle (M-wave). An elevated H/M ratio is often used as a measure of spasticity, although it does not tell us whether this change relates to an increase in motoneuron excitability, a change in afferent transmission to the motoneuron, or both possibilities.[23]

Ashworth Scale

The Ashworth Scale[75] and Modified Ashworth Scale[76] are biomechanical tests that evaluate muscle tone and stretch reflexes elicited by movement. One of five (or six) grades is assigned by the evaluator depending on the amount of resistance the evaluator experiences to passive movement and where in the movement resistance occurs (*see* Table 18-3).

Consistent evaluation by one individual becomes critical because spasticity varies across joints. Responses change with the speed of limb movement, the range of the movement, and the number of joint movements that are made. Contractures may limit the range of movement that is possible at a joint. Therefore, in the presence of contractures, grades generated using the Ashworth Scale or Modified Ashworth Scale may result in values that do not reflect the behavior of the spastic muscle.[77] Furthermore, there can be changes in the structural properties of the spastic muscle that increase its stiffness. In the clinic, it is questionable whether these passive changes in muscle can be distinguished from stretch reflex activity that arises from neural processes and is velocity dependent.[78]

Tardieu Scale

Defining the neural component of spasticity may be feasible with another biomechanical test, the Tardieu Scale (see Table 18-4), which involves passive movement of the joint through its range at three different velocities. The intensity and duration of the muscle reaction to each stretch is rated on a 5-point scale, along with the joint angle at which the muscle reaction is first felt[79] (for an English description, see Scholtes et al[80]). To reduce the time involved in this assessment, the Tardieu scale was modified to measure the joint angle at which muscle contraction was encountered in response to a fast velocity stretch (see Boyd and Graham[81]). With either test, it is difficult to standardize the velocity of the movement in the clinic. Use of extremes (very slow and very fast velocity of stretch) and a standard test position may improve the repeatability of this assessment method. Compared to the Ashworth Scale, the Tardieu Scale more accurately reflects the behavioral response of the muscle in indi-viduals who have contractures.[77]

Pendulum Test

The pendulum test is also a biomechanical measure of spasticity. This test assesses the responsiveness of knee

Table 18-3

Ashworth Scale and Modified Ashworth Scale

Score	Ashworth Scale	Score	Modified Ashworth Scale
0	No increase in muscle tone	0	No increase in muscle tone
1	Slight increase in muscle tone, with the limb "catching" when it is flexed and extended	1	Slight increase in muscle tone, manifested by a catch and release or by minimal resistance at the end range of motion when the affected part(s) is flexed or extended
		2	Slight increase in muscle tone, manifested as a catch, followed by minimal resistance throughout the remainder (less than half) of the range of movement
2	More marked increase in tone, but limb easily flexed	3	More marked increase in tone through most of the range of movement, but the limb is easily moved
3	Considerable increase in tone; passive movement difficult	4	Considerable increase in muscle tone; passive movement difficult
4	Limb rigid in flexion and extension	5	Tested extremity rigid in flexion and extension

extensor muscles to rapid, gravity-assisted stretch. The individual is positioned supine on a mat table such that the knee is flexed and the lower legs hang over the edge of the table. The examiner grasps the heel of one foot, extends the knee, and then releases the heel, allowing the lower part of that leg to swing. The excursion of the first swing (the knee joint angle at which contraction of the quadriceps first causes reversal from knee flexion to knee extension) has been shown to be a good indicator of the level of spasticity, and this measure is preferable to using the number or duration of oscillations as the indicator of spasticity level.[82] This test has been shown to be a

Table 18-4

Tardieu Scale

Score	Intensity and Duration of Reflex	Score	Velocity of Stretch
0	No reflex		
1	Only visible contraction	1	Slow
2	Contraction with a short catch	2	Under gravity
3	Contraction lasting a few seconds or fatigable clonus after a few seconds	3	Rapid
4	Contraction lasting a few seconds or sustained clonus, not even for a few seconds	Range-of-motion	Joint angle at which reflex assessed and velocity used

reproducible,[83] valid, and sensitive measure for assessment of spasticity in the clinic.[82,84] Application of the pendulum test to assess the responsiveness of muscles other than the quadriceps muscle may be difficult, however.

The Spinal Cord Assessment Tool for Spastic Reflexes

The Spinal Cord Assessment Tool for Spastic reflexes (SCATS) is a clinical tool intended to quantify the magnitude and duration of reflex responses to imposed movement or stimulation.[85] The SCATS includes assessments of the response of the soleus muscle to imposed stretch (clonus), stimulation of the foot to evaluate the flexor reflex response, and imposed hip and knee extension to examine the extensor response. The test position, stimulus, response type and response scoring criteria are given in Table 18-5. Responses to the SCATS items have been shown to be well correlated with kinematic and EMG data. The SCATS clonus scores and flexor spasm scores correlate with some clinical measures such as the Ashworth scores. The clonus scores are correlated with the Penn spasm frequency scale. The benefit of the SCATS tool is that it allows clinicians to evaluate various motor responses that contribute to the manifestation of spasticity, measures that may be weighted differently, therefore presenting different problems in various individuals. One of the limitations of the SCATS is that the measurement of reflex duration is limited to a maximum of 10 seconds (i.e., a response lasting 10 seconds denotes the highest spasticity level). Some individuals with severe

Table 18-5
The Spinal Cord Assessment Tool for Spastic Reflexes

Test	Position	Stimulus	Response	Rating
Ankle clonus	Supine, stand on medial side of tested limb, hold limb off surface, place one hand under calf and the other grasping ball of foot	Rapid, passive dorsiflexion movement of the ankle	Clonic bursts of soleus muscle Observe/record duration	0—no reaction 1—mild, <3 sec 2—moderate, 3–10 sec 3—severe, >10 sec
Flexor spasm	Supine, tested limb with hip and knee at 0 degree flexion	Pinprick of 1 sec duration to medial arch of foot	Excursion of great toe into extension Ankle dorsiflexion Knee/hip flexion Observe/record ROM	0—no reaction 1—mild, <10 degree extension of great toe **or** <10 degrees knee/hip flexion 2—moderate, 10–30 degrees knee/hip flexion 3—severe, >30 degrees knee/hip flexion
Extensor spasm	Supine, contralateral limb extended, stand on lateral side of tested limb, hold limb in 90–110 degree knee/hip flexion, one hand cupping heel, the other on the posterior calf	Passive extension of knee and hip simultaneously	Quadriceps muscle contraction, superior displacement of the patella Observe/record duration	0—no reaction 1—mild, <3 sec 2—moderate, 3–10 sec 3—severe, >10 sec

spasticity have longer duration responses, so 10 seconds may not be a sufficient duration to identify intervention-related changes in these individuals or to allow distinctions to be made among individuals with severe spasticity.

Penn Spasm Frequency Scale and Snow Scale

The Penn Spasm Frequency Scale (see Table 18-6) consists of one of five numerical scores that are primarily assigned according to the frequency of muscle spasms per hour.[86] The Snow Scale rates spasm number by day.[87] These scales largely assume that it is the number of these involuntary contractions that makes them problematic. Contraction intensity may also disrupt everyday activities, but the terms *mild* or *full* spasms are not clearly defined in the Penn scale. Similarly, the duration of the contractions, the type of contraction (e.g., the repeated, rhythmic contractions of clonus), or the combination of muscles that contract may determine whether or not a task is disrupted. Moreover, what one individual with SCI considers a spasm, another may not. These scales also depend on the individual's recollection of the events. Given that most SCIs involve both sensory and motor deficits, it is possible that the individual may not perceive some of the spasms. Along these lines, individuals report that spasms can disrupt sleep,[5,7] but if the individual is not awakened by spasms, then he or she would not report these events. Objective assessments of muscles as they spasm are needed. To objectively quantify activity in paralyzed muscles, long-term recordings (24 hours) of

EMG activity have been initiated.[71] These data can be correlated to subjective spasm ratings to define what a spasm is, to quantify what features of the involuntary contractions disrupt function, and to verify the reliability of spasm frequency scales. To our knowledge, no assessment of the reliability of these spasm frequency scales has been published.

The Hoffman Reflex

The *Hoffman reflex* (or *H-reflex*) is the response of a muscle to stimulation of the sensory component of its nerve. While many reflex circuits likely contribute to the H-reflex, it is thought that the Ia reflex (i.e., the monosynaptic stretch reflex) makes a significant contribution to the response.[88] For this reason, the H-reflex is considered the electrophysiological equivalent of the monosynaptic stretch reflex. Since the monosynaptic stretch reflex is thought to make a considerable contribution to spasticity, numerous rehabilitation-related studies have used the H-reflex as an indirect measure of spasticity.[89-91] Because of its widespread use, it is important to have knowledge of the H-reflex test. However, this approach is not without significant limitations,[92-95] not the least of which is that electrically evoked responses (i.e., H-reflex amplitude) often do not correlate with the responses evoked with mechanical activation of the reflex (i.e., muscle stretch in response to tendon tap).[96-98]

The procedure for measuring H-reflex amplitude involves electrical stimulation of a mixed nerve and recording both the reflex (indirect) and the direct EMG response in the associated muscle. When a stimulus pulse with a long duration is used (i.e., 1 msec pulse duration), the large afferent (sensory) nerve fibers (especially the Ia fibers) respond at a lower threshold (i.e., a lower stimulus intensity) than do the motor (efferent) nerve fibers. The afferent impulses are conveyed to the spinal cord where the Ia afferent fibers synapse with the alpha motoneurons. The excitation of the alpha motoneurons results in excitation of the muscle and an ensuing muscle contraction. This contraction is the *indirect* motor response evoked by reflex activation of the motoneurons via the Ia afferent fibers (and likely other fibers as well).[88] In the soleus muscle, the latency from the onset of the stimulating pulse to the afferent-evoked reflex response in the muscle is approximately 30 to 40 msec (*see* Fig. 18-1A).

In assessing the H-reflex, the stimulation intensity is increased in small increments until the maximal H-reflex (H_{max}) is recorded. As the H-reflex responses approach their maximum amplitude, the motor fibers in the nerve begin to reach threshold in response to the nerve stimulation, resulting in a *direct* motor response (M-response or M-wave) with contraction of the muscle at a latency of approximately 10 msec following the onset of the stimulating pulse (*see* Fig. 18-1B). As stimulus intensity is increased further, the amplitude of the M-wave increases, while the amplitude of the H-reflex decreases. This

Table 18-6
Spasm Frequency Scales

Penn Spasm Frequency Scale	Score	Snow Spasm Frequency Scale
No spasms	0	No spasms
Mild spasms induced by stimulation	1	≤1 spasm per day
Infrequent full spasms, <1 per hour	2	1–5 spasms per day
2–10 spasms per hour	3	5–9 spasms per day
>10 spasms per hour	4	≥10 spasms per day, or continuous contraction

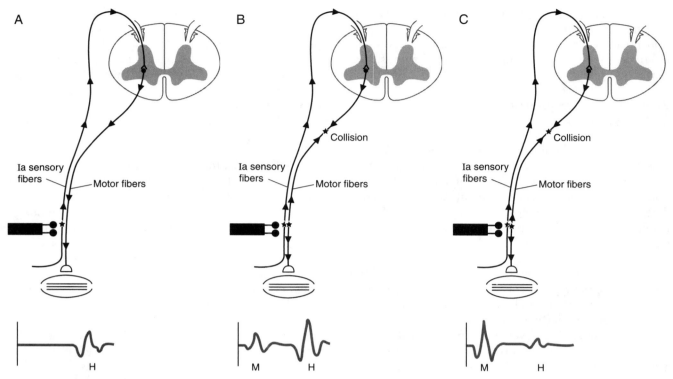

Figure 18-1 Measurement of the H-reflex and M-wave responses. (A) The stimulating electrode is placed near a mixed nerve and stimulus intensity is increased to activate the Ia sensory fibers and elicit a H-reflex in the muscle. (Note H in signal trace below circuit diagram.) (B) As stimulation intensity is increased, it reaches an intensity that begins to active the motor fibers, resulting in an M-wave. (Note M and H in signal trace below circuit diagram.) (C) At high levels of stimulation, there is collision between the antidromic motor-evoked response in the motor nerve and the orthodromic reflex-evoked response. The two signals collide, cancelling each other, and only the orthodromic motor response is observed (M-wave; noted in the signal trace below the circuit diagram.) M = M-wave; H = H-reflex.

decrease in H-reflex amplitude is the result of collision between the afferent-evoked impulses traveling along the motor nerve (Ia afferent fiber to motor neuron to motor nerve) in the direction of the muscle (in the orthodromic conduction direction) and the motor-evoked impulses traveling in the direction of the spinal cord (in the antidromic conduction direction), resulting in signal cancellation (Fig. 18-1C). Therefore, at high stimulus intensities, the reflex-evoked motor response is eliminated, and all that remains is the direct motor response. Figure 18-2 illustrates the recruitment of the H-reflex and the M-wave as stimulus intensity is increased.

The amplitude of the EMG signal associated with the maximal H-reflex represents the amount of muscle that can be recruited via the reflex pathway. However, because muscle atrophy may affect the size of the evoked reflex response, the H-reflex must be normalized to the total available muscle response (maximum M-wave or M_{max}), determined by delivering electrical stimuli of supramaximal intensity to the peripheral nerve. Therefore, the resulting H_{max}/M_{max} ratio (i.e., the H/M ratio) theoretically represents the magnitude of the muscle response that can be elicited via the reflex pathway as a proportion of the total muscle response. Given that spasticity is a form of hyperreflexia, it is not surprising that in individuals with

spasticity the reflex-evoked muscle contraction activates a larger proportion of available muscle, resulting in a larger H/M ratio. Nondisabled individuals typically have an H/M ratio in the range of 0.4 to 0.6, and individuals with spasticity may have ratios that are higher than this. Increased H/M ratios have been reported in individuals with motor complete injury[99–101] and in those with motor incomplete injury.[100,102,103] However, other investigators have found no differences in reflex activity in individuals with SCI compared to nondisabled individuals.[13,104] Hiersemenzel et al[4] demonstrated that while normalized H-reflex responses were greater in individuals with motor complete tetraplegia versus thoracic SCI, overall reflex amplitudes were not different from those of nondisabled individuals.

Management of Spasticity

To Treat or Not to Treat?

Spasticity is a complex phenomenon, and its management is no less complicated. The effects of spasticity can be negative or positive. For example, the spasms associated with spasticity can be strong enough to throw an individual out of a chair. Spasticity may interfere with

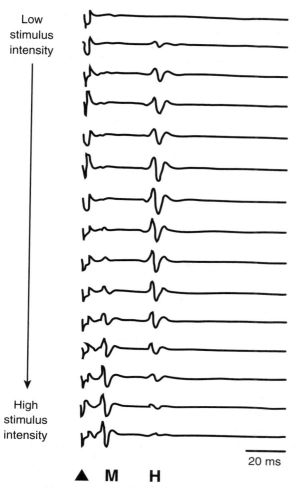

Low
stimulus
intensity

High
stimulus
intensity

20 ms

▲ M H

Figure 18-2. Evoked response in the muscle to increasing levels of electrical stimulation to a mixed nerve. At low levels of stimulation, only the H-reflex is observed at a latency of approximately 30 to 40 msec after the stimulus onset. As stimulus intensity increases, the motor fibers begins to reach threshold. As the amplitude of the M-wave increases with increasing stimulus intensity, the H-reflex amplitude declines. At the highest levels of stimulation, only the M-wave is observed. ▲ = stimulus artifact; M = M-wave; H = H-reflex.

mobility, positioning, sleep, comfort, and hygiene. Violent spasms may result in friction and/or shearing, which is detrimental to skin health. Contractures resulting from spasticity may make dressing and positioning difficult and painful and may predispose the individual to pressure ulcers. On the other hand, individuals often learn to trigger their spasms in such a way that the contractions augment mobility tasks such as transfers by either providing a brief period of involuntary muscle activity or by facilitating voluntary activation of muscles. Involuntary muscle contractions in individuals with spasticity may preserve muscle mass and contribute to blood circulation. Furthermore, hyperactive reflexes make possible reflexive bladder and bowel function (detailed information on this topic is provided in chapter 15).

There is considerable controversy regarding whether or not spasticity affects an individual's ability to move. Some investigators have demonstrated that reducing spasticity improves the ability to perform functional movements.[105–107] Others have suggested that antispastic (spasmolytic) medications impair functional movements.[108] However, others have concluded that there is little relationship between the level of spasticity and the performance of functional activities.[109,110] Part of this complexity arises because measures of spasticity are typically performed on an individual who is at rest, a neural state that is very different from that which occurs when the individual is moving.[2]

Another controversy relates to the issue of whether physical treatments should be directed at reducing spasticity or whether exercise and training should focus on improving function, with reduced spasticity a beneficial by-product. After stroke, Sahrmann and Norton[111] demonstrated that decreased descending drive rather than resistance from a spastic antagonist muscle is the factor that most limits voluntary movement. Thus, the primary contributor to decreased volitional control in those with upper motor neuron pathology is thought to be weakness rather than spasticity.[112] Furthermore, muscle strengthening increases the capacity for functional activity and does not increase spasticity in those with stroke (for review see Ada et al[113]). The situation may be similar in individuals in whom damage to the spinal cord limits the amount of supraspinal information that reaches the motoneurons in the spinal cord.[114,115]

Finally, it has been argued that spasticity is a functional adaptation that optimizes available control mechanisms in a system in which motor function is impaired.[116,117] This perspective is consistent with the view that physical treatments should be the first line of approach in individuals who have some functional mobility and that pharmacological intervention should only be attempted when these approaches fail to bring relief. In contrast, pharmacological approaches may be the best intervention for those who are immobile.[118]

When spasticity interferes with function more than it aids function, treatment is indicated. Conventional therapy attempts to dampen symptoms of spasticity by physical therapy, medication, or a combination of these strategies. As described by Adams and Hicks,[16] physical treatments may include limb positioning to maintain muscle length (possibly with splints or orthoses), passive stretching of muscle through its range of motion, weight bearing to prolong muscle stretch, or electrical stimulation of muscle or skin. Unfortunately, treatment effectiveness varies, and there is little standardization in its implementation. Here, we will describe the evidence for three of these physical treatment strategies in more detail, in each case emphasizing the need for studies that clarify whether these treatments work and the mechanisms that may underlie treatment effectiveness.

Physical Treatments for Spasticity

Muscle Stretching

Surveys show that more than 40% of spinal cord-injured individuals use stretching exercises to control symptoms of spasticity.[7,119] Stretching is reported to first evoke spasms and then to reduce spasms and tone. Although the clinical recommendation is that stretching be performed on a daily basis,[120] studies have not systematically examined how stretching induces suppression of spastic symptoms. In able-bodied individuals, muscle stretching induces changes in tendon reflexes, H-reflexes, and motor-evoked potentials. These data suggest that there are *short-term* changes in muscle spindle sensitivity, as well as involvement of both presynaptic and postsynaptic processes.[121] Similar processes may occur in individuals with incomplete cord injury. In individuals with spasticity arising from various neurological conditions, repeated movements often cause fatigue of stretch reflexes. Yet, stretch of an antagonist muscle still evokes EMG activity in the agonist in which the stretch reflex had disappeared.[122] Thus, the agonist motoneurons were still capable of reflex activation, suggesting that the reduction in stretch reflexes must involve the afferent pathway to the motoneuron and possibly presynaptic inhibition.[123–125]

Stretching may also have *long-term* consequences on muscle structure. For example, it is known that intermittent stretch of largely immobilized muscle prevents loss of sarcomeres, reduces buildup of connective tissue (although it may not affect soft tissue extensibility), minimizes changes in length–tension relationships, and ameliorates muscle atrophy.[73,120,126–129] After stroke, vigorous dynamic stretching appears to improve muscle strength in spastic muscles, as well as increase range of motion and decrease stiffness.[130] Stretch, together with botulinum toxin (BTX) injection, may also reduce spastic symptoms.[131] Passive stretching also tends to reverse the changes in motoneuron properties that occur with cord transection in rats[47] and normalizes frequency-dependent habituation of the H-reflex.[132,133] Thus, in addition to facilitating the short-term management of spasticity, stretching exercise may have positive influences on other long-term neuromuscular changes that occur after human SCI.

Serial Casting and Bracing

Spastic muscles and their tendons are known to undergo intrinsic structural changes that make them more resistant to stretch,[8–11] possibly contributing to the development of muscle contractures. Serial casting is a technique intended to provide prolonged, progressive stretching to muscles. Serial casting involves the use of a padded cast to hold the joint in the position that allows the shortened muscle to be maximally stretched. The cast is replaced periodically (usually weekly), and each subsequent cast increases the range of motion of the affected joint. In a study of 105 individuals with fixed contractures due to increased muscle tone of cerebral origin (e.g., stroke, traumatic brain injury, cerebral palsy), serial casting was shown to be effective in increasing range of motion of joints in both the upper and lower extremity.[134]

Botulinum toxin injection (discussed below), in combination with serial casting, is becoming increasingly common. However, reported results are mixed. One study concluded that the combined approach is more effective and results in shorter treatment time compared to serial casting alone.[135] Other studies suggest the two approaches are equally effective,[136,137] but the effects of the intervention are maintained for a longer period with BTX injection compared to serial casting[137] and the injections may be preferred over casting for reasons of convenience.[136] Conversely, other studies indicate that there is little to be gained by adding BTX injection to the serial casting intervention.[138,139] One study in children with cerebral palsy concluded that the addition of BTX injections to the serial casting intervention resulted in an earlier return of the treated joint deformity.[139]

Electrical Stimulation

As for other methods of physical intervention, few controlled studies have examined the effects of electrical stimulation on spasticity. Stimuli have been applied locally and directed to specific problems. In these studies, stimulation has been delivered (1) to the agonist muscle to excite Renshaw cells and to increase recurrent inhibition to the same motoneurons. These stimuli will fatigue the muscles, activate cutaneous afferents, and may induce limb movements, factors that are also likely to contribute to reductions in spasticity; (2) to an antagonistic muscle to enhance reciprocal inhibition to the agonist muscle; and (3) to a dermatome belonging to the same spinal segment as a spastic muscle to activate low-threshold afferents in skin that have inhibitory effects on that muscle.[140,140–147]

While some reductions in spasticity following electrical stimulation have been documented, the studies involve small numbers of subjects. For example, in one such study, stimulation of the triceps surae muscle group decreased the reflex response to tendon tap and Ashworth scores. No change in H-reflex excitability was identified.[98] In another small study involving individuals with upper extremity spasticity due to stroke, the investigators concluded that 10 minutes of electrical stimulation was associated with a decrease in peak muscle torque in response to stretch, with the effect lasting 30 minutes after stimulation.[148] There is some indication that electrical stimulation may be as effective as pharmacological interventions at reducing spasticity.[149]

Studies that explore the effects of electrical stimulation on spasticity typically have had no comparison group and may have included combinations of interventions.

Furthermore, the effects have been variable and short-term, and different outcome measures have been used to assess spasticity. The stimulation parameters have also varied widely (pulse type, duration, frequency, intensity, duty cycle, time of delivery). The stimuli may be painful, limiting the individuals who can participate to those who are able to tolerate the stimulation. The mechanisms underlying reductions in spasticity with electrical stimulation have not been explored systematically, but they may relate to changes in reciprocal or presynaptic inhibition, postactivation depression, the mechanical properties of muscles and joints, and activity-related changes in muscle properties. These processes may be slow to change and require long-term studies that show effects from electrical stimulation that exceed the day-to-day variation in spasticity. When coupled with studies that involve functional movements, it is important to be able to discern effects arising from the stimulation itself versus effects from the behavior studied.

Pharmacological Interventions for Spasticity

While physical treatments are typically the first choice for management of spasticity, antispastic (spasmolytic) pharmacological intervention may be indicated when the impact of physical treatments is insufficient. Common medications include baclofen, diazepam, dantrolene, tizanidine (or the closely related medication, clonidine). When spasticity is focal, local treatment with injection of BTX, phenol, or alcohol may be used. Conversely, with more generalized severe spasticity, more invasive interventions, such as an intrathecal pump for baclofen delivery, are options. Unfortunately, there are few clinical trials to substantiate the selection of antispastic (spasmolytic) medication in individuals with SCI. A 2006 systematic review of pharmacological interventions for spasticity after SCI concluded that "there is insufficient evidence to assist clinicians in a rational approach to spasmolytic treatment for SCI."[150] Other issues include the lack of a universally accepted method for assessment of spasticity, limited use of quality of life indicators, little assessment of the effect of medications on the ability to perform activities of daily living, and a lack of studies that compare effectiveness of different medications (i.e., as opposed to comparisons between drug versus placebo). Perhaps most concerning is that there have been no clinical studies of the long-term effectiveness of any of these meds, and it is possible that the nervous system adapts to their use in such a way that chronic use is ineffective in reducing spasticity.

Baclofen

Oral baclofen (Lioresal) acts on the central nervous system at the level of the spinal cord. Baclofen is an agonist of the inhibitory neurotransmitter gamma aminobutyric acid (GABA). It suppresses spinal reflex activity by mimicking the inhibitory effects of this neurotransmitter at the $GABA_B$ receptors. While baclofen has been reported to have both presynaptic effects (at the primary afferent or sensory fibers) and postsynaptic effects on the motoneuron itself,[151] more recent evidence suggests that postsynaptic effects may not be achieved at clinical doses of this medication.[152] Because baclofen acts at the level of the spinal cord, it is the agent with a spinal basis that is considered best suited for spasticity and is the antispastic (spasmolytic) medication most commonly prescribed for management of spasticity in individuals with SCI. However, there have been no clinical trials to substantiate this practice.[150] The accepted maximum daily dosage is considered to be 80 mg to 100 mg (the typical average dose being 40 mg to 60 mg, or 20 mg taken two or three times per day), with peak effects observed 1 to 2 hours after dosing. However, higher dosages are not uncommon. The common use of higher doses is worrisome, as evidence from rats with experimentally induced SCI and spasticity indicates that at higher doses, baclofen *increases* motoneuron excitability rather than having the intended inhibitory effect.[152] Drowsiness is a side effect of oral baclofen and represents one of the most often-cited reasons individuals give for wanting to discontinue its use. Abrupt discontinuation of oral baclofen may be accompanied by side effects such as seizures and should only be undertaken with medical supervision and guidance.

Intrathecal baclofen pumps are an alternative to oral baclofen. This intervention may be appropriate for some individuals with SCI who do not respond well to oral antispastic (spasmolytic) medications or find them to have unacceptable side effects. This intervention involves the insertion of a tube into the subarachnoid space, with the tube routed subcutaneously to connect with a mechanical pump. The pump is typically implanted subcutaneously in the lateral abdominal wall. The advantage of the pump is that it allows the use of lower medication doses (typically 500 to 1000 µg daily) since it is delivered more directly to the central nervous system. In contrast, pump malfunction may result in under- or overdosing of the medication.[83] Furthermore, this is an invasive procedure, and the device may offer a route of entry for infections, including meningitis.[153]

Diazepam (Valium)

Diazepam belongs to the benzodiazepine class of drugs. Like baclofen, these are GABA agonists and therefore act as depressants of central nervous system activity. Diazepam increases presynaptic inhibition through its actions on the $GABA_A$ receptors in the brainstem and spinal cord.[154] The common side effects of diazepam are related to central nervous system depression and include drowsiness as well as adverse effects on attention and memory.[155] In addition, drug dependence may be problematic with long-term use of higher doses. Withdrawal symptoms such as depression, irritability, and agitation have been reported following abrupt discontinuation of diazepam. Maximum dose is considered to be 40 to 60 mg per day.

Dantrolene (Dantrium)

Unlike baclofen and diazepam, which affect the central nervous system, dantrolene (Dantrium) reduces spasticity by limiting the contractile capacity of the muscle. Dantrolene affects the extrafusal muscle fibers by preventing the release of calcium from the sarcoplasmic reticulum and the intrafusal fibers of the muscle spindle by decreasing the sensitivity of the spindle to stretch.[156] In addition to preventing spasticity, dantrolene may also limit the ability to perform voluntary muscle contractions, resulting in weakness during voluntary effort. Other common side effects include drowsiness and dizziness. Possible liver toxicity with dantrolene requires ongoing monitoring of liver function; therefore, this medication may not be appropriate for long-term use. The accepted maximum daily dose of dantrolene is 400 mg (typically 100 mg taken four times per day), but higher doses are reported.

Tizanidine (Zanaflex)

Tizanidine is an alpha-2 adrenergic receptor agonist. It is pharmacologically similar to clonidine, an agent prescribed for its antihypertensive effects. These medications act on the adrenergic system by suppressing the release of both adrenalin and noradrenalin. The spasmolytic effects of tizanidine are derived from its ability to enhance the activity of the descending noradrenergic inhibitory pathways, resulting in both presynaptic and postsynaptic inhibition of reflex muscle activity.[157] The most frequently reported side effects of tizanidine are drowsiness, dizziness, hypotension, nausea, and dry mouth. However, given the antihypertensive effects of alpha-2 adrenergic receptor agonists, tizanidine also has the potential to affect cardiovascular responses to exercise. As with dantrolene, liver function should be monitored during treatment, although no cases of hepatic failure have been reported with tizanidine. Some studies have suggested that tizanidine has pain relief properties in addition to its antispasticity effects.[158] The typical maximum daily dosage of tizanidine is 36 mg.

Chemodenervation via Neuromuscular or Perineural Blockade

The use of agents that prevent the contraction of spastic muscles by damaging the motor nerve fibers or blocking the neuromuscular junction are pharmacological alternatives that have local, rather than systemic effects. By blocking the neuromuscular junction with local injections of BTX or by damaging the nerve with injections of phenol (benzyl alcohol) or ethanol (ethyl alcohol), the electrical signals are incapable of crossing from the nerve to the muscle, thereby preventing muscle contraction. This chemodenervation is intended to decrease the transmission of electrical signals related to spastic, involuntary motor activity, but it affects transmission of signals related to voluntary motor commands as well with the consequence being muscle weakness. Neuronal or neuromuscular blockade is therefore most appropriate when the goal is to inactivate particular focal areas of a muscle or certain small groups of muscles. A published systematic review[159] of studies related to the use of neuronal or neuromuscular blockade for improving upper extremity spasticity in stroke found BTX to be effective at reducing tone and improving passive range of motion. However, it is not possible to draw conclusions from available studies about whether these effects are associated with an improvement in functional status.[159]

BTX is a potent neurotoxin produced by the bacterium *Clostridium botulinum*. The neurotoxin is a proteolytic enzyme that exerts its effects by inhibiting acetylcholine release at the neuromuscular junction, resulting in neuromuscular blockade. It provides temporary results lasting approximately 3 to 4 months, with peak effects beginning approximately 2 weeks after injection. There are two forms of BTX, type A (BTX-A; BOTOX or Dysport) and type B (BTX-B; Myobloc or NeuroBloc). Because Botox is a toxin, side effects include antibody formation when used to treat large muscles or with repeated injections, resulting in resistance to the medication. Therefore, this approach is only appropriate for treatment of small muscles or small areas of larger muscles. Other side effects may include dry mouth, blurred vision, excess weakness, or mild flu-like symptoms. In the United States, BTX-A is approved by the U.S. Food and Drug Administration (FDA) for treatment of blepharospasm (i.e., spasm of the eyelids), cervical dystonia (i.e., severe neck muscle spasms), severe primary axillary hyperhydrosis (i.e., excessive sweating), and for cosmetic improvement in the appearance of facial frown lines. The use of BTX in treatment of spasticity represents an off-label use. In early 2008, the FDA issued a statement in response to reports of systemic adverse reactions, such as respiratory compromise and death from respiratory failure following BTX injection, including the death of children with cerebral palsy being treated for spasticity. The statement indicated that while the FDA was not advising health-care professionals to discontinue the use of BTX, safety data associated with the use of BTX was under review, and that those using these agents should heed label warnings to be alert for adverse reactions.[160]

Phenol (benzyl alcohol) and ethanol (ethyl alcohol) are chemical defatting agents. When injected near a nerve, these agents dissolve the insulating myelin sheath that surrounds the axon. Following demyelination, axons are unable to efficiently conduct electrical signals, resulting in perineural blockade. The effects of phenol/ethanol injection last approximately 6 months, and the extent of effects depends on the size of the area treated and the amount of agent that was injected. Phenol and ethanol also destroy muscle tissue and may result in scar formation in an injected muscle. Scar formation has the potential to make worse any contracture of the treated muscle. Phenol injections for elbow flexor spasticity in individuals with stroke have been reported to improve function.[107] BTX and phenol (or ethyl alcohol) may be used in combination, especially when the intent is to treat a large muscle.

Often, a pretreatment injection of local anesthetic (e.g., lidocaine) will be used to produce a short-term blockade that will allow assessment of the effects of a planned neuromuscular or perineural blockade. The effects of injection are typically evident within a few minutes and persist for up to several hours.[18] During the period of the transient blockade, it may be possible to gain insight regarding issues such as what muscle is most problematic, whether the muscle shortening is due primarily to hyperreflexia or to contracture, what is the true functional capacity of the antagonist muscle, and whether function is likely to be improved by a more permanent blockade.

Different Features of Spasticity Do Not Necessarily Covary

Most studies have been unable to show significant correlations between problematic spasticity and alterations in spinal inhibition, muscle tone, or muscle spasms. For example, evaluations of tone, tendon reflexes, and plantar responses performed at rest correlate poorly with subject reports of spasm frequency and severity.[161] Correlation between tonic stretch reflexes and the briskness of tendon jerks are low.[162] Exaggerated tendon jerks or increased resistance to passive stretch do not predict the contribution of spasticity to disorders of voluntary movement or gait.[69,163] No correlation between the degree of spasticity when measured as an Ashworth score and reduced reciprocal inhibition has been identified.[58] However, Crone et al[63] concluded that there is a linear relationship between impaired agonist–antagonist reciprocal inhibition and hyperactive soleus stretch reflexes. This likely signifies generalized impairment of spinal reflex modulation, consistent with the concept that spasticity is a multifactorial phenomenon.

The lack of significant correlations between these various parameters could result from many factors. First, there is variability in muscle- and reflex-related parameters, even when measured in nondisabled indi-viduals. Data are often compared across subjects with SCI, which introduces variability due to differences in severity and completeness of the injuries and the specific areas of the cord that are damaged. Physical factors such as temperature and humidity, as well as alertness and emotional state, may influence the responsiveness of nerves and muscles. There are likely to be differences in the type of therapy provided, when the therapy was initiated, and for how long it is continued. These factors argue strongly for examination of numerous parameters of spasticity over time in the same injured individual. Furthermore, not only will the damage and possible neural repair change neural circuitry and how it functions, but studies of stroke patients have also shown that behavioral experience is a potent modulator of post-injury cortical plasticity.[164] How

therapy, or lack of it, changes behavior after spinal injury is only just beginning to be explored. Changes can be expected at various levels (e.g., cortex, brainstem, cord, muscle[165]) and are likely to involve multiple mechanisms. Our limited knowledge in these areas suggests a need to evaluate many signs of spasticity in response to controlled therapeutic interventions.

There remains much to learn about the natural history of spasticity, in part because the assessment tools available in the clinic are poor. There are many important questions that remain: Do spastic symptoms reflect the response of the nervous system to the inactivity imposed by neuropathology? Can early activity prevent the onset of spasticity? What are the long-term outcomes of current treatments for spasticity? How do these outcomes change when the individual exercises? Are there optimal forms of activity to ameliorate spasticity? How frequently must they be performed? These and many other important questions remain to be answered.

Summary

Spasticity is a form of hyperreflexia and is associated with exaggerated responses to afferent input, particularly muscle stretch. A large proportion of individuals living with SCI experience spasticity, and the involuntary muscle contractions associated with spasticity may have a considerable impact on the individual's quality of life. Spasticity may restrict daily activities, inhibit or disrupt movements, and result in pain, fatigue, and/or contractures. The factors that contribute to spasticity after SCI include alterations in supraspinal modulation of spinal reflex activity, reorganization of spinal circuits, and changes in the mechanical properties of the spastic muscles themselves. There are numerous clinical assessment tools available to characterize and quantify spasticity; however, these tools are often poorly correlated with subjective reports of the experience of spasticity or with the functional significance of spasticity. Spasticity has been treated clinically with physical therapy interventions and pharmacological interventions, with varying degrees of success reported in the literature. It seems clear that studies directed at answering basic questions related to spasticity are needed.

REVIEW QUESTIONS

1. How does spasticity differ from rigidity? Include in your answer the types of pathology that result in each form of impairment.
2. What abnormal motor behaviors are typically associated with spasticity?
3. In what situation(s) may an individual use their spasticity in a useful way?

4. What are the limitations of the Ashworth scale as a measure of spasticity?
5. How is electrical stimulation useful to reduce spasticity?
6. What are some of the issues that may arise from use of baclofen as an antispastic (spasmolytic) pharmacological intervention for spasticity?

REFERENCES

1. Lance JW. Symposium synopsis. In: Feldman RG, Young RR, Koella WP, editors. *Spasticity: Disordered Motor Control.* Chicago, IL: Year Book Medical; 1980. pp. 485–494.
2. Dietz V. Spastic movement disorder. *Spinal Cord.* 2000;38: 389–393.
3. Sheean G. The pathophysiology of spasticity. *Eur J Neurol.* 2002;9:S3–S9.
4. Hiersemenzel LP, Curt A, Dietz V. From spinal shock to spasticity: Neuronal adaptations to a spinal cord injury. *Neurology.* 2000;54:1574–1582.
5. Sköld C, Levi R, Seiger A. Spasticity after traumatic spinal cord injury: Nature, severity, and location. *Arch Phys Med Rehabil.* 1999;80:1548–1557.
6. Young RR. Spasticity: A review. *Neurology.* 1994;44: S12–S20.
7. Little JW, Micklesen P, Umlauf R et al. Lower extremity manifestations of spasticity in chronic spinal cord injury. *Am J Phys Med Rehabil.* 1989;68:32–36.
8. Mirbagheri MM, Barbeau H, Ladouceur M et al. Intrinsic and reflex stiffness in normal and spastic spinal cord injured subjects. *Exp Brain Res.* 2001;141:446–459.
9. Mirbagheri MM, Settle K, Harvey R et al. Neuromuscular abnormalities associated with spasticity of upper extremity muscles in hemiparetic stroke. *J Neurophysiol.* 2007;98: 629–637.
10. Fridén J, Lieber RL. Spastic muscle cells are shorter and stiffer than normal cells. *Muscle Nerve.* 2003;27:157–164.
11. Lieber RL, Runesson E, Einarsson F, Friden J. Inferior mechanical properties of spastic muscle bundles due to hypertrophic but compromised extracellular matrix material. *Muscle Nerve.* 2003;28:464–471.
12. Dietz V, Trippel M, Berger W. Reflex activity and muscle tone during elbow movements in patients with spastic paresis. *Ann Neurol.* 1991;30:767–779.
13. Calancie B, Broton JG, Klose KJ et al. Evidence that alterations in presynaptic inhibition contribute to segmental hypo- and hyperexcitability after spinal cord injury in man. *Electroencephalogr Clin Neurophysiol.* 1993;89:177–186.
14. Woolacott AJ, Burne JA. The tonic stretch reflex and spastic hypertonia after spinal cord injury. *Exp Brain Res.* 2006;174:386–396.
15. Sanger TD, Delgado MR, Gaebler-Spira D et al. Classification and definition of disorders causing hypertonia in childhood. *Pediatrics.* 2003;111:e89–e97.
16. Adams MM, Hicks AL. Spasticity after spinal cord injury. *Spinal Cord.* 2005;43:577–586.
17. Biering-Sørensen F, Nielsen JB, Klinge K. Spasticity-assessment: A review. *Spinal Cord.* 2006;44:708–722.
18. Gracies JM, Elovic E, McGuire J et al. Traditional pharmacological treatments for spasticity. Part I: Local treatments. *Muscle Nerve Suppl.* 1997;6:S61–S91.
19. Gracies JM, Nance P, Elovic E et al. Traditional pharmacological treatments for spasticity. Part II: General and regional treatments. *Muscle Nerve Suppl.* 1997;6:S92–S120.
20. Gracies JM. Pathophysiology of spastic paresis. I: Paresis and soft tissue changes. *Muscle Nerve.* 2005;31:535–551.
21. Gracies JM. Pathophysiology of spastic paresis. II: Emergence of muscle overactivity. *Muscle Nerve.* 2005;31: 552–571.
22. Nielsen JB, Crone C, Hultborn H. The spinal pathophysiology of spasticity—From a basic science point of view. *Acta Physiol Scand.* 2007;189:171–180.
23. Pierrot-Deseilligny E, Burke D. *The Circuitry of the Human Spinal Cord: Its Role in Motor Control and Movement Disorders.* Cambridge, England; Cambridge University Press; 2005.
24. Taricco M, Pagliacci MC, Telaro E et al. Pharmacological interventions for spasticity following spinal cord injury: Results of a Cochrane systematic review. *Europa Medicophysica.* 2006;42:5–15.
25. Thomas CK, Ross BH. Distinct patterns of motor unit behavior during muscle spasms in spinal cord injured subjects. *J Neurophysiol.* 1997;77:2847–2850.
26. Dietz V, Ketelsen UP, Berger W et al. Motor unit involvement in spastic paresis. Relationship between leg muscle activation and histochemistry. *J Neurol Sci.* 1986;75: 89–103.
27. Hagbarth KE, Wallin G, Löfstedt L et al. Muscle spindle activity in alternating tremor of Parkinsonism and in clonus. *J Neurol Neurosurg Psychiatry.* 1975;38:636–641.
28. Hagbarth KE, Wallin G, Lofstedt L. Muscle spindle responses to stretch in normal and spastic subjects. *Scand J Rehabil Med.* 1973;5:156–159.
29. Szumski AJ, Burg D, Struppler A et al. Activity of muscle spindles during muscle twitch and clonus in normal and spastic human subjects. *Electroencephalogr Clin Neurol.* 1974; 37:589–597.
30. Thomas CK, Westling G. Tactile unit properties after human cervical spinal cord injury. *Brain.* 1995;118: 1547–1556.
31. Magladery JW, McDougal DB, Jr. Electrophysiological studies of nerve and reflex activity in normal man. I. Identification of certain reflexes in the electromyogram and the conduction velocity of peripheral nerve fibres. *Bull Johns Hopkins Hosp.* 1950;86:265–290.
32. Curt A, Keck ME, Dietz V. Clinical value of F-wave recordings in traumatic cervical spinal cord injury. *Electroencephalogr Clin Neurol.* 1997;105:189–193.
33. Tsai CT, Chen HW, Chang CW. Assessments of chronodispersion and tacheodispersion of F waves in patients with spinal cord injury. *Am J Phys Med Rehabil.* 2003;82:498–503.
34. Butler JE, Thomas CK. Effects of sustained stimulation on the exciteility of motoneurons innervating paralyzed and control muscles. *J Appl Physiol.* 2003;94:567–575.
35. Hager-Ross CK, Klein CS, Thomas CK. Twitch and tetanic properties of human thenar motor units paralyzed by chronic spinal cord injury. *J Neurophysiol.* 2006;96:165–174.
36. Bennett DJ, Li Y, Siu M. Plateau potentials in sacrocaudal motoneurons of chronic spinal rats, recorded in vitro. *J Neurophysiol.* 2001;86:1955–1971.
37. Bennett DJ, Sanelli L, Cooke CL et al. Spastic long-lasting reflexes in the awake rat after sacral spinal cord injury. *J Neurophysiol.* 2004;91:2247–2258.

38. Bennett DJ, Hultborn H, Fedirchuk B et al. Synaptic activation of plateaus in hindlimb motoneurons of decerebrate cats. *J Neurophysiol.* 1998;80:2023–2037.

39. Hultborn H, Malmsten J. Changes in segmental reflexes following chronic spinal cord hemisection in the cat. II. Conditioned monosynaptic test reflexes. *Acta Physiol Scand.* 1983;119:423–433.

40. Stein RB, Brucker BS, Ayyar DR. Motor units in incomplete spinal cord injury: Electrical activity, contractile properties and the effects of biofeedback. *J Neurol Neurosurg Psychiatry.* 1990;53:880–885.

41. Thomas CK, Zijdewind I. Fatigue of muscles weakened by death of motoneurons. *Muscle Nerve.* 2006;33:21–41.

42. Collins DF, Burke D, Gandevia SC. Large involuntary forces consistent with plateau-like behavior of human motoneurons. *J Neurosci.* 2001;21:4059–4065.

43. Gorassini M, Yang JF, Siu M et al. Intrinsic activation of human motoneurons: Possible contribution to motor unit excitation. *J Neurophysiol.* 2002;87:1850–1858.

44. Nickolls P, Collins DF, Gorman RB et al. Forces consistent with plateau-like behaviour of spinal neurons evoked in patients with spinal cord injuries. *Brain.* 2004;127:660–670.

45. Gorassini MA, Knash ME, Harvey PJ et al. Role of motoneurons in the generation of muscle spasms after spinal cord injury. *Brain.* 2004;127:2247–2258.

46. Zijdewind I, Thomas CK. Motor unit firing during and after voluntary contractions of human thenar muscles weakened by spinal cord injury. *J Neurophysiol.* 2003;89:2065–2071.

47. Beaumont E, Houlé JD, Peterson CA et al. Passive exercise and fetal spinal cord transplant both help to restore motoneuronal properties after spinal cord transection in rats. *Muscle Nerve.* 2004;29:234–242.

48. Cope TC, Bodine SC, Fournier M et al. Soleus motor units in chronic spinal transected cats: Physiological and morphological alterations. *J Neurophysiol.* 1986;55:1202–1220.

49. Hochman S, McCrea DA. Effects of chronic spinalization on ankle extensor motoneurons. II. Motoneuron electrical properties. *J Neurophysiol.* 1994;71:1468–1479.

50. Faist M, Mazevet D, Dietz V et al. A quantitative assessment of presynaptic inhibition of Ia afferents in spastics. Differences in hemiplegics and paraplegics. *Brain.* 1994;117:1449–1455.

51. Nielsen J, Petersen N, Crone C. Changes in transmission across synapses of Ia afferents in spastic patients. *Brain.* 1995;118:995–1004.

52. Schindler-Ivens S, Shields RK. Low frequency depression of H-reflexes in humans with acute and chronic spinal-cord injury. *Exp Brain Res.* 2000;133:233–241.

53. Field-Fote EC, Brown KM, Lindley SD. Influence of posture and stimulus parameters on post-activation depression of the soleus H-reflex in individuals with chronic spinal cord injury. *Neurosci Lett.* 2006;410:37–41.

54. Nielsen J, Crone C, Hultborn H. H-reflexes are smaller in dancers from The Royal Danish Ballet than in well-trained athletes. *Eur J Appl Physiol Occup Physiol.* 1993;66:116–121.

55. Rémy-Néris O, Denys P, Daniel O et al. Effect of intrathecal clonidine on group I and group II oligosynaptic excitation in paraplegics. *Exp Brain Res.* 2003;148:509–514.

56. Downes L, Ashby P, Bugaresti J. Reflex effects from Golgi tendon organ (Ib) afferents are unchanged after spinal cord lesions in humans. *Neurology.* 1995;45:1720–1724.

57. Morita H, Shindo M, Momoi H et al. Lack of modulation of Ib inhibition during antagonist contraction in spasticity. *Neurology.* 2006;67:52–56.

58. Crone C, Nielsen J, Petersen N et al. Disynaptic reciprocal inhibition of ankle extensors in spastic patients. *Brain.* 1994;117:1161–1168.

59. Perez MA, Field-Fote EC. Impaired posture-dependent modulation of disynaptic reciprocal Ia inhibition in individuals with incomplete spinal cord injury. *Neurosci Lett.* 2003;341:225–228.

60. Boorman G, Hulliger M, Lee RG et al. Reciprocal Ia inhibition in patients with spinal spasticity. *Neurosci Lett.* 1991;127:57–60.

61. Okuma Y, Mizuno Y, Lee RG. Reciprocal Ia inhibition in patients with asymmetric spinal spasticity. *Clin Neurophysiol.* 2002;113:292–297.

62. Ashby P, Wiens M. Reciprocal inhibition following lesions of the spinal cord in man. *J Physiol.* 1989;414:145–157.

63. Crone C, Johnsen LL, Biering-Sorensen F et al. Appearance of reciprocal facilitation of ankle extensors from ankle flexors in patients with stroke or spinal cord injury. *Brain.* 2003;126:495–507.

64. Pearson KG, Collins DF. Reversal of the influence of group Ib afferents from plantaris on activity in medial gastrocnemius muscle during locomotor activity. *J Neurophysiol.* 1993;70:1009–1017.

65. Edamura M, Yang JF, Stein RB. Factors that determine the magnitude and time course of human H-reflexes in locomotion. *J Neurosci.* 1991;11:420–427.

66. Yang JF, Fung J, Edamura M et al. H-reflex modulation during walking in spastic paretic subjects. *Can J Neurol Sci.* 1991;18:443–452.

67. Morita H, Crone C, Christenhuis D et al. Modulation of presynaptic inhibition and disynaptic reciprocal Ia inhibition during voluntary movement in spasticity. *Brain.* 2001;124:826–837.

68. Knutsson E, Martensson A, Gransberg L. Influences of muscle stretch reflexes on voluntary, velocity-controlled movements in spastic paraparesis. *Brain.* 1997;120: 1621–1633.

69. McLellan DL. Co-contraction and stretch reflexes in spasticity during treatment with baclofen. *J Neurol Neurosurg Psychiatry.* 1977;40:30–38.

70. Given JD, Dewald JP, Rymer WZ. Joint dependent passive stiffness in paretic and contralateral limbs of spastic patients with hemiparetic stroke. *J Neurol Neurosurg Psychiatry.* 1995;59:271–279.

71. Thomas CK, Onate L, Ferrell S et al. *Muscle Spasms after Human Spinal Cord Injury.* IBRO World Congress of Neuroscience, Motor Control at the Top End Satellite Meeting. Melbourne, Australia, July 12–17, 2007. pp. 49.

72. Savolainen J, Vaananen K, Puranen J et al. Collagen synthesis and proteolytic activities in rat skeletal muscles: Effect of cast-immobilization in the lengthened and shortened positions. *Arch Phys Med Rehabil.* 1988;69:964–969.

73. Coutinho EL, DeLuca C, Salvini TF et al. Bouts of passive stretching after immobilization of the rat soleus muscle increase collagen macromolecular organization and muscle fiber area. *Connect Tissue Res.* 2006;47:278–286.

74. Ada L, O'Dwyer N, O'Neill E. Relation between spasticity, weakness, and contracture of the elbow flexors and upper limb activity after stroke: An observational study. *Disabil Rehabil.* 2006;28:891–897.

75. Ashworth B. Preliminary trial of carisoprodol in multiple sclerosis. *Practitioner*. 1964;192:540–542.

76. Bohannon RW, Smith MB. Interrater reliability of a modified Ashworth scale of muscle spasticity. *Phys Ther*. 1987;67:206–207.

77. Patrick E, Ada L. The Tardieu Scale differentiates contracture from spasticity whereas the Ashworth Scale is confounded by it. *Clin Rehabil*. 2006;20:173–182.

78. Vattanasilp W, Ada L, Crosbie J. Contribution of thixotropy, spasticity, and contracture to ankle stiffness after stroke. *J Neurol Neurosurg Psychiatry*. 2000;69:34–39.

79. Tardieu G, Shentoub S, Delarue R. Research on a technic for measurement of spasticity. *Revue Neurol*. 1954;91:143–144.

80. Scholtes VA, Becher JG, Beelen A et al. Clinical assessment of spasticity in children with cerebral palsy: A critical review of available instruments. *Dev Med Child Neurol*. 2006;48:64–73.

81. Boyd RN, Graham HK. Objective measurement of clinical findings in the use of botulinum toxin type A for the management of children with cerebral palsy. *Eur J Neurol*. 1999;6:S23–S35.

82. Fowler EG, Nwigwe AI, Ho TW. Sensitivity of the pendulum test for assessing spasticity in persons with cerebral palsy. *Dev Med Child Neurol*. 2000;42:182–189.

83. Dykstra D, Stuckey M, DesLauriers L et al. Intrathecal baclofen in the treatment of spasticity. *Acta Neurochir Suppl*. 2007;97:163–171.

84. Nance PW, Bugaresti J, Shellenberger K et al. Efficacy and safety of tizanidine in the treatment of spasticity in patients with spinal cord injury. North American Tizanidine Study Group. *Neurology*. 1994;44:S44–S51.

85. Benz EN, Hornby TG, Bode RK et al. A physiologically based clinical measure for spastic reflexes in spinal cord injury. *Arch Phys Med Rehabil*. 2005;86:52–59.

86. Penn RD, Savoy SM, Corcos D et al. Intrathecal baclofen for severe spinal spasticity. *N Engl J Med*. 1989;320:1517–1521.

87. Snow BJ, Tsui JK, Bhatt MH et al. Treatment of spasticity with botulinum toxin: A double-blind study. *Ann Neurol*. 1990;28:512–515.

88. Burke D, Gandevia SC, McKeon B. Monosynaptic and oligosynaptic contributions to human ankle jerk and H-reflex. *J Neurophysiol*. 1984;52:435–448.

89. Matthews WB. Ratio of maximum H reflex to maximum M response as a measure of spasticity. *J Neurol Neurosurg Psychiatry*. 1966;29:201–204.

90. Stokic DS, Yablon SA. Neurophysiological basis and clinical applications of the H-reflex as an adjunct for evaluating response to intrathecal baclofen for spasticity. *Acta Neurochir Suppl*. 2007;97:231–241.

91. Sehgal N, McGuire JR. Beyond Ashworth. Electrophysiologic quantification of spasticity. *Phys Med Rehabil Clin N Am*. 1998;9:949–79, ix.

92. Crone C, Johnsen LL, Hultborn H et al. Amplitude of the maximum motor response (Mmax) in human muscles typically decreases during the course of an experiment. *Exp Brain Res*. 1999;124:265–270.

93. Crone C, Hultborn H, Mazieres L et al. Sensitivity of monosynaptic test reflexes to facilitation and inhibition as a function of the test reflex size: A study in man and the cat. *Exp Brain Res*. 1990;81:35–45.

94. Crone C, Nielsen J. Methodological implications of the post activation depression of the soleus H-reflex in man. *Exp Brain Res*. 1989;78:28–32.

95. Misiaszek JE. The H-reflex as a tool in neurophysiology: Its limitations and uses in understanding nervous system function. *Muscle Nerve*. 2003;28:144–160.

96. Morita H, Petersen N, Christensen LO et al. Sensitivity of H-reflexes and stretch reflexes to presynaptic inhibition in humans. *J Neurophysiol*. 1998;80:610–620.

97. Leis AA, Kronenberg MF, Stetkarova I et al. Spinal motoneuron excitability after acute spinal cord injury in humans. *Neurology*. 1996;47:231–237.

98. Goulet C, Arsenault AB, Bourbonnais D et al. Effects of transcutaneous electrical nerve stimulation on H-reflex and spinal spasticity. *Scand J Rehabil Med*. 1996;28:169–176.

99. Little JW, Halar EM. H-reflex changes following spinal cord injury. *Arch Phys Med Rehabil*. 1985;66:19–22.

100. Shemesh Y, Rozin R, Ohry A. Electrodiagnostic investigation of motor neuron and spinal reflex arch (H-reflex) in spinal cord injury. *Paraplegia*. 1977;15:238–244.

101. Nakazawa K, Kawashima N, Akai M. Enhanced stretch reflex excitability of the soleus muscle in persons with incomplete rather than complete chronic spinal cord injury. *Arch Phys Med Rehabil*. 2006;87:71–75.

102. Phadke CP, Wu SS, Thompson FJ et al. Soleus H-reflex modulation in response to change in percentage of leg loading in standing after incomplete spinal cord injury. *Neurosci Lett*. 2006;403:6–10.

103. Nakazawa K, Kawashima N, Akai M. Enhanced stretch reflex excitability of the soleus muscle in persons with incomplete rather than complete chronic spinal cord injury. *Arch Phys Med Rehabil*. 2006;87:71–75.

104. Schindler-Ivens SM, Shields RK. Soleus H-reflex recruitment is not altered in persons with chronic spinal cord injury. *Arch Phys Med Rehabil*. 2004;85:840–847.

105. Latash ML, Penn RD, Corcos DM et al. Effects of intrathecal baclofen on voluntary motor control in spastic paresis. *J Neurosurg*. 1990;72:388–392.

106. Corcos DM, Gottlieb GL, Penn RD et al. Movement deficits caused by hyperexcitable stretch reflexes in spastic humans. *Brain*. 1986;109 Pt 5:1043–1058.

107. McCrea PH, Eng JJ, Willms R. Phenol reduces hypertonia and enhances strength: A longitudinal case study. *Neurorehabil Neural Repair*. 2004;18:112–116.

108. Nielsen JF, Sinkjaer T. Peripheral and central effect of baclofen on ankle joint stiffness in multiple sclerosis. *Muscle Nerve*. 2000;23:98–105.

109. O'Dwyer NJ, Ada L, Neilson PD. Spasticity and muscle contracture following stroke. *Brain*. 1996;119 Pt 5:1737–1749.

110. Ada L, Vattanasilp W, O'Dwyer NJ et al. Does spasticity contribute to walking dysfunction after stroke? *J Neurol Neurosurg Psychiatry*. 1998;64:628–635.

111. Sahrmann SA, Norton BJ. The relationship of voluntary movement to spasticity in the upper motor neuron syndrome. *Ann Neurol*. 1977;2(6):460–465.

112. Kamper DG, Fischer HC, Cruz EG et al. Weakness is the primary contributor to finger impairment in chronic stroke. *Arch Phys Med Rehabil*. 2006;87:1262–1269.

113. Ada L, Dorsch S, Canning CG. Strengthening interventions increase strength and improve activity after stroke: A systematic review. *Aust J Physiother*. 2006;52:241–248.

114. Thomas CK, Zaidner EY, Calancie B et al. Muscle weakness, paralysis, and atrophy after human cervical spinal cord injury. *Exp Neurol.* 1997;148:414–423.

115. Gregory CM, Bowden MG, Jayaraman A et al. Resistance training and locomotor recovery after incomplete spinal cord injury: A case series. *Spinal Cord.* 2007;45:522–530.

116. Dietz V, Sinkjaer T. Spastic movement disorder: Impaired reflex function and altered muscle mechanics. *Lancet Neurol.* 2007;6:725–733.

117. Dietz V. Proprioception and locomotor disorders. *Nat Rev Neurosci.* 2002;3:781–790.

118. Dietz V. Gait disorder in spasticity and Parkinson's disease. *Adv Neurol.* 2001;87:143–154.

119. Sköld C. Spasticity in spinal cord injury: Self- and clinically rated intrinsic fluctuations and intervention-induced changes. *Arch Phys Med Rehabil.* 2000;81:144–149.

120. Harvey L, Herbert R, Crosbie J. Does stretching induce lasting increases in joint ROM? A systematic review. *Physiother Res Int.* 2002;7:1–13.

121. Guissard N, Duchateau J. Neural aspects of muscle stretching. *Exerc Sport Sci Rev.* 2006;34:154–158.

122. Burke D, Gillies JD, Lance JW. The quadriceps stretch reflex in human spasticity. *J Neurol Neurosurg Psychiatry.* 1970;33:216–223.

123. Burke D, Andrews CJ, Gillies JD. The reflex response to sinusoidal stretching in spastic man. *Brain.* 1971;94: 455–470.

124. Devanandan MS, Eccles RM, Yokota T. Muscle stretch and the presynaptic inhibition of the group Ia pathway to motoneurones. *J Physiol.* 1965;179:430–441.

125. Devanandan MS, Eccles RM, Yokota T. Depolarization of afferent terminals evoked by muscle stretch. *J Physiol.* 1965;179:417–429.

126. Harvey LA, Herbert RD. Muscle stretching for treatment and prevention of contracture in people with spinal cord injury. *Spinal Cord.* 2002;40:1–9.

127. Houle JD, Morris K, Skinner RD et al. Effects of fetal spinal cord tissue transplants and cycling exercise on the soleus muscle in spinalized rats. *Muscle Nerve.* 1999;22:846–856.

128. Tidball JG. Mechanical signal transduction in skeletal muscle growth and adaptation. *J Appl Physiol.* 2005;98: 1900–1908.

129. Williams PE, Catanese T, Lucey EG et al. The importance of stretch and contractile activity in the prevention of connective tissue accumulation in muscle. *J Anat.* 1988;158:109–114.

130. Chung S, Bai Z, Rymer WZ et al. Changes of reflex, nonreflex and torque generation properties of spastic ankle plantar flexors induced by intelligent stretching. *Conf Proc IEEE Eng Med Biol Soc.* 2005;4:3672–3675.

131. Giovannelli M, Borriello G, Castri P et al. Early physiotherapy after injection of botulinum toxin increases the beneficial effects on spasticity in patients with multiple sclerosis. *Clin Rehabil.* 2007;21:331–337.

132. Kiser TS, Reese NB, Maresh T et al. Use of a motorized bicycle exercise trainer to normalize frequency-dependent habituation of the H-reflex in spinal cord injury. *J Spinal Cord Med.* 2005;28:241–245.

133. Reese NB, Skinner RD, Mitchell D et al. Restoration of frequency-dependent depression of the H-reflex by passive exercise in spinal rats. *Spinal Cord.* 2006;44:28–34.

134. Pohl M, Ruckriem S, Mehrholz J et al. Effectiveness of serial casting in patients with severe cerebral spasticity: A comparison study. *Arch Phys Med Rehabil.* 2002;83: 784–790.

135. Booth MY, Yates CC, Edgar TS et al. Serial casting vs combined intervention with botulinum toxin A and serial casting in the treatment of spastic equinus in children. *Pediatr Phys Ther.* 2003;15:216–220.

136. Flett PJ, Stern LM, Waddy H et al. Botulinum toxin A versus fixed cast stretching for dynamic calf tightness in cerebral palsy. *J Paediatr Child Health.* 1999;35:71–77.

137. Corry IS, Cosgrove AP, Duffy CM et al. Botulinum toxin A compared with stretching casts in the treatment of spastic equinus: A randomised prospective trial. *J Pediatr Orthoped.* 1998;18:304–311.

138. Verplancke D, Snape S, Salisbury CF et al. A randomized controlled trial of botulinum toxin on lower limb spasticity following acute acquired severe brain injury. *Clin Rehabil.* 2005;19:117–125.

139. Kay RM, Rethlefsen SA, Fern-Buneo A et al. Botulinum toxin as an adjunct to serial casting treatment in children with cerebral palsy. *J Bone Joint Surg Am.* 2004;86: 2377–2384.

140. Bajd T, Gregoric M, Vodovnik L et al. Electrical stimulation in treating spasticity resulting from spinal cord injury. *Arch Phys Med Rehabil.* 1985;66:515–517.

141. Franek A, Turczynski B, Opara J. Treatment of spinal spasticity by electrical stimulation. *J Biomed Eng.* 1988;10: 266–270.

142. Mirbagheri MM, Ladouceur M, Barbeau H et al. The effects of long-term FES-assisted walking on intrinsic and reflex dynamic stiffness in spastic spinal-cord-injured subjects. *IEEE Trans Neural Syst Rehabil Eng.* 2002;10: 280–289.

143. Robinson CJ, Kett NA, Bolam JM. Spasticity in spinal cord injured patients: 1. Short-term effects of surface electrical stimulation. *Arch Phys Med Rehabil.* 1988;69: 598–604.

144. Robinson CJ, Kett NA, Bolam JM. Spasticity in spinal cord injured patients: 2. Initial measures and long-term effects of surface electrical stimulation. *Arch Phys Med Rehabil.* 1988;69:862–868.

145. Daly JJ, Marsolais EB, Mendell LM et al. Therapeutic neural effects of electrical stimulation. *IEEE Trans Rehabil Eng.* 1996;4:218–230.

146. van der Salm A, Veltink PH, Ijzerman MJ et al. Comparison of electric stimulation methods for reduction of triceps surae spasticity in spinal cord injury. *Arch Phys Med Rehabil.* 2006;87:222–228.

147. Vodovnik L, Bowman BR, Hufford P. Effects of electrical stimulation on spinal spasticity. *Scand J Rehabil Med.* 1984;16:29–34.

148. Dewald JP, Given JD, Rymer WZ. Long-lasting reductions of spasticity induced by skin electrical stimulation. *IEEE Trans Rehabil Eng.* 1996;4:231–242.

149. Aydin G, Tomruk S, Keles I et al. Transcutaneous electrical nerve stimulation versus baclofen in spasticity: Clinical and electrophysiologic comparison. *Am J Phys Med Rehabil.* 2005;84:584–592.

150. Taricco M, Adone R, Pagliacci C et al. Pharmacological interventions for spasticity following spinal cord injury. *Cochrane Database Syst Rev.* 2000;CD001131.

151. Yang K, Wang D, Li YQ. Distribution and depression of the GABA(B) receptor in the spinal dorsal horn of adult rat. *Brain Res Bull.* 2001;55:479–485.

152. Li Y, Li X, Harvey PJ et al. Effects of baclofen on spinal reflexes and persistent inward currents in motoneurons of chronic spinal rats with spasticity. *J Neurophysiol.* 2004;92:2694–2703.

153. Wunderlich CA, Krach LE. Gram-negative meningitis and infections in individuals treated with intrathecal baclofen for spasticity: A retrospective study. *Dev Med Child Neurol.* 2006;48:450–455.

154. Abbruzzese G. The medical management of spasticity. *Eur J Neurol.* 2002;9 Suppl 1:30–34.

155. Rich JB, Svoboda E, Brown GG. Diazepam-induced prospective memory impairment and its relation to retrospective memory, attention, and arousal. *Hum Psychopharmacol.* 2006;21:101–108.

156. Leslie GC, Part NJ. The effect of dantrolene sodium on intrafusal muscle fibres in the rat soleus muscle. *J Physiol.* 1981;318:73–83.

157. Delwaide PJ, Pennisi G. Tizanidine and electrophysiologic analysis of spinal control mechanisms in humans with spasticity. *Neurology.* 1994;44:S21–S27.

158. Elovic E. Principles of pharmaceutical management of spastic hypertonia. *Phys Med Rehabil Clin North Am.* 2001;12:793–816, vii.

159. van Kuijk AA, Geurts AC, Bevaart BJ et al. Treatment of upper extremity spasticity in stroke patients by focal neuronal or neuromuscular blockade: A systematic review of the literature. *J Rehabil Med.* 2002;34:51–61.

160. Early Communication about an Ongoing Safety Review Botox and Botox Cosmetic (Botulinum toxin Type A) and Myobloc (Botulinum toxin Type B) website at http://www.fda.gov/cder/drug/early_comm/botulinium_toxins.htm.

161. Priebe MM, Sherwood AM, Thornby JI et al. Clinical assessment of spasticity in spinal cord injury: A multidimensional problem. *Arch Phys Med Rehabil.* 1996;77:713–716.

162. Fellows SJ, Ross HF, Thilmann AF. The limitations of the tendon jerk as a marker of pathological stretch reflex activity in human spasticity. *J Neurol Neurosurg Psychiatry.* 1993;56:531–537.

163. Dietz V, Quintern J, Berger W. Electrophysiological studies of gait in spasticity and rigidity. Evidence that altered mechanical properties of muscle contribute to hypertonia. *Brain.* 1981;104:431–449.

164. Nudo RJ. Mechanisms for recovery of motor function following cortical damage. *Currt Opin Neurobiol.* 2006;16:638–644.

165. Wolpaw JR. The education and re-education of the spinal cord. *Prog Brain Res.* 2006;157:261–280.

166. Johnson RL, Gerhart KA, McCray J et al. Secondary conditions following spinal cord injury in a population-based sample. *Spinal Cord.* 1998;36:45–50.

167. Maynard FM, Karunas RS, Waring WP. Epidemiology of spasticity following traumatic spinal cord injury. *Arch Phys Med Rehabil.* 1990;71(8):566–569.

168. Noreau L, Proulx P, Gagnon L et al. Secondary impairments after spinal cord injury: A population-based study. *Am J Phys Med Rehabil.* 2000;79:526–535.

169. Westgren N, Levi R. Quality of life and traumatic spinal cord injury. *Arch Phys Med Rehabil.* 1998;79:1433–1439.

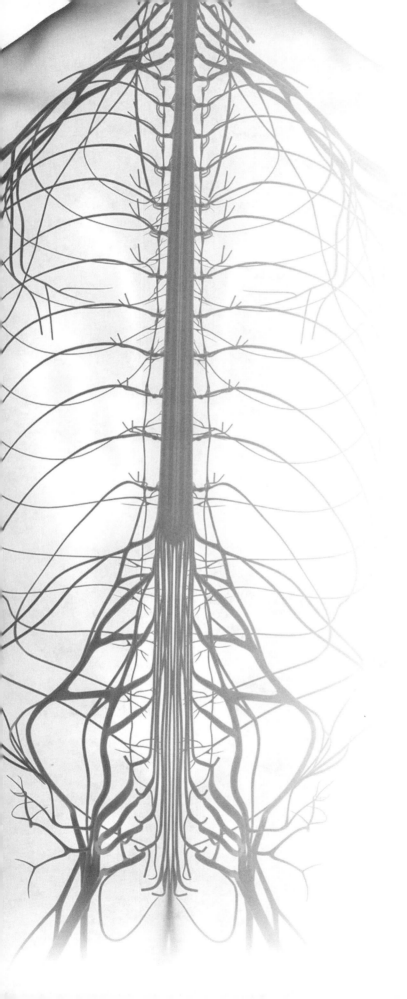

III

Beyond Basic Function

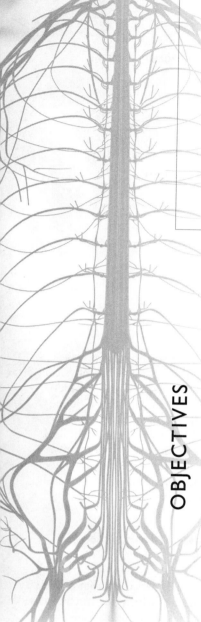

Physical Activity and Sport Participation After Spinal Cord Injury

19

Kathleen A. Curtis, PT, Ph.D.

After reading this chapter, the reader will be able to:

OBJECTIVES

- Analyze the associated health risks of physical inactivity in an individual with a spinal cord injury (SCI)
- Discuss the roles of rehabilitation professionals in recommending sport and physical activity participation, health promotion, prevention, and performance enhancement for persons with SCIs
- Establish guidelines for safe and effective physical activity, fitness, training, and sport participation, including principles of exercise prescription and specificity of exercise
- Access print and online resources to describe the scope of opportunities for physical activity and sport for persons with disabilities
- Identify equipment and multimedia resources that support physical activity and fitness for persons with disabilities
- Identify organizational and community resources that promote physical activity or provide recreational and competitive sport opportunities for persons with disabilities
- Discuss strategies for prevention and reoccurrence of the most common athletic injuries and disability-specific medical conditions in athletes with SCI
- Contrast functional and medical athlete classification systems used in competitive sport for athletes with disabilities

Introduction

With increasing awareness of the influence of lifestyle choices on long-term outcomes in the general population, there is an expanding body of knowledge about the long-term health risks faced by the sedentary individual with spinal cord injury (SCI). The first records of sport in wheelchairs appeared in the post-World War II era, involving veterans who had been hospitalized with their war injuries. Since then, we have seen marked changes in the equipment, health care, and performance of athletes with SCI. Even with these significant advances, most persons with SCI fail to meet levels of physical activity recommended by the World Health Organization.[1]

The impact of a sedentary lifestyle is amplified in individuals with SCI due to unique metabolic factors that increase their risk for diabetes mellitus and heart disease.[2,3] Obesity is a major problem in the population with SCI, with the prevalence of overweight and obesity among veterans with SCI estimated at 65.8% and 27.9%, respectively.[4]

Several authors have pointed to the need for health promotion and prevention of secondary disability in the population with SCI.[5,6] Others have noted that health promotion needs after SCI are the same as in the general population, but information on health promotion is not frequently received from health providers.[7] Over 20 years ago, the role of rehabilitation professionals in promoting safe participation in wheelchair sports was identified.[8] Faced with a national physical inactivity crisis and a growing body of evidence that places the individual with SCI at high risk for cardiovascular disease, rehabilitation professionals must play a key role in promotion of life-long physical activity and prevention of secondary disability in this vulnerable population.

The purpose of this chapter is to present the latest evidence regarding health risks associated with physical inactivity in individuals with SCI; to discuss the role of the rehabilitation professional in promoting physical activity, fitness, training, and recreational and competitive sports for this population; and to provide guidelines for safe and effective physical activity participation. Furthermore, this chapter will identify available physical activity, sport, and equipment resources; provide strategies to prevent initial onset and to limit the reoccurrence of the most common injuries and medical conditions; and introduce athletic classification systems for athletes with disabilities.

Secondary Health Risks Associated With Sedentary Lifestyle

Evidence has accumulated in the last 15 years that points to a host of health risks associated with poor nutrition, social isolation, and sedentary lifestyle in individuals with SCI. Physical activity after SCI may be limited by loss of voluntary motor control, as well as autonomic dysfunction, altered metabolism, and temperature regulation disorders.[9] Although all these factors warrant our consideration when prescribing exercise, this chapter will primarily focus on the current body of knowledge that supports the importance of and access to physical activity and sport participation for individuals with SCI.

A sedentary lifestyle is characterized by reduced activity, associated deconditioning, loss of lean tissue mass (e.g. muscle), and early-onset of muscle fatigue on exertion. This phenomenon often leads, in a downward spiral, to further deconditioning, with further loss of total lean tissue mass. When caloric intake exceeds energy expenditure, excess body fat tissue accumulates, also making activity more difficult.

This is even further complicated when individuals who attempt to increase physical activity in a deconditioned state then experience chronic musculoskeletal injuries and subsequent loss of joint mobility, eventually leading to even less physical activity. The "weekend warrior" who uses a wheelchair is just as vulnerable to the risks of going from chronic inactivity to sudden activity as is the weekend athlete in the general population. There are many health problems as well as a host of metabolic disturbances associated with a sedentary lifestyle in individuals with SCI.

Cardiovascular Disease

Recent studies show that the risk of cardiovascular disease (CVD) in persons with SCI is higher than in the general population. This includes coronary heart disease, hypertension, cerebrovascular disease, valvular disease, and dysrhythmia.[10] We are just beginning to understand the many factors that increase risk of CVD in persons with SCI. Chapter 16 includes a complete discussion of these risks.

Risk factor modification through weight, lipid, and glucose control is critical. Physical activity plays an important part in addressing these health concerns.

Obesity

Overweight and obesity are also associated with a sedentary lifestyle. Although evidence indicates that overweight and obesity are present in over 40% of the population with SCI, researchers report that fewer than 5% are counseled to lose weight.[11]

Body mass index (BMI) is frequently used to estimate body fat in the general population: BMI equals weight in kilograms divided by height in meters.[12] Measurement of obesity in SCI by calculation of BMI tends to underestimate body fat due to shifts in lean body mass following injury.[12] Although persons with SCI may not look obese, investigators have noted that they are likely to carry large amounts of fat tissue. For example, a recent study documented that in comparison to a group of age-, height-, and weight-matched able-bodied adults, total lean tissue mass averaged 8.9 kg lower and total fat mass was 7.1 kg higher in the SCI group.[12]

Evidence indicates that BMI also underestimates percentage of body fat in children with SCI. Children with SCI show lower total lean tissue mass and a lower resting metabolic rate than do matched able-bodied controls, and they may be predisposed to relative gains in body fat.[13]

Musculoskeletal System Disorders

Musculoskeletal system disorders are another complication of physical inactivity. Chronic musculoskeletal pain, weakness with muscle imbalance, deconditioning, joint contracture, and overuse syndromes all influence daily life in persons with SCI. There is a high prevalence (over 70%) of chronic upper extremity pain associated with long-term wheelchair use.[14–16] Overuse disorders such as tendonitis and carpal tunnel syndrome are also common

in the population with SCI.[17–21] Upper extremity pain, especially at the shoulder, is often associated with muscle imbalance and impingement syndromes.

Muscle imbalance is characterized by overstretched, weaker musculature opposed by stronger and tighter opposing musculature. Several investigators have found muscle imbalance between shoulder adductors and abductors to be associated with a higher risk of rotator cuff disorders.[22–23] This is often the case when strengthening programs emphasize the anterior shoulder musculature, such as the pectoral, anterior deltoid, biceps, and triceps muscles, and neglect to strengthen scapular adductors, such as the rhomboids, middle trapezius, posterior deltoid, and external rotator muscles. Although others have found that increased shoulder muscle strength decreases risk for shoulder pain,[24] it is critical to focus on the development of symmetrical muscle strength on both sides of the shoulder joint.

The level of SCI involvement may also increase risk of muscle imbalance and joint contracture of the extremities or spine. Innervation of musculature on only one side of a joint, such as the combination of a strong biceps muscle and weaker or paralyzed triceps muscle, increases risk of loss of joint mobility. Similarly, the combination of strong hip flexor muscles and weak or paralyzed hip extensor muscles may result in hip flexion contracture. Muscle imbalance in the trunk and spinal musculature may lead to scoliosis, especially among individuals with pediatric-onset SCI. In addition to loss of spinal mobility and postural deviations, individuals with scoliosis may also experience skin breakdown and pulmonary and cardiovascular system complications.[25]

Another musculoskeletal complication, *osteoporosis*, characterized by an increased bone resorption rate, decreased bone density, and increased fracture risk, is often seen in people with SCI. Findings of a recent study showed that 61% of a sample of 41 men with SCI screened using dual-energy absorptiometry had bone density levels consistent with osteoporosis; another 19% were osteopenic. Over one-third of these men (34%) reported a history of fracture since SCI.[26] An individual with SCI who has osteoporosis and lacks protective sensation is at high risk for an unrecognized fracture. Additional details related to bone health after SCI are discussed in Chapter 3.

Emotional Health

Lastly, social participation greatly influences emotional and mental health and quality of life. Overall, persons with SCI experience an increased prevalence of psychosocial dysfunction, leading to social isolation, depression, and substance abuse.[27] Investigators have documented that almost 30% of individuals with SCI report depression.[28]

Clearly, individuals with SCI experience increased risk of many secondary and comorbid conditions that are related to their injuries, their lifestyles, and physical activity levels. In the following section, current knowledge regarding the impact of physical activity and nutrition on the prevalence of secondary conditions in SCI will be reviewed.

Preventing Secondary Conditions in SCI: Physical Activity and Health Promotion

A substantial body of evidence indicates that physical activity promotes physical and emotional well-being and prevents multisystem decline and medical complications.[9] For example, investigators have found that programs of regular physical activity raise HDL-C,[29] reduce shoulder pain,[30,31] and reduce the incidence of rehospitalization.[32,33] Findings of one study showed that rates of hospitalization for kidney infections and skin breakdowns were three times greater for nonathletes than for athletes.[33]

The aging process may actually be accelerated by diminished physiological reserves and escalating demands on functioning body systems.[34] Advocates for physical activity have stressed the importance of physical activity in long-term health promotion.[35]

The Role of the Rehabilitation Professional

Rehabilitation professionals are uniquely positioned to assume roles in recommending, monitoring, and supporting healthy choices and lifestyles for their clients with SCI. As Rimmer,[35] a leader in promoting physical activity among persons with disabilities, noted, "For rehabilitation to play a role in the long-term maintenance and enhancement of physical functioning among people with disabilities, increasing participation in various types of physical activity must be a part of the recovery and maintenance continuum."

The rehabilitation professional has an important role in screening for preventable secondary conditions[36] and in engaging in productive discussions with individuals with SCI, their caregivers, and their supporters to minimize the health risks associated with the onset and progression of these conditions. Professional roles from which rehabilitation professionals may influence physical activity in the population with SCI include those of a care provider; an educator for consumers or health professions education students; a consultant to community recreation, fitness, or sports facilities; or even a classifier or volunteer for organized wheelchair sport.[8,37]

Rimmer also advocated for rehabilitation professionals to expand their roles to include community-based fitness:

Health promotion for people with disabilities must become a major focus for the new millennium. In the long run, preventing secondary health conditions by empowering people with disabilities to take control of their own health will be more cost-effective, and certainly more humane, than watching people with disabilities decline in function from a lack of good health maintenance. Health-care professionals should join in this collective effort to enrich the lives of people with disabilities. It could truly be an exciting era if rehabilitation professionals extend their services into community-based fitness centers and facilitate the promotion of good health practices for the more than 50 million Americans with disabilities.[5]

Although rehabilitation involvement in sport and physical activity for people with SCI stemmed from its *therapeutic* value to post-World War II veterans, the disability sport movement in recent years has clearly focused more on *performance* and has included the involvement of many more professionals from the sport world, including coaches, exercise scientists, sports medicine professionals, sports psychologists, and equipment specialists. Ironically, the movement has come full circle; it is evident that a physically active lifestyle is beneficial for *everyone* to prevent long-term disease and disability, including athletes, ex-athletes, and nonathletes with and without SCI. However, rather than considering physical activity to be *therapeutic*, it is more productive to consider it in the context of *health promotion*.

Health Promotion and Prevention

There are many definitions for *health promotion*. The following definition is particularly appropriate to the discussion of physical activity in persons with SCI:

Health promotion is a strategy for improving the health of the population by providing individuals, groups and communities with the tools to make informed decisions about their well-being. Moving beyond the traditional treatment of illness and injury, health promotion efforts are centered primarily on the social, physical, economical and political factors that affect health, and include such activities as the promotion of physical fitness, healthy living and good nutrition.[38]

Prevention

Prevention is closely related to health promotion. Prevention strategies are classified as (1) *primary* or *universal*, (2) *secondary* or *selective*, and (3) *tertiary* or *indicated*. Primary or universal strategies are targeted to prevent occurrences in the general population. Secondary strategies target an at-risk population to prevent occurrences of a health problem. Tertiary strategies target individuals in whom adverse outcomes or problems have already occurred. There are clearly roles for secondary and tertiary prevention in individuals with SCI. For example, many athletes with SCI report reinjury after musculoskeletal injury, most likely due to inadequate conditioning in the recovery period, which then increases risks for chronic musculoskeletal dysfunction.[39] Ongoing participation in physical activity, fitness, and conditioning activities are essential to preventing secondary conditions, even among elite athletes.

With the identification of health promotion as a key need for people with disabilities, leaders in physical activity and disability have advocated a paradigm shift from disability prevention to prevention of secondary conditions (e.g., obesity, hypertension, shoulder injuries, CVD, pressure sores).[5] Recent efforts by researchers, funding agencies, health-care providers, and consumers have focused attention on health promotion for the millions of Americans with disabilities to reduce secondary conditions in order to maintain functional independence, to provide an opportunity for leisure and enjoyment, and to enhance the overall quality of life by reducing environmental barriers to good health.[5]

Adopting a Healthy Lifestyle

Regular physical activity is critical to living a healthy life after SCI. It is, however, just one of many health-related actions that is important to promote (Box 19-1). Together with healthy nutrition, attention to safety issues, skin protection, tobacco cessation, regular medical and dental care, stress management, and disability-specific screening for secondary conditions ensures that persons with SCI are most able to participate fully in their work, social, and personal lives.[40]

Promoting Participation in a Physically Active Lifestyle

Evidence indicates that the most frequently cited reasons that persons with disabilities participate in physical activity and sport include fitness, fun, health, competition, and social contact. Participation is strongly influenced by friends and peers.[41] In addition to exploring sources of peer and social support, an assessment of an individual's interests, cognitive and physical abilities, and needs for adaptive equipment or assistance to engage in activity and/or sports will be helpful. Figure 19-1 shows a

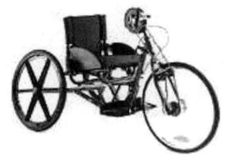

Figure 19-1. Hand cycles provide the wheelchair user with an alternative for upper body exercise.

handcycle that would be appropriate for community participation.

There are multiple options for leisure activity and sport participation. Table 19-1 provides examples of the broad variety of physical activities and organized sport in which people with SCI can participate. Some competitive sports are well organized and offer local, regional, national, and international competition. Others exist only in certain countries and haven't developed fully. Many offer both recreational and competitive opportunities.

So What's the Problem? Overcoming Barriers to Physical Activity Participation

Despite the many options available, evidence shows that the population with SCI is largely sedentary.[1] There are multiple perceived barriers to adopting regular physical

---

Box 19-1
Ten Steps for Staying Healthy After SCI

1. Healthy Eating: Consume a nutritious, low-fat, high-fiber, high-complex carbohydrate diet with vitamin and mineral supplements as needed. Drink at least 2 liters of water or noncarbonated, low-sugar beverages per day.

2. Aerobic Exercise: Engage in moderate intensity aerobic exercise for 15 to 60 minutes at least three times per week.

3. Stretching: Include a regular routine of daily stretching exercises for arms, legs, and spine to maintain joint range of motion and flexibility.

4. Muscle Building: Include resistive exercises to maintain or increase muscle mass in functioning muscles as part of your exercise regime at least twice weekly.

5. Accident Prevention: Observe safety precautions to prevent falls and fractures, skin abrasion, and accidental injuries to insensitive feet and legs.

6. Monitor Skin: Safeguard your skin from excess pressure with weight shifting and regular use of a wheelchair cushion. Monitor skin carefully for signs of breakdown and treat pressure areas immediately. Protect your skin from sunburn and skin cancer by using sunscreen on all exposed areas when outdoors.

7. Stop Smoking: Stop smoking cigarettes, pipes, and cigars. Discontinue using smokeless tobacco products.

8. Regular Medical/Dental Care: Plan and schedule an annual medical examination, including screening examinations for urinary tract function, hypertension, diabetes, cholesterol and triglycerides, and colon, breast, or prostate cancer. See your dentist regularly, no less frequently than every 6 months.

9. Emotional Health: Promote emotional health in your personal and work relationships; find ways to monitor and manage stress. Restrict consumption of caffeine and alcohol.

10. Observe And Report Changes: Form a partnership with your health care provider. Monitor and report changes in weakness, loss of sensation, swelling, posture, or pain to your healthcare provider. **Don't wait** until you have a serious problem to take action.

Adapted from: Curtis KA. Health smarts. Part 6. Slowing down the hands of time: Extending your athletic career and your life. *Sports 'n Spokes.* 1996;22(6):53–60.

Table 19-1
Physical Activity and Sport Options for Persons With SCI

Activity/Sport	Organizations	Website Links
Alpine Skiing/Snowboarding	United States Ski and Snowboard Association International Paralympic Committee—Winter Sports	http://www.ussa.org http://www.paralympic.org
Archery	International Archery Federation International Paralympic Committee—Summer Sports: Archery	http://www.archery.org http://www.paralympic.org
Athletics (track, field, road racing)	USA Track and Field	http://www.usatf.org
Aviation	Freedom's Wings International International Wheelchair Aviators	http://www.freedomswings.org http://www.wheelchairaviators.org
Baseball/Softball	National Wheelchair Softball Association (NWSA)	http://www.wheelchairsoftball.org
Basketball	Canadian Wheelchair Basketball Association National Wheelchair Basketball Association International Wheelchair Basketball Federation	http://www.cwba.ca http://www.nwba.org http://www.iwbf.org
Billiards	National Wheelchair Pool Players Association (NWPA)	http://www.nwpainc.org
Boating	PVA/boating and fishing	
Boccia	International Paralympic Committee	http://www.paralympic.org
Bowling (also see Lawn Bowling below)	American Wheelchair Bowling Association	http://www.awba.org
Canoeing/Kayaking	National Center on Physical Activity and Disability	http://www.ncpad.org
Curling (Wheelchair)	International Paralympic Committee—	http://www.paralympic.org
Cycling	United States Handcycling Federation	http://www.ushf.org
Dance	Wheelchair Dance Sport International Paralympic Committee—	http://www.wdance.com/ http://www.paralympic.org
Equestrian	North American Riding for the Handicapped Association International Paralympic Committee—	http://www.narha.org http://www.paralympic.org
Fishing	PVA/boating and fishing	http://www.pva.org
Hockey Ice Sledge Hockey	National Wheelchair Hockey League International Paralympic Committee—	http://www.thewchl.com http://www.paralympic.org
Nordic Skiing	International Paralympic Committee—	http://www.paralympic.org

Table 19-1

Physical Activity and Sport Options for Persons With SCI—cont'd

Activity/Sport	Organizations	Website Links
Outdoor Adventures (horseback riding, kayaking, camping, canoeing, rock climbing, scuba, white water rafting, deep sea fishing, snow skiing, skydiving, water skiing)	Casa Colina Outdoor Adventures Breckenridge Outdoor Education Center (B.O.E.C) Craig Hospital Therapeutic Recreation National Ability Center (outdoor sports)	http://www.casacolina.orgcenters/adventures.shtml http://www.boec.org http://www.craighospital.com/InfoResources/craigsTRecPrograms.asp http://www.nac1985.org
Physical Activity Resources	National Center for Physical Activity and Disability	http://www.ncpad.org
Powerlifting	International Paralympic Committee—	http://www.paralympic.org
Sailing	International Foundation for Disabled Sailing International Association For Disabled Sailing Options for Sailors with Disabilities	http://ifds.org http://www.sailing.orgdisabled http://www.footeprint.com/sailingweb
Scuba	Handicapped Scuba Association International International Association for Handicapped Divers (IAHD)	http://www.hsascuba.com http://www.iahdeurope.org
Swimming (Competitive)	USA Swimming—Swimmers-Disability International Paralympic Committee—Summer Sports	http://www.usaswimming.org http://www.paralympic.org
Table Tennis	International Paralympic Committee—	http://www.paralympic.org
Target Shooting	Amateur Trap Shooting Association Shooting Canada	http://www.shootata.com/ http://www.targetshooting.ca
Triathlon	International Triathlon Union	http://www.triathlon.org
Water-Skiing	USA Water Ski	http://www.usawaterski.orgpages/divisions/WSDA
Wheelchair Fencing	International Wheelchair Fencing Committee International Paralympic Committee—	http://www.iwfencing.com/ http://www.paralympic.org
Wheelchair Rugby	United States Quad Rugby Association International Paralympic Committee— International Rugby Board	http://www.quadrugby.com http://www.paralympic.org http://www.irb.com
Wheelchair Sports (archery, athletics, track and field, road racing, shooting, swimming, table tennis, and weightlifting for junior and adult competitors)	Canadian Wheelchair Sports Association Wheelchair Sports USA	http://www.cwsa.ca http://www.wsusa.org

Continued

Table 19-1
Physical Activity and Sport Options for Persons With SCI—cont'd

Activity/Sport	Organizations	Website Links
Wheelchair Tennis	United States Tennis Association International Tennis Federation International Paralympic Committee—	http://www.usta.com/playnow/wheelchair.aspx http://www.itftennis.com/wheelchair/ http://www.paralympic.org
Winter And Outdoor Sports (including skiing, snowboarding, sled hockey, bobsled, and more)	National Ability Center (outdoor sports) International Paralympic Committee—	http://www.nac1985.org http://www.paralympic.org Select Winter Sports

activity in individuals with disabilities. Perceived barriers include fatigue, lack of resources or information, little direction from health-care providers, as well as structural barriers.[42,43] Findings of a 10-city qualitative study showed 10 major categories of barriers and facilitators to physical activity among people with disabilities (*see* Table 19-2).[44]

Inclusive Fitness. The tasks of recognizing and addressing these barriers are critically important in facilitating

behavior change to include physical activity in persons with SCI. For example, easy access to an exercise environment that provides inclusive fitness equipment may attract people with all types of disabilities. The Inclusive Fitness Initiative (IFI), funded by lottery profits in the United Kingdom, is an example of policy-focused action intended to reduce barriers to physical activity among people with disabilities. IFI standards include principles of accessible facilities, criteria for inclusive fitness equipment, qualifications of staff with appropriate training

Table 19-2
Major Categories of Barriers and Facilitators to Physical Activity in People With Disabilities[44]

Category	Definition
Built and natural environment	Barriers or facilitators relating directly to aspects of the built or natural environment
Cost/economic	Barriers or facilitators relating to the cost of participating in recreation/fitness activities or costs associated with making facilities accessible
Equipment	Accessibility of exercise and recreation equipment
Guidelines, codes, regulations, and laws	Issues related to the use and interpretation of laws and regulations concerning accessibility of information, particularly building codes and the Americans with Disabilities Act (ADA)
Information	Access of information both within the facility (e.g., signs, brochures) and in facility brochures and advertisements
Emotional/psychological	Physical, emotional, or psychological barriers to participation in fitness and recreation activities among persons with disabilities
Knowledge, education, and training	Barriers and facilitator regarding the education and training of professionals in the areas of accessibility and appropriate interactions involving people with disabilities
Perceptions and attitudes	Perceptions and attitudes of both professionals and nondisabled individuals toward accessibility and persons with disabilities

Table 19-2

Major Categories of Barriers and Facilitators to Physical Activity in People With Disabilities[44]—cont'd

Category	Definition
Policies and procedures	Barriers imposed by the implementation of facility or community-level rules or regulations
Resource availability	Needed resources that would allow persons with disabilities to participate in fitness and recreation activities, including transportation and adaptive equipment

Reprinted from: Rimmer JH, Riley B, Wang E, Rauworth A, Jurkowski J. *Physical activity participation among persons with disabilities: Barriers and facilitators. Am J Prev Med.* 2004;26(5):419–425.

and skills, and descriptions of appropriate, inclusive marketing strategies.[45]

There are multiple resources available that identify and promote inclusive fitness equipment and resources. Table 19-3 lists some examples of inclusive fitness equipment and multimedia resources. These products are commercially available for individuals, rehabilitation centers, fitness facilities, schools, and community centers. Figure 19-2 shows a piece of equipment that can be used easily and adjusted independently by an individual with tetraplegia. Multimedia resources such as exercise videos may also serve as valuable educational tools for both clients and staff.

Table 19-3

Selected Examples of Inclusive Fitness Equipment and Multimedia Resources

Type of Equipment	Manufacturer	Product and Features
Strength training equipment	Pulse Fitness Systems, Inc. http://www.pulfit.com	Access by Pulse Fitness Systems manufactures eight different upper extremity weight machines designed with seats that swivel to the side, allowing access to individuals using wheelchairs.
Strength training equipment	Equalizer Exercise Machines http://www.equalizerexercise.com	The Equalizer machines provide universal access in a multistation, multiexercise unit.
Strength training equipment	Bowflex http://www.bowflex.com	The Bowflex Versatrainer is specially designed for people with limited mobility or different physical abilities. From strength training to cardiovascular to rehabilitative exercises, the VersaTrainer accommodates wheelchair users. Adapted hand grips are available.
Strength training equipment	GPK, Inc. http://www.gpk.com/upprtone.htm	Uppertone is a specialized exercise system that allows people with C4–C5 and below tetraplegia to do strength training, make adjustments, including resistance, without hand grip strength, cuffs, or assistance.
Strength training equipment	Cybex http://www.cybexintl.com	A variety of inclusive fitness/weight training machines with swing-away seats accommodating wheelchair access are offered.
Strength training equipment	RehaMed, Int. LLC http://www.grouprmt.com	(See Vitaglide below under upper body aerobic exercise.)

Continued

Table 19-3

Selected Examples of Inclusive Fitness Equipment and Multimedia Resources—cont'd

Type of Equipment	Manufacturer	Product and Features
Upper body aerobic exercise	Biodex Medical Systems, Inc. http://www.biodex.com	This upper body cycle has removable or large swivel seat; adapted hand grips.
Upper body aerobic exercise	McLain Cycle Products, Otsego, MI Distributor: http://www.accesstr.com	McLain Wheelchair Roller, or "The Bug Roller," is a ramped wheelchair roller system that allows for muscular and cardiovascular conditioning; accommodates all chair sizes; portable and easy to store.
Upper body aerobic exercise	RehaMed, International, LLC http://www.grouprmt.com	Vitaglide Pro Wheelchair Fitness Machine uses a repetitive, linear push-pull motion for both upper trunk and shoulder strengthening, as well as cardiovascular conditioning. Adjustable resistance and height; equipped with a built-in roll-away seat that is easily moved into position for non-wheelchair users; optional gloves and tri-post adaptors for tetraplegia.
Upper body aerobic exercise (handcycles)	Sunrise Medical http://www.sunrisemedical.com

Eagle Sportschairs http://www.eaglesportschairs.com | Quickie handbikes offer a variety of models and sizes for adults and children.

Eagle Sportschairs offers handcycles for both adults and children. |
Full body seated exercise	No Boundaries Mobility, LLC http://www.noboundariestv.com	The Active/passive trainer is a bicycle-type exerciser with adjustable height, speed, resistance, and range of motion; offers a manual mode and a powered mode that provides assistance to propel pedals. Special features include an antispasm mechanism, auto-reverse, and bi-directional pedals.
Full body seated exercise	NuStep http://www.nustep.com	The NuStep recumbent cross trainer is ergonomically designed to provide simultaneous upper and lower body conditioning for muscles and cardiovascular system, without stress on hips, knees, or shoulders.
Full body seated exercise	Rand-Scot Inc. http://www.saratoga-intl.com/saratoga/	Saratoga cycles are available for arm-only, leg-only, or combined arm and leg cycling. Available with adapted hand grip options, ankle-stabilizing boots, or ankle-toe straps.
Full body seated exercise	Thoele Manufacturing, Inc. Montrose, IL Distributed by: http://www.accesstotr.com	Pedal in Place is a bicycle-like exerciser that can be pedaled by hands, feet, or both.
Exercise videos	Christopher and Dana Reeve Paralysis Resource Center http://www.paralysis.com (Produced by the National Center for Physical Activity and Disability)	*Exercise Program for Individuals with Spinal Cord Injuries: Paraplegia* (VHS/DVD) *Exercise Program for Individuals with Spinal Cord Injuries: Tetraplegia* (VHS/DVD) Exercise video are available including 25 minutes with warm-up, upper body aerobics, strength training, cool down, and stretching.

Table 19-3

Selected Examples of Inclusive Fitness Equipment and Multimedia Resources—cont'd

Type of Equipment	Manufacturer	Product and Features
Exercise videos	Comprehensive listing of exercise videos at http://www.sci-health.org/library/videos.php *Armchair Aerobics* *I Want Those Arms* *Lisa Ericson's Seated Aerobic Workout* *Richard Simmons Sit Tight* *Secrets of a Great Body Upper Body Workout* *Sexy Arms* *Shortcuts: Tone and Tighten Arms and Shoulders in Minutes* *TAEBO* *The Firm Fat Blaster* *The Firm Upper Body* *The Firm Cross Trainers Super Cardio* *The Firm Cross Trainers Upper Body Split* *Yoga Health*	This comprehensive listing of exercise tapes/DVDs have been reviewed by people with SCIs (with tetraplegia and paraplegia) and people with limited mobility who are exercising from a seated position. Some of the tapes/DVDs were developed for people with SCI or persons with limited lower body strength, and some are upper body workouts for people without disabilities.

Getting Started in Physical Activity, Recreational, and Competitive Sports

Designing a Fitness or Conditioning Program

A fitness program can be designed to improve strength, endurance, or flexibility. There are key principles of safety, intensity, frequency, duration, and specificity that must be considered when planning a fitness or conditioning program for a person with SCI. Following these principles will ensure identification of risks, provide an appropriate starting point and structure for progression, and facilitate the achievement of desired outcomes.

Screening

A physician and physical therapist should screen the client with SCI for occult and known conditions that may require further evaluation and treatment, precautions, monitoring, or modified participation to avoid injury or exacerbation. Recommended diagnostic tests include (1) an exercise stress test to determine a peak heart rate and oxygen consumption (VO$_2$ peak); (2) a bone mineral density (BMD) scan to screen for fracture risk; (3) a pulmonary function test (PFT) to identify

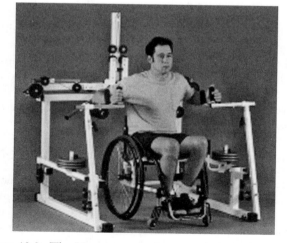

Figure 19-2. The Uppertone can be set up independently by a person with tetraplegia to perform 16 different strengthening exercises.

ventilatory parameters that may interfere with exercise; and (4) blood tests, including a lipid panel and a glucose test.[46–48] Further investigation is needed to identify a threshold BMD level that predicts fracture risk in SCI.

Exercise Prescription

An *exercise prescription* is based on established principles of exercise training. Training requires an *overload*, which is achieved at a specified intensity, duration, and frequency of exercise. Normal activities of daily living are generally insufficient in intensity or not sustained long enough to reach overload conditions.

The program should also incorporate principles of *specificity* of training. Training outcomes are largely related to the types of activities employed as the training stimulus. Training has an effect on muscle fibers, metabolic systems, and respiratory and cardiovascular systems. Training effects are both peripheral (size and metabolism within muscle fibers) and central (efficiency of cardiovascular, respiratory, and oxygen delivery systems). Although there is a transfer of conditioning from activities involved in training to other activities, especially among individuals who are deconditioned, inclusion of anaerobic and aerobic exercise will provide greater peripheral and central benefits, respectively. Therefore, for optimal results, the program should include both anaerobic and aerobic training.

The selection of training activities may also be most beneficial if it is specific to functional needs. For example, there has been evidence that training using arm cranking does not improve either wheelchair propulsion or upper extremity function. However, keep in mind that the inclusion of specific exercises may prevent musculoskeletal disorders from developing. For example, sufficient flexibility of the shoulder girdle and the strength of key posterior shoulder muscle groups may be of critical importance in preventing shoulder pain that will ultimately interfere with function.[30]

Warm Up and Cool Down

Essential parts of the exercise program before either anaerobic or aerobic exercise include a gradual warm-up and cool-down routine. Spending 10 minutes to slowly begin exercise will ensure optimal peripheral and myocardial blood flow at the onset of more strenuous exercise. A cool-down of similar duration should be followed by stretching and flexibility exercises.

Anaerobic Training

Anaerobic training is used to develop strength, power, or speed. *Anaerobic training* involves exercises less than 2 minutes in duration, overloading muscles with short-duration high loads. Anaerobic training is generally carried out using weight stations, free weights, or elastic bands for resistance. The *intensity* of anaerobic training is planned by determination of one repetition maximum (1-RM), the load that an individual can lift for one and only one repetition of an exercise. To minimize the risk of injury in untrained lifters, 1-RM can be predicted by using a sub-maximal load that can be lifted for 4 to 10 repetitions.[49]

There are many on-line web-based calculators that provide conversions from a sub-maximal performance to an estimated 1-RM load. One should use caution when using these, however, as they have been developed from studies on individuals with healthy, innervated muscle. Recent evidence supports that 1-RM can even be estimated from as few as four to six repetitions of a submaximal load.[49] In any case, the recommended intensity of anaerobic exercise is then determined by calculating a range from 50% to 80% of 1-RM.[46] The recommended duration of anaerobic training is two to three sets of 10 repetitions of each exercise. The recommended frequency of anaerobic training is two times per week.[46]

Aerobic Training

Aerobic training is used to develop endurance. *Aerobic* activities that use large muscle groups offer the best mode of exercise to improve cardiorespiratory conditioning. Upper body physical activities that are considered aerobic include arm cycling, continuous wheelchair propulsion (outside or indoors on rollers), hand-biking, swimming, chair aerobics, rowing, and kayaking. Walking, running, and cycling are also aerobic exercise options for people who are able to use their legs. The recommended intensity of aerobic exercise should be great enough to reach a *target heart rate (THR)*, a range that reflects the sum of the *resting heart rate (RHR)* and 40% to 80% of the *heart rate reserve (HRR)*. The heart rate reserve is calculated by subtracting the resting heart rate from the *maximum* or *peak heart rate (MHR)*, found during a stress test, often done using arm cycle ergometry.

$$HRR = MHR - RHR$$

If an exercise stress test has not been performed, the THR should be set at 20 to 30 beats above the RHR.[46]

The Karvonen formula is used to calculate the target exercise heart rate range. To use this formula, the therapist must know the MHR and the RHR.

$$THR = [(MHR - RHR) \times 40\% \text{ to } 80\%] + RHR$$

The lowest levels of intensity (e.g., 40%) are used for those individuals who are most deconditioned, and intensity is slowly progressed toward the higher levels over weeks of exercise. The recommended duration should be 30 minutes of continuous aerobic exercise. Exercise should be done at least two to three times per week.[46] If aerobic and anaerobic training are done on different days, it is possible to alternate aerobic training 3 days per week with anaerobic training twice per week. Box 19-2 illustrates how THR is calculated in two individuals with SCI.

Physical activity at submaximal rates (60% to 75% of MHR) can be continued at a safe rate for a long period of time. A good guideline as to appropriate intensity is the

---

Box 19-2
Target Heart Rate Calculation

Case 1: Stanley is a 50 year-old male with T-12 paraplegia (ASIA A). Weight 220, height 5 feet 10 inches; 33 years post-injury

Maximal heart rate (MHR) = 160; resting heart rate (RHR) = 90

Exercise target heart rate (THR) range = [(MHR – RHR) × 40% to 80%] + RHR

MHR – RHR = 160 – 90 = 70

40% (MHR – RHR) = .40 × (70) = 28

80% × (MHR – RHR) = .80 × (70) = 56

Exercise target heart rate (THR) range = (RHR + 28) to (RHR + 56) = (90 + 28) to (90 + 56) = 118 to 146 beats per minute

Case 2: Julia is a 30-year-old woman with C-7 tetraplegia (ASIA A). Weight 120, height 5 feet 6 inches; 7 years post-injury

Maximal heart rate (MHR) = 120; resting heart rate (RHR) = 60

Exercise target heart rate (THR) range = [(MHR – RHR) × 40% to 80%] + RHR

MHR – RHR = 120 – 60 = 60

40% (MHR – RHR) = .40 × (60) = 24

80% × (MHR – RHR) = .80 × (60) = 48

Exercise target heart rate (THR) range = (RHR + 24) to (RHR + 48) = (60 + 24) to (60 + 48) = 84 to 106 beats per minute

---

ability to carry on a conversation during the physical activity. If exercise is so intense that it is not possible to converse without shortness of breath, it's time to decrease the intensity or the pace.

Flexibility

Although it is possible to stretch during the warm-up phase, the most effective prolonged stretching should be done after exercise. The pectoral, biceps, triceps, wrist extensor, and wrist flexor muscles are all included in stretching recommendations. In addition, stretching into shoulder flexion, horizontal abduction, and internal and external rotation is important to maintain shoulder range of motion, especially following strenuous exercise.[50,51] It is important to note that athletes with disabilities often exhibit muscle imbalance, with stronger tight muscle groups and opposing overstretched, weaker muscles. The goal of stretching is to achieve an optimal length–tension relationship, minimizing stretching of overstretched weaker muscles and achieving full range of the stronger opposing muscle groups. Typically, in athletes with disabilities who have innervated upper extremity musculature, the pectoral, biceps, shoulder internal rotator, and adductor muscles tend to be stronger and tighter. In contrast, the shoulder external rotator and scapula adductor muscles tend to be weaker and overstretched.

Benefits of Training

Aerobic training contributes to function and health by reducing the resting heart rate and increasing stroke volume, resulting in greater central efficiency. By becoming more fit, aerobic capacity is increased. The energy costs of daily activity then become a smaller percentage of the maximum capacity, thus leaving a greater energy reserve to carry out daily activities. Recent evidence also indicates that arm-cranking exercise has a positive effect in raising blood levels of HDL-C, but has minimal effects on total cholesterol and triglycerides in either persons with SCI or in able-bodied subjects.[29] Additionally, with increased lean body mass (e.g., muscle), the resting metabolic rate is higher, requiring more energy and facilitating reduction in body fat stores and weight loss efforts. In addition, reduced pain, greater energy, and improved quality of life have all been reported as beneficial outcomes of regular physical activity in persons with SCI.[52]

Adherence is a major issue in sustaining new exercise habits, as in any health behavior change. Peer support and social engagement provide key motivation. In addition, supervised exercise seems to support and sustain physical activity behavior change in individuals with SCI. In fact, half of the participants with SCI in a controlled exercise trial failed to continue when the supervised program concluded. Those who did not continue subsequently reported lower quality of life and higher pain and stress levels.[52]

Ensuring Safe Physical Activity and Sport Participation

Injuries and Illnesses of Athletes with SCI

There have been a number of studies that have examined the injuries and illnesses of athletes with SCI.[53–56] Similar to the general population, athletes with SCI experience athletic injuries related to the specific risks and demands of their sport. Table 19-4 compares the results of four surveys of injuries and medical conditions reported by adult and pediatric wheelchair athletes.

Track, road-racing, and wheelchair basketball present the highest risk for injuries among athletes who compete in wheelchairs.[53,54] Overuse injuries of the shoulder, elbow, and wrist occur frequently. Athletes who report a training history that includes more hours per week and a longer duration generally report more injuries than do

Table 19-4
Common Injuries of Wheelchair Athletes[57]

Type of Injury	128 Adult Athletes, All Sports (% of 291 Reported Injuries)[55]	90 Adult Athletes, All Sports (% of 346 Reported Injuries)[56]	69 Pediatric Track Athletes (% of Athletes Reporting)[57]	19 Elite Athletes (% of 50 Reported Injuries)[58]
Soft tissue injuries	33	32	34	52
Blisters	18	25	77	6
Lacerations/ abrasions	17	27	38	24
Decubitus/ pressure areas	7	3	14	Not reported
Arthritis/joint inflammation	5	1.5	Not reported	Not reported
Fractures	5	2	6	6
Hand weakness/ numbness	5	Not reported	Not reported	Not reported
Bruises/ contusions	Not reported	8	41	10
Temperature regulation disorders	3	Not reported	49	Not reported
Head injury/ concussion	2	2	Not reported	Not reported
Dental injury	1	1	Not reported	Not reported
Dislocation	Not reported	<1	Not reported	Not reported
Eye injury	Not reported	<1	Not reported	Not reported
Wheel burns	Included with lacerations	Not reported	71	Not reported
Other illness	Not reported	Not reported	Not reported	2

Adapted from: Curtis KA, Gailey RS. The athlete with a disability. In: Zachazewski J, Quillen W, Magee D, editors. *Athletic Injuries and Rehabilitation*. Philadelphia, PA: W.B. Saunders; 1996.

those who have a shorter duration and less-intense training history.[53] The most common injuries to athletes competing in wheelchairs are soft tissue injuries of shoulder, elbow, wrist, abrasions and contusions of arms and hands, and blisters of the hands.[53–56]

Preventing Common Athletic Injuries

Athletes with SCI are at risk for the same types of injuries that athletes without disabilities experience, such as overuse injuries, strains, sprains, abrasions, lacerations, and joint trauma.

Soft Tissue Injuries of Upper Extremities

Wheelchair propulsion involves specific repetitive upper extremity motion and therefore stresses the shoulder, elbow, and wrist joints. Overuse injuries such as rotator cuff injuries, bicipital tendonitis, shoulder impingement syndromes, epicondylitis (tennis elbow), extensor carpi radialis tendonitis, and carpal tunnel syndrome are common problems in athletes with SCI who compete in wheelchairs.[22,25,53]

It is important to understand the biomechanical requirements of wheelchair propulsion. The wheelchair push stroke stresses development of the pectoral, anterior deltoid, triceps, and biceps muscles. This often results in upper extremity muscle imbalance with increased strength and tightness in these muscle groups and weaker, over-stretched posterior shoulder musculature. This pattern of posterior muscle weakness and anterior muscle tightness may cause postural deviations, such as forward head (lower cervical flexion, upper cervical extension) and rounded shoulders (scapula elevation, protraction, and forward tilt, often with internal rotation of the humerus) while sitting.

Although some evidence indicates that shoulder pain among wheelchair users is less common in athletes than in nonathletes,[31] many athletes with SCI experience chronic soft tissue problems of the upper extremities. Consider the demands of wheelchair propulsion during a busy competitive season. While wheelchair basketball players often practice and play in excess of 15 to 20 hours per week, elite road racers often train total distances in excess of 100 miles per week.

Wheelchair users frequently engage in overhead activity to carry out daily activities. The need to reach overhead, combined with muscle imbalance, often leads to *impingement syndrome*.[22] Rotator cuff impingement syndrome has been associated with comparative weakness of the humeral head depressors (shoulder rotator and adductor muscles) in comparison to shoulder abductors and flexors in wheelchair users.[22]

There are roles for both stretching and strengthening in addressing impingement syndrome. Specific stretching exercises should emphasize flexibility in shoulder flexion, extension, horizontal abduction, and external rotation, and achieve full length of the triceps and biceps muscles, since they are two-joint muscles. Strength training exercises should emphasize restoring balance at the shoulder and scapular muscles. Usually, these exercises are most beneficial if they focus on strengthening of the posterior shoulder, including posterior deltoid, latissimus dorsi, external rotator, rhomboids, and middle and lower trapezius muscles. Shoulder pain can be reduced significantly by achieving muscle balance (Fig. 19-3).[30]

Standard guidelines of acute management of soft tissue injuries, such as RICE (rest, ice, compression, and elevation), also apply to the musculoskeletal injuries sustained by persons with SCI. Preventive taping and applications of cold after participation and anti-inflammatory medications may help athletes with chronic soft tissue problems control exercise-associated inflammation. Effective management of chronic musculoskeletal conditions is critical to prevent reinjury, further complications, and secondary disability in this population.

Degenerative Joint Disease

Most long-term wheelchair users eventually experience degenerative joint disease of the upper extremities. In addition to degenerative joint disease, osteonecrosis of the

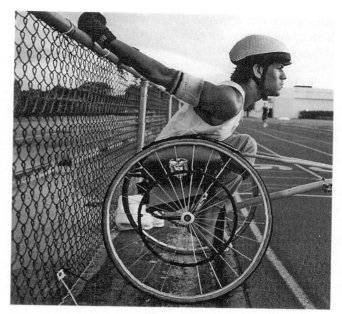

Figure 19-3. Wheelchair track athlete stretching the biceps by extending both elbow and shoulder.

shoulder has been reported in wheelchair users.[58] The demands of upper extremity weight bearing and constant shoulder use are thought to precipitate the development of chronic shoulder problems. Intra-articular pressures have been reported to be two and one-half times greater than arterial pressure during wheelchair transfers.[59]

Abrasions and Contusions

Wheelchair users often sustain abrasions and lacerations from incidental contact with the wheelchair parts.[53] Wheelchair racers frequently experience friction burns on the medial surface of the upper arms from repeated contact with the large tires during the down stroke when pushing a racing wheelchair. Others have abrasions from contact with the back of the racing wheelchair at the sacrum. Novice athletes, who don't have equipment that is specific for sports, often use wheelchairs with brakes located adjacent to the wheelchair push rim. Traumatic thumb injuries may occur from contact with the brake during wheelchair propulsion.

There are simple protective measures to take to prevent these types of injuries. The upper arm is protected from accidental contact with wheelchair tires by wearing protective gear. Wearing gloves may eliminate hand injuries. Bicycle-type helmets help prevent head injury in event of collision. All wheelchair parts or sharp surfaces that could accidentally result in a contact injury should be covered or removed.

Blisters

Blisters can be a problem for both novice and experienced wheelchair athletes. Athletes report blisters of the fingers and thumb related to continuous contact with the wheelchair rim required during wheelchair propulsion. Thick calluses may form on the palm of the hand. These calluses are prone to dry out, crack, and result in painful fissures that are open to infection.

To prevent these problems, athletes should clean their hands frequently and file calluses with a pumice stone. Open cracks or fissures, blisters, and other abrasions should be treated with antibiotic creams and covered with Band-Aids or dressings as appropriate. Athletes should wear gloves routinely for both training and competition. Leather batting gloves or handball gloves are easily adapted and reinforced for wheelchair pushing by applying layers of tape to the areas of highest pressure. Custom-designed leather mitts with reinforced neoprene are also widely used in wheelchair road racing (Fig. 19-4).

Preventing Disability-Specific Medical Problems

In addition to the specific hazards of injury from sport participation, there are other disability-specific conditions that athletes with SCI often experience. It is important to evaluate each person individually to be able to devise the best strategies for prevention of secondary conditions during physical activity or sport participation.

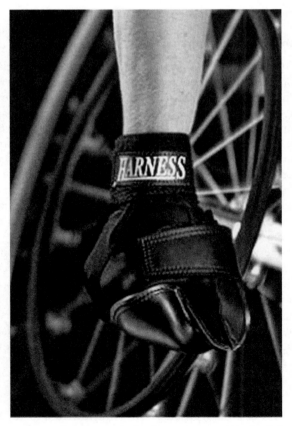

Figure 19-4. Custom-made leather mitts provide both hand protection and traction for the track- and road-racing athlete.

Lack of Protective Sensation

Persons with SCI often lack the protection provided by pressure, temperature, and pain sensation. Insensitive areas are vulnerable to skin breakdown, ulceration, and infection. Therefore, insensitive skin must be inspected frequently.

If persistent redness of the skin is noted over a bony prominence, the athlete should relieve all pressure from sitting or clothes or equipment until the redness resolves and normal skin color returns. These areas are at risk for ulceration and may progress to serious infections. Athletes with open pressure sores should not participate in training or competition and should sit as little as possible to prevent additional pressure damage.

Bones in insensitive areas are often osteoporotic and may fracture from a trivial injury. Since the athlete with SCI may lack sensation of pain that would accompany a bone fracture, any evidence of an abnormal body position, bruising, edema, or grinding sensations with movement calls for a radiographic assessment to rule out a fracture.

Temperature Regulation Disorders

Environmental exposure to heat and cold often provide unique challenges to the athlete with a SCI. Although able-bodied athletes may also experience thermal injuries, the athletes with SCI are even more susceptible due to sensory impairments, sympathetic nervous system dysfunction, and inadequate physiological mechanisms for cooling or warming. With poor sensation and relatively lower blood flow to the skin and deep tissues, the lower extremities are more susceptible to both sunburn and frostbite. Exposure to heat or cold may cause serious deep tissue damage. Similarly, healing of a burn or frostbite injury in the paralyzed lower limb tends to be slow and difficult.

Individuals with SCI should take particular care when skin is in contact with metal equipment, asphalt surfaces, and artificial turf, which heat up in the sun and may burn the person without sensation. Dependent edema of the lower extremities can also be a problem, especially in hot climates, due to inadequate venous return.

Individuals with SCI may experience problems with regulation of core body temperature due to a loss of normal blood flow regulation via the central nervous system. Athletes with tetraplegia often report heat and cold intolerance.[53] These athletes are unable to perspire below the level of the cervical SCI. Furthermore, some medications used for pain, depression, allergy, bladder dysfunction, high blood pressure, and other problems may also interfere with normal perspiration. Since both hypothermia and hyperthermia are potentially fatal conditions, it is important to know how to recognize and prevent these conditions.

Hypothermia

Hypothermia is a potentially fatal condition because it may result in cardiac arrhythmias and dysfunction of other body systems. Early symptoms include weakness, fatigue, and a decreased shivering response, followed by collapse and unconsciousness.

Cold and wet conditions are especially dangerous and increase risk of hypothermia. An athlete with SCI may lack sensation to feel cold extremities. Furthermore, the athlete may lack normal physiological mechanisms to conserve heat, such as goose bump production, shivering, and circulatory shunting for warming. After training or competition, the athlete should change out of cold or wet garments and ensure that there is no post-exercise lowering of the body temperature. Medically supervised rewarming is the recommended treatment for athletes with SCI who experience hypothermia.

The following general principles will aid in the prevention of hypothermia in the athlete with SCI:

- Protective clothing should be sufficient to keep the athlete comfortable during the activity. Multiple layers of clothes will trap air between the layers. Cotton and polypropylene fabrics are recommended for the innermost layer to carry moisture away from the body because cooling will occur more rapidly if the skin surface is wet.
- The athlete should wear a hat or helmet when training or competing in cold weather because 25% of heat loss occurs from the head.
- Adequate hydration is critical, and thirst is often an inaccurate indicator in cold conditions.

Hyperthermia

Intolerance to heat is exacerbated by the environmental temperature and humidity. Some mild symptoms of heat illness are characterized by muscle cramps in exercising muscles after exercising in the heat. More severe symptoms of heat exhaustion are headache, nausea, vomiting, lightheadedness, weakness, cramps, and general malaise. With progression to heat stroke, the athlete's body temperature may rise dangerously high, and he or she is at risk for multiple organ damage. He or she may become confused or disoriented, may faint, and often stops sweating normally.

Athletes with SCI, especially tetraplegia, should exercise extreme caution when the sum of the outdoor temperature in degrees Fahrenheit and percentage of humidity exceeds 150. Excessive humidity prevents cooling of the body by normal sweating, and high ambient temperatures prevent heat dissipation from the body to the environment. This is further complicated because athletes with tetraplegia above the level of the first thoracic segment (T-1) do not sweat below the level of the neurological lesion and therefore will not be able to lower their body temperature by this form of heat exchange.

Athletes must be educated that thirst is an unreliable indicator of hydration in hot environments. Athletes should drink water continuously, regardless of thirst. Optimal hydration guidelines are to drink at least 1 liter

(about a quart) of water 1 to 2 hours before competition or training and 1/2 liter (16 oz) of water 30 minutes before the event. Fluid replacement should continue at a rate of at least 250 cc (8 oz) every 10 to 15 minutes during training or competition. Cool water is the best form of fluid replacement for events lasting less than 1 hour. Glucose/electrolyte and carbohydrate polymer solutions may be beneficial in events lasting over 1 hour, as they delay the onset of fatigue. Solutions should be of a concentration of less than 10%; a concentration of 6% to 8% is ideal. If the athlete drinks electrolyte solutions or soda, he or she should dilute the solution two times more than is recommended or drink 2 cups of water for each cup of soda or electrolyte solution consumed. Alcoholic beverages and caffeine-containing beverages should be avoided because they will cause further dehydration. Some athletes with disabilities restrict water intake because of bladder incontinence. Coaches need to ensure that athletes have access to adequate bathroom facilities.

In addition to hydration, seeking shade and wearing protective clothing are the best means to prevent heat exposure. Athletes should be provided access to well-ventilated, shady areas. Additional preventive measures, such as spraying a mist of cool water on the exposed surface of the face, neck, upper trunk, and arms, may also be helpful in facilitating cooling.

Sunscreens should be used whenever athletes will be exposed to the sun. Sunburn is a risk to athletes with SCI, especially in areas without sensation, as there are often concomitant circulatory changes to the skin. Even though sunscreens will protect against sunburn, they may increase risk of heat intolerance by impeding sweating and impairing cooling, especially in athletes who do not perspire normally. To prevent this, athletes should use sunscreen only on those areas exposed to the sun.

Any athlete showing signs of heat intolerance should be removed to a shaded, cool, well-ventilated area and be treated for heat illness. Medical attention is essential to cool the athlete as quickly as possible. Fluid replacement and cooling at the neck, groin, and armpits are often adequate to reverse symptoms, although more extensive treatment may be indicated.

Bladder Dysfunction

Athletes with SCI often have a neurogenic bladder. Bladder infections, bladder stones, and bladder obstruction are common when the bladder does not empty properly or completely. To prevent recurrent bladder infection, athletes should ensure adequate fluid intake and have access to clean areas to avoid contamination during handling and use of catheters and connecting tubing and bags.

Bladder obstruction may precipitate autonomic dysreflexia, and blood pressure can rise dangerously high, increasing risk of cerebral hemorrhage. Exercise may exacerbate these problems. Some athletes with tetraplegia have found that the concomitant rise in blood pressure and release of catecholamines enhance performance and intentionally simulate a temporary bladder obstruction to cause autonomic dysreflexia, a practice called *boosting*.[60–63] This is very dangerous and should never be practiced in training or competition due to the unpredictable risk of uncontrollable hypertension. The International Paralympic Committee has officially banned athletes from voluntarily inducing autonomic dysreflexia during competition.[64]

Postural Hypotension

Athletes with SCI may experience postural hypotension with rapid position changes due to sympathetic nervous system dysfunction that does not accommodate for the shift in blood volume or effects of medications. Athletes who have hypotension may experience lightheadedness or fainting. This is usually rectified by positioning. If an athlete in a wheelchair experiences lightheadedness due to hypotension, the individual should be assisted to a recumbent position or the wheelchair tipped back to help return blood flow to the brain. Gentle pressure on the abdomen with deep breathing may also be helpful. Table 19-5 includes a summary of prevention and treatment strategies to address the most common injuries and disability-specific medical conditions of athletes with SCI.

Table 19-5
Injuries and Disability-Specific Medical Conditions of Athletes With SCIs

Problem	Prevention	Treatment
Chronic overuse syndromes (shoulder impingement, tendonitis, bursitis, carpal tunnel syndrome)	Use taping, splinting, protective padding; proper wheelchair positioning; good technique. Employ posterior shoulder and scapula muscle strengthening. Use regular stretching into shoulder flexion, horizontal abduction, and external rotation.	Rest. Apply injury-specific principles of care; selective strengthening, muscle balancing, flexibility; analysis of technique.
Overexertion (muscle strains)	Warm up and stretch; use proper conditioning and equipment.	Rest, gradual progression of exercise program.
Falls, physical contact (sprains, contusions)	Observe equipment safety. Use appropriate padding for sport. Use appropriate sport-specific spotting. Use qualified assistance/guides for athletes.	Apply injury-specific principles of care. Check for signs of fracture in athletes without movement or sensation.
Blisters	Encourage callous formation. Use protecting taping, gloves, padding, cushioning, adequate clothing.	Apply injury-specific principles of care; be aware of areas that lack sensation; adjustments of clothing or protective gear.
Abrasions/lacerations	Be aware of areas that lack sensation. Check equipment for sharp or abrasive surfaces; wear protective clothing. Use cushions or towels in all transfers. Use mats on hard surfaces. Camber wheelchair wheels.	Apply injury-specific principles of care.
Decubitus ulcers and burns	Check equipment for sources of pressure or friction. Use adequate cushioning; proper weight shifting; dry clothing. Take special precautions for areas without sensation. Inspect skin frequently. Use good nutrition and hygiene.	Bed rest if necessary to remove all pressure from a weight-bearing surface. Open wound care as necessary.

Table 19-5

Injuries and Disability-Specific Medical Conditions of Athletes With SCIs—cont'd

Problem	Prevention	Treatment
Temperature regulation disorders (hyperthermia)	Minimize exposure to direct sun; provide shade. Wear adequate clothing for insulation and maintain hydration. Spray externally with water to help cooling. Avoid hot and humid conditions.	Remove from ambient conditions. Cool immediately. Seek medical assistance.
Temperature regulation disorders (hypothermia)	Minimize exposure. Wear adequate clothing, keeping head covered. Maintain hydration. Avoid exposure to cold and wet conditions.	Cover and seek medical assistance.
Autonomic dysreflexia (precipitous increase in systolic blood pressure and pounding headache in individuals with high thoracic and cervical SCI)	Empty bowel/bladder fully. Be aware that inducing autonomic dysreflexia ("boosting") has been reported as a means to improve performance. This is a very dangerous practice.	Lift to sitting position. Search for source of stimulus, usually full bladder or bowel. Attempt to relieve condition. This is a medical emergency.
Orthostatic hypotension	Wear elastic stockings or corset supports to aid venous return; avoid heat.	Recline in wheelchair or on ground/bed. Encourage deep breathing.
Seizures (previously diagnosed seizure disorders)	Avoid stress, dehydration, extremes of temperatures, and fatigue. Take seizure medications as prescribed (especially when traveling).	Turn on side; protect head and keep airway open by jaw thrust. Avoid putting objects in the mouth.
Unexplained fever (often urinary tract infections)	Drink fluids; practice good hygiene for self-catheterization.	Seek medical treatment and evaluation of source of fever.
Allergies (bee sting, drug)	Notify medical personnel at competition site of potential problem. Be prepared.	Seek medical treatment as needed.
Eye injuries	Use protective eyewear, goggles/safety glasses.	Apply injury-specific principles of care.

Adapted from: Curtis KA, Gailey RS. The athlete with a disability. In: Zachazewski J, Quillen W, Magee D, editors. *Athletic Injuries and Rehabilitation*. Philadelphia, PA: W.B. Saunders; 1996.

Classification of Athletes With Disabilities

Classification systems are intended to provide a means to ensure more equitable competition by making it more likely that training and athletic skills, not degree of physical disability, differentiates competitors. Athletes of a similar level of disability are grouped together in a *classification* designated for competition by sport. In individual sports, such as track and field or swimming, athletes in the same classification compete against each other. In contrast, in team sports, athletes in various classifications compete as a team in designated combinations.

Classification systems also serve to ensure that athletes with the most severe disabilities will not be excluded from the sport, especially in team sports.

Evolution From Medical to Functional Classification Systems

Prior to the 1980s, classification systems for athletes with disabilities were based solely on an examination of voluntary movement and neurological function. These classification systems presented multiple problems. They classified athletes within a disability group for all sports in which they competed, regardless of the relative functional advantages of having neurological function or mobility for a particular sport. For example, athletes who compete in wheelchair track events require considerably less trunk rotation for performance than do athletes who compete in sports such as wheelchair basketball.

Furthermore, there were arbitrary divisions between classification groups that did not reflect parallel advantages in performance across all sports. Some classification groups were very large and included athletes with a tremendous range of trunk and lower extremity function. In the United States, even today, the National Wheelchair Basketball Association (NWBA) continues to use a three-point medical classification system.[65] In contrast, international wheelchair basketball competition uses a functional system that includes four classifications and intermediate point values for athletes who do not fit well into one of the four classification groups.[66]

It is important to note that sport for athletes with disabilities also includes athletes with other disabilities besides SCI. Athletes with other disabilities such as post-polio paralysis, cerebral palsy, multiple sclerosis, and amputation often compete in wheelchairs. In a study to determine the equity of the classification system for athletes who compete in wheelchairs, data identifying the various disabilities of athletes who were finalists in each classification group were collected at a national multi-sport, multidisability championship. The study found that finalist groups comprised a disproportionate number of athletes with post-polio paralysis and athletes with amputations compared to the distribution of athletes with these types of disabilities in the organization's membership.[67] Athletes with SCI, spina bifida, and cerebral palsy were underrepresented in the finalist groups. This provided further evidence supporting a need to change.

As classification systems and sport organizations evolved over time, athletes within one disability group were prevented from competing against athletes from other disability group, as each disability sport organization (DSO) held separate national championships for their athletes. Even at world championship events, amputees using wheelchairs competed in different classification groups than did athletes with paraplegia using wheelchairs for each event in a track competition. By the 1988 Seoul Paralympic Games, this division of athletes by classification and by disability group resulted in over 40 different 100-meter races being run! This was both confusing and time-consuming for meet organizers, athletes, and spectators.

Although dissatisfaction with classification systems still remains, arbitrary divisions by disability seemed counter to the advancement of sport for athletes with disabilities. In the mid-1980s a sport scientist, an athlete, and a physical therapist collaborated to develop and revise the first classification system based on observation of an athlete's functional movement during actual wheelchair basketball competition, rather than the athlete's neurological level.[66] The classification system used a biomechanical analysis of the athlete's ability to rotate the trunk in a horizontal plane, bend forward in the sagittal plane, and bend from side to side in the coronal plane while seated in the wheelchair. An example of the principle of *volume of action*, used in the International Wheelchair Basketball Federation classification system is illustrated in Figure 19-5.

Other sports followed during the late 1980s and 1990s in an effort to consolidate athletes from multiple disability groups in their sport, rather than segregate competitions by athlete disability. Sport-specific functional classification systems have now developed for many sports, with medical personnel, sports scientists and technical experts, former athletes, and coaches as members of the classification team. Some multidisability sports differentiate disability groups, such as those with visual impairment from sighted competitors. Others use different classification groups for sitting and standing competitors. For example, classification systems in Alpine and Nordic skiing use a system that incorporates the type of adaptive ski equipment used and comparative data from the performance of athletes from all classification groups on the course to determine the winning performance. Classification systems are expected to continue to evolve further. Table 19-6 shows the types of classification systems currently used for various competitive sports. Additional information on classification systems is available at http://www.paralympic.org.

Classification Team

Rehabilitation professionals have traditionally been involved as classifiers in most sport organizations for athletes with disabilities. Traditional classification involved physical and disability assessment, often requiring that the classifier have expertise in neurology and orthopedics. Although these traditional observations still play a part in some functional classification systems, the observation of movement during performance in the sport is paramount.

The role of the classifier in the era of functional classification is to observe movement during performance in sports competition. Analysis of movement during sport performance is a skill critical to becoming a classifier.

Equipment Considerations

Equipment for sport competition is specialized and often expensive. There are lightweight wheelchairs for road racing and track competition (Fig. 19-6) and more mobile wheelchairs for wheelchair basketball, tennis, and rugby athletes. Athletes often construct heavier, more stable chairs and stands for field competition. Rules govern the dimensions and characteristics of sport equipment. An everyday wheelchair is not appropriate for

VOLUME OF ACTION

The key element of classification is the observation and assessment of each player's "volume of action."

The **Volume of Action** of a player is described as:

The limit to which a player can move voluntarily in any direction, and with control return to the upright seated position, without holding the wheelchair for support or to aid the movement. The volume of action includes all directions, and describes the position of the ball when held with both hands.

In the seated position, there are several "planes of movement" available. Although these planes have biomechanical names, in order to simplify the definition, they will be referred to as follows:

The **vertical plane**: rotating the trunk to face left or right while maintaining an upright postion (A)

The **forward plane**: bending the trunk forward, reaching the hands toward the feet and returning to upright (B)

The **sideways plane**: leaning the trunk to the left or right without movement in the forward plane and returning to upright (C)[66]

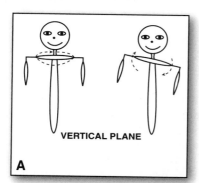
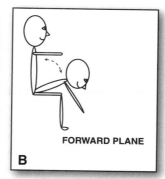
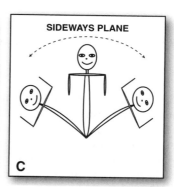

Figure 19-5. Volume of action provides a framework for observation of a wheelchair basketball player's functional movement during participation.

Table 19-6
Selected Classification Systems for Athletes With Disabilities

Sport	Classification System
Alpine and Nordic skiing	Three disability classes, based on athlete participation in blind (with a guide), standing, and sitting competitions.
Athletics (track and field)	Three classifications for athletes with visual impairment; seven classes for ambulatory athletes; seven classes for seated athletes
Basketball (wheelchair)	Three-class system (United States only) based on neurological function; four-class IWBF system based on functional trunk movement in wheelchair. Combined classification points of players on court limited by playing rules.
Cycling	Blind athletes compete on tandem cycle with sighted pilot. Leg cycling uses a four functional classes based on use of lower limbs in cycling. Handcycling uses a three-division, eight-classification system based on trunk and lower limb function.
Powerlifting	Competition by weight classes.
Shooting	Two-class system for athletes who do and do not require the use of a shooting stand for competition; a separate classification for athletes with visual impairment.

Continued

Table 19-6
Selected Classification Systems for Athletes With Disabilities—cont'd

Sport	Classification System
Swimming	Ten-class integrated system, with different classifications for breaststroke, backstroke, and freestyle
Table Tennis (seated and standing)	Five-class system for seated athletes, based on upper extremity and trunk function; five-class system for standing athletes
Tennis (wheelchair)	Two-class system, creating separate classification for athletes with tetraplegia or upper limb involvement.
Volleyball (sitting and standing)	For sitting volleyball: All players must sit; there is only a classification by minimal disability. Standing athletes play using nine-class system. Combined classification points of players on court limited by playing rules.
Wheelchair dance sport	Twp-class system based on ability to control wheelchair, extend arms, and rotate trunk.
Wheelchair rugby	Seven-class system, combining motor/sensory function and movement tests.

sport participation and, in most cases, is not allowed due to the hazards to the athlete, potential damage to the playing surface, and hazards to other competitors.

Equipment innovation has contributed greatly to improved performance. The technology involved in lightweight wheelchair design has used many principles and some hardware from bicycle technology. Athletes have led wheelchair design innovations. The first sub-5-minute wheelchair mile pace was reached in the late 1970s using a standard everyday wheelchair with athlete-designed adaptations. With widespread use of advanced racing technology and specialized training techniques, the current world record for the 1500 km is now less than 3 minutes (2:56.61, a 2001 record set by Franz Nietlispach of Switzerland.)[68]

Established athletes and sport programs can often provide equipment on a trial basis for novice participants. However, equipment is best fitted individually to each athlete and is specific for the sport and events in which they participate. There are specific measurement guidelines that are published by equipment vendors and wheelchair manufacturers. Care should be taken to ensure that there is proper cushioning and protection on all surfaces. In addition, protective gear, such as helmets and gloves, will ensure safe and enjoyable competition. See "Sources of Lightweight High-Performance Wheelchairs (Court Chairs)" and "Sources of Handcycles for Wheelchair Users" in Case Study 19-1.

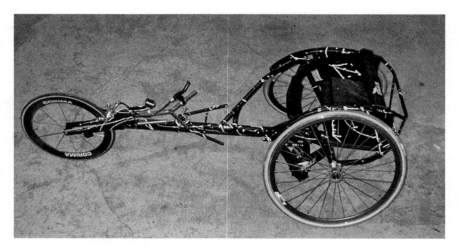

Figure 19-6. Specialized lightweight wheelchairs are used for track and road-racing competition.

CASE STUDY 19-1   Introducing Sports to Individuals With SCI

Background

Anton, a 17-year-old high school senior, sustained a T-12/L-1 vertebral fracture/dislocation with T-12 paraplegia, American Spinal Injury Association Impairment Scale B (AIS B), 2 months ago in an automobile accident. Following a spinal fusion with internal fixation, his recovery was uneventful, and he quickly became independent in most activities of daily living and most wheelchair mobility activities. He is 6 feet 4 inches tall and weighs 180 pounds.

One day, while in the rehabilitation center, he saw a bunch of guys in lightweight wheelchairs out on the basketball court outside his window. He slowly wheeled himself out by the court in his hospital wheelchair. One of the guys passed him the ball. He awkwardly caught it and felt stiff and uncoordinated, so different from just a few months ago when he led his high school team to the state championship. He took a breath and released the ball, taking a shot from his favorite spot in 3-point range. His shot fell short of the basket by 10 feet. One of the guys in the wheelchair commented, "Not bad for a rookie. Hey, we've got spot for a Class II like you!" Anton, embarrassed at his "air ball," wondered, "What is a Class II?" He returned to physical therapy, and his physical therapist gave him a flyer about wheelchair basketball and told him about a game next week where the team he just met would play their rivals from another city.

What do rehabilitation professionals need to know in order to inform their clients about organized sports opportunities? How can rehabilitation professionals introduce wheelchair sports to their clients and patients?

Although it is too early in Anton's recovery for him to participate actively in wheelchair basketball competition, he can prepare for and begin to socialize in this new athletic world. Let's learn a bit more about him.

Interview

Anton lives with his parents and is the oldest in a family of four children. The family lives in a suburban area. There are no stairs to enter or in the single-story home. Some doorways are narrow, and a paved driveway is sloped at 30-degree angle to street below. There are accessible sidewalks around the home. His family is supportive and wants to help him in any way they can.

He lives 3 miles from the high school where he was previously an active student, excelling in sports and involved in community service activities. He had recently purchased a used automobile, which was totally destroyed in the accident. It is unlikely that he will be licensed to drive soon due to pending legal issues.

Anton enjoys sports, especially basketball and track. Has been playing basketball since he was 4 years old. He likes to watch sports on television and live. He planned to go to college on a basketball scholarship. Has many friends and enjoys volunteering in the Boys' Club in sports programs.

Physical Assessment

Anton has full active-motion bilateral upper extremities and cervical spine. Strength is within normal limits. His thoracolumbar mobility was not tested due to post-surgical precautions. There is no active motion of bilateral lower extremities except for trace (1/5) hip flexion and poor (2/5) quadratus lumborum function bilaterally. Lower extremity tone is flaccid.

Anton is independent in wheelchair propulsion and level transfers, including chair to bed and chair to chair transfers. He showers with shower chair. He has not attempted independent chair to automobile or floor to chair transfers yet. He is able to perform pressure relief weight shift independently using shoulder/scapula depression.

Considerations

Anton has expressed an interest in participating in wheelchair sports, especially basketball. His therapist makes a list of the issues they must discuss:

1. Equipment
2. Wheelchair basketball contacts
3. Classification
4. Upcoming events
5. Training opportunities
6. Injury prevention
7. Overcoming barriers to participation

Equipment

From the equipment perspective, the best choice for Anton is a solid frame court chair. There are a number of manufacturers, including Quickie (Sunrise Medical), Top End (Invacare), Eagle, Colours in Motion, Kuschall, and more. An everyday wheelchair will not work well for sports and may actually be a detriment to his training.

Court chairs are ultralightweight (often 18 to 23 pounds), are more responsive due to cambered wheels, and may provide greater trunk stability with adjustments such as dropping the rear portion of the seat. In addition, court chairs have solid frames, plastic spoke guards, footrest covers that protect the floor, and straps that keep the athlete's feet on the footrests. For optimal performance, court chairs should be customized for the individual's height and width, leg length, and trunk stability. With a T-12 SCI, Anton is going to be most stable with his thighs and knees strapped together and possibly use a elasticized trunk support (often sold as motorcycle kidney belts) to provide greater trunk stability. Strapping his legs together prevents him from falling forward, as holding the legs in adduction substitute to some extent for nonfunctioning gluteal muscles. Some court chairs come with such support available.

In addition, court chairs need to meet specific criteria for competition to be in compliance with the rules of the NWBA, the U.S. national governing body for wheelchair basketball (see the boxed text).

Continued

CASE STUDY 19-1   Introducing Sports to Individuals With SCI—cont'd

National Wheelchair Basketball Association Section 24

The wheelchair used in tournament and league competition shall meet the following requirements:

1. The height of the seat rail must be no more than 21 inches. Measurement must be made from ground or court to the top of the seat rail bar (highest point) with player in the chair.
2. That part of the footrest or roll bar that projects forward the farthest and that would be the first point of contact with another wheelchair in head-on contact must be at a height of not more than 5 inches from the ground or court.
3. A strap must be attached firmly and drawn taut to the telescope bar of the footrest platform. This strap shall measure no less than 1.5 inches in width, and the bottom of the strap must be attached within 6 inches of the footrests. In the case of all players, this strap should be drawn taut so that a foot may not be used as a brake.
4. Use of a cushion is condoned, being of common understanding that it is for therapeutic reasons specifically. As such, it shall be composed of any therapeutic material as made by popular manufacturers and shall not exceed 4 inches at its highest point (thickness) for Class I and II players, nor more than 2 inches at its highest point (thickness) for Class III players. Pneumatic cushions and contoured cushions are permissible, providing they are commercially manufactured for therapeutic use and do not exceed thickness restrictions (above). Cushions composed of nontherapeutic materials, such as hard (nonpliable) rubber, wood, or other solid composition, shall not be acceptable. In all situations, the decision of the officials shall be final.
5. Each chair must be equipped with a roll bar, or the foot platforms must be adequately covered on their undersides to ensure against damage to the playing surface.
6. The footrest must have rounded or smooth corners. Door bumpers, knobs, projections of folding footrest, or other projection from the body of the footrest, which may readily become entangled in the wheels and/or spokes of another chair or used to hook and/or hold an opponent, shall not be allowed.
7. Any chair equipped with either a horizontal bar behind the backrest or push handles extending to the rear must have these areas sufficiently padded so as to prevent injury to another player.
8. A chair is permitted to have anti-tip casters attached to the underside or rear of the chair. The lowest point of the anti-tip caster cannot exceed 1 foot from the floor nor can any part of the anti-tip caster project from the chair rearward so that it would extend past any part of the rear wheels.

Source: National Wheelchair Basketball Association. NWBA Official Rules Casebook 2007–2008. Available at: http://www.nwba.org. Accessed August 26, 2008.

For court chair options, see the table titled "Sources of Lightweight High-Performance Wheelchairs (Court Chairs)."

Wheelchair Basketball Contacts

There are a number of contacts for wheelchair basketball players. The best place to start is the NWBA directory of teams, which is available online at www.nwba.org. The client should call a team and watch a practice, a game, or a tournament. Getting connected is an important step.

Sometimes rehabilitation centers host teams, and some colleges and universities also offer intercollegiate teams for student athletes. Talented young athletes may be able to participate in intercollegiate sports and even earn a scholarship.

Joining an NWBA team will involve getting classified.

Classification

Sport-specific classification varies by national organization. The United States uses a system that is not used elsewhere in the world. It may be helpful to establish athlete classification as soon as possible because a player's role on the team may vary with classification status due to the limitations placed on combinations of players of various classifications on the floor. The NWBA classification system follows:[69]

Class I. Complete motor loss at T-7 or above or comparable disability where there is total loss of muscle function originating at or above T-7.

Class II. Complete motor loss originating at T-8 and descending through and including L-2, where there may be motor power of hips and thighs. Also included in this class are amputees with bilateral hip disarticulation.

Class III. All other physical disabilities as related to lower extremity paralysis or paresis originating at or below L-3. All lower extremity amputees are included in this class except those with bilateral hip disarticulation (see Class II).

CASE STUDY 19-1   Introducing Sports to Individuals With SCI—cont'd

Sources of Lightweight High-Performance Wheelchairs (Court Chairs)

Manufacturer	Product	Features
Sunrise Medical North American Headquarters 7477 East Dry Creek Parkway Longmont, Colorado, 80503 USA (800) 333-4000 (303) 218-4590 Main Fax http://www.sunrisemedical.com	Quickie All Court Chair	Features a patented center-of-mass adjustment. All Court adjusts to match each user's unique center-of gravity and seat angle requirements. Used by both recreational and elite athletes. Comes in Titanium as well. Approximately 24 pounds.
Eagle Sports Chairs bewing@bellsouth.net 2351 Parkwood Rd, Snellville, Georgia, 30039 USA phone: 770-972-0763 fax: 770-985-4885 http://www.eaglesportschairs.com	Basketball Chair	Fully welded solid frame, aluminum or titanium, with pivoting fifth wheel, anti-pick bars, and quick release, heat-treated wheels. It is 100% custom built and weighs approximately 16 to 20 pounds.
Invacare One Invacare Way P.O. Box 4028 Elyria, Ohio 44036 USA http://www.invacare.com/	Invacare Top End Transformer All Sport	Fully adjustable and a good choice for teams and athletes who are just starting out. It features adjustable front and rear seat-to-floor heights, center of gravity, footrest height, angle and fore/aft position, back angle, and height and is equipped with an adjustable/removable swivel anti-tip bar and an easy-to-remove offensive wing or bumper. Weighs approximately 23 pounds.
Colours in Motion 860 E. Parkridge Avenue Corona, CA 92879 USA Tel: 951-808-9131 Fax: 951-808-9949 Toll Free: 800-892-8998 http://www.colourswheelchair.com	Swish basketball wheelchair	Multiple adjustments and options. Wide range of nylon upholstery choices and chair colors.

Anton's classification is easily determined. With T-12 motor function, he clearly falls into Class II.

Upcoming Events

Those interested in attending NWBA games should check out the team's schedule for the season, which roughly approximates NCAA playing schedules. In addition, there are often pre-season tournaments in September through October and post-season tournaments during the spring and summer months.

Training Opportunities

Year-round training is optimal to keep in condition and provide flexibility, strength, and power for on-court performance. Strengthening programs should emphasize the posterior shoulder musculature to minimize risk for shoulder

Continued

CASE STUDY 19-1 Introducing Sports to Individuals With SCI—cont'd

impingement syndromes. Power for 3-point shooting can be developed by plyometrics. Training for optimal reach for defensive blocking and rebounds should take place in the sport wheelchair. General conditioning should emphasize a base of endurance with additional anaerobic training added for additional speed and power. Wheelchair mobility exercises should include control both with and without the basketball. Skills in dribbling, passing, and shooting should all be developed with the support of an experienced coach.

Injury Prevention

Conditioning is at the foundation of an injury prevention program. It is important that athletes develop good habits, including a warm-up (slow pushing for 10 minutes around the court, followed by light stretching) and cool-down (3 to 5 minutes of slower-paced activity, followed by stretching). A strengthening program should emphasize (1) scapular retraction and horizontal shoulder abduction (Fig. 19-7), scapular depression and shoulder adduction (Fig. 19-8), and (Fig. 19-9) external rotation. Triceps muscle strengthening may be of value in push stroke power and shooting reach. Such exercises can be done easily with resistive bands.

Stretching is a critical component of the exercise routine, including stretches of the shoulder internal rotator (Fig. 19-10), biceps (Fig. 19-11), triceps, pectoralis major (Fig. 19-12), wrist extensor, and finger flexor muscles.

Scapular retraction:
• Hold elastic band out in front of you with arm straight.
• With arm at chest level, pull one arm back in a rowing motion.
• Return elastic band slowly to starting position.
• Do 3 sets of 15 repetitions.
• Repeat with other arm.

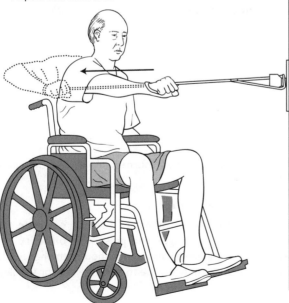

Figure 19-7. Scapular retraction and shoulder horizontal abduction exercise using elastic bands.

Shoulder adduction:
• Position wheelchair so that your side is toward the door with elbow straight.
• Pull your arm down toward your side to produce tension in the elastic band while keeping your elbow straight and thumb pointed down.
• Do 3 sets of 15 repetitions.
• Repeat with other arm.

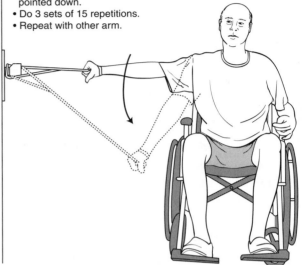

Figure 19-8. Scapula depression and shoulder adduction exercise using elastic bands.

External rotation:
• With elbow firmly against side and bent to 90 degrees, allow elastic band tension to rotate your hand to your stomach.
• Keeping elbow at side and bent 90 degrees, pull hand away from stomach.
• Do 3 sets of 15 repetitions.
• Repeat with other arm.

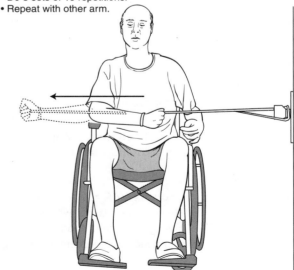

Figure 19-9. Shoulder external rotation exercise using elastic bands.

CASE STUDY 19-1   Introducing Sports to Individuals With SCI—cont'd

Internal rotator stretch:
- With elbow at side and bent to 90 degrees, lean slightly foreward or rotate away from arm until a firm strech is felt about the front of the shoulder.
- Do 5 repetitions holding for 15 seconds each.
- Repeat with other arm.

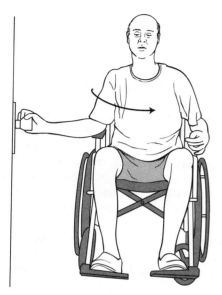

Figure 19-10. Stretching the shoulder internal rotator muscles using a doorway.

Biceps stretch:
- Position arm 45 degrees away from side, elbow straight, and biceps muscle facing forward.
- Lean slightly forward or rotate away from arm until a good stretch is felt in the biceps muscle.
- Do 5 repetitions holding for 15 seconds each.
- Repeat with other arm.

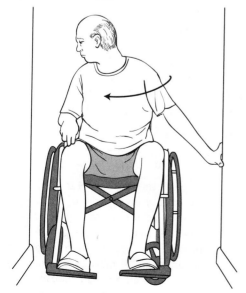

Figure 19-11. Stretching the biceps muscle using a doorway.

Pectoralis major stretch:
- With elbow at shoulder height and bent to 90 degrees, lean slightly forward until a firm stretch is felt in the chest region.
- Do 5 repetitions holding for 15 seconds each.
- Repeat with other arm.

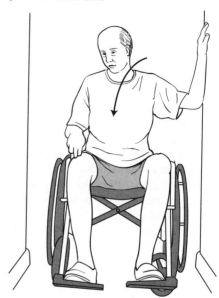

Figure 19-12. Stretching the pectoralis major muscle using a doorway.

Overcoming Barriers to Participation

Obviously, availability of an existing wheelchair basketball program (or other organized sports and recreation program) is necessary. Most large cities have such programs. In addition, transportation may be an issue. Arranging transportation with another player or finding a way to involve other family members may help. Cost of equipment is often an issue and may require special planning to purchase new or used equipment.

Social support is often a major factor in continuing participation. A visit by experienced players to the rehabilitation center was a critical first step in recruiting Anton. Once involved, the atmosphere of being part of a team and having a coach provided a natural support system that encouraged him to participate and facilitated his involvement in both competitive and related social events. Lastly, home modifications, such as widening doors or customizing a shower, may make life in general much easier, which, of course, facilitates participation in outside activities.

Outcomes

Anton first attended a tournament being held in his local community just 9 weeks after his injury. Although he still was limited in his twisting and bending to allow for spinal fusion healing, he was able to attend some practices and begin training with the team. He found a player about his size who offered him a used court chair to begin training. He became so enthusiastic about the sport that he soon

Continued

CASE STUDY 19-1   Introducing Sports to Individuals With SCI—cont'd

ordered his own wheelchair and arranged for some friends to go to practices with him and to become statisticians for the team. He enrolled as a member of the NWBA team and was officially classified as a Class II. Because of his height, he played forward on the team. He played a few minutes in his first game just 7 months after his injury. His friends, family, and rehabilitation team all were in attendance. Even better, his team won!

CASE STUDY 19-2   Exercise Prescription: Chronic Shoulder Pain With Muscle Imbalance, Obesity, and Deconditioning

Background

Sylvia is a 50-year-old married woman with T-10 paraplegia (AIS A), 15 years post-injury. She currently weighs 170 pounds and is 5 feet 5 inches tall. She uses a lightweight manual wheelchair. She reports chronic shoulder pain and often wakes up if she sleeps on her side on either shoulder. She has noticed that the pain occurs with strenuous activity, while pushing her wheelchair on rough terrain or inclines, performing nonlevel transfers, or reaching overhead.

Sylvia wants to lose weight and get in shape. She has slowly gained weight over the last 15 years, adding a few pounds every year. She was recently diagnosed with type 2 diabetes, which is controlled by diet. She is taking quinapril (ACE inhibitor) to control her blood pressure and Naprosyn (NSAID) to relieve shoulder pain.

Interview

Sylvia works full-time in a medical supply business with her husband. Her once active lifestyle has become much less so with the heavy demands of work. She lives in a single-story home in a suburban area with her husband and two teenage children. Her shoulder pain limits her ability to reach or lift objects overhead and to transfer from low to higher surfaces. She routinely drives a van with a lift, but can drive a two-door sedan and load her lightweight wheelchair independently.

Sylvia would prefer to exercise with her husband and children in either a gym or on the bike path near their home. She also enjoys swimming.

Sylvia would like to lose 15 pounds and relieve her shoulder pain.

Physical Assessment

On a monitored submaximal exercise test using an arm cycle ergometer, her peak heart rate was 150; her resting heart rate is 90. Her resting blood pressure is 128/85.

She has full active motion of elbows, wrists, and hands. Active-assisted shoulder flexion and abduction reaches 150 degrees bilaterally, with tightness and discomfort at the end range. Shoulder external rotation also shows tightness at end range, with available motion to only 70 degrees bilaterally. Cervical spine motion shows limitation in lower cervical extension, with difficulty bringing her head into a neutral position over her upper trunk.

She sits in her wheelchair in lumbo-thoracic flexion, with forward-rounded shoulders and a forward head posture. Her scapulae are protracted and shoulders are internally rotated.

Sylvia shows normal motor function of the upper extremities and no voluntary control in lower extremities or lower trunk. She shows a strength imbalance, with normal strength (5/5) of her pectoral muscles and poor strength (2+/5) in the rhomboid, middle, and lower trapezius and shoulder external rotator muscles. Her sitting balance without hand support is poor, and she has difficulty responding to trunk perturbation, especially from behind.

She is independent in a lightweight everyday wheelchair on level surfaces and small curbs. She is independent in wheelchair to bed, to toilet, and to car transfers. She drives a van with a lift and frequently transports her children to sports events and soccer.

Considerations

Sylvia has been cleared by her physician to begin a program of moderate physical activity. Her therapist considers the following issues:

1. Exercise prescription
2. Equipment needed
3. Training opportunities
4. Injury prevention
5. Overcoming barriers to participation

Exercise Prescription

The exercise program should include strength, flexibility, and endurance training.

For aerobic training we use the Karvonen formula to set a target heart rate. Her heart rate reserve may be calculated by plugging in the data from her exercise test.

$$HRR = MHR - RHR \text{ or } HRR = (150 - 90) = 60$$

Calculating a range of 40% to 80% of HRR = 24 to 48.

$$HRR_{40\%} + RHR = 24 + 90 = 114$$
$$HRR_{80\%} + RHR = 48 + 90 = 138$$

Therefore, her target heart rate is 114 to 138. Since she is quite deconditioned, the lower end of the range will probably be sufficient to achieve a training effect. In addition, exercising in the lower end of the range will also help with gradual weight loss. Her target will be to complete two 12-minute periods (or 25 to 30 minutes continuously) of aerobic exercise 3 days a week. She can choose from arm cycling, continuous wheelchair propulsion (outside or

CASE STUDY 19-2   Exercise Prescription: Chronic Shoulder Pain With Muscle Imbalance, Obesity, and Deconditioning—cont'd

indoors on rollers), hand-biking, swimming, chair aerobics, rowing, and kayaking.

For strength and anaerobic training, we determine 1-RM by looking at how much weight Sylvia can lift for each desired muscle group for four to five repetitions. For example, she lifts 10 pounds in a scapula retraction exercise five times before fatiguing. On a 1-RM calculator, we find that 1-RM will be 11 pounds. From that calculation, one can establish a goal of 50% of 1-RM, or 5 pounds. Her exercise prescription would be to complete two to three sets of 10 repetitions of each exercise twice weekly at an intensity of 50% of 1-RM. As her strength increases, it will be necessary to recalculate 1-RM. An easy on-line calculator is available at: http://www.timinvermont.com/fitness/orm.htm.

Muscle groups on which to focus during training in order to correct muscle imbalance include triceps, scapular retraction, latissimus dorsi, and shoulder external rotators (see Figs. 19-7, 19-8, and 19-9). The already strong pectoral muscles must be stretched to allow the opposing muscles to assume their normal resting position. A program can be designed for use in the gym using weights or at home using resistive bands.

Since Sylvia currently lacks active range of motion of her arms, it is important that she improve flexibility and muscle balance as she undertakes a training program. At a minimum, she should include flexibility exercises that include range of motion of her cervical spine (lower cervical extension with upper cervical flexion, cervical rotation, and lateral flexion), scapulae, shoulders, elbows, wrists, and fingers. It will be particularly important to emphasize stretching of pectoral, shoulder internal rotator, biceps, and wrist and finger flexor muscles (see Figs. 19-10, 19-11, and 19-12).

Equipment Needed

Although Sylvia has used a manual wheelchair for many years, she will benefit from a seating evaluation with wheelchair adjustments to enhance her balance and to provide for better thoraco-lumbar support. Refer to Chapter 8 for additional discussion related to seating.

Sylvia is interested in getting a handcycle for use outdoors. There are several choices, depending on whether she wants a free-standing handcycle or a dock-on style that provides an attachment for the wheelchair. There are also stationary hand bikes for indoor use (see the table "Sources of Handcycles for Wheelchair Users").

Sources of Handcycles for Wheelchair Users

Manufacturer	Product	Features
Invacare Top End One Invacare Way P.O. Box 4028 Elyria, Ohio 44036 USA http://www.invacare.com	Excelerator (free-standing)	A stable and maneuverable upright three-wheel handcycle that is capable of speeds up to 15 mph. The Shimano shifter allows for easy navigation of hills or level terrain. The design includes a 7-speed Shimano hub and reverse braking. These features allow you to keep your hands on the handles at all times.
Prime Engineering Corporate Headquarters 4202 Sierra Madre Fresno, CA 93722 559-276-0991 800-827-8263 Fax 800-800-3355 http://www.primeengineering.com	Coaster Hand Bike (freestanding)	A 21-speed handcycle that offers racing technology to the recreational rider. Combines high-grade components with optimum maneuverability for a comfortable, high-performance ride. This design allows a seat level transfer from a wheelchair, facilitating ease of transfer and use. Quick release axles and the unique two-piece frame allow for easy transportation in a car, eliminating the need for a van. Adjustable seat depth accommodates riders of various heights without the need for modification.
Sunrise Medical Quickie North American Headquarters 7477 East Dry Creek Parkway Longmont, Colorado, 80503 USA (800) 333-4000 (303) 218-4590 Main Fax http://www.sunrisemedical.com	Quickie Mach 2 (free standing)	A versatile choice for the rider looking to exercise or take a family ride on a favorite path. Smooth operation with easy shifting, easy-to-use coaster brake. Easy to back up. 3- or 7-speed. Angle-adjustable, flip-up footrests and a sliding seat for easier transfers. Mix and match short and standard frame lengths and crank assemblies for precise fit. Seat depth adjustment for your changing needs.

Continued

CASE STUDY 19-2   Exercise Prescription: Chronic Shoulder Pain With Muscle Imbalance, Obesity, and Deconditioning—cont'd

Sources of Handcycles for Wheelchair Users

Manufacturer	Product	Features
Sunrise Medical Quickie (see above)	Quickie Cyclone (dock-on handcycle attaches to an every-day wheelchair)	Transforms an everyday wheelchair into a handcycle. The Cyclone attaches and detaches quickly and easily to most wheelchair makes and models. Available in 7-speed.

Training Opportunities

There are ample training opportunities in most communities. It is important for Sylvia to look for fitness facilities that have universally accessible exercise equipment or to purchase her own equipment for home use. The table "Guidelines for Selection of a Fitness Facility" lists factors to consider should she choose a fitness facility.[70]

Guidelines for Selection of a Fitness Facility

Location	How close is the health club or fitness center to home or work? If you choose a facility that is close by to your daily activities, you'll be more likely to use it.
Hours	Check the hours to be sure it will be open at the times you will most likely exercise (early morning, late evening, weekend hours).
Environment	Check for cleanliness of equipment, floors, and locker room. Does it appear to be climate-controlled and well-ventilated? Is this a place you will enjoy spending your time?
Cost	Most clubs require a fixed membership fee and then a monthly fee. Be sure to ask exactly what is included in the fees. Extras, such as staff time, child care, classes, or pool use often require additional fees. Request a discount on your membership fees/dues if areas are not accessible. Some clubs offer family or joint memberships to couples, partners, or friends. Ask if the membership fee can be waived. Read the fine print in the contract. Avoid signing up for a multi-year membership.
Equipment	Is the equipment usable by persons in wheelchairs? Universal access is becoming a design standard. Are there activities and equipment that can be adapted for your unique health needs? Are there aquatic facilities and exercise classes?
Accessibility	Are there other wheelchair users who use the facility? Is the facility and equipment accessible? For wheelchair users, is there a wheelchair ramp to access the swimming pool for flexibility exercises or aquatic aerobics? Are the hallways wide enough for wheelchair mobility? Is there an elevator? Are lockers, restrooms, and shower facilities wheelchair accessible?
Classes	Find out what kinds of classes are available and when. Make sure that the times match your availability.
Friendly, well-trained employees	Do staff members say hello and smile? Do they work with clients, offering tips and encouragement? Is personal training an option? What are the qualifications of the fitness center personnel? The American College of Sports Medicine, the National Strength and Conditioning Association, and the National Academy of Sports Medicine are reputable organizations that provide certification tests for fitness professionals.
Reputation	Chat with other members of the fitness center, friends, and family about their experiences at the facility. Check with your local Better Business Bureau before signing a contract with the club to see if any complaints have been registered against the facility.
Take a tour	Try to schedule your tour at a time you would normally use the facility. How crowded is it? Is parking readily available? Are there accessible spaces? Are the entrances and exits well marked and easy to negotiate with ramps and easy-to-open doors? Are there clear paths between pieces of equipment? Can you easily maneuver? Does the equipment look well-maintained? If a facility declines to give you a tour, look elsewhere. Use this time to ask questions and assess your comfort with the other clients and staff, as well as the cleanliness and accessibility of the facilities.

Adapted from: National Center for Physical Activity and Disability. Exercise/Fitness: Choosing a Fitness Center. Available at: http://www.ncpad.org/exercise/fact_sheet.php?sheet=359. Accessed August 26, 2008.

CASE STUDY 19-2   Exercise Prescription: Chronic Shoulder Pain With Muscle Imbalance, Obesity, and Deconditioning—cont'd

Injury Prevention

Participation in a regular fitness program is a key step toward injury prevention, in addition to the preventative exercises detailed in Case Study 19-1. She is also, in all likelihood, quite deconditioned and will need to start slowly and build her strength and endurance gradually.

Sylvia should be sure to use caution when transferring from the wheelchair to the handcycle. She should use a bicycle helmet and protective gear as needed. Sunscreen and proper hydration are essential when exercising outdoors. She also should be careful of being sure her feet and lower extremities are placed and held in a stable position on the handcycle and not at risk of accidentally dragging on the ground.

Overcoming Barriers to Participation

Common barriers to participation are fatigue, lack of accessible facilities, and structural barriers. Others include time, money, and not knowing what to do. It will be important to start slowly and seek guidance from exercise professionals when she begins her program. Perhaps her physical therapist can offer some guidelines at the fitness center.

In addition, it will be important for her to fit her program into a daily schedule and calendar these activities in the same way she would for her business appointments. Consistency is the key to success. Commitment to participation by the rest of the family can also help Sylvia achieve her fitness goals.

Outcomes

Sylvia's physician was delighted to hear that she was pursuing a fitness program. Sylvia found a local fitness facility that offered a family membership and gave her a discount since she was unable to use the aerobic training equipment. She began working with a personal trainer for the first few sessions until she felt comfortable doing her stretching and strengthening routine on her own. She was able to successfully use a number of upper extremity machines and visited the gym either at lunchtime or in the evening on the days she was not riding. When unable to visit the gym, she used resistive bands at home to keep up with shoulder strengthening exercises for her scapula retraction and external rotator and shoulder adductor muscle strength. Her shoulder pain no longer interfered with her sleep, and she now found inclined wheelchair propulsion and nonlevel transfers easier and less painful to perform.

She chose a Quickie Cyclone because it could be attached to her everyday wheelchair. It was easy to transport to the bike path near her home and allowed her adequate mobility on both inclines and flat surfaces. She chose to ride in the evening, three times a week, with a friend or family member. She began with 8- to 10-minute rides after a 5-minute warm-up and quickly progressed each week, adding 1 to 2 minutes. She monitored her heart rate during rest and water stops and exercised at a pace to remain within her heart rate range. At the end of 6 weeks, she was able to ride for 30 minutes without stopping.

After exercising for 6 weeks, she had lost 5 pounds, as well as an inch off her waist. Her resting heart rate had dropped to 72. Her blood pressure remained under control, and her physician asked her to continue exercise for another 6 months, and they would work to discontinue the hypertension medication. She reported that she felt better, looked better, and had much more energy. She vowed to never let herself return to her sedentary lifestyle.

Summary

Individuals with SCI face a host of health risks associated with poor nutrition, social isolation, and a sedentary lifestyle. Physical inactivity increases risk of multisystem disease and secondary conditions. Regular physical activity is a key component of a wellness and health promotion program for persons with SCI. Individuals with higher levels of fitness derive multiple benefits in their daily lives, including reduced fatigue and greater ease of performance of daily activities.

Recreational and competitive sport has evolved with specialized equipment, sophisticated training, and widespread opportunities for participation. Rehabilitation professionals play key roles in health promotion, particularly in stressing the importance of and access to lifelong physical activity and safe sport participation for individuals with SCI.

REVIEW QUESTIONS

1. Many individuals with SCI report a sedentary lifestyle. What secondary conditions may result from physical inactivity? How do these chronic conditions develop? How does physical activity prevent or ameliorate these conditions?

2. What are three roles that rehabilitation professionals can play in encouraging physical activity and sports participation after SCI?

3. What are the evaluative criteria one should use before prescribing a conditioning or fitness program for an individual with SCI? What findings would indicate a need for close monitoring and/or medical supervision of the fitness program?

4. Design a conditioning program for the following individuals. Include possible exercises, appropriate

intensity, duration, and frequency. Include equipment recommendations and safety considerations.

a. Kevin is a 25-year-old man with C-7 tetraplegia, 5 years post-injury (AIS A). He weighs 140 pounds, height 5 feet 10 inches. He had skin problems over his sacrum that have now resolved. However, his skin in this area remains quite thin and fragile. He wants to compete in road racing. You have performed a submaximal exercise test using arm cycle ergometry. His peak heart rate was 118; his resting heart rate is 56. His resting blood pressure is 100/60.

b. Stan is a 45-year-old man with T-4 paraplegia (AIS C), 25 years post-injury. He weighs 200 pounds and is 5 feet 7 inches tall. He was referred for a progressive conditioning program following a coronary artery bypass graft 6 weeks ago. He has been cleared by his cardiologist for supervised upper extremity exercise. You have performed a submaximal exercise test using arm cycle ergometry. His peak heart rate was 140; his resting heart rate is 70. His resting blood pressure is 110/70. He is taking beta blockers to control his blood pressure and heart rate.

5. You have been asked by a local fitness facility to consult regarding the purchase of inclusive fitness equipment. They would like to advertise their facility as being "wheelchair-friendly." What will you include in your discussion with the manager of the facility?

6. A local high school coach approaches you regarding a young man with a SCI who wants to play wheelchair tennis. To what resources can you refer the coach to facilitate participation in competitive sport?

7. A race organizer has added a wheelchair division to a well-known 10-K race held in your city and has attracted some experienced wheelchair athletes to enter. He wants to provide the wheelchair racers with an early start. The city police will need to control traffic as the first racers cross the major intersections toward the end of the course. What information can you provide regarding how long it will take for the elite wheelchair racers to complete the course?

8. A successful wheelchair basketball team is seeking your advice to prevent and treat common athletic injuries and disability-related medical problems experienced by the team. They have asked you to give a talk on sport-related injury prevention and to provide them with some exercises they can incorporate in their warm-up routine.

9. Estimate the likely classification using the NWBA classification guidelines (in this chapter) for the following individuals:

a. Mary Ann, T-5 paraplegia (AIS A)

b. Joseph, T-12/L-1 fracture; cauda equina injury resulting in L-4 motor level, L-3 sensory level

c. Kevin, T-10 motor level (AIS B) with sacral sensory sparing.

REFERENCES

1. Buchholz AC, McGillivray CF, Pencharz PB. Physical activity levels are low in free-living adults with chronic paraplegia. *Obes Res.* 2003;11(4):563–570.

2. Bauman WA, Spungen AM. Carbohydrate and lipid metabolism in chronic spinal cord injury. *J Spinal Cord Med.* 2001;24(4):266–277.

3. Bauman WA, Spungen AM. Metabolic changes in persons after spinal cord injury. *Phys Med Rehabil Clin North Am.* 2000;11(1):109–140.

4. Gupta N, White KT, Sandford PR. Body mass index in spinal cord injury—A retrospective study. *Spinal Cord.* 2006;44(2):92–94.

5. Rimmer JH. Health promotion for people with disabilities: The emerging paradigm shift from disability prevention to prevention of secondary conditions. *Phys Ther.* 1999;79(5):495–502.

6. Stuifbergen AK. Building health promotion interventions for persons with chronic disabling conditions. *Fam Community Health.* 2006;29Suppl 1:28S–34S.

7. Warms CA, Belza BL, Whitney JD et al. Lifestyle physical activity for individuals with spinal cord injury: A pilot study. *Am J Health Promot.* 2004;18(4):288–291.

8. Madorsky JG, Curtis KA. Wheelchair sports medicine. *Am J Sports Med.* 1984;12(2):128–132.

9. Nash MS. Exercise as a health-promoting activity following spinal cord injury. *J Neurol Phys Ther.* 2005;29(2):87–103, 106.

10. Groah SL, Weitzenkamp D, Sett P et al. The relationship between neurological level of injury and symptomatic cardiovascular disease risk in the aging spinal injured. *Spinal Cord.* 2001;39(6):310–317.

11. Johnston MV, Diab ME, Chu BC et al. Preventive services and health behaviors among people with spinal cord injury. *J Spinal Cord Med.* 2005;28(1):43–54.

12. Jones LM, Legge M, Goulding A. Healthy body mass index values often underestimate body fat in men with spinal cord injury. *Arch Phys Med Rehabil.* 2003;84(7):1068–1071.

13. Liusuwan A, Widman L, Abresch RT et al. Altered body composition affects resting energy expenditure and interpretation of body mass index in children with spinal cord injury. *J Spinal Cord Med.* 2004;27 Suppl 1:S24–S28.

14. Curtis KA, Drysdale GA, Lanza RD et al. Shoulder pain in wheelchair users with tetraplegia and paraplegia. *Arch Phys Med Rehabil.* 1999;80(4):453–457

15. Dyson-Hudson TA, Shiflett SC, Kirshblum SC et al. Acupuncture and Trager psychophysical integration in the treatment of wheelchair user's shoulder pain in individuals with spinal cord injury. *Arch Phys Med Rehabil.* 2001;82(8):1038–1046.

16. Salisbury SK, Nitz J, Souvlis T. Shoulder pain following tetraplegia: A follow-up study 2–4 years after injury. *Spinal Cord.* 2006;44(12):723–728.

17. Boninger ML, Robertson RN, Wolff M et al. Upper limb nerve entrapments in elite wheelchair racers. *Am J Phys Med Rehabil.* 1996;75(3):170–176.

18. Goodman CM, Steadman AK, Meade RA et al. Comparison of carpal canal pressure in paraplegic and nonparaplegic subjects: Clinical implications. *Plast Reconstr Surg.* 2001;107(6):1464–1471; discussion 1472.

19. Burnham R, Chan M, Hazlett C et al. Acute median nerve dysfunction from wheelchair propulsion: The development of a model and study of the effect of hand protection. *Arch Phys Med Rehabil.* 1994;75(5):513–518.

20. Burnham RS, Steadward RD. Upper extremity peripheral nerve entrapments among wheelchair athletes: Prevalence, location, and risk factors. *Arch Phys Med Rehabil.* 1994;75(5):519–524.

21. Jackson DL, Hynninen BC, Caborn DN et al. Electrodiagnostic study of carpal tunnel syndrome in wheelchair basketball players. *Clin J Sport Med.* 1996;6(1):27–31.

22. Burnham RS, May L, Nelson E et al. Shoulder pain in wheelchair athletes. The role of muscle imbalance. *Am J Sports Med.* 1993;21(2):238–242.

23. Sinnott KA, Milburn P, McNaughton H. Factors associated with thoracic spinal cord injury, lesion level, and rotator cuff disorders. *Spinal Cord.* 2000;38(12):748–753.

24. van Drongelen S, de Groot S, Veeger HE et al. Upper extremity musculoskeletal pain during and after rehabilitation in wheelchair-using persons with a spinal cord injury. *Spinal Cord.* 2006;44(3):152–159.

25. Vogel LC, Krajci KA, Anderson CJ. Adults with pediatric-onset spinal cord injury: Part 2: Musculoskeletal and neurological complications. *J Spinal Cord Med.* 2002;25(2):117–123.

26. Lazo MG, Shirazi P, Sam M et al. Osteoporosis and risk of fracture in men with spinal cord injury. *Spinal Cord.* 2001;39(4):208–214

27. Groah SL, Stiens SA, Gittler MS et al. Spinal cord injury medicine. 5. Preserving wellness and independence of the aging patient with spinal cord injury: A primary care approach for the rehabilitation medicine specialist. *Arch Phys Med Rehabil.* 2002;83 Suppl 1:S82–89–S90–98.

28. Dryden DM, Saunders LD, Rowe BH et al. Depression following traumatic spinal cord injury. *Neuroepidemiology.* 2005;25(2):55–61.

29. El-Sayed MS, Younesian A. Lipid profiles are influenced by arm cranking exercise and training in individuals with spinal cord injury. *Spinal Cord.* 2005;43(5):299–305.

30. Curtis KA, Tyner TM, Zachary L et al. Effect of a standard exercise protocol on shoulder pain in long-term wheelchair users. *Spinal Cord.* 1999;37(6):421–429.

31. Fullerton HD, Borckardt JJ, Alfano AP. Shoulder pain: A comparison of wheelchair athletes and nonathletic wheelchair users. *Med Sci Sports Exerc.* 2003;35(12):1958–1961.

32. Curtis KA, McClanahan S, Hall KM et al. Health, vocational, and functional status in spinal cord injured athletes and nonathletes. *Arch Phys Med Rehabil.* 1986;67(12):862–865.

33. Stotts KM. Health maintenance: Paraplegic athletes and nonathletes. *Arch Phys Med Rehabil.* 1986;67(2):109–114.

34. Capoor J, Stein AB. Aging with spinal cord injury. *Phys Med Rehabil Clin North Am.* 2005;16(1):129–161

35. Rimmer JH. Exercise and physical activity in persons aging with a physical disability. *Phys Med Rehabil Clin North Am.* 2005;16(1):41–56.

36. Curtis KA, Hall K. Spinal cord injury community follow-up—The role of the physical therapist. *Phys Ther.* 1986;66:1370–1375.

37. Curtis KA. Health smarts Part 4. Providing sports medicine services for athletes with disabilities. *Sports 'n Spokes.* 1996;22(4):67–73.

38. Public Health Agency of Canada website. Glossary of Terms. Available at: http://www.phac-aspc.gc.ca/vs-sb/glossary_e.html. Accessed September 14, 2007.

39. Taylor D, Williams T. Sports injuries in athletes with disabilities: Wheelchair racing. *Paraplegia.* 1995;33(5):296–299.

40. Curtis KA. Health smarts Part 6. Slowing down the hands of time: Extending your athletic career and your life. *Sports 'n Spokes.* 1996;22(6):53–60.

41. Wu SK, Williams T. Factors influencing sport participation among athletes with spinal cord injury. *Med Sci Sports Exerc.* 2001;33(2):177–182.

42. Scelza WM, Kalpakjian CZ, Zemper ED et al. Perceived barriers to exercise in people with spinal cord injury. *Arch Phys Med Rehabil.* 2005;84(8):576–583.

43. Harrison T. Health promotion for persons with disabilities: What does the literature reveal? *Fam Community Health.* 2006;29 Suppl 1:12S–19S

44. Rimmer JH, Riley B, Wang E et al. Physical activity participation among persons with disabilities: Barriers and facilitators. *Am J Prev Med.* 2004;26(5):419–425.

45. Inclusive Fitness Initiative website. Inclusive Fitness Standards. Available at: http://www.inclusivefitness.org. Accessed May 24, 2006.

46. Myslinski MJ. Evidence-based exercise prescription for individuals with spinal cord injury. *J Neurol Phys Ther.* 2005;29(2):104–106.

47. Nash MS, Jacobs PL, Mendez AJ et al. Circuit resistance training improves the atherogenic lipid profiles of persons with chronic paraplegia. *J Spinal Cord Med.* 2001;24(1):2–9.

48. Jacobs PL, Nash MS. Exercise recommendations for individuals with spinal cord injury. *Sports Med.* 2004;34(11):727–751.

49. Dohoney P, Chromiak JA, Lemire D et al. Prediction of one repetition maximum (1-RM) strength from a 4-6 RM and a 7-10 RM submaximal strength test in healthy young adult males. *J Exerc Physiol.* [serial online]. 2002;5(3),54–59. Available at http://faculty.css.edu/tboone2/asep/Dohoney.pdf. Accessed September 14, 2008.

50. Curtis KA. Wheelchair sports medicine—Part III: Stretching routines. *Sports 'n Spokes.* 1981;7(3):16–18.

51. Curtis KA. Health smarts Part 2. Strategies and solutions for wheelchair athletes-common injuries of wheelchair athletes: Prevention and treatment. *Sports 'n Spokes.* 1996;22(2):13–19.

52. Ditor DS, Latimer AE, Ginis KA et al. Maintenance of exercise participation in individuals with spinal cord injury: Effects on quality of life, stress, and pain. *Spinal Cord.* 2003;41(8):446–450.

53. Curtis KA, Dillon DA. Survey of wheelchair athletic injuries: Common patterns and prevention. *Paraplegia.* 1985;23(3):170–175.

54. McCormack DAR, Reid DC, Steadward RD et al. Injury profiles in wheelchair athletes: Results of a retrospective survey. *Clin J Sport Med.* 1991;1:35–40.

55. Wilson PE, Washington RL. Pediatric wheelchair athletics: Sports injuries and prevention. *Paraplegia.* 1993;31(5):330–337.

56. Ferrara MS, Davis RW. Injuries to elite wheelchair athletes. *Paraplegia.* 1990;28(5):335–341.

57. Curtis KA, Gailey RS. The athlete with a disability. In: Zachazewski J, Quillen W, Magee D, editors *Athletic*

Injuries and Rehabilitation. Philadelphia: W.B. Saunders; 1996.

58. Barber DB, Gall NG. Osteonecrosis: An overuse injury of the shoulder in paraplegia: Case report. *Paraplegia*. 1991;29(6):423–426.

59. Bayley JC, Cochran TP, Sledge CB. The weight-bearing shoulder. The impingement syndrome in paraplegics. *J Bone Joint Surg-Am*. 1987;69(5):676–678.

60. Bhambhani Y. Physiology of wheelchair racing in athletes with spinal cord injury. *Sports Med*. 2002;32(1):23–51.

61. Schmid A, Schmidt-Trucksass A, Huonker M et al. Catecholamines response of high performance wheelchair athletes at rest and during exercise with autonomic dysreflexia. *Int J Sports Med*. 2001;22(1):2–7.

62. Wheeler G, Cumming D, Burnham R et al. Testosterone, cortisol, and catecholamine responses to exercise stress and autonomic dysreflexia in elite quadriplegic athletes. *Paraplegia*. 1994;32(5):292–299.

63. Harris P. Self-induced autonomic dysreflexia ('boosting') practised by some tetraplegic athletes to enhance their athletic performance. *Paraplegia*. 1994;32(5):289–291.

64. Wheelchair Track and Field (WTFUSA) USA. Competition Rules for Track and Field and Road Racing. In: *Official Rulebook of the Member Organizations of Wheelchair Sports, USA, 2006*. Available at: http://www. wsusa.org/Sports/2006WTFUSA.pdf. Accessed July 21, 2006.

65. National Wheelchair Basketball Association. *Official Rules and Casebook 2003-2004*. Available at: http://www.nwba. org. Accessed July 29, 2006.

66. International Wheelchair Basketball Federation. *A Guide to IWBF Functional Classification System for Wheelchair Basketball Players*. Available at http://www.iwbf.org/pdfs/ ClassificationManual_2004_final.pdf. Accessed July 9, 2006.

67. Weiss M, Curtis KA. Controversies in medical classification of wheelchair athletes. In Sherrill C, editor. *Sport and Disabled Athletes*. 1984 Olympic Scientific Congress Proceedings, Vol. 9. Champaign, IL: Human Kinetics; 1986.

68. International Paralympic Committee—Athletics. T54 1500 m Records page. Available at: http://www.ipc-athletics.org. Accessed July 29, 2006.

69. National Wheelchair Basketball Association. Player Classification. *NWBA Official Rules and Casebook 2006-7*. Available at: http://www.nwba.org. Accessed May 15, 2007.

70. National Center for Physical Activity and Disability. *Exercise/Fitness: Choosing a Fitness Center*. Available at: http://www.ncpad.org/exercise/ fact_sheet.php?sheet=359. Accessed May 27, 2007.

Adaptive Driving After Spinal Cord Injury $\quad$ 20

Judi Sue Hamelburg, PT, CDRS

After reading this chapter, the reader will be able to:

OBJECTIVES

- Describe the role of the driver rehabilitation specialist
- Describe the options available to assist with grip on the steering wheel
- Understand the availability of different types of hand controls
- Understand the importance of adequate dynamic balance in a moving vehicle
- Discuss the multitude of vehicle options
- Understand the impact that cognitive and visual deficits have on driving
- Appreciate the complexity of driving issues for the individual with SCI

Introduction

Driving goes beyond the transportation realm in today's society; for many, it is a rite of passage from adolescence to adulthood. Therefore, the loss of driving privileges has emotional, social, and financial ramifications. The consequences of losing the privilege of driving imbue driving with significance well beyond the use of the brake and accelerator pedal. But in today's populous cities, where traffic is congested and wheelchair-accessible public transportation may be limited, safety must be the first and foremost consideration when performing a driving evaluation.

The *driver rehabilitation specialist* is a relatively new role in North America and Europe. In the United States and Canada, the Association of Driver Rehabilitation Specialists is the professional organization that provides education and certification examinations to therapists in the field of driver assessment and training. Finding a qualified therapist is a critical step to start the process. While many people believe that the individual with disability will know what will best suit his or her needs, most people with limits in functional capacity are not aware of what their options are and often rely on a salesperson or others who have limited knowledge to make these decisions. The therapist will have no financial interest in the individual's purchase and have an extensive knowledge of the medical issues necessary for decision making. Yet, the individual with disability is an integral part of the evaluation and decision-making process, and his or her desires and needs must be addressed whenever possible.

Although long-time drivers think of driving as a simple task, the effort is truly quite complex. A driver must be able to execute multiple tasks simultaneously, including observing the signs and signals, visually tracking the roadway, moving the steering wheel as much (or as little) as is required for a given situation, and applying the brake or accelerator with adequate speed and pressure. Accomplishing all this while driving at 30, 40, 50, or 60 miles per hour requires multiple skills and coordination! Speed is a critical component in this equation. The faster the car is moving, the less time is available to acquire and process critical information, and the shorter the time available to take the necessary action.

Critical Components of the Driving Task

Vision

Vision may be affected in the individual with spinal cord injury (SCI) in many different ways. The eye may be injured in the trauma that damaged the spinal cord. Medications and trauma may affect the clarity of the individual's visual acuity.[1] Visual perceptual and visual-processing issues fall into the cognitive realm. Visual and cognitive deficits may result when there is a whiplash injury.[2] Results from studies indicate that cognitive deficits occur quite frequently with SCI in the absence of documented brain injury.[3–7]

Important elements of vision include peripheral vision, depth perception, and ability to visually scan all areas of the visual field. A driver rehabilitation specialist is qualified to perform screening tests to identify problems with vision and/or visual perception. For example, the *confrontation test* is an informal screening test used to detect and grossly define peripheral and/or large central visual field defects. The *cancellation test* is a measure of neglect, organizational process, and attention. For more complex cases, the client will be referred to a neuro-optometrist for evaluation.

Steering

In an individual with SCI, determining whether there remains sufficient grip strength and dexterity to manipulate the steering wheel is important. If hand controls will be required for the accelerator and brake function due to lower extremity weakness, paralysis, or spasticity, the functional capacity of the upper extremities is critical. If the individual will be a two-handed driver, then a great amount of grip strength will not be required as the wheel will be handed off from the left to the right hand, never requiring a large amount of gripping power. But if the individual will steer with only one hand, then good grip function with the hand available for steering is critical as significant gripping power on the wheel will be required.

In addition to grip strength, shoulder and arm strength must be adequate to turn the wheel in a moving vehicle quickly and repeatedly. Both muscle strength and endurance must be considered when addressing steering issues. There are a number of options available to assist steering in individuals who have deficits of upper extremity strength. Low-effort and zero-effort steering assistive devices may be needed with some individuals, but these systems cannot be installed in all vehicles. There are a number of options for gripping and steering and the most common of these are reviewed next.

Options for Gripping and Steering

Spinner Knob. A spinner knob (Fig. 20-1) is a round knob attached to the steering wheel to provide an additional handle on the wheel; this is the most common grip device used by individuals with paraplegia. The spinner knob is small and partially flattened and therefore does not intrude into the driver's compartment. To manipulate the steering wheel with a spinner knob requires that the individual have a grip capacity that is close to fully functional.

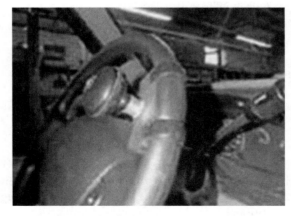

Figure 20-1. Spinner knob steering device.

Tri-Pin Steering Device. The tri-pin steering device (Fig. 20-2) consists of foam or plastic pins. The wrist is placed between two of the pins, and a third pin stabilizes the web space of the thumb to provide stability on the steering wheel. This device configuration allows the individual to turn the wheel using the shoulder and elbow. The tri-pin steering device is probably the most common steering device used by individuals with tetraplegia; it provides a functional grasp of the wheel in individuals having wrist extension but little or no grip function. This device is adjusted to fit each individual for optimal control. Some manufacturers include an optional disk over the thumb peg to keep the web space from inadvertently sliding off the pin.

V-grip Steering Device. The V-grip steering device (Fig. 20-3) is similar to the tri-pin device, except it has only two pins. A fairly significant amount of wrist control, as well as some grip strength, is needed to use this device. It is adapted to the individual by adjusting one bolt.

Palm-Grip. The palm-grip steering device (Fig. 20-4) is an open C-shaped cuff with a plastic platform on which

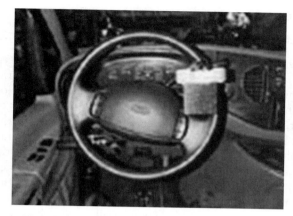

Figure 20-4. Palm-grip steering device.

to rest the wrist. This device is suitable for the individual with some active finger flexion who is able to use the hand in a pronated position.

Wrist Splint Steering Devices. The wrist splint steering device (Fig. 20-5) is generally the most efficient option for individuals in whom active control of the wrist is absent. Some wrist splint steering devices are available off the shelf. Most often, if the device is used with an individual who has fair or poorer C6 function, specially designed versions of his or her own successful hand splints or creative modifications of splints will be needed.

Accelerating and Braking

Many different styles of hand controls are available for acceleration and braking. The best general rule for determining which device to use is based on functional ability and simplicity. However, an individual with long legs who owns a small sports car may need a more creative approach to meet his or her specific needs. The more simple mechanical devices have a lower cost and less chance of failure if properly installed due to their uncomplicated design. The more complex a hand mechanism control, the greater the cost, the greater the cost of upkeep, and the higher the risk of failure.

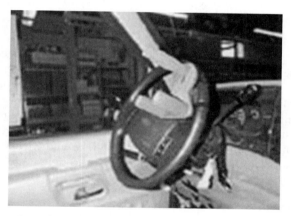

Figure 20-2. Tri-pin steering device.

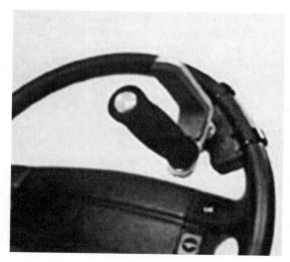

Figure 20-3. V-grip steering device.

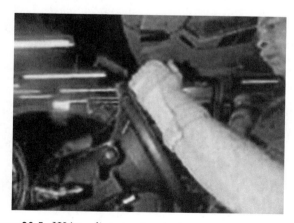

Figure 20-5. Wrist splint steering device.

Options for Accelerating and Braking

Push-Right Angle Hand Controls

Push-right angle hand controls (Fig. 20-6) are a type of mechanical control that is mounted to the steering column under the steering wheel. A handle extends out from the steering column, either to the right or to the left, for operation of the accelerator and brake with either the right or left hand. Pushing forward engages the brake with a direct link through a brake rod to the existing brake pedal. Pulling down toward the lap from the neutral position engages the accelerator pedal through a geared mechanism. The handle may be adapted with a "quad grip"; this is a U-shaped handle with a foam wrist support and side hand guard that provides more wrist support than standard right-angle controls. Most hand controls are installed on the left side for left-hand operation for several reasons:

1. If controls are on the left, the brake can be easily applied and the gears changed with the right hand.
2. With hand controls on the left, it is quite easy to reach the turn signal by lifting the hand momentarily off the accelerator prior to applying the brake.
3. The gear selector and radio are on the right side, and fitting hand controls around these obstacles is challenging.

Hand control installation on the right-hand side for accelerator and brake function is typically done when the individual does not have sufficient strength or shoulder range of motion to steer the vehicle with the right hand. Less strength and range of motion are required to use hand controls than to steer. For this reason, if the strength of one upper extremity is adequate to steer, and strength of the other upper extremity is not, then often the hand controls will be installed on the side of the weaker upper extremity.

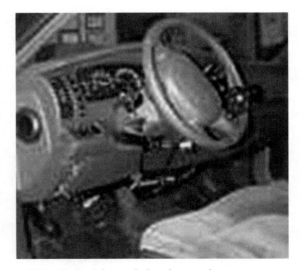

Figure 20-6. Push-right angle hand control.

Push-Pull Hand Controls

Push-pull hand controls are another type of mechanical hand control. As with the push-right angle hand controls, push-pull hand controls may also be mounted to the steering column with bolts. Alternatively, these may be mounted on the floor in a van. When the driver pulls the handle of the push-pull hand control toward himself or herself, it causes acceleration through a chain or cable-type assembly. Pushing the handle forward toward the dashboard puts direct pressure on the brake through a rod. The steering column-mounted push-pull hand control offers some advantages as well as some disadvantages compared to the push-right angle hand control.

1. The push-pull hand control does not allow the individual to accidentally accelerate as the brake is applied.
2. Depending upon the manufacturer and the installer, the push-pull hand controls may require more effort than push-right angle controls. When strength and fatigue are issues, this is a consideration.
3. The push-pull hand control can sometimes work in a vehicle with limited space above the legs, whereas there may be insufficient space for the excursion required for acceleration with a push right-angle device.

The floor-mounted push-pull hand control is most frequently used in vans due to installation space needs. Used in a van, the floor-mounted push-pull device gives the same advantages as when used in a car, with less effort required due to changes in leverage. Push-rocker style hand controls are a related mechanical hand control that is steering column mounted. Push-rocker style devices require a direct push forward to brake and a rocking motion to engage the accelerator through a geared mechanism.

Vacuum-Assisted Hand Controls

Vacuum-assisted hand controls offer a motorcycle-style twist accelerator. More cost and upkeep are required of these controls compared to other devices, but they offer an advantage in cases where the size of vehicle or length of legs limits the available space. Full hand strength is generally required to use this style of hand control.

High-Tech Driving Systems

Electronic acceleration and braking systems, as well as electronic small steering wheels, horizontal steering wheels, and joystick systems for driving represent a specialty within the field of driver rehabilitation. Use of these devices requires the knowledge of a highly qualified expert who has the equipment to evaluate the individual's specific needs and test his or her ability to use these devices. High-tech devices tend to be more costly and are more prone to breakdown than are the low-tech, mechanical alternatives.

Balance and Postural Control Devices

For individuals with inadequate sitting balance and postural control, support may be provided through wedges, lumbar supports, lateral stabilizers, chest straps, or a combination of these aids. It is critical that balance be stable throughout the learning process. It is not uncommon for an individual to stop using these devices several months or years after the end of the training program. Once the individual has learned to counterbalance using head or trunk leans, he or she may, or may not, continue with the prescribed equipment. For individuals driving a car, cross-legged sitting and a slight recline of the seat may adequately assist balance without the need for equipment. However, most individuals with SCI who do not have functional muscle strength above the T7 spinal level will require some type of balance assistance equipment.

Vehicle Selection and Options

Wheelchair Issues

Most individuals who require vehicle modification following SCI will use a wheelchair as the primary means of mobility. There are a number of questions related to the wheelchair and wheelchair transport that must be considered as part of the vehicle selection and modification process. Is the wheelchair appropriate for the individual's current vehicle and needs? If a new wheelchair is to be ordered, will the individual be able to load the new wheelchair into the car independently? Can it be loaded with a loading device onto the roof, into the bed of a truck, or into the passenger area of a van? Will the wheelchair interface with a van tie-down?

Vehicle Selection

Vehicle selection must be addressed early during the driver rehabilitation process. An individual must consider whether it will be feasible to use the current vehicle, or if a new vehicle will be required. If it is necessary to purchase a new vehicle, an assessment of the individual's ability to use this vehicle should be made based on how well the individual does driving the vehicle when it (or a very similar one) is fitted with different assistive device options. There is an additional set of issues that must be considered when determining the selection of a vehicle. Can the individual safely and independently get into and out of the vehicle? Can the wheelchair be loaded into and out of this vehicle? Will the current vehicle accept the equipment that the individual will use for the accelerator and brake? Can the individual steer this vehicle? Can reduced-effort steering be added to the vehicle? Can the individual fit his or her family into this vehicle with the wheelchair loaded? Can the individual secure small children in car seats safely in this vehicle? Family size and age

of children may play a role in these choices. For example, a single parent with two young children in his or her care may wish for the low-cost solution of a two-door car, but having to load a wheelchair into the rear seat along with an infant may make this impossible.

The combination of a car with a rooftop loader (Fig. 20-7) and a folding frame wheelchair may represent one viable alternative. On the other hand, a more costly option of a van may be safest for the children. After entering the van from a lift or a ramp (Fig. 20-8) into the midsection of the van, the children can be secured in car seats and the wheelchair can be tied down to the floor behind the driver's seat. In a different case, an individual without young children may find loading a rigid frame wheelchair into a car to be a good solution. The individual must be able to independently assemble and disassemble the chair for this to be a viable option. An individual's ability to transfer safely into a car is critical for car use to be safe. The use of a transfer board may work well in the early stages, but for maximum flexibility and ease, it is recommended that the individual be taught and encouraged to perform this transfer without a transfer board. When using a transfer board, if the board slides out, it often lands under the car, making it difficult for the individual to retrieve it independently.

The individual's ability to load a wheelchair into the vehicle is another consideration. Although a rooftop wheelchair loader and carrier may be a good solution for a folding wheelchair, there are no rooftop-loading devices for rigid frame wheelchairs. While there are devices that load the wheelchair onto the rear bumper, this requires that the individual be able to walk from the

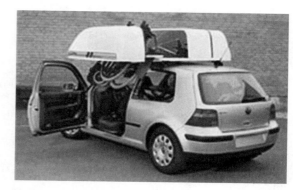

Figure 20-7. Car with a rooftop loader.

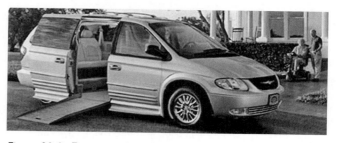

Figure 20-8. Ramp-equipped minivan.

rear of the vehicle to the front seat, which may not be possible. Devices that can load a chair into the backseat area of a truck or minivan may be good options for some individuals. Loading arms are available that place power and manual wheelchairs into the bed of a truck (Fig. 20-9).

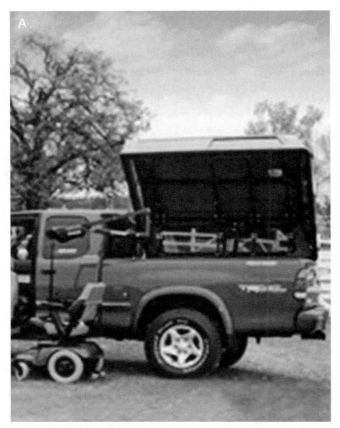

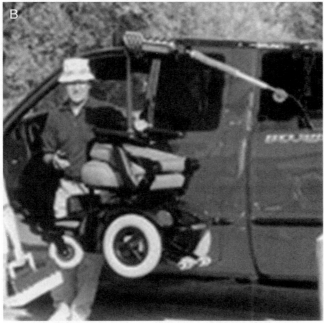

Figure 20-9. Truck with wheelchair loader (A); loading a wheelchair into a truck (B).

Power wheelchairs or scooters are usually not easily loaded into a car due to their excessive weight. Vans are generally most useful for accommodating motorized wheelchairs or scooters. However, lowered-floor minivans with ramps and full-size vans with lifts are among the most costly vehicle options.

Equipment Selection

Once the issue of vehicle selection has been settled, the selection of assistive devices must be considered. Selection of devices is based on an assessment of the individual's functional capacity and knowledge of the devices that are best suited to compensating for the individual's functional limitations. Many costly errors have been made when a person guesses at what can be made functional. A solution that works well for one individual may not work well for another with a similar functional level, as each individual has different needs and abilities. For this reason, providing the individual with the opportunity to try different assistive devices and evaluating his or her ability to use them is the optimal approach to device selection.

Financial Considerations

Adding hand controls to an individual's current automatic transmission vehicle may cost $1000. Purchasing and equipping a van for an individual with C5 tetraplegia may cost up to $100,000. When assisting with vehicle and device selection for individuals with SCIs, the level and severity of injury will provide a great deal of information about their equipment needs. For individuals with complete tetraplegia above the C5 level, there is currently no equipment available to permit driving. An individual with C5 tetraplegia may require hand controls with reduced-effort steering or braking equipment. Some individuals with less strength or with limitations in active range of motion may require electronic controls, such as a joystick for the gas and brake and a joystick or small electronic wheel for steering. Due to the costliness of electronic equipment and its breakdown rate being higher than mechanical controls, the use of electronic assistive devices for driving should be reserved for times when there are no other viable options.

Special Considerations for Driving an Adapted Van

Driving from the wheelchair in a van should be considered an option only when transfers cannot be accomplished safely (Fig. 20-10). The wheelchair-seated driver must contend with a number of issues that may not be problems for a person who drives from a car seat.

Some of the most critical of these issues are the Federal Motor Vehicle Safety Standards (FMVSS),[8] the laws for safety equipment that govern the automotive industry in the United States. All original equipment on a motor vehicle must comply with these laws. FMVSS

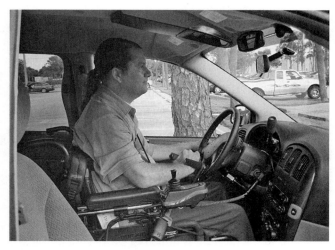

Figure 20-10. Wheelchair-seated van driver.

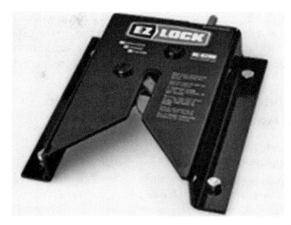

Figure 20-11. EZ Lock wheelchair securement and docking system.

include specifications intended for the safety and protection of the vehicle occupant in a collision; these specifications pertain to seat angles, safety belt angles of pull, and seat back angles. The most pertinent of these standards are reviewed below.

a. **Seat safety:** Original van seats from the vehicle manufacturer must meet FMVSS. They must have a specific seat angle and seatbelt-to-hip angle. They must include upper thoracic protection and provide a head restraint for whiplash protection. Wheelchairs are not designed with these criteria in mind, as they are designed for home and community mobility. Many wheelchairs have low-slung backs with no upper thoracic or neck protection. Therefore, using the wheelchair as a van seat should only occur when there is no other option available.

b. **Securing the wheelchair in position:** Securing the wheelchair into the driver's station floor is critical. If a wheelchair is not properly secured, the weight of the chair will add to the weight of the person, propelling the driver into the dashboard and windshield with an even greater force than an unrestrained person in a car seat. Specialized crash-tested wheelchair securement and docking systems are available (Fig. 20-11). However, due to differences in wheelchair design, these securement systems cannot be safely placed on every wheelchair.

c. **Lap and shoulder harnesses:** Modifications to harness devices are frequently necessary when the van's driver seat is removed to allow an individual to drive from a wheelchair. The lap and shoulder harness are attached to the vehicle wall, but the receptacle for the seatbelt securement system is typically attached to the seat itself. When the seat is removed, the seatbelt buckle receptacle is also removed. It is possible to add a receptacle to the adjacent front passenger seat, but as these passenger seats are removable, this is not the preferred solution. Rather, a stanchion (an upright

metal post) can be bolted to the floor with the free end holding the seatbelt buckle receptacle. The stanchion is placed so that the pull of the belt across the lap is sufficient for restraining the pelvis in the event of impact. The height of the stanchion is essential for optimal safety and function. If the stanchion is too high, the lap portion of the seatbelt will not hold the ilium, and in a collision, the pelvis may slide under the belt, resulting in leg injuries. If the stanchion is too low, the individual may be unable to release it quickly in an emergency.

d. **Visibility:** The eye ellipse (optimal position for visibility through the windshield) must be considered when working with a wheelchair-seated driver. A particularly small individual may not be able to see over the steering wheel if the wheelchair floor-to-seat height positions the driver too low in a van. More commonly, the wheelchair's floor-to-seat height positions an individual too high for proper visibility through the windshield. Although a raised roof may provide for adequate head clearance, it does not raise the windshield to improve visibility. Lowering the wheelchair height, or alternatively, lowering the vehicle floor, are options to consider.

e. **Leg clearance:** The amount of space available under the steering wheel must be considered for tall or large individuals who drive while seated in a wheelchair. This problem may also arise with chairs that are too high in the floor-to-seat measurement.

f. **Specificity of the driver's station:** Usually, only one wheelchair can be fitted to the driver's station. When an individual uses both a power wheelchair and a manual wheelchair, generally speaking, only one chair can be fitted into the wheelchair securement system for driving. Due to the size and configuration differences between manual and power wheelchairs, these are rarely interchangeable. Thus, wheelchair breakdowns are also problematic for driving and will render the wheelchair-seated driver dependent on another to drive. A van's driver's seat removed for a wheelchair-seated driver may be replaced into the driver's station to allow another driver to operate the van. However, van seats are heavy and can be difficult to maneuver.

Individual-Specific Considerations for Adapted Driver Education

A simple, straightforward assessment of an adapted driver by a qualified therapist will require a minimum of 2 hours. A complex assessment for individuals with tetraplegia may take more than 1 day. Driver training may last for several weeks. Ultimately, all issues must be identified and addressed for the safety of both the individual and the public.

Neuromuscular Control Issues Affecting Driving Function

Many individuals recover substantial motor function in the first post-injury year. Therefore, for individuals who are evaluated for driving early after injury, waiting may be the best option if driving is not possible during the first evaluation. Some individuals, especially those with tetraplegia, may not be physically or emotionally prepared for driving during the first year after injury. In general, the higher the level of injury, the more time from onset of injury may be required prior to driving.

Impairments of Balance and Postural Control

Sitting balance must be stable for turns and curves in a moving vehicle. If balance is inadequate, an individual may fall over in a turn, losing vehicular control. When the driver loses control of sitting balance, he or she may pull on the steering wheel to regain balance and thereby compromise steering control. Impaired balance function and postural control will be obstacles that need to be addressed for individuals with higher levels of SCI. In individuals with paraplegia below the T8 level of injury, balance is usually sufficient for the individual to independently maintain proper upright posture (assuming that the individual has received adequate rehabilitation care).

Spasticity and Muscle Spasms

Spasticity is a problem for many individuals with SCI and can seriously complicate the driving task, thereby creating an unsafe driving environment. Issues related to involuntary muscle activity as the vehicle turns are not uncommon and can be a source of great anxiety for the driver. When the vehicle turns, the resulting forces passively move the body; spasms are often triggered by this movement and may cause a loss of balance.

Lower extremity extensor spasms may interfere with the foot accelerator and brake pedals. Equipment is available to block these pedals to prevent them from being

inadvertently depressed. In extreme cases, flexor spasms may clamp the legs onto the steering column, blocking the use of hand controls for braking or accelerating and blocking movement of the steering wheel. This interference with the devices can lead to serious problems for vehicular control. Teaching the individual to slow down in situations that may trigger spasms (or loss of balance), such as when the vehicle turns, rounds curves, or goes over bumps, may assist in maintaining vehicular control.

Brown-Sequard Syndrome

As discussed in Chapter 1, in individuals with Brown-Sequard injuries, motor function and discriminative sensory function are spared on one side, but sensations of pain and temperature are impaired on that same side of the body. Sensory deficits in the arm can often be overcome with training, but sensory loss in the lower extremity can significantly affect driving ability.

Equipment for individuals with Brown-Sequard injuries may be minimal or may be similar to that used by an individual with hemiplegia, such as a spinner knob or left accelerator pedal. At times, these individuals may do well using one foot to accelerate and the other to brake.

Central Cord Syndrome

In individuals with central cord syndrome, there may be significant deficits of upper extremity strength that limit hand and arm function as discussed in Chapter 1. These individuals may also have some involvement of the legs. This clinical presentation poses many different problems. Positioning to optimize available shoulder function is critical. If the seat is positioned closer to the steering wheel, then steering is easier, but use of foot pedals for acceleration and braking may consequently be more difficult due to limited space to move the legs. Conversely, moving the seat farther back often optimizes lower extremity function, but requires more effort and may increase fatigue in the upper extremities.

If the individual recovers full hand function, a spinner knob may be used. Some individuals will be able to steer adequately without an assistive device. The individuals with tetraplegia or higher levels of paraplegia will require some balance assistance, at least in the early stages of driving. Cross-legged sitting may help with both balance and spasticity control.

Heterotopic Ossification

Heterotopic ossification is a common complication in individuals with SCI.[9] Ossification of soft tissues surrounding the hips and knees can significantly interfere with positioning and balance. Ossification may also interfere with steering if it involves the elbows or shoulder joints. Creative positioning solutions may be needed and may require that the individual use a wheelchair when driving a van.

SCI With Concurrent Brain Injury

The incidence of concurrent brain injury with SCI is well documented in the literature.[2–7] Often, these injuries are a direct result of the trauma due to the head hitting an object; the spine sustains a fracture while the brain is contused. Impairments may be due to the acceleration–deceleration within the cranium during the trauma.[2] Cognitive impairment may also occur in individuals with SCI in whom no confirmed head trauma is known.[3]

Cognitive deficits may include memory loss such that an individual cannot respond to common traffic signs.

Drifting out of the traffic lane may occur due to visual-perceptual or spatial-perceptual problems. Poor judgment, lack of attention, and difficulties dividing attention may also cause danger on the road. Cognitive deficits will slow the progress of learning a new task, such as the use of hand controls.[10]

As with any driver, high-risk behaviors such as drug or alcohol abuse, issues with depression, attention deficit, and learning disability must also be considered.[11–13] High-risk driving behaviors must be addressed and corrected. Fear of driving may also be an issue for the individual.

CASE STUDY 20-1   Individual With Low Paraplegia

Willie is a 23-year-old man with a T12 incomplete paraplegia sustained 15 months prior to his evaluation and training for driving. He was injured in a motor vehicle accident. At the time of his accident, he had been driving, but he had never been licensed to operate a motor vehicle. He reported that he was working as a barber, living with friends, and using drugs and alcohol recreationally. After his injury, he returned home to live with his mother. Willie arrived for the evaluation accompanied by his mother. She had obtained funding for the evaluation and driver training through a state-sponsored program to assist people with brain injuries and SCIs.

Evaluation of function revealed the following:

1. Sensation was intact to T12 and impaired below this level.
2. Willie had normal (5/5) strength in both upper extremities.
3. Willie was able to overcome gravity in movements of his lower extremities (i.e., at least fair [3/5] strength), but spasticity rendered these movements very slow. He was unable to use his lower extremities to assist with driving at the time of his evaluation, but he could use them to assist with transfers and wheelchair loading.
4. Willie was usually able to maintain balance while moving from one position to another, but lower extremity spasms threw him off balance at times.
5. Mild incoordination was noted in the right upper extremity as evidenced by poor performance on a test requiring rapid alternating movements (i.e., pronation/supination). Normal coordination was noted in the left upper extremity.
6. Reaction time was normal for both upper extremities.

7. Vision tests indicated 20/25 acuity, good color vision to red/green, and full peripheral fields to confrontation testing.
8. Cancellation tests showed disorganized visual scanning and visual perceptual deficits.
9. Traffic sign testing resulted in 16 correct answers of 18 questions in 5 minutes.

Based on this evaluation the driver rehabilitation specialist determined that Willie should be able to drive following participation in the adapted driver education program. Willie was required to obtain a learner's permit. Willie's mother reported that Willie was a "self-taught" driver and had been a risk taker on the road. Willie reported that he wanted to do things "the right way now."

Willie's vehicle was equipped with a push-right angle hand control with a foam grip, mounted on the left, with a horn button mounted on the handle. The goals of the adapted driver education program were for Willie to accomplish the following:

1. Learn to use hand controls in all traffic settings
2. Learn remedial driver education and defensive driving strategies
3. Learn to load, unload, assemble, and disassemble his wheelchair, placing it into the rear seat of a two-door vehicle.

After 14 hours of in-vehicle training (in addition to independent time spent reading the materials in a driver education book), Willie was able to obtain a full driver's license with hand control restrictions.

CASE STUDY 20-2   Individual With Tetraplegia

Sean is a 40-year-old man with a C5 tetraplegia. He had been involved in a motor vehicle collision as an unrestrained rear seat passenger. His injury was 9 years prior to his enrolling in the adapted driver education program. He had considered adapted driver education soon after his rehabilitation stay, but concerns about his strength and fear of spasms kept him from participating at that time. He was

independently mobile in a power wheelchair with tilt-in-space features.

Evaluation of his function revealed the following:

1. Strength testing indicated
   • anterior deltoids, middle deltoid, and posterior deltoids showed normal (5/5) strength;
   • biceps strength was normal (5/5);

Continued

CASE STUDY 20-2   Individual With Tetraplegia—cont'd

- no triceps contraction was noted (0/5);
- pectoral strength was good (4/5);
- wrist extension was good (4/5); and
- no contraction of the wrist flexors or finger flexors was noted (0/5 for each).

2. No lower extremity function was noted.
3. Sitting balance was poor
4. Vision was intact to acuity screening, contrast sensitivity, color perception, and depth perception. Visual fields were full to confrontation screening.
5. No visual perceptual or spatial perceptual deficits were identified on testing.

While Sean's family had used a 1998 Dodge Caravan ramp-equipped minivan conversion to transport him, a new vehicle was purchased by Sean for his own driving. He opted to purchase a 2006 Dodge Caravan. The equipment required included the following:

1. A 10-inch lowered floor
2. Power door openers on the rear sliding doors and rear hatch
3. Fully automatic wheelchair ramp
4. Mechanical kneel mechanism (to decrease the angle of the ramp)
5. Remote controls for door and ramp
6. Wheelchair tie-down with front stabilizer for securement of his power wheelchair in the driver's station
7. Additional wide-angle mirrors added to the side view mirrors of the vehicle
8. Push-right angle hand controls (mounted on the left) with offset foam quad grip and a horn button
9. Tri-pin steering device
10. Zero-effort steering
11. Factory seatbelt extension
12. Rigid floor-mounted seatbelt stanchion
13. Vinyl floor covering added over the carpeting, to allow the power chair to operate better and with less damage
14. Electric parking brake
15. Tab adapters to allow operation of the windshield washers and wipers, as well as air conditioner controls
16. Chest restraint for balance assist
17. Quad-style key adapter

Sean was working full time as an accountant; therefore, his driver evaluation and training was paid for by the state division of vocational rehabilitation. The vehicle was purchased by Sean, but the state program paid to equip the vehicle for his use. Once the vehicle conversion was completed, Sean was able to participate in adapted driver education program.

Issues that arose during training included:

1. Balance losses due to spasms on turns.
2. Anxiety on turns.
3. Fatigue due to low endurance. Fatigue was due to both decreased muscular and decreased cardiorespiratory endurance.

To minimize the disruption of balance during turns, Sean was taught to counterbalance the movement of his body during turns by moving his head in the opposite direction (in much the same way a bicyclist or motorcyclist would during a turn). After 22 hours of training, all issues had been resolved and Sean was licensed with the hand controls in his van.

Summary

Driving is an important skill for independent mobility in both city and rural areas. Although mass transit may be available for the general public in an urban setting, it is often inaccessible by the wheelchair user. And if mass transit is accessible, pushing a wheelchair several blocks in the rain or snow may make this transportation option unsafe. There are many options available to make driving a safe and efficient experience. A thorough evaluation of the individual's physical resources and needs will assist in determining what equipment is optimal. Education, training, and supervised practice are recommended to develop safe driving skills with specialized equipment and to ensure safe and independent driving for most clients after SCI.

REVIEW QUESTIONS

1. What type of therapist assists disabled clients with driving issues?
2. What are three types of devices used to assist with grip on the steering wheel?
3. What are three types of hand controls available to assist with acceleration and braking?
4. Why is balance an issue for drivers with SCI?
5. What types of vehicles can be used by the SCI client? List pros and cons for each vehicle option.
6. What could be the effects of a concurrent brain injury on the SCI driver?

REFERENCES

1. Devinsky O, D'Esposito M. *Neurology of Cognitive and Behavioral Disorders.* New York: Oxford Press; 2004. pp. 122–159.

2. Torres F, Shapiro SK. Electroencephalograms in whiplash injury. *Arch Neurol* 1961;5:28–35.

3. Davidoff GN, Roth EJ, Richards JS. Cognitive deficits in spinal cord injury: Epidemiology and outcome. *Arch Phys Med Rehabil.* 1992;73(3):275–284.

4. Holly LT, Kelly DF, Counelis GJ et al. Cervical spine trauma associated with moderate and severe head injury: Incidence, risk factors, and injury characteristics. *J Neurosurg.* 2002;96(3) Suppl:285–291.

5. Michael DB, Guyot DR, Darmody WR. Coincidence of head and cervical spine injury. *J Neurotrauma.* 1989;(3): 177–189.

6. Davidoff G, Thomas P, Johnson M et al. Closed head injury in acute traumatic spinal cord injury: Incidence and risk factors. *Arch Phys Med Rehabil.* 1988;69(10):869–872.

7. Sommer JL, Witkiewicz PM. The therapeutic challenges of dual diagnosis: TBI/SCI. *Brain Injury.* 2004;18(12): 1297–1308.

8. U.S. Department of Transportation National Highway Traffic Safety Administration. Federal Motor Vehicle Safety Standards and Regulations Booklet. HS808 878. Washington, DC: Office of Communications and Consumer Information (NPO–502).

9. Banovac K, Sherman AL et al. Prevention and treatment of heterotopic ossification after spinal cord injury. *J Spinal Cord Med.* 2004;27(4):376–382.

10. Ylvisaker M. *Traumatic Brain Injury Rehabilitation: Children and Adolescents.* 2nd edition. Boston: Butterworth-Heinimann; 1988. pp. 181–191.

11. Kolakowsky-Hayner SA, Gourley EV III, Kreutzer JS et al. Post injury substance abuse among persons with brain injury and persons with spinal cord injury. *Brain Injury.* 2002;16(7):583–592.

12. Turner AP, Bombardier CH, Rimmele CT. A typology of alcohol use patterns among persons with recent brain injury or spinal cord injury: Implications for treatment matching. *Arch Phys Med Rehab.* 2003;84(3)358–364.

13. Ylvisaker M. *Traumatic Brain Injury Rehabilitation: Children and Adolescents.* 2nd edition. Boston: Butterworth-Heinemann; 1988. pp. 181–191.

Sexuality After Spinal Cord Injury

21

Stacy Elliott, MD

After reading this chapter, the reader will be able to:

OBJECTIVES

- Appreciate that sexuality is a very high priority for persons with spinal cord injuries (SCI)
- Understand the mind–body interaction in sexual function and expression
- Understand the underlying neurophysiology of sexual response and genital physiology, including assessment measures
- Apply the principles of sexual reflexes to predict the changes in sexual functioning depending on the level of lesion after SCI
- Understand the comprehensive changes to sexuality outside of sexual functioning and fertility
- Review therapies currently available to men and women with acquired sexual dysfunctions and their applicability to the SCI population

Introduction

If you had a spinal cord injury (SCI), what would be a higher priority for you, to be able to walk again or to have sex? Most able-bodied persons would imagine that being able to walk again would be the function most desired. Thirty years ago, a survey of veterans with SCI noted that sex was a lower priority than the use of lower or upper limbs for individuals with paraplegia and tetraplegia,[1] and for many years a negative perception existed that persons with SCI were asexual. Fortunately, this myth is slowly being dissipated, since the conscious rehabilitative emphasis on ability versus disability, the advent of oral erection enhancement medication in the late 1990s, and research clarifying the priorities of the SCI population have changed the attitude of health-care professionals and the public about sexuality after SCI. Now, when surveyed about what gain of function was most important to their quality of life,[2] men and women with SCI said sexuality is a major priority, placing it above the return of sensation, walking, and bladder and bowel function. Of 681 participants (approximately 25% female), the majority of individuals with paraplegia felt regaining sexual function was their *highest priority*, and it was the *second highest* priority for individuals with quadriplegia (preceded only by regaining hand and arm function). In a more recent survey, the majority (86%) of male and female participants with SCI stated that their injury had altered their sexual sense of self and that improving their sexual function would improve their quality of life.[3,4]

The purpose of this chapter is to illustrate how changes to sexuality following SCI can be assessed and therapeutically managed in a comprehensive way to promote long-term gain rather than short-term solutions. The physiology of sexual function will be reviewed, followed by a discussion of specific changes to sexual function in men and women after SCI. A comprehensive approach to dealing with sexuality, a complex interaction of mind and body, will be presented to illustrate how sexual rehabilitation has the unique ability to continue to undergo evolution and expression after SCI, even when motor or sensory recovery has reached its full potential.

The Mind–Body Interaction

Sexuality is much more than the performance of sexual acts. General health, emotions, feelings, self-confidence, and a sense of sexual self-esteem are all involved in the capacity to experience what is known collectively as sexual arousal. Both subjective and objective observations can be made of psychological (fantasy, interpretation of body stimuli) and physical (feeling of pelvic vasocongestion and tension in the genital area or sexual responsiveness in nongenital areas) arousal.

After SCI, the vast majority of men and women find it difficult to become physically aroused, and in addition, more women (74.7%) than men (48.7%) have difficulty becoming psychologically aroused.[3,4] New sexual sensations must be learned because differing and adaptive capacities for psychological and physical sexual arousal occur after SCI. Of 286 men and women with various levels and completeness of SCI, slightly over one-half of the men and two-thirds of the women stated they could feel a buildup of sexual tension in their head during stimulation, and about half of both could feel it in their body.[3] Loss of physical sensory and motor options forces an appreciation of the power of "brain or cerebral sex." Such focus on cerebrally initiated sexual response results in "neuroplasticity" and development of adapted sexual experience. This phenomenon is best explained with a computer analogy: the "software" can still be intact and adaptable despite the "hardware" being altered after SCI.[5] Research studies are just beginning to address the potential of "sensory substitution,"[6] where sexual sensations can be rerouted via brain circuitry to be recognized in insensate areas once more. In the medical treatment of sexuality after SCI, the mind–body interaction cannot be overlooked by the clinician or the therapeutic value of this potential is lost.

Neurophysiology of the Sexual Response and the Effect of SCI

Vision, hearing, smell, taste, fantasy, and cerebral evaluation of skin and visceral stimulation constitute sexual triggers in the brain. These signals are modulated by general health status, hormones, emotions, and feelings of safety in the sexual situation. For sexual arousal to begin, a generated neuronal signal is coordinated in the limbic system, hypothalamus, and other midbrain structures and is carried distally through the brainstem and spinal tracts. This signal is usually inhibitory, until excitatory signals dominate and instigate the triggering of spinal reflexes for sexual function. Descending signals are relayed to the various spinal nuclei to release spinal sexual reflexes, and in some cases, these spinal nuclei can activate spinal cord systems directly.[7] SCI, depending on the completeness, will interfere with these descending autonomic messages in varying degrees. Furthermore, persons with SCI and concomitant brain injury may not have the same degree of cerebral modulation, causing some alterations in sexual desire or function and/or promoting atypical sexual behaviors.

Numerous components of the somatic and autonomic nervous system are involved in sexual behaviors and in the highly coordinated mechanisms of sexual arousal, ejaculation (in men), and orgasm. Neurotransmitter release precipitates increased heart and respiratory rate, sexual flush and perspiration, increased muscle tone and piloerection, pupil dilatation, and increased sensitivity to erogenous zones that occur with sexual arousal.[8] Certain neurotransmitters relaying sexual signals may be excitatory in the brain, but inhibitory in the periphery or vice versa.[9] Such complexity helps explain the wide variation of sexual effects of medications and emotions on sexual functioning. In addition, SCI may have a major effect on the ascending sensory signals coming from physical stimulation (decreasing positive sexual feedback), on muscle tone and spasticity, and, in persons with higher lesions, can exaggerate respiratory and cardiovascular reflexes secondary to the lack of neural control and descending autonomic regulation (autonomic dysreflexia, or AD).[10]

In able-bodied individuals, sexual arousal involves coordinated participation of all three nervous systems: *sacral parasympathetic* (pelvic), *thoracolumbar sympathetic* (hypogastric and lumbar sympathetic chain), and *somatic* (pudendal) nerves.[11] The activity of the vasoconstrictor preganglionic neurons (mainly sympathetic) becomes suppressed, and vasodilatory preganglionic neurons (primarily parasympathetic) become activated, leading to penile or clitoral tumescence. Activation of the somatic motor neurons causes contraction of the pelvic floor muscles.[12] The relative contribution of each of these three systems is altered in a unique way in with each individual with SCI.

Genital Physiology in Men and Women

It appears that men and women have similar genital physiology (clitoral pharmacology and histology parallels that of penile tissue), although external appearance and subjective and objective interpretation of individual arousal mechanisms can be very different.[13] In men, the visible male penis consists of a body composed of three parts: bilateral corpora cavernosal bodies and a ventral corpus spongiosum through which the urethra passes. The glans penis is the distal expansion of the corpus spongiosum. Entering the body, the corpora converge into a penile bulb, then diverge to form two crura that attach to the ischial rami.[14] When signals (via mental sexual arousal and touch) initiate smooth muscle relaxation in the erectile bodies, the cavernosal bodies fill with arterial blood and widen and elongate (penile tumescence). A fibroelastic stocking (the tunica albuginea) surrounds the corpora cavernosa and stretches with tumescence until finally, limited by its expansibility, it occludes the emissary veins that pierce it (veno-occlusive mechanism), effectively ceasing venous outflow. Blood flow exchange is virtually stopped, intracavernosal pressure increases, and penile rigidity ensues. Contraction of the pelvic floor muscles (bulbospongiosus and ischiocavernosus muscles) further enhances intracavernosal pressure and penile rigidity.[15] Loss of arousal, ejaculation, or orgasm cause reversal of the events, leading to detumescence.

Similarly, women also have erectile tissue, including the clitoris and glans clitoris. The clitoris consists of two corpora cavernosa that enter the body and diverge as two crura, similar to men. The three closely related structures of the clitoris, distal urethra, and vagina (although the last two are not erectile in nature) appear to be the locus of sexual function and orgasm.[13] Clitoral tissues and other erectile tissues deep in the vulva undergo tumescence and engorgement, but the clitoris cannot attain the same rigidity as the male structures due to the thinner tunica albuginea and ineffective veno-occlusive mechanism.[13] Pelvic floor contractions add to the pelvic tension and vasocongestion in women.

Erection depends on the relaxation of corporal smooth muscle, and this relaxation is primarily initiated by the nitric oxide (NO) pathway in both men and women. NO and other neurotransmitters act as modulators for erectile smooth muscle, encouraging contraction or relaxation (flaccidity and erection, respectively). NO is released from nerve endings upon initiation of sexual arousal from the brain, but healthy endothelial tissue is another source of NO.[11] While neuronal NO is the primary source of NO for erectile function, the endothelial source of NO may take more of a role after SCI.[16] With sexual arousal in women, vaginal lubrication, a transudate from vasocongestion of the pelvis, appears. With continued arousal, the vagina also elongates and the uterus elevates, lifting and ballooning the deep (distal) vagina.[8] These physiological changes to the genitalia are necessary for the vagina to comfortably accommodate an erect male penis for the act of sexual intercourse. Recent magnetic resonance scans of human intercourse have illustrated these mechanics.[17]

Orgasm is acknowledged as a pleasurable feeling accompanying the release of body and pelvic tension and vasocongestion as well as the visceral awareness of smooth muscle contractions of internal genitalia (including uterine or prostatic contractions). However, very little is known about the specific neurology of orgasm. There is evidence of a pattern generator in the spinal cord for ejaculatory/orgasmic function in both male and female rats.[18–21] This evidence suggests that genital orgasm is a pelvic reflex requiring an intact sacral reflex and that this reflex, when triggered, is accompanied by sensory perception. In able-bodied individuals, supraspinal inhibition can inhibit the reflex, or alternatively, supraspinal activation and/or practice can augment the reflex. "Genital orgasm" most likely reflects an intricate coordination of several nervous systems involved in generating a local pelvic reflex[22–24]. However, orgasm is likely dependant on hormonal and psychogenic modulation, since men and women with SCI can be orgasmic without genital stimulation (recognized as a "nongenital orgasm"), and in men, ejaculation is not always necessary for orgasm to occur.[23,25] That said, the chance of orgasm post-injury is positively correlated with having genital sensation.[3,26]

Physiological measurements in men at ejaculation and in men and women at orgasm have more recently become available.[27–32] Significant changes to blood pressure, heart rate, vaginal vasocongestion, and bulbocavernosus and abdominal muscle tension have been noted at ejaculation and/or orgasm.[30,31,32] However, the assessment of the intactness of the descending autonomic pathways may prove crucial in the prediction of orgasmic capacity after SCI.[25,31] Neural tracts outside of the central nervous system may also be involved: Whipple and Komisaruk[33] have demonstrated a genitospinal visceral afferent pathway in women with upper SCI that bypasses the spinal cord and projects directly to the brain during orgasm. Recent research by this group using functional magnetic resonance imaging (fMRI) has complemented their earlier positron emission testing-MRI studies,[34] showing how vaginal-cervical stimulation in women ($n = 4$) with complete SCI at or above T10 activates the inferior region of the nucleus tractus solitarii (NTS), the region of the medulla oblongata to which the vagus nerves project. Three women with complete SCI achieved orgasm with vaginocervical stimulation and the specific brain areas elucidated were not previously documented in other sexual studies using fMRI.[34] So far, this pathway has not been investigated in men with SCI.

Spinal Cord Arousal Pathways

There are basically two distinct control mechanisms that induce male penile erection and female clitoral tumescence and vaginal lubrication: the *psychogenic pathway*, located between T11 and L2 in the spinal cord, and the *reflex pathway*, located in the sacral cord (S2–S4).

In the *psychogenic pathway*, mental stimuli (fantasy, images, smells, etc.), along with the brain's evaluation of remaining sensory inputs from the genitalia and other erogenous zones that can ascend spinal pathways, contribute to form a sexual trigger. This resulting signal descends from the brain, activates the genital parasympathetic neural pathways, and (probably) simultaneously inhibits sympathetic outflow.[35] This pathway routes through the sympathetic chain coming off the thoracic spinal cord (T11–L2) to travel via the hypogastric nerves, with the final common pathway being the cavernous nerve containing both parasympathetic and sympathetic fibers. Studies have shown the neurological ability to achieve psychogenic arousal after SCI can be predicted in both males and females[27,29,36] by the degree to which the combined ability to perceive surface sensation to pinprick and light touch in the T11–L2 dermatomes is preserved. This observation suggests that similar neurological pathways for the control of mental sexual arousal exist for men and women. In men, the sympathetic nervous system has also been shown to maintain erections after injury to the parasympathetic pathways,[11] because the hypogastric nerve can act as an accessory pro-arousal pathway when a sacral spinal cord lesion precludes the usual pathways.[37] Men and women with injuries to their sacral cord or cauda equina are often dependant on these intact psychogenic pathways via the hypogastric nerve to elicit erection and vaginal lubrication.

The *reflex pathway* for erection and vaginal lubrication share similar neurology in both sexes (S2–S4). Being a reflex, both the afferent and efferent limbs must be at least partially physiologically intact for activation to occur, and therefore this pathway may be affected by injury to the conus medularis. For men with SCI, the tactile-dependent afferent limb is composed of the dorsal nerve of the penis, which continues via the pudendal nerve to reach the spinal cord. The efferent limb, arising from the sacral parasympathetic center and continuing through to the cavernous nerve in the penis, contains both autonomic and somatic inputs.[11,35] SCI, especially a complete injury above the sacral level, will not only preserve the reflex, but may even enhance it[11] due to loss of tonic inhibitory control that reduces the sensory threshold and onset of erectile responses.[12] If the pudendal or pelvic nerve is destroyed or the sacral spinal cord injured, activation of this reflexogenic pathway for erection and vaginal lubrication may be lost.

The arousal pathways are altered by SCI in a number of ways. The heightened reflexogenic erectile response in men with cervical lesions is demonstrated by reflex erections to nonsexual touch, such as catheterization or chafing from clothing ("spontaneous" erections), and is usually not amenable to higher center control. Although a lesion between the psychogenic and reflexogenic pathways would seem protective for both types of erections,[38] actually, these erections are unreliable, probably due to loss of reinforcing intraspinal connections between the two pathways. Men with sacral injuries who are dependant on psychogenic pathways to maintain their erection can activate the fibers of the sympathetic chain, triggering seminal emission (see below) and possibly loss of erection. To have this happen while maintaining intense mental focus on arousal, results in frustration and feelings of worthlessness.[39]

Injury to the conus terminalis damages sacral nerves but leaves intact thoracolumbar psychogenic pathways, whereas in contrast, a cauda equina lesion damaging only peripheral nerves may include some fibers originating from the lumbar area, potentially interfering with psychogenic arousal.[38]

There are many invasive and noninvasive tests to assess penile hemodynamics and neurophysiology, including color/Doppler penile or clitoral ultrasound, nocturnal penile tumescence, vaginal pulse amplitude, sacral reflex testing, pudendal evoked responses, electromyography of the anal or urethral sphincter, and autonomic clinical function testing.[40–42] However, these tests are usually not necessary in order to pursue practical therapeutic management. A clinical test called the bulbocavernosus reflex, a polysynaptic response elicited by low-threshold pudendal sensory fibers, demonstrates that tactile stimulation to the glans penis or clitoris that results in pelvic floor contraction is predictive of an intact sacral reflex. A good summary of neurological testing for erectile capacity for men with SCI is available in other writings.[38]

Ejaculation in Men

The ejaculatory reflex, consisting of seminal emission and propulsatile ejaculation (also called expulsion or ejection) is commonly disrupted by SCI.[5] Central ejaculatory control originates from hypothalamic nuclei within the limbic system of the brain, and several neurotransmitters are involved, including serotonin (5-hydroxytryptamine receptors are the key players).[43] The ejaculation reflex, primarily an autonomic process with somatic input, consists of sensory afferent signals (coming from the genitalia and from mental arousal) processed in the brain which then descend down the spinal cord as an efferent signal to two spinal centers, T10–L2 for emission and S2–S4 for propulsatile ejaculation (ejection). Emission involves primarily sympathetically mediated sequential contraction of the bladder neck and accessory sexual organs (prostate, seminal vesicles, vas deferentia, and epididymis) such that ejaculate is deposited in the posterior urethra. Propulsatile ejaculation is primarily controlled by the parasympathetic nervous system along with efferent somatic fibers emerging from S2–S4 that innervate the striated pelvic floor muscles, particularly the ischiocavernosus and bulbocavernosus. These contractions, along with the bladder neck closure and the relaxation of the external urinary sphincter, propel the semen forward out the urethral meatus (*antegrade ejaculation*). The penile shaft and glans are usually at maximal rigidity at this time. Marked elevation of blood pressure, heart, and respiration, myotonic muscle spasm, perspiration, and orgasm usually accompany ejaculation.[8]

After SCI, either interrupted descending signals or lower motor neuron (LMN) damage may result in altered ejaculation (including retrograde ejaculation) or no emission nor propulsatile ejaculation (*anejaculation*). In neurologically intact men, marked elevation of blood pressure, heart, and respiration, myotonic muscle spasm, perspiration, and orgasm usually accompany ejaculation.[8] In men with lesions higher than T6, these cardiovascular responses are often exaggerated, resulting in severe blood pressure elevations, bradycardia and/or arrhythmias, and AD.[31,32]

Changes to Sexual Functioning After SCI

Male Sex Functioning After SCI

Changes to Erection

Erection potential after SCI depends on the level and completeness of injury and also whether the injury is an upper motor neuron (UMN) lesion or LMN lesion. In general, a review of older studies stated the incidence of reported erections after SCI to be 69% to 87%.[44] More recent studies show erectile capacity from either reflexogenic or psychogenic sources to be 80% to 100%.[38] These estimates are from observations or self-report, with validated measures of erectile function usually being

reserved for interventional studies for erection enhancement therapies. For this reason, it is important to remember that the erection capacity reported in surveys may not reflect whether the erection is of sufficient quality or duration to allow for predictable intercourse. This is a practical reality and source of dissatisfaction for many men with SCI, and it is the reason why, despite "being able" to have an erection, erection enhancement is often used.

Erectile function after SCI is determined by injury level and severity, and whether the the injury involves an UMN or LMN lesion. Men with complete UMN lesions above T11 retain reflexogenic erections, and those with complete LMN lesions are dependent on psychogenic erections, as long as there is some degree of preservation of neurological function in the T11–L2 region of the cord.[45] Men with incomplete lesions retaining some neurological function in the T11–L2 cord should be able to have psychogenic as well as reflexogenic erections if it is an UMN lesion, but only psychogenic erections if it is an incomplete LMN lesion.[45]

Completeness of injury also has a great influence on erectile function after SCI; almost all men with cervical or high thoracic lesions are expected to get an erection regardless of completeness of injury (mainly reflexogenic, but may be a combined psychogenic and reflexogenic, if incomplete). Complete injuries remove the natural supratentorial inhibition on the spinal reflexes and allow for unheeded, or even enhanced, reflexogenic erections; incomplete injuries may allow remaining descending inhibitory control to negatively affect the erection quality if the circumstances are not ideal (i.e., if there is poor mental arousal or if the situation is anxiety ridden). Since more recent injuries are most often incomplete rather than complete SCI lesions, especially below the cervical level, this may explain the unreliability of erection quality.[38]

A number of other factors related to erectile function are also changed after SCI. Erections may not last long enough or be dependable for sexual intercourse. For men with SCI, the sexual position, relative fullness of the bladder, and pressure on the erect penis or glans will influence whether the erection is suddenly lost to a greater extent than that seen in uninjured men. In one study, approximately 62% of men with SCI stated that although they could get erections without erection enhancement aids, they were not reliable, with only 13% saying they could get a firm erection that lasted.[26] Only the presence of spasticity during sexual activity and/or the presence of genital sensation, not the level of injury or experiencing symptoms of AD, correlated positively with the reliability of erections.[26] Irrespective of the SCI, erectile dysfunction may be compounded by concomitant medical disorders (i.e., diabetes, hypertension, hyperlipidemia) or medications typically used in the rehabilitation setting, such as antidepressants, antihypertensives, antispasmodics, and urological drugs, such as alpha-blockers and anticholinergics.

Changes to Ejaculation

Most men wish to ejaculate after SCI, not for fertility reasons, but for pleasure and sexual intimacy.[26] Some men use ejaculation to reduce spasticity.[46] The chance of ejaculation after SCI has been variously quoted from 12% to 15%[47] up to 48%[26] in men with all levels of SCI. After SCI, the most common ejaculatory problem is that of anejaculation (absence of both seminal emission and propulsatile ejaculation). Like erection, ejaculation capacity depends on the level of lesion and completeness of injury. In men with SCI above T11, 75% reported erections, but only 10% reported ejaculation.[46] Men with higher lesions require more physical sources of stimulation compared to men with lower lesions, who achieve ejaculation through psychogenic arousal pathways.[49] The chance of ejaculating is better if psychogenic erections are attainable, able to be retained, and if there is direct penile manipulation versus intercourse.[44,48] Some men experience distressing severe premature or even spontaneous emission after injury at the T12–L1 level.[50]

Ejaculation by natural sexual means is rare in men with complete UMN lesions (4%), infrequent (18%) in complete LMN lesions, infrequent (32%) in men with incomplete UMN lesions, and most frequent (70%) in men with incomplete LMN lesions.[44] A recent report on 81 male study subjects with varying levels and completeness of injury stated 91% were able to reach ejaculation, with 30% doing so by natural stimulation (versus assisted by penile vibrostimulation or medication).[30] Men with complete lesions tend to be less successful ejaculating with sexual practices than those men with incomplete lesions,[51,52] probably because in the latter, the remaining descending pathways can promote ejaculation when the mental stimulus is sexually arousing. This finding may not be the case for specialized vibrator use in the sperm retrieval clinic.[5] For men with complete injuries, the lack of mental interference from remaining inhibitory pathways provoked by embarrassment or anxiety in a clinical setting may be beneficial to trigger the ejaculation response using a vibrator, whereas in those with incomplete injuries the mental interference may a disadvantage in this setting.

In men with SCI, erection is not necessary for ejaculation to occur, although the chance of ejaculation seems to be enhanced by the presence of improved erectile quality.[53] Direct penile stimulation may be more successful than sexual intercourse[54] in provoking ejaculation, with vibrostimulation being successful in over 75% of men with injury above T6.[5] Nocturnal emissions are also more prevalent (11% to 13%) in adult men with SCI than without.[54] Ejaculation is almost always accompanied by specific signs of abdominal and lower limb spasm, chest tightening, urethral spasm, and signs of mild to severe AD,[5,30,31] although these cardiovascular changes are not always noted by the individual with SCI (silent AD). Furthermore, ejaculation is usually antegrade, but may be retrograde, or both,[55] and may or may not be accompanied by orgasmic sensation.[23] During vibrostimulation for sperm retrieval, erection may be enhanced or hindered by the strong stimulus; however, fullness of the glans is often noted just prior to ejaculation regardless of the rigidity of erection.[5,56,57]

Changes to Male Orgasm

Various studies have found 42% to 68% of men self-describe the presence of orgasmic sensation (described as either the same or altered from pre-injury state) after SCI.[44,19,20] Men with incomplete injuries appear more likely to reach orgasm than men with complete injuries.[52]

Men with complete LMN injury affecting the sacral segments are significantly less likely than men with any other level and degree of SCI to achieve orgasm.[23] Although orgasm and ejaculation most often occur together (approximately 90% of the time), men with SCI may experience a disconnection between the two.[23,24] After SCI, some men, especially those with no genital sensation, acquire orgasmic sensations through nongenital stimulation (e.g., "eargasms"), likely related to sensory remapping via brain neuroplasticity, or in some cases, adapted AD. One study focusing on genital stimulation suggested that the climactic experience of ejaculation seems related to the subjective experience of AD, with fewer orgasmic sensations reported when AD was not noticed, pleasurable sensations when mild to moderate AD was experienced, and unpleasant or painful sensations when severe AD was reported.[30]

Female Sexual Functioning After SCI

Changes to Female Arousal

In one large survey by the Kinsey Institute,[47] about one-half of the women experienced vaginal lubrication and only a third experienced orgasm after SCI. Most studies on women with SCI have concentrated on the contributions of the psychogenic and reflex pathways in generating genital sexual arousal in women with varying levels of SCI by focusing on individual subjective reports as well as objective measurements of vaginal congestion using vaginal photoplethysmography or vaginal pulse amplitude,[60,61] heart rate, respiratory rate, and blood pressure readings.[62]

In one survey, women with complete UMN SCI, when asked to arouse themselves manually, used genital stimulation to achieve reflex lubrication. Those women with complete LMN injuries at S2–S5 did not choose this method, but some (25%) could obtain psychogenic lubrication through their intact lumbosacral cord.[62] Sensory perception in the T11–L2 dermatomes is associated with the ability to achieve psychogenic lubrication,[27] whereas reflex arousal in women appears to be dependent on intact sacral pathways, similar to reflex erection in men.

Changes to Female Orgasm

After SCI, women's ability to reach orgasm is impaired compared to that of able-bodied women.[52,63] While over 90% of women with SCI reported being orgasmic pre-injury,[3] only 30% to 50% of these women with varying levels and completeness of SCI were able to attain self-defined orgasm after injury. The likelihood of attaining orgasm is better if genital sensation is retained.[3,47,64] Two other variables that predicted a higher chance of reaching orgasm after SCI were greater sexual knowledge and higher sex drive.[47] In general, compared to pre-injury experience, the incidence of orgasm after SCI generated by self or partner stimulation is decreased, the time required to attain orgasm is increased,[24,47,65] and the orgasm may not be as intense.[66] Breast stimulation, mechanical genital stimulation (clitoral or cervical vibrators), and the stimulation of hypersensitive areas around the level of injury and other erogenous sensate areas, are often employed[47] to reach orgasm after SCI.

As with other aspects of sexual function, orgasm in women with SCI is influenced by level and completeness of injury. Women with incomplete lesions attain orgasm more frequently than women with complete lesions, regardless of level of injury.[47] Women with cervical lesions are less likely to achieve orgasm than individuals with thoracic and lumbosacral lesions.[67] Orgasm is less likely to be experienced if there is complete disruption of the sacral reflex arc (such as occurs with conus medullaris injuries).[24,64,68] Only 17% of women with complete LMN injuries affecting the S2–S5 spinal segments reached orgasm using genital stimulation as compared to 59% of women with other levels and degrees of injury.[62]

Female Reproductive Issues

Men suffer more severe fertility consequences than do women after SCI due to the interference with erectile and ejaculation capacity and poor semen quality. The issues around fertility in men after SCI will be covered in Chapter 22. In women with SCI, because the capacity for fertility is maintained, issues around birth control and birth control precautions are more applicable to women with SCI than men with SCI, unless the man is ejaculating. For birth control, most men with SCI use condoms, but if maintaining an erection is an issue, especially related to lack of sensation, condoms are often abandoned.[69] However, condom use is required for safe sex practices.

About 40% to 75% of women surveyed post-injury used some form of birth control,[67] with oral contraceptives, progesterone patch, or intrauterine device being used most commonly.[3] Difficulties with genital sensation and poor hand function interfere with the use of vaginal barrier birth control methods, and thrombosis secondary to immobility makes the use of oral contraceptives a risk. Immediately following injury, amenorrhea may occur, lasting on average 4 to 5 months.[66,67,70] After this initial delay in menstruation following traumatic SCI, fertility in women is believed to be unaffected. Interestingly, 15% of the female participants in one survey thought their injury had negatively affected their fertility, and 22% felt that their injury had negatively altered their changes of being a mother.[3]

Pregnancy is associated with increased risks and complications, such as increased incidence of urinary tract infections (UTIs), changes in bladder management, increased risk for skin breakdown, difficulty with transfers due to increasing maternal weight, increased risk for deep vein thrombosis, delayed bowel emptying, pedal edema, spotting, fatigue, and thrombophlebitis.[66,67,70] Labor and delivery must be monitored, since, depending on the level of lesion, labor may or may not be felt or may present differently than in noninjured women.

Premature cervical dilation and labor are more common in women with SCI as compared to the general population,[71] as are Caesarian sections and vacuum and forceps extractions.[67] Women with SCI also deliver lower birth-weight infants, the etiology of which is not clearly understood.[59] The risk of AD during induction of labor must be differentiated from preeclampsia and may require special anesthetic measures.[71,72] There are reports of cerebral intraventricular hemorrhage[73] with resultant neurological deficits and death[21] associated with unrecognized AD during labor or delivery. The risk of AD can be reduced by the use of epidural anesthesia to block the reflex arc or by Caesarian section to hasten delivery.[75,76] Breastfeeding in women with SCI above T4 may be interfered with due to loss of nipple (suckling afferent) innervation, but active mental imaging and relaxation techniques, as well as oxytocin nasal spray, may facilitate the let-down reflex for milk ejection[77] in women with higher-level lesions.

The Comprehensive Approach to Sexuality After SCI

What Happens to Sexual Satisfaction and Practices After SCI?

Sexual satisfaction is reportedly lower in both men and woman after SCI,[52,78] but the majority of those surveyed (72%) are satisfied with current life circumstances.[79] Not surprisingly, factors significantly related to sexual satisfaction include the relationship with the partner, ability to move, and mental well-being.[78] In general, the frequency of sexual activity decreases after injury in both men and women, as does sexual desire, although men's sexual desire consistently remains higher (or even remains at pre-injury levels) than women's.[52,67,80,81] General factors predicting higher sexual satisfaction scores for both sexes include having a higher education, higher income, and younger age, whereas lower scores are associated with bed sores, uncontrolled bladder, flexor spasms, and UTIs.[81]

Most studies do not distinguish between heterosexual and other sexual orientations, thus there is no information with regard to potential sexual issues in persons with SCI who are not heterosexual or who may have gender identity issues. In sexual rehabilitation, respecting sexual triggers and gender preferences without judgment, as long as they are not harmful to the person or his or her partner, is important. When appropriate, safe sexual practices and birth control must be mentioned when discussing sexual issues.

Factors affecting men and women after SCI are both physiological and psychosocial. Women with new injuries felt they were less sexually attractive, questioned their ability to perform in a sexually satisfying role, and thought they were viewed by others as less attractive.[80,82] Over time and with experience with their changed bodies, women became more comfortable with their sexuality and developed improved sexual self-esteem.[82,83] In one study, the primary reason women with SCI sought sexual activity was the need for intimacy; however, the second most commonly cited reason was to keep a partner.[3] A more recent survey found that the 92% of women having intercourse felt their main difficulties were positioning during foreplay (72.4%) and intercourse (77.0%), vaginal lubrication (65.5%), and spasticity (63.2%). The least reported difficulty was vaginal pain with intercourse (18.4%).[3] Women with cervical injuries had the greatest difficulties. Additionally, 28.7% of women participated in anal penetration post-injury. Factors affecting sexual satisfaction in both sexes include urinary incontinence, UTIs, spasticity, pain, fecal incontinence, AD, and altered genital sensation, as well as altered body image, sexual desire, quality of the intimate relationship, perceived partner satisfaction, and level of social and vocational activity.[65,67,80,84,85]

After SCI, the majority of men remain sexually active or interested in sexual activity. The level and extent of injury has not been found to affect the frequency of sexual activity.[52] Similarly, in another large study, despite considerable variation in levels of genital sensation, orgasmic capacity, and erectile function in men with SCI, none of these variables predicted sexual behavior, enjoyment, or satisfaction.[59] The authors did point out that these findings did not mean these variables were not important. For men, sexual satisfaction was influenced by perceived partner satisfaction with the sexual relationship, relationship satisfaction, sexual desire, concerns about not satisfying a partner, and decreased erectile function.[52,59,86]

Changes to Sensation and Sexual Stimulation Preferences After SCI

After SCI, there may be a loss or alteration of normal sensory pathways. Forms of genital stimulation may include hand, oral, penile-vaginal, or penile-anal intercourse, and assistive aids, including vibrators and sex toys. For women after SCI, pelvic anesthesia and poor hand function dictate different masturbatory attempts, including heightened use of breast and nipple stimulation and vibrators.[47] After SCI, only half of men with SCI attempt to self-stimulate; those who do masturbate do so primarily by hand stimulation to the penis, but upon finding this effort does not result in ejaculation or orgasm (even if an erection was provoked), they may abandon this method.[47] In both men and women with SCI, especially when genital stimulation is altered, extra-genital stimulation can be as critical for arousal as is genital stimulation, if not more so.

Being involved in a sexual relationship is not synonymous with having sexual intercourse. However, in most surveys, the majority of men and women with SCI still participate in sexual (penetrative) intercourse, but at a lower frequency compared to pre-injury. Older surveys state that between 67% and 72% of women with SCI participated in sexual intercourse[59,72] whereas only 61% to 63% of men with SCI did.[52,86] Why the frequency of intercourse for men with SCI declines compared to pre-injury may be due to fewer opportunities, unreliable erections, or noncoital activities being viewed more favorably.[45]

Other Factors Affecting Sexual Satisfaction After SCI

There may be other factors associated with SCI that indirectly affect sexual function, often to a significant degree. For some, this can even result in years of sexual avoidance or sabotaged relationships. The discomfort triggered and the fear associated with AD brought on by high arousal (and/or ejaculation and orgasm), the frustration with mobility issues, and the fear of incontinence during sexual activity are the primary sexual concerns for many persons with SCI, although sensory issues (i.e., hypersensitivity and paresthesias), genital hygiene issues, spasm, pain, and other SCI-related functional issues can also influence sexuality.

Autonomic Dysreflexia

AD is a condition of episodic hypertension triggered by noxious and non-noxious afferent stimuli below the level of the lesion of the spinal cord. It is characterized by headache, upper body flushing and sweating, nausea, photophobia, bradycardia, and cardiac arrhythmias.[32] Typically found in persons with SCI above T6, AD may have serious consequences, including intracerebral hemorrhage and death.[87] Common stimuli below the level of the lesion eliciting this response are pain, pressure sores, distension or inflammation of the bladder or gastrointestinal tract, muscle spasm,[88]induction, labor, delivery, breast-feeding,[71,89] and sexual activity.[90] AD is known to occur during sperm retrieval and ejaculation in men and other sexual activity leading to excessive movement or high arousal states in men and women with SCI.[5,30]

Whether or not AD is symptomatic, or if so, if it is tolerated, is individualized.[30] The knowledge that ejaculation is imminent can be both positive and negative: it may be accompanied by a sense of pleasurable release or orgasm, or may be dreaded if it predictably provokes significant AD. About 10% to 32% of men and women with all levels of SCI experience AD during sexual stimulation, with this figure increasing to 50% in those with cervical injuries.[66,91] AD interfered with the motivation to have sex in 28% of women and 16% of men in a recent survey of persons with SCI.[3,26] For a small percentage of men and women, the symptoms of AD can be pleasant or arousing.[30,91]

Mobility Issues

The ability to transfer onto a bed, hold or turn a partner, or engage in various sexual positions can regulate motivation to participate in sexual relationships. However, reduction in physical options can also inspire creative sexual alternatives and emphasize emotional intimacies. The extent of mobility after SCI dictates the level of independence in social engagement and sexual activities. For men and women with SCI, spasticity was noted to occur 26% to 38% of the time while engaged in sexual activity.[59,83] Treatments for spasticity, especially intrathecal baclofen, have been noted to interfere with erection and ejaculation in men and possibly interfere with orgasm in women.[84,92,93]

Bladder and Bowel Issues Influencing Sexuality

Bladder and bowel issues are seen as major factors influencing sexual pursuit, willingness, and sexual satisfaction after SCI. The risk of incontinence per se during sexual activity and the time taken to manage these concerns prior to leaving the house, socializing, or getting ready for sexual activity further deter the chance of sexual activity. Potential odors or visible external collection apparatus can affect the interest of a person with SCI or his or her partner. Thus, bladder and bowel issues may persuade people with SCI (women more than men) to avoid seeking sexual activities with a partner.[3,20] For women with quadriplegia who have significant difficulties with intermittent catheterization or indwelling catheters, improved quality of life and sexuality may be achieved with the use of continent urinary diversions (e.g., umbilical stoma) that also improve their body image and independence.[94] Like bladder issues, bowel incontinence can be anxiety provoking for women with SCI who resume sexual activity,[66] and bowel issues were ranked second only to urinary accidents as an area of concern following injury.[80]

Current Therapeutic Approaches

Sexual rehabilitation is far more than providing medical options to enhance functioning. The cornerstones to sexual rehabilitation of the person with SCI are *maximization* of existing and/or remaining function of both the mind and body and *adapting* to the remaining limitations

with an *optimistic, open attitude*.[5] Following these rehabilitation principles will result in better therapeutic results, since the mind-body interaction is respected. The clinician also has to remain open and non-judgmental and recognize sexuality as important as any other area of rehabilitation after SCI. Unfortunately, resistance to dealing with sexuality after SCI or other chronic debilitating neurological conditions still exists in certain rehabilitation centers and/or long-term care homes.[95]

Treatment for Arousal Difficulties in Women With SCI

In contrast to treatments for men with SCI, there are no approved medications for sexual difficulties in women with SCI. The use of phosphodiesterase (PDE5) inhibitors, revolutionary oral medications that enhance or amplify the signal for cavernosal smooth muscle relaxation and erectile response in men, have not been shown to be effective in able-bodied women with sexual dysfunction. Only a small, but statistically significant, increase in subjective arousal and borderline significance on vaginal pulse amplitude was noted in women with SCI who used the medication.[96] Alternately, there seems to be some evidence that cognitive-based therapies and the use of sympathetic nervous system manipulation in those women with impaired, but not absent, ability to achieve psychogenic genital vasocongestion may be of benefit.[28] Topical prostaglandin preparations used to enhance genital arousal have not yet been tried in women with SCI.

Based on the theory that orgasm is a spinal cord reflex, studies examining the efficacy of either vibrostimulation or clitoral vacuum stimulation procedures are underway.[28] For women, the use of vibrators has been helpful, and the site of effective stimulation may vary from around the area of injury, to the clitoris, inside the vagina, or on the cervix. Eros Therapy, a vacuum device inducing clitoral vascular engorgement, is the only U.S. Food and Drug Administration cleared-to-market device available by prescription to treat female sexual dysfunction and may prove to be of benefit in increasing orgasmic responses in women with SCI.[97] Theoretically, by initiating the bulbocavernosus reflex and vasocongestion, this therapy may also improve sensory awareness in those women with some pelvic floor sensory preservation.

Treatment for Erectile Dysfunction in Men With SCI

For men with SCI, treatment of erectile dysfunction has been shown to improve men's relationships and quality of life and also that of their partners.[98,99] Despite many gratifying sexual options not dependant on erection, being able to get an erection is important for most men post-injury.[98] Currently the medical options for erectile dysfunction include the following:

1. Oral medications that indirectly relax the penile smooth muscle and enhance an erection attained from sexual stimulation, such as the PDE5 inhibitors Viagra (sildenafil), Levitra (vardenafil), and Cialis (tadalafil)
2. Injectable medications that directly relax the penile smooth muscle, creating an erection (prostaglandin E1 penile injections PGE1; compounded or Caverject), and other injectable combinations, typically of papaverine and phentolamine[100–106]
3. Topical agents for penile smooth muscle relaxation (prostaglandin, minoxidil, and nitroglycerine)[107–111]
4. Intraurethral preparation of PGE1 (MUSE)[112,113]
5. Mechanical methods such as vacuum devices and penile rings[114,115]
6. Surgical penile implants[116]

Practical issues such as visual acuity, hand function, bladder management, ability to independently prepare for use of these various options, partner acceptance and assistance, and cost all influence the choice of which therapy to use. First-line treatments in the SCI population are noninvasive oral therapies and mechanical devices, with second choices being intracavernosal injections, followed by surgical options.[117] One survey[20] of men with SCI demonstrated the diversity of erection enhancement currently used: while 23.1% used nothing, 60% of the men had tried using some type of erection enhancement or drug, including Viagra (20.6%), penile injections (7.5%), Cialis (5.5%), penile ring at base (3.5%), vacuum device (3%), Levitra (2.5%), penile prosthesis (1.5%), or other (1%).[20]

Approximately 1000 men with SCI have been investigated in a series of randomized and nonrandomized controlled studies of the various PDE5 inhibitors. The range of efficacy varies from 75% to 85%, with a pooled estimate of efficacy of Viagra of 79%.[114] Phosphodiesterase

inhibitors require a source of NO to work. Studies have shown conflicting results on men with higher and lower lesions; some show there is no difference in efficacy,[119,120] while others suggest that those men with LMN lesions and poor reflexogenic erections may not respond as well to the PDE5 inhibitors due to poorer NO sources.[5,121,122] One study suggests that men with incomplete lesions do better with the PDE5 inhibitors than with complete or higher level lesions.[16] Men with SCI who take PDE5 inhibitors notice more frequent or enhanced spontaneous erections in nonsexual situations when the drug effect is still present.

Absence of both psychogenic and reflexogenic erections (confirmed by urodynamic and electrophysiological findings) seems to exclude successful treatment with sildenafil,[37] and presumably the other PDE5 inhibitors as well. Tadalafil, based on its long half-life, allowed the majority of men with SCI to achieve normal sexual functioning up to 24 hours after dosing compared to the shorter-lasting sildenafil.[123] In general, headache (10% to 15%) and flushing (6% to 10%) were noted to be the most common side effect for men with SCI using the PDE5 inhibitors, followed by dyspepsia, nasal congestion, dizziness, and visual disturbances (mostly under 5%), and a slight decrease in blood pressure. In all studies[31,124,125] except one,[126] it was felt that the decrease in blood pressure had no significant clinical implications, even in individuals who were naturally hypotensive (high level lesions). Other oral therapies, including Apomor-phine (a dopamine-receptor agonist) and 4-aminopyridine (a potassium channel-blocking agent noted for increasing neurotransmitter release at neuroneuronal sites), were not effective in the SCI population.[127,128] Table 21-1 evaluates the remaining nonoral options.

Talk-oriented therapy should be integral to any of the pharmaceutical approaches, since an understanding of

Table 21-1
Erection Enhancement Techniques for Men With SCI

	Method of Action	Therapeutic Recommendations	Pros	Cons
Oral phosphodiesterase-5 inhibitors Viagra, Levitra, Cialis	Indirectly enhances penile smooth muscle relaxation but requires sexual stimulation to trigger effect (genital and mental; NO-cGMP pathway)	Allow 1/2-1 hour before sexual stimulation. High fat meals with Viagra and Levitra will slow absorption. Start with low dose in hypotensive quadriplegics and young men (good erectile tissue). Nitrate use contraindicated.	Efficacy ~80%. Noninvasive. Helps enhance erectile response and maintain erections in sexual situations. May use daily.	Side effects (up to 15% of men) include headaches, facial flushing, nasal stuffiness, blurred vision with high doses (Viagra) or myalgia (rare). May have unwanted spontaneous erections (reflexogenic).

Table 21-1
Erection Enhancement Techniques for Men With SCI—cont'd

	Method of Action	Therapeutic Recommendations	Pros	Cons
		Window of opportunity for Viagra and Levitra 1-12 hours, with Cialis up to 48 hours.		
Intracavernosal Injection (ICI) (PGE1, papaverine, phentolamine)	Directly causes smooth muscle relaxation (cAMP pathway) by placement of medication within penile tissue.	Start with small doses (5 μg of PGE1) in SCI population. Proceed with home dosing increments of no more than 5 μg. Technique critical for best efficacy.	Neurogenic population ICI sensitive. Rigid erection, reliable results if technique good.	Invasive. Complications 15% to 30%: bruising, pain, priapism (short term), fibrotic nodule or penile curvature (long term).
Topical medications (PGE1, papaverine, nitroglycerin, minoxidil)	Smooth muscle relaxants placed on the penile skin.	Absorption into cavernosal bodies interfered with by tunica albuginia and poor retrograde venous flow.	Noninvasive.	Not effective for this population.
Intraurethral PGE1 (Medicated Urethral System for Erection; MUSE)	Absorption through the urethra to the corpora cavernosa via retrograde venous flow.	Technique critical: must be sitting or standing, and after application, roll the penis between the hands for 1 minute to distribute medication.	Less invasive, easier than ICI. Familiarity with catheters a help.	Not effective for this population.
Vacuum Device & Penile Rings	Cylinder and vacuum attachment draw in (primarily venous) blood for penile tumescence: erection maintained by ring at base of penis. Lubricant required.	Correct placement and seal of device important.	Reversible. No mediation required. Can use more than once per day and as backup for failed oral or ICI attempts.	Technically may be cumbersome Erection may swivel on its base due to lack of internal tumescence. SCI men may not feel pain of forgotten ring placement and may lead to anoxia of the penile tissues.
Surgical Implants	Replacement of the corpora cavernosal bodies with flexible or inflatable implants.	Appropriate only for those men who have failed above methods. Improved devices on the market.	Reliable erection. Assists with condom drainage apparatus.	Not reversible. Major surgery. Infection and extrusion higher in SCI population. Will not cause tumescence of glans penis.

how the specific therapy works in the psychosocial context is critical for motivation, compliance, partner acceptance, and success. Another approach is *cognitive-behavioral* therapy based on perineal muscle activity to optimize the effect of glans penis stimulation on the resulting erections. Restricted to those men with incomplete SCI injuries who have some perineal innervation, it has been demonstrated that through home exercises using biofeedback and the bulbocavernosus reflex, significant improvements in average and maximal tumescence were attained as well as maintained over time.[129] There may be similarities between this bulbocavernosus reflex training for men and that for women with SCI, which may be somewhat mimicked by the Eros Therapy vacuum device.

Treatment for Ejaculatory Disorders in Men With SCI

For men with SCI, the chance of having an orgasm is higher if ejaculation occurs, and with vibrostimulation, rates of ejaculation substantially improve in men with SCI above T6.[5,30] An intact lumbosacral reflex is required for ejaculation induced by vibrostimulation and is most reliably triggered by specific vibrator amplitudes and speed[55] not reproducible with self or partner sexual stimulation. The safe use of vibrostimulation at home in conjunction with high sexual arousal and positive partner influences may promote ejaculation and/or orgasm. Since AD is a serious issue, men with SCI above T10 wishing to ejaculate for the first time using vibrostimulation should do so in a clinic setting under cardiovascular monitoring. Such monitoring will also identify silent AD and avoid false reassurance that ejaculatory practices are safe just because the man feels little effect of the hypertension.[130] Severe dysreflexia is not only life threatening, but it can also cause sexual avoidance[90] and impair relationships. That said, sexual rehabilitation should emphasize the potential of self-exploration and self-ejaculation (30), and the use of prophylactic medication for hypertension can be helpful in some cases.

In one study, Levitra (vardenafil), besides improving erectile function in men with SCI, significantly improved ejaculation success rates (19% vs 10% in the placebo group) and self-confidence,[53] but it was not elucidated which men, according to their level or degree of completeness of injury, most benefited. Sudafed, an over-the-counter decongestant drug, may be used to enhance the sympathetic ejaculatory response but, due to its hypertensive properties, must be used with caution in individuals with higher SCI[5] as it could worsen AD. Similarly, mididrone, an alpha-stimulating drug, has been shown to assist ejaculatory potential in selected patients.[30] Finally, the rare but distressing problem of severe premature emission after injury at the T12–L1 level is very difficult to treat, but slight improvement has been noted with phenoxybenzamine, terazoin, or prazosin.[50]

Orgasmic Therapies and Sexual Gratification for Men and Women With SCI

Men and women with SCI wish and deserve personal gratification in their sexual experiences. Achieving good control over bladder and bowel issues during sexual experiences, changing or managing the timing of medications that may interfere with sexual function and responsiveness, reducing spasticity and pain during sexual activities, and being proactive regarding the management of AD will maximize the sexual experience. With caution to AD, the use of vibrators can be helpful on the clitoral area of women (although cervical and intravaginal insertion may also be helpful) and glans penis of men. We are currently developing a male and female version of a vibrator designed for those with disability.

For some persons with SCI, acquiring the ability to interpret or "mold" the cardiovascular and autonomic symptoms or use spasms to enhance arousal may assist in the attainment of orgasm. Ejaculation can improve the chances of experiencing orgasmic sensations.[30] Interestingly, in the vardenafil study in men, 16% of men receiving vardenafil and 8% receiving placebo felt orgasm "almost always" or "always" in the latter part of the study as compared to 4% and 6% at baseline, respectively.[53] However, for both men and women, the physical and mental abandonment required to promote orgasm may conflict with the realistic fears of negative consequences (i.e., AD, pain, urinary incontinence).

There is little literature regarding the subject of orgasmic pleasure after SCI because little is known about the genesis of orgasm, even in persons without neurological changes. A clear definition of orgasm is still elusive in the medical literature, although it is quite clear to most individuals themselves! This discrepancy is most evident in persons who sustained an SCI before having experienced an orgasm: he or she is harder pressed to pursue the socially revered "orgasm" without a memory of what it should feel like. For the previously experienced, the altered but recognizable pleasurable physiological changes and their mental interpretation are all reframed in a changed body after SCI. For example, cognitive reframing has been shown to maximize sexual perceptions in men with SCI.[30] Learning new signals from sensate areas, allowing (over time) the interpretation of previously non-erotic areas to take on more sexual significance, and allowing the emotional intimacy of the moment to be of higher import has, anecdotally, seemed to work for those who feel they have attained orgasm after SCI. This transition may be difficult or unattainable, but aside from physical assistance such as sexual aids (i.e., vibrators), clinical experience dictates factors such as quality of pre-injury orgasmic experience, an attitude of sexual openness, lack of depression, and falling in love to be positive influences on orgasmic potential after SCI.

For young men, especially, this transition is initially more difficult, since the usual instant pleasure from genital stimulation and reliable ability to ejaculate and experience orgasm may immediately disappear after injury. Some men and women, on the other hand, may have been more in tune with the components of nongenital sexual arousal and those of intimacy-based sexual expression prior to injury, allowing for a smoother transition after SCI. The chance of experiencing orgasm after SCI is improved if a longer-term, highly significant, and trusted partner with whom to experiment has been available.[83] Individuals with SCI, if single, need to be motivated to pursue their own sensuality, to use sexual aids, and to focus on the ability of the brain to promote sexual arousal and release.

In spite of this, orgasmic experiences are still elusive to many after SCI, and the philosophies of Tao and Tantric sexual practices, with their emphasis on mind transcendence, have been particularly useful adjuncts for enhancing sexuality in men and women with SCI.[25,131] For many men and women with SCI, the process of learning to enhance one's sexual responsiveness increases with time, self-experimentation, positive partner sexual experience, emotional intimacy, and general open-mindedness.[25, 30, 82,83]

Summary

In both men and women with SCI, the primary reason for pursuing sexual activity is the desire for intimacy, and for the vast majority , improving sexual function is important in improving overall quality of life The human quality of being sexual is not altered by SCI. The barriers are in the perception of one's own sexuality or in the ignorant views of others. That is why some persons with SCI have excellent sexual adjustment: they take the challenge and expand, rather than shrink, their sexual potential. Programs directed at modifying, enhancing, or amplifying body signals by physical touch and the power of the mind have been in the repertoire of sexual therapy for years to assist men and women after any type of mental or physical injury. SCI is a model for neurological sexual potential.

Clinicians working in the area of sexual health have many anecdotal stories of men and women with SCI who have found new and creative ways (sometimes even defying neurology as we know it) to enjoy the sexual responsivity of their new bodies and enhanced emotional and sexual intimacy. Working in the area of sexuality after SCI demands an open view of possibilities and respect for the experiences of these individuals, allowing them to teach us. The whole context of the person must be considered when assessing and assisting sexual potential.

To work in the area of sexual rehabilitation, a comprehensive, multidisciplinary approach is needed. Following the sexual rehabilitation principles of *maximization, adaptation and remaining open and optimistic* are critical in successful rehabilitation. This means not reaching first to pharmacological or surgical solutions, but rather *assessing* (after doing a good history and physical examination) the potential based on the current understanding of neurophysiology and respectfully *listening* to the experience to date of the person before mutually deciding what sexual areas should be addressed as a priority. Sexual rehabilitation is one area of medicine where individuals with disability truly are the greatest teachers, since sexual growth goes beyond the limits of hard-wired motor and sensory recovery and rehabilitation in this area goes beyond the traditional medical model.

As health-care providers, we have a role to educate and inform ourselves in the area of sexual function and sexuality in order to meet the sexual and fertility rehabilitative needs of persons with SCI, regardless of their age or care facility. With greater openness about the importance of sexuality to people with SCI, and the concomitant development of evidence-based treatments, the number of health-care providers actively involved in sexual rehabilitation is increasing.

A woman researcher, who has a spinal injury herself, noted the huge challenges faced by persons after SCI, and observed that every aspect of life is altered. While the need for intimacy is universal, it is especially so after such a devastating injury. In her studies, the impact of SCI specifically on sexuality was enough to significantly lower perceived quality of life. While the search for "cure" for SCI is vitally important, those therapeutic treatments to induce neuronal regeneration in the chronically injured spinal cord are not at the stage of being readily applicable or successful in humans as of yet. Persons with SCI are living longer lives, and today, the priorities persons with SCI identify as enabling them to enhance their day-to-day function and quality of life should be considered paramount when choosing the direction of future research. Knowing that men and women with SCI have a high desire for intimacy and that sexuality and sexual function is a major, important priority in their lives should be sufficient justification for increased research funding in the area of sexuality after SCI. In the meantime, sexuality is an integral and meaningful part of being human and should be embraced with curiosity and respect by health-care professionals as an essential part of rehabilitation after SCI.

REVIEW QUESTIONS

1. Beyond performance, what personal factors contribute to sexual satisfaction for persons after SCI?
2. What are the two control mechanisms/pathways involved in penile erection in men and clitoral tumescence/vaginal lubrication in women, and how may the function of the associated pathways be predicted after SCI?

3. What are the roles of the supraspinal and spinal centers in the control of orgasmic and ejaculatory function in men, and how is this function affected by SCI?

4. What two factors are the primary determinants of potential for erectile function in men with SCI, and what is the proportion of men with SCI who have preservation of erectile function?

5. Is erectile capacity or ejaculatory capacity more likely to be affected in men with SCI, and how does level of injury influence these functions?

6. What are the pathways associated with sexual arousal in women, and how are these pathways affected by SCI?

7. What factors contribute to the likelihood of achieving orgasm in women with SCI?

8. How does spinal cord injury affect reproductive function in women with SCI?

9. According to survey results, what proportion of men and women continue to participate in penetrative sexual intercourse following SCI?

10. What treatments are available to enhance arousal in women and erectile capacity in men with SCI?

REFERENCES

1. Hansen AM. Towards independence for paraplegics. *Can Nurse.* 1976;72(12):24–31.

2. Anderson K. Targeting recovery: Priorities of the spinal cord injured population. *J Neurotrauma.* 2004;21(10):1371–1383.

3. Anderson KD, Borisoff JF, Johnson RD et al. Spinal cord injury influences psychogenic as well as physical components of female sexual ability. *Spinal Cord.* 2006.

4. Anderson KD, Borisoff JF, Johnson RD et al. The impact of spinal cord injury on sexual function: Concerns of the general population. *Spinal Cord.* 2006.

5. Elliott S. Sexual dysfunction and infertility in men with spinal cord disorders. In: Lin V, editor, *Spinal Cord Medicine: Principles and Practice.* 5th edition. New York: Demos Medical Publishing, Inc.; 2003. pp. 349–365.

6. Borisoff J. Personal communication. Neil Squire Society, Brain Interface Lab, GF Strong Rehabilitation Center. Vancouver, British Columbia, Canada.

7. Marson L. Central nervous system control. In: Carson C, Kirby R, Goldstein I, editors. *Erectile Dysfunction.* Oxford, UK: ISIS Medical Media; 1999. pp. 73–88.

8. Masters WH, Johnson VE. *Human sexual response.* Boston: Little, Brown and Co. pp. 174–176.

9. Bradford A, Meston CM. The impact of anxiety on sexual arousal in women. *Behav Res Ther.* 2006;44:1067–1077.

10. Krassioukov AV, Fehlings MG. Effect of graded spinal cord compression on cardiovascular neurons in the rostro-ventro-lateral medulla. *Neuroscience.* 1999;88(3):959–973.

11. Chuang AT, Steers WD. Neurophysiology of penile erection. In: Carson C, Kirby R, Goldstein I, editors. *Textbook of Erection Dysfunction.* Oxford, UK: ISIS Medical Media Inc.; 1999:59–72.

12. McKenna, K. The brain is the master organ in sexual function: Central nervous system control of male and female sexual function. *Int J Impot Res.* 1999;11(Supp 1): S48–S55.

13. O'Connell HE, Sanjeevan KV, Hutson JM. Anatomy of the clitoris. *J Urol.* 2005;174:1189–1195.

14. Roberts KP, Pryor JL. Anatomy and physiology of the male reproductive system. In: Hellstrom W, editor. *Male Infertility and Sexual Dysfunction.* New York: Springer-Verlag, Inc.; 1997. pp. 1–21.

15. Shetty SD, Farah RN. Anatomy of erectile function. In: Carson C, Kirby R, Goldstein I, editors. *Erectile Dysfunction.* Oxford, UK: ISIS Medical Media; 1999. pp. 23–30.

16. Derry F, Hultling C, Seftel AD et al. Efficacy and safety of sildenafil citrate (Viagra) in men with erectile dysfunction and spinal cord injury: A review. *Urology* 2002;60:49–57.

17. Willibrord Weijmar S, van Andel P, Sabelis I et al. Magnetic resonance imaging of male and female genitals during coitus and female sexual arousal. *Brit Med J.* 1999;319:1596–1600.

18. Truitt WA, Coolen LM. Identification of potential ejaculation generator in the spinal cord. *Science.* 2002;29:1566–1569.

19. Carro-Juarez M, Cruz SI, Rodriguez-Manzo G. Evidence for the involvement of a spinal pattern generator in the control of genital motor pattern of ejaculation. *Brain Res.* 2003;975:222–228.20.

20. Carro-Juarez M, Rodriguez-Manzo G. Alpha-adrenergic agents modulate the activity of the spinal pattern generator for ejaculation. *Int J Impot Res.* 2006;18:32–38.

21. Carro-Juarez M, Rodriguez-Manzo G. Evidence for the presence of the spinal pattern generator involved in the control of the genital ejaculatory pattern in the female rate. *Brain Res.* 2006;1084(1):54–60.

22. Sipski, ML, Alexander CJ, Rosen RC. Orgasm in women with spinal cord injuries: A laboratory based assessment. *Arch Phys Med Rehab.* 1995;76(12):1097–1102.

23. Sipski ML, Alexander CJ, Gomez-Marin O. Effects of level and degree of spinal cord injury on male orgasm. *Spinal Cord.* 2006:44(12):796–804.

24. Alexander M,Rosen RC. Spinal cord injuries and orgasm: A Review *J Sex Marital Ther.* 2008;34:308–324.

25. Elliott S. Ejaculation and orgasm: Sexuality in men with SCI. *Top Spinal Cord Inj Rehabil.* 2002;8(1):1–15.

26. Anderson KD, Borisoff JF, Johnson RD et al.Long-term effects of spinal cord injury on sexual function in men: implications for neuroplasticity. *Spinal Cord.* 2007;45(5): 338–48.

27. Sipski ML, Alexander CJ, Rosen RC. Physiological parameters associated with sexual arousal in women with incomplete spinal cord injury. *Arch Phys Med Rehabil.* 1997;78: 305–313.

28. Sipski ML, Arenas A. Female Sexual Function after spinal cord injury. In: Weaver LC, Polosa C, eds. Progress in *Brain Research.* Amsterdam, NL: Elsevier B.V.; 2006;152: 441–447.

29. Sipski M, Alexander C, Gomez-Marin O, Spalding J. The effects of spinal cord injury on psychogenic sexual arousal in males. *J Urol.* 2007;177(1):247–51.

30. Courtois F,Charvier K,Leriche A et al. Perceived Physiological and Orgasmic Sensations at Ejaculation in Spinal Cord Injured Men. *J Sex Med.* 2008;5:2419–2430.

31. Sheel W, Krassioukov A, Inglis T, Elliott S. Autonomic dysreflexia during sperm retrieval in spinal cord injury influence of lesion level and sildenafil citrate. *J Applied Physiol.* 2005;99(1):53–58.

32. Claydon VE, Elliott SL, Sheel AW et al. Cardiovascular responses to vibrostimulation for sperm retrieval in men with spinal cord injury. *J Spinal Cord Med.* 2006;29:207–216.

33. Whipple B, Komisaruk BR. Brain (PET) response to vaginal-cervical self-stimulation in women with complete spinal cord injury: Preliminary findings. *J Sex Marital Ther.* 2002;28(1):79–86.

34. Komisaruk BR, Whipple B, Crawford A, Liu WC, Kalnin A, Mosier K. Brain activation during vaginocervical self-stimulation and orgasm in women with complete spinal cord injury: fMRI evidence of mediation by the vagus nerves. *Brain Res.* 2004: 22;1024(1–2):77–88.

35. Giuliano FA, Rampin O, Benoit G Jardin A. Neural control of penile erection. *Uro Clin North Am.* 1995;22(4):747–66.

36. Sipski ML, Alexander CJ, Rosen RC. Physiological parameters associated with psychogenic sexual arousal in women with complete spinal cord injuries. *Arch Phys Med Rehabil.* 1995;76:811–818.

37. Schmid DM, Schurch B, Hauri D. Sildenafil in the treatment of sexual dysfunction in spinal cord injured patients. *Eur Urol.* 2000;38:184–193.

38. Courtois FJ, Charvier KF, Leriche A et al. Sexual function in spinal cord injured men. I. Assessing sexual capacity. *Paraplegia.* 1993;31:771–784.

39. Szasz, G. Sexual health care. In: Zejdlik C, editor. *Management of the Spinal Cord Injured.* Monterey, CA: Wadsworth Health Sciences Division; 1983. pp. 125–152.

40. Richenberg J, Richards D. Radiological diagnosis of venous leakage. In: Hellstrom W, editor. *Male Infertility and Sexual Dysfunction.* New York: Springer-Verlag Inc.; 1999. 225–232.

41. Patel U, Lees WR. Pharmacological testing: Doppler. In: Hellstrom W, ed. *Male Infertility and Sexual Dysfunction.* New York, NY: Springer-Verlag; 1999:207–220.

42. Beck, RO. Investigation of male erectile dysfunction. In: Fowler CJ, editor. *Neurology of Bladder, Bowel and Sexual Dysfunctions.* Boston: Butterworth-Heineman Ltd.; 1999. pp. 145–160.

43. Giuliano F, Clément P. Serotonin and premature ejaculation: from physiology to patient management. *Eur Urol.* 2006 Sep;50(3):454–66.

44. Bors E, Comarr AE. Neurological disturbances of sexual function with special reference to 529 patients with spinal cord injury. *Urol Surv.* 1960;10:191–222.

45. Beneveto BT, Sipski ML. Neurogenic bladder, neurogenic bowel and sexual dysfunction in people with spinal cord injury. *Phys Ther.* 2002;82(6):601–612.

46. Laessoe L, Nielson JB, Biering-Sorenson F et al. Antispastic effect of penile vibration in men with spinal cord lesion. *Arch Phys Med Rehabil.* 2004;85:919–924.

47. Donohue J, Gebhard P. The Kinsey Institute/Indiana University report on sexuality and spinal cord injury. *Sex. Disabil.* 1995;13(1):7–85.

48. Talbot HS. The sexual function in paraplegia. *J Urol.* 1955;73:91.

49. Courtois FJ, Charvier K, Raymond D et al. Self-induced ejaculation and orgasmic potential in spinal cord injured men. *Christopher Reeve Foundation Spinal Cord Symposium: A Dialogue Between Grant Holders and the Community They Serve.* Boston, MA, September 16–18, 2005. Short Hills, NJ: Christopher Reeve Foundation.

50. Kuhr CS, Heiman J, Cardenas D et al. Premature emission after spinal cord injury. *J Urol.* 1995;153:429–431.

51. Yarkony GM. Enhancement of sexual function and fertility in SCI males. *Am J Phys Med Rehabil.* 1990;69(2)81–87.

52. Alexander CJ, Sipski ML, Findley TW. Sexual activities, desire, and satisfaction in 20 males pre- and post-spinal cord injury. *Arch Sex Behav.* 1993;22(3):217–228.

53. Giuliano F, Rubio-Aurioles E, Kennelly M et al. Vardenafil Study Group. Vardenafil improves ejaculation rates and self-confidence in men with erectile dysfunction due to spinal cord injury *Spine.* 2008;33(7):709–715.

54. Talbot HS. The sexual function in paraplegia. *J Urol.* 1955;73:91.

55. Ohl DA, Sonksen J. Penile vibratory stimulation and electroejaculation. In: Hellstrom W, editor. *Male Infertility and Sexual Dysfunction.* New York: Springer-Verlag, Inc.; 1997. pp. 219–229.

56. Szasz G, Carpenter C. Clinical observations in vibratory stimulation of the penis in men with spinal cord injury. *Arch Sex Behav.* 1989;8:461–474.

57. Sonksen J, Biering-Sorensen F, Kristensen JK. Ejaculation induced by penile vibratory stimulation in men with spinal cord injuries. The importance of vibratory amplitude. *Paraplegia.* 1994;32:651–660.

58. Phelps G, Brown M, Chen J et al. Sexual experience and plasma testosterone levels in male veterans after spinal cord injury. *Arch Phys Med Rehabil.* 1983;64:47–52.

59. Phelps J, Albo M, Dunn K et al. Spinal cord injury and sexuality in married or partnered men: Activities, function, needs and predictors of sexual adjustment. *Arch Sex Behav.* 2001;30(6):591–602(12).

60. Rosen RC, Beck JF. Genital blood flow measurement in the female: Psychophysiological techniques. In: Rosen RC, Beck JF, editors. *Patterns of Sexual Arousal.* New York: Guilford Press; 1988. pp. 78–107.

61. Laan E, Everanerd W. Physiological measures of vaginal vasocongestion. *Int J Impot Res.* 1998;10(Suppl 2):S107–S110.

62. Sipski ML, Alexander CJ, Rosen RC. Sexual arousal and orgasm in women: Effect of spinal cord injury. *Ann Neurol.* 2001;49:35–44.

63. Lundberg PO. Physiology of female sexual function and effect of neurologic disease. In: Fowler CJ, editor. *Neurology of Bladder, Bowel and Sexual Dysfunction.* Boston: Butterworth-Heinemann Ltd.; 1999. pp. 33–46.

64. Sipski ML. Central nervous system based neurogenic female sexual dysfunction: Current status and future trends. *Arch Sex Behav.* 2002;31:421–424.

65. Ferrerio-Velasco ME, Barca-Buyo A, Salvador DeLaBarrera S. Sexual issues in a sample of women with spinal cord injury. *Spinal Cord.* 2005;43(1):51–55.

66. Charlifue SW, Gerhart KA, Menter RR et al. Sexual issues of women with spinal cord injuries. *Paraplegia.* 1992;30:192–199.

67. Jackson AB, Wadley V. A multicenter study of women's self-reported reproductive health after SCI. *Arch Phys Med Rehabil.* 1999;80:1420–1428.

68. Kiekens C, Spiessens C, Duyck F et al. Pregnancy after electroejaculation in combination with intracytoplasmic sperm injection in a patient with idiopathic anejaculation. *Fertil Steril.* 1996; 66(5):834–836.

69. Mona LR, Krause JS, Norris FH et al. Sexual expression following spinal cord injury. *NeuroRehabil* 2000;15:121–131.

70. Axel SJ. Spinal cord injured women's concerns: Menstruation and pregnancy. *Rehabil Nurs.* 1982;(7):10–15.

71. Sipski ML. The impact of spinal cord injury on female sexuality, menstruation and pregnancy: A review of the literature. *J Am Paraplegic Soc.* 1991;14(3);122–126.

72. Burns AS, Jackson AB. Gynecological and reproductive issues in women with spinal cord injury. *Phys Med Rehab Clin N Am.* 2001;12(1):183–99.

73. McGregor JA, Meeuwsen J. Autonomic hyperreflexia: A mortal danger for spinal cord-damaged women in labor. *Am J Obstet Gynecol.* 1985;151(3):330–333.

74. Abouleish E. Hypertension in a paraplegic parturient. *Anesthesiology.* 1980;53:348–349.

75. Yarnovy GM, Chen D. Sexuality in patients with spinal cord injury. *Phys Med Rehabil.*1995;9:325–343.

76. Pereira, L. Obstetric management of the patient with spinal cord injury. *Obstet Gynecol.* Surv. 2003;58(10):678–687.

77. Cowley, KC. Psychogenic and pharmacological induction of the let-down reflex can facilitate breast-feeding by tetraplegic women: A report of 3 cases. *Arch Phys Med Rehabil.* 2005;86:1261–1264.

78. Reitz A, Tobe V, Knapp PA et al. Impact of spinal cord injury on sexual health and quality of life. *Int J Impotence Res.* 2004;16:167–174.

79. Kennedy P, Lude P, Taylor N. Quality of life, social participation, appraisals and coping post spinal cord injury. A review of four community samples. *Spinal Cord.* 2006;44:95–105.

80. White MJ, Rintala DH, Hart KA et al. Sexual activities, concerns and interests of women with spinal cord injury living in the community. *Am J Phys Med Rehabil.* 1993; 72(6):372–378.

81. Sharma SC, Singh R, Dogra R et al. Assessment of sexual functions after spinal cord injury in Indian patients. *Int J Rehabil Res.* 2006;29:17–25.

82. Ekland M, Lawrie B. How a woman's sexual adjustment after sustaining a spinal cord injury impact sexual health interventions. *SCI Nursing.* 2004;21(1):14–19.

83. Tepper MS, Whipple B, Richard E et al. Women with complete spinal cord injury: A phenomenological study of sexual experiences. *J Sex Marital Ther.* 2001;27:615–623.

84. Forsythe E, Horsewell JE. Sexual rehabilitation of women with spinal cord injury. *Spinal Cord.* 2006;44:234–241.

85. Pentland W, Walker J, Minnes P et al. Women with spinal cord injury and the impact of aging. *Spinal Cord.* 2002;40:374–387.

86. White MJ, Rintala DH, Hart KA et al. Sexual activities, concerns and interests of men with spinal cord injury. *Am. J Phys Med Rehabil.* 1992;71:225–231.

87. Krassioukov AV, Claydon VE. The clinical problems in cardiovascular control following spinal cord injury: An overview. In: Weaver LC, Polosa C, editors. *Prog Brain Res.* Amsterdam, Netherlands: Elsevier BV; 2006. pp. 152, 223–229.

88. Weaver LC, Polosa C, editors. Autonomic dysfunction after spinal cord injury. *Prog Brain Res.* Amsterdam, Netherlands: Elsevier; 2006:152:1–453.

89. Pope CS, Markenson GR, Bayer-Zwirello LA et al. Pregnancy complicated by chronic spinal cord injury and history of autonomic hyperreflexia. *Obstet Gynecol.* 2001; 97(5):802–803.

90. Elliott S, Krassioukov A. Malignant autonomic dysreflexia following ejaculation in spinal cord injured men. *Spinal Cord.* 2006;44(6):386–392.

91. Anderson KD, Borisoff JF, Johnson RD et al. The impact of spinal cord injury on sexual function: Concerns of the general population. *Spinal Cord.* 2006.

92. Denys P, Mane M, Azouvi P et al. Side effects of chronic intrathecal baclofen on erection and ejaculation in patients with spinal cord lesions. *Arch Phys Med Rehabil.* 1998; 79:494–496.

93. Meythaler JM, Steers WD, Tuel SM et al. Continuous intrathecal baclofen in spinal cord spasticity. A prospective study. *Am J Phys Med Rehabil.* 1992;71:321–327.

94. Moreno JG, Chancellor MB, Karasick S. Improved quality of life and sexuality with continent urinary diversion in quadriplegic women with umbilical stoma. *Arch Phys Med Rehabil.* 1995;76:758–762.

95. Bethan, JE. "Sexual Activity in Long-Term Care." PhD Thesis. Vancouver: Department of Philosophy, Faculty of Graduate Studies in Interdisciplinary Studies. University of British Columbia, Vancouver; 2005

96. Sipski ML, Rosen RC, Alexander CJ et al. Sildenafil effects on sexual and cardiovascular responses in women with SCI. *Urology.* 2000;55:812–815.

97 Billups KL. The role of mechanical devices in treating female sexual dysfunction and enhancing the female sexual response. *World J Urol.* 2002;20:137–141.

98. Hultling CP. Partner's perception of the efficacy of sildenafil citrate (Viagra) in the treatment of erectile dysfunction. *Int J Clin Pract.* 1999;Suppl 102:16–18.

99. Hultling C, Guiliano F, Quirk F et al. Quality of life in patients with spinal cord injury receiving Viagra (sildenafil citrate) for the treatment of erectile dysfunction. *Spinal Cord.* 2000;38:363–370.

100. Spahn M, Manning M, Juenemann KP. Intracavernosal therapy. In: Carson C, Kirby R, Goldstein I, editors. *Textbook of Erectile Dysfunction.* Oxford, UK: ISIS Medical Media; 1999. pp. 345–353.

101. Bernard F, Lue TF. The role of the urologist and patient in autoinjection therapy for erectile dysfunction. *Contemp Urol.* 1990;2:21–26.

102. Sidi AA, Cameron JS,Dykstra DD, Reinberg Y, Lange PH. Vasoactive Intracavernous Pharmacotherapy for the Treatment of Erectile Impotence in Men with Spinal Cord Injury. *J Urol.* 1987;138:539–542.

103. Watanabe T, Chancellor MC, Rivas DA, et al. Epidemiology of current treatment for sexual dysfunction in spinal cord injured men in the USA model spinal cord injury centers. *J Spinal Cord Med.* 1996;19:186–189.

104. Zaslau S, Nicolis C, Galea G, Britanico J, Vapnek JM. A Simplified pharmacologic erection program for patients with spinal cord injury. *Spinal Cord Med.* 1999;22:303–307.

105. Dietzen CJ, Lloyd LK. Complications of intracavernous injections and penile prostheses in spinal cord injured men *Arch Phys Med Rehabil.* 1992;73:652–655.

106. Lloyd LK, Richards JS. Intracavernous pharmacotherapy for management of erectile dysfunction in spinal cord injury. *Paraplegia.* 1989;27:457–464.

107. Kim ED, El-Rashidy R, McVary KT. Papaverine topical gel for the treatment of erectile Dysfunction. *J Urol.* 1995;153:361–365.

108. Kim ED, McVary KT. Topical prostaglandin-E1 for the treatment of erectile Dysfunction. *J Urol.* 1995;153: 1828–1830.

109. Sonksen J, Biering-Sorensen F. Trancutaneous nitroglycerin in the treatment of erectile dysfunction in spinal cord injured. *Paraplegia.* 1992;30:554–557.

110. Chancellor MB, Rivas PA, Panzer DE, Freedman MK, Staas WE, Jr. Prospective comparison of topical minoxidil to vacuum constriction device and intracorporeal

papaverine injection in treatment of erectile dysfunction due to spinal cord injury. *Urology.* 94:43;365–369.

111. Beretta G, Saltarelli O, Marzotto M et al. Transcutaneous minoxidil in the treatment of erectile dysfunctions in spinal cord injured men. *Acta Eur Fertil.* 1993;24:27–30.

112. Bodner DR, Haas CA, Krueger B et al. Intraurethral alprostadil for treatment of erectile dysfunction in patients with spinal cord injury. *Urology.* 1999;53:199–202.

113. Waldbaum J, Chen D, Nussbaum SB et al. Use of transurethral alprostadil to treat erectile dysfunction in spinal cord injured patients. *Arch Phys Med Rehabil.* 1998;79:1184. (Abstr.)

114. Zasler ND, Katz PG. Synergist erection system in the management of impotence secondary to spinal cord injury. *Arch Phys Med Rehabil.* 1989;70:712–771.

115. Denil J, Ohl DA, Smythe C. Vacuum erection device in spinal cord injured men: Patient and partner satisfaction. *Arch Phys Med Rehabil.* 1996;77:750–753.

116. Shah PJR. Spinal cord injury. In: Carson C, Kirby R, and Goldstein I, editors. *Textbook of Erection Dysfunction.* Oxford, UK: ISIS Medical Media Inc.; 1999. pp. 59–72.

117. Ramos AS, Samso JV. Specific aspects of erectile dysfunction in spinal cord injury. *Int J Impot Res.* 2004;16 Supp 2: S42–S45.

118. DeForge D, Blackmer J, Moher D et al. *Sexuality and Reproductive Health Following Spinal Cord Injury.* Evidence Report/Technology Assessment No. 109. Prepared by the University of Ottawa Evidence-Based Practice Center under Contract No. 290-02-0021. AHRQ Publication No. 05-E003-2. Rockville, MD: Agency for Healthcare Research and Quality; 2004.

119. Giuliano F, Hultling C, El Masry WS et al. Randomized trial of sildenafil for the treatment for erectile dysfunction in spinal cord injury. *Ann Neurol.* 1999;46:15–21.

120. Sanchez Ramos A, Vidal J, Jaurequi ML et al. Efficacy, safety and predictive factors of therpeutic success with sildenafil for erectile dysfuntion in patients with different spinal cord injuries. *Spinal Cord.* 2001;39:637–643.

121. Raviv G, Heruti RJ, Katz H et al. Clinical experience with Viagra in spinal cord injured patients. *Eur Urol.* 2000; 37 Suppl 2:81. (Abstr.)

122. Holmgren E, Giuliano F, Hultling C et al. Sildenafil (Viagra) in the treatment of erectile dysfunction (ED) caused by spinal cord injury (SCI): A double bind, placebo-controlled, flexible-dose, two way crossover study. *Neurology.* 1998;50:A127. (Abstr.)

123. Del Poplo G, Marzi VL, Mondaini N et al. Time/duration effectiveness of sildenafil versus tadalafil in the treatment of erectile dysfunction in male spinal cord-injured patients. *Spinal Cord.* 2004;42:643–648.

124. Sipski M, Alexander C, Guo X et al. Cardiovascular effects of sildenafil in men with SCIs at and above T6. *Top Spinal Cord Inj Rehabil.* 2003;8(3)26–34.

125. Garcia-Bravo AM, Suarez-Hernandez D, Ruiz-Fernandez MA et al. Determination of changes in blood pressure during administration of sildenafil (Viagra) in patients with spinal cord injury and erectile dysfunction. *Spinal Cord.* 2006;44:301–308.

126. Ethans KD, Casey AR, Schryvers OI et al. The effects of sildenail on the cardiovascular response in men with spinal cord injury at or above the sixth thoracic level. *J Spinal Cord Med.* 2003;26(3):222–226.

127. Strebel RT, Reitz A, Tenti G et al. Apomorphine sublingual as a primary or secondary treatment for erectile dysfunction in patients with spinal cord injury. *BJU Int.* 2004;93:100–104.

128. Potter PJ, Hayes KC, Segal JL et al. Randomized double-blind crossover trial of fampridine-SR (sustained release 4-aminopyridine) in patients with incomplete spinal cord injury. *J Neurotrauma.* 1998;15:837–849.

129. Courtois FJ, Mathieu C, Charvier KF et al. Sexual rehabilitation for men with spinal cord injury: Preliminary report of behavioral strategy. *Sex Disabil.* 2001;19(2): 149–157.

130. Ekland MB, Krassioukov AV, McBride KE, Elliott SL. Incidence of autonomic dysreflexia and silent autonomic dysreflexia in men with SCI undergoing sperm retrieval: implications for clinical practice. *J Spinal Cord Med.* 2008;31(1):33–39.

131. Tepper, M. Personal Communication. Via sexualhealth.com (owned and operated by the Sexual Health Network, Inc.). Pennsylvania, PA. 2001.

Fertility After Spinal Cord Injury 22

Nancy L. Brackett, PhD, HCLD
Emad Ibrahim, MD

Introduction

Spinal cord injury (SCI) occurs most often to young men at the peak of their reproductive health. In the United States, 80% of new injuries occur to men between the ages of 16 and 45.[1] Around the world, similar statistics are found.[2-6] The most common causes of SCI are motor vehicle accidents, violence, sports-related injuries, and falls.[1] It is assumed that more men than women are injured because men engage in more risk-taking behavior that leads to injury. The actual cause for the disproportionately high percentage of injured men, however, is unknown. Recent evidence suggests that sex hormones may play a role in this discrepancy; that is, estrogen may be neuroprotective and/or that testosterone may be neurotoxic after injury.[7,8]

Following SCI, fertility is severely impaired in men, but not in women. For example, 90% of men with SCI cannot father a child via sexual intercourse.[9] Women with SCI, however, can conceive and deliver children with nearly the same success rate as the general population.[10] Reproductive function is of great importance to men with SCI.[11,12] Regaining sexual function has been identified as the highest priority among individuals with paraplegia.[11] Most men with SCI require medical assistance to father children due to impairments in erection, ejaculation, and semen quality.[13]

Given the fact that sexual function and fertility are of paramount importance to men with SCI, it is critical that these topics be included as part of any standard rehabilitation curriculum for clients. In addition, rehabilitation professionals should continually educate themselves with current and accurate information on these topics and be prepared to discuss these topics with their clients. Clients will request this information at different times during their recovery. Some clients wish to know this information immediately after injury, and other clients may not request this information for months or years. As with other questions regarding rehabilitation, clients typically first query a therapist or nurse, rather than a physician. It is therefore vital that rehabilitation professionals be ready to discuss these topics whenever they are brought up. Discussion of sexual and fertility issues may be uncomfortable for some caregivers as well as for some individuals with SCI. In those instances, the caregiver should at least be knowledgeable about professionals in their community who can act as a backup resource for additional education and/or management.

Treatments for Erectile Dysfunction

The same treatments used for treatment of erectile dysfunction in noninjured men are used for treatment of erectile dysfunction in men with SCI. Most men with SCI respond well to oral administration of phosphodiesterase-5 inhibitors (PDE-5 inhibitors), including Viagra (sildenafil citrate), Levitra (vardenafil HCL), and Cialis (tadalafil).[14-16] Men with SCI who do not respond well to oral PDE-5 inhibitors may respond better to medications injected into the corpus cavernosum of the penis, such as Caverject (alprostadil) or Trimix (a mixture of papaverine/regitine/prostaglandin E-1; Fig. 22-1). Other therapies for erectile dysfunction include MUSE, an acronym for medicated urethral system for erections (a pellet of alprostadil inserted into the penile urethra), vacuum erection devices (Fig. 22-2), or a surgically implanted penile prosthesis (Fig. 22-3).

Treatments for Anejaculation

The majority of men with SCI are *anejaculatory*, that is, unable to ejaculate during sexual intercourse.[17] Methods are available to improve or overcome anejaculation in

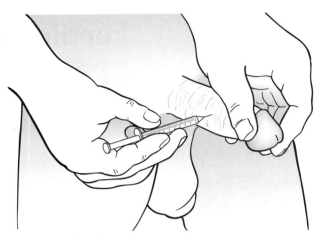

Figure 22-1. Intracavernous injections are effective remedies for erectile dysfunction in men with SCI.

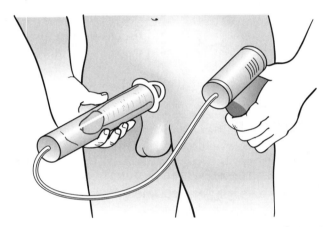

Figure 22-2. This example of a vacuum erection device is one of the available therapies for erectile dysfunction in men with SCI.

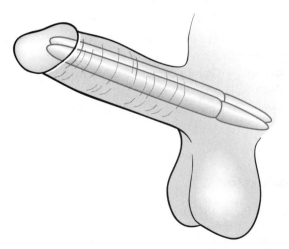

Figure 22-3. Penile implants are indicated for erectile dysfunction in some men with SCI who are unresponsive to other methods. Risks of this therapy include infection and, in nonsensate men, inability to detect erosion of the penile implant through the skin.

men with SCI. The choice of the method depends on the purpose of the ejaculation. The primary purposes of ejaculation in men with SCI are (1) to retrieve sperm for use in assisted reproductive technologies or (2) for sexual pleasure. Several methods are available to retrieve sperm for assisted reproductive technologies, including penile vibratory stimulation (PVS), electroejaculation (EEJ), surgical sperm retrieval, and prostate massage.

Penile Vibratory Stimulation

PVS is usually recommended as the first line of treatment for anejaculation in men with SCI.[18,19] PVS involves placing a vibrator on the dorsum or frenulum of the glans penis (Fig. 22-4).[20] Mechanical stimulation produced by the vibrator recruits the ejaculatory reflex to induce ejaculation.[21] This method is more effective in men with an intact ejaculatory reflex, that is, men with a level of injury T10 or above (88% success rate) compared to men with a level of injury T11 and below (15% success rate).[22]

Unlike the methods of EEJ, surgical sperm retrieval, and prostate massage, PVS may be performed at home by some couples. Couples should first be evaluated in a clinic prior to trying PVS at home. The evaluation should include assessment for risk of autonomic dysreflexia, assessment for optimal stimulation parameters to induce safe ejaculation in the given individual, and demonstration that the man and/or his partner can perform the procedure properly.[20] Autonomic dysreflexia (AD) is a risk for any method of sperm retrieval in men with a level of injury T6 and above,[23] (see Chapter 1). Briefly, AD is a potentially life-threatening medical complication that can occur in individuals injured at or above T6. AD is an uninhibited sympathetic reflex response of the nervous system to an irritating stimulus below the level of injury. Symptoms of AD include hypertension, bradycardia, sweating, chills, and headache. In some cases, AD can lead to dangerously high blood pressure levels, and this

complication can lead to stroke, seizure, or even death. Symptoms of AD can be well-managed or prevented by oral administration of nifedipine.[23]

PVS may be attempted using any of a number of commercially available devices sold over the counter as wand massagers. One of the most effective commercially available vibrators is the Ferti Care (Multicept, Denmark), engineered specifically for inducing ejaculation in men with SCI (Fig. 22-5). The advantage of this vibrator is its ability to deliver high-amplitude stimulation, 2.5 mm excursions of the vibrating head, at a frequency of 90 to 100 hertz. These stimulus parameters were found to be most effective for ejaculatory success in men with SCI.[24]

If a man is unable to ejaculate with a high-amplitude vibrator, then auxiliary methods may be employed to facilitate ejaculation with PVS, such as application of two vibrators (Fig. 22-6),[25] use of abdominal electrical stimulation in addition to PVS (Fig. 22-7),[26] or oral

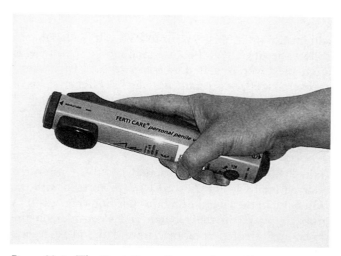

Figure 22-5. The Ferti Care vibrator, pictured here, was engineered specifically for ejaculation of men with SCI.

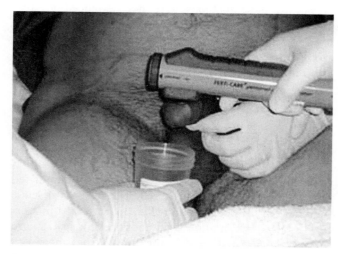

Figure 22-4. Penile vibratory stimulation is recommended as the first line of treatment for anejaculation in men with SCI.

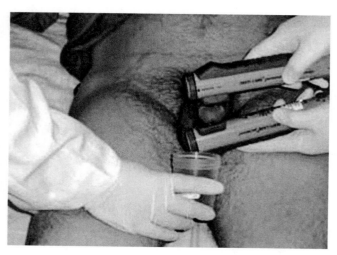

Figure 22-6. Individuals who cannot respond to PVS with one vibrator may respond to PVS with two vibrators.

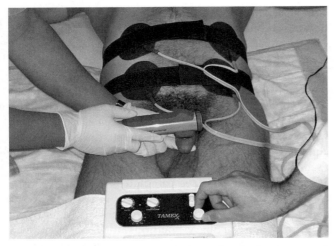

Figure 22-7. PVS, in combination with abdominal electrical stimulation using a commercially available device, has been shown to be successful in some men who do not respond to PVS alone.

administration of Viagra prior to PVS.[27] It is advisable to collect sperm via PVS because total motile sperm yields are highest with this method compared to EEJ, surgical sperm retrieval, or prostate massage.[28,29] Higher yields of total motile sperm allow for the use of a wider range of assisted reproductive technologies.[30,31]

Electroejaculation

Individuals who cannot respond to PVS are often referred for EEJ (Fig. 22-8). EEJ is performed with the man lying in the lateral decubitus position (Fig. 22-9). A probe is placed in the rectum, and electrodes on the probe are oriented anteriorly toward the prostate and seminal vesicles. Current delivered through the probe stimulates nerves that lead to emission of semen.

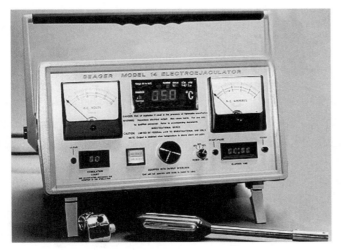

Figure 22-8. EEJ is a method used to retrieve semen when PVS fails.

The method of EEJ was first developed in the 1930s for use in veterinary medicine[32] and modified in the 1980s for use in humans.[33,34] Prior to the development of the high-amplitude vibrator in the mid-1990s, EEJ was the most common method of semen retrieval in men with SCI due to its higher success rate compared to PVS. Currently, EEJ is recommended as a second choice for those individuals who have failed to achieve semen retrieval via PVS. PVS is the preferred method because EEJ is more invasive, preferred less by men, and results in a lower yield of total motile sperm in the antegrade fraction.[28,29]

Prostate Massage

Prostate massage has been used to collect semen from men with SCI for use in insemination.[35,36] The physician inserts a gloved finger into the man's rectum and massages the seminal vesicles and prostate. In a recent report by Engin-Ustun and colleagues, prostatic massage was used in 10 men with the resulting sperm retrieval leading to two pregnancies (20% pregnancy rate).[37] It is not clear when this method is indicated in men with SCI. Some practitioners may not have PVS or EEJ equipment, and in these cases, prostate massage may be useful. The rationale for doing prostate massage is that sperm are stored in the ampulla of the vas deferens and, in men with SCI, are sequestered in the seminal vesicles as well.[38] The practitioner, therefore, attempts to mechanically push the sperm out through the ejaculatory ductal system.

Surgical Sperm Retrieval

Surgical sperm retrieval is a method of retrieving sperm from reproductive tissue (Fig. 22-10). A variety of techniques may be used, including testicular sperm extraction (TESE), testicular sperm aspiration (TESA), microsurgical epididymal sperm aspiration (MESA), percutaneous epididymal sperm aspiration (PESA), and aspiration of sperm from the vas deferens.[39-45] Unlike the methods discussed previously, these methods were not developed to treat anejaculation. Instead, these methods were originally developed to retrieve sperm from men without SCI who were azoospermic, that is, men who had no sperm in their ejaculate. Further exploration of this topic is found in Box 22-1.

Semen Quality in Men With SCI

Men With SCI Have Abnormal Semen Quality

With the advent of PVS and EEJ, data have accumulated on semen quality in men with SCI. The majority of these men have a distinct semen profile characterized by normal total sperm numbers but abnormally low sperm motility.[21,46-48] Furthermore, the sperm from men with SCI are "fragile"; they lose motility and viability faster than sperm from noninjured controls.[49]

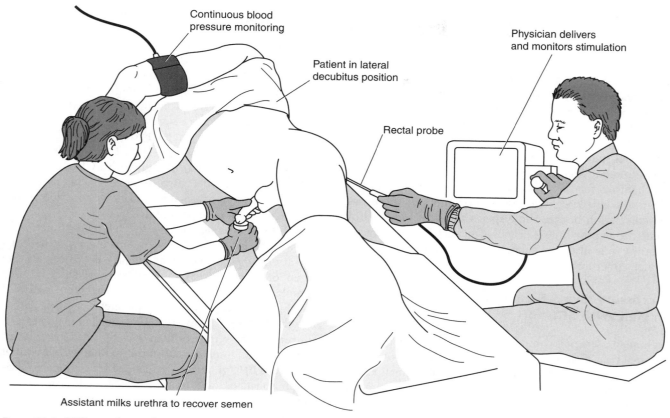

Figure 22-9. EEJ must be performed by a specially trained physician. EEJ is effective in retrieving semen in 95% of men with SCI.

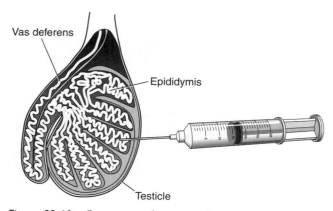

Figure 22-10. Sperm may be surgically removed from men with SCI. Use of surgical sperm retrieval in men with SCI is controversial.

Semen Profiles of Men With SCI Are Not Related to Lifestyle

Historically, there had been no precedent for understanding the cause of abnormal semen quality in men with SCI. Initial investigations tended to focus on lifestyle factors such as elevated scrotal temperature from sitting in a wheelchair,[50] infrequency of ejaculation,[51] methods of bladder management,[52] and methods of assisted ejaculation[28] as the

BOX 22-1
Advanced Concepts

Using surgical sperm retrieval for men with SCI is controversial. A recent survey[22] indicates that some practitioners are using surgical sperm retrieval as the first option of treatment for an ejaculation in men with SCI. The primary reasons given by these practitioners for not offering PVS or EEJ were lack of equipment and/or lack of training in these techniques.[22] It is unclear why practitioners are not being trained in the techniques of PVS and EEJ. One possible reason is that anejaculatory men with SCI represent only a small fraction of the male infertile population, whereas azoospermic men represent a much larger proportion of men with infertility. Thus, physicians may possess the necessary equipment for, and become adept at, performing the procedures that are appropriate for the majority of their client population. Another possible reason for not offering PVS or EEJ is the issue of reimbursement, as PVS and EEJ result in lower reimbursement than surgical sperm retrieval. In addition, the low yield of total motile sperm obtained by surgical sperm retrieval commits the couple to the most expensive assisted reproductive technology—intractyoplasmic sperm injection (ICSI).

cause for low sperm motility. Studies showed that such factors could not entirely account for the problem. For example, scrotal temperature was similar in injured and noninjured men (Table 22-1),[50] frequent ejaculation did not improve low sperm motility,[48,51,53] and sperm motility remained subnormal despite some improvements by method of bladder management[52] and some improvements by method of assisted ejaculation (Table 22-2).[28,29]

With lifestyle factors apparently not the cause of abnormal sperm parameters in men with SCI, attention then turned to secondary physiological factors as possible mechanisms for this condition. Again, this line of investigation yielded negative results. For example, there was no correlation between low sperm motility and level of injury, time post-injury, or age of subject.[48,55] Low sperm motility was also not related to hormone levels[56,57] or urinary tract infections.[52]

Accessory Gland Function Is Abnormal in Men With SCI

In humans, semen is composed of fluids primarily from the seminal vesicles and prostate gland. Examination of semen from men with SCI shows numerous abnormalities in addition to abnormal sperm parameters. For example, 27% of men with SCI have brown-colored semen that does not become normally colored with repeated ejaculations.[58] The brown color is not simply hematospermia, but instead indicates a dysfunction of the seminal vesicles.[58] Additional evidence of seminal vesicle dysfunction is the finding that men with SCI show an abnormal pattern of transport and storage of sperm in the seminal vesicles.[38]

In addition to dysfunction of the seminal vesicles in men with SCI, there is also evidence of prostate gland dysfunction in these men. Prostate-specific antigen (PSA) was higher in the blood (Fig. 22-11A) but lower in the semen (Fig. 22-11B) of men with SCI compared to healthy, age-matched control subjects.[59] This pattern of PSA expression indicates a secretory dysfunction of the prostate gland in men with SCI.

Additional evidence of accessory gland dysfunction in men with SCI is found in studies showing abnormal concentrations of various biochemical substances in the semen of men with SCI versus control subjects. For example, compared to able-bodied men, men with SCI have higher concentrations of platelet-activating factor acetylhydrolase,[60] and reactive oxygen species.[61–63] Conversely, the semen of men with SCI has lower levels of fructose, albumin, somatostatin (in men with lesions at or above T6),[64] glutamic oxaloacetic transaminase, alkaline phosphatase,[65] and transforming growth factor-beta 1 compared to the semen of able-bodied men.[66]

Table 22-1
Comparison of Temperatures (°C) Between Subjects With SCI and Control Subjects

	Room Temperature	Oral Temperature	Scrotal Temperature	Difference Between Oral and Scrotal Temperature
	Mean ± standard error of the mean			
SCI	22.6 ± 0.23	37.0 ± 0.06	35.4 ± 0.09	1.6 ± 0.09
Control	20.2 ± 0.18	37.0 ± 0.07	35.7 ± 0.16	1.3 ± 0.17

Scrotal temperature was not elevated in men with SCI. Group means were compared by analysis of variance. Adapted from Brackett NL, Lynne CM, Weizman MS, et al. Scrotal and oral temperatures are not related to semen quality, or serum gonadotropin levels in spinal cord injured men. *J Androl.* 1994;15:614–619.

Table 22-2
Comparison of Semen Quality By Method of Ejaculation

	Masturbation: SCI Men n = 15	PVS: SCI Men n = 106	EEJ: SCI Men n = 90	Controls: n = 56
Count / cc x 10[6]	114.1 ± 24.6***	104.5 ± 8.1***	65.0 ± 7.7*	84.7 ± 6.2
% Motile sperm	29.0 ± 4.7**, ***	26.0 ± 1.7**, ***	14.8 ± 1.4*, **	63.6 ± 2.5*

*Significantly different from masturbation in SCI men. **Significantly different from controls. ***Significantly different from EEJ. Means were compared by analysis of variance. Adapted from Brackett NL, Lynne CM. The method of assisted ejaculation affects the outcome of semen quality studies in men with spinal cord injury: a review. *NeuroRehab.* 2000;15:89–100.

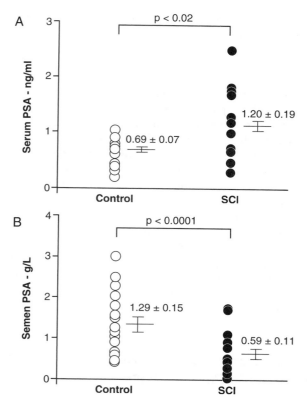

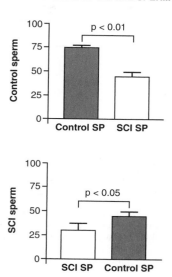

PERCENT OF MOTILE SPERM

Figure 22-12. Seminal plasma from men with SCI inhibited sperm motility of non-SCI men, indicating that seminal plasma contributes to low sperm motility in men with SCI. Adapted from Brackett NL, Davi RC, Padron OF, et al. Seminal plasma of spinal cord injured men inhibits sperm motility of normal men. *J Urol.* 1996;155:1632–1635.

Figure 22-11A,B. The prostate gland is dysfunctional in men with SCI as evidenced by higher concentrations of PSA in the blood (A) and lower concentrations of PSA in the semen (B) of men with SCI compared to control subjects. Adapted from Lynne CM, Aballa TC, Wang TJ, et al. Serum and semen prostate specific antigen concentrations are different in young spinal cord injured men compared to normal controls. *J Urol.* 1999:162;89–91.

Seminal Plasma From Men With SCI is Toxic

Evidence of abnormal accessory gland function in men with SCI led to studies investigating the role of the seminal plasma as a contributing factor to the abnormal sperm parameters found in these men. The studies showed that the seminal plasma of men with SCI is toxic to normal sperm. For example, when seminal plasma of men with SCI was mixed with sperm from normospermic men, a rapid and profound impairment to normal sperm motility occurred (Fig. 22-12).[67] Furthermore, sperm unexposed to the seminal plasma (i.e., aspirated from the vas deferens) had significantly higher motility than sperm in the ejaculate of these men (Fig. 22-13).[68] These findings introduced the concept of an abnormal seminal plasma environment as a cause of impaired sperm motility in men with SCI.

Men With SCI Have Leukocytospermia

One of the most pronounced abnormalities in men with SCI is *leukocytospermia*, which is an abnormally high concentration of white blood cells (WBCs) in the semen (Fig. 22-14).[69–71] Leukocytospermia has been studied in

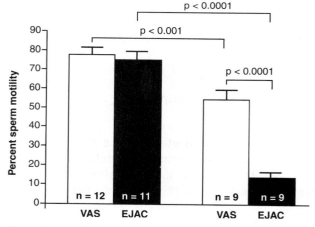

Figure 22-13. In each of 12 men with SCI, sperm motility was 2 to 13 times higher when obtained from the vas deferens than from the ejaculate. The net result was that mean sperm motility was significantly higher when obtained from the vas deferens versus the ejaculate (two bars on right side of graph). In contrast, in control subjects, there was little difference in sperm motility between the two sites (two bars on left side of graph). This study provided definitive evidence that seminal plasma was a major contributor to low sperm motility in men with SCI.[68] The individual data clearly showed that in each SCI subject, sperm motility was much higher in the vas deferens than in the ejaculate. Although the vas deferens-aspirated sperm from these men generally had lower motility than that of controls, suggesting that some epididymal or testicular factor may also have a role in decreasing sperm motility, the major decrease in motility was obviously due to contact with the seminal plasma. These results represented a major step toward understanding the source of poor sperm motility in men with SCI. Adapted from Brackett NL, Lynne CM, Aballa TC, et al. Sperm motility from the vas deferens of spinal cord injured men is higher than from their ejaculates. *J Urol.* 2000;164:712–715.

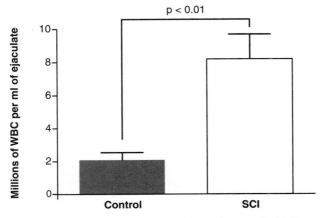

Figure 22-14. Most men with SCI have abnormally high concentrations of WBCs in their semen. This condition is termed *leukocytospermia*. Adapted from Basu S, Lynne CM, Ruiz P, et al. Cytofluorographic identification of activated T cell subpopulations in the semen of men with spinal cord injuries *J Androl* 2002;23:551–556.

non-SCI men, especially with respect to its relationship with genitourinary tract infections and infertility.[52] These studies have established that cellular elements, in general, may be related to abnormal sperm parameters,[72–75] but the sperm–leukocyte interaction is not clearly understood.[74,76] Low sperm motility in men with SCI does not seem to be caused simply by local infection of the genitourinary tract. In these men, treatment of genitourinary infections with antibiotics does not result in improved sperm motility.[52]

Men With SCI Have Immune Abnormalities

There is ample experimental evidence that individuals with SCI suffer from immune regulatory dysfunction.[57,77–79] Typically, their circulating lymphocytes demonstrate suppressed responses to challenges that stimulate cell division (standard mitogen challenges), have reduced ratios of specific WBCs, show reduced natural killer cell responses, and have altered responses to exercise challenges. The conclusion of these studies is that autonomic nervous system dysfunction results in alterations of the normal operations of the immune response, possibly via the interruption of sympathetic innervation of the lymphatics and spleen, the normal hypothalamic–pituitary–adrenal axis, or normal neurologic feedback from the periphery on these systems. The relationship of these findings to any disease state is unclear. In examining the semen of men with SCI during routine semen analysis, nearly all have an elevated number of WBCs.[69] Flow cytometric analysis of the semen of these men has shown the presence of large numbers of activated T-lymphocytes.[69] Activated T-lymphocytes are known to secrete cytotoxic cytokines.[80] It is well known that activated T-lymphocytes can exert a damaging effect on other cells by cytotoxic cytokines.[80–83]

Cytokines Contribute to Low Sperm Motility in Men With SCI

Cytokines play an important role in the function of the immune system,[80] but elevated concentrations of cytokines can be harmful to sperm.[84–86] It is possible that the activated T-lymphocytes observed in semen of men with SCI are secreting cytokines that impair sperm motility. It is hypothesized that semen cytokine concentrations are abnormal in men with SCI. Basu et al[66] measured levels of 10 cytokines in the seminal plasma of men with SCI versus age-matched, healthy, non-SCI control subjects. The results showed that compared to control subjects, concentrations of 5 of the 10 cytokines were elevated in the seminal plasma of men with SCI.[66] Furthermore, interfering with the actions of specific cytokines by addition of monoclonal antibodies directly to the semen improved sperm motility in men with SCI.[87] This treatment represented the first intervention that significantly improved sperm motility in men with SCI.

Reproductive Options for Couples With a Male Partner With SCI

Intravaginal Insemination at Home

The majority of men with SCI cannot ejaculate during sexual intercourse and require some form of technical or medical assistance to father a child. The least invasive and least expensive of the assisted reproductive options is intravaginal insemination, sometimes called "in-home insemination." It is advisable for couples to be evaluated in a clinic prior to attempting intravaginal insemination at home. The clinic should evaluate the male partner to determine the optimal method for safe and effective ejaculation. This evaluation should assess the male partner with SCI for risk and management of autonomic dysreflexia. The evaluation should also determine the optimal method of inducing ejaculation, such as use of one vibrator,[20] two vibrators,[88] abdominal electrical stimulation plus PVS,[26] or oral medications such as Viagra prior to PVS.[27] The clinic should also evaluate the semen quality of the male partner with SCI. While minimum numbers of total motile sperm have not been established for successful pregnancy using intravaginally inseminated sperm from men with SCI, the clinic should discuss guidelines regarding the number of intravaginal insemination cycles that will be attempted prior to choosing more advanced methods of assisted conception.

The female partner should be evaluated for the absence of any tubal or uterine pathology and for the presence of normal ovulatory cycles. She should also be counseled regarding methods of ovulation prediction at home. Insemination should occur at the time of ovulation. If the male partner with SCI cannot ejaculate during intercourse, the couple may collect his semen by PVS into a clean specimen cup. The semen is then drawn into the barrel of a syringe.

The syringe is inserted deep into the vagina, similar to a tampon. Once the syringe is in place, the semen is delivered into the vagina by pushing on the plunger of the syringe. Some clinics advise the female to remain recumbent for 15 to 30 minutes following insemination to allow gravity to help keep the semen in the vagina; however, there are no data to indicate if this recumbent position increases the probability of pregnancy.

There are reports in the literature of the successful use of intravaginal insemination to achieve pregnancy in couples with a male partner with SCI (see Table 22-3). Sonksen et al[89] reported a 25% pregnancy rate per couple for 16 couples undergoing PVS and vaginal self-insemination. Basal body temperature was used to predict ovulation timing and multiple ovulation cycles were required within a period of 2 years. Löchner-Ernst et al[90] reported a total of 60 pregnancies in 35 couples with male partners with SCI. Of these, 37 pregnancies occurred in 22 couples who performed semen collection and insemination at home, and 23 pregnancies occurred in 13 couples after intravaginal insemination in the clinic, but the study did not provide details on the proportion of couples that achieved pregnancy. Additionally, the study did not provide details about the ovulation cycles needed for this outcome, such as the number of cycles or whether the female partner took fertility drugs to produce multiple eggs per cycle.

Nehra et al[91] reported pregnancies in 5 of 8 couples (63% pregnancy rate) following PVS and intravaginal or cervical self-insemination during multiple ovulation cycles. Dahlberg et al[92] reported 12 pregnancies in 8 couples after PVS and intravaginal insemination during multiple

cycles using luteinizing hormone kits for timing of ovulation. Couples attempted intravaginal insemination at home approximately six times before going on to more advanced assisted reproductive technologies. Elliott[13] reported 28 infants born to 31 couples, with almost half of the couples conceiving at home using PVS.[13]

Rutkowski et al[93] retrospectively reviewed outcomes of infertility management in their male clients with SCI. The clinic used PVS or EEJ as semen retrieval techniques. Intravaginal insemination was attempted in 17 couples. A total of six pregnancies were achieved in 45 cycles. Five of these pregnancies occurred in 23 cycles of PVS (22% pregnancy rate per cycle), and one pregnancy occurred in 22 cycles of EEJ (5% pregnancy rate per cycle).

Hultling[94] reported on 19 couples who tried PVS and intravaginal insemination at home. Eight of the 19 couples (42%) conceived.

Intrauterine Insemination

Intrauterine insemination (IUI) has been used to achieve pregnancy in couples with a male partner with SCI (see Table 22-4). IUI involves collecting semen from the male partner and processing the semen in a laboratory to separate the sperm from the semen and to isolate the motile from the nonmotile sperm. In men with SCI, semen to be used in IUI is usually collected by PVS or EEJ. The processed sperm is placed inside the uterus of the woman (Fig. 22-15). IUI can be performed during unstimulated cycles where no fertility drugs are prescribed to the woman or during stimulated cycles where fertility drugs are prescribed to stimulate the production of eggs and/or to stimulate ovulation.

Table 22-3

Summary of Studies Using Intravaginal Insemination in Couples With Male Partners With SCI

Author, Year	Couples (n)	Cycles (n)	Pregnancies (n)
Sonksen et al, 1997[89]	16	ND	4
Löchner-Ernst et al, 1997[90]	35	ND	60
Nehra et al, 1996[91]	8	ND	5
Dahlberg et al, 1995[92]	8	≤48*	12
Elliott et al, 2003[13]	31	ND	14*
Rutkowski, et al, 1999[93]	17	45	6
Hultlig et al, 1997[94]	19	ND	8

The total number of couples, the total number of attempts at pregnancy (cycles), and the total number of pregnancies are summarized for each study.
(n) = number, ND = no data.
*Data estimated from information in study.

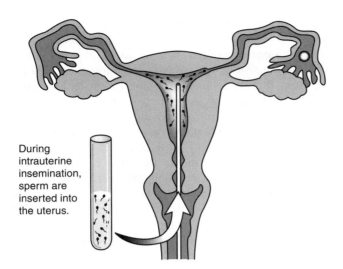

During intrauterine insemination, sperm are inserted into the uterus.

Figure 22-15. IUI has been used successfully to achieve pregnancy in couples with SCI male partners.

Sonksen et al[89] reported the results of 17 IUI cycles in 4 couples. The women received medications to stimulate ovulation in 14 of the 17 cycles. PVS and EEJ were used as semen retrieval methods. Median total sperm count was 65 million (range 100,000 to 480 million) with a median motility of 13% (range 1% to 60%). Three pregnancies occurred in 2 of the 4 couples (i.e., 1 couple had 2 pregnancies), for a 50% pregnancy rate per couple and a 17.6% pregnancy rate per cycle.

Nehra et al[91] reported no pregnancies in 11 natural (no fertility drugs) cycles of IUI, but achieved 5 pregnancies in 13 couples after 25 cycles of IUI in which medications were administered to stimulate ovulation. Dahlberg et al[92] reported 9 pregnancies in 15 couples where IUI was tried for 4 to 6 cycles (≤90 cycles).

Ohl et al[95] studied 121 consecutive couples who used EEJ in combination with assisted reproductive technology in the treatment of anejaculatory infertility. For those couples that did not conceive within 3 to 6 cycles of IUI, GIFT or IVF procedures were recommended. Eighty-seven of the 121 couples had male partners with SCI. In 479 cycles of EEJ with IUI in these couples, 41 pregnancies were obtained. This outcome represents an 8.6% pregnancy rate per cycle and 32.2% pregnancy rate per couple.

Ohl et al[95] concluded that the type of fertility drug used to stimulate egg production and/or ovulation, the method of monitoring, and timing of insemination did not affect IUI cycle fecundity. No multiple gestations were observed with natural cycle IUI procedures. In comparing ranges of motile sperm counts and IUI cycle fecundity, the authors suggested that clients with counts of <4 million total motile sperm should proceed directly to high-level assisted reproductive technologies, since below this threshold the pregnancy rate per cycle decreased sharply to 1.1%. Based on cost-effectiveness estimation between IUI and IVF, they recommended that

Table 22-4
Summary of Studies Using Intrauterine Insemination in Couples With Male Partners With SCI

Author, Year	Couples (n)	Cycles (n)	Pregnancies (n)	Medications Used in Study
Sonksen et al, 1997[89]	4	17	3	CC/hCG
Nehra et al, 1996[91]	13	25	5	None/CC/hMG
Dahlberg et al, 1995[92]	15	≤ 90*	9	CC/hMG
Ohl et al, 2001[95]	87	479	41	CC/hMG/hCG/LA
Pryor et al, 2005[96]	10	19	6	CC/hCG
Rutkowski et al, 1999[93]	5	10	3	ND
Taylor et al, 1999[35]	14	92	11	ND
Chung et al, 1996	10	50	5	CC/hCG
Heruti et al, 2001[98]	15	33	4	ND

The total number of couples, the total number of attempts at pregnancy (cycles), and the total number of pregnancies are summarized for each study. Medications used in the study are listed. Some women had multiple cycles with different medications.

(n) = number; CC = clomiphene citrate; hCG = human chorionic gonadotropin; hMG = human menopausal gonadotropin; LA = leuprolide acetate; ND = no data.
*Data estimated from information provided in study.

couples should attempt 3 to 6 cycles of IUI before proceeding to IVF. When inseminated total motile sperm counts were greater than 40 million, the pregnancy rate per cycle was 17.6%. They concluded that an IUI program can be successful and cost-effective in men with SCI.

Some studies discussed whether semen specimens were obtained by antegrade (out the tip of the penis) versus retrograde (into the bladder) ejaculation. Men with SCI often experience retrograde ejaculation due to discoordination between the external urinary sphincter and the bladder neck, which, in normal circumstances, ensures that the ejaculate flows forcefully out the end of the urethra. Pryor et al[96] reviewed outcomes in 10 couples undergoing IUI. Ejaculates were obtained by PVS in two clients and by EEJ in nine clients. Retrograde samples with <5 million motile sperm were not used if the antegrade sample had >5 million motile sperm. Six pregnancies were achieved in 10 couples after 19 cycles of IUI when the women received human chorionic gonadotropin (hCG) to stimulate ovulation. No pregnancies occurred in 19 unstimulated cycles of IUI in 5 couples. Also, there were no pregnancies in the same 5 couples when the women received a combination of clomiphene citrate (CC) plus hCG to stimulate ovulation. Pryor's study, like Ohl's[95] underlined the vital role that semen quality plays in the chances for pregnancy and the importance of semen preparation techniques that isolate the most motile sperm for insemination. This study again emphasized the consideration of cost in assisted fertility procedures and also suggested that initial conception attempts should be made by IUI if adequate numbers of motile sperm are available.

Rutkowski et al[93] reviewed pregnancy results with IUI. In 5 couples who had EEJ and IUI, 3 pregnancies were achieved during 10 cycles. This outcome represents a 30% pregnancy rate per cycle, which was an improvement over the 13% pregnancy rate per cycle obtained with intravaginal insemination. The authors emphasized that conventional insemination techniques such as IUI will remain an important option in couples with male partners with SCI, particularly in health-care systems where IVF procedures such as intracytoplasmic sperm injection (ICSI) are beyond the financial reach of many couples.

Taylor et al[35] studied 19 couples with an anejaculatory male partner with SCI. Semen was obtained with PVS, PVS plus prostate massage, or EEJ. Assisted reproduction treatments offered were IUI, GIFT, and ICSI. Men with motile sperm were first offered IUI. The pregnancy rate per cycle for IUI was 12% (11 pregnancies out of 92 cycles). Of the 14 couples treated with IUI, 6 achieved at least 1 pregnancy (42.9%). The authors suggested that sperm numbers within the normal range with at least 10% good progressive motility can be used for timed IUI with washed concentrated sperm, a procedure they characterize as "relatively inexpensive and minimally invasive."

Chung et al[97] reported their experience with EEJ combined with IUI or IVF. Female partners received clomiphene citrate 50 mg/day (for 3 to 7 days) during IUI cycles to improve pregnancy rates. EEJ was performed on the day of insemination, and both antegrade and retrograde specimens were processed by swim-up technique. A total of 50 IUIs were performed in 10 couples, resulting in 5 pregnancies in 3 couples, with 2 couples conceiving twice. Pregnancy thus occurred in 30% of the couples and in 10% of the IUI cycles. One couple failed to conceive after 8 cycles of IUI, but successfully delivered twins after IVF.

Heruti et al[98] studied 15 couples with male partners with SCI who underwent assisted reproductive technology. Semen was collected by EEJ in all men. Four pregnancies were achieved after 33 cycles of IUI for a pregnancy rate per couple of 28.6%.

In Vitro Insemination/Intracytoplasmic Sperm Injection

Advanced assisted reproductive technologies are available when fertilization is not possible or not indicated by intravaginal insemination or IUI. IVF is a procedure in which sperm are placed in a laboratory dish with retrieved ova. The sperm–ova mixture is then placed in an incubator for up to 5 days. Sperm are allowed to fertilize the ova. Embryos that develop to the highest-quality blastocyst stage are then placed into the uterus of the woman. Transfer of high-quality blastocysts are associated with higher pregnancy rates compared to transfer of poorly formed blastocysts.[99] This method whereby sperm are allowed to fertilize the eggs is termed *conventional IVF* (Fig 22-16).

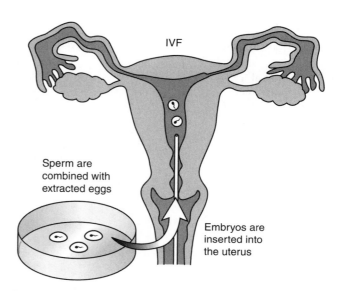

IVF

Sperm are combined with extracted eggs

Embryos are inserted into the uterus

Figure 22-16. Example of conventional IVF in which sperm and eggs are mixed together in a laboratory dish. Sperm are allowed to fertilize the eggs. Well-developed embryos are transferred to the uterus.

When the number of motile sperm is too low for conventional IVF, the method of ICSI is often used to achieve fertilization. ICSI is a procedure in which a single sperm is injected directly into the egg (Fig. 22-17).

IVF and ICSI have been used to achieve pregnancy in couples with male partners with SCI (Table 22-5). Hultling et al[94] reported a longitudinal descriptive study on the benefit of IVF in cases of anejaculatory infertility due to SCI and the results achieved by ICSI. Sperm were retrieved through PVS or EEJ. If sperm quality was judged to be sufficient, conventional IVF was performed. If sperm quality was very poor, ICSI was performed. Twenty-five couples underwent 52 cycles. Total sperm counts ranged from 0.01 to 978 million. Although the fertilization rate improved from 30% with conventional IVF to 88% with ICSI, there was no difference in pregnancy rate between the two methods. A total of 16 clinical pregnancies were established leading to 11 deliveries, for a pregnancy rate of 56% per couple.

Heruti et al[98] reported 18 pregnancies after 68 cycles of IVF/ICSI in 20 couples. Sonsken et al[89] reported 3 pregnancies in 10 cycles of IVF/ICSI in 8 couples. Brinsden et al[100] reported on the treatment of 35 couples with a male partner with SCI. Sperm was obtained by EEJ. Eighteen clinical pregnancies were obtained in 85 cycles of IVF. The pregnancy rate per treatment cycle was 18 out of 85, or 21.2%. The pregnancy rate per couple was 18 out of 35, or 51.4%.

Shieh et al[101] reported on 9 couples undergoing 11 cycles of ICSI. Nine pregnancies were achieved (1 pregnancy per couple). Seven of the couples achieved pregnancy in 8 cycles of EEJ and ICSI. One couple achieved pregnancy in 2 cycles of PVS and ICSI, and one couple achieved pregnancy with donor sperm and ICSI.

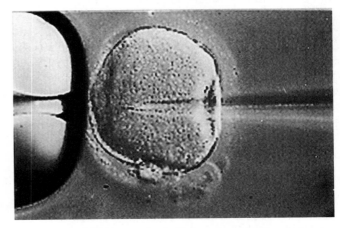

Figure 22-17. ICSI is a method of injecting sperm directly into an egg. This method is used to increase the chance of fertilization.

Table 22-5
Summary of Studies Using IVF/ICSI in Couples With Male Partners With SCI

Author, Year	Couples (n)	Cycles (n)	Pregnancies (n)	Medications Used in Study
Hultling et al, 1997[94]	25	52	18	GnRH/hMG/FSH/hCG
Heruti et al, 2001[98]	20	68	15	ND
Sonksen et al, 1997[89]	8	10	3	GnRH/hMG/hCG
Brinsden et al, 1997[100]	35	85	18	GnRH/hMG/FSH
Shieh et al, 2003[101]	9	11	9	GnRH/hMG/FSH
Löchner-Ernst et al, 1997[90]	11	ND	13	ND
Nehra et al, 1996[91]	12	15	6	LA/hMG/FSH/hCG
Dahlberg et al, 1995[92]	9	14	4	CC/hMG
Rutowski et al, 1999[93]	21	42	8	ND
Taylor et al, 1999[35]	15	40	12	ND

The total number of couples, the total number of attempts at pregnancy (cycles), and the total number of pregnancies are summarized for each study. Medications used in the study are listed. Some women had multiple cycles with different medications.

(n) = number; GnRH = gonadotropin releasing hormone agonist; hMG = human menopausal gonadotropin; hCG = human chorionic gonadotropin; ND = no data; LA = leuprolide acetate; FSH = follicle stimulating hormone; CC = clomiphene citrate.

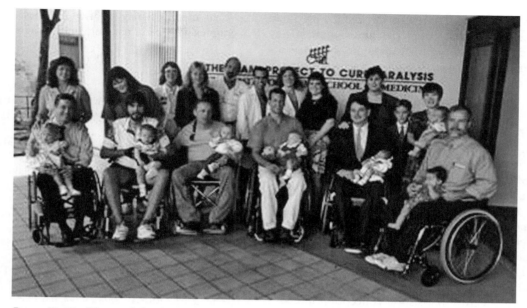

Figure 22-18. Photo of the first seven babies born at the Miami Project to Cure Paralysis Male Fertility Program, including one set of twins (far right). All of these couples met and got married after the man's injury. One man, (second from right) had a child from a previous marriage prior to his SCI. To date, over 150 babies have been born with the help of this program.

Löchner-Ernst et al[90] reported on 13 pregnancies (two sets of twins) in 11 couples using IVF and ICSI. Semen was obtained by PVS or surgical sperm retrieval. Nehra et al[91] reported pregnancy rates in 12 couples. GIFT was performed in 5 couples, and 4 achieved pregnancy in 8 cycles for a 50% pregnancy rate per cycle and 80% pregnancy rate per couple. ICSI was performed in 7 couples, resulting in 2 pregnancies in 7 cycles for a 29% pregnancy rate per cycle and a 29% pregnancy rate per couple.

Dahlberg et al[92] reported on pregnancy outcomes in 9 couples. Four couples had 6 cycles of IVF with sperm obtained by PVS or EEJ. Two pregnancies were achieved by this method. Two pregnancies were also achieved in five couples who had 8 cycles of IVF with sperm obtained from the vas deferens. Taylor et al[35] achieved 12 pregnancies in 15 couples undergoing 40 cycles of GIFT or ICSI. Six of 7 couples achieved 7 pregnancies (2 pregnancies in one couple) in 18 cycles of GIFT. Three of 8 couples achieved 5 pregnancies (3 pregnancies in one couple) in 22 cycles of ICSI (Fig. 22-18.).

Although definitive studies have not yet been performed, pregnancy outcomes using sperm from men with SCI seem to be similar to those using sperm from non-SCI clients with male-factor infertility. Similar pregnancy rates are found between the two groups for IUI, conventional IVF, and ICSI.[89,101,102] Although there are some studies showing impaired sperm function in men with SCI,[47,103] these functional impairments apparently do not lower pregnancy rates in couples. These findings may reflect the increasing ability of laboratory-assisted reproductive technologies to overcome all forms of male infertility.[104,105]

Selection of Assisted Reproductive Technology Approach

Recent improvements in the treatment of male-factor infertility *in general* have led to a problem for couples with male partners with SCI *in particular*. The ejaculates of many of these men are not being examined as a source of sperm for Assisted Reproductive Technology (ART) procedures. Instead, sperm are being retrieved directly from their testes or epididymides as a first line of treatment for anejaculation. This development has resulted in many centers recommending ICSI as a first line of treatment for assisted conception to couples with an SCI male partner. For many such couples, the cost of ICSI is prohibitive. ICSI is currently the most invasive of the available ART options.

The risks to the female partner and the incidence of multiple gestations are significantly higher with IVF compared to IUI procedures.[106] If ICSI is the only treatment option offered to couples, many will not attempt biologic parenthood. This outcome will impede rather than encourage progress in treatment of infertility in these couples.

Studies have shown that semen may be easily obtained by PVS or EEJ in 95% of men with SCI. Centers cite lack of familiarity, training, or equipment as the primary reasons for not offering these procedures.[22] It is understandable that centers may not want to invest a large sum of money to purchase EEJ equipment to use in a small number of cases. The majority of men with SCI, however, can ejaculate easily with a low-cost vibrator.

A recent study[22] showed that (1) the majority of men with SCI have reasonable yields of total motile sperm in their ejaculates and (2) IUI has been successfully used to achieve pregnancy in these couples. It is recommended that centers continue (or begin) to examine semen as a source of sperm and consider IUI as a treatment option for assisted conception in couples with SCI male partners.

Summary

Young men make up the overwhelming majority of individuals with SCI. Fertility is severely impaired in men with SCI due to erectile dysfunction, ejaculatory dysfunction, and semen abnormalities. The same treatments that are effective for erectile dysfunction in the general population are effective for treatment of erectile dysfunction in the SCI population. These treatments include oral PDE-5 inhibitors, intracavernous or intraurethral injections of alprostadil, vacuum erection devices, and penile implants. Similarly, the same treatments that are effective in assisting conception in couples with non-SCI male-factor infertility are effective in assisting conception in men with SCI male-factor infertility. These treatments include IUI, IVF, and ICSI.

The most apparent differences in male-factor infertility symptoms between men with SCI and non-SCI men are the high occurrences of anejaculation and atypical semen profiles in men with SCI. Methods are available to assist ejaculation in men with SCI. These treatments include PVS and EEJ. Using surgical sperm retrieval as the first line of treatment for anejaculation in men with SCI is currently controversial.

Most men with SCI have a unique semen profile characterized by normal sperm concentration, but abnormally low sperm motility and viability. Abnormal accessory gland function, possibly due to disinnervation of the prostate gland and seminal vesicles, may lead to abnormalities in the seminal plasma, which contribute to this condition. Despite abnormal sperm parameters, pregnancy outcomes using sperm from men with SCI seem to be similar to pregnancy outcomes using sperm from non-SCI men. Future studies in the field of infertility in men with SCI should focus on improving natural ejaculation and improving semen quality in these men.

REVIEW QUESTIONS

1. What conditions contribute to infertility in men with SCI?
2. What methods may be used to treat erectile dysfunction in men with SCI?
3. What methods may be used to retrieve sperm in men with SCI?
4. What is the predominant defect in semen quality in men with SCI?
5. What causes poor semen quality in men with SCI?
6. What methods may be used to assist conception in couples with male partners with SCI?

REFERENCES

1. National Spinal Cord Injury Statistical Center. Spinal cord injury. Facts and figures at a glance. *J Spinal Cord Med.* 2005;28:379–380.
2. O'Connor P. Incidence and patterns of spinal cord injury in Australia. *Accident Anal Prev.* 2002;34:405–415.
3. Kuptniratsaikul V. Epidemiology of spinal cord injuries: A study in the Spinal Unit, Siriraj Hospital, Thailand, 1997–2000. *J Med Assoc Thailand.* 2003;86:1116–1121.
4. Mena Quinones PO, Nassal M, Al Bader KI et al. Traumatic spinal cord injury in Qatar: An epidemiological study. *The Middle East Journal of Emergency Medicine.* 2002;1:1–5.
5. Kondakov EN, Simonova IA, Poliakov IV. The epidemiology of injuries to the spine and spinal cord in Saint Petersburg, Russia. *Zhurnal Voprosy Neirokhirurgii Imeni N-N-Burdenko.* 2002;2:50–53.
6. Exner G, Meinecke FW. Trends in the treatment of patients with spinal cord lesions seen within a period of 20 years in German centers. *Spinal Cord.* 1997;35:415–419.
7. Farooque M, Suo Z, Arnold PM et al. Gender-related differences in recovery of locomotor function after spinal cord injury in mice. *Spinal Cord.* 2006;44:182–187.
8. Sipski ML, Jackson AB, Gomez-Marin O et al. Effects of gender on neurologic and functional recovery after spinal cord injury. *Arch Phys Med Rehabil.* 2004;85:1826–1836.
9. Kolettis PN, Lambert MC, Hammond KR et al. Fertility outcomes after electroejaculation in men with spinal cord injury. *Fertil Steril.* 2002;78:429–431.
10. Sipski ML. The impact of spinal cord injury on female sexuality, menstruation and pregnancy: A review of the literature. *J Am Paraplegic Soc.* 1991;14:122–126.
11. Anderson KD. Targeting recovery: Priorities of the spinal cord-injured population. *J Neruotrauma.* 2004;21:1371–1383.
12. White MJ, Rintala DH, Hart KA et al. Sexual activities, concerns, and interests of men with spinal cord injury. *Am J Phys Med Rehabil.* 1992;71:225–231.
13. Elliott S. Sexual dysfunction and infertility in men with spinal cord disorders. In: Lin V, editor. *Spinal Cord Medicine: Principles and Practice.* New York: Demos Medical Publishing; 2003. pp. 349–365.
14. Padma-Nathan H, Giuliano F. Oral drug therapy for erectile dysfunction. *Urol Clin North Am.* 2001;28:321–334.
15. Sanchez RA, Vidal J, Jauregui ML et al. Efficacy, safety and predictive factors of therapeutic success with sildenafil for erectile dysfunction in patients with different spinal cord injuries. *Spinal Cord.* 2001;39:637–643.
16. Derry FA, Dinsmore WW, Fraser M et al. Efficacy and safety of oral sildenafil (Viagra) in men with erectile dysfunction caused by spinal cord injury. *Neurology.* 1998;51:1629–1633.
17. Brown DJ, Hill ST, Baker HW. Male fertility and sexual function after spinal cord injury. *Prog Brain Res.* 2006;152:427–439.
18. Brackett NL, Ferrell SM, Aballa TC et al. An analysis of 653 trials of penile vibratory stimulation on men with spinal cord injury. *J Urol.* 1998;159:1931–1934.

19. DeForge D, Blackmer J, Garritty C et al. Fertility following spinal cord injury: A systematic review. *Spinal Cord.* 2005;43:693–703.

20. Brackett NL. Semen retrieval by penile vibratory stimulation in men with spinal cord injury. *Hum Reprod Update.* 1999;5:216–222.

21. Sonksen J, Ohl DA. Penile vibratory stimulation and electroejaculation in the treatment of ejaculatory dysfunction. *Int J Androl.* 2002;25:324–332.

22. Kafetsoulis A, Brackett NL, Ibrahim E et al. Current trends in the treatment of infertility in men with spinal cord injury. *Fertil Steril.* 2006;86:781–789.

23. Sheel AW, Krassioukov AV, Inglis JT et al. Autonomic dysreflexia during sperm retrieval in spinal cord injury: Influence of lesion level and sildenafil citrate. *J Appl Physiol.* 2005;99:53–58.

24. Sonksen J, Biering-Sorensen F, Kristensen JK. Ejaculation induced by penile vibratory stimulation in men with spinal cord injuries. The importance of the vibratory amplitude. *Paraplegia.* 1994;32:651–660.

25. Brackett NL, Kafetsoulis A, Ibrahim E et al. Application of 2 vibrators salvages ejaculatory failures to 1 vibrator during penile vibratory stimulation in men with spinal cord injuries. *J Urol.* 2007;177:660–663.

26. Kafetsoulis A, Ibrahim E, Aballa TC et al. Abdominal electrical stimulation rescues failures to penile vibratory stimulation in men with spinal cord injury: A report of two cases. *Urol.* 2006;68:204–211.

27. Giuliano F, Rubio-Aurioles E, Kennelly M et al. Efficacy and safety of vardenafil in men with erectile dysfunction caused by spinal cord injury. *Neurology.* 2006;66:210–216.

28. Brackett NL, Padron OF, Lynne CM. Semen quality of spinal cord injured men is better when obtained by vibratory stimulation versus electroejaculation. *J Urol.* 1997;157:151–157.

29. Ohl DA, Sonksen J, Menge AC et al. Electroejaculation versus vibratory stimulation in spinal cord injured men: Sperm quality and patient preference. *J Urol.* 1997;157:2147–2149.

30. Wainer R, Albert M, Dorion A et al. Influence of the number of motile spermatozoa inseminated and of their morphology on the success of intrauterine insemination. *Hum Reprod.* 2004;19:2060–2065.

31. van der WL, Naaktgeboren N, Verburg H et al. Conventional in vitro fertilization versus intracytoplasmic sperm injection in patients with borderline semen: A randomized study using sibling oocytes. *Fertil Steril.* 2006;85:395–400.

32. Gunn RMC. Fertility in sheep: Artificial production of seminal ejaculation and the characteristics of the spermatozoa contained therein. *Australian Commonwealth Council of Scientific and Industrial Research.* 1936;94:1–5.

33. Brindley GS. Electroejaculation and the fertility of paraplegic men. *Sex Disabil.* 1980;3:223–229.

34. Halstead LS, VerVoort S, Seager SW: Rectal probe electrostimulation in the treatment of anejaculatory spinal cord injured men. *Paraplegia.* 1987;25:120–129.

35. Taylor Z, Molloy D, Hill V et al. Contribution of the assisted reproductive technologies to fertility in males suffering spinal cord injury. *Aust N Z J Obstet Gynaecol.* 1999;39:84–87.

36. Marina S, Marina F, Alcolea R et al. Triplet pregnancy achieved through intracytoplasmic sperm injection with spermatozoa obtained by prostatic massage of a paraplegic patient: Case report. *Hum Reprod.* 1999;14:1546–1548.

37. Engin-Uml SY, Korkmaz C, Duru NK et al. Comparison of three sperm retrieval techniques in spinal cord-injured men: Pregnancy outcome. *Gynecol Endocrinol.* 2006;22:252–255.

38. Ohl D.A., Menge A, Jarow J. Seminal vesicle aspiration in spinal cord injured men: Insight into poor semen quality. *J Urol.* 1999;162:2048–2051.

39. Craft I, Tsirigotis M. Simplified recovery, preparation and cryopreservation of testicular spermatozoa. *Hum Reprod.* 1995;10:1623–1626.

40. Tsirigotis M, Pelekanos M, Beski S et al. Cumulative experience of percutaneous epididymal sperm aspiration (PESA) with intracytoplasmic sperm injection. *J Assist Reprod Genet.* 1996;13:315–319.

41. Haberle M, Scheurer P, Muhlebach P et al. Intracytoplasmic sperm injection (ICSI) with testicular sperm extraction (TESE) in non-obstructive azoospermia—Two case reports. *Andrologia.* 1996;28 Suppl 1:87–88.

42. Kahraman S, Ozgur S, Alatas C et al. High implantation and pregnancy rates with testicular sperm extraction and intracytoplasmic sperm injection in obstructive and non-obstructive azoospermia. *Hum Reprod.* 1996;11:673–676.

43. Craft I, Tsirigotis M, Courtauld E et al. Testicular needle aspiration as an alternative to biopsy for the assessment of spermatogenesis. *Hum Reprod.* 1997;12:1483–1487.

44. Westlander G, Hamberger L, Hanson C et al. Diagnostic epididymal and testicular sperm recovery and genetic aspects in azoospermic men. *Hum Reprod.* 1999;14:118–122.

45. Chiang H, Liu C, Tzeng C et al. No-scalpel vasal sperm aspiration and in vitro fertilization for the treatment of anejaculation. *Urol.* 2000;55:918–921.

46. Linsenmeyer TA. Male infertility following spinal cord injury. *J Am Paraplegic Soc.* 1991;14:116–121.

47. Denil J, Ohl DA, Menge AC et al. Functional characteristics of sperm obtained by electroejaculation. *J Urol.* 1992;147:69–72.

48. Brackett NL, Nash MS, Lynne CM. Male fertility following spinal cord injury: Facts and fiction. *Phys Ther.* 1996;76:1221–1231.

49. Brackett NL, Santa-Cruz C, Lynne CM. Sperm from spinal cord injured men lose motility faster than sperm from normal men: The effect is exacerbated at body compared to room temperature. *J Urol.* 1997;157:2150–2153.

50. Brackett NL, Lynne CM, Weizman MS et al. Scrotal and oral temperatures are not related to semen quality or serum gonadotropin levels in spinal cord-injured men. *J Androl.* 1994;15:614–619.

51. Laessoe L, Sonksen J, Bagi P et al. Effects of ejaculation by penile vibratory stimulation on bladder reflex activity in a spinal cord injured man. *J Urol.* 2001;166:627.

52. Ohl DA, Denil J, Fitzgerald-Shelton K et al. Fertility of spinal cord injured males: Effect of genitourinary infection and bladder management on results of electroejaculation. *J Am Paraplegic Soc.* 1992;15:53–59.

53. Siosteen A, Forssman L, Steen Y et al. Quality of semen after repeated ejaculation treatment in spinal cord injury men. *Paraplegia.* 1990;28:96–104.

54. Brackett NL, Lynne CM. The method of assisted ejaculation affects the outcome of semen quality studies in men with spinal cord injury: A review. *Neurorehabil.* 2000;15:89–100.

55. Brackett NL, Ferrell SM, Aballa TC et al. Semen quality in spinal cord injured men: Does it progressively decline post-injury? *Arch Phys Med Rehabil*. 1998;79:625–628.

56. Brackett NL, Lynne CM, Weizman MS et al. Endocrine profiles and semen quality of spinal cord injured men. *J Urol*. 1994;151:114–119.

57. Naderi AR, Safarinejad MR. Endocrine profiles and semen quality in spinal cord injured men. *Clin Endocrinol*. 2003;58:177–184.

58. Wieder JA, Lynne CM, Ferrell SM et al. Brown-colored semen in men with spinal cord injury. *J Androl*. 1999;20:594–600.

59. Lynne CM, Aballa TC, Wang TJ et al. Serum and seminal plasma prostate specific antigen (PSA) levels are different in young spinal cord injured men compared to normal controls. *J Urol*. 1999;162:89–91.

60. Zhu J, Brackett NL, Aballa TC et al. High seminal platelet-activating factor acetylhydrolase activity in men with spinal cord injury. *J Androl*. 2006;27:429–433.

61. Padron OF, Brackett NL, Sharma RK, et al. Seminal reactive oxygen species and sperm motility and morphology in men with spinal cord injury. *Fertil Steril*.1997;67:1115–1120.

62. de Lamirande E, Leduc BE, Iwasaki A et al. Increased reactive oxygen species formation in semen of patients with spinal cord injury. *Fertil Steril*. 1995;63:637–642.

63. Rajasekaran M, Hellstrom WJ, Sparks RL et al. Sperm-damaging effects of electric current: Possible role of free radicals. *Reprod Toxicol*. 1994;8:427–432.

64. Odum L, Sonksen J, Biering-Sorensen F. Seminal somatostatin in men with spinal cord injury. *Paraplegia*. 1995;33:374–376.

65. Hirsch IH, Jeyendran RS, Sedor J et al. Biochemical analysis of electroejaculates in spinal cord injured men: comparison to normal ejaculates. *J Urol*. 1991;145:73–76.

66. Basu S, Aballa TC, Ferrell SM et al. Inflammatory cytokine concentrations are elevated in seminal plasma of men with spinal cord injuries. *J Androl*. 2004;25:250–254.

67. Brackett NL, Davi RC, Padron OF et al. Seminal plasma of spinal cord injured men inhibits sperm motility of normal men. *J Urol*. 1996;155:1632–1635.

68. Brackett NL, Lynne CM, Aballa TC et al. Sperm motility from the vas deferens of spinal cord injured men is higher than from the ejaculate. *J Urol*. 2000;164:712–715.

69. Basu S, Lynne CM, Ruiz P et al. Cytofluorographic identification of activated T-cell subpopulations in the semen of men with spinal cord injuries. *J Androl*. 2002;23:551–556.

70. Aird IA, Vince GS, Bates MD et al. Leukocytes in semen from men with spinal cord injuries. *Fertil Steril*. 1999;72:97–103.

71. Trabulsi EJ, Shupp-Byrne D, Sedor J et al. Leukocyte subtypes in electroejaculates of spinal cord injured men. *Arch Phys Med Rehabil*. 2002;83:31–33.

72. Diemer T, Huwe P, Ludwig M et al. Urogenital infection and sperm motility. *Andrologia*. 2003;35:283–287.

73. Omu AE, Al-Qattan F, Al-Abdul-Hadi FM et al. Seminal immune response in infertile men with leukocytospermia: Effect on antioxidant activity. *Eur J Obstet Gyn R B*. 1999;86:195–202.

74. Maegawa M, Kamada M, Irahara M et al. A repertoire of cytokines in human seminal plasma. *J Reprod Immunol*. 2002;54:33–42.

75. Henkel R, Schill WB. Sperm separation in patients with urogenital infections. *Andrologia*. 1998;30:91–97.

76. Rossi A, Aitken R. Interactions between leucocytes and the male reproductive system. The unanswered questions. In: Ivell and Holstein, editors. *The Fate of the Male Germ Cell*. New York: Plenum Press; 1997. pp. 245–252.

77. Cruse JM, Lewis RE, Dilioglou S et al. Review of immune function, healing of pressure ulcers, and nutritional status in patients with spinal cord injuyr. *J Spinal Cord Med*. 2000;23:129–135.

78. Popovich PG, Jones TB. Manipulating neuroinflammatory reactions in the injured spinal cord: Back to basics. *Trends Pharmacol Sci*. 2003;24:13–17.

79. Kawashima N, Nakazawa K, Ishii N et al. Potential impact of orthotic gait exercise on natural killer cell activities in thoracic level of spinal cord-injured patients. *Spinal Cord*. 2004;42:420–424.

80. Parham P. *The Immune System*. New York: Garland Science; 2005.

81. Hoek JB, Pastorino JG. Cellular signaling mechanisms in alcohol-induced liver damage. *Semin Liver Dis*. 2004;24:257–272.

82. Yamaoka J, Kabashima K, Kawanishi M et al. Cytotoxicity of IFN-gamma and TNF-alpha for vascular endothelial cell is mediated by nitric oxide. *Biochem Biophys Res Commun*. 2002;291:780–786.

83. van Soeren MH, Diehl-Jones WL, Maykut RJ et al. Pathophysiology and implications for treatment of acute respiratory distress syndrome. *AACN Clinical Issues*. 2000;11:179–197.

84. Kocak I, Yenisey C, Dundar M et al. Relationship between seminal plasma interleukin-6 and tumor necrosis factor alpha levels with semen parameters in fertile and infertile men. *Urol Res*. 2002;30:263–267.

85. Eggert-Kruse W, Boit R, Rohr G, et al. Relationship of seminal plasma interleukin (IL) -8 and IL-6 with semen quality. *Hum Reprod*. 2001;16:517–528.

86. Sikka SC, Champion HC, Bivalacqua TJ et al. Role of genitourinary inflammation in infertility: Synergistic effect of lipopolysaccharide and interferon-gamma on human spermatozoa. *Int J Androl*. 2001;24:136–141.

87. Cohen DR, Basu S, Randall JM et al. Sperm motility in men with spinal cord injuries is enhanced by inactivating cytokines in the seminal plasma. *J Androl*. 2004;25:922–925.

88. Brackett NL, Kafetsoulis A, Ibrahim E et al. Application of two vibrators salvages ejaculatory failures to one vibrator during penile vibratory stimulation of men with spinal cord injuries. *J Urol*. 2007;177:660–663.

89. Sonksen J, Sommer P, Biering-Sorensen F et al. Pregnancy after assisted ejaculation procedures in men with spinal cord injury. *Arch Phys Med Rehabil*. 1997;78:1059–1061.

90. Löchner-Ernst D, Mandalka B, Kramer G et al. Conservative and surgical semen retrieval in patients with spinal cord injury. *Spinal Cord*. 1997;35:463–468.

91. Nehra A, Werner M, Bastuba, Title C et al. Vibratory stimulation and rectal probe electroejaculation as therapy for patients with spinal cord injury: Semen parameters and pregnancy rates. *J Urol*. 1996;155:554–559.

92. Dahlberg A, Ruutu M, Hovatta O. Pregnancy results from a vibrator application, electroejaculation, and a vas aspiration programme in spinal-cord injured men. *Hum Reprod*. 1995;10:2305–2307.

93. Rutkowski SB, Geraghty TJ, Hagen DL et al. A comprehensive approach to the management of male infertility following spinal cord injury. *Spinal Cord*. 1999;37:508–514.

94. Hultling C, Rosenlund B, Levi R et al. Assisted ejaculation and in-vitro fertilization in the treatment of infertile spinal cord-injured men: The role of intracytoplasmic sperm injection. *Hum Reprod.* 1997;12:499–502.

95. Ohl DA, Wolf LJ, Menge AC et al. Electroejaculation and assisted reproductive technologies in the treatment of anejaculatory infertility. *Fertil Steril.* 2001;76:1249–1255.

96. Pryor JL, Kuneck PH, Blatz SM, et al. Delayed timing of intrauterine insemination results in a significantly improved pregnancy rate in female partners of quadriplegic men. *Fertil Steril.* 2001;76:1130–1135.

97. Chung PH, Verkauf BS, Eichberg RD et al. Electroejaculation and assisted reproductive techniques for anejaculatory infertility. *Obstet Gynecol.* 1996;87:22–26.

98. Heruti RJ, Katz H, Menashe Y et al. Treatment of male infertility due to spinal cord injury using rectal probe electroejaculation: The Israeli experience. *Spinal Cord.* 2001;39:168–75.

99. Balaban B, Urman B, Sertac A et al. Blastocyst quality affects the success of blastocyst-stage embryo transfer. *Fertil Steril.* 2000;74:282–287.

100. Brinsden PR, Avery SM, Marcus S et al. Transrectal electroejaculation combined with in-vitro fertilization: Effective treatment of anejaculatory infertility due to spinal cord injury. *Hum Reprod.* 1997;12:2687–2692.

101. Shieh JY, Chen SU, Wang YH et al. A protocol of electroejaculation and systematic assisted reproductive technology achieved high efficiency and efficacy for pregnancy for anejaculatory men with spinal cord injury. *Arch Phys Med Rehabil.* 2003;84:535–540.

102. Brackett NL, Abae M, Padron OF et al. Treatment by assisted conception of severe male factor infertility due to spinal cord injury or other neurological impairment. *J Assist Reprod Genet.* 1995;12:210–216.

103. Buch JP, Zorn BH. Evaluation and treatment of infertility in spinal cord injured men through rectal probe electroejaculation. *J Urol.* 1993;149:1350–1354.

104. Maduro MR, Lamb DJ. Understanding new genetics of male infertility. *J Urol.* 2002;168:2197–2205.

105. Isidori A, Latini M, Romanelli F. Treatment of male infertility. *Contraception.* 2005;72:314–318.

106. Winston RM, Hardy K. Are we ignoring potential dangers of in vitro fertilization and related treatments? *Nat Cell Biol.* 2002;4:s14–s18.

Assistive Technology 23

K. Rao Poduri, MD

Thomas Cesarz, MD

After reading this chapter, the reader will be able to:

OBJECTIVES

- Discuss the latest advancements in adaptive technology for mobility
- Discuss the use of adaptive technology for performing activities of daily living
- Discuss assessment of the individual and the individual's need for assistive technology
- Understand how to select the appropriate assistive device based on the assessment of the individual and the individual's needs
- Describe available adaptive technology for recreational activities

OUTLINE

Introduction

Technology now gives increased independence to many individuals with spinal cord injury (SCI) in their homes, at work, and in recreational activities. The purpose of this chapter is to assist the clinician by briefly reviewing the traditional assistive technology devices available and then highlighting some of the newer devices, with an emphasis on the process of device selection and their practical use.

Assistive technology is defined by the 1988 Technology Related Assistance for Individuals with Disabilities Act as "any item, piece of equipment, or product system, whether acquired commercially off the shelf, modified, or customized, that is used to increase, maintain, or improve functional capabilities of individuals with disabilities."[1] The assistive technology field is expanding, with countless devices in a market that generate $2.87 billion in U.S. sales.[2] How do we sort through them and match the right device to the individual?

Relying on the literature for an answer regarding a specific device's clinical efficacy will be ineffective, as rarely will there be mention of the product being considered. Some products do have published studies to inform the clinician, while other studies focus on categories of devices rather than specific products. One such survey of civilians and veterans found that the most frequently owned devices fall into categories of (1) manual or powered mobility and independent living, (2) prosthetics and orthotics, (3) assistive computer technology, and (4) augmentative and alternative communication devices (AACD).[1] Several of these device categories will be covered in this chapter, with a focus on newer devices and technologies. Included is a discussion of devices identified as being most important to employment, including powered environmental control devices and ambulatory support devices.[1]

Members of a rehabilitation team strive to help individuals with SCI overcome the functional loss that occurs with injury to the spinal cord. Assistive devices play a key role in the lives of these individuals as they provide a bridge to maximum independence. Prior to the injury, the individual functions automatically and spontaneously to satisfy desires and daily needs, from activities as physically simple as turning in bed to those as complex as walking. After a SCI, activities once taken for granted are now seemingly out of reach. However, with the deliberate introduction of assistive devices, many lost functions may be regained.

The importance of conducting a thorough assessment of the individual's needs and priorities cannot be overemphasized. Before recommending a particular device, the rehabilitation specialist must assess the individual's remaining abilities, function, desires, and potential. The practicality of using the device and the three Cs—comfort, cosmesis, and cost—will dictate if the device matches the individual's needs.

A brief review of SCI and the expected impairments for an individual with complete tetraplegia is necessary in order to lay a foundation for the use of assistive technology to aid the individual. For levels C1–C3, there is paralysis of all four limbs and ventilator dependence. At the C4 level, scapular elevation and some diaphragmatic innervation is gained, and the individual may be off the ventilator. With the C5 level, some arm and shoulder movements are available. At C6, wrist extension is gained, and at C7–C8 elbow extension is added. The lower the level of SCI, the more distal are the upper limb functions added. With lesions at C8 and below, nearly complete functional independence is the typical goal and expected outcome of adaptive devices.[3] Excellent in-depth discussions of expected functional outcomes and recommended equipment are already available.[3,4] Assessment for assistive technology should include medical history, physical capability, functional ability, community accessibility, and lastly, funding resources.

Mobility and Exercise

In this section, advances across a spectrum of technology, from orthoses to functional electrical stimulation to an advanced mobility device, is discussed. Wheelchairs are discussed elsewhere in this book. Many of the devices discussed here do not provide functional ambulation, but do offer physiological benefits. There are many devices available to promote mobility in persons with SCI. Many of the devices listed above are addressed in other chapters. We will describe a few advanced mobility devices here.

Functional Electrical Stimulation

Functional electrical stimulation (FES) is the activation of muscles via electrical stimulation for the purpose of performing a functional activity. Activating a muscle by application of electrical stimulation is not new. What is challenging is making the contractions safe, functional, and practical for everyday use. Some recent uses of FES for people with SCI are explored in this section. A comprehensive survey of FES in SCI is described in Creasey et al.[5] FES is beneficial for various activities such as standing, sitting, and walking.

Sitting and Standing

A study of 15 individuals with T6–T11 paraplegia showed that standing assisted by FES causes greater heart rate and VO$_2$ uptake than passive standing in frame, showing promise for cardiorespiratory conditioning.[6] Another study has shown that FES reduces orthostatic hypotension and presyncopal symptoms upon standing in individuals with tetraplegia. Mean duration of standing without orthostatic hypotension increased from 31.2 minutes to 45.4 minutes, a statistically significant difference.[7] FES may be considered an adjunct method for increasing the duration of standing upright, with the hope of reaping benefits such as increased participation in therapies and weight-bearing.

A recent study demonstrated that FES may be useful for control of the seated posture in paraplegics by contraction of the hip and trunk muscles.[8] This may ultimately lead to a more physiologic posture and a greater range for reaching.

Standing and Walking: Parastep

Parastep (Sigmedics, Inc., Fairborn, Ohio) is an FES system that uses skin surface electrodes to stimulate the nerves and muscles. It can be used by individuals with paraplegia who have intact lower extremity innervation. Pairs of electrodes are placed bilaterally over quadriceps and gluteal muscles for hip and knee extension for standing. Another pair of electrodes is placed over the common peroneal nerve to elicit a flexion withdrawal response for stepping. The hip and knee extensor excitation is tonically "on" until the individual triggers stepping via a switch on the walker. Stimulus levels may be adjusted at each site to achieve the appropriate level of current. The device was approved by the U.S. Food and Drug Administration in 1994 and became eligible for Medicare reimbursement in 2004.

An early study with 16 individuals with thoracic level paraplegia found that Parastep allows the ability to stand

and achieve short-distance ambulation, but there is great variation between users. The authors comment that Parastep "is severely limited as a substitute for pre-injury walking ability,"[9] but point out that Parastep might have other uses, such as improving physical and mental health.[9] In this study, which lacked controls, 15 subjects trained on the Parastep three times weekly for 32 sessions, with arm ergometry testing before and after the Parastep use, as a measure of cardiovascular fitness.[10] There was a significant increase in peak VO_2, time to fatigue, and peak workload.[10]

One study measured femoral bone density both before and after 32 sessions with Parastep and found no significant change in bone mineral density associated with its use.[11] However, Parastep has been suggested to improve emotional state, with increased self-confidence and decreased depression scores after 32 sessions of use.[12]

The activity that occurs with Parastep is intense enough to result in adaptive changes in the peripheral vasculature similar to those seen in physically trained individuals without SCI.[13] One criticism of the Parastep is that it may be too strenuous. A case study of an individual with T5–T6 AIS A paraplegia found that standing with the Parastep requires a continuous quadriceps contraction, whereas standing with lower extremity bracing (an advanced reciprocating gait orthosis [ARGO]), requires no muscle effort at all. In ambulation, the Parastep uses more energy than a wheelchair or ARGO (with or without concurrent FES).[14]

Advanced Personal Mobility

Overcoming environmental barriers is a key goal of the therapeutic partnership between the individual with SCI and the rehabilitation specialist. The wheelchair permits some freedom of mobility on flat surfaces, but unramped changes in terrain still pose a challenge. Within an individual's home environment, accessibility to multiple floors is often impossible without major redesign of the house itself. An elevator is a logical solution, but the cost is frequently prohibitive. Additionally, elevators allow only movement up and down one specific flight of stairs rather than all stairs in general. One potential solution to the problem posed by stairs is the iBOT (Fig. 23-1).[17] The iBOT is a four-wheeled chair controlled by hand with a joystick. It has various functional modes, including stair climbing. A survey of four men with SCI who used the iBOT found that the balance function, in which the seat is raised with only two of four wheels on the ground, was one of the most frequently used functions. In using the balance function, the individual is raised upward to reach high shelves and to talk to others at eye level. The ability to adjust seat height and angle provides the opportunity to be more comfortable at a given work station. All four of the users noted that they liked being able to speak to someone at eye level. The feature that the participants liked least was the high level of the seat in the standard position.

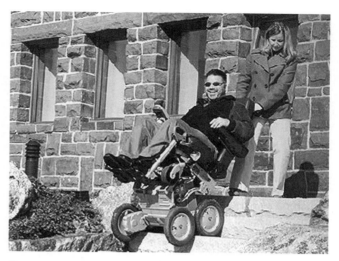

Figure 23-1. INDEPENDENCE iBOT 4000 Mobility System. (Courtesy of Independence Technology LLC, a Johnson & Johnson company, Warren, NJ. http://www.independencenow. com/ibot/stair.html)

Overall, the individuals with tetraplegia had a more positive impression of the iBOT than those with paraplegia.[15]

A thorough assessment of both the individual and the environment is necessary to determine compatibility with the iBOT. The rosiest portrait painted of the iBOT is of a personal robot suit; the most realistic view is that it has limitations, including limited maneuverability in some indoor environments and no power-controlled weight shift.[16] By shifting their weight in the wheelchair, individuals redistribute pressure on their skin, lessening the risk for pressure ulcers. If an individual lacks the strength to change positions, a power-controlled weight shift helps to perform this task.

Electronic Aids to Daily Living

This chapter will focus only on electronic aids to daily living (EADLs). EADLs help individuals with SCI control their environment and perform actions other than the traditional activities of daily living (ADLs). Devices to assist with upper extremity function (and ADLs) will be addressed elsewhere in this book.

Increasing Control of the Environment Through Electronic Aids

Electronic aid to daily living is a newer term that takes the place of *environmental control unit*, because the latter term technically refers to furnace thermostats.[18] EADL refers to a device used to group the control of multiple items in the individual's environment. Various terms and abbreviations have been used in the literature to describe these devices. For the sake of simplicity, to help avoid confusion, and in keeping with the current terminology, the term *EADL* will be used here, even if the cited literature uses a different term for these devices.

EADLs have a history dating back to the 1950s when Possum (patient-operated selector mechanism) was used by individuals with polio and cerebral palsy. Initially, bulky EADL designs were streamlined over ensuing decades, and as the science of electronics advanced, the current units developed to be the size of a television remote control.[19] The basic design is one in which the individual activates a switch in the control unit that signals the desired external device.[19] The control switch, whether it is a sip and puff, joystick, or even a voice-recognition device, will activate a unit that gives a visual or auditory feedback to the individual, indicating what to switch on or what to turn off.[20] Signals are sent by a variety of forms, including infrared, ultrasound, radio waves, or conventional electric wires.[20] Typical devices that are controlled are as follows: [19]

- Intercoms
- Doors (electronic lock)
- Alarms
- Lights
- Television/entertainment systems
- Electronic page turners
- Computers, telephones

Note that the individual can control electronic devices as well as traditionally nonelectronic devices, such as doors that have been instrumented. EADL can be used for simple on/off toggling, as well as for control of devices that use infrared input, such as a remote-controlled television, entertainment system, etc. EADL devices use either published codes for the infrared device or are trained (similar to a universal remote control) to work the infrared device. Items such as the telephone and hospital bed are often directly connected to the EADL rather than controlled remotely (Fig. 23-2).[21] Computer keyboards can also be instrumented for this type of control.[18]

Fitting EADL to the Individual

Choosing the appropriate EADL switching device is crucial.[19] The individual must be able to use it with ease within his or her functional capability, making it one of the most important considerations in EADL implementation. If the individual cannot use the EADL, then the goal of improved function has not been achieved.

Evaluation of the individual's motor strength, endurance, and coordination, as well as sensation, vision, and hearing is crucial when selecting the best fit of the control switch for the EADL. Input control may be binary (sip and puff) or computer operated or via voice recognition. The control must be easy to operate. If the user fatigues, he or she may not be able to call for help.[22]

Yet another option for interaction is a headset that, when activated by the tongue, sends an infrared beam to a communication board displaying selectable icons of environmental goals. By turning head and neck, items are activated, and interaction with the environment becomes

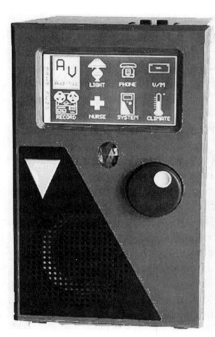

Figure 23-2. EADL. (Courtesy of Angel ECU, Port Saint Lucie, FL. http://www.angelecu.com)

possible. A study comparing nonspeaking individuals with tetraplegia with nondisabled subjects found that there was no significant difference between the groups in terms of accuracy and time spent interfacing with the control board. It appears this technology is a viable option for EADL interaction.[23]

EADLs assist in various domains, including communication, education, leisure, self-care, and household management. Using EADLs requires cognition adequate for remembering the proper use of the device and performing correct sequences to obtain the desired result.[24]

Benefits

Benefits of EADLs are numerous: increased security, independence, and recreational involvement are seen with EADL use.[20] Additionally, EADLs can decrease caregiver burden.[19]

EADLs have a role in the care of an individual with an SCI in the hospital setting, living in chronic care facility, or in a community dwelling. Introducing EADLs early in the hospital course can provide motivation and a sense of empowerment.[25] A Canadian study of 15 hospitalized individuals with disability affecting all limbs (four individuals had SCI) assessed independence before and after installation of the EADLs. Once installed, the systems were used most frequently for personal comfort (adjusting lights and fan) and recreation (television, radio, stereo). After installation, both individuals and hospital staff noted improvements. Individuals were more independent. Prior to the EADLs, they had requested about an hour's worth of care, but with the EADLs, they gave themselves about 2 hours of care. Staff felt less frustrated and felt the EADLs reduced demands on their time.[26]

An American study surveyed individuals with tetraplegia who used EADLs. Benefits in the domains of communication, security and health, and recreation were perceived as being the most important outcomes of EADL use. Use of a telephone was the most important function, with television ranked second. This is consistent with the Canadian study. The EADLs allowed individuals to manage themselves for longer periods without assistance from another person. In this 1989 study, EADLs were not directly contributing to employment, as none of the individuals who worked (19%) used the EADL for work tasks.[27] Since the time of this study, the field of assistive technologies has made significant progress toward getting individuals with SCI back into the workforce with the help of EADLs. Most of the high-level tetraplegics are cognitively intact and of an age where gainful employment is society's expectation.[25]

A study was undertaken to compare the functional and psychosocial status of EADL users and nonusers with tetraplegia. The groups were demographically similar, including employment status. Similar levels of functional dependence were found for self-care and mobility. The EADL users were twice as likely to live alone, and they also were significantly more independent with their EADLs, a finding consistent with the suitability of EADLs for assisting with telephone, computer, and door opening. Clearly, EADL technology is of benefit.[28] As the SCI individual's reach into the world is extended by EADL equipment, it is important that they are not cast adrift by equipment failure. Backup systems and alarms to signal malfunctions are essential.[25]

Funding

A survey of occupational therapists found that poor funding for assistive technology devices impeded access to them.[20] The most frequently denied pieces of durable medical equipment are ranked as follows: (1) manual wheelchair, (2) power wheelchair, (3) shower and commode chairs, and (4) EADL. Lack of policy coverage is the primary reason for refusal to pay, with lack of documentation of medical necessity second.[20]

Brain–Computer Interface: Switching Mechanism of the Future

A brain–computer interface (BCI) senses and conveys brain signals to a device outside the body that can then interact with the environment. Signals include electroencephalograph (EEG), electric activity from beneath the cranium, individual neuron activity, and magnetoencephalography. The detected brain signals can ultimately interact with a computer cursor, a prosthetic limb, or the individual's own limb.[29]

Most BCI devices used with humans have used EEG signals. EEG detects alpha and beta rhythms over the sensorimotor cortex when those regions are not engaged in sensory input or motor output. Actual or imagined movement will change these rhythms, making thoughts of movement detectable by the EEG machine. Slow cortical potentials are another pattern detected on EEG that individuals can learn to control. The P300 potential (for parietal, 300 msec peak) occurs in response to infrequent or highly significant stimuli, including visual or auditory input. The BCI system makes use of this phenomenon because it displays different items or symbols to a user; once the individual sees the desired objects, a P300 potential will be activated within the brain, which is then sensed and relayed to an output device.[35]

EEG's main advantage lies in its noninvasive nature. The disadvantage is that it has limited fidelity and spatial specificity, requiring longer training periods for users to achieve control. Additionally, the electrodes are prone to mechanical and electrical interference from events outside the user's brain. Of course, long-term application of electrodes to the scalp is problematic.[29] Electrocorticography (EcoG) uses a grid placed within the cranium, either in the subdural or epidural region, and compared to EEG, it detects detailed information from specific anatomic regions.[29] EcoG signal has been used in BCI, but clinical trials are needed to evaluate it.

To date, studies with humans have taken place in very controlled situations, which circumvent some of the issues that a user will face, such as the application of the BCI if it is external (EEG electrodes) and how to turn it on and off once it is applied. Experiments have not mimicked the distractions of the real world in which individuals will ultimately have to control their brain waves in order to use the BCI[29] in the presence of competing distractions in the environment.

Vocation and Recreation

Vocation and Assistive Computer Technology

The computer, now ubiquitous for its importance in work, communication, and recreation, is a key target of adaptive technology. Since the rise of the Internet, access to computers enables access to the world. Providing equal access to information through computers has even been described as being "morally imperative," because our society's function has grown intertwined with computer function.[30] Stephen Hawking, the prominent astrophysicist, reliant on wheelchair for mobility due to motor neuron disease, presents an example of the powers of adaptive computer technology. Using adaptive computer technology, he has written papers and books that have advanced humanity's understanding of the universe.[31]

The traditional keyboard features keys that respond immediately when pressed, and if held down, they will continue to generate strings of symbols. Individuals with SCI may experience difficulty with this system because, when using a mouthstick or other adaptation, they may rest their hands on the keyboard and inadvertently depress a key for too long, generating multiple symbols instead of a single one. Some of these potential problems can be addressed within the computer itself by adjusting the auto-repeat rate and by using the slow keys feature. When the slow keys feature is activated, it requires that a key be depressed for a certain period before its effect is registered, thereby circumventing the effects of brief, unintentional key pressings.[18] On-screen keyboards are another option, typically operated by mouse or an equivalent tool.[18] Keyguards may be placed over the keyboard, rendering the keyboard into rows of wells upon which the individual rests his or her arm and then uses gross proximal musculature to push a pen attached to the hand into the keyholes.[31]

Another computer input device that can be adapted is the computer mouse. They are already available in many sizes, shapes, and configurations, including the trackball and touchpad. A head-pointing mouse uses infrared light and is a good option for users without hand control. The user wears a small reflector, typically on his or her head, which is moved to reflect the infrared light that is detected by a camera. These movements are converted to the mouse cursor movements. The clicking feature of the mouse is incorporated by fixing the beam on the desired point for a period of time. This design feature, known as *dwell-clicking*, frees the individual from the need to make any upper limb movements at all.[18]

Alternative forms of data input are sometimes sought. Speech recognition has held promise and ideally is one of the fastest ways of conveying data, but its use in practice has been frustrating. Many people who have tried speech recognition do not continue using it. Morse code, once learned, can be used to sip and puff words at a rate greater than 20 per minute, but it is not often suggested as an alternative by clinicians. Two reasons for this are that past Morse systems were somewhat expensive and that Morse code can seem challenging to those unfamiliar with it.[18]

For those with the least voluntary movement, a scanning system of input is a good choice. Scanning involves a system highlighting different options in series, with the user selecting, with some action, the desired option when it is highlighted.[18]

Many of the devices already discussed assist with computer use for either recreation or vocation. Employment rates after SCI range from 13% to 69%, depending on the study.[32] Even though 69% are employed, there are still 31% unemployed. Employment benefits the individual, as it is related to higher quality of life and improved survival, and society, as it does not have to fully support the injured person. Manual labor opportunities may be limited after SCI, but telecommuting is a viable option for typists, accountants, and other professionals. There is a need for accessibility and independent use of computers for the SCI individuals.[32] Vocational training is essential to maximize an individual's use of a particular assistive technology.[33]

Table 23-1 describes assistive technology as it applies to the level of SCI and their costs.

Recreational Aids

Individuals with SCI are at increased risk for cardiovascular diseases and are prone to rapid loss of musculoskeletal function at a severely deconditioned level.[34] A regular exercise program would benefit these individuals, but poor accessibility and barriers limit such activity. Sedentary lifestyles, low level of activity, and decreased fitness compound these problems. The benefits of exercise include cardiovascular fitness; increased strength, endurance, muscle and bone mass; decrease of body fat; and reversal of insulin resistance. The benefits of increasing muscle strength and endurance and cardiovascular fitness will enable individuals with SCI to engage in recreational activities. Individuals that engage in regular exercise activities improve their fitness to a degree that enables them to participate in recreational activities. Similarly, fitness and health, along with quality of life improve when the SCI population engages in recreational activities, just as in the case of the general population.

SCI should not preclude participation in the same recreational activities enjoyed prior to the injury. With appropriate resources and assistive technology, an individual with SCI can access many recreational and sports activities. When assessing individuals for recreation, the same principles apply as for the able bodied individuals. If a sports activity is available to a noninjured person, the chances are that it is available to the SCI individual as well. Most recreational activities are accessible to the SCI individuals with or without adaptations.

With the passage of the Americans with Disabilities Act,[35] access to public facilities, including recreational sites, is required for disabled individuals. This has clearly enabled individuals with disabilities, including those with SCI, to participate in many recreational activities.

SCI affects young and active individuals (mean age at onset 26 years), and recreational activities are vital for their well being. Ability to participate in exercise and recreational activities is limited by the level of injury, motor function, and motivation. Increased energy demands required to participate in exercise and recreational activities may demotivate individuals with SCI. Encouragement, opportunities, adaptive equipment, training, and maintenance of health are all critical for participation in recreational activities.

Latest Advances in Assistive Technology for Recreational Activities

For many recreational activities, adaptations are required based on the level of injury and functional ability of the individual. Some of the sporting activities need minimal adaptations, while competitive sports that include wheelchairs require special modifications. Recreational activities

Table 23-1
Assistive Technology as it Applies to the Level of SCI and Their Costs

Technology	Neurological Level	Cost ($)
Low Tech		
Mouthstick	C3–C4	33–60
Dorsal wrist splints, long Wanchick splints, ratchet splints, typing stick, right angle pocket	C5	6–43
Wanchik Typer, universal cuffs, Slip-On Typing Aid/keyboard aid, Clear View Typing Aid, weaving typing stick between fingers	C6	1–30
Ergorest forearm supports (to support shoulder musculature; can be attached to wheelchair armrest).	C5–C6	140
Overhead slings (shoulder support)	C5	100–205
Accessibility options (standard Windows feature)		
StickyKeys	C3–C6	0
FilterKeys (adjust time key must be held down before repeating)	C4–C6	0
Mouse keys (control mouse using numeric keypad)	C3–C5	0
Computer Workstation Needs		
Height-adjustable workstation, deskalators (low tech), modular furniture, manually adjustable and power height-adjustable tables	C3–C6	50–2000
Adjustable keyboard trays	C3–C6	40–500
Adjustable monitor arms or monitor stands	C3–C6	15–200
Alternative keyboards:		
Small modules (Space Saver, Mini-Thin, Wireless, Little Fingers, USB mini)	C3–C6	30–100
Small Membrane or stylus (EKEG Mini, Magic Wand)	C3–C5	475–2000
Keyboards with built-in trackballs	C5–C6	50–105
Notetakers (AlphaSmart 3000, DreamWriter, Link)	C6–C8	200–300
Mouse Alternatives		
Trackballs (Kensington, Ergo-Trackball, Evolution Mouse Trak, Roller Plus, Roller II)	C4–C8	50–400
Mouth-controlled joystick (QuadJoy)	C4–C5	600
Touchpads (Easy Cat, Smart Cat, Cruise Cat)	C6–C8	50–80
Head-pointing mice (Tracer, HeadMouse, Tracker, Smart NAV, Headmaster)	C3–C6	300–2840
Software Applications		
On-screen keyboards (ScreenDoors, Keystrokes, REACH Interface Author, IMG's OnScreen, SofType, Wivik). Use with head-pointing mice.	C3–C5	95–495
Mouse emulators (Dragger, Gus!, Dwell Cursor, MagicCursor, Qpointer Keyboard, Joystick-to-Mouse, Click It). These take the place of the mouse. Can be switch operated or used with a head-pointing mouse.	C3–C5	50–195
Speech recognition (Dragon Naturally Speaking, Dragon Dictate, Qpointer Voice, ViaVoice)	C3–C6	200–700

Adapted with author's permission from McKinley W, Tewksbury MA, Sitter P et al. Assistive technology and computer adaptations for individuals with spinal cord injury. *Neurorehabilitation.* 2004;19(2):141–146.

are vital, and the available assistive technology and designs make participation possible.

Recreational activities include gardening, photography, reading, and sports, to name a few. In the area of sports, motor function is the limiting factor, and ability to participate depends on the function spared after the injury. Common sports include fishing, bowling, golf, swimming, and sailing. Less common sports activities include karate, horseback riding, mountain climbing, water skiing, scuba diving, sky diving, flying, hunting, and snorkeling.[34]

The number of adaptations required for recreational activities depends upon the level of SCI. The higher the level of lesion, the greater the number of adaptations required. Most recreational activities are accessible to all levels of SCI. Environmental modifications remove barriers, and personal adaptations provide independence to the individuals.

All these activities require certain amount of adaptation to the equipment. The amount varies from minimal to maximal for paraplegics versus tetraplegics when it comes to a specific sport such as bowling.

Many organizations exist for recreational sports in the United States and many of them have websites (Table 23-2).[36] There are many modifications that are required for wheelchairs for sporting activities. Tennis wheelchairs, basketball wheelchairs, quad rugby chairs, and racing wheelchairs are all available.

When SCI individuals engage in exercise and recreational activities, they are prone to injuries and trauma more than able-bodied individuals. Since most paraplegics depend on their upper extremities for their mobility and recreational activities, their shoulders are frequently affected with pain and trauma. Rotator cuff and overuse injuries are also common.[37–39]

Extensive precautions should be exercised to prevent additional damage to the already compromised function in individuals with SCI. With proper selection of the sports activity, adequate training, education, and early intervention after injury, the SCI population will be able to enjoy recreational activities to their fullest potential.

With the advent of technology in the form of Internet, cable TV, and their availability and easy access, people with disabilities can live active lives. Researchers in the Rehabilitation Engineering Research Center (RERC) through the National Institute of Disability and Rehabilitation Research (NIDRR) have been working on Recreational technologies (RecTech) by analyzing how the emerging technologies may be used to provide more enjoyable opportunities for individuals with disabilities

Table 23-2
U.S. Organizations for Recreational Sports

Activities	Website
American Canoe Association	www.acanet.org
Bowling—American Wheelchair Bowling Association	www.amwheelchairbowl.qpg.com
Billiards—National Wheelchair Billiards	www.nwpainc.com
Camping—National Park Services, Office of Special Programs	www.nps.gov
Disabled Sports—USA	www.dsusa.org
Flying—International Wheelchair Aviators	www.wheelchairaviators.org
Freedom's Wings International	www.freedomswings.org
Fishing—Paralyzed Veterans of America	www.pva.com
Handicapped Scuba Association	www.hsascuba.com
Horseback Riding—North American Riding for the Handicapped Association	www.narha.org
Hunting—NRA Disabled Shooting Services	www.nrahq.org
POINT—Paraplegics on Independent Nature Trips	www.turningpoint1.com
Sailing—National Ocean Access Project	www.dsusa.org
Special Olympics International	www.specialolympics.org
U.S. Rowing Association	www.usrowing.org
U.S. Wheelchair Swimming, Inc.	www.wsusa.org
Water Sports—American Water Ski Association	www.usawaterski.org
Wheelchair Sports—USA	www.wsusa.org

and SCI.[36] Recreational technologies (or RecTech) focuses on enhancing universal design features of equipment programs, and facilities. RecTech encourages collaboration between disabled individuals, entrepreneurs, industry professionals, researchers and exercise physiologists to increase access and participation in exercise and recreational activities. Key Activities of RERC Rectech are described as to "identify existing and needed recreational and fitness technologies for people with disabilities" and to "determine feasibility, efficacy, and safety of various recreational and exercise technologies in improving health and function for people with disabilities."

Rimmer and Schiller describe four essential components for enjoyable recreational activities. They are access, participation, adherence, and health and function. Technology for a healthier lifestyle, as they called it, includes these four elements. There is a logical progression through these elements in that the most basic is *access*. Access includes environmental as well as specific sports-related adaptations. Also included in the area of access is availability of information and awareness of the recreational programs. There are many adaptations to allow SCI individuals to take part in sports and recreation. However, many people are totally unaware that they exist.

The next step is the ability of the SCI individual to *participate* in the activities. Having the appropriate equipment with suitable adaptations is the key for participation. Hence, there is a need for sports or leisure activity-specific adaptations in relation to the individual's level of lesion.

The third element is *adherence*. Barring ill health and lack of motivation, adherence to exercise or participation in recreational activities depends on the availability of full access, which enables those with SCI to participate. There should be many options in sporting activities, just as there should be several locations to promote adherence. Again, access leads to adherence.

Lastly, *health and function* dictate the success of the above three elements. Participation in recreational activities poses additional demands on the energy requirements. Repetitive motions in a particular activity might even cause injuries to parts of the body such as shoulders and wrists.

Additionally, there is a great need for information technology to partner with assistive technology. There are online resources with regard to adaptive recreation technology. There is a recreation technology and sports database that can be accessed at www.rechtech.org. The database has specific classifications for exercise, sports, and recreation and is subdivided into categories based on the activities desired, such as fitness, recreation, and sports. These subcategories are described as equipment adaptations and personal adaptations. The equipment adaptations address specific activity-related equipment, such as bowling ramps, wheelchairs, etc. Personal adaptations refer to adaptations made by the individual to function with the disability. Auto-configuration is the process whereby the recreational equipment adjusts to the requirements of the individual. Here are some examples of the adaptive equipment available for various recreational activities.

Examples of some of the commonly used recreational assistive technology are as follows.

1. The Strong Arm Rod Holder for fishing (Fig. 22-3). Fishing is enjoyed by SCI individuals with a simple device called the Strong Arm Holder. This device is particularly useful for individuals with tetraplegia with little or no hand or wrist function. There are other devices available to hold the fishing rod for cutting and tying the fishing line.
2. The Sure Hands Wheelchair-to-Water Pool Lift for access to pools (Fig. 23-4). Swimming is an enjoyable sport and can be used for therapeutic purposes as well a recreation. The Sure Hands Wheelchair-to-Water Pool Lift enables the SCI individual access to swimming pools. Several lifting mechanisms, such as hydraulic, drive, or geared lifts, are available on the market. All of these lifts are equipped with various seating options and head, chest, and leg supports.
3. Aquatic wheelchairs for beaches and pools (Fig. 23-5). There are aquatic wheelchairs available for use on sandy beaches and around swimming pools. Beach wheelchairs may be manual or power operated, whereas pool chairs operate manually. Beach wheelchairs have extrawide wheels, known as balloon wheels, which enable them to move over sand. Regular wheelchairs can be converted to beach wheelchairs by adding balloon wheels.
4. The Sit-Ski for water skiing (Fig. 23-6). SCI individuals participate in water skiing more frequently than any other sport. Sit-Ski is a practical adaptation that allows the user to sit while skiing. The skis are equipped with body and leg supports to help the user sit in place.

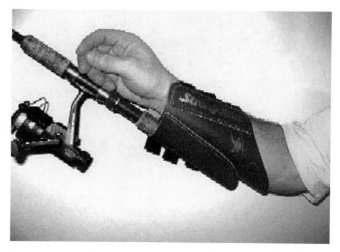

Figure 23-3. The Strong Arm Rod Holder from Access to Recreation straps to the wrist and forearm to enable persons with limited or no grip to fish.[40] (Courtesy of Access to Recreation, Inc., Newbury Park, CA. http://www.acesstr.com)

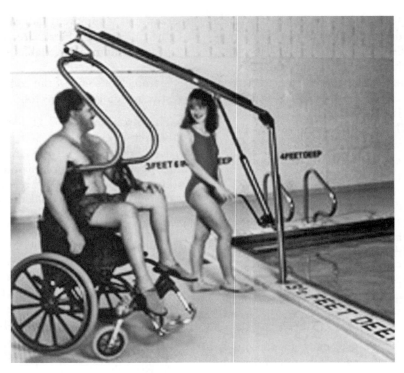

Figure 23-4. The SureHands Wheelchair-to-Water Seat Sling (with body support) from SureHands Lift & Care Systems is a motorized pool lift that transfers an individual from a wheelchair to the water.[41] (Courtesy of SureHands Lift & Care Systems, Pine Island, NY. http://www. surehands.com)

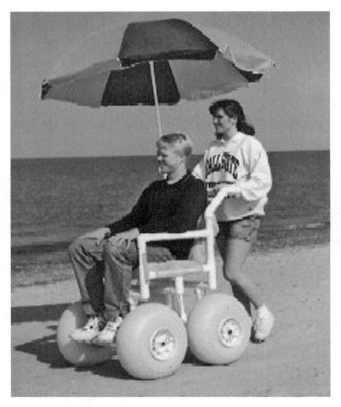

Figure 23-5. The All Terrain Chair from Assistive Technology, Inc. is a beach wheelchair with balloon wheels for moving on sand.[42] (Courtesy of Assistive Technology, Inc., Elkhart, IN.)

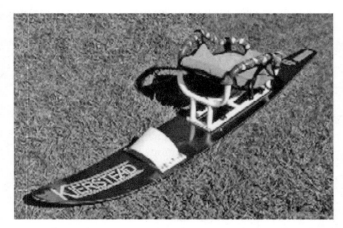

Figure 23-6. The Sit-Ski from Kierstead Water Skis allows individuals to water ski in a seated position while being held securely in place by a custom-fitted cage.[43] (Courtesy of Liquid Access, Melbourne, FL. http://www.liquidaccess.org)

CASE STUDY 23-1 Home and School With High Tetraplegia

A 19-year-old woman has C2 AIS A tetraplegia after a gunshot wound. She was living with her parents in a ranch-style house and attending college prior to her injury. She now is on a ventilator. She would like to continue to live with her parents and pursue study in molecular biology. What adaptive equipment would you recommend to assist with her living and vocational goals?

CASE STUDY 23-2 Computer and Sports With Paraplegia

A 43-year-old fast-food restaurant manager has sustained a T12 AIS A paraplegia after a snowmobile accident. He has always enjoyed computers and would like your help in providing adaptive equipment to change careers. Additionally, he wants to remain active, especially in his preferred realms of winter and aquatic sports. He wants to know if adaptive equipment is available for his recreational interests.

Summary

Assistive technology devices are critical for maximizing the independence of those with SCI. With thorough evaluation and diligent device selection, a more fulfilling life is possible, including many pre-injury pursuits such as employment and recreation.

REVIEW QUESTIONS

1. How does level and completeness of injury influence your choice of equipment for a patient?
2. How do differing vocational goals lead to different equipment choices?
3. If an individual has no upper limb movement, what devices would you suggest to facilitate interaction with the environment?
4. What would you recommend for ambulation to an individual with paraplegia?
5. What options does a nonambulatory individual have for negotiating a multilevel dwelling?

REFERENCES

1. Hedrick B, Pape TL-B, Heinemann AW et al. Employment issues and assistive technology use for persons with spinal cord injury. *J Rehabil Res Dev.* 2006;43(2):185–198.
2. Cooper RA. Bioengineering and spinal cord injury: A perspective on the state of the science. *J Spinal Cord Med.* 2004;27(4):351–364.
3. Consortium for Spinal Cord Medicine CPG. *Outcomes following traumatic spinal cord injury: Clinical practice guidelines for health-care professionals.* Washington, DC: Paralyzed Veterans of America; 1999.
4. Kirshblum S. Rehabilitation of spinal cord injury. In: DeLisa J, Gans BM, Walsh NE, editors. *Physical Medicine and Rehabilitation: Principles and Practice.* Vol. 2. 4th edition. Philadelphia: Lippincott Williams & Wilkins; 2005. pp. 1715–1751.
5. Creasey GH, Ho CH, Triolo RJ et al. Clinical applications of electrical stimulation after spinal cord injury. *J Spinal Cord Med.* 2004;27(4):365–375.
6. Jacobs PL, Johnson B, Mahoney ET. Physiologic responses to electrically assisted and frame-supported standing in persons with paraplegia. *J Spinal Cord Med.* 2003;26(4):384–389.
7. Chao CY, Cheing GL. The effects of lower-extremity functional electric stimulation on the orthostatic responses of people with tetraplegia. *Arch Phys Med Rehabil.* 2005;86(7):1427–1433.
8. Wilkenfeld AJ, Audu ML, Triolo RJ. Feasibility of functional electrical stimulation for control of seated posture after spinal cord injury: A simulation study. *J Rehabil Res Dev.* 2006;43(2):139–152.
9. Klose KJ, Jacobs PL, Broton JG et al. Evaluation of a training program for persons with SCI paraplegia using the Parastep 1 ambulation system. Part 1. Ambulation performance and anthropometric measures. *Arch Phys Med Rehabil.* 1997;78(8):789–793.
10. Jacobs PL, Nash MS, Klose KJ et al. Evaluation of a training program for persons with SCI paraplegia using the Parastep 1 ambulation system. Part 2. Effects on physiological responses to peak arm ergometry. *Arch Phys Med Rehabil.* 1997;78(8):794–798.
11. Needham-Shropshire BM, Broton JG, Klose KJ et al. Evaluation of a training program for persons with SCI paraplegia using the Parastep 1 ambulation system. Part 3. Lack of effect on bone mineral density. *Arch Phys Med Rehabil.* 1997;78(8):799–803.
12. Guest RS, Klose KJ, Needham-Shropshire BM et al. Evaluation of a training program for persons with SCI paraplegia using the Parastep 1 ambulation system. Part 4. Effect on physical self-concept and depression. *Arch Phys Med Rehabil.* 1997;78(8):804–807.
13. Nash MS, Jacobs PL, Montalvo BM et al. Evaluation of a training program for persons with SCI paraplegia using the Parastep 1 ambulation system. Part 5. Lower extremity blood flow and hyperemic responses to occlusion are augmented by ambulation training. *Arch Phys Med Rehabil.* 1997;78(8):808–814.
14. Spadone R, Merati G, Bertocchi E et al. Energy consumption of locomotion with orthosis versus Parastep-assisted gait: A single case study. *Spinal Cord.* 2003;41(2):97–104.
15. Cooper RA, Boninger ML, Cooper R et al. Preliminary assessment of a prototype advanced mobility device in the work environment of veterans with spinal cord injury. *Neurorehabilitation.* 2004;19(2):161–170.
16. Kirshblum S. New rehabilitation interventions in spinal cord injury. *J Spinal Cord Med.* 2004;27(4):342–350.
17. Independence Technology LLC. http://www.independencenow.com/ibot/stair.html. Accessed September 2, 2008.

18. Anson D. Computers and EADL access for individuals with spinal cord injury. *Top Spinal Cord Inj Rehabil.* 2006; 11(4):42–60.

19. Wellings DJ, Unsworth J. Fortnightly review. Environmental control systems for people with a disability: an update. *BMJ.* 1997;315(7105):409–412.

20. Holme SA, Kanny EM, Guthrie MR et al. The use of environmental control units by occupational therapists in spinal cord injury and disease services. *Am J Occup Ther.* 1997;51(1):42–48.

21. Angel ECU. http://www.angelecu.com/index.htm. Accessed September 4, 2008.

22. Dickey R, Shealey SH. Using technology to control the environment. *Am J Occup Ther.* 1987;41(11):717–721.

23. Chen SC, Tang FT, Chen YL et al. Infrared-based communication augmentation system for people with multiple disabilities. *Disabil Rehabil.* 2004;26(18):1105–1109.

24. Lange ML. The future of electronic aids to daily living. *Am J Occup Ther.* 2002;56(1):107–109.

25. Platts RG, Fraser MH. Assistive technology in the rehabilitation of patients with high spinal cord lesions. *Paraplegia.* 1993;31(5):280–287.

26. Symington DC, Lywood DW, Lawson JS et al. Environmental control systems in chronic care hospitals and nursing homes. *Arch Phys Med Rehabil.* 1986;67(5):322–325.

27. McDonald DW, Boyle MA, Schumann TL. Environmental control unit utilization by high-level spinal cord injured patients. *Arch Phys Med Rehabil.* 1989;70(8):621–623.

28. Rigby P, Ryan S, Joos S et al. Impact of electronic aids to daily living on the lives of persons with cervical spinal cord injuries. *Assist Technol.* 2005;17(2):89–97.

29. Leuthardt EC, Schalk G, Moran D et al. The emerging world of motor neuroprosthetics: A neurosurgical perspective. *Neurosurgery.* 2006;59(1):1–14; discussion 11–14.

30. Grodzinsky FS. Equity of access: Adaptive technology. *Sci Eng Ethics.* 2000;6(2):221–234.

31. Hawking, S. "My experience with ALS." http://www.hawking.org.uk/disable/dindex.html. Accessed December 28, 2006.

32. Poole CJ, Millman A. ABC of medical computing. Adaptive computer technology. *BMJ.* 1995;311(7013):1149–151.

33. McKinley W, Tewksbury MA, Sitter P et al. Assistive technology and computer adaptations for individuals with spinal cord injury. *Neurorehabilitation.* 2004;19(2):141–146.

34. Nash MS, Horton JAI. Recreational and therapeutic exercise after spinal cord injury. In: Kirshblum S, Campagnalo DI, DeLisa J, editors. *Spinal Cord Medicine.* Philadelphia: Lippincott Williams & Wilkins; 2002. pp. 331–347.

35. Americans with Disabilities Act of 1990. 42nd United States Congress, 2101 note.

36. Remmir J.H. and Schutler W.J. Future directions in exercise and recreation technology for people with spinal cord injury and other disabilities: Perspectives from the Rehabilitation Engineering Research Center on Recreational Technologies and Exercise Physiology for People with Disabilities. *Topics in Spinal Cord Injury Rehabilitation.* Volume 11, No # 4, 2006, 82–93.

37. Pentland WE, Twomey LT. Upper limb function in persons with long term paraplegia and implications for independence. Part I. *Paraplegia* 1994;32:211–218.

38. Burnham R, Chan M, Hazlett C et al. Acute median nerve dysfunction from wheelchair propulsion: The development of a model and study of the effect of hand protection. *Arch Phys Med Rehabil.* 1994;75:513–518.

39. Burnham RS, Steadward RD. Upper extremity peripheral nerve entrapments among wheelchair athletes: Prevalence, location, and risk factors. *Arch Phys Med Rehabil.* 1994;75:519–524.

40. ABLEDATA. Strong Arm Rod Holder. http://www.abledata.com/abledata.cfm?pageid=113583&top=0&productid=87074&trail=0. Accessed September 3, 2008.

41. ABLEDATA. The SureHands Wheelchair-to-Water Pool Lift (with the Body Support) from SureHands Lift & Care Systems. "Fact Sheet." www.abledata.com/abledata_docs/Aquatic_Sports.txt. Accessed September 3, 2008.

42. ABLEDATA. All Terrain Chair (Model ATC 100). http://www.abledata.com/abledata.cfm?pageid=113583&top=0&productid=80545&trail=0. Accessed September 3, 2008.

43. ABLEDATA. Competition Sit-Ski. http://www.abledata.com/abledata.cfm?pageid=113583&top=0&productid=125685&trail=0. Accessed September 3, 2008.

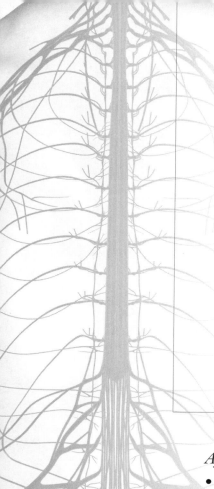

Special Considerations in the Rehabilitation of Children With SCI

24

John Kuluz, MD

Heakyung Kim, MD

Denise Dixon, PhD

Amer Samdani, MD

Manuel Gonzalez-Brito, DO

M.J. Mulcahey, PhD

After reading this chapter, the reader will be able to:

OBJECTIVES

- Describe how the epidemiology and pathophysiology of spinal cord injury (SCI) differ between children and adults
- Describe the medical sequelae of SCI in children
- Discuss the management of spasticity in children with SCI
- Describe the spinal column complications of SCI in children
- Describe the psychological effects of SCI on children and their families
- Discuss the management of the upper extremities in children with SCI
- Describe the available orthotic options for standing and walking for children with SCI
- Discuss the selection of wheelchairs for children with SCI
- Discuss the challenges of discharge planning and school reentry after SCI in children

Introduction

Management of children with spinal cord injury (SCI) presents unique acute and long-term medical, surgical, psychological, and rehabilitative challenges. As with other severe, chronic diseases in children, SCI affects the entire family, and as such, requires that care be directed not only to the affected child, but also to all members of the child's family. Advancements in medicine, technology, and public policy related to disabilities have combined to increase the expectation of improved outcome and quality of life. With provision of timely and appropriate interventions during acute, subacute, and long-term rehabilitation and good general pediatric, as well as SCI-focused, medical care, children with SCI can participate in a full range of social, educational, recreational, and interpersonal activities and become productive members of society as adults. In this chapter, we review the important aspects of SCI in children that will enable therapists, nurses, physicians, and other specialists to help children achieve these goals.

Epidemiology and Pathophysiology of SCI in Children

The Incidence of Pediatric SCI

Pediatric SCI is a relatively uncommon disease that each year affects approximately 1500 to 2000 children younger than 18 years of age in the United States. Of the 10,000 to 11,000 cases of SCI annually, only 5%[1] occur in children younger than 10 years old, the time at which the spine approaches adult size and rigidity.[1,2] The incidence varies between countries, ranging from 0.5 to nearly 3 cases per 100,000 children per year.[3] The U.S. incidence is estimated to be 1.99 per 100,000.[4] As with other forms of childhood trauma, gender and race play important roles. Boys are almost twice as likely as girls to experience SCI, with an incidence in boys of 2.79 per 100,000 versus 1.15 per 100,000 in girls. While most cases of pediatric SCI occur in Caucasians, the incidence in African Americans and Hispanics has been rising steadily over the last two decades. The etiology of SCI in children includes motor vehicle accidents (MVA; 56%), falls (14.2%), gun violence (9.2%), and sports injuries (7.7%). As one would expect, etiology of SCI is very much age dependent, with younger children sustaining injuries due to MVAs and falls, whereas violence and sports-related injuries are more common causes of SCI in older children and adolescents.

Anatomical and Biomechanical Features of the Pediatric Spinal Cord and Column

The pediatric spinal cord and spinal column have anatomical and biomechanical differences compared to adults that predispose children to different mechanisms of injury and result in a unique injury profile.[5–8] Young children have a large occiput and increased laxity of their spinal ligaments, making the spine less rigid and more mobile. This mobility allows for stretching and torsional forces on the spinal cord, even with minor trauma, particularly in the cervical region. In comparison to their adult counterparts, children with SCI tend to have a higher percentage of upper cervical and thoracic spine injuries,[9,10] higher susceptibility to delayed onset of neurological deficits,[11] greater percentage of complete SCIs,[12–14] and higher incidence of SCI without radiographic abnormality (SCIWORA).[15]

SCI Without Radiographic Abnormality

The term *SCIWORA* was coined prior to the availability of magnetic resonance imaging (MRI), when x-rays and computerized tomography (CT) scans failed to show SCI, for example, fractures, misalignment, dislocation, etc., despite the presence of a SCI. Pang[15] first described the condition in 1982 and estimated the incidence of SCIWORA to be 30% to 40% of all pediatric cases of SCI. Children have unique features that result in hypermobility of the spinal column, leading to distraction injury following trauma, as discussed above.[16,17] In addition, the intervertebral discs have a high water content, allowing them to stretch considerably without rupture.[18] Furthermore, the facet joints are horizontal and the vertebral bodies are wedged anteriorly, allowing increased forward slippage, which can stretch the spinal cord.[15–17] These features make the pediatric spine malleable and, in combination with a large occiput, result in stretch or distraction injury to the spinal cord after trauma. According to this theory, SCIWORA results from excessive stretch or torsional stress on the relatively nonelastic spinal cord tissue, owing to the fact that the spinal column can stretch as much as five to eight times more than the spinal cord.[19] In contrast, the adult spine is rigid and more likely to fracture and cause damage to the spinal cord via direct tissue trauma.

The implication of the biomechanical differences between adults and children is that the spinal cord pathology in SCIWORA is a result of stretching and torsional forces and not due to direct tissue trauma. However, in a more recent review of the MRI findings in SCIWORA, Pang[20] found that 18 of 50 children who presented with SCIWORA had either minor hemorrhage, major hemorrhage, or disruption of the spinal cord, and all but 2 of these children had severe or complete deficits 6 months post-injury. All 23 SCIWORA children with normal cords as seen upon MRI made a complete recovery, whereas 9 children with "edema only" upon MRI recovered to normal or mild disability. The author concluded that children with suspected SCI need MR imaging of the spine to completely rule out SCI and that SCIWORA may result from torsional stretch injuries. In most cases SCIWORA also includes a significant component of direct tissue injury from contusional or compressional forces.

Determining whether the SCI is classified as complete or incomplete using the American Spinal Cord Injury Association (ASIA) Impairment Scale (AIS) is important.[21] Occasionally, however, correct assessment may not be possible if the child is unconscious, heavily sedated, intubated, or in spinal shock. Additionally, some children, particularly preschool children, may require repeat exams due to inconsistencies in the child's response to sensory stimulation and lack of response to commands. Mulcahey et al[22] found that the motor and sensory components of the AIS scale were inappropriate for infants and toddlers under age 4 and that children below age 10 became anxious and stressed by the pinprick exam. Despite these deficiencies, an AIS classification determination should be attempted in all children with SCI and described in detail in the medical record (*see* Chapter 6).

Physiology of Injury and Repair in the Immature Spinal Cord

Basic science research into the molecular pathophysiology of traumatic injury to the immature spinal cord is limited. At distinct stages of fetal and neonatal development, the reparative and regenerative capabilities of the spinal cord are much greater than later in development.[22–24] Neonatal and juvenile animals display greater plasticity and functional recovery than their adult counterparts.[25–28] For unknown reasons, the regenerative qualities of the immature spinal cord abruptly disappear during later development. For example, after complete transection of the thoracic spinal cord in 1-week-old neonatal opossum, complete recovery of sensorimotor function and normal walking occurs. This regenerative capacity declines by 2 weeks and disappears by 1 month of age. The greater ability to recover in the younger opossum may be due to differences in inflammatory cellular and molecular responses.[27]

In addition to superior repair and recovery following SCI, there is evidence that in the developing spinal cord the cellular and molecular environment is less inhibitory to axon regeneration in comparison to the adult. Injury to the adult spinal cord disrupts cells and compromises the blood–brain barrier, causing extensive cellular damage and interruption of ascending and descending axonal tracts. The initial trauma is the source of the primary injury, but it also causes a secondary tissue response, including activation of astrocytes and invasion of foreign cells from the periphery. The combination of primary and secondary insults results in progressive cellular death of both neuronal and non-neuronal cells.[29–31] Within days after injury, severed axons begin to sprout, but growth usually stops at the injury site. Intense activation of astrocytes results in the formation of a glial scar. Reactive astrocytes of the mature nervous system inhibit axon regeneration by forming a glial scar at the injury site.[32–34]

In contrast, reactive astrocytes of developing animals do not appear to be inhibitory, and there is enhanced regeneration of axons after SCI. In short, the immature spinal cord has a greater capacity to repair, recover, and permit regeneration following traumatic injury. These findings represent some of the most promising and compelling aspects that are unique to pediatric SCI, and they have important implications for repair of SCI across all ages.

Medical Sequelae of SCI in Children

Clinical and animal studies have shown that every organ system may be affected adversely after SCI, depending on the level and severity of injury. Other associated traumatic injuries can add to or augment organ system dysfunction, especially in the first few weeks after SCI. The respiratory and cardiovascular systems are commonly affected in those with either cervical injuries or upper thoracic injuries, and children with SCI may have life-threatening conditions both acutely and chronically. Optimal outcome for the child with SCI after the acute hospitalization requires a multidisciplinary team that includes a pediatric rehabilitation specialist, a pediatrician for primary and general medical care, and multiple pediatric subspecialists appropriate to the child's complications. This team may include a pediatric neurosurgeon and/or orthopedic spine surgeon, otolaryngologist, pulmonologist, urologist, gastroenterologist, nutritionist, and wound care team. While respiratory management and cardiovascular response to SCI are discussed in other chapters, those approaches with special importance for children with SCI are reviewed in the following section.

Pain

One of the most important issues in caring for children with SCI is pain control. Children with SCI often experience significant pain during the acute period after injury and during later stages of recovery. While very little has been written about this sequel of SCI in children, anecdotal evidence suggests that the incidence, distribution, and etiology of pain in children is similar to that in adults (for a more detailed discussion of pain *see* Chapter 17).

Management of pain in children in general is complex, risky, and very challenging. Pain management in children with SCI is even more difficult because of the potential for synergistic effects of SCI and pain medications on vital organ functions such as consciousness, breathing, airway patency, blood pressure control, heart rate, etc. Inadequate treatment of pain can increase metabolism, temperature, diencephalic storming, spasticity, psychological impairments, sleep disturbances, and parental as well as child satisfaction. On the other hand, overtreatment of pain can cause excessive sedation, weakness, nausea, vomiting, pruritis, constipation, urinary retention, depressed mood, and narcotic addiction, as well as respiratory and hemodynamic compromise. All of these problems interfere with recovery and prevent effective rehabilitation. For the pharmacological management of pain in children, anesthesiologists and pediatric conscious sedation specialists emphasize the importance of monitoring for acute and delayed side effects of the various pain medications rather than the choice of the medication itself, although both are obviously very important.

Choosing an analgesic depends on the type and severity of pain as well as many other constitutional factors within the child. Using drugs with few or minimal side effects, such as acetaminophen or nonsteroidal anti-inflammatory agents, and progressing to more potent agents, such as narcotics and anesthetics if the pain persists are always advisable. Unfortunately, these medications are rarely effective for neuropathic pain, which results from injury, inflammation, or dysfunction in the peripheral or central nervous system, and occurs commonly in the setting of SCI. Pharmacological options for children with neuropathic pain mostly consist of the off-label use of antiepileptic drugs, antidepressants, and, most recently, botulinum toxin. A large component of the pain experience in children can be psychogenic in nature; therefore, anxiolytics and sedatives, as well as nonpharmacological relaxation techniques, may be beneficial in managing and preventing pain in children with SCI.

Effects of SCI on the Pediatric Airway and Respiratory System

Vocal cord dysfunction, direct tracheal injury, and diaphragm weakness or paralysis are common with upper cervical SCI and predispose the child to recurrent hypoxemia and overt respiratory failure. Respiratory management is discussed in detail in Chapter 14 and evaluation of the respiratory system is discussed in the web-based supplement chapter. For children sustaining injuries at or above C6, early tracheostomy can be lifesaving and hastens the transition from acute care to the rehabilitation unit. The safest approach is to have all children with cervical injuries evaluated completely for airway injury and dysfunction and for diaphragmatic paresis or paralysis, which may be unilateral. In children with abnormal findings, a more conservative approach to weaning from mechanical ventilation and tracheal decannulation is prudent. Children rarely have respiratory difficulties when SCI is at L1 or lower; however, above L1, intercostal muscle paralysis can lead to weak cough, airway secretion buildup, and recurrent atelectasis. Incentive spirometry, upright positioning, chest physical therapy, frequent suctioning, and early mobilization are the cornerstones of respiratory care. Other helpful mechanical strategies include the insufflator and exsufflator (CoughAssist; Emerson, Cambridge, MA). The vibratory vest, which has not been studied in children with SCI, has been shown to increase sputum production and to be well tolerated in children with cystic fibrosis[35] (respiratory management of the individual with SCI is discussed in detail in Chapter 14). Theophylline, a phosphodiesterase inhibitor that increases intracellular cyclic AMP, has been shown experimentally to improve diaphragm function in animals with hemitransection of the cervical cord, suggesting both direct and indirect beneficial effects on the diaphragm and the respiratory system as a whole.[36,37] Currently, there is insufficient evidence to support the routine use of theophylline in individuals with SCI and diaphragm dysfunction, although in refractory cases it may be beneficial.[38]

Another bedside technique for individuals with SCI who have weak respiratory muscles and poor cough is the assisted cough, which involves a forceful push on the upper abdomen at the end of a deep inspiration to mimic a true cough. To maintain lung compliance, an "air-stacking exercise" is recommended. Providing deep insufflation can be achieved via glossopharyngeal breathing (GPB), volume-cycle ventilator, or manual resuscitator. These techniques are appropriate for children with or without a tracheostomy. GPB is a technique that involves rapidly taking small gulps of air, specifically six to nine gulps of 60 to 200 ml, using the tongue and pharyngeal muscles to project the air past the glottis into the lung. This approach can increase vital capacity, which allows for assistance in cough, improvement in voice audibility, and ventilatory-free time in children with minimal vital capacity.[39–41] Like limb articulations and other soft tissues, the lungs and chest wall require regular range of motion exercise and stretching to prevent chest wall contractures and lung restriction from muscle weakness. This concern is critical in children with SCI because lung growth peaks in the early teenage years and vital capacity reaches a plateau at 19 years of age.[42] Continuous monitoring of pulmonary function is important over time, as changes may be observed, for example, in the development of a progressive scoliotic curve.

Special Challenges for the Ventilator-Dependent Child

Very little has been published in the medical literature about the management and outcome of children with SCI who require mechanical ventilation. DeVivo et al[43] described data from the model systems for SCI, which demonstrated a 1-year survival rate of 49.7% for the entire population of mostly young to middle-aged adults with ventilator-dependent SCI. However, if the child survived the first year, then the 14-year cumulative survival rate was over 60%. Improvements in emergency and critical care and rehabilitative medicine have certainly contributed to a reduction in short-term mortality over the last decade.[44]

Despite improved survival rates, young children on chronic ventilatory support are at high risk of early death compared to older children and adults due to lower cardiorespiratory reserves, smaller and more easily occluded tracheostomy tubes, and inability to communicate their discomfort when they are poorly ventilated or oxygenated

or when the ventilator malfunctions. Hospital charges for ventilator-dependent children in the pediatric ICU in a large urban hospital are between $6000 and $10,000 per day, whereas caring for the same child in the rehabilitation unit costs approximately one-third this amount. Cost reductions and improved quality of life for the child and family have motivated some children's hospitals to establish specially prepared units for these and other ventilator-dependent children, and they have proven to be very successful as well as safe.[45] Ideally, a brief stay in this type of intermediate care unit should be included in the progression from acute to rehabilitative care in order to determine if the child is ready, from a medical standpoint, to be transferred to the rehabilitation unit.

To progress toward independence from the ventilator, the child with upper cervical SCI must meet certain criteria before weaning is attempted, including nonparadoxical diaphragm motion on fluoroscopy, tidal volume of a minimum of 2 to 3 cc/kg, negative inspiratory force of -5 to -10 cm H_2O, and relatively normal blood gases on room air (oxygen saturations >92% to 94% and $PaCO_2$ <45 to 50 mm Hg).[46] The most important principles to adhere to when weaning are to (1) individualize the process for the child and family, (2) decrease ventilator support slowly, (3) monitor the effects of reducing ventilator support on respiratory function and ability to participate in rehabilitation therapies, and (4) return to previous settings if unsuccessful (i.e., do not rush or force the process). In an excellent review of the experience of DuPont Children's Hospital in progression of care in children who are ventilator dependent, Padman et al describe a step-by-step care pathway for ventilator-dependent children with SCI from the intensive care unit through inpatient rehabilitation and the discharge process.[46] Successful discharge and long-term home ventilation require an experienced team of pediatric pulmonologists, rehabilitation specialists, primary care pediatricians, and family members who are all deeply committed to providing the labor-intensive home care and close medical follow-up these children require.[47,48] High quality of life can be achieved in children who are ventilator dependent, but only if medical complications are kept to a minimum and good preventative care is provided.[49,50]

Cardiovascular Responses to SCI

During the acute response to SCI, a sympathetic stress response occurs, followed by variable degrees of cardiovascular disturbances, which can lead to secondary insults to the injured cord as well as to other organs throughout the body. Spinal or neurogenic shock following traumatic SCI is a well-recognized yet poorly investigated and reported phenomenon.[51,52] *Neurogenic shock* is defined as a state of inadequate tissue oxygen delivery with resultant end-organ failure following SCI above the sixth thoracic vertebra. This situation occurs because the sympathetic outflow and cardiac accelerators are located at T1–T5 and because sufficient sympathetic output is inhibited with injuries above this level, resulting in widespread vascular paresis. The most common result is hypotension, while the heart rate response is variable. Tachycardia predominates in the immediate post-injury period, whereas bradycardia occurs at later stages. Bradycardia results from the loss of sympathetic input and eventual development of unopposed vagal tone.[53–56] These acute cardiovascular changes are usually managed successfully with fluids and vasopressors such as dopamine. If they persist, they can significantly limit participation in rehabilitation. Occasionally, salt supplementation, additional fluid boluses, or oral alpha agonists will be needed until blood pressure control and feedback mechanisms are reestablished after SCI.

One of the most dangerous late complications of SCI is autonomic dysreflexia (AD), which is characterized by a sudden exaggerated reflex increase in blood pressure, sometimes accompanied by bradycardia, in response to a noxious stimulus originating below the level of injury. AD occurs in 48% to 85% of all SCI individuals with injury at T6 and above, but the true incidence in children is unknown. A strong painful stimulus is transmitted to the spinal cord through the sensory nerves. The etiology and pathophysiology of AD are discussed in Chapter 1. Clinical manifestations of AD in children may be more subtle or vague because of developmental, cognitive, and verbal communication variations.[54] Therefore, both children with SCI and their caretakers, including family, school teachers, school nurses, coaches, and community-based health-care providers, should be educated on the prevention, detection, and management of AD. Furthermore, the child or adolescent who is susceptible to AD should wear a medical alert bracelet or carry an identification card.[58]

Prevention of Venous Thromboembolism

Incidence of venous thromboembolism (VTE) in the pediatric population with SCI is less than that in the adult population.[59] The risk of clinically significant VTE, including deep venous thrombosis (DVT) and pulmonary embolism (PE), in children with SCI younger than 14 years of age is very low (1.1%). However, the incidence in the adolescent population is 4.8%, which is closer to the reported 5.4% incidence in adults with SCI.[60] The incidence of VTE is higher in the first few weeks after injury.[61,62] Anticoagulation is the mainstay of prevention and therapy for VTE after SCI. Unfractionated heparin is the most frequently used anticoagulant for the initial treatment of VTE in children because of its short half-life. Low-molecular-weight heparin (LMWH) is now increasingly being used because its pharmacokinetic properties are more predictable than unfractionated heparin or oral anticoagulants, thereby minimizing the frequency of monitoring and its associated costs. LMWH can be administered subcutaneously,

thereby eliminating the need for venous access. Children with uncomplicated venous thrombosis are usually treated for 3 to 6 months. There is increasing evidence that individuals with clot progression while on therapy, completely occlusive clots on presentation, or persistently high levels of inflammatory markers are at risk for treatment failure and may benefit from a longer duration of anticoagulation therapy or placement of a vena caval filter.[63]

Management of Neurogenic Bladder

Immediately after SCI, the bladder is areflexic because of loss of sympathetic input that occurs normally between T10 and L2. Initial management includes placing an indwelling Foley catheter to prevent bladder overdistention followed shortly by a program of frequent chronic intermittent catheterizations (CICs). However, children on IV fluid may need CIC too frequently, resulting in increased risk of urinary tract infection compared to using an indwelling Foley catheter. Strict recording of daily intake and output should be continued throughout inpatient rehabilitation. CIC is best started at 4-hour intervals and can be adjusted according to voiding and residual volumes obtained. Frequency of CIC is calculated based on a child's ideal bladder capacity for age as follows: between 2 and 12 years of age, the formula is (age + 2) × 30 ml; children older than 12 years old have an adult-sized bladder, with a capacity of 350 to 450 ml. For example, for an 8-year-old child whose daily fluid intake is 1800 ml, ideal bladder capacity is (8 + 2) × 30 = 300 ml.[64] Fluid loss through skin and lungs is approximately 30% of maintenance fluid intake, or 600 ml in this example. Therefore, this child will need CIC four times daily (1200 ÷ 300), or every 6 hours, to prevent bladder overdistention. Timed voidings and fluid management are important in managing neurogenic bladder and preventing renal injury.

Intermittent catheterization can be initiated as early as 3 years of age, and self-catheterization can be begun when the child is developmentally 5 to 7 years old.[65] Training the child who is physically capable of self-catheterizing not only ensures good bladder care, but also promotes the child's independence in self-care. To avoid frequent urination from hyperreflexic voiding, which can cause vesicoureteral reflux and hydronephrosis, anticholinergics (e.g., imipramine, ditropan) may be considered to relax the bladder wall. Dosing for anticholinergics will be determined as the child becomes continent between CICs. Children with limited bladder capacity who are unresponsive to anticholinergics may be candidates for bladder augmentation. One form of bladder augmentation, a continent catheterizable conduit (the Mitrofanoff procedure), consists of creating a conduit using the appendix or a segment of small bowel that connects the bladder to a stoma, either through the umbilicus or lower abdominal wall.[66] This procedure allows children with upper extremity function that is too limited for CIC to catheterize independently. Also, surgically implanted functional electrical stimulation devices are currently being used to augment the function of the bowel and bladder.[67]

Prophylactic antibiotics should be given to children with recurrent and severe urinary tract infections, obstructive uropathy, or compromised renal function, including vesicoureteral reflux hydronephrosis. Children with asymptomatic bacteriuria are generally not treated unless they have compromised renal function; treatment should be limited to symptomatic children. The use of fluoroquinolones may be contraindicated in children due to possibility of cartilage damage.[68] In summary, neurogenic bladder management is important in the prevention of infection and renal injury, and continence is essential for adolescents to move on to the challenge of living an independent and satisfying adult life.

Management of Neurogenic Bowel

Gastrointestinal motility may cease for several days after acute SCI or as a result of trauma. (See Chapter 15 for detailed coverage of this topic.) Children with SCI should receive prophylactic H_2 blockers or proton pump inhibitors to reduce the risk of stress ulceration and gastrointestinal bleeding, although the duration of the need for this therapy is unknown. Enteral feeding may be started orally or via an enteral feeding tube as soon as the child is hemodynamically stable. Because of lack of neural control, a bowel program should be instituted as soon as the child begins receiving enteral nutrition. The goal of the bowel program is regular bowel movements and continence without impaction.[69] A bowel program may be initiated with timed toileting by simply placing the child on a commode or toilet at the same time every day and encouraging him or her to bear down. The use of digital stimulation, stool softeners, laxatives, suppositories, or enemas may be needed to ensure regular elimination. Every effort must be made to assist the child or adolescent to become as independent as possible with his or her bowel management program.[68] Timing the bowel regimen appropriately to maximize the effect of the gastrocolic reflex (approximately 30 minutes to 1 hour after meals) is important.

The goal of bowel management in infants and toddlers is prevention of constipation or stool impaction. A bowel program is usually initiated at approximately 3 years of age.[70] Components of success include regularity, consistency, privacy, proper seating, and patience. A child should be placed on a potty chair regularly for brief periods of time, while the parent or guardian instructs him to "bear down." School-aged children may be able to perform a bowel program with assistance and should be encouraged to assume self-care. Adolescents should be proficient at performing or directing their bowel program. In addition to the many psychosocial issues related to adolescence, managing a bowel program can be an additional emotional stress. Because the need to be

accepted by peers may conflict with the need to attend to self-care, adolescents may not take the time to perform their bowel program. Parents and guardians must gradually relinquish responsibility of bowel management to the child, while remaining observant for lapses in self-care.[68]

Nutritional Needs

The nutritional needs of children with SCI must be adequately assessed and met in order to ensure appropriate weight gain, wound healing, and physical strength needed to participate in rehabilitation and self-care. This is best accomplished through consultation with a trained pediatric nutritionist. It is not uncommon for children to refuse to eat because of oral aversions or behavioral/psychological maladaptation to their disabilities. In this instance, if efforts of speech therapists and child psychologists fail to improve oral intake, tube feedings may be needed. It is often prudent to place a gastrostomy tube early in the acute period following severe SCI, for feeding and medication administration, especially if a tracheostomy is needed or if swallowing difficulties are anticipated.

Skin Care

Skin care is an essential component in the care of children and adolescents with SCI. Pressure ulcers are a serious and, unfortunately, common complication in this population and can develop in individuals with either acute or chronic SCI. Children or adolescents with pressure ulcers may need to be immobilized, hospitalized, or may require surgical repair. Furthermore, it may lead to additional complications, such as sepsis, osteomyelitis, and malnutrition.[71] In addition to the financial cost to families, the loss in terms of school, work, and opportunity is extensive. Therefore, preventative measures are very important and include frequent weight shifting, proper seating equipment, and an adequate wheelchair cushion; the goal is to prevent friction and shear forces, which are the main cause of pressure ulcer development. Thermal injuries may also occur to insensate areas. Prevention includes avoiding hot car heaters, radiators, hair dryers, curling irons, and hot plates or cups placed in the lap.

Heterotopic Ossification

Heterotopic ossification (HO), the formation of true bone at ectopic sites, is the most common orthopedic complication after SCI. Incidence of HO in pediatric SCI is between 3% and 18%, compared with 20% to 50% in adult SCI.[72,73] The most common site is around the hip joint. Less-frequent locations include the knee, elbow, and shoulder. The average onset of HO in the pediatric SCI population is reported as 14 months after injury, compared with 1 to 4 months after injury in the adult SCI population. The etiology of HO after SCI remains unknown. Fever is an early symptom, followed by joint swelling and pain that ultimately may limit joint range of motion. Differential diagnosis for HO includes DVT, cellulitis, fracture, impending ulcer, and septic arthritis. Increased inflammatory markers such as erythrocyte sedimentation rate (ESR), C-reactive protein (CRP), and serum alkaline phosphatase can be found in the early stages of HO. However, urinary levels of prostaglandin E2 (PGE2) have been shown to increase concomitantly with the progression of HO.[74] Bone scintigraphy is the most commonly used diagnostic study to detect HO in its early stages and typically becomes positive 2 to 3 weeks after the first appearance of soft tissue swelling. The first phase of the test represents the blood flow, the second phase shows blood pooling in hypervascular areas, and the third phase is a whole-body scan obtained 4 hours after administration of a radioactive test substance. The first two phases indicate perfusion and relative vascularity of the lesion.

Hyperemia is a precursor of the ossification process; therefore, bone perfusion measurements are important for early detection of HO as well as for monitoring the maturity of HO. Pharmacological prophylaxis to prevent HO is not routinely recommended in children due to relatively lower risk of HO in this population and the potential complications from editronate disodium (the most commonly used treatment for HO used in adults), including rachitic-like changes (outward bowing of long bones, pseudofractures, and thin, weak, painful bones).[75] Management of HO in children with SCI is otherwise similar to that in adults. Surgical resection of HO may be recommended when HO limits joint motion. Typically, this would occur 1 to 1.5 years after developing HO, once the heterotopic bone has fully matured, as supported by a normalized bone scan and laboratory values such as alkaline phosphatase.

Disorders of the Hip

In contrast to their adult counterparts, children frequently develop hip complications as a result of SCI.[76] Hip disorders in children with SCI range in severity and chronicity. These disorders include subluxation/dislocation, contractures, pathological fractures, septic arthritis, and HO (discussed above). Nonseptic hip subluxation/dislocation is the most common hip problem in children with SCI and occurs as a complication of both spastic and flaccid paralysis, although spasticity considerably increases the risk after SCI as in other neuromuscular disorders.[77] *Subluxation* is the term used when there is less than complete covering of the femoral head by the acetabulum, and *dislocation* is defined as having no contact between these two articular surfaces. In one study of children with SCI, aseptic hip subluxation/dislocation had an incidence of 82%.[77] Hip instability was also found to be related to age at onset of injury and time since injury.[78] Studies have shown that as many as 90% of children with SCI before age 10 years develop hip subluxation or dislocation, whereas less than 10% of children who sustain SCI after age 10 have this complication.[79] Subluxation and dislocation may occur unilaterally or bilaterally and are usually diagnosed radiographically.[80] Pathological hip fractures in children with SCI have a prevalence of 10% to 20%.[81] Up to 47% of long bone fractures in these children involve the hip joint.[82]

Individuals with hip complications may develop significant pain, difficulty with sitting, or challenging perineal hygiene. Hip disorders in children with SCI may also contribute to the formation of pelvic obliquity, which can lead to scoliosis, and skin breakdown. The management and prevention of hip disorders in children with SCI is controversial and should be directed by a team of pediatric orthopedic specialists with experience in this unique patient population. Preventative measures may be implemented early after SCI, but there are little data proving that these measures affect long-term outcome. Such conservative care often includes careful stretching, range of motion, control of spasticity, and prophylactic bracing.[83]

Management of hip fractures in children with SCI often presents challenges. Splinting and immobilization with soft tissue dressing and limited casting to prevent skin breakdown are currently recommended.[83] Providing individual family-oriented educational programs is important in order to emphasize the importance of safety, nutrition, equipment training, and preventative measures.

Surgical intervention for hip dislocation is even more controversial and is usually reserved for those children in whom a functional improvement in ambulation is a realistic goal. It is important to note that surgical intervention may not be definitive and does not necessarily prevent recurrent dislocations. In plegic children, since little functional benefit is expected, surgical reduction is not recommended.[84,85] Young age is also thought to reduce the chance of successful change in functional ambulation with surgical hip reduction.[77] Children with lower extremity paresis from incomplete SCI who are using functional electrical stimulation (FES) may benefit from the improved hip stability afforded by surgical reduction.[86–88] Gait analysis can assist in determining normal ambulatory patterns and the treatment modality best suited for the child.[89]

Spasticity

Here we address those aspects of spasticity that are of special consideration for children with SCI. (*See* Chapter 18 for detailed coverage of this topic.) Spasticity develops after a period of spinal shock, although there is no clear relationship between the duration or severity of spinal shock and the timing or severity of spasticity symptoms. Spasticity was defined by Lance in 1980[90] as "...a motor disorder characterized by a velocity-dependent increase in tonic stretch reflexes (muscle tone) with exaggerated tendon jerks, resulting from hyperexcitability of the stretch reflex, as one component of upper motor neuron syndrome." According to research results, 65% to 78% of sample populations with chronic SCI (≥1 year post-injury) have symptoms of spasticity.[91,92] Approximately 50% of children with SCI have spasticity that tends to be common in those with incomplete lesions.[93] Spasticity usually has a negative impact on the child's quality of life and can cause joint contractures, pressure ulcers, difficulty with care, negative self-image, pain, and an inability to participate in rehabilitation.

Management of spasticity in children must be individualized and, in general, should begin with less risky, conservative interventions and progress to the more aggressive and therefore risky options as indicated by the response to treatment. Spasticity management may include conservative physical rehabilitation modalities, pharmacologic interventions, injections for chemodenervation, intrathecal baclofen, and surgery. The number of these approaches is likely due to the fact that the syndrome can have various presentations, each with its own specific etiology. Therefore, appropriate therapy for children with SCI whose spasticity is diffuse often includes combination therapy instituted by a multidisciplinary rehabilitation team.

Pharmacological Interventions

For spasticity that impairs functioning and is refractory to conservative management, oral medications may be sufficient. Baclofen is commonly the initial drug of choice, although compliance and the potential for substance abuse of this and other drugs must be considered when using it in adolescents. Other pharmacologic agents that may be beneficial in the management of spasticity include diazepam, clonidine, and tizanidine. In addition, although not formally approved for use in spasticity, antiepileptic medications such as gabapentin may prove beneficial. Because of the potential effects on developing cognitive skills in children, use of antispasticity medications in childhood must be monitored closely.

Chemodenervation

For localized spasticity, chemodenervation with botulinum toxin (BTX) injections are an option, and the literature supports its use for treatment of spasticity in individuals with SCI.[94,95] By preventing release of acetylcholine at the neuromuscular junction, BTX reduces muscular activity in a dose-dependent manner. There is a body weight-dependent maximal dose that must not be exceeded if toxicity is to be avoided; the recommended safe total-body dose is 12 U/kg for BTX-A (Botox), or up to 400 U per person every 3 months, whichever is less.[96] However, experienced clinicians have reported that they regularly exceed the recommended maximal dose under certain circumstances without noting harmful effects.[97,98] Side effects are rare but include mild, generalized weakness, urinary incontinence, constipation, and dysphagia in more vulnerable individuals such as children. Contraindications

for BTX use include a history of disease affecting the neuromuscular junction, such as myasthenia gravis, and the use of aminoglycoside antibiotics and nondepolarizing muscle relaxants, since these medications can potentiate the action of BTX. Specifically in the SCI population, BTX injections are used most frequently to aid the control of bladder function.[99,100]

Intrathecal Baclofen Pumps

For diffuse spasticity that is unresponsive to oral agents, intrathecal baclofen is an option. Recent literature has shown that, by using an implanted pump, small amounts of intrathecal baclofen (Lioresal; Medtronics Inc., Minnea-polis, MN) can be delivered efficaciously to the cerebrospinal fluid in individuals with severe spasticity.[101] Theoretically, when the drug infuses intrathecally, the spinal sensory nerve activity will be decreased, resulting in a decrease in the excitatory drive to the spinal motor nerve that is thought to be the primary source of the hyperreflexia underlying the spasticity. Electrophysiologic studies[102–105] have confirmed a strong inhibition of lower limb mono- and polysynaptic potentials after intrathecal administration of baclofen. The intrathecal delivery allows a more potent antispasticity effect with decreased side effects.

Each candidate should undergo an intrathecal baclofen trial before pump placement. During the first trial, adults with SCI receive a 50 mcg bolus intrathecally. Onset of action occurs at approximately 1 hour after administration, with peak effect at 4 hours in most individuals. Loss of effect occurs by 8 hours. A successful result from an intrathecal baclofen trial is considered to have occurred if the administration is associated with a two-point decrease in the individual's modified Ashworth score or Penn spasm score. If the first trial is not successful, then a second trial with 75 mcg is attempted, which can be followed by a third trial with 100 mcg, if needed. If there is no effect from the third trial, implantation of the pump is not recommended. Following a successful trial, pumps are implanted under the abdominal wall or fascia, with a trend toward using the subfascial site in young children to prevent wound and skin complications.[106] The tip of the catheter is typically placed at the level of T10–T12 for individuals with paraplegia. In individuals with tetraplegia, to better control upper extremity spasticity, the catheter tip has recently been advanced to higher levels within the spinal canal (e.g., C5–T2).[107] The starting dose of the pump is generally recommended to be twice the effective trial dose, unless a prolonged effect (more than 8 hours) of the trial dose was seen. The intrathecal baclofen dose needs to be increased gradually by 5% to 20% per adjustment. Adjustments can be made every 24 hours or as tolerated. The average maintenance dose for the treatment of spinal origin spasticity is 400 to 600 mcg per day. There are no accepted guidelines for pediatric trial doses at this time.

Complications of baclofen pump placement include local and systemic infection, cerebrospinal fluid leakage and seroma around the pump, wound dehiscence, and catheter disconnection and migration.[108,109] Complications of intrathecal pumps occur more commonly in children than in adults[110] Following baclofen pump implantation, catheter dislodgement, kinking, or leakage may cause acute baclofen withdrawal. Adverse effects of abrupt cessation of intrathecal baclofen, such as rebound spasticity, agitation, itching, fever, seizures, and severe end-organ damage may be avoided if the problem is identified and managed in a timely fashion. Such adverse events can escalate to a life-threatening situation if not handled appropriately in the early stages. Therefore, emergent intervention is required. Individuals or parents and caregivers of children with an intrathecal baclofen pump should be instructed to administer oral baclofen when withdrawal is suspected until a complete pump evaluation is performed. In the event of acute baclofen withdrawal, severe agitation and muscle rigidity can be managed with intravenous benzodiazepines to decrease severe spasticity and agitation, thereby reducing the risk of developing rhabdomyolysis, which can subsequently impair renal function. Excessive doses can occur during trials or after pump refills. Symptoms of baclofen overdose include respiratory depression and arrest, drowsiness, dizziness, nausea, hypotension, and weakness. This overdosing should be managed by stopping the pump and beginning supportive care.

In summary, an intrathecal baclofen pump can be an effective treatment for severe diffuse spasticity, with potential for dramatic quality of life improvements and only a small number of significant complications. Long-term benefits and complications, however, need to be monitored in this complex population.

Hyercalcemia

A frequent cause of nonspecific gastrointestinal complaints in adolescents with SCI is hypercalcemia, which would usually manifest within the first 3 months post-injury. Hypercalcemia affects 10% to 23% of persons with SCI and is most common in young males.[111] Clinical symptoms and signs are nausea, vomiting, abdominal pain, poor appetite, polydipsia, and mental status change. The increase in bone turnover characteristic of growing children, combined with increased bone resorption seen in acute SCI, might be responsible for the high incidence of hypercalcemia in this population. Intravenous hydration and administration of furosemide are the recommended treatment, as they facilitate renal excretion of calcium and typically provide symptom relief within 3 to 4 days. Subcutaneous calcitonin may also be considered if these methods are ineffective. Prolonged hypercalcemia is associated with the development of urinary tract lithiasis (calcium oxalate "stones") and ultimately renal failure.[111]

Osteoporosis

There is rapid loss of trabecular bone in the lower extremities and pelvis in individuals with SCI, and homeostasis is reached by approximately 16 months post injury, with bone mass at 50% to 70% of normal and near fracture threshold.[88] Bone loss also occurs in the upper extremities of individuals with tetraplegia, but spinal density is relatively preserved. The bone loss is due to enhanced osteoclastic activity with relative hypercalcemia, hypercalciuria, and suppression of the parathyroid hormone–vitamin D axis. Bone loss continues over subsequent years due to aging. Fracture diagnosis in individuals with SCI is difficult because of the absence of pain. The child typically presents with a swollen limb, malaise, and a low-grade fever, and x-rays reveal a fracture. Fracture management most commonly consists of nonoperative care, including joint immobilization with well-padded splinting or casting. Immobilization time varies based on the type and location of the fracture and is followed by range of motion exercises.[112] Surgical intervention may be considered when conservative methods cannot control rotational deformity or when adequate immobilization cannot be achieved. Prophylactic anticoagulant therapy to prevent deep vein thrombosis should be considered in all individuals with SCI and lower limb fractures for perhaps 7 to14 days.[113]

Management of the Spine

The paralyzed, skeletally immature child is at a high risk for developing a spine deformity. These deformities occur as a result of a variety of factors, including asymmetric truncal weakness, injury to growth plates leading to asymmetric growth, post-laminectomy deformity, and chronic instability at the site of the injury. Furthermore, such deformities may be compounded by the presence of osteoporotic bone, spasticity, and posttraumatic syringomyelia. The incidence of scoliosis in children is close to 100% if SCI occurs prior to the pubertal growth spurt.[116]

Spinal column stability must be fully addressed prior to undertaking a program of rehabilitation. This examination requires obtaining anteroposterior and lateral views of the spine in the region of injury as well as full spine x-rays. These images will provide baseline films for documenting the development of progressive spinal deformity. The full spine x-rays also allow an opportunity to detect noncontiguous fractures that may have been overlooked during the inpatient admission. In a large series of more than 800 individuals with traumatic spinal fractures, approximately 6.4% harbored noncontiguous spine fractures.[116] Radiographic signs of potential instability include motion on flexion-extension x-rays, hardware breakage or pullout, and failure to observe a solid bony fusion. Clinically, the individual may complain of persistent pain or paresthesias with activity. If any suspicions arise, a CT scan of the area of interest will better address the presence of pseudoarthrosis.

Many children will have a brace at the time they begin the rehabilitative phase of care. The duration of brace wear is highly variable and depends on the type of injury, the quality of the fixation obtained, and surgeon preference. Generally, the cervical spine is immobilized for 3 months and the lumbar spine for 6 months. The thoracic spine is generally braced for a shorter time because of the additional support provided by the rib cage. Improved instrumentation techniques, in particular pedicle screw fixation, have shortened the time that most surgeons require the individual to wear a brace.

Mehta et al[117] studied the effect of bracing on development of scoliosis in 123 skeletally immature children. Forty-two children presented with a curve of less than 10 degrees. Twenty-nine out of 42 were braced. Only 13 (45%) of the 29 children who were braced eventually required surgical intervention in comparison to 77% (10 of 13) of the nonbraced group who went on to spinal fusion. A similar trend was observed for children who presented with curves between 10 and 20 degrees. In addition, the braced group demonstrated a longer time period to surgical fusion, thus allowing for maximal truncal growth. Instituting bracing in skeletally immature children who present with complete SCI is therefore recommended. The brace most commonly used is the thoracolumbosacral orthosis (TLSO). There are currently no good data supporting the length of time each day that the brace should be worn, but longer lengths of time appear better and a minimum of 12 hours per day is required. In-brace x-rays should be obtained to document the effectiveness of the brace (ideally the curve should reduce by 50%). Subsequently, x-rays are obtained at 4- to 6-month intervals to assess for curve progression. If curve progression is documented or if the curve exceeds an angle of 50 degrees, then surgical intervention is contemplated.

The decision to undergo surgical correction is based on assessment of the overall curve angle, sitting posture, and development of pressure sores. The objectives of surgical intervention are to obtain correction and balance the spine over the pelvis, to distribute sitting skin pressure equally, and to minimize pressure ulcers. The surgical procedures involve fusing the spine from T1 or T2 down to the pelvis. In this way, the pelvic obliquity, which is often present, is adequately addressed. These procedures can be successfully done using either sublaminar wires or pedicle screw constructs.

Children with SCI have decreased nutritional and respiratory reserves. Thus, they have an increased risk of postoperative complications, including wound infection, respiratory difficulties, and failure to form a solid fusion. Postoperative activity restrictions depend on the quality of fixation that has been attained. Children with SCI are often restricted from performing independent transfers or operating a manual wheelchair for 6 months after surgery. However, if strong fixation is attained, then the length of time of these restrictions may be reduced.

Psychological Care of the Child and Family

The psychological care of children with SCI represents one of the most important aspects of the multidisciplinary team approach to rehabilitation of the child with SCI. As psychological factors tend to impact every aspect of rehabilitation, children and their families may require a long-term psychological treatment plan. Despite the great need for research in this field, there remains a dearth of information specific to the management of the psychological care of children with SCI. Some authors have described the psychosocial adjustment to pediatric SCI, focusing primarily upon the longer-term adjustment of children and adolescents in the outpatient setting.[118] Little information is available regarding the acute inpatient phase, specifically during the period of time immediately following injury.

Comparison of Response to SCI in Children Versus Adults

Children and their parents tend to vary greatly with regard to their response and adjustment to the trauma. The interactions of health-care providers who serve pediatric SCI patients often leave lasting impressions and can influence the emotional adjustment of the child or adolescent. In many children's hospitals, medical and rehabilitation teams have the benefit of the services of mental health professionals who specialize in pediatric critical care and rehabilitation. However, in settings that lack such integration of mental health care, members of the inpatient team will need to obtain the skills necessary to minimize psychological distress and maximize the coping abilities of the child and family.

The psychological care of children with SCI and their families evolves during the acute hospitalization, inpatient rehabilitation, and throughout the child's life. Treatment is complex, as multiple factors affect the child's and family's ability to cope and adapt to this life-altering injury. Children will benefit most from psychological and social support interventions that are appropriate to their age, developmental level, and level of perceived family functioning,[119,120] all of which may change over time. Fortunately, children with SCI often demonstrate remarkable long-term resilience. One study revealed that adults with SCI who sustained their injury during childhood (versus adulthood) reported significantly better health-related quality of life and expressed better performance in physical functioning than did individuals who had sustained their injury in adulthood.[121] Another study determined that greater life satisfaction remained associated with higher level of education, income, satisfaction with employment, and social and recreational opportunities.[122] Level of injury, age at injury, and duration of injury failed to correlate with life satisfaction, while a greater number of medical complications remained associated with lower life satisfaction.[122] Adults who sustained SCI during childhood demonstrate greater satisfaction with their adult life if rehabilitation strengthened their psychosocial, educational, vocational, and long-term medical well-being.[122] Improvements in the acute medical management of SCI have resulted in enhanced functional capacities of children and adolescents, with resultant improvements in quality of life.[123,124]

Managing Stress and Anxiety in the Pediatric Intensive Care Unit

SCIs may involve protracted stays in a pediatric intensive care unit, particularly with cervical injuries requiring ventilatory support. Upon awakening in the intensive care unit, the child will experience a plethora of unfamiliar sights, sounds, and medical interventions that often are painful and that can exacerbate feelings of anxiety and fear. Children tend to react with a range of emotional and behavioral responses.[125] They may withdraw, regress, cry or scream inconsolably, become irritable, aggressive, nonadherent, and refuse to eat or communicate. In some cases, passive suicidal ideation may present as nonadherence with treatment. In other cases, children may demonstrate more active suicidal ideation and behaviors, perhaps by engaging in self-destructive behaviors. Psychological interventions that acknowledge the child's fear and anxiety in a calm and resolute manner can help the child to cooperate with medical interventions. During episodes of acute emotional distress, the child is usually not ready to hear the implications of the injury or even explanations regarding medical interventions. While seemingly paradoxical, acknowledging distress in an empathic manner will typically help the child to calm down, after which time the child may become more receptive to the intervention. However, occasionally the empathic approach will worsen emotional reactions in some children. In these instances, the health provider can only remain resolute, while "riding the wave" of emotional distress reactions demonstrated by the child. A clinical child psychologist can be a tremendous resource for the health-care team in cases of behaviorally challenged children with SCI.

Psychological Preparation of the Child and Family for Rehabilitation

The pediatric rehabilitation unit is often viewed by parents as the place where their child will learn to walk again. Parents may enter this phase of treatment with very high expectations regarding the outcomes of treatments. Whenever possible, efforts to conduct direct communication between the parents and members of the rehabilitation care team prior to transfer can help to reduce unrealistic expectations and set more reasonable goals for the inpatient stay. The transfer to the rehabilitation unit may increase fear and anxiety in both children and their parents, especially with regard to the child's medical safety and overall stability. Because of this possibility, the rehabilitation team should monitor the child more frequently during the first few days and until the child has successfully transitioned to the new environment. Increased assessment of vital signs, twice daily physician rounds, and more frequent discussions with the child and family about the treatment plan can all facilitate this transition process.

Whether verbalized or not, the question regarding their child's potential to walk again is foremost on the minds of all parents. This question cannot be answered with any degree of certainty, especially during the acute hospital phase. While supporting the child's and parents' initial feelings of hope for the best outcome possible, members of the health-care team need to firmly yet gently remind them that complete recovery may not happen. If and when the long-term prognosis is declared, the child and parents may experience intense feelings of grief and despair, which may require increased support from staff and other family members. Focusing on the "here and now" with great care and sensitivity during this delicate time can often facilitate the coping process.

When the child confronts the longer-term implications of the injury, he or she may plaintively ask, "Why me?" for the first time. The child may perceive the injury as punishment for real or imagined mistakes[125] and may withdraw while combating feelings of intense rage, grief, and/or humiliation.[125] Psychological interventions provide the opportunity to process thoughts and feelings such as anger, sadness, depressed mood, feelings of self-blame or blame toward others who failed to protect the child from the injury. One psychological intervention includes asking the child, "If we could know *why* you were injured, would it help you to feel better, or would it make a difference in how angry/hurt/upset/sad/depressed you feel *right now*?" This intervention serves to empathize with the child's emotional distress and provides a forum through which to gain a better appreciation of any attributions of cause for the injury that the child may have previously internalized. Following this initial response, the child may demonstrate difficulty with coping with the physical changes in appearance accompanied by the SCI.[125]

Posttraumatic Stress Disorder in Children

Posttraumatic stress disorder (PTSD) occurs commonly in children and parents after life-threatening injuries, particularly when injuries involve violence.[126] Experiences in the trauma center and intensive care unit even after relatively mild trauma can activate PTSD or, more specifically, in some cases induce an acute stress disorder in children.[127] Symptoms include nightmares or daytime flashbacks, insomnia, apathy, detachment from others, restricted range of feelings and interests, difficulty concentrating, exaggerated startle response, and increased anxiety, all of which can inhibit participation in rehabilitation and long-term self-care. The symptoms of PTSD or acute stress disorder symptoms are different in children than in adults. These symptoms among children with SCI include acting younger than their age, increased somatic complaints, and excessively worrying about dying.[128,129] Parental PTSD may impact their ability to provide appropriate care and support for their child.[126] Thus, the evaluation and treatment of PTSD, as well for other anxiety and mood disorders, including depression, in the child and parents remain important in their overall care. While cognitive-behavioral therapy has been shown to be effective in PTSD and should be tried first, psychopharmacological management may be helpful, particularly when depression and other mood disorders are present.[130]

The child and family's response to SCI may result in changes in the parent–child relationship, such that the parent may set fewer limits, discipline unacceptable behavior less, or become overprotective. The child or adolescent may respond with inappropriate behavior, such as rebelling against the parent or refusing to adhere to self-care or medical treatment regimens.[131] The health professional can intervene by reassuring the parent that the child will benefit most from parenting that focuses directly on dealing with the behavior versus the injury. Setting boundaries and enforcing discipline provides the child with a feeling of security and safety at a time when the child feels most insecure and out of control. As many children experience fear of abandonment, at least one parent or other family member should remain at bedside as much as possible and be directly involved in the medical care and rehabilitative therapies of the child, including venipuncture, imaging procedures, dressing changes, and physician and nursing rounds. Integrating the parent as a member of the medical/rehabilitative team also facilitates parental feelings of usefulness, rebuilds their confidence in their role as a parent, and lays the foundation for greater parental participation in the child's rehabilitation and lifelong care following discharge.

Interventions for Parents and Caregivers of Children With SCI

Interventions for parents should match their apparent coping style and level of psychological distress. If a psychologist is not available, then the medical staff will need to assess whether the parent is using an emotion-focused versus information-focused coping style. The former will seek more emotional comfort in response to the trauma, while the latter will seek more information regarding prognosis and treatment course. Parents may struggle with guilt about not protecting the child from harm, frustration with the health-care delivery system, and denial and anger regarding the long-term prognosis. As these intense feelings may result in difficulties with comprehending medical information, staff should take care to ensure that all information and training are presented effectively. Information stated in short, easy-to-understand language that avoids medical jargon can facilitate comprehension and acceptance of the current prognosis and treatment plan. The health provider may need to respond to the same questions repeatedly, with the understanding that acute psychological distress impairs the ability to attend to, process, and recall information.

Health-care professionals, especially those in resuscitation or intensive care settings, but also in rehabilitation centers, may find themselves confronting their own discomfort regarding SCI and paralysis. Managing these feelings is an integral component of maintaining professional boundaries. For example, individuals who place a high priority on physical activities and sports may have difficulty with confronting the child's immobility. Such feelings may cause an individual to either disengage completely or to become inappropriately overinvolved in the care of the child and family and could lead to breaches in professionalism. If left unchecked, these feelings may hinder the ability to serve as an effective leader or member of the medical team. Any of these psychological reactions have the potential to negatively affect the relationship between the individual with SCI and the health care provider and deserve careful attention on the part of the health-care professional. All who deal with the child and family must understand that children and adolescents who experience SCI can demonstrate remarkable resilience and positive coping if afforded proper psychosocial care and appropriate opportunities for educational, social, recreational, and occupational success.[122]

Management of the Upper Extremities in Children With SCI

The upper extremity of children with tetraplegia has features similar to adult-onset SCI, with a few notable exceptions.[132] Because of their small trunk size, younger children with tetraplegia are able to reach their mouths with elbow flexion and little shoulder forward flexion; in essence, everything they need to access is within their immediate workspace. Since the requirements for active range of shoulder forward flexion and abduction is minimal in young children, they are at great risk for significant shoulder contractures. The functional significance of active shoulder range of motion may not be appreciated until the children grow and are no longer able to reach their mouths. Similar to recommendations for range of motion of the hip, active or active-assisted range of motion of the shoulder at each diaper change, or at least three times a day, will prevent future problems in activity performance.

Splinting

The hands of infants and toddlers are too small to benefit from commercially available splints and adaptive equipment.

Custom-made splints for function can be fabricated to assist in grasping of bottles, cookies, and age-appropriate toys. For very young children, when mouthing of the hand or when teething occurs, the insensate hand is at risk for breakdown, and protection splints may be required. A problematic secondary complication of SCI in children injured before 5 years of age with midcervical SCI is metacarpal-phalengeal (MCP) extension deformities. Prophylactic nighttime splinting should be prescribed prior to the onset of the deformity so limitations in the future will be avoided.

Tendon Transfers

In cases of SCI, the principle of tendon transfer is that if there are two or more preserved muscles that perform the same function, one of those muscles can be transferred to provide a distal function without compromise to the original function. For example, when all three muscles that flex the elbow have been preserved, the brachioradialis can be transferred to the wrist for restoration of active wrist extension. The principles of tendon transfers and other soft tissue reconstruction procedures that are described in Chapter 10 are also applicable to children.[133,134]

For children and youths with C5 level SCI, tendon transfers and/or upper limb FES systems increase independence by reducing the amount and level of support required by a personal care attendant. The number and type of activities that can be accomplished are also broader for those with C5 SCI after tendon transfers and/or FES. Importantly, children with complete C5 SCI will continue to require two hands for activities because of the loss of thumb control, even with tendon transfers and FES. In contrast, through tendon transfers or FES, children with complete C6 SCI gain unilateral and bimanual function. In addition, for these children, upper limb reconstruction reduces or eliminates the need for adaptive equipment, thereby enabling children to become more spontaneous throughout the day and exert less effort to complete a task. Because of the significance of hand function for self-care, school, and play activities, these interventions are recommend for children with SCI prior to entering first grade and, for those injured during childhood and adolescence, at the time of neurological stability, even if stability occurs within 6 months of the injury.

Task-Oriented Practice and Training

Task-oriented training has emerged as a promising rehabilitation paradigm in SCI. Task-oriented training is a term used to describe an exercise program that focuses on repeated practice of task-oriented activities. Task-oriented training stimulates and recruits the central pattern generators of the spinal cord to assist with voluntary control of movement. While adult reports on body-supported treadmill training and cycling have been published, little work has been done with children. (See Chapter 13, regarding locomotor training, and Chapter 11, regarding upper extremity training, for an extensive review of the adult literature in this area.)

Functional Electrical Stimulation

Perhaps the highest level of evidence supporting task-oriented training in children is emerging from work done at the Shriners Hospital for Children in Philadelphia. Lauer et al[135] in Philadelphia have enrolled 30 children into a randomized controlled trial designed to study the outcomes of FES-assisted cycling, passive cycling, and other FES exercise. Children participated in the exercise for 1 hour, three times per week at home. To date, data are available on 12 children, and the report suggests trends toward increases in bone mineral density (BMD), strength, and cardiovascular parameters. Children in the FES-assisted active cycling group had the greatest improvements in these parameters compared to children in the passive cycling and other FES exercise groups. In addition, a fasting blood lipid profile was performed, and in all cases, serum triglyceride decreased, which could improve long-term cardiovascular status. While these data are only preliminary, the trends are promising.

Training in Activities of Daily Living

Activities of daily living (ADLs), including feeding, dressing, bathing, transferring, grooming, and community activities, need to be relearned in order for the child to regain independence. Bladder self-catheterization should be included in these activities. For young children, teaching may be incorporated into play activities. By the age of 5, children with paraplegia are usually capable of being independent in the majority of self-care activities with supervision. Children with high level SCI should be taught how to direct a caregiver to assist them with these various activities.

Orthotic Options for Standing and Walking

When designing orthotics for children with SCI, many factors must be considered, including developmental level, potential growth, functional status, and cognitive abilities. The type of orthosis needed depends on the age of the child, the level of SCI, and the presence of deformities. Children with complete SCI at the level of C7 and above are wheelchair dependent. Some children with upper thoracic lesions may ambulate with a hip-knee-ankle-foot orthosis (HKAFO) or reciprocal gait orthosis (RGO) and use a walker or crutches for transfers. RGOs are used by children with lesions at the level of L2 or higher. It provides more energy-efficient reciprocal gait for individuals with active hip flexion. RGOs can be initiated in children as young as 15 to 18 months old. A thoracolumbosacral orthosis (TLSO) may also be indicated for improving trunk support and postural alignment.

Children with a T12–L1 level of SCI injury can walk using HKAFOs and crutches, with a swing-through gait pattern. Children with SCI at the level of L3 or below typically become community ambulators and may use a knee-ankle-foot orthosis (KAFO) with crutches or a cane. Children with SCI below L4 walk using only an ankle-foot orthosis (AFO) without any assistive devices. In general, children are more likely to be active ambulators compared with adults because of their small size, higher energy levels, and less concern for cosmesis.[69] Parapodia, mechanical support systems for the trunk and lower extremities, allow children with SCI to stand without upper extremity weight bearing, thereby allowing them to perform activities using both hands. Parapodia can be used in children as young as 9 to 12 months of age, and they typically outgrow it by 7 to 10 years of age.[59]

Wheelchairs for Children With SCI

A wheelchair should be provided for the child with SCI as soon as possible after injury. There are many different types of wheelchairs, including standard, powered, recliner, tilt in space, standing, and seat elevator. Even children who are expected to be household ambulators will usually need a wheelchair for long distances and for greater independence at school and in the community. Children with high level tetraplegia will require a power wheelchair, as they are unable to self-propel a manual wheelchair with their upper extremities. Children as young as 2 years of age can be trained to use a power wheelchair under supervision.[136] Most children with tetraplegia and paraplegia should be fitted for a wheelchair by age 3 to 4. The chair should be customized to fit the individual child, and seating posture is examined biomechanically. The wheelchair should be adjustable to accommodate for growth, orthoses, and ventilators. Furthermore, wheelchair training should be done on several different types of surfaces, from flat or level to curbs to rougher terrain. (This is discussed in greater detail in Chapter 8.)

Discharge and Disposition

Discharge planning should begin even before the child is admitted to the rehabilitation unit. Members of the rehabilitation team will arrange for an on-site home visit to prepare for the child's discharge. Many home modifications need to be completed prior to the child leaving the hospital to make the home wheelchair accessible. These modifications include building a wheelchair ramp, removing high curbs, modifying the bathroom with handle bars or a tub bench, and adjusting the height of the toilet seat to facilitate transfers without assistance. Additionally, if the child needs to climb stairs, a stair glider or elevator may be considered. Alternatively, creating a first floor setup (bedroom and bathroom) may be easier and more affordable.

For children who will require complex medical and nursing care at home, another option is a transitional medical home care or step-down nursing care unit. The child with SCI is ready for discharge when (1) he or she can continue the same recovery rate with less intensive therapy as an outpatient, (2) the child and family have met inpatient educational goals regarding care, (3) equipment and other supplies needed for care of the child have been delivered to the home, and (4) appropriate provisions have been made for transport to and from school, the outpatient rehabilitation center, and medical and surgical clinics for follow-up care.

School Reentry for Children With SCI

Preparation for school reentry begins while the child with SCI is relearning mobility and self-care skills during inpatient rehabilitation. Allowing the child to attend school or resume schoolwork in the hospital during inpatient rehabilitation is ideal. The rehabilitation team should evaluate the child's school and correct any architectural barriers. School staff and students need to be educated about SCI, and parents or caregivers should be informed of the ongoing need for therapeutic services at school. Furthermore, in some instances, a child may elect to switch from private to public school, where therapies and modification of architectural barriers are guaranteed. In many cases, a brief period of homebound schooling is instituted for the first few months after discharge from inpatient rehabilitation so that the child can continue to participate in intensive outpatient rehabilitation, accommodations can be made in the school, and parents can become more comfortable with allowing their child to return to school, particularly from a safety standpoint.

Concerns for the Older Child With SCI

As children with SCI grows into adolescence, or for children who are injured in adolescence, they face the same issues as do their nondisabled peers; the pressure to "fit in" becomes even greater at this stage of life. With appropriate counseling and education, children with SCI can have happy and fulfilling lives.

Sexuality and Fertility

Sexuality is considered in detail in Chapters 21 and 22. Children with SCI and their caregivers need to be informed about how SCI affects sexuality and fertility and what interventions, if any, are available that can restore normalcy in these areas. The information needs to be developmentally appropriate and presented in an optimistic fashion. Parents need to know that children with SCI may begin to ask direct questions about sexuality at ages as young as 8 years of age. Sexual counseling for adolescents should be done without parents or caretakers present. By the teenage years, these discussions may include specific information, such as birth control methods. Teenage peer group discussions about dating and self-esteem may also prove helpful. Furthermore, teenagers may benefit from having mentors with SCI who can facilitate discussions of this type with humor and real-life experiences.

Women with SCI are affected less than men with regards to fertility and sexual activity. Women can be assured that SCI results in only minor or possibly even no abnormalities or delays in onset or resumption of menstruation, and that fertility is spared[114] Conversely, most men with SCI have decreased ejaculatory function, which contributes greatly to decreased fertility. In addition, the semen of men with SCI contains a lower percentage of motile sperm, and the number of sperm produced decreases with time following injury. Recent research shows the average motility rate of sperm in semen samples collected from men with SCI is 20% compared to 70% in able-bodied men.[115]

Driving

For older children who are eligible to drive, a referral is made to a driving center that has the personnel, experience, and equipment to train and assess individuals for safe driving. One method of training requires the individual to first master safe-driving skills in a virtual driving simulator before proceeding to real road conditions. Modifications will need to be made to the car, including hand controls, seat and seatbelt design, wheelchair lift, and remote or voice-activated controls.

CASE STUDY 24-1   SCIWORA in a Three-year-old Child With Tetraplegia

This case study demonstrates many of the features of SCI that are unique to children. A 3-year-old boy sustained acute tetraplegia secondary to a fall from less than 3 feet. On arrival at the hospital, he had no sensory or motor function below C4. He was immediately intubated and placed on mechanical ventilation. CT scans and plain x-rays showed no cervical abnormality, which, together with tetraplegia on exam, confirmed the diagnosis of SCIWORA. The MRI showed signal abnormalities and diffuse swelling from C2 to T4. He did not require surgical intervention and was placed in a cervical collar for 3 months. His neurological exam did not change, and when weaning was attempted, he became diaphoretic and very anxious. A tracheostomy was performed for chronic ventilatory support, and a nasogastric tube was placed for nutritional support, with the hope that his oral intake would improve later. A Foley catheter was placed initially, followed by institution of intermittent catheterization every 4 hours. Vitamin C and hippuric acid were given to prevent urinary tract infection. He later required ditropan to prevent bladder spasms. The bowel program consisted of stool softeners and one-half of a bisacodyl suppository every other day. Anticoagulants were not given. Skin care consisted of turning every 2 hours and close surveillance for pressure-related injuries. A pediatric psychologist evaluated the child and family and remained heavily involved throughout the hospitalization. The child protection team was consulted because of the unusual nature of the injury, and they concluded that the injury was indeed accidental. Psychosocial evaluation revealed that the father was incarcerated and the mother had abandoned the child to the grandmother's care. It was discovered that he had been made a ward of the state previously. After 6 weeks in the pediatric ICU, he was transferred to the pediatric rehabilitation unit on ventilator support.

On arrival at the rehabilitation unit, the most important and difficult problem to address was the child's depressed psychological state. He was severely withdrawn and cried constantly. He made no attempt to speak and refused to take anything by mouth, including medications. He refused to participate in any form of therapy. He was felt to be too young for antidepressant medication and that his depressed mood and anxiety were situational and not due to organic mental illness. A gastrostomy tube was placed because of severe oral aversion, and the nasogastric tube removed. Initial attempts to liberate him from mechanical ventilation were successful in reducing the settings on the ventilator (4 breaths per minute), but he experienced easy fatigability, recurrent hypoxemia, atelectasis, and greater psychological stress. Weaning trials were abandoned, and the ventilator settings were increased (10 breaths per minute), which greatly improved his mood and endurance. It was decided to slow down the pace of his rehabilitation and to focus on reducing his fear and anxiety and improving his mood. He was moved to a bed by a large window, and his room was redecorated with toys, dolls, Sesame Street posters, etc. Family members and friends, especially other children, were encouraged to spend more time at the bedside. He was taken on field trips, to movies, and to the swimming pool, and was allowed to ride a pony for his birthday (with maximal assistance). He improved gradually. Two months after admission, he took his first oral intake—a gummy bear. He later progressed to a single French fry for lunch and dinner. He learned to ask to be suctioned and manually ventilated when needed.

Psychological support included calm, consistent, and frequent reassurances to the child that he would be kept safe, that he would not be alone or abandoned, and that everyone in the rehabilitation unit cared about him and wanted to make him well so he could go home. Acute anxiety and fear of abandonment occurred frequently, especially at the conclusion of family visits when family members left the hospital. The child participated in creating his daily schedule

CASE STUDY 24-1   SCIWORA in a Three-year-old Child With Tetraplegia—cont'd

of activities, including rehabilitation, and boundaries were set and adhered to. Punishment for misbehaving consisted of time out. Family members experienced tremendous grief and required intensive counseling and support.

Speech therapists focused on providing extra- and intra-oral stimulation to reduce his feeding aversion and to encourage oral feeding. In addition, he was trained to vocalize while on the ventilator. He was able to produce short utterances that, despite being characterized by reduced vocal loudness, were intelligible enough for him to be able to communicate orally. Voice output was assisted with lengthening the inspiratory time of each ventilator breath to 2 seconds. The family was trained to provide stimulation for his oral aversion as well as cueing to improve speech production. The occupational therapists concentrated on teaching him how to use a mouthstick to activate toys, turn pages, color, brush paint, and use a computer. Considerable time was spent educating the child and family on SCI topics such as range of motion, positioning, nutrition, skin care, bowel and bladder management, and splinting, among other topics. Physical therapy goals consisted of family education to prevent and limit issues with skin and skeletal deformity through positioning, splinting, and range of motion activities and teaching skills to become independent with bed mobility, transfers, and wheelchair mobility. He had no sustained spasticity, but later developed paroxysms of spontaneous, sustained clonus of the lower extremities, which resolved with low-dose baclofen. Goals consisted of becoming independent with wheelchair mobility both indoors and outdoors using a mouth joystick for the power wheelchair. A standing frame was used for weight bearing of lower

extremities for 1 hour three to five times per week, using chest, waist, and leg straps as well as lateral hip supports. An abdominal binder was used during the day for trunk support and to enhance respiratory function. The recreation therapist taught him power wheelchair skills in the community through campus hikes, community skills trips, and attending a ventilator-assisted day camp. He also experienced going into the pool and playing with other children. Additionally, he learned to use the sip and puff controller to operate computer games such as Nintendo and was taught to direct others to assist him to meet his recreational and leisure needs.

Discharge planning consisted of home modifications, setting up 24-hour nursing, having the home nurses do a shift in the rehabilitation unit to learn his care, ordering and delivery of equipment and supplies to the home, training family members in CPR and in the use of all of his equipment, and scheduling medical return visits for follow-up care. He was eventually discharged home on 24-hour ventilator support 14 months after the initial injury.

This case illustrates many of the challenges in the rehabilitation of children with SCI. As with other chronic diseases of childhood, empowering the child and family to manage the disease at home is critical to a successful outcome, yet still there can be unforeseeable complications. This case also makes clear how much effort is required on the part of the rehabilitation, general pediatric, and pediatric subspecialty teams. The African saying, "it takes a village to raise a child" certainly applies to the level of support required to provide children with SCI and their families the opportunity to regain an acceptable quality of life.

Summary

Rehabilitation of the child with SCI often presents problems not seen in adults with similar injuries. Promising results from basic science and clinical research suggest that children have greater potential for recovery of function compared to their adult counterparts. These data strengthen the argument for allocating greater resources to pediatric SCI research and clinical care of children with SCI. A comprehensive, multidisciplinary child- and family-oriented approach to the acute- and long-term care of children with SCI is needed to combat this devastating injury and improve quality of life for affected individuals. Injury prevention, early intervention, and preventative strategies against secondary complications are needed to reduce the long-term personal and societal costs of this disease.

REVIEW QUESTIONS

1. What are the different consequences for injury to spinal vertebrae in children compared to adults, and why do they occur?
2. What are the medical sequelae of SCI in children?
3. What are the risk factors for development of hip disorders that may occur after SCI in children, and how may these be prevented?
4. What are the factors that affect the decision to place an intrathecal baclofen pump in children with SCI, and what are the potential complications associated with this intervention?
5. What are the spinal deformities that may develop in children with SCI, and why do these occur?
6. Describe a comprehensive discharge plan for a child with SCI, including family and home readiness and a plan for school reentry.

REFERENCES

1. Reynolds R. Pediatric spinal injury. *Curr Opin Pediatr.* 2000;12(1):67–71.
2. Nobunaga AI, Go BK, and Karunas RB. Recent demographic and injury trends in people served by the Model Spinal Cord Injury Care Systems. *Arch Phys Med Rehabil.* 1999;80(11):1372–1382.
3. Augutis M, Abel R, and Levi R. Pediatric spinal cord injury in a subset of European countries. *Spinal Cord.* 2006;44(2):106–112.
4. Vitale MG, Goss JM, Matsumoto H et al. Epidemiology of pediatric spinal cord injury in the United States: Years 1997 and 2000. *J Pediatr Orthop.* 2006;26(6):745–749.
5. Birney TJ, and Hanley EN Jr. Traumatic cervical spine injuries in childhood and adolescence. *Spine.* 1989;14:277–282.
6. Dickman CA, Rekate HL, Donntag VK et al. Pediatric spinal trauma: Vertebral column and spinal cord injuries in children. *Pediatr Neurosci.* 1989;15:237–256.
7. Hadley MN, Zabramski JM, Browner CM et al. Pediatric spinal trauma: Review of 122 cases of spinal cord and vertebral column injuries. *J Neurosurg.* 1988;68:18–24.
8. Ruge JR, Sinson GP, McLone DG et al. Pediatric spinal injury: The very young. *J Neurosurg.* 1988;68:25–30.
9. Hasue M, Hoshino R, Omata S et al. Cervical spine injuries in children. *Fukushima J Med Sci.* 1974;20:115–123.
10. Hill SA, Miller CA, Kosnik EJ et al. Pediatric neck injuries: A clinical study. *J Neurosurg.* 1984;60:700–706.
11. Zike K. Delayed neuropathy after injury to the cervical spine in children. *Pediatrics.* 1959;24:413–417.
12. Bresnan MJ, Abroms IF. Neonatal spinal cord transection secondary to intrauterine hyperextension of the neck in breech presentation. *J Pediatr.* 1974;84:734–737.
13. Kewalramani LS, Kraus JF, Sterling HM. Acute spinal-cord lesions in a pediatric population: Epidemiological and clinical features. *Paraplegia.* 1980;18:206–219.
14. Ohry A, Rozin R, Brooks ME. Pediatric spinal cord injuries in Israel. *Isr J Med Sci.* 1985;21:526–528.
15. Pang D, Willberger JE Jr. Spinal cord injury without radiographic abnormalities in children. *J Neurosurg.* 1982;57:114–129.
16. Townsend EH Jr, Rowe ML. Mobility of the upper cervical spine in health and disease. *Pediatrics.* 1952;10:567–573.
17. Sullivan CR, Bruwer AJ, Harris E. Hypermobility of the cervical spine in children. A pitfall in the diagnosis of cervical dislocation. *Am J Surg.* 1958;95:636–640.
18. Henrys P, Lyne ED, Lifton C et al. Clinical review of cervical spine injuries in children. *Clin Orthop.* 1977;129,172–176.
19. Leventhal HR. Birth injuries of the spinal cord. *J Pediatr.* 1960;56:447–453.
20. Pang D. Spinal cord injury without radiographic abnormality in children, 2 decades later. *Neurosurgery.* 2004;55(6):1325–1342.
21. Maynard FM Jr, Bracken MB, Creasey G et al. International standards for neurological and functional classification of spinal cord injury patients (revised 1996). *Spinal Cord.* 1997;35:266–274.
22. Mulcahey MJ, Gaughan J, Betz RR et al. The international standards for neurological classification of spinal cord injury: Reliability of data when applied to children and youths. *Spinal Cord.* 2007;45:452–459.
23. Kunkel-Bagden E, Dai HN, Bregman BS. Recovery of function after spinal cord hemisection in newborn and adult rats: Differential effects on reflex and locomotor function. *Exp Neurol.* 1992;116(1),40–45.
24. Nicholls J, Saunders N. Regeneration of immature mammalian spinal cord after injury. *Trends Neurosci.* 1996;19(6):229–234.
25. Saunders NR, Kitchener P, Knott GW et al. Development of walking, swimming, and neuronal connections after complete spinal cord transection in the neonatal opossum, Monodelphis domestica. *J Neurosci.* 1998;18(1):339–355.
26. Bernstein DR, Stelzner DJ. Plasticity of the corticospinal tract following midthoracic spinal injury in the postnatal rat. *J Comp Neurol.* 1983;221:382–400.
27. Van den Aardweg GJ, Hopewell JW, Whitehouse EM. A new model of radiation-induced myelopathy: A comparison of the response of mature and immature pigs. *Int J Radiat Oncol Biol Phys.* 1983;29(4):763–770.
28. Saunders NR, Deal A, Knott GW et al. Repair and recovery following spinal cord injury in a neonatal marsupial (Monodelphis domestica). *Clin Exp Pharmacol Physiol.* 1995;22(8):518–526.
29. Wang XM, Basso DM, Terman JR et al. Adult opossums (*Didelphis viirginiana*) demonstrate near normal locomotion after spinal cord transection as neonates. *Exp Neurol.* 1998;151(1):50–60.
30. Osterholm JL. The pathophysiological response to spinal cord injury: The current status of related research. *J Neurosurg.* 1974;40:5–33.
31. Senter HJ, Venes JL. Loss of autoregulation and posttraumatic ischemia following experimental spinal cord trauma. *J Neurosurg.* 1979;50:198–206.
32. Dusart I, Schwab ME. Secondary cell death and the inflammatory reaction after dorsal hemisection of the rat spinal cord. *Eur J Neurosci.* 1994;6:712–724.
33. Anderson DK, Howl DR, Reier PJ. Fetal neural grafts and repair of the injured spinal cord. *Brain Pathol.* 1995;5(4):451–457.
34. Giovanini MA, Reier PJ, Eskin TA et al. Characteristics of human fetal spinal cord grafts in the adult rat spinal cord: Influences of lesion and grafting conditions. *Exp Neurol.* 1997;148(2):523–543.
35. Kluft J, Beker L, Castagnino M et al. A comparison of bronchial drainage treatments in cystic fibrosis. *Pediatr Pulmonol.* 1996;22:271–274.
36. Nantwi KD, Goshgarian HG. Effects of chronic systemic theophylline injections on recovery of hemidiaphragmatic function after cervical spinal cord injury in adult rats. *Brain Res.* 1998;789(1):126–129.
37. Nantwi KD, Goshgarian HG. Adenosinergic mechanisms underlying recovery of diaphragm motor function following upper cervical spinal cord injury: Potential therapeutic implications. *Neurol Res.* 2005;27(2):195–205.
38. Bascom AT, Lattin CD, Aboussouan LS et al. Effect of acute aminophylline administration on diaphragm function in high cervical tetraplegia: A case report. *Chest.* 2005;127(2):658–661.
39. Montero JC, Feldman DJ, Montero D. Effects of glossopharyngeal breathing on respiratory function after

cervical cord transection. *Arch Phys Med Rehab.* 1967; 48(12):650–653.

40. DiPasquale PA. Exhaler class: A multidisciplinary program for high quadriplegic patients. *Am J Occup Ther.* 1986;40:482–485.

41. Bach JR, Rogers B, King A. Noninvasive respiratory muscle aids: Intervention goals and mechanism of action. In Bach JR, editor. *Management of Patients with Neuromuscular Disease.* Philadelphia: Hanley & Belfus; 2004. pp. 211–269.

42. Padman R, Alexander M, Thorogood C et al. Respiratory management of pediatric patients with spinal cord injuries: Retrospective review of the duPont experience. *Neurorehab Neural Re.* 2003;17(1):32–36.

43. DeVivo MJ, Ivie CS III. Life expectancy of ventilator-dependent persons with spinal cord injuries. *Chest.* 1995; 108(1):226–232.

44. Strauss DJ, Devivo MJ, Paculdo DR et al. Trends in life expectancy after spinal cord injury. *Arch Phys Med Rehabil.* 2006;87(8):1079–1085.

45. Ambrosio IU, Woo MS, Jansen MT et al. Safety of hospitalized ventilator-dependent children outside of the intensive care unit. *Pediatrics.* 1998;101(2):257–259.

46. Padman R, Alexander M, Thorogood C et al. Respiratory management of pediatric patients with spinal cord injuries: Retrospective review of the duPont experience. *Neurorehabil Neural Re.* 2003;17(1):32–36.

47. Gilgoff RL, Gilgoff IS. Long-term follow-up of home mechanical ventilation in young children with spinal cord injury and neuromuscular conditions. *J Pediatr.* 2003; 142(5):476–480.

48. Wilson S, Morse JM, Penrod J. Absolute involvement: The experience of mothers of ventilator-dependent children. *Health Soc Care Community.* 1998;6(4):224–233.

49. Noyes J. Health and quality of life of ventilator-dependent children. *J Adv Nurs.* 2006;56(4):392–403.

50. Noyes J. Comparison of ventilator-dependent child reports of health-related quality of life with parent reports and normative populations. *J Adv Nurs.* 2007;58(1):1–10.

51. Kasssioukov A, Claydon VE. The clinical problems in cardiovascular control following spinal cord injury: An overview. *Prog Brain Res.* 2006;152(14):223–229.

52. Ditunno JF, Little JW, Tessler A et al. Spinal shock revisited: A four-phase model. *Spinal Cord.* 2004;42(7):383–395.

53. Bravo G, Guizar-Sahagun G, Ibarra A et al. Cardiovascular alterations after spinal cord injury: An overview. *Curr. Med Chem.* 2004;2:133–148.

54. Teasell RW, Arnold JM, Krassioukov A et al. Cardiovascular consequences of loss of supraspinal control of the sympathetic nervous system after spinal cord injury. *Arch Phys Med Rehabil.* 2000;81:506–516.

55. Balridge BR, Burgess DE, Zimmerman EE et al. Heart rate-arterial blood pressure relationship in conscious rat before vs. after spinal cord transection. *Am J Physiol Regul Integ Comp Physiol.* 2002;283:R748–R756.

56. Tibbs PA, Young B, McAllister RG et al. Studies of experimental cervical spinal cord transection, Part I: Hemodynamic changes after acute cervical spinal cord transection. *J Neurosurg.* 1978;49:558–562.

57. Consortium for Spinal Cord Injury Medicine. *Acute Management of Autonomic Dysreflexia: Individuals with Spinal Cord Injury Presenting to Health-Care Facilities.* 2nd edition. 2001; Jackson Heights, NY, Eastern Paralyzed Veterans Association.

58. Hickey KJ, Vogel LC. Autonomic dysreflexia in pediatric spinal cord injury. *SCI Nurs, Pediatr Perspect.* 2002;19(2): 82–84.

59. Vogel LC, Betz RR, Mulcahey MJ. Spinal cord medicine. In: Kirshblum S, Campagnolo DI, Delisa A., editors. *Pediatric Spinal Cord Disorders.* Philadelphia: Lippincott Williams & Wilkins; 2002. pp. 438–470.

60. Jones T, Ugalde V, Franks P et al. Venous thromboembolism after spinal cord injury: Incidence, time course, and associated risk factors in 16,240 adults and children. *Arch Phys Med Rehabil.* 2005;86(12):2240–2247.

61. Merli G, Herbison G, Ditunno J et al. Deep vein thrombosis: Prophylaxis in acute spinal cord injured subjects. *Arch Phys Med Rehabil.* 1988;69:661–664

62. Geerts W, Code K, Jay R et al. A prospective study of venous thromboembolism after major trauma. *N Engl J Med.* 1994;331:1601–1606.

63. Monagle P, Chan A, Massicotte P et al. Antithrombotic therapy in children: The Seventh ACCP Conference on Antithrombotic and Thrombolytic Therapy. *Chest.* 2004; 126:645S–687S.

64. Berger RM, Maizels M, Moran GC et al. Bladder capacity (ounces) equals age (years) plus 2 predicts normal bladder capacity and aids in diagnosis of abnormal voiding patterns. *J Urology.* 1983;129(2):347–349.

65. McLaughlin JF, Murray M, Van Zandt K et al. Clean intermittent catheterization. *Dev Med Child Neurol.* 1996;38(5): 446–454.

66. Mitrofanoff P. Trans-appendicular continent cystostomy in the management of the neurogenic bladder. *Chir Pediatr.* 1980;21(4):297–305.

67. Brindley GS, Polkey CE, Rushton DN. Sacral anterior root stimulators for bladder control in paraplegia. *Paraplegia.* 1982;20(6):365–381.

68. Vogel LC, Hickey KJ, Klaas SJ et al. Unique issues in pediatric spinal cord injury. *Orthop Nurs.* 2004;23(5): 300–308.

69. Nelson VS. Spinal cord injuries. In: Molnar GE, Alexander MA, editors. *Pediatric Rehabilitation.* Philadelphia: Hanley & Belfus; 1999. pp. 269–288.

70. Gleeson RM. Bowel continence for the child with a neurogenic bowel. *Rehabil Nurs.* 1990;15:319–321.

71. Vogel LC. Medical management of pressure ulcers. In: Betz RR and Mulcahey MJ., editors. *The Child with a Spinal Cord Injury.* Rosemont, IL: American Academy of Orthopaedic Surgeons; 1996. pp. 293–304.

72. Betz RR. Orthopedic problems in the child with spinal cord injury. *Top Spinal Cord Inj Rehabil.* 1997;3:9–19.

73. Garland DE. A clinical perspective on common forms of acquired heterotopic ossification. *Clin Orthop.* 1991;263: 13–29.

74. Schurch B, Capaul M, Rossier A. Prostaglandin E2 measurements: Their value in the early diagnosis of heterotopic ossification in spinal cord injury patients. *Arch Phys Med Rehabil.* 1997;78:687–691.

75. Silverman SL, Hurvitz EA, Nelson VS et al. Rachitic syndrome after disodium etidronate therapy in an adolescent. *Arch Phys Med Rehabil.* 1994;75:118–120.

76. Yoshimura O, Takayanagi K, Kawaguchi K et al. Spinal cord injures in children observed over many years. *Hiroshima J Med Sci.* 1996;45(1):37–41.

77. Rink P, Miller F. Hip instability in spinal cord injury patients. *J Pediatr Orthop.* 1990;10(5):583–587.

78. Vogel LC, Krajci KA, Anderson CJ. Adults with pediatric-onset spinal cord injury: Part 2: Musculoskeletal and neurological complications. *J Spinal Cord Med.* 2002;25(2): 117–123.

79. McCarthy JJ, Chafetz RS, Betz RR et al. Incidence and degree of hip subluxation/dislocation in children with spinal cord injury. *J Spinal Cord Med.* 2004;27 Suppl 1:S80–S83.

80. Tan JB, Smith EJ, Newman JH. Superolateral subluxation of the femoral head prosthesis: An indication of joint sepsis. *Injury.* 1990;21(2):115–116.

81. Betz RR, Mulcahey MJ, Smith BT et al. Implications of hip subluxation for FES-assisted mobility in patients with spinal cord injury. *Orthopedics.* 2001;24:181–184.

82. Freehafer AA, Mast WA. Lower extremity fractures in patients with spinal-cord injury. *J Bone Joint Surg-Am.* 1965;47:683–694.

83. McCarthy JJ, Betz RR. Hip disorders in children who have spinal cord injury. *Orthop Clin North Am.* 2006;37(2): 197–202, vi–vii.

84. McCarthy JJ, Weibel B, Betz RR. Results of pelvic osteotomies for hip subluxation or dislocation in children with spinal cord injury. *Top SCI Rehabil.* 2000;6S:48–53.

85. Faflik J, Bik K, Lipczyk Z. An evaluation of surgical outcomes in luxation and subluxation of the hip joint in children with cerebral palsy. *Ortop Traumatol Rehabil.* 2002;4(1): 15–20.

86. Betz RR, Mulcahey MJ, Smith BT et al. Implications of hip subluxation for FES-assisted mobility in patients with spinal cord injury. *Orthopedics.* 2001;24(2):181–184.

87. Johnston TE, Betz RR, Smith BT et al. Implanted functional electrical stimulation: An alternative for standing and walking in pediatric spinal cord injury. *Spinal Cord.* 2003;41(3):144–152.

88. Johnston TE, Finson RL, Smith BT et al. Functional electrical stimulation for augmented walking in adolescents with incomplete spinal cord injury. *J Spinal Cord Med.* 2003;26(4):390–400.

89. Smith PA, Hassani S, Reiners K et al. Gait analysis in children and adolescents with spinal cord injuries. *J Spinal Cord Med.* 2004;27 Suppl 1:S44–S49.

90. Lance JW. Symposium synopsis. In: Feldman RG, Young RR, Koella WP, editors. *Spasticity: Disorder Motor Control.* Chicago: Mosby Yearbook; 1980:17–24.

91. Maynard FM, Karunas RS, Waring WP III. Epidemiology of spasticity following traumatic spinal cord injury. *Arch Phys Med Rehabil.* 1990;71(8):566–569.

92. Levi R, Hultling C, Seiger A. The Stockholm Spinal Cord Injury Study. 3. Health-related issues of the Swedish annual level-of-living survey in SCI subjects and controls. *Paraplegia.* 1995;33(12):726–730.

93. Vogel LC. Spasticity: Diagnostic workup and medical management. In: Betz RR and Mulcahey MJ, editors. *The Child with a Spinal Cord Injury.* Rosemont, IL: American Academy of Orthopaedic Surgeons;1996. pp. 261–268.

94. Kirshblum S. Treatment alternatives for spinal cord injury related spasticity. *J Spinal Cord Med.* 1999;22(3):199–217.

95. Adams MM, Hicks AL. Spasticity after spinal cord injury. *Spinal Cord.* 2005;43(10):577–586.

96. Graham HK, Aoki KR, Autti-Ramo I et al. Recommendations for the use of botulinum toxin type A in the management of cerebral palsy. *Gait Posture.* 2000;11:67–79.

97. Goldstein EM. Safety of high-dose botulinum toxin type A therapy for the treatment of pediatric spasticity. *J Child Neurol.* 2006;21(3):189–192.

98. Ramachandran M, Eastwood DM. Botulinum toxin and its orthopaedic applications. *J Bone Joint Surg Br.* 2006; 88(8):981–987.

99. Schurch B, de Seze M, Denys P et al. Botulinum toxin type A is a safe and effective treatment for neurogenic urinary incontinence: Results of a single treatment randomised, placebo controlled 6-month study. *J Urology.* 2005;174:196–200.

100. Klaphajone J, Kitisomprayoonkul W, and Sriplakit S. Botulinum toxin type A injections for treating neurogenic detrusor overactivity combined with low-compliance bladder patients with spinal cord lesions. *Arch Phys Med Rehabil.* 2005;86:2114–2118.

101. Loubser PG. Akman NM. Effects of intrathecal baclofen on chronic spinal cord injury pain. *J Pain Symptom Manage.* 1996;12(4):241–247.

102. Azouvi P, Roby-Brami A, Biraben A et al. Effect of intrathecal baclofen on the monosynaptic reflex in humans: Evidence for a postsynaptic action. *J Neurol Neurosurg Psychiatry.* 1993;56:515–519.

103. Kroin JS, Penn RD, Beissinger RL et al. Reduced spinal reflexes following intrathecal baclofen in the rabbit. *Exp Brain Res.* 1984;54:191–194.

104. Latash ML, Penn RD, Corcos DM et al. Short term effect of intrathecal baclofen in spasticity. *Exp Neurol.* 1989;103:165–172.

105. MacDonnel RAL, Talalla A, Swash M et al. Intrathecal baclofen and the H reflex. *J Neurol Neurosurg Psychiatry.* 1989;52:1110–1112.

106. Maynard, F M. Immobilization hypercalcemia following spinal cord injury. *Arch Phys Med Rehabil.* 1986;67: 41–44.

107. Kopell, BH, Sala, D, Doyle, WK et al. Subfascial implantation of intrathecal baclofen pumps in children: Technical note. *Neurosurgery.* 2001;49(3):753–757.

108. Albright, AL, Turner, M, and Pattisapu, JV. Best-practice surgical techniques for intrathecal baclofen therapy. *J Neurosurg.* 2006;104 Suppl 4:233–239.

109. Gooch JL, Oberg WA, Grams B et al. Care provider assessment of intrathecal baclofen in children. *Dev Med Child Neurol.* 2004;46:548–552.

110. Gooch JL, Oberg WA, Grams B et al. Complications of intrathecal baclofen pumps in children. *Pediatr Neurosurg.* 2003;39:1–6.

111. Vender JR, Hester S, Waller JL et al. Identification and management of intrathecal baclofen pump complications: A comparison of pediatric and adult patients. *J Neurosurg.* 2006;104:9–15.

112. Freehafer AA. Limb fractures in patients with spinal cord injury. *Arch Phys Med Rehabil.* 1995;76(9):823–827.

113. Bick RL. International concensus recommendations. Summary statement and additional suggested guidelines. *Med Clin North Am.* 1998;82:613–633.

114. Anderson CJ, Vogel LC, Willis KM et al. Stability of transition to adulthood among individuals with pediatric-onset spinal cord injuries. *J Spinal Cord Med.* 2006; 29(1):46–56.

115. Amador MJ, Lynne CM, Brackett NL. *A Guide and Resource Directory to Male Fertility Following Spinal Cord Injury/ Dysfunction.* Miami: Miami Project to Cure Paralysis. 2004.

116. Keenen TL, Anthony J, Benson DR. Non-contigous spinal fractures. *J Trauma.* 1990;30(4):489–491.

117. Mehta S, Betz RR, Mulcahey MJ et al. Effect of bracing on paralytic scoliosis secondary to spinal cord injury. *J Spinal Cord Med.* 2004;27 Suppl 1:S88–S92.

118. Warschusky, S. et al. Psychosocial factors in rehabilitation of a child with a spinal cord injury. In: Betz RR and Mulcahey MJ, editors. *The Child with a Spinal Cord Injury.* Rosemont, IL: American Academy of Orthopaedic Surgeons; 1996. pp. 471–482.

119. Merenda LA, The pediatric patient with SCI—not a small adult. *SCI Nurs.* 2001;18(1):43–44.

120. Keen TP, Nursing care of the pediatric multitrauma patient. *Nurs Clin North Am.* 1990;25(1):131–141.

121. Kannisto M, Merikanto J, Aaranta H et al. Comparison of health-related quality of life in three subgroups of spinal cord injury patients. *Spinal Cord.* 1998;36(3):193–199.

122. Vogel LC et al. Long-term outcomes and life satisfaction of adults who had pediatric spinal cord injuries. *Arch Phys Med Rehabil.* 1998;79(12):1496–1503.

123. Pontari MA et al. Improved quality of life after continent urinary diversion in pediatric patients with tetraplegia after spinal cord injury. *Top Spinal Cord Injury Rehabil.* 2000; Suppl 6:25–29.

124. Dixon PJ et al. Recovery of functional independence in children with spinal cord injury. *SCI Psychosocial Process.* 2001;14(2):68–73.

125. Warschusky S, Kewman DG, Bradley A et al. Pediatric neurological conditions. In: Roberts MC, editor. *Handbook of Pediatric Psychology.* New York: Guilford Press; 2003. pp. 380–385.

126. Boyer BA Knolls ML, Kafkalas CM, et al. Prevalence and relationships of posttraumatic stress in families experiencing pediatric spinal cord injury *Rehabil Psychol.* 2000;45(4): 339–355.

127. Ostrowski SA, Christopher NC, van Dulmen MH et al. Acute child and mother psychophysiological responses and subsequent PTSD symptoms following a child's traumatic event. *J Trauma Stress.* 2007;20(5):677–687.

128. Perry BD, Azad I. Posttraumatic stress disorders in children and adolescents. *Curr Opin Pediatr.* 1999;11(4): 310–316.

129. Pfefferbaum B. Posttraumatic stress disorder in children: A review of the past 10 years. *J Am Acad Child Adolesc Psych.* 1997;36(11):1503–1511.

130. Cohen J, Berliner L, March J. Treatment of children and adolescents. In: Foa EB, Keane TM, Friedman MJ, editors. *Effective Treatments for PTSD: Practice Guidelines from the International Society for Traumatic Stress Studies.* New York: Guilford Press; 2000. pp. 330–332.

131. Iannaccone S. Pediatric aspects of spinal rehabilitation. *J Neurol Rehabil.* 1994.8(1):41–46.

132. Mulcahey MJ. An overview of the upper extremity in pediatric spinal cord injury. *Top Spinal Cord Injury Rehabil.* 1997;3(2):48–55.

133. Mulcahey MJ. Rehabilitation and outcomes of upper extremity tendon transfer surgery. In: Betz RR, Mulcahey MJ, editors. *The Child with Spinal Cord Injury.* Rosemont, IL: American Academy of Orthopaedic Surgeons; 1996. pp. 419–448.

134. Mix CM, Specht DP. Achieving functional independence. In: Braddom RL, Buschbacher RM, Dumitru D et al., editors. *Physical Medicine and Rehabilitation.* Philadelphia: W.B. Saunders;1996. pp. 514–530.

135. Johnston TE, Smith BT, Oladeji O, Betz RR, Lauer RT. Outcomes of a home cycling program using functional electrical stimulation or passive motion for children with spinal cord injury: a case series. *J Spinal Cord Med.* 2008;31(2):215–221.

136. Butler C, Okamoto G, McKay T. Powered mobility for very young children. *Dev Med Child Neurol.* 1983;25:472.

Index

Note: Page numbers followed by f indicate figures; t, tables; b, boxes.